Clinical Measurement of Speech and Voice

Second Edition

CLINICAL MEASUREMENT OF SPEECH AND VOICE

Second Edition

R. J. BAKEN, PH.D.

ROBERT F. ORLIKOFF, PH.D.

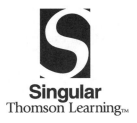

Singular
Thomson Learning™

Singular Publishing Group
Thomson Learning
401 West A Street, Suite 325
San Diego, California 92101-7904

Singular Publishing Group publishes textbooks, clinical manuals, clinical reference books, journals, videos, and multimedia materials on speech-language pathology, audiology, otorhinolaryngology, special education, early childhood, aging, occupational therapy, physical therapy, rehabilitation, counseling, mental health, and voice. For your convenience, our entire catalog can be accessed on our website at *http://www.singpub.com*. Our mission to provide you with materials to meet the daily challenges of the ever-changing health care/educational environment will remain on course if we are in touch with you. In that spirit, we welcome your feedback on our products. Please telephone (**1-800-521-8545**), fax (**1-800-774-8398**), or e-mail (*singpub@singpub.com*) your comments and requests to us.

Typeset in 10/12 Palatino by D&G Ltd.
Printed in Canada by Transcontinental Printing

Library of Congress Cataloging-in-Publication Data

Baken, R. J. (Ronald J.) 1943-
    Clinical measurement of speech and voice / R.J. Baken, Robert F.
Orlikoff. –2nd ed., rev. and expanded.
      p   cm.
    Includes bibliographic references and indexes.
    ISBN 1-56593-869-0 (soft cover : alk. paper)
    1. Speech disorders—diagnosis.   2. Voice disorders—Diagnosis.
3. Speech—Measurement. 4. Voice—Measurement. I. Orlikoff,
Robert F. II. Title.
    [DNLM: 1. Speech Production Measurement.   WV 501 B167c 1999]
RC423.B28   1999
616.85'5075—dc21
DNLM/DLC
For Library of Congress
                                                     99-24709
                                                         CIP

CONTENTS

Appendixes

Preface to the First Edition

Several years ago a group of doctoral candidates in speech pathology urged Dr. Carol Wilder and me to organize and lead a seminar that would provide a formal framework for consideration of the state of the art of speech and voice diagnosis. As a group, we were strongly committed to clinical practice as well as to research in diagnostic and therapeutic methods. We also shared an interest in various facts of speech science. It seemed like an interesting and potentially useful undertaking, and so we met each week for a semester. We argued philosophies, debated viewpoints, proposed paradigms. But mostly we dug into the literature to see whether it could be mined for nuggets of methodology—founded on viable theory and validated by adequate research—that could be refined and cast into a cohesive whole of diagnostic and therapeutic procedure, at least in some small corner of the vast realm of communicative disorders.

As so often happens in academe, we had hardly begun when the semester ended. But we had found a lot of useful material. And we reached a consensus that, indeed, the resources were there to sharpen diagnoses and perhaps greatly improve therapy. Our discussions uncovered plausible reasons why so much of what was in the literature should have achieved so little application.

Rather than let the issues die, I volunteered to write a brief report of our findings and conclusions. I did, but the resulting document clearly was not good enough or long enough to do the subject any real justice. So I began drafting a more complete version, that grew and developed a life of its own and became this book. It is, in some very real ways, a belated report to my erstwhile students—now my colleagues—on our seminar.

Although this book deals with a considerable array of instrumentation, it is different from the few "speech instrumentation" texts that have appeared so far. One of my primary goals has been to cull, from the literature of speech pathology and related fields, assessment methods that can be said to be "objective" and valid. Another major goal was to summarize methods that offer relatively precise measurement of physiologic events during speech or of characteristics of the speech signal itself. The objective was to consider methods and techniques that are consistent with our present understanding of speech processes on the one hand and with acceptable engineering principles on the other. The prime emphasis has been on techniques that are applicable in the context of speech rehabilitation settings. Occasionally, more complex or more invasive methods have been included, either because they are common tools of researchers or because, in instances of real need, they may be done by physicians or other technical personnel available to the speech clinician.

Almost everything discussed in this book depends on instrumentation, so there is a very heavy emphasis on "machines." Where different instruments are available to achieve the same objective, they are considered and compared. Because I have always believed that valid use of instrumentation requires a clear understanding of operating principles, there are sometimes-lengthy explanations of what is inside the various "black boxes." For the same reason, there is a separate chapter on the elementary principles of electronics. Finally, there are occasional microtutorials on important, but sometimes overlooked, aspects of the physiology or acoustics of speech.

There is no point in informing the reader about tests that can be performed without also providing information about what the test results should look like. Therefore, tabulations of data that approximate "norms" for the various test methods have been provided wherever possible. They are intended to serve as guidelines to interpretation of test results.

There is only passing reference to microcomputers. This is not meant to denigrate them or to deny that they are in fact the wave of the future. And it is emphatically not because the author hates them (at least not most of the time). Rather, the decision to forego discussion of microcomputers was based on the observation that, at least for the present, they are doing no more in the domain of diagnosis and appraisal than what more traditional analog methods do. They can usually do it faster, often do it more conveniently, and—on occasion—can do it much better. But what they do is not different. And, the computer takes its input from the same analog instrumentation discussed in this book, so it seemed better to stick with what a clinician—or computer—must do to obtain data rather than to devote a great deal of space to consideration of computer function and mechanics. Fortunately, a great many other books are starting to appear on that subject.

The organization of this book posed genuine problems. Many test methods are useful for a wide range of disorders, so that a division of the text by classes of pathology did not seem optimal. But there are exceptions to this rule, and so, for example, there are separate chapters on laryngeal and velopharyngeal dysfunction. A glance at the table of contents will show that no general principle was found to divide the material of the book into chapters. The organization may be inscrutable (in places, even to the author!), but it is hoped that reference to the index will allow a reader to find whatever is needed.

The text is very liberally sprinkled with references. Their function is not so much to assure that what is presented is "true," but rather to guide the reader to more complete explanations and to the original data. (Despite the size of the book, a great deal has been left out.) Sometimes references have been included for historical purposes; we have too often forgotten where we came from and to whom we owe what we have.

Although the title page recognizes just one author, in fact many people contributed to this undertaking in diverse but important ways. My wife, Joan, considered this book another of my esoteric hobbies and was good natured and understanding throughout its gestation. She and Dr. Jeannette Fleischner (whom some think is my alternative spouse) spent untold hours listening to my meanderings in the arcane lore of speech pathology and to my all-too-frequent groaning when the work was going badly. And, somehow, they usually managed to keep smiling.

A number of my colleagues read major segments of the first versions and offered helpful comments and insights. Among them are Drs. Elizabeth Allen, Steve Cavallo, Ray Daniloff, Kathy Harris, Honor O'Malley, Nick Schiavetti, Phil Schneider, and Carol Wilder. Bob Orlikoff gamely tried out segments of the book on the unsuspecting graduate students in his course on clinical laboratory techniques and broke the news of their responses to me as gently as possible. Dr. Ed Mysak, chairman of my department, was very encouraging and tolerant of the many quirks in my work style that developed as the book matured. Dr. Miriam Goldberg often applied those psychological insights for which she has gained a worldwide reputation, doing a wonderful portrayal of the gadfly to my reluctant role of Io. She managed to apply frequent motivating prods where she thought they would do the most good.

Finally, my doctoral students suggested revisions in the text, relishing the opportunity to do unto me as I often do unto them. They also volunteered—with somewhat less enthusiasm—to be subjects as I tested out various methods and procedures. I know how much happier they will be now that I can, once again, devote all my creative energies to the task of making their lives more interesting.

Ad
Secundam Editionem
Praefatio

The preface is the only place in a book where the authors can escape the literary conventions, scholarly tone, and editorial requisites of textbook style, kick off their mental shoes, sit back, and talk to their readers as informally as their publisher's blood pressure medication and attorneys will allow. Those of our colleagues who know us will understand that this is not an opportunity we can pass up. (Especially one of us.)

It is, of course, gratifying to know that there is a demand for a second edition of this book. That an update was widely called for, and that it required so many changes and additions, speaks loudly about the progress of the field of communicative rehabilitation in the past several years.

Speech and voice measurement has become very respectable. It's even chic! It gets a listing in the program of every professional meeting—and at a few it's even taken seriously. Objective measurement is now an accepted part of clinical practice. In some settings it's an integral part of every clinical undertaking. In a few it's held to be indispensable. There are some clinical programs that make serious attempts to educate their students about it.

The Introduction of the first edition argued the case for measuring speech and voice, rather than simply describing how it sounded. It seems unnecessary to do that now. Anyone reading this book is likely to already be convinced (or to be a helpless student whose instructor is convinced).

At least some of the reasons for this sudden embrace of objective measurement are easily discerned, even if their relative importance is difficult to assign. Theory has advanced, and viewpoints have changed in some corners of the discipline. Speech and voice functions are more widely recognized as motor behaviors with acoustic consequences, and they are better understood from a physiologic point of view. As a result, many observations that were once meaningful primarily to the laboratory researcher are now seen to have direct clinical relevance. Another factor, particularly salient in the United States, is the inherent distrust by third-party insurers of the professionals whom they pay. Understandably, clinicians have felt constrained to offer objective evidence that a patient's symptoms exist and that the proffered diagnosis is valid. And, of course, data are also required to document the beneficial effects of treatment. Then, too, we live in a technological age—socially and clinically—in which the addition of a little technology to the clinical setting provides a sense of validation.

But most important, it would seem, is the fact that measurement is now clinically feasible. That is not to say that it was previously an impossible task, but it was difficult. Or at least time consuming, bothersome, and in general too inconvenient to warrant the expenditure of time and effort for the benefit that was formerly to be gained.

The development of miniature electronic systems changed that. As a result, sophisticated electronic measurement systems could be (relatively) simply designed and built, cheaply sold, and easily used. Equally important, and more obvious, was the fact that ultraminiature integrated circuits created the personal computer—the first universal machine for home and office. Put the two together, and every clinician can have, in a square meter of clinic space, a laboratory as powerful as any that existed 40 years ago. Quantified observations of speech function and acoustic characterization of the speech product can be had at the click of a mouse.[1]

Clearly, we are excited and enthusiastic about the growing role of speech and voice measurement on communicative rehabilitation. We are, however, also seriously concerned about some aspects of it. Professional training and education are not keeping pace with the growing potential of technological advances. We badly

---

[1]The convenience of today's microcomputers is perhaps only fully appreciated by those who recognize the term "batch processing."

need, but have thus far not had, effective leadership on the educational front. Too often, clinical measurement practice is determined by what a computer program does, rather than by what clinicians determine to be valid or useful. We have been too willing to overlook questionable procedures or undocumented "norms" that are built into the software that they buy. In the service of our patients we will need to be more sophisticated and more skeptical.

But this new edition of *Clinical Voice and Speech Measurement* is a statement of our continuing optimism about the role of objective acoustic and physiologic observation in clinical practice. Our rationale in writing it is unchanged from that set forth in the preface to the first edition, which we hope the reader will peruse both as a guide to our present purposes and as an indication of how the emphasis has changed.

In this edition, as in the first, we have proceeded in the belief that users must be knowledgeable about the techniques they employ and the systems they use. As a result, this edition, like its predecessor, devotes considerable space to the technological details of measurement systems and to their theoretical background. We have expanded the data tables to include findings that have appeared since the first edition and have, where appropriate, given greater consideration to computer-specific details. We regret that, despite considerable effort, we have still not come up with a logical basis for this volume's overall organization and so we ask the reader's indulgence in reliance on the index to find what is needed. Finally, we ask our readers to consider the numerous references to the professional and technical literature as a salute to all those who have provided the knowledge base upon which our professional work rests.

In addition to all those whose substantial contributions were acknowledged in the first edition, we recognize with gratitude the continuing support and help of many of our colleagues. Special thanks are due to Drs. Ben Watson and Rick Roark, of New York Medical College, whose expert advice in speech science and electrical engineering, respectively, was important at many stages of the work. Thanks, also, to Dr. James Dembowski, for his editorial efforts, and Ms. Janet Rovalino and the speech pathology staff of the New York Eye and Ear Infirmary who tolerated disruptions of their clinical routine and honored requests for clinical data for the sake of this book. Dr. Steven Schaefer, Chair of the Department of Otolaryngology at the New York Eye and Ear Infirmary, was particularly supportive and uncomplaining of the chaos that the department's voice scientist and his buddy from Memorial Sloan-Kettering occasionally wrought in his bailiwick.

Thanks also to Dr. Jatin Shah, Chair of the Head and Neck Service at Memorial Sloan-Kettering Cancer Center, and to Dr. Dennis Kraus, Head of the Speech, Hearing and Rehabilitation Center at the same institution, for their unswerving toleration of the second author's book-related activities. There was often much to tolerate. The second author also expresses particular gratitude to his wife, Jennifer, and his children, Russell, Emily, and Erica, for their love and support, with apologies for the months of late nights while this book took form.

Finally, the first author wants to express his appreciation of his coworker. His talent, organization, and sensitivity made a second edition possible. Its best parts are his.

R. J. Baken
Woodstock, New York

Bob Orlikoff
West Windsor, New Jersey

In memoriam

Dr. Joan W. Baken

1945-1995

Nobis cum semel occidit brevis lux
Nox est perpetua una dormienda.
                                        —*Catullus*

1

Introduction

This book addresses ways of "measuring" speech and voice. More precisely, it deals with the means available for determining what the various parts of the speech system are doing to generate a given product and with the ways of describing the acoustic result, in a quantitative manner whenever possible. It is intended for all medical and rehabilitative professionals who evaluate and treat disorders of voice and speech, but its primary audience is the speech pathologist, with whom responsibility for communicative rehabilitation ordinarily rests.

Ever since the birth of their discipline, speech pathologists have relied heavily—and in many cases exclusively—on their highly trained ears for judgments of speech acceptability. When something sounded wrong, auditory perception typically formed the basis of a diagnosis. Based on careful listening, clinicians would commonly make judgments such as "inadequate velopharyngeal closure," "vocal fold hyperfunction," or "inadequate breath support." Now, nothing in this book is meant to deny the importance of listening skills in dealing with communicative disorders. The very first step in diagnosis, after all, is the determination of whether or not a problem exists, and almost all speech and voice problems signal their presence by acoustic cues that may be quite subtle. There is, as yet, no instrument, no technique, no computer, that can begin to match the human auditory system for detecting acoustic variations or for determining whether they reflect a variety of normal speech or something amiss in the speech system.

Yet there has always been a strong current in the professional literature, a point of view distinctly articulated from the very beginning, that listening is not enough, that a clinician's perceptions cannot provide the sole and universal basis for mapping and guiding the course of the therapeutic enterprise. That current has grown ever stronger and, in just the few years since this book's first edition, has become an overpowering tide that has reshaped the landscape of the clinical world. The inadequacy of unaided perception is readily apparent and has come to be widely accepted. But, especially for those approaching the study of communicative disorders for the first time, some words of explanation may be in order.

A major problem with listening as a diagnostic method is that the human auditory system is inherently configured for dealing with the speech signal as a whole entity, and for detecting linguistically relevant features in it. It is this highly evolved aptitude that makes it so efficient in speech communication. Unfortunately, from the speech pathologist's point of view, auditory processing often does not leave the listener with a conscious awareness of the acoustic details that have combined to produce a given perception. Yet it is commonly the individual acoustic components, the ingredients, as it were, of the speech product, that require evaluation. It is the specific defective aspects of the speech signal that must be the target of therapy.

Furthermore, a feature perceived is not necessarily a component characterized. The ear is too easily

1

fooled. Pitch peculiarities, for example, may be due more to the resonance properties of the vocal signal than to the oscillatory rate of the vocal folds. Perceived hypernasality may have its origin in abnormal velar timing rather than in inadequate velar closure.

Worse, there is the problem of *degrees of freedom.* Almost any speech sound, normal or otherwise, can be produced in a variety of ways. There is often no means, on the basis of listening alone, to be sure of exactly what the vocal tract is doing to produce a given output. The problem here is analogous to that of fixing a stereo system that has become distorted and noisy. The trouble might be in any of a number of places: in the tape transport, the playback head, the amplifier, or the speakers. Listening to the system can provide hints about where to look for the trouble, but only careful testing of the several components can really pinpoint the source of the difficulty and indicate appropriate solutions.

Dealing with aberrant mechanisms is really what speech and voice rehabilitation is about. While the therapist's goal is to establish an adequate signal, the therapist's actions must be focused on aberrant function. The speech signal is not, in itself, an entity. It is simply the product of speech system physiology. As such, speech or voice are not available for manipulation; only the structures and processes that produce them are. The therapist's role is to change function, and to do so physiologic abnormalities must first be identified and characterized.

So, it is a major tenet of this book that objective observation and measurement of the speech signal and of its physiologic bases is a sine qua non of effective practice. Specifically, the advantages of speech and voice measurement include:

■ increased precision of diagnosis, with more valid specification of abnormal functions that require modification;

■ more positive identification and documentation of therapeutic efficacy, both for short-term assessment (is a given approach modifying the abnormal function?) and long-term monitoring (how much has speech behavior changed since the inception of therapy?);

■ expansion of options for therapeutic modalities. Most measurement techniques offer a means of demonstrating to the patient exactly what is wrong, and they can often provide feedback that is therapeutically useful.

Historically, there have been strong disincentives to the incorporation of objective measurement methods into the diagnostic and therapeutic undertaking. Speech pathology was—and quite often still is—considered a branch of the social and behavioral disciplines. The intrusion of technology and "machines" into the patient-therapist relationship was viewed as disruptive, if not deleterious. A social-sciences model of clinical education left many therapists ill equipped to deal with the technology and poorly prepared to undertake the requisite application of biologic and physical science. Then, too, the requisite instrumentation requires a significant (although not overwhelming) capital investment, which could not be justified when the advantages to be gained were only dimly perceived.

Many clinicians were alienated from the technologic and scientific end of the profession, and some of the blame for this must be laid at the feet of the research community. Although there are notable exceptions, most speech scientists (and even many clinical investigators) have not taken the trouble to ensure that their methods and findings are accessible to clinical practitioners. While mathematics may be the best language for the expression of many complex concepts, translations into more common prose are possible and obviously useful, even if some precision and subtlety are lost in the process. But "popularization" has not been held in high regard by scientists, and has not been encouraged by the research journals (which scientists commonly control). Compounding the problem is the fact that, at least in the United States, the national professional association that effectively controls the education of speech pathologists pays only scant attention to the technological awareness and research literacy of candidates seeking its professional seal of certification.

Finally, the adoption of technology has been impeded by the fact that relevant and important information is scattered throughout a large number of different sources, often highly specialized, published by many different professional groups. It is unreasonable to expect any working professional to winnow the haystack of literature looking for needles of methodologic utility.

But the most important inhibition was, perhaps, the sheer inconvenience of the measurement undertaking. Early clinicians and researchers commonly had to spend hours obtaining data about speech system function. In the 1920s, for instance, it took several hours of work to produce a record of the fundamental frequency characteristics of just a few seconds of speech. The process involved generating a record of the speech waveform on moving film, developing the film, projecting it and measuring the wavelengths by hand, tabulating the results, and deriving the summary means, wave-to-wave variations, and other measures of interest. The recent past saw great improvements in methodologic "friendliness," but the gathering of numerous samples with separate and distinct instruments whose connections needed to be independently set up, whose settings had to be individually adjusted, and whose outputs needed to be separately deciphered, still left the process a time-consuming and physically inconvenient chore.

Much of that has changed. The growing importance of communicative rehabilitation in the medical setting has provided the impetus for the more biologically oriented approach to communicative disorders that has gained favor in a segment of the professional community and, in a handful of cases, in a small number of professional training programs. The rationale for acoustic and physiologic assessment has accordingly been increasingly legitimized. The medical model, and its third-party payment system, has also fueled a growing emphasis on documentation of the need for and efficacy of treatment. The requirement of objective documentation justifies capital investment in appropriate technology. The needs of the external clinical world have pushed training programs to begin to add science and technology studies to their curricula, with the result that clinicians are at least a little more comfortable with the rationales for, methods of, and interpretational procedures required for speech and voice measurement.

But more than anything else, the horizon has been altered by the personal computer, the "universal machine." Thanks to a proliferation of commercially available computer systems it has suddenly become easy to get measures, to generate numbers, to derive indices of function. In fact, it is becoming the "in" thing to do. The proverbial pendulum is definitely swinging the other way. That has not, unfortunately, been an unmitigated good.

The problem is that the proliferation of plots, tabulation of ratios, elaboration of quotients, and extraction of indices does not inevitably indicate better diagnosis, deeper insight, or improved intervention. Data are valuable only to the extent that they are relevant to the problem at hand, are valid and reliable, and are interpretable. Several principles—"rules," if you will—therefore need to inform the clinician's use of speech and voice measurements.

1. The purpose of testing and measurement is not to describe speech or voice, but to characterize abnormalities of vocal tract function. Insight into function is the foundation for inferring causes; the causes, in turn, are the bases of the diagnosis and the indicators of the treatment. Therefore, to be useful, **measurements must have a known (or at least a very likely) and specific relationship to recognized aspects of speech system physiology.**

2. **A measurement must have clear relevance.** That is, it must be able to demonstrate features of vocal tract functioning that are known—or at the very least, strongly believed—to be implicated in dysfunction. The ease with which computers can acquire data and calculate results is not in itself a rationale for doing so. The unsupported belief that an observation might be meaningful, or its utility in other fields of endeavor, are not adequate justifications for its employment. It must have a compelling, specific, and testable hypothetical justification.

3. **A measurement method should have a "history" in the literature.** Its performance in the hands of others, in different settings, with various kinds of cases, verifies and qualifies its utility.

4. **Measurements must be thoroughly understood.** While electronic systems make measurement easy, they also make it covert. The details of data acquisition and processing may therefore remain a mystery. But not to know how a measurement is done is not adequately to know what the result means. It also implies that threats to validity are not specifically appreciated and so the quality of the result cannot be assessed. It is therefore critical that the user understand the theoretical and technical details of the system being used.

5. **Never trust a computer completely.** In the "old days" measurement was done by hand and signals were evaluated by eye. Although tedious, this forced a confrontation with the data's quality. One knew if the data were acceptable, whether they had any peculiarities that might interfere with analysis and, of paramount importance, whether they had characteristics that—while perhaps not relevant to the specific measure to be applied—were instructive about the nature of the clinical problem at issue. Computers, for all their speed and arithmetic accuracy, are stupid machines. They process what they are given, good or bad, meaningful or nonsensical. They have no sense of the significant. The data should be examined by a professional.

6. **Measurement should be limited to situations in which it is likely to be useful.** If a test does not sharpen the clinical picture or guide clinical intervention, then its use is a waste of time, effort, and resources.

There is, finally, one overriding principle. Because the sole value of a measurement is in its interpretation, **measurements can be no better than the knowledge and skills of the clinician who chooses and obtains them.**

It is in the hope of refining that knowledge and of sharpening those skills that this book has been written.

2

Analog Electronics

Until just a few years ago, information about the world was almost always presented to us in the form of an analogy. The length of a column of mercury *is analogous to* the temperature of the air. The motion of the clock's hands *is analogous to* the passage of time, and their position represents—*is analogous to*—the time that has elapsed since some reference starting event. Similarly, the position of a point on an oscilloscope screen is an analogy for the oral air pressure. Measurement instruments almost always work by presenting the magnitude of some phenomenon that is hard for us to observe (like pressure, flow, or heat) in terms of a variable that is easier for us to deal with (such as position, voltage, or length). Instruments that work this way are described as **analog** devices.

In principle, it is possible to manipulate information in analog form[1] but in practice it is usually far more convenient for us to deal with numbers. This is especially true when complex processing or transformations are required (spectral analysis is an example) or when the measurement results must be communicated to others or transported to different systems for further analysis. Devices that operate on numbers or whose output is numerical are said to be **digital**.

Both analog and digital systems are critical to speech and voice measurement. We will begin the consideration of this fundamental area by dealing with the basic principles of electrical flow in analog circuits. Chapter 3 will then consider elementary aspects of number systems and digital logic and will explore some of the simpler ways in which electrical circuits can be used to perform digital chores.

PRINCIPLES OF ANALOG ELECTRONICS

Electronics is the medium through which measurements are made. Ingenious mechanical means of observing the action of the speech system were devised in the early days of the profession (for example, Stetson, 1928; Stetson & Hudgins, 1930; Scripture, 1902), but modern instrumentation is almost always electronic. This development is not the result of any perverse desire on the part of scientists and engineers to mystify or to confuse their professional public. It simply reflects the fact that electronic circuits can perform measurement functions much faster and more accurately than mechanical systems can, while interfering far less with the process being evaluated. In fact, in most cases only electronic circuits are capable of doing the job at hand.

Using an electronic instrument does not by any means guarantee valid or reliable measurements. Far from it. Any instrument or circuit must be used in ways that are consistent with its characteristics, with its capabilities, and, quite often, with its quirks. Failure to do so may compromise the validity of the information obtained, often to the point of seriously misleading the unsuspecting user. If they are to obtain maximally useful evaluations of their patients' speech behaviors, clinicians will need to know at least a little about electronics. This is not to imply that they must become biomedical engineers: a little understanding, creatively applied, goes a remarkably long way.

The need to deal with electronic theory seems often to provoke either panic or despair. On the assumption that these reactions are elicited by the mathematical approaches commonly employed, this chapter will try to develop an understanding of the most basic electrical phenomena by relying on more intuitive explanations. The objective is not to train the reader to design circuits (although, due to the easy availability of pre-fabricated integrated circuits, it is remarkably easy to do so today) as much as to develop enough understanding to use those that are available intelligently, productively, and creatively. It is the intent of this very cursory review to provide just enough background to understand the instrumentation and methods discussed later. Many basic textbooks are available for those who are motivated (or driven by necessity) to delve more deeply into this area.

Electricity: Current, Voltage, and Resistance

In the simplest sense, electricity is the flow of electrons from a place where they are abundant to a region where they are relatively scarce. The path that the electrons follow is called a **circuit**. Nothing moves without being pushed, so the electrons obviously must be driven by some force. Each electron has a negative charge. Since like charges repel, the electrons stuffed into some region will tend to push away from each other. It is this mutual repulsion that provides the pushing force. The more crowded with electrons a space is, the greater the mutual repulsion will be. Therefore, if there is a path that they can follow, electrons will flow from a zone of relatively tight electron packing (which results in a relatively large repulsive force) to an area where the packing is not so dense (and the outward pushing force is therefore less). Electron flow will con-

---

[1] In fact, computers that operate on purely analog principles have a long history and still find use in special circumstances.

tinue until the electron concentration is equalized in the two areas. One can imagine an analogous situation involving two identical balloons, one fully inflated (having tight packing of air molecules) and the other blown up only slightly (and therefore having less crowding of the air molecules). If the two balloons are connected by a tube, air will flow out of the fully inflated one into the less inflated one. When both have the same density of air molecules the airflow will stop.

In the everyday world of practical electronics, the source of electrons is called a *power supply*. It might be a device that plugs into a wall outlet or it might be a simple battery. Whatever its form, it has a region where electrons are abundant and a region where electrons are scarce. There is some way of connecting wires to each region. The electrons cannot flow from one zone to another inside the power supply. The only route for them to take in order to equalize the imbalance is via an external device that the user connects to the terminals. Hence, a power supply provides a flow of electrons for activating electronic devices.

The flow of electrons is called *current*. The symbol for current is **I**. It is measured in *amperes* (A). One ampere (1 A) represents the flow of a given number of electrons every second. (The number happens to be about 6.02×10^{23}. It is of importance to physicists and chemists, but doesn't really matter to the user of electronic instrumentation.) The pressure, or force, pushing the electrons is called *voltage* or *potential* (symbol, **E**), measured in **volts**.[2] It is the difference in electrical pressure between two points. Current and voltage in an electrical circuit are equivalent to flow and pressure in a plumbing system. Just as the flow through a pipe might be measured in liters per minute, current is quantified in amperes. The pressure of water in a pipe might be described in terms of kilograms per square centimeter, and in the same way the electrical pressure in a wire is described in volts.

All other things being equal, the greater the voltage (difference in pressure between two points) the greater the flow between the two points will be. One is directly proportional to the other: $I \propto E$.

Direct and Alternating Current

There is a fundamental distinction to be made between electron flows that are steady (or that change only *very* slowly) and those that vary from one instant to the next. Steady flow is called *direct current* (DC) while variable electron flow is known as *alternating current* (AC). The distinction is important because there are several electronic components whose charac-

teristics vary depending on whether, and how fast, the current is changing. In fact, it is this property that makes such components useful. (More will be said about this later.)

It is easy to understand DC. It might be exemplified by current in a flashlight: After the switch is turned on electrons flow at a constant rate—out of one pole of the battery, through the lamp, and back to the battery's other pole—until the switch is turned off again. Except for the instants when the switch is moved (and current flow suddenly begins or ends) the current through the flashlight is DC.

There are two common misconceptions about AC that may interfere with understanding basic electronic circuits. First, current in an AC circuit does not necessarily reverse direction from time to time. Reversal is the case in many systems, but it is not reversal that makes them AC devices. What characterizes AC is not changes in the *direction* of the current flow, but changes in the *amount* of current. Second, the changes in flow need not be periodic. That is, there is no requirement that there be a regular waveform. Any current change, according to any pattern or following no pattern at all, makes an AC signal.

Because information can only be conveyed by a change in some quantity it is not surprising that most useful electronic devices are built around AC circuits. However, AC signal processing is much more complex than the handling of DC signals. To facilitate understanding of the most basic aspects of electrical circuits discussion of the more complex phenomena of AC will be deferred until later.

BASIC PRINCIPLES OF DIRECT CURRENT

Conductors, Insulators, and Resistance

Differences in atomic structure permit electrons to pass through some materials more easily than through others. Substances through which electrons can move with relative ease are called *conductors*. Most metals are good conductors. This is why copper and aluminum, which are excellent but reasonably priced conductors, are used to make wire. On the other hand, it is very difficult to get current to flow through some other materials, including wood, air, glass, and many plastics. These substances are called *insulators*. Under normal conditions all materials, even the best conductors, present *some* impediment to the flow of electricity. That impediment is referred to as *resistance* (R) and it is measured in *ohms* (symbol: Ω). A good conductor has very low resistance; an insulator has very high resistance. At a given voltage (driving force, pressure)

---

[2] There is a difference between voltage and potential. In essence, it is the difference between the actual and the ideal. Any electronics text can provide further information about this distinction, but it will not concern us here.

more current will flow through a low resistance than through a high resistance. In other words, current is inversely proportional to resistance: $I \propto \dfrac{1}{R}$.

Ohm's Law

Taking the relationships between current and voltage ($I \propto E$) and between current and resistance,

$$I \propto \frac{1}{R},$$

a general rule of electrical flow can be formulated: **Current is proportional to voltage and inversely proportional to resistance.** This principle is known as *Ohm's Law*. It is the foundation upon which most of the field of electronics rests. If the units used to measure resistance (R), current (I), and potential or voltage (E) are properly chosen (and they have been!), then Ohm's law can be stated as an equation:

$$I = \frac{E}{R}.$$

Expressed in words, the equation says that flow (current, in amperes) is equal to the pressure (voltage, in volts) divided by impediment to flow (resistance, in ohms). This relationship can be manipulated algebraically to derive two alternate forms:

$$R = \frac{E}{I}$$

(resistance equals voltage divided by current) and

$$E = IR$$

(voltage equals current times resistance).

This last form of Ohm's law has a very significant implication that may not be immediately apparent. It really says that a voltage (pressure difference) *results from* the flow of current through a resistance. That is, when a flow of electrons encounters an obstacle (a resistance) the electrical pressure will be higher on the "upstream" side of the resistance than on the "downstream" side. The voltage (or pressure) "drops" across the resistance. If there is no resistance between two points then there can be no voltage difference between them.

A couple of examples will demonstrate the usefulness of even these simple electronic principles.

1. According to the manufacturer's specification sheet, a transducer for sensing intraoral air pressure has a resistance of 300 Ω. It can tolerate a current through it of no more than 0.5 A. (Greater currents may destroy it.) Can the transducer be safely connected to the 20-V power supply available in your clinic?

The problem is to find out how much current will flow through the pressure transducer when 20 V is applied to it. We need to determine the current (I). Therefore:

$$I = \frac{E}{R} = \frac{20 \text{ V}}{300 \text{ }\Omega}$$

$$I = 0.067 \text{ A}.$$

The 20-V supply on hand will not overpower the transducer and can be safely used.

2. The manufacturer of a flow sensor recommends that it be heated by a current of 0.1 A. The heater element has a resistance of 250 Ω. How much voltage is needed to provide the necessary heating?

We are interested in determining the voltage (E) that produces a current (I) of 0.1 A through the heater's resistance (R) of 250 Ω. Therefore:

$$E = IR = (0.1 \text{ A})(250 \text{ }\Omega)$$

$$E = 25 \text{ V}.$$

Proper heating will require a 25-V power supply.

Power

Another important concept can be derived from Ohm's Law. Both pressure and flow represent the energy that is available to do work in any system. In electrical terms, the voltage drop and the current determine the **power** (P) being used or dissipated. Power, then, is

$$P = EI$$

(power equals voltage times current). Power is measured in *watts* (W).

Because voltage, current, and resistance are all related to each other there are a number of formulae by which power can be calculated, depending on which variables are known in a given situation. For instance, because $E = IR$ we can substitute IR for E in the power equation. That is

$$P = EI$$

but since $E = IR$

$$P = (IR)I$$

which can be simplified to

$$P = I^2R.$$

Similarly,

$$P = EI$$

but since $I = \dfrac{E}{R}$

$$P = E\left(\dfrac{E}{R}\right)$$

which can be simplified to

$$P = \dfrac{E^2}{R}.$$

Power may be dissipated as sound pressure, light, or motion, among other forms. Mostly, however, power is lost as heat. Sometimes generating heat is the goal (as was the case for the flow-transducer heater), but usually it is only a by-product. Many electronic systems are housed in ventilated cases so that the waste heat can be carried away easily.

Ohm's law, then, relates four electrical quantities: current, voltage, resistance, and power. By using algebraic substitutions again, a number of forms of Ohm's law can be derived to express any one of the quantities in terms of the others. All of the alternative forms are summarized in Table 2–1.

Schematic Diagrams

It is very much easier to describe an electronic circuit by means of a diagram than to use words to explain how its various elements are connected to each other. For this reason more-or-less standardized symbols are used according to a generally agreed upon set of rules to generate what are called "schematic diagrams." Some of the basic principles of reading them are considered here in order to facilitate further consideration of electronic circuits.

Figure 2–1 is a set of schematics for a very simple electrical circuit: two lamps connected to a source of DC current.[3] In Figure 2–1A, the flow of current is from the +10 V side of the source (which might be a battery) through a switch.[4] After the switch the current pathway has two branches: part of the total current flowing from the source flows through lamp 1, and part flows through lamp 2. The circuit paths merge again to carry the current to the 0 V side of the DC source, completing the circuit. Note the symbols used for the DC supply, the lamps, and the switch. Straight lines represent wires (or other conductors). The layout of the schematic diagram is intended to make the circuit easy to understand. It does not necessarily have any rela-

Table 2–1. Summary of Ohm's Law

Current	Voltage
$I = \dfrac{E}{R}$	$E = IR$
$I = \dfrac{P}{E}$	$E = \dfrac{P}{I}$
$I = \sqrt{\dfrac{P}{R}}$	$E = \sqrt{PR}$

Resistance	Power
$R = \dfrac{E}{I}$	$P = EI$
$R = \dfrac{P}{I^2}$	$P = \dfrac{E^2}{R}$
$R = \dfrac{E^2}{P}$	$P = I2R$

I = current in amperes
R = resistance in ohms
E = potential across R in volts
P = power in watts

tionship to the actual physical placement of the wiring that would be used in building the circuit. The circuit diagrammed in Figure 2–1B is identical in every way to the one shown in Figure 2–1A, although it looks different on the page. In each case the current flow is from the source, through a switch, through one of two branches that includes a lamp, and back via a final single path to the power supply.

In complex circuits many elements may share a common current path back to the power source. In order to simplify their diagrams the convention shown in Figure 2–1C has been adopted. The triangular marker indicates a "common" connection, a single point or wire in the actual circuit to which the marked points are connected. In reading these diagrams all points marked with this triangular symbol should be considered to be joined together.

Ground

The common return path for current in a circuit is often referred to as the circuit's **ground**, a term that goes

---

[3] Since "DC" stands for "direct current" the term "DC current" is redundant. However, the usage is common, as is the term "AC current."

[4] In point of fact, of course, current flows from the negative pole to the positive pole of the electrical supply. The error about direction dates from the earliest days of research on electricity. For most purposes, however, it does no harm to treat the circuit as if current flows from positive to negative. Sometimes this "wrong-way" flow is referred to as "conventional current."

back to the very early days of electronics. Ground is commonly the metal chassis on which an instrument is built, and the metal parts of the instrument case are often attached to the ground for safety (see "Electrical Safety," this chapter). These days it is not uncommon for the ground of a circuit to be physically connected to the earth itself by a separate wire (the third contact on a three-prong plug), but this is not usually true for older devices, in which the ground is "floating"—unconnected to anything that is actually in contact with the earth.

Series and Parallel Circuits

Figure 2–2 shows the two basic ways in which components can be arranged in any circuit. In Figure 2–2A the current path is through a set of elements (in this case, light bulbs) in sequence. Each electron traveling around this *series circuit* must pass through every component. The electrons are like cars traveling bumper-to-bumper along a single-lane road through a series of towns. Each car must go through each town in sequence, and all the cars must travel at the same rate, which is the overall speed of traffic. In a series circuit, then, all the electrons (cars) move at the same speed everywhere in the circuit (road). In electronic terms, the current in a series circuit is everywhere the same.

In a *parallel circuit*, on the other hand, there are alternative paths that the electrons can travel. Some of the electrons in Figure 2–2B go through lamp 1, while others are routed through lamp 2. If the lamps have different resistances then the current through the two branches of the circuit will be different. The total current flowing from the power source is the *sum* of the currents through lamps 1 and 2 in the parallel circuit. This contrasts with the series circuit, in which the current from the power source is the same as the current through either lamp 1 or lamp 2, since the current in a series circuit is everywhere the same.

Most real circuits are combinations of series and parallel arrangements. The circuit depicted in various ways in Figure 2–1 provided an example of this, although it was not mentioned. The switch in that circuit is in *series* with the lamps, while the two lamps are themselves connected in *parallel*. Since all of the current flows through a series element, opening the switch in Figure 2–1 interrupts the current to both lamps, turning them both off. On the other hand, if lamp 1 should burn out, lamp 2 will be unaffected because it represents an alternative current path through which electrons can flow without going via lamp 1 first.

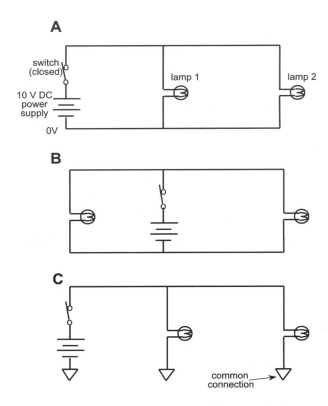

Figure 2–1. Three ways of diagramming the same simple circuit.

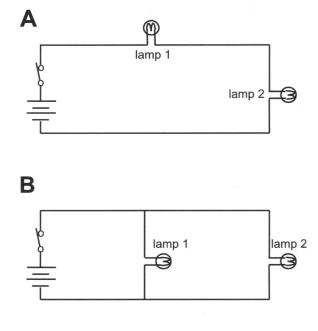

Figure 2–2. Series **(A)** and parallel **(B)** lamp circuits.

Resistance Networks

While some amount of resistance is inherent in all circuit components (even if, like wires, they are excellent conductors) circuit function usually depends on having exact amounts of resistance at specific places. This is arranged by using *resistors*, components which are characterized by specific amounts of resistance. Resistors can be made of many different materials—carbon powder, special metal wire, carbon films, and so forth—to optimize them to meet different requirements (such as stability in the face of temperature change, or minimization of aging effects). They are available with values ranging from a fraction of an ohm to several million ohms. (The value of a resistor is most commonly marked on it in the form of a series of colored bands.) Resistors dissipate power (Ohm's law: P = I²R), and they are designed to handle different amounts of power without overheating. The conventional schematic symbols for resistors are shown in Figure 2–3.

Series and Parallel Resistance. Each resistor represents a certain impediment to the flow of current. When resistors are arranged in series, as in Figure 2–4A, the current must pass through all of them, and the total resistance encountered by the electrons will be the sum of all the resistances in the series. Therefore, given a set of resistors in series, $R_1, R_2, R_3, \dots , R_n$, the total resistance is

$$R_{series} = R_1 + R_2 + R_3 + \dots + R_n.$$

The total resistance of a set of resistors connected in parallel may be somewhat less easy to grasp. Consider the very simple circuit of Figure 2–4B which (except for the absence of a switch) is the same as the parallel lamp circuit of Figure 2–1B. Here, however, resistors R_1 and R_2 have taken the place of the light bulbs. We will need to evaluate the current through each of them (I_1 and I_2) as well as the total current (I_T) flowing from the power supply. The circuit of Figure 2–4B is rearranged to the form of Figure 2–4C to facilitate the evaluation. It is clear from the rearrangement that R_1 and R_2 are both directly connected to the voltage supply, V. Therefore, according to Ohm's law, the current through R_1 must be

$$I_1 = \frac{V}{R_1}.$$

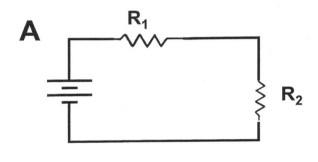

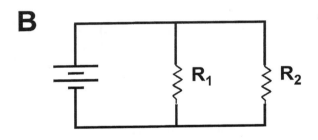

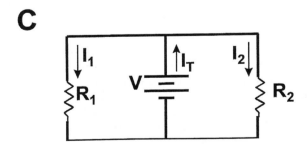

Figure 2–4. Total resistance of series and parallel circuits. **(A)** series resistance: $R_T = R_1 + R_2$. **(B)** parallel resistance, $R_T = \dfrac{R_1 R_2}{R_1 R_2}$. **(C)** is a rearrangement of **(B)**.

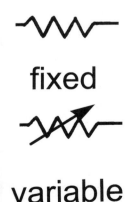

fixed

variable

Figure 2–3. Resistor schematic symbols.

Similarly, current through R_2 must be

$$I_2 = \frac{V}{R_2}.$$

The total current (I_T) from the supply must be equal to the sum of these two currents, so that

$$I_T = I_1 + I_2 = \left(\frac{V}{R_1} + \frac{V}{R_2}\right).$$

As the power supply "looks out" at the circuit it sees its voltage, V, causing a current flow of I_T amperes. Therefore, from the point of view of the supply, the resistance of the total circuit must be

$$R_T = \frac{V}{I_T}$$

which can be reduced to

$$R_T = \frac{1}{\frac{1}{R_1} + \frac{1}{R_2}}.$$

This relationship can be generalized to any number of resistors in parallel. The total resistance of n resistors is equal to the reciprocal of the sum of the reciprocals of the resistances:

$$R_T = \frac{1}{\frac{1}{R_1} + \frac{1}{R_2} + \ldots + \frac{1}{R_n}}.$$

In the case of only two resistors a little mathematical manipulation provides a more convenient formula:

$$R_T = \frac{R_1 R_2}{R_1 + R_2}.$$

The need to evaluate the sum of resistances in series and parallel frequently arises, as a simple example can illustrate. Many audio amplifiers provide several different connections for loudspeakers or earphones. Very often there are three, labeled "4 ohms," "8 ohms," and "16 ohms." These designations refer to the resistance of the speaker (or earphones) to be hooked up to the amplifier. Most speakers have a resistance of 8 Ω. If only one is to be wired to a single connection on the amplifier, it should obviously be wired to the 8 Ω output. But suppose that two sets of earphones (one for the patient, the other for the clinician) are to be used to listen to some audio material. Each earphone set, according to its label, has a resistance of 8 Ω. In order for both listeners to hear the same material, the two sets of earphones must obviously be connected to the same output. This means that current coming from the amplifier can follow either of two alternate paths. That is, the earphones will be in paral-lel. To which of the amplifier's three connectors should both earphones be wired: 4 Ω, 8 Ω, or 16 Ω?

Since the earphones are to be connected in parallel, the total of their resistances must be

$$R_T = \frac{R_1 R_2}{R_1 + R_2}.$$

Therefore,

$$R_T = \frac{(8 \times 8)}{(8 + 8)} = \frac{64}{16} = 4\ \Omega.$$

Since the total resistance of the paralleled devices is 4 Ω, the audio output should be taken from the 4 Ω connection on the amplifier.

Voltage Dividers and Potentiometers. Figures 2–5A shows a simple circuit in which two resistors are connected in series to a power supply. Measurement points are provided at the positive side of the supply (point A), at the junction of the two resistors (point B), and at the negative side of the supply (point C) to allow the voltage differences between several points in the circuit to be determined. The total voltage of the circuit (V_T) is the 10 V provided by the supply. (This is the voltage difference between measurement points A and C.) The total resistance of the circuit is $R_T = R_1 + R_2$, which is $100 + 400 = 500\ \Omega$. Current through the series resistances must therefore be

$$I_T = \frac{E}{R_T} = \frac{10\ V}{500\ \Omega} = 0.02\ A.$$

Now, since this is a series circuit, the current must everywhere be the same. That means that the current through R_1 equals the current through R_2 equals 0.02 A. Ohm's law states that current interacts with resistance to produce a voltage difference across a resistor. The voltage difference (or drop) produced by the 100 Ω of R_1 must be $V_1 = IR_1 = 0.02\ A \times 100\ \Omega = 2\ V$. This is what a voltmeter connected to point A and point B would read. On the other hand, the voltage created by the 400 Ω of R_2 is $V_2 = IR_2 = 0.02\ A \times 400\ \Omega = 8\ V$. A voltmeter connected to points B and C would show this much voltage. Note that the two voltages, from A to B and from B to C, total 10 V. This is as it should be, since the total voltage drop in the circuit (the voltage difference between the two poles of the power supply) must occur across the total of the resistive elements in the circuit. What the resistive circuit has done is to split the total available voltage provided by the supply into two parts. For this reason this circuit arrangement is called a *voltage divider*. Any number of resistors can be included in series to allow the total available voltage to be split into as many smaller voltages as there are

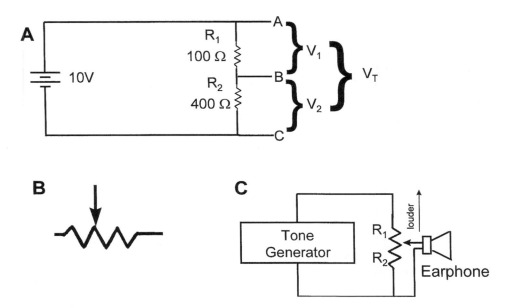

Figure 2–5. **(A)** Voltage divider circuit. **(B)** Schematic symbol for a potentiometer. **(C)** The potentiometer as a variable voltage divider in an intensity-control function. R_1 and R_2 are resistors, V_1 and V_2 are the voltages across R_1 and R_2, and V_T is the total voltage. A and C are measurement points at the positive and ground side of the power supply, B is a measurement point at the junction of the two resistors.

resistors in series. The analysis of voltage division by any number of resistors is the same as the evaluation for the circuit of Figure 2–5.

There is a simpler way of describing (or, for that matter, of calculating) the voltage drops in a voltage divider. Note that, in Figure 2–5, R_1 is 1/5 of the total resistance and the voltage drop across it is 1/5 of the total applied voltage. Similarly, R_2, which accounts for 4/5 of the total resistance in the circuit, produces a voltage drop that is equal to 4/5 of the applied voltage. To generalize, in a voltage divider the voltage drop across a resistor is to the total applied voltage as the resistance in question is to the total resistance. That is, V_x : $R_x = V_T$: R_T. Therefore, the voltage across a given resistor R_x is

$$V_X = \frac{R_X}{R_T} V_T .$$

Because any given circuit is likely to need a great many different voltages at different places, fixed voltage-divider networks are quite common. However, there is often a need for *variable voltage division*. For instance, a clinician might want to use a sine-wave generator to produce a tone to be matched by the patient's phonation. The voltage produced by the generator might produce too loud a tone when it is fed to a set of earphones. A voltage divider between the gen-

erator and earphones would reduce the voltage, and thereby the tone intensity, but perhaps by too much. In order to adjust the sound intensity to suit the needs of the moment an *adjustable* voltage divider network is needed.

Variability is easily provided by a device known as a **_potentiometer_**, shown in Figure 2–5B. Usually it is made of a resistive element (perhaps a strip of carbon film or a resistive wire winding) that is contacted by a "wiper." The two ends of the resistive element correspond to points A and C of the voltage divider, while the wiper is point B. The wiper contact really separates the total resistance of the potentiometer into two resistances and, because the wiper can be moved along the resistive element, the two resistances may be adjusted to any ratio. If the tone generator and earphone are connected as in Figure 2–5C the patient could control the sound intensity over a continuous range simply by adjusting a knob on the potentiometer shaft. This use of a potentiometer is familiar to anyone who has ever adjusted a radio's volume.

The Wheatstone Bridge. One of the most useful and widely employed circuits in electronic instrumentation is called the Wheatstone bridge.[5] It lies at the heart of many measurement devices including, for example, pressure gauges (see Chapter 8, "Air Pressure") and motion transducers (Chapter 12,

---

[5] Named for its creator, Sir Charles Wheatstone (1802–1875), better known in less technological circles as the inventor of the concertina.

"Speech Movements"). Given its importance in so many measurement applications, it seems worthwhile to examine it in some detail here.

As shown in Figure 2–6A, the Wheatstone bridge is a purely resistive network and so can be analyzed at this point in our discussion. To simplify slightly, the Wheatstone bridge produces a voltage that is proportional to the change in the resistance of R_x, which could be a sensing element in a pressure gauge, for instance.

In Figure 2–6B the circuit has been redrawn, and the resistors assigned values to facilitate analysis. The two schematics show exactly the same circuit, except that a meter has been added in Figure 2–6B so that the circuit output can be measured. (We will assume that the meter does not allow any current to flow between points 1 and 2. In other words, the meter is considered to have infinite resistance. Any detector that *does* allow a meaningful current to flow across the bridge behaves like a resistor connecting the two sides, greatly altering circuit function. In real-life situations, of course, points 1 and 2 would more likely be connected to an amplifier or other electronic detection system. Anything

connected across the bridge must meet the requirement of essentially infinite resistance if the bridge circuit is to function correctly.) It is worth noting at this point that, while the circuit we are considering has a DC "excitation" (supply) voltage, a Wheatstone bridge will work just a well with any sort of AC signal. Indeed, this is one of its major attractions.

The redrawn bridge circuit looks very much like two voltage dividers, connected in parallel to a voltage source. One of the resistors (R_x) is variable. (In use, the variable resistor would be a strain gauge or other sensing device whose resistance changes in response to some phenomenon in which we are interested.) For the moment, let us assume that the variable resistance has the same value as the other resistors. If this is so, then the two voltage dividers are identical, and the voltage drops across each of their resistors must be the same. Therefore, the meter connected to points 1 and 2 sees no voltage difference and registers 0 V. The bridge is said to be "balanced." But suppose that something happens to change the resistance of R_x. (Perhaps a pressure has been applied to the gauge that R_x represents.) Now the two voltage dividers are *not* the

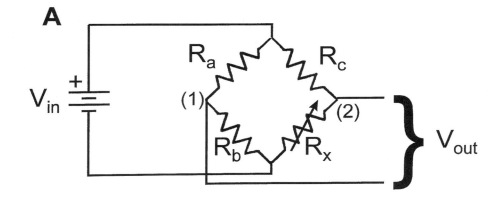

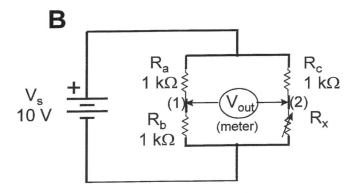

Figure 2–6. The Wheatstone bridge. **(A)** as commonly drawn in schematics. **(B)** redrawn (with the addition of a meter) for analysis. R_a, R_b, and R_c are constant resistances, while R_x is variable.

same (the bridge is said to be *unbalanced*) and the voltage at point 1 is no longer the same as the voltage at point 2. The meter now detects a voltage difference. The greater the disparity between R_x and the other resistors in the bridge, the greater the voltage that will be seen by the meter.

Figure 2–7 illustrates the relationship between the variation of R_x and the output of the bridge circuit of Figure 2–6. Note that the voltage across the bridge is directly and fairly linearly related to the value of R_x over a usable, if narrow, range of resistances.

It should be noted, of course, that the output of a simple voltage divider circuit, in which one of the resistances is the variable R_x, would also vary as R_x changed. So the reasonable question is, why use a four-resistor

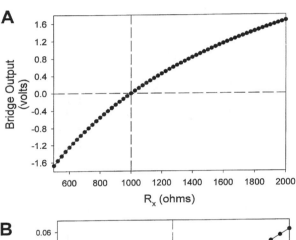

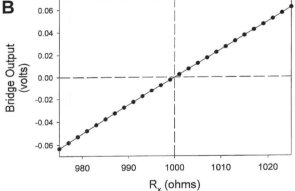

Figure 2–7. Output of the Wheatstone bridge of Figure 2–6. When the variation of Rx is large (as in A) it is clear that the output of a Wheatstone bridge is not a linear function of its value. However, over a much smaller range of R_x values (as in B) the linearity of the bridge output is sufficiently good for almost all purposes. (The dashed lines indicate the bridge's condition at balance, when all resistors have the same value.)

Wheatstone bridge, that requires careful matching of its elements, when a two-resistor circuit would do? The answer lies in the fact that the voltage divider produces a real voltage (equal to one half of the supply voltage) when both resistors are equal, and there is no way in which the divider's output can ever be zero. The bridge, on the other hand, produces an output of 0 V when all of its resistors are of equal value and, as R_x increases above zero, while the output becomes increasingly less than zero as R_x becomes less than the other resistances. Centering the output symmetrically about 0 V is a real advantage in most electronic systems, and largely accounts for the preference for the Wheatstone bridge and its relatives.

From an applied point of view, the value of the Wheatstone bridge lies in the fact that many sensing devices have detecting elements whose resistance changes as a function of the variable of interest. By including the resistive detector in a Wheatstone bridge, its resistance change is converted into a voltage change, centered at 0 V, that can be used by analysis circuits or display devices, such as oscilloscopes, amplifiers, chart recorders, and the like. There are many variations of the basic Wheatstone bridge. For example, diagonally opposite resistors in the bridge are commonly both active—that is, they both vary as a function of the phenomenon being sensed—doubling the sensitivity of the bridge. Other resistors are often added to regulate current or to provide a means of calibration. These modifications are discussed in Geddes and Baker (1989) and in most basic electronics textbooks.

BASIC PRINCIPLES OF ALTERNATING CURRENT

In the real world most signals are *time dependent*: something about them changes with time. Such signals constitute **alternating current** or AC. It is worth repeating here that, despite the usual meaning of the term "alternating" there is no requirement that the flow of current or the polarity of the voltage actually reverse. Any change with time makes a signal AC.

The simplest kind of time variation is the sine wave, the basic building block of all other periodic waves (see Chapter 7, "Sound Spectrography"). And the simplest kind of sine wave is, in fact, one in which the current actually does reverse direction (which implies that the driving voltage reverses direction). A simple sine wave of this type will be used to elucidate some of the basic characteristics of AC signals and the ways in which AC differs from DC.

---

[6] Technically, of course, a signal that shows voltage, rather than current, change, should be referred to as "alternating voltage." However sloppy, application of the term "alternating current" even to voltage changes is well established.

AC Current and Voltage

Because an AC signal is continuously changing, a simple measure of voltage or current is inadequate to describe it completely. Its frequency and phase, with which speech pathologists are already familiar, must also be specified. The fact that the amplitude of an AC signal is constantly changing creates problems in describing the voltage or current, since any single reading is valid for only one point in time. To cope with this several standard measures have been adopted. They are illustrated in Figure 2–8.

Instantaneous AC. The *instantaneous current* or *voltage* is the amplitude of the wave at a given point in time. To distinguish this value from a more global, overall measure it is generally symbolized by a lowercase letter. Hence, instantaneous voltage is e, while instantaneous current is i.

Peak-to-Peak AC. *Peak-to-peak current* or *voltage* of the wave is the difference between its most negative and its most positive values. In other words, it is the height of the wave from the bottom of a trough to the top of a peak. In Figure 2–8 the peak-to-peak voltage is $2V_{p-p}$.

Peak AC. The *peak current* or *voltage* is defined as the amplitude of the wave above (or, equivalently, below) the zero-voltage or zero-current line. In Figure 2–8 the peak voltage is $1V_p$.

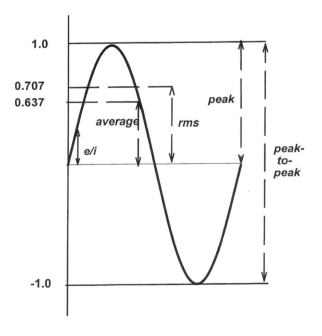

Figure 2–8. Relationship among AC measures of voltage or current.

Average AC. It is often useful to have an overall average of all of the instantaneous voltages or currents. A problem with taking the simple average of all of the instantaneous values should be obvious: If the waveform is symmetrical about the zero point, the average of all the negative- and positive-signed points must equal zero. The way around this is, of course, to limit the averaging process to half of the cycle—that is, to either a positive or a negative alternation. Then, when the averaging is performed (by a process known in the calculus as integration) the average value (V_A or I_A) *of a sine wave* will be equal to 0.637 times its peak amplitude. (It must be strongly emphasized that this particular ratio of the average value to peak amplitude is valid only for a sine wave!)

Root-mean-square (RMS) current or **voltage.** Perhaps the most common specification of an AC signal is its *equivalent* or *effective amplitude*. This is the amplitude that a DC voltage (or current) would need to be in order to deliver the same power as a given AC signal. Since power is proportional to the square of the voltage or current, deriving the equivalent amplitude involves (in theory) taking the square of the amplitude of the wave at every point in time, finding the average or mean of these squared values, and then finding the square root of the mean. Hence, this amplitude measure is referred to as the *root-mean-square* value, commonly denoted *RMS*. In practice, of course, there is no real need to do the mathematics (which is specified by the calculus of integration). For a sine wave (but *only* for a sine wave) the RMS voltage (or current) will be equal to the peak voltage (or current) times 0.7071. Thus, if the peak voltage of a particular sine wave is 1.00V, its RMS voltage will be $0.7071V_{RMS}$. This indicates that the power delivered by a sine wave of 1 V peak amplitude is equal to the power that would be delivered by a DC flow at 0.7071 V in the same circuit.

It is important to re-emphasize that the constant 0.7071 is valid only for the relationship between a sine wave and a DC signal. If the waveform being evaluated is not a sine wave, some other ratio will apply. If the waveform is complex it may not be possible to determine exactly what the constant should be. This last point is of importance to the speech pathologist, who has frequent occasion to measure the amplitude of complex periodic waves, such as speech signals. A problem arises because most meters (whether digital or analog) actually determine average voltage (or current) and then apply a correction factor to derive RMS values. But the correction factor is valid only for sine waves, not for complex waveforms. The difference between the scale reading and the actual RMS value can be substantial. For complex waves a "true RMS" meter (that actually performs the required calculation)

Table 2–2. Relationship among AC voltage and current values.

To derive*:	Multiply Peak by	Multiply Average by	RMS
Peak	—	1.57	1.41
Average	0.637	—	0.9
RMS	0.707	1.11	—

*Example: To derive the *average* equivalent of a measured *RMS* voltage, multiply RMS voltage by 0.9.

is needed. Table 2–2 provides the appropriate values by which to multiply readings to convert voltage (or current) readings from one form to another. The conversions are fully valid only for sine waves, but can provide useful approximations in other, carefully-considered, circumstances.

DC Bias

Very often the current or voltage of an AC signal does not, in fact, reverse direction. An example of a sine wave for which this is the case is shown in Figure 2–9. What is happening here is that the waveform is alternating around some middle value that is not zero. (In Figure 2–9 a dotted line has been drawn at the level of that central value.) A moment's reflection reveals that the central value is equivalent to a DC signal. The AC wave, then, really represents the addition of a varying voltage (an AC signal) to a DC level. The AC wave is said to be associated with a **DC bias**. To completely specify the wave of Figure 2–9 we need to state not only its amplitude (peak, RMS, or average) but also the DC bias associated with it. It is possible to remove this bias, but doing so requires the use of reactive circuit devices, which are considered in the next section.

Reactance

A prime difference between DC and AC circuits is the fact that AC circuits are subject to the effect of **reactance**. This special property is due to energy storage by circuit elements. (In fact, several electronic components are designed to optimize their energy-storage capabilities so as to take advantage of this property.) The storage itself is fully analogous to that which occurs in mechanical systems: the work done in stretching a rubber band, for instance, is stored by its elasticity, to be unleashed later when the rubber band is let go. Similarly, a pendulum swings because the

energy of the starting push is saved as momentum. The electrical analogs of elasticity and momentum are called **capacitance** and **inductance**, respectively. They are embodied in devices known as **capacitors** and **inductors**. Capacitance and inductance affect the flow of alternating current by means of capacitative and inductive **reactance**.

It is inherently very difficult to miniaturize inductors to a size that makes them well-suited for use on ordinary circuit boards, so their use is uncommon in the situations with which we need to be concerned. Accordingly, the discussion to follow will focus on capacitance.

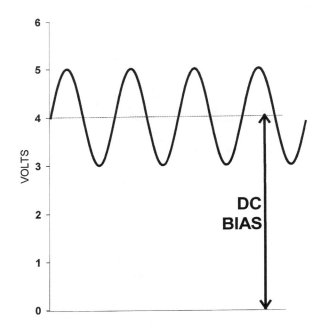

Figure 2–9. A sine wave signal in which the current does not reverse direction. The voltage varies by about 1 volt above and below a nonzero "center" value, indicated by the dashed line. This "DC bias" amounts to about 4 volts for this signal.

Capacitance

A capacitor stores electrons. It is constructed of two metallic plates that face each other but are separated by a very thin layer of insulating material, called the *dielectric*, as shown in Figure 2–10. When the plates are connected to a DC voltage, electrons flow until their packing into the dielectric under one plate becomes dense enough to produce a voltage that equals the driving voltage. The accumulation of electrons under one plate causes the electrons near the opposing plate to be driven away (since like charges repel). They are pushed to the other pole of the DC source. During the period when electrons are being packed into one region and driven away from the facing region of the dielectric there is an electron flow (current) in both of the wires that connect the capacitor to the DC source. (Note, however, that the electrons do not cross the insulating barrier in the capacitor.) It doesn't take very long for as many electrons to be packed into the dielectric as the applied voltage can force it to hold, and when the maximal packing has been achieved the flow stops, even though the DC voltage is still acting. If, at this point, the capacitor is disconnected from the voltage supply, the electrons remain in the dielectric, leaving the plates charged to the same voltage as the original driving source.

The unit of capacitance (C) is the *farad* (F). It describes how many electrons can be stored under the plate for every volt of packing pressure. That is, capacitance is a measure of the storage capability of the capacitor. (One farad represents an enormous electron-storage capability.) Actual capacitors have values ranging from several picofarads (pF, 10^{-12} farads) to a few hundreds of microfarads (µF, 10^{-6} farads). Capacitance increases with the area of the metal plates. (Increasing the size of the plates increases the electron storage area, allowing more electrons to be packed in.) It can also be increased by making the insulating layer between the metal plates thinner. This allows the electrons on one side of the dielectric more efficiently to repel electrons from the other side. In practice, the metal "plates" take many forms—foil or metallic coatings, for example—while the dielectric can be paper, ceramic, mica, air, or a layer of metal oxide. The three layers are usually rolled up or molded to occupy the smallest possible volume.

TIME CONSTANT

Let us consider a simple circuit, composed of a switch, a 1 V power source, a 100 000 Ω resistor, and a 2 µF capacitor, as in Figure 2–11A. We put a meter into the circuit to measure the current (I_C), and observe the voltage across the capacitor (V_C). In Figure 2–11B the voltage applied to the circuit is shown in the upper plot, while the lower one shows the voltage across the capacitor and the current flowing into it.

As long as the switch is open (denoted by negative time on the data plots), no voltage is applied to the circuit, so there is no current flowing in the circuit, and no voltage across the capacitor. At time 0 the switch is closed, and 1 volt is applied to the circuit. The current instantly rises to the value predicted by Ohm's law: I = E/R = 1 V/100 000 Ω = 0.000001 A = 10 µA. The voltage across the capacitor, however, does not instantly change to its final value. The capacitor is "elastic"—it *absorbs* the electrons—and so the pressure (voltage) in it lags behind the current flow into it. As time passes, however, the packing of electrons in the capacitor gets greater and greater, and so the voltage across the capacitor rises. As the electron packing increases, however, it becomes harder and harder to pack more electrons in (just as it gets harder and harder to continue to blow up a balloon). In a sense, this is seen by the circuit as an increasing resistance to flow into the capacitor, and so the current gets less and less.

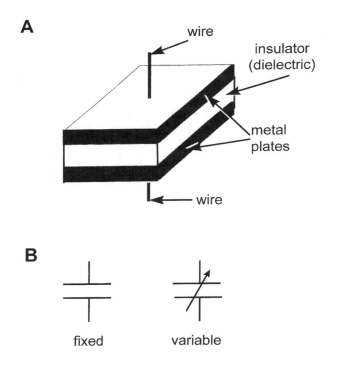

A

wire

insulator (dielectric)

metal plates

wire

B

fixed   variable

Figure 2–10. Construction (A) and schematic symbols (B) of a capacitor.

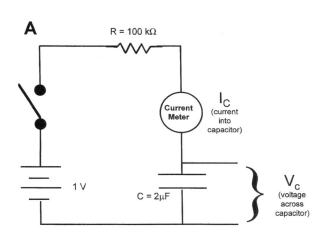

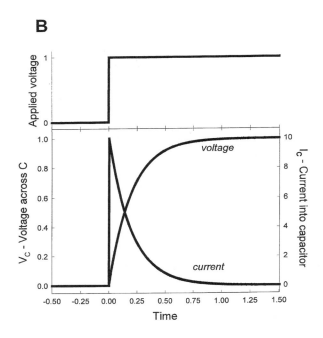

Figure 2–11. (A) A simple circuit to measure the current (I_C) and to observe the voltage across the capacitor (V_C). (B) The voltage applied to the circuit is shown in the upper plot, while the lower one shows the voltage across the capacitor and the current flowing into it.

The "sluggishness" of the system is measured by its *time constant*, the value of which is a function of the capacitance and the series resistance. Specifically, the voltage across a capacitor following the application of a driving voltage (at time 0) is

$$v_o = V_s (1 - e^{\text{t-RC}})$$

where v_o is the voltage across the capacitor;

V_s is the applied voltage;

t is time in seconds after application of the voltage;

R is the series resistance in ohms;

C is the capacitance in farads.

The product "RC" in this relationship is the time constant of the circuit. For the circuit of Figure 2–11 the time constant is RC = 100 000 Ω x 2 x 10^{-6} F = 0.20 s. In one time constant the voltage (or current) change will amount to 63% of the difference between its present and final value. That is, in the example circuit of Figure 2–11, at the end of the first time constant the voltage will have risen to 0.63(1 V – 0 V) = 0.63 V. In the

next RC interval the change will be 0.63(1 V – 0.63 V) = .233 V, and so on. Thus, we expect the following voltages at the end of each time constant:

RC interval	Change in voltage	Cumulative Change
1	0.63	0.63
2	0.233	0.863
3	0.086	0.949
4	0.032	0.981
5	0.011	0.992
6	0.005	0.997
7	0.002	0.999

In principle, the voltage across the capacitor will never arrive at its final value. But, after 5 time constants an approximation will have been reached that will suffice for almost all everyday purposes.

PHASE LAG

Figure 2–12 repeats the circuit of Figure 2–11A, except that the switch has been removed and the DC source is replaced by a sine-wave generator that produces a 1000 Hz wave with a peak voltage of 1 V. We again monitor the current through the circuit and the voltage across the capacitor. Figure 2–13 plots the results. (Voltage is represented by a heavy line, and current by a lighter one.)

Ohm's law states that current is proportional to voltage, and therefore we would expect that the current would rise and fall in step with the voltage. But that is not what happens in this—or in any reactive—circuit. The energy-storing property of the capacitor is producing asynchrony of voltage and current: they are out of phase with each other. In fact, the phase difference is 90°, and the current *leads* the voltage.

Reactance, Frequency Dependence, and Impedance

The phase difference between the voltage and current produces a special problem if we want to calculate the "resistance" of the capacitor. The standard Ohm's law relationship, R = E/I, cannot be valid because, given the timing difference, the calculated R would vary depending on exactly when in the cycle it was measured. What this suggests is that, although the capacitor presents an impediment to current flow, that impediment is something other than that created by a resistance.

The AC equivalent of resistance is called **reactance**. Like resistance, it is measured in ohms. But, in contrast to resistance, reactance is a vector quantity.

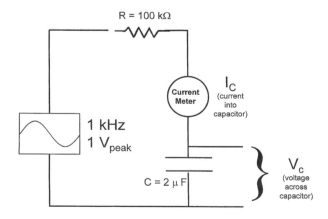

Figure 2–12. The same circuit shown in Figure 2–11A, except that the switch has been removed and the DC source is replaced by a sine-wave generator that produces a 1000 Hz wave with a peak voltage of 1 V.

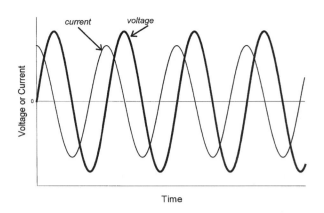

Figure 2–13. A plot of the current (thin line) through the circuit shown in Figure 2–12 and the voltage (thicker line) across the capacitor.

That is, it has both magnitude (expressed in ohms), and direction (expressed as phase angle). Another important characteristic of reactance is that it is frequency-dependent. The reactance of a capacitor, (X_c, expressed in ohms) is

$$X_C = \frac{1}{2\pi fRC}$$

where f = frequency in hertz

C = capacitance in farads

R = resistance in ohms.

(The quantity $2\pi f$ is called the *angular velocity* of the wave. Note that it is often symbolized, in the literature of physics and electrical engineering, as ω.) Thus, in the circuit of Figure 2–12, where f = 1 kHz and C = 2 µF, the magnitude of the capacitive reactance is

$$X_c = 1/2\pi(1000)(2 \times 10^{-6}) = 1 / 0.01257 = 79.6 \ \Omega.$$

If the frequency of the sine wave generator were lowered to 500 Hz, then the reactance would be

$$X_c = 1/2\pi(500)(2 \times 10^{-6}) = 1 / 0.00628 = 159.2 \ \Omega.$$

Reactance is linearly proportional to frequency.

Because X_c, the capacitive reactance, is a vector quantity we cannot simply add the values of the series R and C to obtain a total that is equivalent to the "resistance" of the circuit. When reactance is involved, we speak therefore not of resistance but of **impedance**, symbolized **Z**, which is the *vector* sum of R and X_c. That is,

$$Z = \sqrt{X_c^2 + R^2}$$

In our example, the impedance of the circuit must be

$$Z = (X_c^2 + R^2)^{1/2} \approx (80^2 + (10^5)^2)^{1/2}$$

$$= (6400 + 10^{10})^{1/2}$$

$$\cong 10\,000\ \Omega.$$

If the sine-wave frequency were 500 Hz, and the reactance therefore about 160 Ω, then the impedance of the circuit would be

$$Z = (X_c^2 + R^2)^{1/2} \approx (160^2 + (10^5)^2)^{1/2}$$

$$= (25600 + 10^{10})^{1/2}$$

$$= 316227\ \Omega$$

which is a very significant impedance difference indeed!

FILTERS

The dependence of capacitative reactance, X_c, and hence of impedance, Z, on the frequency of the AC wave allows us to construct circuits that are frequency selective. These circuits are known as *filters*.

Low-Pass Filters

The RC circuit that we have been using as an example can be pressed into service again to evaluate how filters work. We will assume that, this time, R = 10 kΩ, and that C = 0.02 μF. In Figure 2–14 we also rearrange the circuit schematic to better suit our present purposes. Notice that, when drawn this way, the RC circuit looks very much like a voltage divider. In fact, it *is* a voltage divider. However, instead of using two resistors, it uses a resistance—whose value of 10 000 Ω is fixed and constant—and the reactive equivalent of resistance, the capacitative reactance, whose value changes with the frequency of the AC voltage source. We may evaluate the characteristics of the circuit, and begin by assuming that the AC source produces a 1000 Hz output with a voltage of $1\,V_{rms}$.

At 1000 Hz the reactance of the capacitor, X_c, is

$$X_c = 1/2\pi fC$$

$$= 1/2\pi(1000)(.02 \times 10^{-6})$$

$$= 1 / 1.2566$$

$$X_c = 7957\ \Omega.$$

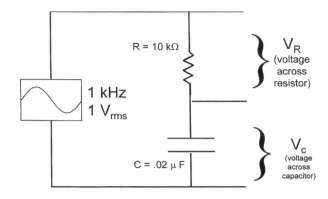

Figure 2–14. A simple resistor-capacitor filter circuit.

To a 1000 Hz voltage, then, the capacitor looks like a 7957 Ω resistor (with a phase shift!). For a voltage divider, the voltage that appears across any element is proportional to that element's share of the total resistance. But in the RC "voltage divider," the voltage that appears across the capacitor is proportional to the capacitor's share of the impedance. So first one must calculate the impedance of the circuit:

$$Z = \sqrt{R^2 + X_C^2}$$

$$Z = \sqrt{10000^2 + 7957^2}$$

$$Z = 12779\ \Omega.$$

The voltage, V_R, that will appear across the resistor, given an input voltage of V_{in}, is

$$V_R = V_{in}\left(\frac{X_C}{Z}\right)$$

$$= 1\,(7957\ /\ 12779)$$

$$= 0.623\ V.$$

Now, if the input frequency drops to, let us say, 250 Hz, the same calculations show that X_c will rise to 31830 Ω, and the impedance of the circuit, Z, will be 33364 Ω. The output across the capacitor will rise to 0.954 V. If the calculation is repeated for several other input frequencies values of Table 2–3 result.

And if we plot these results, as in Figure 2-15, we can see the relationship between input frequency and output voltage, referred to as the circuit's *transfer function*.

Up to a certain point (roughly 100 Hz in our circuit), the output voltage seems hardly to be affected at all by the frequency. But as the frequency gets higher

---

[7] It does not matter whether we measure the voltage as RMS, peak, average, or peak-to-peak, as long as we use the same measure at both input and output.

Table 2–3. Reactance, impedance, and voltage across the capacitor of the circuit of Figure 2–14 at different frequencies.

Frequency (Hz)	X_c (Ω)	Z (Ω)	VC
10	795775	795838	0.999
50	159155	159468	0.998
100	79577	80203	0.992
200	39788	41026	0.969
500	15915	18796	0.847
796	10000	14142	0.707
800	9947	14104	0.705
1500	5305	11320	0.469
2500	3183	10494	0.303
3000	2652	10345	0.256
3500	2273	10255	0.222
4500	1768	10155	0.174
5500	1446	10104	0.143
6500	1224	10074	0.122
7500	1061	10056	0.106
8500	936	10043	0.093
10000	795	10032	0.079
30000	265	10003	0.027
50000	159	10001	0.016
100000	79	100000	0.008

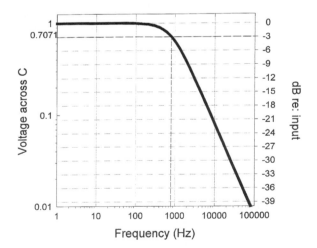

Figure 2–15. The transfer function of the circuit shown in Figure 2–14.

the voltage across the capacitor decreases at an accelerating rate until (at roughly 1000 Hz) the decrease in the output voltage as the frequency rises becomes steady. The circuit passes sine waves below a certain *cut-off frequency* essentially without loss, but higher frequencies are increasingly attenuated. The circuit, therefore, discriminates *against* low frequencies and *in favor of* high frequencies. It is therefore called a *high-pass filter*.

The *cut-off frequency* (f_{co}) of the circuit is defined as the frequency at which the output is attenuated by 3 dB. In other words, it is the frequency at which the output voltage is 0.7071 times the input voltage, which implies that the power of the signal is reduced by half (see Chapter 5, "Speech Intensity"). (Dashed lines in the figure show the relationship of the cutoff frequency to the output.) Beyond this frequency the output voltage diminishes at the rate of 6 dB for every octave of increase (doubling) of the input frequency. The *roll-off* of the circuit is thus said to be 6 dB/octave.

Examination of the data plot shows that the cut-off frequency is roughly 800 Hz. It is easy enough to calculate the value. Since the output across the capacitor at the cut-off frequency has half the power of the input, the reactance of the capacitor at that frequency must account for half of the circuit's impedance. The only other component of the impedance is the resistor. Hence, at the cut-off frequency, the reactance of the capacitor, X_c, must equal the resistance, R. Therefore, at f_{co}, $\dfrac{1}{2\pi f_{co}C} = R = R$. Simple algebraic rearrangement, then, shows that

$$f_{co} = \frac{1}{2\pi RC}$$

where R is in ohms

C is in farads.

Therefore, the exact cutoff frequency of the circuit of Figure 2–14 is

$$f_{co} = \frac{1}{2\pi(10^4)(.02 \times 10^{-6})}$$

$$f_{co} = 795.8 \text{ Hz.}$$

High-Pass Filters

If the RC circuit is really just a special voltage divider, then it stands to reason that whatever part of the input voltage does not appear across the capacitor must appear across the resistor. This suggests that, if we were to look at the output of the circuit across R instead of across C we would obtain a reciprocal function. That is, when the output is taken across the resistor in Figure 2–14, the circuit will discriminate against low frequency inputs and in favor of high-frequency inputs. It will be, in short, a *high-pass filter*. Table 2–4 shows the voltage across the resistor at several frequencies.

When these data are plotted (Figure 2–16) it is clear that indeed the cutoff frequency is still about 795 Hz, but taking the output across the resistor makes the circuit a high-pass filter. In short, the only difference between a high-pass and a low-pass RC circuit is in where one takes the output.

We are not limited to a single filter "section." That is, the output of a filter can be applied to a second filter stage. If the filter stages are identical, then the output will have the almost the same f_{co} as a single-section circuit, but the roll-off will be doubled,

Table 2–4. Reactance, impedance, and voltage across the resistor of the circuit of Figure 2–14 at different frequencies

Frequency	$X_c(\Omega)$	$Z(\Omega)$	VR
10	795775	795838	0.012
100	79577	80203	0.125
200	39788	41026	0.244
500	15915	18796	0.532
800	9947	14104	0.709
1500	5305	11320	0.883
2500	3183	10494	0.953
3000	2652	10345	0.967
3500	2273	10255	0.975
4500	1768	10155	0.985
5500	1446	10104	0.989
6000	1326	10087	0.991
8000	994	10049	0.995
10000	795	10031	0.997
30000	265	10003	0.999
50000	159	10001	0.999
100000	79	10000	1.00

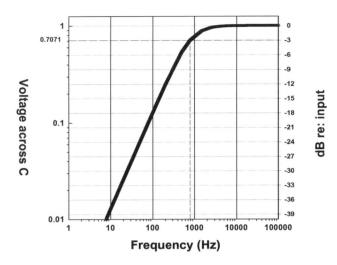

Figure 2–16. Transfer function of the circuit shown in Figure 2–14 when the output is taken across the resistor.

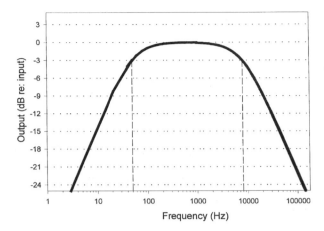

Figure 2–17. **(A)** The transfer function of a simple band-pass filter, with a highpass cutoff frequency of 50 Hz and a lowpass cutoff frequency of 8000 Hz. **(B)** Reversing the highpass and lowpass cutoff frequencies creates a band-reject filter.

to 12 dB/octave. The result is a filter that is twice as *selective*. One might think that the trick could be extended to as many sections as might be needed, to obtain, for instance, a filter with a 72 dB/octave roll-off. Unfortunately, the interaction among the sections quickly becomes very significant, so the process does not work very well. More selective filters require more complex "active" circuits, which have amplifiers to isolate the filter sections.

Band-Pass and Band-Reject Filters

At least conceptually, it is possible apply the output of a high-pass filter to the input of a low-pass filter.[8] If f_{co} of the high-pass circuit is lower than that of the low-pass circuit, then all frequencies between the two cut-off frequencies—referred to as the **pass band**—will be passed with essentially no loss. The circuit is therefore a **band-pass filter**. On the other hand, making f_{co} for the high-pass section higher than f_{co} for the low-pass section creates a circuit that suppresses frequencies between the two cut-off points, in the **reject band**. This is a **band-reject** filter. The transfer functions for a band-pass and a band-reject filter (using the same cut-off frequencies for both) are shown in Figure 2–17.

Filters are very common, and extremely important, circuits. They are used to limit the frequency content of a signal so as ensure that it falls within a range acceptable for further processing (as by A/D converters, see Chapters 3 and 4), to emphasize frequencies within a range of particular interest (as is done in sound spectrography, see Chapter 7) and, very often, to remove unwanted signal components (often noise).

A Note on Filtering

Filtering may be accomplished by appropriate mathematical manipulation of data.[9] (Of course, the signal must first have been converted to digital form.) *Digital filtering* can be tailored to meet the particular exigencies of almost any situation. It also offers great flexibility, because the characteristics of a digital filter can be altered simply by changing a few parameters in the filtering program. Furthermore, digital filters can provide transfer functions which are not easily achieved with standard electronic components. Finally, digital filtering has a sort of "with it" aura about it. In the computer-dominated environment of the clinical sciences it enjoys a kind of "state-of-the-art" reputation.

---

[8] While one could, in theory, simply connect RC sections such as have been used for examples in the present discussion, in actual practice a number of considerations enter into the design of practical band-pass filters that make them somewhat more complex. Any elementary textbook of electronics can provide guidance along these lines.

[9] Discussion of basic principles of digital filtering is available in many introductory textbooks, such as Jackson (1996). For consideration of specific problems of design of complex filters for voice and speech research see Hillenbrand and Houde (1996) and the ensuing discussion by Roark (1997) and Hillenbrand and Houde (1997).

Nonetheless, analog filtering is very much here to stay. It is very much easier and far more efficient to do needed filtering (and needed it almost always is) "on line" than to depend on a computer to perform necessary filtering of the signal after the fact. Figure 2–18 provides an example of the utility of on-line filtering. An electroglottographic (EGG) recording was made of a slightly dysphonic patient who, because of neuromotor problems, has significant movement in the perilaryngeal region. The movement produced intermittent perturbations of the EGG baseline. Since these are of very low frequency compared to the F_0 of phonation, they can be removed by high-pass filtering. (High-pass filtering rejects low frequency components in the signal.) The filtering was done with a cutoff frequency of 70 Hz. The figure shows how the baseline was stabilized without significant alteration of the individual EGG waveforms.

It is important to recall, however, that filtering constitutes a distortion of the original signal. This may

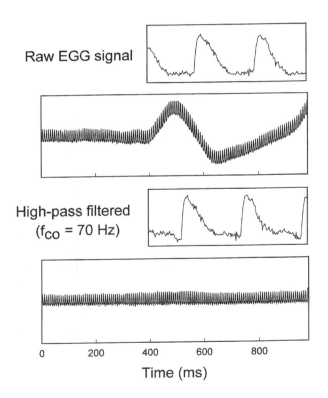

Raw EGG signal

High-pass filtered (f_{CO} = 70 Hz)

Time (ms)

Figure 2–18. The longer record at the top is of an EGG signal whose baseline shifts very significantly as a result of laryngeal movement in the neck. High pass filtering, with a cutoff frequency of 70 Hz, restores baseline stability (bottom record), making the signal useful for extraction of data such as fundamental frequency. The shorter traces are expanded segments of the longer records, and show that the filtering has not altered the EGG waveshape enough to interfere with clinical interpretation.

be an important consideration when qualitative assessment of signal characteristics is required. The filter attenuates frequencies beyond its cutoff frequency, and, equally important, most filters cause signal components of different frequencies to be "phase-shifted" by different amounts. In other words, the time relationships among the various frequency components of the signal are seriously altered. Attenuation of some components results in a change in the signal's power spectrum (see Chapter 7, "Sound Spectrography"). The phase shifting leaves the power spectrum unchanged, but results in a potentially significant change in the shape of the signal waveform.

Inductance

A magnetic field surrounds any wire through which current is flowing. The strength of that magnetic field is proportional to the current. As the current changes, the magnetic field enlarges and contracts. Conversely, a conductor placed in a magnetic field will have a current generated in it (or a voltage produced across it) whenever the strength of the magnetic field changes. Considering the magnetic and electrical phenomena together, it should be clear that a conductor carrying a current not only produces a magnetic field, but is itself caught in the very field that it itself produces. Whenever the current in the conductor changes, the resulting expansion or contraction of the magnetic field will induce a current in the conductor that is producing the field in the first place. The induced current will be in a direction that is *opposite to* the direction of the original current. (This is referred to as Lenz's law.) Therefore, a conductor is caught in a sort of "Catch-22" situation: Any change in the current through it causes an alteration of its magnetic field that opposes the change.

It is precisely this effect—self-opposition to change of current—that an inductor exploits. It does so by storing some of the energy of the electrical flow in the form of a magnetic field. If the current increases, some of its energy is withdrawn to enlarge the field, leaving less energy to push the electrons and therefore slowing the rate of current increase. If, on the other hand, the current diminishes, the magnetic field becomes smaller, returning energy to the conductor and helping to push the electrons along, thereby partially making up for the diminished driving force. In short, an inductor represents electrical momentum: it tends to keep electrons moving when the force pushing them lessens, and it opposes their rapid acceleration when the pushing force increases. The momentum effect in an electrical system is called *inductance*, symbolized **L**.

Inductors are generally made of a coil of wire, since the coiling concentrates the magnetic field, making the device more effective. This makes them rather bulky and has severely limited their usefulness in today's highly miniaturized circuits. They remain the heart of magnetic-detection devices, such as tape-recording heads (see Chapter 4, "General-Purpose Tools"). They are also used in some transducers, such as variable-reluctance pressure gauges (see Chapter 8, "Air Pressure"), the Respitrace™, and Articulograph™ (see Chapter 12, "Speech Movements").

Only a changing magnetic field can induce a current in a wire. Therefore, an inductor only interacts with a current that is varying. In other words, an inductor affects only AC. Furthermore, the faster the rate of change of the current the more strongly it is affected by the inductance. Since *rate of change* is another way of describing frequency, the degree to which a given inductance influences a signal depends on the signal's frequency.

INDUCTIVE REACTANCE

The unit of inductance is the **henry** (H)[10], and the opposition to change in the current is referred to as the **inductive reactance**, X_L. Like capacitative reactance, considered earlier, it is measured in ohms. Whereas the reactance of a capacitor is inversely proportional to frequency, X_L increases with frequency:

$$X_L = 2\pi fL.$$

As was the case with capacitative reactance, X_L causes a phase shift, but one which is the reverse of that seen with capacitance. That is, an inductance causes the current to lag behind the voltage by 90°. Similarly, in a circuit with a resistive and inductive element, the total impediment to current is expressed as the impedance,

$$Z = \sqrt{R^2 + X_L^2}.$$

Inductors can be viewed as *inverse capacitors*. That is, their reactance changes in a manner that is the reverse of that seen in inductors, and the phase lag is opposite to that of capacitors.

Inductive Filters

Just as was the case with capacitance, inductance can be used to construct frequency-selective circuits, or filters. The cutoff frequency (the frequency at which the output has one-half the power of the input) of a resis-tor-inductor circuit is that frequency at which the resistance equals the inductive reactance. That is, the frequency at which $R = X_L = 2\pi fL$. By algebraic manipulation, then, the cutoff frequency of a resistor-inductor filter is $f_{co} = 2\pi RL$.

The circuit of Figure 2–19 is a typical RL single-stage filter. Given that the inductor's reactance increases with frequency, more and more of the input voltage will appear across the inductor as the frequency of the input signal rises. This, then, is a high-pass filter. (Note how the inductive circuit is an inverted form of the equivalent high-pass capacitative filter in which the output would be taken across the resistor.) The cutoff frequency must be

$$f_{co} = 2\pi RL$$

$$= 2\pi(10\ 000)(.001267)$$

$$\approx 796\ Hz.$$

This filter, then, is exactly the functional equivalent to that of Figure 2–14. Taking the output across the resistor would produce a low-pass filter with the same cutoff frequency, and it would be exactly the functional equivalent of a capacitative low-pass filter.

Mutual Inductance and Transformers

The changing magnetic field that surrounds an inductor can induce a current in any conductor that lies within it. If a second inductive coil is placed near one that is carrying an alternating current, a current will be induced in it. The current in the second coil, however, produces its own magnetic field, and this, in turn, affects the first coil. The inductors influence each other. This situation is referred to as *mutual inductance*. The effect can be used to transfer electrical power from one circuit to another in a device called a **transformer**, illustrated in Figure 2–20.

The two inductor coils are wound on a single (usually iron) form, or core. The one carrying the input signal is called the primary coil, while the one in which a current is induced is designated the secondary coil. All other things being equal, the relationship between the applied and induced voltages is a function of the ratio of the number of turns in the two coils. If, for example, the primary coil has 10 turns of wire and the secondary has 20 turns, the voltage induced across the secondary coil will be twice the voltage applied to the primary. In other words, the voltage can be determined from the *turns ratio*: $N_{secondary}/N_{primary}$, where N is the

---

[10] One henry is defined as the amount of inductance that will generate a potential of 1 V when the current is changing at the rate of 1 ampere per second.

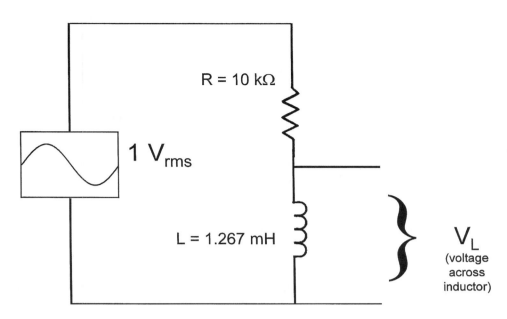

Figure 2-19. A resistor-inductor high-pass filter. This circuit is functionally equivalent to that of Figure 2–14.

number of turns in the coil. The voltage across the secondary coil ($V_{secondary}$) is simply

$$V_{secondary} = V_{primary}\left(\frac{N_{secondary}}{N_{primary}}\right).$$

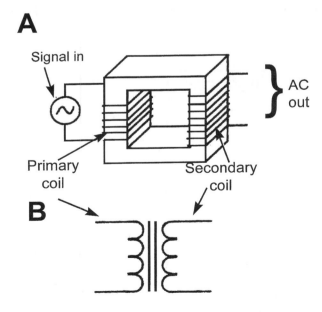

Figure 2-20. Simplified plan of transformer construction (**A**) and its schematic symbol (**B**).

If the secondary coil has more turns than the primary ($N_{secondary}/N_{primary}) > 1$) the output voltage is greater than the input voltage and the transformer is of the *step-up* type. Fewer turns in the secondary than in the primary coil ($N_{secondary}/N_{primary} < 1$) results in a *step-down* transformer whose output voltage is less than the input voltage. When both coils have the same number of turns the output and input voltages are (in the ideal case) the same.

Transformers serve many functions. Obviously they are useful for converting AC voltage to the levels needed for circuit operation. For example, most modern instruments are designed to operate in the range of 5 to 20 V DC. Yet the standard wall outlet in the United States provides about 120 V AC. The voltage mismatch is almost always resolved by a transformer in the power supply that is built into an instrument. (How AC is converted to DC is discussed later.) It is not uncommon for a single device to require several different operating voltages. An oscilloscope, for instance, needs low voltages for its amplifier circuits, but several hundred volts for its display tube. Different voltages can be obtained from a transformer with several secondary coils, each having an appropriate number of turns.

Only the *changes* in primary coil current can induce a current in the secondary coil. If an AC signal having a DC bias is applied to the primary, only the changing (AC) portion of the signal will be effective in producing a secondary-coil voltage. The output of the transformer will therefore be free of the DC bias. Hence, transformers also see service as "DC blockers."

Finally, because there is no physical connection between the circuits of the primary and secondary coils, transformers are often used to isolate devices from the main power supply, particularly in cases where the instrument's circuitry makes physical contact with a patient. In electroglottography, for instance, a very weak current must be passed through the neck (see Chapter 10, "Laryngeal Function"). The presence of transformers at appropriate points in the electroglottograph circuit ensures that the neck-current supply is in no way connected to the wall outlet. If the very worst were to happen, and something were to go catastrophically wrong with the instrument, the patient would be protected from the large current capability of the wall outlet by the isolation provided by a transformer.

Loading and Impedance Matching

Thus far, in all the situations in which we have measured the output of a circuit we have tacitly assumed that connecting a measuring device (such as a voltmeter or oscilloscope) to the output has no effect on circuit function. This is not really the case. Some current flows out of the circuit to any device that is connected to it. Therefore, anything connected to the circuit behaves like an impedance in parallel with it. This has important implications in instrumentation.

Consider, for example, a situation that is extremely common in clinical practice. The clinician wants to observe a patient's vocal waveform and so connects a microphone to an amplifier, and then connects an oscilloscope to the amplifier's output, as diagrammed in Figure 2–21. But the amplifier has a capacitor in series with its output; its function is to block any DC that the amplifier might create from being transmitted to the next instrument.

Now, the signal from the amplifier is not merely "applied" to the oscilloscope. A certain amount of signal current actually flows into it. That is, the amplifier "sees" the oscilloscope's input connection as a parallel resistor. Therefore, we can show the oscilloscope as a "load resistor" (R_L) connected to the amplifier. Notice that, viewed in this way, the capacitor in the amplifier and the load resistor of the oscilloscope form a capacitative high-pass filter. Recalling that the cutoff frequency of a filter is the one at which capacitative reactance (X_C) is the same as the resistance (R_L), and remembering too that X_C rises as frequency decreases, it is clear that the cutoff frequency of the transmission filter must be high if the oscilloscope allows a lot of current to flow (that is, if R_L is small). If the input impedance of the oscilloscope were even lower, more low-frequency components in the complex signal coming from the amplifier would be attenuated and lost to the oscilloscope, which would therefore show an increasingly distorted version of the speech signal. Clearly, in situations such as this one, the higher the input impedance of the oscilloscope the better. That is, the oscilloscope should represent a minimal "load" on the amplifier. (Loading can also have very serious consequences for the fidelity of microphones, a problem that is discussed in Chapter 4, "General-Purpose Tools").

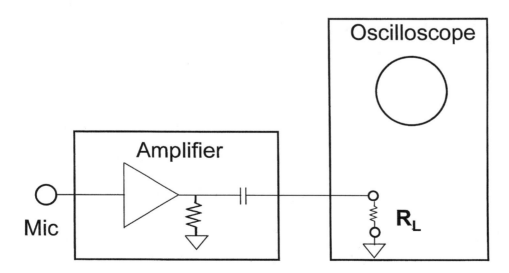

Figure 2–21. Effect of load resistance. Note that the capacitance at the output of the amplifier and the internal "load" resistance (R_L) of the oscilloscope form a high-pass filter. As R_L decreases the cutoff frequency of this filter increases, causing greater signal distortion.

Distortion of the signal is perhaps the most serious consequence of connecting excessive loading, but it is certainly not the only one. Consider the situation diagrammed in Figure 2–22. A voltage divider has been designed to deliver 5 V from a 10 V source, as shown. To verify that the circuit is correctly designed and connected, it is tested by connecting a voltmeter across R_2. Now, the voltmeter draws current, which is to say that it has an internal resistance (R_L). When the voltmeter is connected across R_2 the voltage-divider circuit is changed because it now consists of R_1 and the parallel sum of R_2 and R_L. If the voltmeter is a good one, R_L will be very large, say 250 kΩ. A bit of calculation shows that the parallel combination of $R_2 = 5$ kΩ and $R_L = 250$ kΩ is 4902 Ω. In this case, connection of the voltmeter changes the voltage divider circuit to the equivalent of 5 kΩ and 4902 Ω in series. The voltage across the modified R_2 will be 4.95 V, which is what the meter will read. While less than the voltage divider's theoretical output of 5.00 V, this is not a bad estimate. However, if a cheap voltmeter were used, one with a very low R_L of, say, 10 kΩ, the $R_2 + R_L$ combination becomes only 3333 Ω, and the meter will read only 4.00 V. In short, the "loading" by the meter will have reduced the output of the voltage divider by 20%. In this situation one might be tempted to believe that there was something wrong with the voltage divider, when the problem actually lies with the inadequate input resistance of the voltmeter.

The lesson in all of this is that the input impedance of one circuit must be suitable in terms of the output impedance of the device to which it will be connected. (Any standard textbook of electronics will provide guidance about determining "suitability.") The input and output impedances of the instruments that the clinician will use are generally indicated on the devices themselves or in their operating manuals. This information should be used when setting up equipment arrays.

SEMICONDUCTOR DEVICES

There are some substances whose inherent properties make them fall somewhere near the middle of the insulator–conductor continuum. Such materials, called *semiconductors*, are the foundation of the miniaturization revolution in electronics. Silicon (Si) and germanium (Ge) are the most common semiconductors. After small amount of "dopant" substances (such as gallium or arsenic) are added, the electrical properties of crystals of these elements can be changed in a known way by varying the voltage applied to them. This is the basis of the transistor and of all the devices related to it. The physics of semiconductors, which rests on quantum theory, is far too complex for consideration here, although adequate discussions can be found in most basic electronics textbooks. For the present purposes it will be sufficient to accept on faith that these devices perform as described.

Diodes

Diodes (Figure 2–23) behave as good conductors when current flows through them in one direction (when they are said to be *forward biased*) but they act as insulators when the current reverses (and they are *reverse*

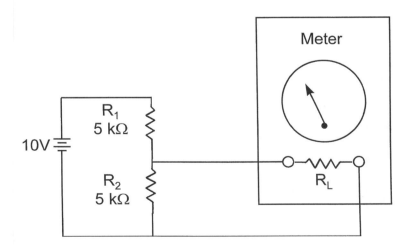

Figure 2–22. Loading of a voltage divider by a meter. The meter's internal resistance (R_L) is connected in parallel with R_2 of the voltage divider, changing its net value. If R_L is very large the effect is negligible, but a small value of R_L will seriously alter the voltage divider's characteristics.

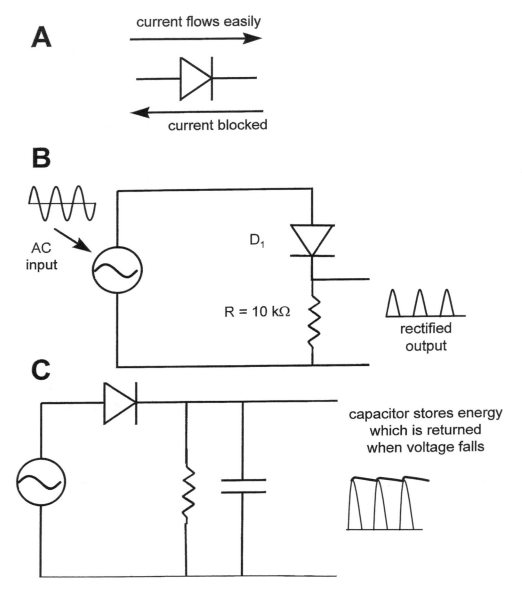

Figure 2–23. The semiconductor diode. **(A)** Symbol and current-flow characteristics. **(B)** Half-wave rectifier. The diode functions much like a resistor whose value depends on the direction of current. **(C)** Using a "filter capacitor" to store charge reduces the ripple at the rectifier's output.

biased). That is, they are electrical one-way valves. This is an extremely useful property, and finds widespread use for "rectification." Consider the circuit shown in Figure 2–23B, in which a diode is wired in series with a resistor to a sine-wave generator. During one alternation of the sine wave the current will flow in the direction indicated by the solid line. The diode is a good conductor of current in this direction, and hence presents very little resistance—certainly less than the 10 kΩ of the resistor. Consequently, most of the voltage drop in the resistor-diode "voltage divider" occurs across the resistor. By monitoring the output across the

resistor, as shown, the positive alternation of the sine wave will be detected. During the sine wave's negative alternation the current goes the other way, in the direction indicated by the dashed line. The diode is a very poor conductor in this direction, and behaves as a very large resistance—much greater than 10 kΩ. Therefore, most of the voltage drop during the negative alternation will occur across the diode itself, with very little observable across the resistor. Monitoring the output across the resistor will indicate almost no voltage during a negative alternation. When the current again reverses, the voltage will appear mostly across the resistor. The diode-resistor circuit, known as a ***half-wave rectifier***, has converted the bidirectional AC into a unidirectional flow of half sine waves, sometimes called *pulsating DC*. A half-wave rectifier is usually terminated with a capacitor, as in Figure 2–23C. The capacitor creates a low-pass filter. It stores energy during the voltage peaks and returns it when the voltage falls. The DC pulses are averaged out, or smoothed. Except for some residual ripple, the original AC signal has been converted to DC.[11] This is obviously useful in deriving the DC needed to power instruments from the AC supplied at the wall outlet. Rectification is also the basis of deriving information from an amplitude-modulated wave and so is an important function of carrier amplifiers (see Chapter 4, "General-Purpose Tools").

Transistors

Since its invention in the 1940s, the transistor has almost completely replaced the vacuum tube as an amplifying element. A host of related semiconductor devices has since evolved to meet special needs.

Among them are FETs, MOSFETs, thyristors, SCRs, and many others, with new ones constantly appearing on the market. It is patently impossible to consider all of these here. The description that follows will be limited to the "bipolar" transistor, which is the classic type, the one originally developed at Bell Telephone laboratories that ushered in the transistor era. Even for this single type, our discussion will have to be a very superficial one.

Transistors are made of the semiconductor elements silicon or germanium. By the addition of impurities to crystals of these metals they can be made into conductors of either electrons (N-type semiconductors) or positive charges (called "holes", P-type semiconductors). A transistor is constructed by making a sandwich of these two types of "doped" semiconductors, as shown in Figure 2–24A. Depending on what kind of material is in the center of the sandwich, a transistor is of either the PNP or NPN type. A connecting wire is attached to each layer in the sandwich. The layers are designated the *emitter* (e), the *base* (b), and the *collector* (c). (The standard schematic symbols for NPN and PNP transistors are shown in Figure 2–24B.)

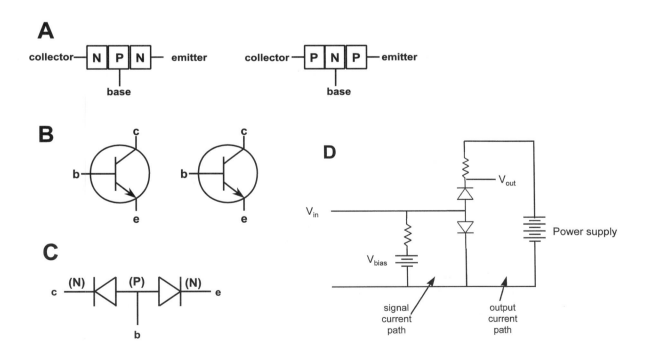

Figure 2–24. Transistors. **(A)** Three-layer, two-junction structure. **(B)** Standard schematic symbols. **(C)** An NPN transistor considered as back-to-back diodes. **(D)** Diode model of a very simple amplifier circuit.

---

[11] There are many more sophisticated circuits that perform rectification more efficiently or with less residual ripple. Consult any electronics text for details.

A junction of P and N materials forms a diode. The bipolar transistor has two such junctions and, therefore, can be represented (Figure 2–24C) as two diodes connected back-to-back. The device can be wired to voltage sources, as shown for the diode model of an NPN transistor in Figure 2–24D, to provide amplification. (The very same wiring would work for a PNP transistor if the polarity of the batteries were reversed.) When connected as shown to the power supply, the collector diode is reverse biased so that it behaves as a very poor conductor. Hence, very little current flows through it from the power supply. The emitter diode is forward biased and creates a path for current from the base if, and only if, there is enough voltage there to push the current through a slight inherent electronic barrier. A small "bias" voltage is applied to the base to insure that current can always flow through the base-emitter pathway. The input signal to be amplified (V_{in}) is also applied to the base, so that the current injected into the base of the transistor is the combined bias current and signal current. Now, it turns out that a current flow into the base alters the conduction properties of the collector-base junction. That is, the diode representing the collector is no longer reverse-biased as it was in the absence of a base current. (This is one of the phenomena that must be taken on faith in this discussion.) Therefore, within certain limits, the greater the current injected into the base, the more conductive the collector–emitter pathway becomes for current coming from the power supply. The greater the current in the collector, the greater the voltage drop produced by the resistor (R_C) in the collector line. This voltage can be tapped as shown. The current in the collector-emitter path is much greater than the current flowing into the base. The voltage drop across the resistor is, therefore, a much larger version of the base voltage. In short, amplification is achieved.

In the circuit shown there are two current paths: signal (+ bias) current flows through the base-emitter loop, while output current travels via the collector and emitter. The emitter is shared by both circuits, which is why this particular configuration is known as a *common emitter* circuit. Other arrangements (common base and common collector) are possible and see service in special situations. Somewhat more detailed consideration of amplifiers (and of a few of the problems that must be addressed in designing practical circuits) is provided in Chapter 4, "General-Purpose Tools").

INTEGRATED CIRCUITS

By adding appropriate impurities to it, the silicon that makes transistors can also be used to create resistors, diodes, and even capacitors. Hence, it is possible, by carefully controlling where different impurities are deposited, to create transistors and all the other elements of a fully functional circuit on a single piece of silicon crystal. Such a circuit then is monolithic (literally, made of a single stone) and integrated. Modern techniques of photoreproduction have made it possible to make such integrated circuits (ICs) very small indeed, packing tens of thousands of transistors and other necessary support components into an area of a few tenths of a square centimeter. The IC "chip" is housed in a case to facilitate handling, and the result is a complete plug-in circuit.

There are literally thousands of different ICs available: memories, microcomputer processors, audio amplifiers, complete instrumentation amplifiers, and so on. Because they are produced by automated processes in very large quantities their cost is almost always very low. The variety is staggering, and more appear each week. The important of this lies in the fact that complete, customized, instrumentation systems can now be constructed with very little need for highly developed engineering skills. Even the neophyte, having chosen the appropriate ICs, can assemble complex electronic systems that are not only better than much of what was available in the "old days" of discrete components, but are very much cheaper as well. Speech pathologists should make an effort to familiarize themselves with the range of ICs available and to experiment with using them as building blocks in circuits they need.

ELECTRICAL SAFETY

At some time or other, everyone has suffered an electric shock. We all know from experience that electricity can be unpleasant. And occasional press reports of people who were accidentally electrocuted have made us all aware that carelessness with current can be lethal. It goes without saying that the instrumentation used by the speech professional should not expose a patient to risk. Electrical safety must be a serious professional concern.

To understand where danger lurks and how to minimize risk it is necessary to understand how the power company delivers its product to us via the electrical "mains" and how we tap into it in our clinics and labs.

The first thing to consider is that the zero reference against which the voltage of the mains is measured is the potential of the earth itself. This is because we, and everything around us, are all connected to the earth and, under normal conditions, we are all at just about the same potential—at least in theory. Also, the earth is an enormous conductor—so big, in fact, that we assume that any amount of current could be injected into it without significantly altering its voltage.

Power is sent out from the utility's generator along three wires, each of which carries current at very high voltage (Figure 2–25). The wires are said to be "hot." A fourth cable at the power plant is attached to a very large metal plate sunk deep into the earth. This true ground connection, the "cold" side of the current-delivery system, will be part of the pathway by which current returns to the generator.

Somewhere between the electric company's cables (under the streets or on poles) and the outlets in our walls is a transformer system. It combines the current on the three cables and reduces their voltage to produce the "hot" lines that feed the building's electrical distribution system. The voltage difference between these two wires is 220V. A "neutral" wire, connected to the power company ground wire and to another ground just outside the building, travels with the hot wires. Each of the hot wires in our buildings has a voltage of 110V with respect to the neutral wire. One of the contacts in each outlet in the walls is connected to one of the 110 V wires; the other is connected to the neutral wire.

It is important to recognize that the neutral contact in the outlet is NOT ground. The wire that connects it to true ground can be quite long, and it has a real resistance. Now, electricity flows from the hot side of the outlet, through any electrical device that is turned on, and back to ground through the neutral wire. So the neutral line is carrying all of the current being used by all of the active devices (appliances, light bulbs, whatever) that feed into it. Obviously, this can be quite a bit of current. And Ohm's law states that the current interacts with the neutral wire's resistance to generate a voltage. Therefore, the so-called neutral wire can have a voltage significantly above zero.

Now consider a patient using a tape recorder in a therapy room. Wires connected to the wall outlet bring power to the recorder. So, inside the instrument there is a hot wire (at 110V) and a neutral wire, ostensibly at 0 V. The metal framework inside the tape recorder serves as the internal "ground" for the instrument; through it current is returned to the neutral wire which carries the "spent" current back to ground and thence to the power plant.

Something goes wrong inside the tape recorder: the insulation on a wire cracks, and suddenly the metal frame is in contact with 110V. So are the control knobs on the tape recorder and maybe even the metal case on the microphone. When the patient touches a metal part on the tape recorder current flows through him as it seeks a path to the 0 V of ground. The resistance of the human body is only moderate, but the resistance of furniture, floors, concrete building supports and the like, which are in series with the patient in the return-to-ground pathway, is fairly high. So not much current is likely to flow through the patient; he might feel a slight tingle. Bad enough, but if the patient happens to be in contact with a relatively low-resistance path to ground (such as another piece of equipment) then a relatively large current will pass through him, and he may experience quite a jolt. The situation is getting worse. If the pathway to ground is

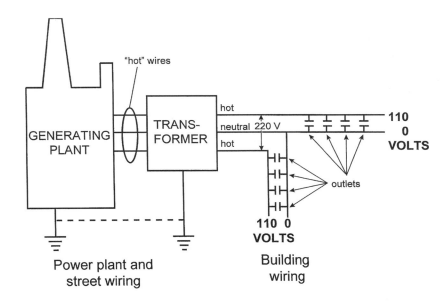

Figure 2–25. Electrical power distribution from utility company.

really quite conductive (a radiator pipe) a truly large current might result, with terrible consequences. The scenario is not a likely one, but it is certainly possible. How do we guard against it?

The most important protection is to connect a very low resistance pathway to ground to the exposed parts of all electrical devices. This is why three-prong plugs and outlets are now the rule. The third (round) contact is to a wire that is separately grounded. It does not ordinarily conduct any current to speak of, so its voltage is really zero. The exposed parts of electrical devices are connected to this ground lead so that, if anything goes wrong, current finds it very easy to travel to ground through it, sparing people the experience of being unwilling conductors.

If your facility has the old two-prong electrical outlets, have them changed by an *electrician*. Never use three-prong "adapters" if there is any way to avoid them. If you must use them, be very certain that the green "ground" wire on the adapter is in excellent contact with a good ground. And, if you have to use adapters, use the equipment connected to them with caution.

Even better protection is afforded by *ground fault interrupters (GFIs)*. These devices, installed in the wall outlet box, monitor the current going to and coming back from any device plugged into them. If the two are not equal, some current must be going somewhere else—not a good sign! When a difference exists the GFI reacts in just a few milliseconds and cuts off the current, thus preserving people from electrical danger. GFIs are a particularly good idea—and are commonly required by building codes—where outlets are near plumbing fixtures and other excellent pathways to ground. They cost very little, and are a worthwhile safety investment.

Most instruments are provided with fuses. When too much current is drawn, the wire in a fuse melts, opening the circuit and cutting off power to the device. The prime purpose of the fuse is to protect the equipment, but they might also limit the amount of current that can pass through a person accidentally connected,

through a fault inside the instrument, to the power line. **Do not substitute larger fuses for the ones specified by the manufacturer**. If the fuse blows there is likely to be something wrong with the equipment. Have it checked and repaired.

See to it that patients are not in contact with an external low-resistance path to ground. Do not use metal tables, or seat patients near pipes, or have ungrounded outlet boxes within reach.

While it may seem a bit paranoid, the best advice is to trust no one about electrical supplies. Hardware stores sell cheap testers that can be plugged into outlets and that indicate if the ground connection is faulty or if the hot and neutral wires have been reversed. Every outlet should be tested and any faults immediately corrected.

REFERENCES

Geddes, L. A., & Baker, L. E. (1989). *Principles of applied biomedical instrumentation* (3rd ed.). New York: John Wiley.

Hillenbrand, J., & Houde, R. A. (1996). Creating filters with arbitrary response characteristics for use in hearing and speech research. *Journal of Speech, Language, and Hearing Research, 39*, 390–395.

Hillenbrand, J., & Houde, R. A. (1997). Comments on finite impulse response filters. *Journal of Speech, Language, and Hearing Research, 40*, 408–409.

Jackson, L. B. (1996). *Digital filters and signal processing* (3rd ed.). Boston, MA: Kluwer.

Roark, R. M. (1997). The frequency sampling method of digital filter design: Comments on Hillenbrand and Houde (1996). *Journal of Speech, Language, and Hearing Research, 40*, 405–409.

Scripture, E. W. (1902). *Experimental phonetics*. New York: Scribners.

Stetson, R. H. (1928). Motor phonetics. *Archives Néderlandaises de la Phonétique Expérimentale, 3*, 1–216. (Reprinted in an expanded edition as: Kelso, J. A. S., & Munhall, K. G. [Eds.] [1988], *R. H. Stetson's motor phonetics: A retrospective edition*. Boston, MA: College-Hill.)

Stetson, R. H., & Hudgins, C. V. (1930). Functions of breathing movements in the mechanism of speech. *Archives Néderlandaises de la Phonétique Expérimentale, 5*, 1–30.

3

Digital Systems

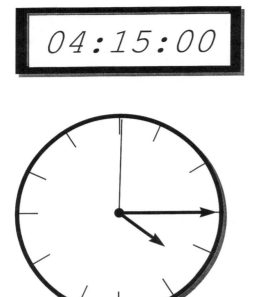

Figure 3–1. Digital and analog clocks showing the same time.

Analog and digital devices differ in critical ways, one of which is clearly exemplified by the familiar digital and analog (dial face) clocks, such as those of Figure 3–1, which show the same time. The relevant question, of course, is "What time is it?" The digital clock says that it is 4:15:00—precisely and exactly four fifteen. But is it? The analog clock's second hand is actually just a bit past the "0" tick mark, so it is telling us that the time is actually a bit *later* than 4:15:00, but not so much as a full second later. In fact, if we were to look more closely at the circumference of the analog clock (say with a magnifying glass) we might see that the time is really 4:15:00.3+. If we enlarged the scale again, we might determine how much time the "+" represented. In fact, in theory we could enlarge the scale again and again to get ever more precise readings of the time. We can do so because analog data are continuous —there are no gaps between adjacent "values" (positions, lengths, voltages) so, at least in principle, we can always read the clock face (or thermometer, or pressure gauge) to whatever degree of precision we might need.

We pay a price for this readily available precision, of course. Because the information (in our example, the time) is ever changing, we never know what the time—really, exactly, precisely—is! That's because the time keeps changing while we're trying to read the clock face. By the time we've made our observation the time has changed, and our observation is no longer truly valid.

The digital clock, on the other hand, is very definite about the time. It clearly and unquestioningly states that it is 04:15:00. And it will say that until the time changes to 04:15:01. We get an unambiguous reading during the intervals between updates of the time shown. Information in digital systems comes in discrete, discontinuous packets. There are no intermediate values, and it is not possible to read the system with some kind of magnifying glass to obtain greater precision from the output. Certainty is bought at the expense of precision.

The fact is that we live in an analog environment. At ordinary scales of time and distance, natural phenomena are continuous. Our instrumental sensors, therefore, are generally analog devices. If we want to manipulate the measured values in a numerical form we will need to digitize the analog signals that our instruments provide. The process of analog-to-digital conversion (generally denoted simply as "*A/D*") is pivotal and foundational to all of the computer processing that we do.

PRINCIPLES OF DIGITAL DATA

Number Systems

We normally count in groups of multiples of ten, each group allotted a "decimal place" in our numeric notation. Although such a system might have had its origins in the number of our fingers ("digits") there is nothing inevitable, pre-ordained, or particularly natural about it. Groups of ten simply are (or were!) convenient. Other cultures, in other times, have preferred different schemes. (Modern French distinctly shows the remnants of a counting scheme based on groups of twenty.) For several reasons numerical notations founded on groups of sizes other than ten lend themselves much better to electronic manipulation. Optimal use of the powerful digital devices—especially computers—that are now the mainstay of much of our work therefore requires at least an elementary understanding of number systems and the ways of translating a number from one notation to another. Of particular importance is the number system based on groups of two (the **binary** numbers) but the groups-of-8 (**octal**) and groups-of-16 (**hexadecimal**) number systems will be of considerable use to those who want to maximize their mastery of the computer's capabilities.

THE CONCEPT OF A NUMBER BASE

We say that we usually count in groups of ten. The mathematician, however, indicates the same thing by stating that our everyday numbers are "**base-10**." In situations in which confusion might occur, the base of a number is written as a subscript following it. Thus, 126_{10} is a base-10 number, while 754_8 is a number to the base 8. The base of a number specifies the two critical properties of a numerical expression: the number of symbols (that is, digits) required, and the value of each location, or place, in a string of numerical symbols. While these properties can be succinctly described in mathematical terms, it is more useful to our present purpose to explore them by way of example, and it is most convenient, for the moment, to use our familiar base-10 numbers—which we may refer to as "decimal numbers"—for illustration.

Numerical Symbols

The first characteristic—the number of symbols required—is easily dealt with intuitively. Suppose, as in our decimal system, we group into sets of ten. We already know from long experience with our traditional numbers that we are going to need ten symbols to designate all of the members of each set. The symbols we use are the numerals 0 through 9. If, however, we were to adopt base-5 numbers (that is, if we grouped things into sets of five) we would need five symbols. If we wanted to make our base-5 system look truly different from our traditional numbers, we might choose to use the symbols $\oplus$, $\Diamond$, ∇, $\leftrightarrow$, and $\cup$. We could also use letters to designate our new numerals; perhaps α, β, γ, δ, and ε, even though doing so might appear a bit confusing at first. But, as a matter of convenience, we would probably choose to use our traditional numerals, 0, 1, 2, 3, and 4. The situation is the same if we chose to group by, say, sixteen (that is, base-16, called *hexadecimal*). We are still free to use any graphic designators we want for our numerals, but we'd likely have a preference for the number symbols we're accustomed to. Unfortunately, we only have ten traditional symbols (0 through 9), and we'll need 16 for base-16 numeric representations. So we're forced to augment our supply of digits. Base-16 numbers are, in fact, common in the world of computing, and by (a relatively recent!) tradition, we augment our symbols by using letters to stand in for the numerical symbols we lack. Thus "A_{16}" is equivalent to 10_{10}, "B_{16}" is 11_{10}, and so on through "F_{16}", which equals 15_{10}. The number "$9A5D_{16}$" is perfectly legitimate, even if we don't have words by which to read it aloud.

Decimal Place Values

So accustomed are we to our traditional ("Arabic") number system that we don't think much about how

it really works, even though we have an everyday example of a radically different system in the "Roman" numbers that are sometimes used for special purposes. What, exactly, is the essential difference between "III" and "3", or between "CCVI" and "206" or between "MCMLXXXIX" and "1989"? Consider, for a moment, how the Roman numbers are to be read. "III" is easy. One adds $1+1+1$. "CCVI" is also relatively straightforward: reading left to right, one adds $100+100+5+1$. "MCMLXXXIX" poses difficulties, however, because a complex set of rules comes into play that specify when numbers are to be added and when they are to be subtracted. So MCMLXXXIX is parsed (reading from *right to left*) as $10 - 1 + 10 + 10 + 10 + 50 + 1000 - 100 + 1000$. The system is built on a series of symbols, each of which has a fixed value irrespective of where in the string of symbols it appears. Whether a given symbol is to be added or subtracted from the total depends on a complex interaction between its value and its location relative to its immediate neighbors. Our customary Arabic numerals, by contrast, take on different values depending, in a regular and invariant way, only on where they appear in the string of digits. Thus, reading the number 1989 from right to left, 9 does indeed signify 9, but the 8 really represents 80. The next 9 represents 900, and the 1 really stands for 1000. Hence, we read it as "one thousand nine hundred eighty nine."

The critical feature of our customary numbers is *place value*. Each place (or column) has a value ten times greater than the place to its right. The first column to the right has the place value "1", the next "10", the next "100", and the leftmost column has the place value "1000." We could (and, in fact, we do!) understand "1989" as $(1 \times 1000) + (9 \times 100) + (8 \times 10) + (9 \times 1)$. As we move from right to left each column has a value that is ten times greater. Since $1 = 10^0$, $10 = 10^1$, $100 = 10^2$, and $1000 = 10^3$, another way of putting this is to say that each column represents an *exponent*, or *power of ten*, that is one greater than that of the column to its right. In fact, we could use the exponents as the column designators, as shown in Table 3–1.

Numbers to Bases Other Than 10

In devising a numbering notation we are in no way restricted to powers of 10. Any number base can be used with no changes in the basic method that we normally employ in our everyday decimal system. Suppose, for example, we chose to use a system to the base 4. Then, from right to left, the columns would have the place values shown in Table 3–2. So, in a base-4 system, we find that we do not have the units, tens, hundreds, . . . columns that we are accustomed to, but

Table 3–1. Place-Value Evaluation of an "Arabic" Number

Column designator (power of ten)	3 (=1000)	2 (=100)	1 (=10)	0 (=1)	
Place Value	10^3	10^2	10^1	10^0	
Number	1	9	8	9	
Value	1×10^3	9×10^2	8×10^1	9×10^0	
	1000 +	900 +	80 +	9	= 1989

Table 3–2. Place Values of a Base-4 Numbering System

Column designator	4	3	2	1	0
Place value	4^4	4^3	4^2	4^1	4^0
Decimal equivalent of column value	256	64	16	4	1

rather we have units, fours, sixteens, sixty-fours, two-fifty-sixes, . . . columns.[1]

By way of practice, we might ask what the number 133011_4 is equivalent to in base-10 notation? The problem can be solved simply enough by completing Table 3–3. We find that $133011_4 = 1989_{10}$.

Base-2 (Binary) Numbers

There is no essential conceptual difference between base-2 numbers, called **binary numbers**, and any others. They are, however, more important in modern technology than other non-decimal numbers because they are the numbers with which digital computers work. (There are several reasons for this, which will be discussed later.)

Binary numbers use only two numerical symbols, conventionally 0 and 1. A little reflection shows that the true meaning of 0 (in binary and in all other notations) is "empty"—that is, the column marked by 0 contains nothing. Thus, there is really only one binary digit ("1"). The words "**bi**nary dig**it**" are generally contracted to "**bit**." So a bit is a column (position) in a base-2 number. Consistent with numbers to any other base, each bit (column) has the value of the base raised to an exponent which is the bit-position (column) designator. The bit values of binary number notation are shown in Table 3–4. Thus, 10110_2, for example, is

$$
\begin{aligned}
2^0 \times 0 &= 0 \\
+\ 2^1 \times 1 &= 2 \\
+\ 2^2 \times 1 &= 4 \\
+\ 2^3 \times 0 &= 0 \\
+\ 2^4 \times 1 &= 16 \\
\hline
10110_2 &= 22_{10}
\end{aligned}
$$

Utility and Importance of the Binary Number System. The most obvious reason (but not the only one) for the importance of binary numbers to data processing is that digital computers use binary numbers. The obvious question is, "Why were binary numbers selected?"[2] Recall from the preceding discussion that one could use any symbols to represent the "digits" in a non-base-10 numerical notation. (That we use the digits to which we are accustomed is only because of our familiarity and comfort with them.) Now, in a base-2

---

[1] The terminology seems very clumsy, but that's because we are so habituated to our base-10 system, and also because we are forced to use base-ten terms—the only terms we have—to describe our base-4 numbers.

[2] Interestingly, binary code has a long history, dating back at least to the 17th century and Francis Bacon. For a nontechnical review, see Heath, F. G. (1972). Origins of the binary code. *Scientific American, 227* (2, August), 76–83.

Table 3–3. Evaluation of 133011_4

Column Designator	$4x = N10$
5	$1024 \times 1 = 1024$
4	$256 \times 3 = 768$
3	$64 \times 3 = 192$
2	$16 \times 0 = 0$
1	$4 \times 1 = 4$
0	$1 \times 1 = 1$
Sum of the columns, expressed to base 10:	**1989**

Table 3–4. Place Values of the Binary (base-2) Number System

Bit Number	Exponential Form	Value in base-10
0	2^0	1
1	2^1	2
2	2^2	4
3	2^3	8
4	2^4	16
5	2^5	32
6	2^6	64
7	2^7	128

system, one of only two possible marks can appear in any column. Clearly, the two marks are mutually exclusive: if one appears, the other is excluded. Digital computers work by opening and closing switches.[3] Now, imagine that, instead of using "1" and "0" as the digits of our binary number, we employ the symbols "Y" (for "switch closed") and "N" (for "switch open"). Then we might have a number that looks like:

"Switch" (column) number: 4   3   2   1   0

Switch closed?   Y   N   Y   Y   N

The closed switch ("Y") in the 4th "binary place" has the numerical value of 2^4, or 16_{10}, the 3rd binary place = 0 (because the switch is open), and so on. Adding up the values of the three filled binary places we have $2^4 + 2^2 + 2^1 = 16_{10} + 4_{10} + 2_{10} = 22_{10}$, which we expressed more conventionally before as 10110_2. The importance of this is that the number 10110_2 or 22_{10} represents the setting of a number of switches. Conventionally, each "Y" (switch closed, or "on") is designated by the binary digit "1," and each "N" (switch open, or off) by the binary digit "0." If each switch is permanently associated with a given numerical column, or binary place, then 10110_2 or 22_{10} must represent a *unique* arrangement of switch settings. The computer opens and closes switches as a result of arithmetic operations, and the final switch settings represent numerical answers.

Arithmetic, however, is only a part of the story. And, from the point of view of the computer user, it is not the most important part. (After all, with the exception of those who need to design computers, who cares

---

[3] In the earliest digital electronic computers, the switches were actually electrically-controlled mechanical devices, called relays. Modern computers use transistors as purely electronic switches.

how they represent numbers internally?) The fact is that, through connections available on most analog-to-digital interfaces (discussed later), it is actually possible to connect switches (actually, to apply voltages, which amounts to the same thing) to the input of a computer so as to generate binary numbers. Those switches can represent *conditions*, and the status of the switches can be read as a number.

Suppose, for instance, that a palatograph (see Chapter 12, "Speech Movements") is being used to track tongue-palate contacts during a patient's performance of a speech task. Each contact point on the palatograph's sensing surface is, in fact, a switch. We select four points and connect each to the computer's input so that it represents a given binary place (column) of an input number. Contact of the tongue with a sensing point closes a switch, representing the digit "1." The sensing points (labeled according to their binary positions in the resulting number) might be:

Point 0: Midline, most anterior

Point 1: Near the right first molar

Point 2: Near the left first molar

Point 3: Midline, 1 cm posterior to incisors.

There are thus four input points, each represented by a column in a binary number. Tongue contact is represented by four binary digits. The system is therefore said to generate 4-bit data. (If there were 8 contact points they would generate 8-bit data, and so on. Obviously, the greater the number of data bits the more accurately tongue contact can be characterized.)

The value of representing the pattern of palatal contacts as a binary number can be made clear by a simple example. Suppose that we wish to set up a computer-controlled practice session for a patient. To help achieve the therapeutic goals, the computer is to reward the speaker when, during a carefully-constructed speech task, tongue contact is only at the midline. No reward is provided if there is contact near the molars. Given the binary-place assignments established for the contact points, it is clear that midline contacts will be represented by

Point 0, front midline, alone $= 0001_2 = 1_{10}$

Point 3, midline, 1 cm back, alone $= 1000_2 = 8_{10}$

Points 0 and 3 together $= 1001_2 = 9_{10}$

So all we need to do is to tell the computer to look for the numbers 1, 8, or 9 in the stream of data it receives from the palatograph.

At first glance, using binary, rather than decimal, numbers for this task might seem an unnecessary complication. In fact, however, it's not: the "either it's contacted or it's not" exclusivity of each binary numerical place is critical to the method's success. It means that a given number represents one, and only one, pattern of tongue contact. Imagine, for example, that we had assigned the values 1, 2, 3, and 4, respectively, to our four palatal positions. Would the output number "5" then mean "most anterior midline and 1 cm posterior midline"? It might—but it could also mean "right first molar and left first molar"—exactly the condition we do NOT want to reward. Unless the number is binary there is no way to know unambiguously which points have been contacted.

Now suppose further that, at some point during a speech task, the computer receives the number 11_{10} from the palatograph. What has the computer been told? Eleven$_{10}$ is 1011_2. Thus, there must have been contact with points 0, 1, and 3 but not with point 2. So there was tongue-palate contact in the midline just behind the teeth (point 0), along the right side of the palate (point 1), and along the midline somewhat posterior to the front teeth (point 3). In short, a very asymmetric tongue-palate contact. This contact pattern (in our limited exemplary system) can be represented *only* by the number 11 (1011_2), and 11 can only represent this particular pattern of tongue contact. The ability of the binary number system to represent multiple dichotomous states is one of the reasons that it is so useful, and therefore so important.

As the hypothetical speech task continues other numbers (patterns of tongue contact) will be reported to the computer—12, 7, 4, in fact, any number from 0 to 15 (1111_2) might appear. The task confronting us is how automatically to decipher the meaning of the numbers in terms of palatal contacts. One could, of course, construct a table of equivalents that shows the contact pattern of each number. And then we could look up the pattern in the table as each number is presented to us by the computer. If there are only four contact points this is perhaps a workable method. But many palatographs record from 64 different points, which, in principle, could generate more than 1,800,000,000,000,000,000 possible patterns. Clearly it is not practical to construct such a monstrous table of values. Fortunately, it is quite easy to get the computer to do the deciphering. All that is required is the application of some techniques of **Boolean logic**. It is the ability to apply these operations to binary numbers that is really at the heart of the utility of base-2 numerical representation.

Boolean Logic

Boolean logic is really an arithmetic system for manipulating binary numbers, but it follows very different rules from those learned in elementary school. With its origins in assessing the validity of logical propositions, Boolean arithmetic uses the values "True" (T) and "False" (F). For our purposes (and, indeed, in general practice) T and F are associated with 1 and 0, respectively, which allows us to construct numbers. Boolean operations are "bitwise" procedures. That is, only a single bit (digit) from each of the numbers entering into the operation is used at a time, and the result does NOT carry from one column to another. Obviously, therefore, Boolean arithmetic does not use addition and subtraction (or their derivatives, multiplication and division) in the usual meaning of those terms. Rather the most important Boolean operations are AND, OR, EXCLUSIVE OR (denoted XOR), and NOT. (Small-capital letters are used to distinguish these Boolean names from the lexical meanings of these terms.) The possible results of each operation are summarized in a "truth table."

AND. Given two binary digits, a and b, then a AND $b = 1$ if and only if $a = 1$ and $b = 1$. Under any other circumstances, a AND $b = 0$. One can construct a truth table to show all possible results of the AND operation by listing the possible values of a along one side of the table, the possible values of b along the top edge of the table, and the resulting value of a AND b in the appropriate row and column of the table. The truth table for AND is shown in Table 3–5. The conventional symbol for AND is a dot between the variables: $A \cdot B$ is read "**A** AND **B**."

An application for the AND function is immediately obvious. We can use it—to continue the example of the palatograph—as a test to see if a given point on the palate has been contacted. Suppose, for example, we want to know if the left molar region is being contacted, irrespective of any other points that may also be touched by the tongue. The left molar region has been designated as point 2, which means that it's the second-column bit, so the left-molar region is represented by the number 0100_2. Any time that this region is contacted, the number-2 bit will be equal to 1. (In the jargon of the

Table 3–5. Truth table for AND.

	a	
b	0	1
0	0	0
1	0	1

0 AND 0 = 0,

0 AND 1 = 0,

1 AND 0 = 0,

1 AND 1 = 1.

science, the bit is said to be "high.") If the left-molar region is not touched, this bit must be equal to 0 (it is said to be "low"). To be notified that the left-molar region has been contacted we must have the computer detect when the number-2 bit equals 1 in any of the numbers coming from the palatograph. To achieve this we program the computer to apply the AND function to all of the data values. Since the number we are looking for, 0100_2, is equal to 4_{10}, we ask the computer to perform the operation "$datum$ AND 4" on every number in the stream of data coming from the palatograph.

Assume that, at a given instant, the palatograph reports $datum = 5$ to the computer. Is the left-molar region being contacted? We do the Boolean AND operation on $datum = 5$ as follows:

$$
\begin{array}{ll}
5 \text{ AND } 4 = ? & \\
\quad 0101 & (5_{10}) \\
\text{AND} \quad 0100 & (4_{10}) \\
\hline
\quad 0100 = 4_{10} &
\end{array}
$$

That is, we apply the rule that a AND $b = 1$ if and only if both $a = 1$ and $b = 1$, and we apply the rule to each individual binary place. By using $b = 4$, we are testing

---

[4] A succinct review of Boolean algebra can be found in Garnier, R., & Taylor, J. (1992). *Discrete mathematics for new technology.* New York: Adam Hilger (IOP Publishing, Ltd.).

to see if the number-2 bit is high or, in descriptive terms, if the left molar contact has been touched. (Obviously, one could test for other contact locations by changing the value of b.) The result of the AND operation will be equal to 4 *if and only if* the left-molar-touched condition is true. Therefore, we can instruct the computer as follows:

Take each palatograph datum. AND *it with* 4_{10}. *If the result is* 4_{10} *signal the user, because it means that the left molar area was contacted.*

The technique works just as well with much longer data numbers, so it is no more of a problem to search for a given contact point among 20 or 30 bits (up to the limits of the computer's capabilities) than to detect one out of only four possible contacts, as in our example. Furthermore, we are not restricted to detecting just one contact point at a time; we can search for combinations. If, to use our example yet again, we wanted to know when both of the midline points (points 0 and 3) were touched simultaneously, we could set $b = 1001 = 9_{10}$, perform the AND function on each datum, and know that whenever the result of the AND operation was 9 both points were contacted.

OR. The truth table for the OR function is shown in Table 3–6. The standard symbol for the OR operator is + or $\oplus$. The rule for OR is that, given a and b, then a OR $b = 1$ **if either value is 1 or if both values are 1**. We could have used OR for detection of a specific point of palatographic contact. Let us assume the same detection problem: we want to know if the left-molar region of the palate has been touched. The left-molar region is point number 3, and is represented by the bit in the 2^2 column of the data. So, we remind ourselves, we need to determine if the 2^2 bit equals 1 (that is, is it high). Thus, the number

Table 3–6. Truth Table for OR

		a
b	0	1
0	0	1
1	1	1

we are looking for, embedded in the data, is 0100_2. That is, we need to check for the presence of 4_{10}. Suppose again that the number reported at a given instant by the palatograph is 5. We can use OR to see if this number includes a left-molar contact as follows:

$$
\begin{array}{lr}
 & 5_{10} \\
\text{OR} & 11_{10} \\
\hline
 & 15_{10}
\end{array}
\qquad
\begin{array}{lr}
 & 0101_2 \\
\text{OR} & 1011_2 \\
\hline
 & 1111_2
\end{array}
$$

What we have done is to set all of the possible data bits to 1 **except** for the one we want to test. Since the number we are looking for is 0100_2 (that is, 4_{10}), we thus set $b = 1011$ (11_{10}), and OR it with our datum, $a = 5$. A brief examination of the "arithmetic" shown above demonstrates that the result can be 15 (= 1111_2) if and only if the 2^3 bit of the datum was high. That is, the result can be 15 if and only if the left-molar contact point is signaling that it was touched. So, any time that the result of the OR operation is 15 we have detected the contact that we were looking for.

While one can use the OR operation to test the status (high or low, 1 or 0) of a particular bit, it may result in trouble in certain circumstances. Suppose, for example, that we do not know how many data bits there are going to be. (This situation might easily arise if a program is written to work with several different palatal detectors, each of which has a different number of contact points.) Assume, for the purpose of illustration, that we have two different detectors. On both of them the left-molar contact is signaled by bit 3, but one detector has more than the four contact points we have so far dealt with. Suppose it has eight points. Now suppose that the simple detector *does* indicate a left-molar region contact. That is, it reports the number 4 to the computer, that number being 0100_2. The more complex palatograph, when it is used, also reports a left-molar contact, but in addition it also detects a contact that is not incorporated into the simpler detector system. So it might report the number 36, that is 100100_2, which is 6 bits long. If we use a 4-bit OR operation, the Boolean logic is as follows:

	Simple System	**6-bit System**
Datum	0100	100100
	OR 1011	OR 1011
	1111 (= 15_{10})	101111 (= 47_{10}).

If we use only 4 bits for the OR function, we will not get the "left-molar result" of 15 for the 6-bit system, and thus we will fail to detect a valid contact. Use of the OR operation requires that we know at least what the maximum number of bits in the data is. This requirement may be inconvenient for writing general programs, and thus the AND function is to be preferred in this instance.

XOR. The XOR (*exclusive OR*) function follows essentially the same rule as the OR function, except that the result is 1 if and only if values *a* and *b* are not both 1. That is, 1 XOR 0 = 1, but 1 XOR 1 = 0 (whereas 1 OR 1 = 1). The truth table for XOR is presented in Table 3–7.

NOT. The NOT function is an inverter. It converts a 1 to a 0, and a 0 to a 1. Formally, NOT 1 = 0 and NOT 0 = 1. The NOT function is symbolized by a bar over the value to which it is applied; thus $\bar{A}$ is read NOT A. The NOT truth table presented in Table 3–8.

NOR and NAND. An important use of the NOT function is that it may be combined with OR and AND to create the "inverted" functions NOR (NOT OR) and NAND (NOT AND). The results of applying these "NOTed" functions is the reverse of the expected outputs. For example, NOT(1 AND 1) = NOT(1) = 0. The truth tables are therefore as shown in Table 3–9.

The Boolean logic operators provide us with a language to describe any possible set of circumstances (provided that all of their elements can be expressed as binary—"one-or-the-other"—factors). Of more applicable importance is the fact that the Boolean operators can be used to tell a computer how to recognize a situation of interest (or clinical significance) to us. (Computer languages perform Boolean operations.) If, for instance, we wanted to know when the patient touched points 1 (right first molar) and 2 (left first molar) after *not* having touched palatal point 0 (anterior midline) we could write something like:

Table 3–7. Truth Table for XOR

a

b	0	1
0	0	1
1	1	0

Table 3–8. Truth Table for NOT

A	$\bar{A}$
1	0
0	1

Table 3–9. Truth Tables for NOR and NAND

NOR

a

b	0	1
0	1	0
1	0	0

NAND

a

b	0	1
0	1	1
1	1	0

Let **A** = status of point 1

   B = status of point 2

   C = the previous status of point 0

   Satisfied = (**A** AND **B**) AND NOT **C**

which is the same as:

   Satisfied = (**A** AND **B**) NAND **C**.

   If *Satisfied* = 1 then the prescribed condition has

been met, and the computer would signal us (or would take some action, like rewarding the patient).

DIGITAL ELECTRONICS

Implementation of the binary number system and Boolean logic in electronic circuits is, at least in principle, simplicity itself. All that is really necessary is a series of switches.

AND Gates

The electrical version of the AND gate can serve as a simple example of how circuits can implement Boolean logic. What is required is a set of switches of the on-or-off (closed-or-open) variety. We define the closed (or "on") position as representing digital 1, and the open (or "off") position as digital 0. In an electrical schematic diagram, the switch would look like the circuit in Figure 3–2. A DC supply is connected to a light bulb through two switches, A and B. Illumination of the light bulb is designated "1," while an unlit lamp signals "0." It is clear that, to obtain a 1 at the light bulb (that is, to turn the light bulb on) **both** switches must be in the 1 position, that is, both switches must be closed. Similarly, the bulb cannot light if either or both of the switches is in the 0 position (open). So the truth table for this simple circuit is:

		Switch B position	
		(Closed) 1	(Open) 0
Switch A Position	1 (Closed)	1	0
	0 (Open)	0	0

Thus, the switching circuit implements the function A AND B = C.

The use of mechanically-operated switches in electronic circuits is clearly impractical. (What would perform the physical operation of opening and closing the switches?) But transistors function very well as simple switches, and they can be activated by an applied voltage (see Chapter 2, "Analog Electronics"). A simplified schematic of the same AND circuit using transistors would look like Figure 3–3. The transistors A and B conduct when a voltage is applied to their bases, and, when both transistors are conducting, the voltage at C will be approximately the same as the power-supply voltage. This circuit, then, is an *electrically* operated AND gate. Other logical functions can similarly be implemented with switch circuits.

The fact is, however, that, for a number of reasons, such simple circuits would not really function: actual logic gates are considerably more complex. The complexity is of little concern to the user, however, because each logical element is available as an integrated-circuit "chip" in a small package, ready to be plugged into the larger device of which it is destined to be a part. And, rather than draw all of a given circuit's elements in a circuit diagram, we simply use a single electronic symbol to represent an entire device. The accepted symbols for the more common logical gates are shown in Figure 3–4.

More Complex Functions

Boolean-function circuits are available in a number of "families," of which the most common is probably the "transistor-transistor logic" (TTL) group. All of the circuits in a family have common electrical characteristics, and they are designed to be connected directly to each other. Thus, the output of one or more can serve as the input to another, allowing the development of very complex logic arrays. To make doing so easier, logic gates are often provided with multiple inputs. For example, one can obtain an integrated-circuit 4-input OR gate (which performs the function A OR B OR C OR D) or a 3-input NAND gate (which evaluates NOT (A AND B AND C)).

Consider the following problem, based yet again on the simple electropalatograph that has been considered before. Suppose that the palatograph has six contact points: A—midline, near incisors; B—midline, 2 cm posterior to the incisors; C—at left canine; D—at left 1st molar; E—at right canine; F—at right 1st molar. We want a circuit that will automatically signal the patient whenever there is a lateralized palatal contact. In other words, when there is palatal contact at both points on one side only, without an accompanying midline contact. The logical condition we need to detect, therefore, is ((C AND D) XOR (E AND F)) AND (NOT (A OR B)). The required logic is shown in Figure 3–5.

Logic gate 1 (an AND gate) produces an output if both C and D are contacted; logic gate 2 does the same for contacts E and F. Logic gate 4, an exclusive OR gate, produces an output if and only if one of the two AND gates is responding, but not if both of them are. Thus we have detected whether there is palatal contact at both points on a single side in the absence of a contact on the other side. Logic gate 3, a NOR gate, evaluates the other part of the logical analysis: its output is high if and only if neither of the midline points is being con-

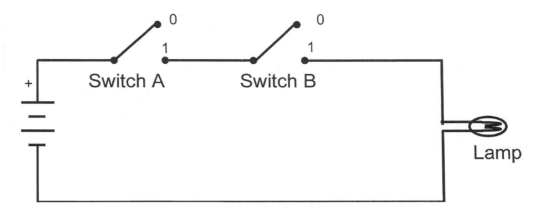

Figure 3–2. Schematic diagram of an AND gate.

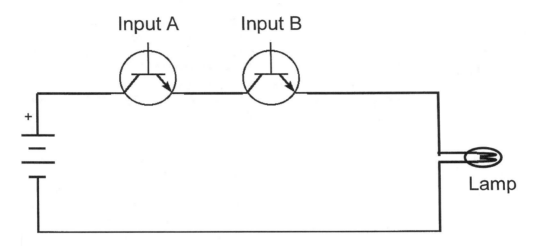

Figure 3–3. Schematic diagram of the same AND circuit shown in Figure 3–2, but using transistors.

tacted. Finally, gate 5, an AND gate, evaluates whether both halves of the set of requirements have been met. That is, it detects whether both of the earlier stages in the circuit are producing a "1." If so, its output goes high, signaling that all conditions are "true," that contact has occurred with both points on one side or the other, but not on both and not at the midline.

INTERFACING THE ANALOG AND DIGITAL WORLDS

Given that natural phenomena (including speech and voice) tend to be analog, and that computers are digital systems, it is clear that there must be some way of converting from one system to the other if computers are to be useful to us in assessing or manipulating the physical world. The processes are referred to as digital-to-analog conversion and analog-to-digital conversion. The latter, it turns out, depends on the ability to perform the former, and so it is most reasonable to begin with digital-to-analog conversion.

Digital-to-Analog Conversion (DAC, D/A)

In principle, digital-to-analog conversion (DAC) is a very simple process. The need for precision and reliability, however, introduces a great many complications into the problem of designing a really useful circuit. Furthermore, there are several different general schemes by which DAC can be achieved. Fortunately, there is no need for most users to design a D/A circuit:

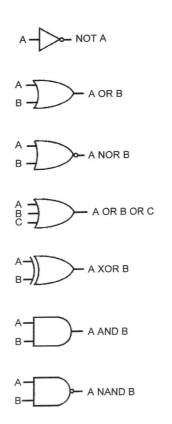

Figure 3–4. Symbols for common logical gates.

excellent integrated devices are widely available at extraordinarily low prices. One common scheme for D/A conversion is considered here in order to provide an introductory understanding of what is involved.

WEIGHTED CURRENT SOURCES

The output of an operational amplifier is proportional to the sum of the currents at its inverting input. Suppose, then, that we had a (binary) digital value being produced by some circuit, as in Figure 3–6A. We assume, for the purposes of illustration, that each digital "1" is represented by a 5 V signal, and each digital "0" by 0 V. Also, although the example circuit involves only 5 bits, the logic of the method can be extended to any reasonable number. In the example the digital circuit has bits 1, 2, and 4 high, so its output represents the number $10110_2 = 14_{10}$. Each of the digital outputs can be applied to the summing point (at the inverting input) of an operational amplifier through its own resistor, and the resistors are scaled such that their values are proportional to powers of 2. That is, if the most significant bit is connected through a resistance of 1 KΩ, then the next less significant bit is associated with a resistance of 2 KΩ, the next lower bit with 4 KΩ, and so forth.

What we achieve by this scheme is to make the current provided to the operational amplifier by each of the digital number's bits proportional to its numeric value. That is, the 1 bit generates a current twice as great as that which would be produced by the 0 bit, the 2 bit's current is four times as large as the 0 bit's, and so forth. In the example of Figure 3–6A, recalling that I = E/R, we can calculate the currents and their sum as follows:

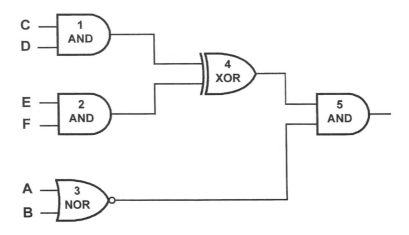

Figure 3–5. The logic required to detect ((C AND D) OR (E AND F)) AND (NOT (A OR B)).

bit 4 = 5 V, I = 5/1 KΩ = 5.0   mA

bit 3 = 0 V, I = 0/2 KΩ = 0.0   mA

bit 2 = 5 V, I = 5/4 KΩ = 1.25 mA

bit 1 = 5 V, I = 5/8 KΩ = 0.625 mA

bit 0 = 0 V, I = 0/16 KΩ = 0.0   mA.

The sum of the currents is 6.875 mA. If, as in Figure 3–6, the feedback resistance, R_f, is 1 KΩ , then the output of the operational amplifier will be –6.875 V. (The output is negative because the operational amplifier is configured as an inverting amplifier.) This analog voltage represents the number 10110_2 or 14_{10}.

Now let us suppose that the digital output increases by one count, so that it is now $10111_2 = 15_{10}$, as in Figure 3–6B. The currents flowing into the operational amplifier are now

bit 4 = 5 V, I = 5/1 KΩ = 5.0   mA

bit 3 = 0 V, I = 0/2 KΩ = 0.0   mA

bit 2 = 5 V, I = 5/4 KΩ = 1.25 mA

bit 1 = 5 V, I = 5/8 KΩ = 0.625 mA

bit 0 = 5 V, I = 5/16 KΩ = 0.3125 mA.

The voltage output from the operational amplifier will thus be –7.1875 V.

If all of the input bits were high (that is, if the number presented by the digital circuit were $11111_2 = 31_{10}$), then the current to the operational amplifier would be 9.6875 mA, and the output of the operational amplifier would be –9.6875 V. We have constructed a 5 bit digital-to-analog converter with a full scale output of –9.6875. Each increase of the numerical input by 1 is represented by an increase of –0.3125 V at the output. (The output scaling can be changed by choosing a different value for R_f.)

Analog-to-Digital Conversion (ADC, A/D)

Analog-to-digital conversion (ADC or A/D) is considerably more complex than DAC. It is also inherently slower. Several different approaches to the problem are in (at least relatively) common use; each generally represents a trade-off between speed and precision. Among A/D types available as off-the-shelf integrated circuits are *tracking* (quite slow but simple), *integrating* (highest resolution but slow operation), *successive approximation* (good speed but somewhat more com-

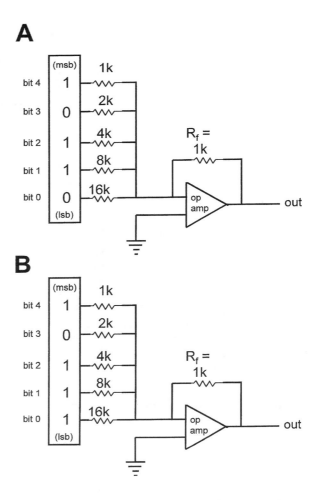

Figure 3–6. A. A digital circuit with bits 1, 2, and 4 high, its output representing the number $10110_2 = 14_{10}$. **B.** The same digital circuit with bits 0, 1, 2, and 4 high, its output representing the number $10111_2 = 15_{10}$.

plex circuitry), and *parallel* (very high speed, but very complex circuitry) A/Ds. The present discussion explores the principles of A/D conversion by examining a simplified "generic" device that is representative of tracking A/D converters. The particular circuit to be considered is schematized in Figure 3–7.

The logic of the system is straightforward. A "clock" circuit continuously produces square waves (in this example, at a frequency of 1 MHz). These can be applied to a counter, whose output represents (in binary) the number of counts tallied since the counter was last reset to zero. The counter's output is applied to a D/A converter, which therefore produces an analog voltage representing this count. This "count" voltage is used as one input to a comparator, whose other input is the signal voltage that is to be converted to a digital

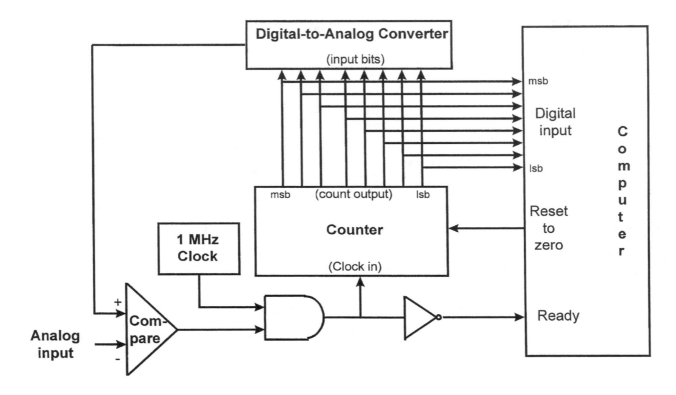

Figure 3–7. Schematic diagram of a simplified "generic" device that is representative of tracking A/D converters.

value. The comparator output can be in one of two states: low (which, in this circuit, indicates that the voltage of the analog signal is greater than the voltage representing the count) or high (meaning that the count voltage exceeds the analog signal voltage). Because of the AND gate clock, pulses can only reach the counter's input when the comparator voltage is high. That is, the count can be incremented only when the "count voltage" does not yet exceed the analog input voltage. When the "count voltage" finally exceeds the analog input voltage the comparator output goes low, which prevents any more pulses from being counted. When this point is reached the count is a number that represents just one bit more than the input voltage, and so a conversion of the analog input to a digital output has been achieved.

When the comparator goes low, signaling that an appropriate binary number has been generated, a signal is sent to the computer telling it that the converter is "ready," that is, that the conversion has been completed. The computer, in turn, reads the counter's number and then sends out a signal that resets the counter to zero, and so the D/A output also falls to zero. This, of course, forces the comparator output to its high state, starting the counting process all over again.

IMPORTANT PARAMETERS OF A/D OPERATION

While there are many parameters that meaningfully characterize A/D operation, those that are most important to the user fall into three groups: digital codes, bit resolution, and sampling rate.

Digital Codes

Binary numbers have no sign. That is, there is no such thing as a negative binary number. But negative voltages often need to be converted to digital form: inspiratory airflow, for example, might be transduced as a negative voltage. Given that all binary numbers are unipolar, the obvious question is *How can negative numbers be accommodated?* There are four common ways.

Offset binary is perhaps the easiest scheme to conceptualize. We can represent negative input values by offsetting them—that is, by adding a constant value of one half the full-scale range (FS/2) to each input so as to force it into the positive range of numbers. Suppose, for example, that an A/D converter has a full-scale range of 0_{10} to 255_{10} (in other words, the counter has 8 bits). Then if we add 128 (one half the full scale range) to each input we guarantee that all output values are positive. Having done this, of course, an A/D value of 128_{10} (or 10000000_2) will represent the "true" 0. To convert from the offset binary representation to the "true" meaning of the number all we need do is subtract FS/2 from each A/D value.

Sign magnitude coding uses the most significant (leftmost) bit of the A/D value to represent the sign of a number while the remaining bits represent its magnitude. Thus, 00111001_2 would be equivalent to 57_{10}, while 10111001_2 would indicate -57_{10}. Unfortunately, of course, 10000000 and 00000000 both represent 0, which makes this method unsuitable for most A/D applications.

2's complementing is perhaps the most complex method conceptually, but it is very easy to implement with digital circuits and is very efficient. To obtain the complement of a binary number one simply changes all of its 0s to 1s and all of its 1s to 0s. The 2's complement is then derived by adding 1 to the complement. The 2's complement then is the negative of the original number. An example may help clarify the process:

Convert $+26$ to -26
Eight-bit number:
$\qquad 00011010_2 \ = \ 26_{10}$
complement $\qquad 11100101_2 = 229_{10}$
complement + 1 $\qquad 11100110_2 = -26_{10}$
Twelve-bit number:
$\qquad 000000011010_2 \ = \ 26_{10}$
complement $\qquad 111111100101_2 = 229_{10}$
complement +1 $\qquad 111111100110_2 = -26_{10}$

If one wishes to use (raw) computer files of A/D values for further processing it is obviously vitally important to determine what representation of negative numbers has been used.

BCD, or **b**inary **c**oded **d**ecimal coding, employs binary numbers to represent the decimal digit in each column of a decimal number. Since any decimal digit (0 through 9) requires at a maximum 4 bits for its binary representation, BCD is a string of 4-bit binary numbers. The number 836_{10}, for example, would be

$$
\begin{array}{ccc}
8 & 3 & 6 \\
| & | & | \\
\end{array}
$$
$$1000\text{-}0011\text{-}0110.$$

BCD coding is very convenient when a digital output needs to drive a digital display (since each four-bit group can be directed to its corresponding display number), but it is clearly ill suited to further mathematical processing. It is also very wasteful of storage space in the computer.

Bit Resolution

The precision with which an analog voltage can be represented by a number is obviously dependent on the largest number that is available. This, in turn, is directly determined by the number of bits used for counting. If only 5 bits are available the maximal range of numbers available is 0 to 64. So each increment of 1 represents 1/64, or 1.56%, of the range. If 8 bits are available the range can be divided into 512 parts, each of which covers 0.19% of the range. Ten bits can divide the range into 2048 parts, and 12 bits into 8192 parts. The greater the number of bits available the smaller the change in the analog voltage that can be detected. In short, the resolution of the A/D converter can be expressed in terms of the number of bits available, and hence one speaks, for instance, of 8-bit resolution, 12-bit resolution, and the like. If FS (full scale) is used to designate the highest voltage that the A/D converter is intended to handle, then the resolution in volts of the converter can be expressed as Resolution = $FS/2^n$. (Table 3–10 lists the resolution of A/D converters of dif-

Table 3–10. Resolution of A/D conversion

Number of bits	Numerical range (base 10)	Resolution in percent
4	0–31	3.125
6	0–127	0.781
8	0–255	0.391
12	0–4095	0.024
16	0–65535	0.0015

---

[5] Adding 1 to 00101 requires a carry operation, just as adding 1 to 09 would require a carry.

ferent bit lengths.) All other things being equal, the greater the number of bits the slower the converter will be, although 10- and 12-bit A/D converters are now widely available that are fast enough for almost all clinical purposes.

Sampling Rate

The fact that greater resolution of an A/D converter is associated with slower A/D speed is simply a function of the fact that, if a greater number of bits are to be used, the counter (in the example we have been considering) must count to higher numbers. In addition to the time required to perform the conversion itself, the converter needs a bit of time to "get itself together"— produce control signals for the computer, transfer results to a storage register so that they are available to the computer, reset itself to zero in preparation for the next conversion, and the like. Still, today's A/D converters are quite fast. It is easy to find an A/D board, at reasonable expense, that is fast enough for almost any clinical need. The question of how fast is fast enough is considered in Chapter 4 ("General-Purpose Tools").

The Digital Manipulation of Signals

Desktop computers have become extraordinarily fast and powerful, making it possible to implement digital processing of signals in systems that are available to the average clinical consumer. An example of the ease with which customized manipulation and analysis of data can be accomplished is provided in Figure 3–8, which is a screen display produced by a software system marketed by Nyvalla DSP of Stockholm, Sweden. The user has connected five icons, chosen from the menu on the right, to construct a band-pass filter. (From left to right, the icons indicate "microphone input—high-pass filter—low-pass filter—amplifier—output.") The parameters associated with each icon (for instance, the gain of the amplifier or the cutoff frequency of a filter) are independently specified by the user. As Figure 3–9 demonstrates, numerous signal-processing functions can be connected to each other in very complex ways to create precisely defined, highly complex, and narrowly specialized analytic instruments to meet almost any need. The ability to imitate analog instruments in this way is an important virtue of computer systems.

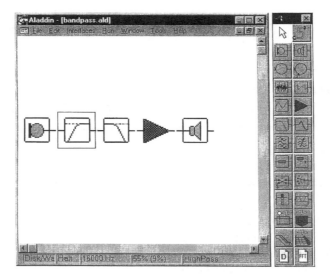

Figure 3–8. A virtual band-pass filter system, as shown on the screen display of the Alladin Interactive DSP™ system by Nyvalla DSP of Stockholm, Sweden. (Courtesy of Dr. S. Ternström.)

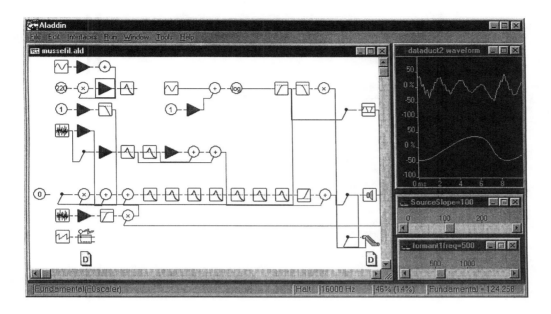

Figure 3–9. Screen display of a complex signal-processing instrument designed using the Alladin Interactive DSP™ system by Nyvalla DSP of Stockholm, Sweden. (Courtesy of Dr. S. Ternström.)

4

General-Purpose Tools

Certain devices are the workhorses of measurement systems. Rather than being specialized for a given task, they are versatile and form the core of most instrumentation arrays. Several are essential to many of the measurement procedures a speech pathologist is called upon to do. They are to the speech clinician what hammers and screwdrivers are to a carpenter: the indispensable general-purpose tools of the trade. The purpose of this chapter is to consider several such devices so that clinicians can select intelligently among the varieties available and use them appropriately. Even in today's computer-centered professional world, in which many integrated digital systems are available (see, for instance, Barlow, Suing, Grossman, Bodmer, & Colbert, 1989; Jamieson, Nearey, & Ramji, 1989; Roark et al., 1990; Rossiter & Howard, 1996), the clinician must, at the very least, decide what is to be connected to the computer input. The decision process is less perilous than it might appear and a little knowledge goes a long way.

ORGANIZATION OF INSTRUMENT ARRAYS

Before moving to a discussion of instrumentation components it is useful to consider the way in which any instrumentation system is organized. In a general sense, any measurement system must do at least three things:

1. First, there must be some means of detecting the phenomenon of interest (motion, pressure, airflow, sound pressure) and converting it into a *signal* that is acceptable for electronic processing. Sound waves, for example, will need to be converted to electrical waves before they can be recorded on tape.

2. Then the system must be equipped to manipulate or modify the signal in a controlled and reliable way and to process it, if necessary, to derive useful information. It is almost always necessary to amplify a signal (make it stronger) but other processing may be needed as well. For instance, it might be necessary to filter the signal to get rid of unwanted components, such as noise.

3. Finally, the electronic signal must be reconverted to a form that can be displayed in a convenient way for evaluation by the user. The signal might be written by a pen writer, or shown on an oscilloscope screen, or converted to a numeric value on a digital indicator.

Almost any instrumentation system will therefore have at least three "stages" of operation. They are diagrammed in Figure 4–1.

A *transducer* converts one form of energy into another. Usually this means translating some phenomenon into an electrical signal. A microphone, for example, converts sound pressure waves into a variable voltage. Hence, a microphone is an "electroacoustic" transducer. Sometimes the transduction is accomplished in more than one stage. In fact, the microphone is really an example of a two-stage process. First the sound pressure is converted to movement of an energy-collecting surface (acoustic-to-mechanical transduction) and then the motion of the energy collector is converted to an electrical signal (mechanical-to-electrical transduction). A microphone is thus composed of a primary transducer (sound-to-motion) and a secondary transducer (motion to voltage or current). The process by which an instrument interfaces with the physical world is known as *input transduction*.

Modification of the signal from the transducer is called *signal conditioning*, a general term that conceals a vast number of processing possibilities. Sometimes the signal needs only to be made larger—amplified—but in other circumstances it may be necessary to derive its fundamental frequency, to eliminate some of its parts, to find the average of its peak amplitudes, to compress it, expand it, code it, and so on. All of these processes (and many others) fall under the heading of "signal conditioning."

Finally, after the signal conditioning, the results of the instrument's processing are made available via

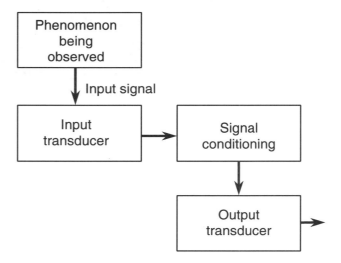

Figure 4–1. Components of an instrumentation system.

output transduction, the process of converting the information from an electrical signal into some form that people can perceive and deal with. Output transduction is the process by which an instrument communicates its "findings" to us, the users.

AMPLIFIERS

The output of most transducers is very small: Strain gauges produce signals in the microvolt range, microphones only a few millivolts. On the other hand, most display devices require significant voltages or currents. The cathode-ray oscilloscope's display tube, for example, needs several volts of input; speaker systems can require currents well in excess of an ampere. In short, most transducers cannot, of themselves, deliver enough power to show us directly what they observe. The discrepancy between what transducers can produce and what analysis or display systems require is resolved by introducing amplification into instrumentation systems. The need is so universal that amplifiers are virtually ubiquitous. It is hard to imagine an electronic device that does not include at least one, and a sophisticated instrument may well have dozens. Aside from those already incorporated into clinical devices, the speech clinician will frequently have occasion to use separate, special-purpose amplifiers for handling audio or physiological systems.

The invention of the transistor, its reduction to virtually microscopic size, and its incorporation into integrated circuits has led to the marketing of hundreds of prefabricated amplifier "building blocks." These permit individuals with only a minimal background in electronics to construct all sorts of special amplifiers to serve their particular needs. But even if one never plans to actually design and build an amplifier, it is important to understand them in order to use them successfully. What amplification is, how it is achieved, and what characterizes the variety of different amplifiers among which the user must choose are discussed in this section. While not every clinician, and perhaps not even most, will need to master all the details, at least a broad familiarity with what follows is important. The success of most measurement procedures rests, at least in part, on the competent use of amplifying devices.

Basic Principles of Amplification

Amplification is the process whereby the magnitude of an electrical signal is increased. The increase may be in voltage, in current, or in both (that is, in power) according to the amplifier's design. In fact, it is common to categorize devices as *voltage amplifiers*, *current amplifiers*, or *power amplifiers* according to which parameter is augmented. Figure 4–2 provides a conceptual schema of what is involved in achieving this.

The diagram underscores the fact that the signal to be amplified is not, itself, magically enlarged. Rather, the input regulates the flow of power from a reservoir by acting on some sort of control valve. For example, we may assume that the reserve in Figure 4–2 represents a source of large quantities of current. Changes of the input signal, which might be a current of only a milliamp or so, cause the control valve to open or close. As the input-signal current increases, the valve is opened wider; as it decreases, the valve closes more and more. Depending on how wide open it is, the valve can permit large amounts of current to flow to the output, and the valve is operated by the small current of the input signal.

In many ways an automobile is a mechanical analog of an amplifier. The power reserve is the gasoline in the tank, while the control valve is the accelerator pedal and the throttle system attached to it. The input signal is the force of the driver's foot on the pedal. As the foot pushes down, more gasoline is fed to the engine from the reservoir, and the engine's power output increases. A very small amount of force (foot pressure) is used to control a large force (engine output) by drawing energy from a reservoir (the gas tank). In some sense, then, the automobile is really an amplifier of foot power.

It is important to remember that the power that moves the car forward does *not* come from the driver's foot; it comes from the gas tank in which the necessary energy has been stored. In an analogous way the out-

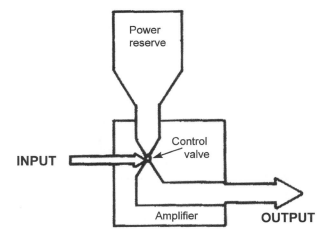

Figure 4–2. Conceptual diagram of an amplifier.

put of an amplifier does not come from the input signal (which serves only as a control function) but from an energy reservoir called the ***power supply***. The control element in an electronic circuit is now almost always a transistor, although older instruments and some very specialized devices use vacuum tubes.

An electronic diagram of Figure 4–2 might look like the circuit shown in Figure 4–3. The control valve is now a transistor. A small input signal is applied between ground and one of the transistor elements (in this case, the *base*) which causes a very small current to flow along the path shown by the solid line. This small input controls the amount of current that the transistor will allow to flow from the reservoir (a battery) through the transistor's *collector* and *emitter* and along the dashed-line current path. The resistor in this part of the circuits develops a voltage proportional to the current through it (Ohm's Law: $E = IR$, see Chapter 2, "Analog Electronics") and this larger voltage is "tapped" to serve as the output.

Real transistors are complex devices, and their use demands that special voltage requirements be met. For this reason practical transistor amplifiers must be more elaborate than the one shown in Figure 4–3 would indicate. Nonetheless, even if the circuit shown is actually impractical, it points up several critical variables in amplifier design or implementation. These, in turn, lie behind the specifications that manufacturers provide for their units.

GAIN

The term ***gain*** describes the amount of amplification achieved by a circuit. It is most conveniently defined as the ratio of output to input. If, for example, an amplifier produces an output of 15 V when the input signal is 0.1 V it is said to have a *voltage gain* of 15/0.1 = 150. Similarly, if a unit produces an output current of 250 mA for an input signal of 2 mA, it has a *current gain* of 250/2 = 125. If the output is smaller than the input, the gain figure will be fractional. In such a case, of course, the circuit is functioning as an attenuator.

Gain is also commonly expressed according to the decibel (dB) scale, already quite familiar to speech and hearing specialists (and reviewed in Chapter 5, "Speech Intensity"). Thus, an amplifier with an output to input voltage ratio of 150 has a gain of (20 log 150) = 43.5 dB, whereas a current gain of 125 represents current amplification of about 42 dB.

The current and voltage gains of a single amplifier are usually quite different, and units are generally designed to optimize one or the other. The selection of an amplifier will then be governed, in the first place, by which parameter—current or voltage—is important, as well as by the amount of gain required. These specifications depend in turn on the use to which the amplifier will be put. Amplifying the output of a microphone for display on an oscilloscope, for instance, will require only a voltage amplifier. Since an oscilloscope is a voltage-sensitive device that draws very little current, adequate voltage gain is vital, but current gain is unnecessary. On the other hand, if the microphone input is to be fed to earphones (perhaps to achieve enhanced auditory feedback) current gain will be very important, because earphones are quite likely to require a great deal of current.

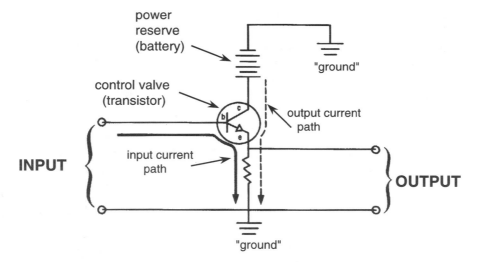

Figure 4–3. A simple amplifier. Input current flows along the path indicated by the solid line, while output current follows the dashed line. The transistor leads are b = base, c = collector, and e = emitter.

AMPLITUDE LINEARITY

An amplifier is said to show amplitude linearity if its gain is constant for all input magnitudes. That is, for a voltage amplifier, the gain should be the same whether the input is 0.01 V or 1.0 V. If the output-to-input ratio is different for different input levels severe distortion of the signal results. Some special amplifiers, however, are designed to be nonlinear. The most common of these is the logarithmic amplifier, in which the output voltage is proportional to the logarithm of the input. This is a useful way of compressing a signal that has very large voltage swings.

The power supply imposes an inherent upper limit on an amplifier's linear range. Consider, for instance, the case of an amplifier that has a gain of 10 and works on a power supply that provides it with 15 V. If a 0.5 V signal is applied to the input, an output of 5.0 V will result. Similarly, a 1.0 V input produces a 10 V output. But what happens if a 2 V signal is applied to the input? The output (under *ideal* circumstances) will be only 15 V, not the expected 20 V. The amplifier's gain drops from 10 to 7.5 when the input is 2.0 V. The reason for this is not hard to understand. Recalling that the amplifier's output is derived from an "energy reservoir" (the power supply), it is clear that the voltage output cannot exceed the reservoir's capacity. If the amplifier has a 15 V supply, it cannot provide an output of more than 15 V, no matter what the gain is supposed to be. The device cannot give what it hasn't got. As the input magnitude increases there will come a point at which the maximum output is reached. Beyond this point, increasing the input does not increase the output. Here the gain (output to input ratio) falls. The amplifier is said to be overloaded or, more precisely, *saturated*.

Figure 4–4 shows the results of amplifier saturation. The sine wave shown at the top of Figure 4–4A has a peak voltage of 2 V. It has been applied to an amplifier that is set for a gain of 10, but the amplifier has only a 15 V power supply. The lower trace of Figure 4–4A shows that the amplifier output "follows" the signal as long as the power supply voltage is not exceeded. When it is, the output remains at maximum until the input voltage falls, when the output again follows the input. The result is severe distortion of a type known (for obvious reasons) as *peak clipping*. This sort of gross distortion is very obvious in a sine wave, but it may be less so when speech or other complex waves are at issue. Note how, in Figure 4–4B, only the very tops of the peaks of the speech waves are lost. These are very rapid events, and the distortion does not seem too severe. In fact, however, the distorted speech waveform may be utterly unsuitable if, for example, analysis such as speech spectrography is planned.

Permitting amplifier saturation and its consequent peak clipping is one of the most common errors made by the novice. Many amplifiers have a meter that shows if they are operating in their linear range. The gain must be set so as to avoid saturation at the greatest expected input amplitude. Figure 4–4B shows that the overload may be fleeting, and thus it may be too rapid to produce a noticeable deflection of the relatively sluggish meter pointer. To avoid clipping occasional peaks of very brief duration, then, amplifiers are usually operated at a gain that is significantly lower than that which produces observable saturation.

FREQUENCY RESPONSE AND BANDWIDTH

Just as the gain of an amplifier should be the same for all input voltages, so it also should be same for any input frequency. That is, a sine wave of 100 Hz should be amplified exactly as much as one of 5 Hz or 25,000 Hz, or, for that matter, of 0 Hz. Unfortunately, for reasons that are beyond the scope of the present discussion, this ideal situation cannot be achieved in practice. (In any case, it is sometimes undesirable to have an amplifier handle all frequencies equally—a concept that will be discussed later.)

It is common to describe an amplifier's response to different frequencies by a graph of gain (in dB) over input frequency. This kind of plot is familiar to anyone

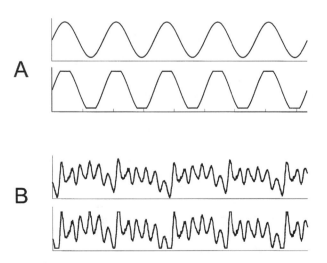

Figure 4–4. Peak clipping due to amplifier saturation. The upper traces show the input signals, while the lower traces are the respective outputs from the amplifier. A. Sine wave. B. Speech wave.

who has worked with hearing aids or similar electroacoustic devices. Figure 4–5A shows an ideal frequency-response curve. Very low and very high frequencies are amplified less than those in the middle of the range, which are amplified with absolute equality. The frequency response of the ideal amplifier, whose characteristics are plotted in Figure 4–5A, would be described as absolutely "flat" over this middle range, with "roll off" at the high and low ends, indicating that beyond certain lower and upper limits the amplifier is less effective. By convention, these limits are taken to be the frequencies at which the gain has fallen by 3 dB. One refers to these as the ***cutoff frequencies*** or, somewhat more descriptively, as the ***3 dB-down*** points. The ***bandwidth*** of the amplifier is then defined as the range between the cutoff frequencies. In Figure 4–5A the cutoff frequencies are 20 Hz and 10,000 Hz, and the bandwidth is therefore 9980 Hz.

The frequency response curve of an actual amplifier is shown in Figure 4–5B. The cutoff frequencies are approximately 40 Hz and 13,000 Hz and, as is typical of real electronic devices, the flatness of the response between those limits is not perfect. For this reason, manufacturers generally specify a tolerance for the gain characteristic. Thus, the amplifier characterized in Figure 4–5B might be said to have a frequency response that is flat ± 2 dB over its bandwidth. Modern components have made it easier to implement electronic designs that achieve excellent frequency response characteristics, and these specifications should be examined before acquiring a unit. It is wise to avoid purchasing any amplification system whose response is unspecified.

INPUT AND OUTPUT IMPEDANCE

The input impedance of an amplifier describes how great a load it imposes on the device providing the input signal. That is, it determines how much current will flow from the signal source into the amplifier. Consider the following example. Suppose one wishes to observe the electromyographic response of the superior orbicularis oris muscle. Appropriate electrodes are attached to the lip over the muscle to sense the voltages accompanying contraction. Since these voltages are very small (much less than a millivolt), considerable amplification will be required to increase their magnitudes to levels suitable for display. It turns out that, while the muscle is a fairly good voltage generator, it is not capable of producing large currents. Therefore, the amplifier that is connected to the electrodes must be capable of using a *very* small current for operating the "control valve" at its input. If the amplifier should draw anything but a minuscule control current it will overtax the generating capacity of the muscle. While this will not damage the muscle, it will probably lower its output voltage very significantly. This implies that drawing too much current may well eliminate the electromyographic voltage that is to be observed. A roughly analogous situation constantly arises in everyday life: voltage drops, and so lights dim, when too much current is drawn from a household electrical outlet. In the same way, it is possible to overload a signal-source by connecting it to an amplifier that draws too much current from it.

The input impedance of an amplifier is a way of quantifying how much current the amplifier will draw from its signal source, since Ohm's law states that current equals voltage divided by the impedance. If, for example, a transducer whose output is 0.01 V is connected to an amplifier with an input impedance of 1 MΩ, a current of 0.01 V / 1,000,000 = 0.00000001 A (1×10^{-8} A or 0.01 μA) will flow into the amplifier. This is unlikely to overload the current-producing capability of most transducers and so would be considered an adequately high input impedance for most transducer amplifiers. Ideally, a voltage amplifier would have an infinite impedance; that is, it would draw no current at all. The laws of thermodynamics tell us that this is an unattainable goal—some current

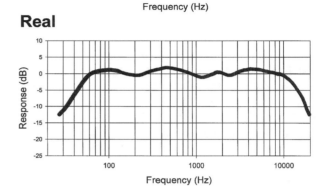

Ideal

Real

Figure 4–5. Frequency response curves of an ideal (top) and a real (bottom) amplifier.

must always flow into the amplifier. But extremely high input impedances are attainable with modern semiconductors, especially with a device known as a field-effect transistor (FET). If needed, for instance, amplifiers can easily be obtained with an input impedance of about 10^{11} (100 billion) ohms.

The inference should not be drawn that a higher input impedance is necessarily better than a lower one. It all depends on the device providing the input signal. Some transducers (certain types of microphones, for instance) have current, rather than voltage outputs. Amplifiers to be used with them should have relatively low input impedances that will permit these currents to flow freely. It is best that the input impedance of an amplifier be matched to the output impedance of the signal source. In a gross sense, this means that the tendency of an amplifier to "absorb" current should match the transducer's capacity to produce it.

The need for appropriate input impedance (either high or low) must be kept in mind when selecting an amplifier for a given job. Transducer manufacturers usually indicate the requirements of their units in this regard, and amplifier suppliers always state the characteristics of their systems. Many audio or general-purpose amplifiers have both high- and low-impedance input connections to accommodate different devices.

At the other end of the amplification process one must consider the amplifier's ability to supply current. This is primarily of importance if the input of the next in a series of connected devices requires large current inputs. Suppose, for instance, that a speech signal is to be amplified and then displayed on an oscilloscope for evaluation. Typically, an oscilloscope has an input impedance on the order of 1 MΩ. This implies that it will not draw significant amount of current from the amplifier, and thus the latter could have a moderately high output impedance without compromising the quality of the oscilloscope display. If, on the other hand, the amplified speech signal is to be fed to a loudspeaker the situation is very different. Speaker systems usually have impedances of about 8Ω, and so they draw very large amounts of current. If the amplifier has an output impedance of, say, 1000Ω it can provide no more than 0.002 A when its output is 2 V. At the same voltage, the speaker would draw 0.25 A, more than 100 times what the amplifier can deliver. With this kind of mismatch the amplifier's output voltage will drop enormously and the output waveform will be terribly distorted.

Amplifier Classification

It is common to describe different kinds of amplifiers by functional category, that is, according to the uses for which they are intended. Audio amplifiers, for example, are optimized for acoustic signals, while electromyography amplifiers are designed to handle certain bioelectric events. It might seem, therefore, that there are a great many different types of amplifiers. In fact, this is not really the case. Despite the myriad specializations for particular purposes that these functional categories represent, almost all amplifiers fall into a few relatively distinct electronic categories. It is important that these electronic distinctions be understood if the actual differences that separate the functional categories are to be appreciated.

ELECTRONIC CLASSIFICATION

Two sets of characteristics can be used to categorize almost any amplifier: response to a DC input and the nature of the reference (zero voltage point) against which the input is measured.

AC and DC Amplifiers

A single-transistor amplifier, such as the one shown in Figure 4–3, usually does not provide sufficient gain for most purposes. Consequently, the output of one transistor is usually used as the input to another, which then further amplifies the signal. A typical circuit of this type, in which the transistor *stages* are *cascaded* is shown in Figure 4–6 in somewhat simplified form. The two stages are identical, and each is of the basic type illustrated in Figure 4–3, although some of the components required for the operation of a real circuit have been added. In spite of the possibly forbidding look of the schematic, it warrants careful consideration.

In this circuit, as in the simpler version of Figure 4–3, the input signal is applied to the base of the transistor. It serves as the control valve that regulates the flow of the power supply's current through the R3–collector–R4 path. This current flow results in a voltage at the R3–collector junction that is larger than, but proportional to, the voltage of the input signal. In short, amplification is obtained. Unfortunately a transistor, by its very nature, is unlikely to be able to handle the input signal in its unaltered form. For instance, the input must exceed a certain minimal voltage before the transistor can use it as a control signal, and (at least in the circuit shown) the actual voltage at the base must never reverse its polarity. It is for these (and other reasons) that R1 and R2 have been added. They serve to guarantee that the base "sees" a given voltage (referred to as the *bias*) to meet the transistor's requirements for linear operation. In reality, the input voltage is *added to* the bias voltage at the base, and the transistor amplifies them both. Therefore, the output of the first stage

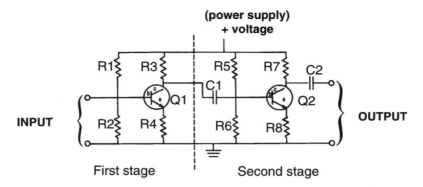

Figure 4–6. A simple two-stage, AC coupled amplifier.

is the amplified version of the sum of the input and bias voltages. The bias voltage is generally much larger than the voltage of the input signal, and if their amplified combination were to be directly applied to the base of the second transistor for further amplification it would be very likely to overload it. The final output would thus be a grossly distorted representation of the original input.

This situation is avoided by connecting the output of the first stage to the input of the second stage through a capacitor, C1. Since a capacitor blocks a steady (DC) current, while passing a changing (AC) current, the amplified form of the steady bias at the input is blocked from passage to the next stage, while the changing voltage of the input is passed along for more amplification. Another capacitor, C2, at the final output, performs a similar function and prevents the bias created for the second stage by R5 and R6 from appearing in the final output.

Connecting the stages of the amplifier with capacitors neatly solves the problem of how to cascade transistors without overload due to bias voltages. The solution is achieved at a price, however: The amplifier will only work for AC inputs. Any steady-state (or even slowly changing) voltage at the amplifier input will be blocked by the coupling capacitors.[1] This is clearly shown in Figure 4–7. The top trace is a square-wave signal applied to the input of an AC coupled amplifier; the lower trace is the amplifier output. The flat portions of the square wave represent (temporarily) steady-state voltages. The output trace shows that the amplifier has, in essence, failed to handle them, while the transitions (changing in voltage) between the steady-state segments are amplified quite well.

There are techniques for canceling out the bias, rather than blocking it. Semiconductor technology has produced transistors that have identical characteristics except that they are, in a sense, mirror images of each other. This reversal applies to their biasing requirements: When the *complementary* transistors are used in successive amplifier stages, the bias of one stage is canceled out by the opposite biasing of the next stage. The final output thus represents simply amplified input, without the bias voltage. With the elimination of DC-blocking elements the circuit is capable of amplifying a DC input.

Amplification of DC inputs is crucial to many physiological measurements. It is not uncommon for the magnitude of a physiological variable (for instance, intraoral air pressure) to change very slowly (by electrical standards). In some cases, such as the evaluation of subglottal pressure, the steady-state period can be

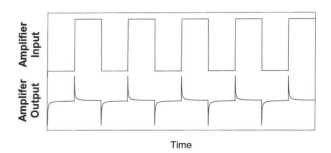

Figure 4–7. Blocking of steady-state (DC) voltages by an AC-coupled amplifier. The unchanging (flat) portions of the square-wave input (top) are blocked, and thus only the transitions appear at the output (bottom).

---

[1]The same end can also be achieved by coupling the stages of the amplifier through transformers, since they also serve to block passage of the DC bias from one stage to the other. The effect on overall amplifier function is essentially the same.

quite long. In these instances the measurement transducer will produce an output that is essentially a DC voltage. Clearly, the amplifier must be capable of handling this situation.

AC amplifiers, then, can deal with AC inputs only, whereas DC amplifiers can handle both AC and DC signals. The logical question is: Why bother with the functionally-restricted AC amplifiers at all? Why not use DC amplifiers for all purposes? The answer is twofold. DC amplifiers are more difficult to design and build. They must, for instance, include compensation for inherent temperature instability. But their problems, with today's technology, are not overly difficult to manage, although the resulting circuits are somewhat more expensive. More important is the fact that many transducers and instrumentation systems produce outputs that have their own useless bias voltages associated with the AC signal of interest. Certain types of microphones, for example, require DC working voltages, and their outputs are composed of a DC voltage plus the changes produced by audio transduction. Since it is only the varying (AC) portion of the microphone output that is of interest, use of an AC amplifier that will ignore the DC bias is obligatory.

Single-Ended and Differential Amplifiers

The amplification techniques discussed thus far have shared an important characteristic that has not been mentioned. Reference to Figures 4–3 and 4–6 shows that, in each case, the input current and output current loop have part of their paths in common. They both feed their current to ground, which serves as the common connection point for both input and output. (The concept of a circuit ground is considered in Chapter 2, "Analog Electronics.") The result of this arrangement is that the amplifier really senses the voltage difference between a single input line and ground, and produces an output voltage that is proportionally "distant" from ground. All of this is a rather elaborate way of saying that the point common to the two portions of the circuit—the input and output loops—serves as a zero reference, with all voltages being measured from that common zero level. An amplifier whose output shares such a common ground reference with its input source is known as a ***single-ended amplifier*** because it senses the voltage on a single "active" input wire.

Unfortunately, a single-ended amplifier is not adequate in those situations (and there are many) in which the input source cannot share a common ground with the amplifier. To see why this might be, consider a simple example.

Certain aspects of labial control are to be evaluated in a dysarthric patient. Electromyography is to be done on two opposing muscles, orbicularis oris and depressor labii inferior, in order to evaluate their coordination. If only single-ended amplifiers are available, the electrode and amplifier arrangement would have to be as shown in Figure 4–8.

The active input of each amplifier is connected to an electrode that picks up the electrical activity of the muscle over which it is positioned. The other input of each amplifier is, of course, connected to a common, neutral reference point—ground. In order for the patient's muscles to serve as an input to the amplifier he must first be connected to the same ground as the amplifier. This is accomplished by connecting a grounded electrode to some site near both of the muscles being examined. A number of problems instantly arise. First, each amplifier is "looking at" the voltage difference between the "ground" electrode and the electrode connected to its active input. From a physiological point of view, there is a vast distance between these two points, a distance within which all sorts of bioelectric events may be happening. Most of them have nothing to do with the activity of the specific muscle being monitored. Because they are all between the active and common electrode, they all contribute (in unpredictable ways) to the voltage seen by the amplifier. If the contributions are unpredictable the final output is uninterpretable. The problem could, of course, be alleviated by moving the common electrode much closer to one of the active electrodes, thereby improving the quality of the signal from one muscle. But that means moving it further from the other electrode, exacerbating the problems of recording from it. If both muscles are to be examined at the same time—as they must be if their coordination is to be evaluated —the difficulties arising from the need to use a common reference point are insoluble. This is one reason why single-ended amplifiers won't do in this situation.

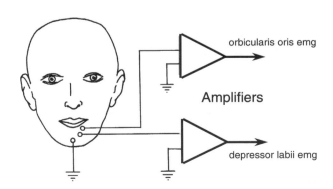

Figure 4–8. Electromyography using single-ended amplifiers.

There is, however, another reason, somewhat more subtle but just as important. The environment in which we do our work is filled with electromagnetic waves: radio signals, electrical noise from motors and lamp dimmers and, most important, radiation from the power lines all around us. The body and the electrode wires serve quite effectively as antennas for all of these. Thus, the electrodes on the muscles also pick up voltages induced by atmospheric electromagnetic radiation. Since the single-ended amplifiers "see" any voltage difference between their inputs and the common ground, they amplify these interfering signals, confounding them with the muscle potentials being examined. Muscular electrical activity is very weak, generally of far lower amplitude than the interfering induced voltages. The electromyographic signals are quite likely to be completely lost in all the electrical noise.

While there are still other problems, these two issues are enough to emphasize the need for an alternative amplification technique. It happens that a solution to all of the problems can be achieved by using what is known as a *differential amplifier*. This type of circuit, in fact, was originally developed by electrophysiologists confronted with the kinds of problems just described.

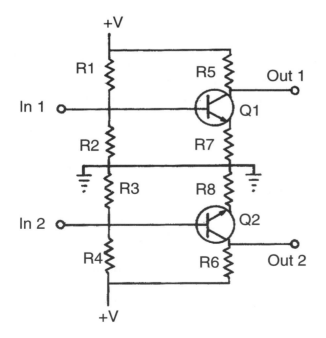

Figure 4–9. A simple differential amplifier. Note that there are actually *two* amplifiers, drawn upside-down with respect to each other. Both are connected to a single ground, but neither input line is grounded.

Put briefly, a differential amplifier is designed to amplify the voltage difference between two active input lines, neither of which (in contrast to the single-ended amplifier) is connected to ground. If, for instance, a differential amplifier with a gain of 100 has an input of 1.00 V at one input connection and 1.01 V at the other, its output will be 1.00 V, which is the difference between the two inputs (1.01 − 1.00 = 0.01) times the gain (100). The way in which this is achieved, although complex in actual implementation, is not difficult to conceptualize, and is schematized in Figure 4–9.

Careful examination shows that this circuit is really very similar to the amplifier shown in Figure 4–6. The key to seeing this is the recognition that there are really two identical amplifiers that have been drawn as mirror images of each other: The bottom amplifier is "upside down" compared to the top one. (This refers only to the way in which the circuits are drawn; it has nothing to do with their function.) Note, for example, the power supply connections, which represent a single power supply connection to two different points, and the location of ground, the common point to which both amplifiers are connected.

What this arrangement provides is a separate amplifier for each input line, making both lines active. Each of the inputs is amplified separately and appears at an output. The resistor networks serve the same function as their counterparts in Figure 4–6. The important fact that both inputs are active confers very significant advantages. Recall that voltage is the difference in electrical pressure between two points. In a single-ended amplifier the two points are an active input and ground, but in the circuit of Figure 4–9, the two points are both active, meaning that they carry meaningful voltages. Taking the output as the difference in voltage between two amplifier outputs (which is what is involved here) yields a major benefit that is best explained by an example.

Consider the situation diagrammed in Figure 4–10. A differential amplifier has been connected to a pressure gauge that has transduced a short period of high intraoral pressure and converted it to a positive voltage pulse on one of its output lines. The two wires from the transducer system, however, serve as antennas and pick up significant noise from the electromagnetic radiation in the environment. The resulting signals that are presented to the amplifier's inputs are depicted. It is clear that both lines have a lot of noise and, because both of the wires have traversed the same space, they have picked up essentially identical noise signals. The voltage pulse representing the intraoral pressure event is present at input 1, but it is clearly contaminated by the noise as well.

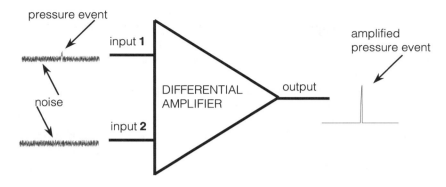

Figure 4–10. Cancellation of a common-mode signal by a differential amplifier.

The differential amplifier looks only at the voltage difference between the two inputs. Since their noise signals are identical, when the voltage at input 2 is subtracted from the voltage at input 1 the noise signals cancel out. What is left is the only voltage feature that is different: the voltage (intraoral pressure) pulse. The physiological event has been recovered from its electrically noisy background.

An identical voltage present at both amplifier inputs is called a ***common mode voltage***. The ability to eliminate such a signal from the final output is a very important feature of differential amplifiers. It is, in fact, very often the prime reason for using them. This capability is quantified by the ***common mode rejection ratio***, or CMRR. In essence, the CMRR is the gain of a common mode signal. That is, it is the ratio of the voltage output to voltage input (V_{out}/V_{in}) for a signal applied to both inputs, usually expressed in dB. Common mode rejection ratios of -85 dB or greater are common in commercially available circuits.

It is important to understand the significance and value of CMRR and, once again, a concrete example may help in clarifying the matter. Consider a differential amplifier with a differential gain of 100 and a CMRR of 90 dB. Suppose that it is operating in an electrically noisy environment with the result that there is a 60 Hz common mode noise signal of 0.1 V at both inputs. At the same time there is a meaningful 0.1 V signal at one input only. The meaningful signal will be amplified by a factor of 100, and so this component appears as $0.1 V \times 100 = 10 V$ at the output. The common mode signal, however, faces a CMRR of 90 dB, signifying an output to input (gain) ratio of about 0.00003. The output for the 60-Hz noise signal is therefore 0.1 V $\times$ 0.00003, or 3 *micro*volts. The signal-to-noise ratio is clearly vastly improved, from a 1-to-1 ratio to greater than 3 million-to-1, or more than 110 dB.

The ability to amplify the voltage difference between two points, neither of which is ground, and to selectively amplify a signal in the presence of relatively high levels of common-mode background noise, makes the differential amplifier very important. It will be encountered often in measurement systems.

FUNCTIONAL CLASSIFICATION

Although all amplifiers can be categorized as AC or DC, single-ended or differential, specific circuits are usually designed for optimal performance with certain kinds of input signals. Therefore, it is common to refer to amplifiers according to their intended function. In some cases the functional description of an amplifier makes its characteristics obvious. For example, one would guess that audio amplifiers, intended to amplify music or speech, are AC, single-ended devices with a flat frequency response from about 50 Hz to more than 15,000 Hz. The first several stages of such a device would probably be voltage amplifiers, but, if speakers are to be connected, the last stage will no doubt be a power amplifier. Other functional descriptions, however, might not be as immediately comprehensible to the nonspecialist. Some of these are briefly described below.

Preamplifiers

Any amplifier designed to accept a small input signal (generally directly from a transducer) and to provide enough gain to make that signal suitable for further electronic processing is called a preamplifier. Often, too, a preamplifier serves the function of matching impedance requirements. A transducer, for example, might need to output its signal into a very high impedance, but the signal conditioning circuits might have a relatively low input impedance. A preamplifier with high input impedance and low output impedance would need to be interposed between the two.

The term "preamplifier" is not rigidly defined, and the circuit referred to can be AC or DC coupled, differential or single-ended. The essential characteristic is that the circuit serve as a first stage "signal conditioner" at the input of a more elaborate array of circuits. For example, the voltage amplifier that boosts a small voltage from a microphone is an audio preamplifier for the power system that drives the loudspeakers.

Bridge Amplifiers

Bridge amplifiers meet the special requirement for amplifying the outputs of bridge-type transducers (see Chapter 8, "Air Pressure"), especially those using DC excitation. These circuits are differential DC amplifiers with high gain, great stability, and high CMRR. Their very large input impedance draws very little current, thus preventing the amplifier from acting as a shunt across the bridge to which it is connected. Bridge amplifiers commonly also provide the required excitation voltage for the transducer.

Carrier Preamplifiers

Carrier preamplifiers are really composed of at least three different circuits housed together for convenience. They incorporate a highly stable oscillator (which serves as the excitation source for a bridge circuit), a high-gain differential AC-coupled amplifier, and a demodulator circuit that extracts the transducer analog voltage from the modulated carrier signal. Together with the transducer, carrier preamplifiers provide for a complete amplitude modulation and demodulation system for generating a voltage analog of an external phenomenon. Carrier preamplifiers are most commonly used with bridge transducers.

Instrumentation Amplifiers

Although the term "instrumentation amplifer" is only loosely defined, in general it is used to describe a precision DC-coupled differential amplifier with very high input impedance, high gain, and very low noise. It is used when a very weak signal must be greatly amplified without "loading" the signal source.

Operational Amplifiers

A special type of high-gain, DC-coupled, differential amplifier whose characteristics are determined by feedback networks is called an *operational amplifier* ("op amp"). While the definition might not immediately suggest it, op amps may well be the most useful circuits ever devised for processing analog signals. There is scarcely any kind of signal modification, from simple amplification to complex mathematical transformation, that these circuits cannot do. (The term *operational amplifier*, in fact, derives from their early use in analog computers, in which they performed the actual mathematical operations.) It is important to remember that op amp circuits do far more than amplify. Addition of a few components to an op amp produces an electronic filter, or an oscillator, a rectifier, voltage summer, integrator, differentiator, comparator, and so on, almost without end.

High-quality operational amplifiers are available as ultraminiature integrated circuits at exceptionally low cost. In many cases it is possible to buy several of them in a single miniature package for well under $2.00. Given their extreme versatility, precision, convenience, and exceptionally low cost, it is not surprising that they have become absolutely ubiquitous. Using them, many laboratories now routinely construct special circuits as needed, overcoming instrumentation problems in a few hours that would have entailed enormous effort, much time, and great expense a couple of decades ago.

It is not possible, in this text, to present a discussion of sufficient depth to make the reader competent at operational amplifier circuit design. Many volumes have been written with that objective in mind: Stout and Kaufman (1976); Walsh, Peyton, and Walsh (1993); Coughlin, Driscoll, and Driscoll (1997); and Franco (1998) are examples. Integrated circuit manufacturers have also produced extensive applications literature. While it takes some effort and time (but very little money) to develop creative skill in the use of op amps, the investment pays off quite handsomely. It takes only a little competence with these devices to permit construction of *usable* precision circuits that can greatly enlarge one's measurement capability. In fact, clinically functional versions of much of the electronic circuitry described throughout this book can be designed (if necessary) and built quite easily with op amps—even by relative novices.

MICROPHONES

Microphones produce an electrical analog of acoustic pressure. They are, by far, the most common input transducer used by the speech pathologist. Perhaps it is because they are so common that they are given so little thought, with the result that their mechanisms and —more important—their characteristics are often poorly understood. This is unfortunate for two reasons: First, there is a truly vast array of microphones available, and a wise choice among them must be based on knowledge rather than on advertising hyperbole. Second, audio reproduction can be no better than the worst of the components through which the audio signal passes. The microphone is the first component, the link between the acoustic world and the audio electronics. If it is not well matched to the audio task on the one hand and to the electronic system on the other, if it is used in ways that are not in keeping with its inherent characteristics, sound reproduction will suffer, perhaps drastically. While casual users might find a poor or noisy audio signal acceptable, the speech pathologist can rarely afford to be so tolerant. Every recording of a patient must be as good as reasonable effort can make it; every transduced speech signal to be analyzed must be as perfect as is reasonably possible. Therefore, the clinician will want to pay particular attention to the choice of microphone. The following material is intended to give basic information in that regard.

Microphone Specifications

There are four different specifications that are most important to the microphone user: sensitivity, impedance, frequency response, and directionality.

SENSITIVITY

A microphone's sensitivity rating quantifies its effectiveness in converting acoustical to electrical energy. The microphone can be considered to be an electrical generator, and *sensitivity* is stated as the amount of electrical power produced for a standard sound pressure input. The rating most commonly used is the electrical output in dB re: 1 mW when the sound pressure input is 10 dynes/cm^2. For audio microphones this value is commonly measured at a frequency of 1000 Hz. Most microphones have sensitivities in the range of -51 to -60 dB, which indicates power outputs of 0.00001 to 0.000001 mW when the microphone is driven by a sound pressure of 10 dynes/cm^2. This is obviously very little power, but audio amplifiers are designed to accept this low level, and so it is perfectly acceptable for ordinary purposes. If the microphone is to be connected directly to some other kind of device, such as an oscilloscope for display of the acoustic waveform, some type of preamplifier will be necessary. If *precisely* known, the microphone's sensitivity rating may be used to determine the sound pressure of an audio signal.

IMPEDANCE

The impedance of a microphone specifies its ability to deliver current to the amplifier or other circuit to which it is connected. Unless one intends to design a special amplifier, the actual current output levels are not overly important. What does matter, however, is the degree to which the impedance of the microphone matches that of the amplifier's input stage. A gross mismatch of the two will significantly reduce microphone sensitivity and increase the noise level. Worse, the mismatch may compromise the microphone's frequency response, with the result that the audio input to the amplifier becomes unacceptably distorted.

Achieving an adequate microphone-to-amplifier impedance match is fortunately not a major problem, thanks to the fact that the audio industry has, by and large, achieved some degree of standardization in this regard. Most microphones have an impedance of approximately 200 Ω and audio amplifiers have been designed around this value. There are exceptions, however, and the impedance rating of a microphone should be checked to be sure that it is suitable for its intended use. Instances of serious mismatch can often be corrected by insertion of a special miniature matching transformer or a resistive "pad" (available at audio stores and from microphone manufacturers) into the amplifier input line. But it is better to have a matched system to begin with.

FREQUENCY RESPONSE

Like a human ear, no microphone is equally sensitive to all audio frequencies. Its *frequency response* is depicted in the equivalent of an audiogram: A given microphone's sensitivity in dB is plotted over frequency. An example is shown in Figure 4–11. This kind of specification should be easily intelligible to any speech pathologist.

Ideally, a microphone would be equally sensitive to all frequencies over (at least) the range of human hearing, from about 20 Hz to approximately 20,000 Hz. While this degree of perfection is not readily achieved, a good quality microphone is usually reasonably close. Thanks to the popular demand that audio reproductions recreate the original acoustic events as precisely as possible, there are many acceptable models among which to choose.

DIRECTIONALITY: THE POLAR RESPONSE

The design of a microphone will strongly affect the variability of its sensitivity to sounds arriving from different directions. The directional sensitivity character-

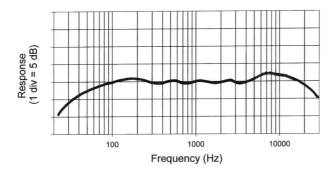

Figure 4–11. A typical frequency-response curve for a high-quality microphone. The response is acceptably flat over the range of human hearing.

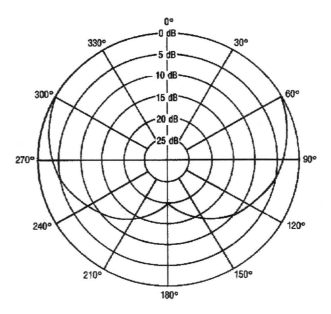

Figure 4–12. A polar-response or directionality plot for a typical microphone. The microphone is assumed to lie in the center of the graph, pointed at the 0° mark. (A microphone having this particular response pattern is said to be "unidirectional.")

istics are typically detailed in a ***polar response*** graph of the type shown in Figure 4–12. The radii on the graph represent the angles from which the test sound arrives. The concentric circles are spaced 5 dB apart. The pattern of the response plot shows the direction(s) from which sound is best picked up. The microphone whose polar response was plotted in Figure 4–12 is most sensitive to sounds coming from the front, within 60° of the microphone's axis. As the sound source moves further to the side, sensitivity falls off. This microphone is least sensitive to sounds coming from directly behind: The response in this direction is 20 dB below that of head-on incidence.

Microphones are often categorized in terms of their directionality characteristics, and several standard patterns are available. The pattern of Figure 4–12 is described as *cardioid* (heart-shaped) and typifies most "unidirectional" microphones. Clearly, this kind of microphone records best those sounds coming from the direction in which the microphone is pointed. Its great advantage is that sound coming from other sources tends to be attenuated. A microphone with a unidirectional sensitivity pattern, then, would be chosen when ambient noise levels are higher than one would like and when the speaker remains in front of the microphone. A unidirectional microphone would normally be used, for example, to obtain a recording of a speech sample from a seated patient.

Figure 4–13 shows the two other common polar response types. The *omnidirectional* microphone (Figure 4–13A) is almost equally sensitive in all directions. It is, therefore, the microphone of choice in those circumstances in which a single microphone must be used to pick up sounds coming from all around it. For recording a child moving around a playroom, for instance, this response pattern may offer significant advantages. On the other hand, extraneous noises

coming from any point in the recording area will be picked up just as clearly as the child's utterances.

Finally, Figure 4–13B shows a *bidirectional* response pattern. The microphone picks up sounds from either side (or from front and back) equally well, but it is very much less sensitive to sound arriving from other directions. This type may be useful in those situations where two speakers (perhaps the therapist and the patient) are facing each other with a microphone between them.

Microphone Mechanisms

There are innumerable methods available whereby sound energy may be converted to an electrical signal. Almost all have been tried in microphones. Some techniques have been found suitable for highly specialized purposes, and a few have proven to be so versatile and easy to implement that they have become the standards for audio transduction. It is with these that we are concerned here.

Almost all microphones have some sort of diaphragm that is exposed to the incoming sound wave. The sound pressure acts on the diaphragm and causes it to move. The diaphragm, then, serves as a collector of

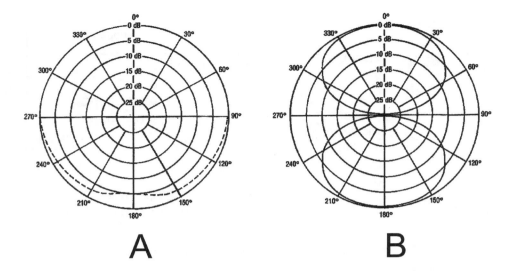

Figure 4–13. Polar response plots of **(A)** an omnidirectional and **(B)** a bidirectional microphone.

acoustic energy; its movement affects an active element that does the actual transduction.

CRYSTAL (PIEZOELECTRIC) MICROPHONES

Crystals of certain substances generate electrical voltages when they are mechanically deformed. The voltage is proportional to the rate of deformation. The phenomenon, known as the *piezoelectric effect*, is used in piezoelectric, or crystal, microphones, in which the movement of the diaphragm is used to deform the crystal. These microphones are very inexpensive, but that is their chief virtue. They do not do a very good job with respect to fidelity because they have a poor low-frequency response and they suffer seriously from frequency nonlinearity. Although they are sometimes provided with recording equipment, they are not suited to the needs of the speech clinician.

DYNAMIC MICROPHONES

Dynamic microphones take advantage of the fact that a voltage is produced across a conductor when it moves through a magnetic field. When, as in a microphone, the conductor's motion is the result of acoustic pressure, the voltage produced will be an analog of the audio input. The most common form of dynamic microphone—the *moving-coil* type—is diagrammed in Figure 4–14. In it a single-layer coil of very fine wire is attached to the sound-collecting diaphragm. This coil is mounted around a cylindrical permanent magnet, with the result that displacement of the diaphragm by a sound wave moves the coil within a magnetic field. As a result, an electric flow through the coil is produced. In a very real sense, this type of microphone is an electrical generator, working on much the same principle as the enormously larger generators that produce power for utility companies.

Because the impedance of the coil is very low, dynamic microphones usually include a transformer within the microphone housing to match them to an amplifier input. On the whole, dynamic microphones are relatively rugged, can be made with excellent frequency-response characteristics, and are moderately sensitive. These features, together with their moderate cost, make them the best all-around choice for routine recording work.

CONDENSER MICROPHONES

The charge on the plates of a capacitor (see Chapter 2, "Analog Electronics") varies as a function of several variables, one of which is the distance separating them. This fact forms the basis of yet another method of acoustic transduction, exploited in the *condenser microphone*.[2]

---

[2] Condenser is the obsolete term for capacitor.

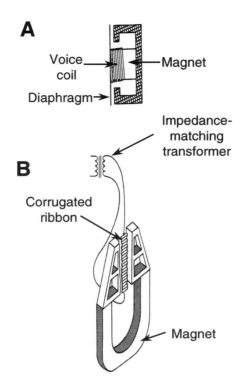

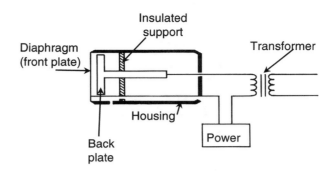

Figure 4–15. Simplified construction of a condenser microphone. The diaphragm and back plate form a capacitor. Movement of the diaphragm changes the capacitance, causing current to flow to or from the power supply through the transformer.

Figure 4–14. Dynamic microphones: **A.** Moving coil. **B.** Ribbon.

The mechanism of a condenser microphone is illustrated (in greatly simplified form) in Figure 4–15. A very thin metallic diaphragm acts as the energy collector and at the same time serves as one plate of a capacitor. The other plate is held rigidly fixed behind, but extremely close to, the diaphragm. A power supply maintains a fairly significant voltage difference between the two plates. Since they are a pair of conductors separated by an insulator (air), the microphone elements form a capacitor that stores a charge imposed by the power supply. When the diaphragm moves in or out under the pressure of sound waves the distance between the plates changes by a microscopic amount. This is sufficient, however, to significantly alter the capacitance of the system, which means that the charge-storage capability changes, causing electrons to flow to or from the plates. The current is made to flow through a transformer that is part of the power-supply circuit. The transformer's primary coil generates a voltage proportional to the magnitude of the current flow, which is transferred to the microphone amplifier by the transformer's secondary coil.

The condenser microphone has a flat response over a wide frequency range, excellent stability, fairly high sensitivity, and very little self-generated internal

noise. For these reasons it is the transducer of choice for precision measurement of sound pressure and for similarly demanding transduction tasks. It is, for example, the type of microphone used by audiologists for calibration of audiometric equipment.

A good condenser microphone usually costs more than other types, and it also has certain drawbacks. First, it will not tolerate abuse. Physical shock can easily damage the capacitor elements or their positioning, as can exposure to high-pressure bursts, such as powerful puffs of air, directed at the diaphragm. Second, there is the extra complication of a separate power supply which, in practice, means that a special preamplifier must be used. These factors often rule out the use of condenser microphones for everyday purposes. On the other hand, the fidelity of their audio transduction more than compensates for their problems where precision is of prime concern.

ELECTRET MICROPHONES

Some of the problems of the condenser microphone are solved by a special type of microphone that uses an ***electret*** as one of the capacitor elements. An electret is a device that retains an electric charge indefinitely. Although the principle has been known for over 150 years, it is only in the past few decades that electret materials suitable for microphone use have been available. Current electret microphones use a thin, metal-plated plastic membrane that permanently holds a charge, which is applied to it in the manufacturing process. The permanence of the charge eliminates the need for a special power supply for the microphone. In essence, the power supply is built in. There is, however, a small problem: The resultant electret capacitor will function only when connected to an amplifier with an *extremely* high input impedance. The most effective way to deal with this requirement is to make a special preamplifier part of the microphone itself. Modern transistor devices make this easy to achieve, but it means that the electret microphone will still need an external power supply—not for the capacitor, which is permanently charged, but for the transistor in the preamplifier. Despite this, the electret condenser microphone's advantage is a significant one, because powering a transistor requires only very low voltages, which means that a miniature battery will suffice. Furthermore, these microphones can be made very small, making them very useful as probe microphones (Villchur & Killion, 1975; Harford, 1980, 1981).

CONTACT MICROPHONES (ACCELEROMETERS)

There are instances in which one is interested in only a specific aspect of the speech signal, such as its fundamental frequency. Occasionally one might need simply an indication of the presence or absence of speech, as in reaction-time determination. In these cases the use of a contact microphone, or accelerometer, should be considered. These devices are specially designed to pick up acoustic signals, or vibrations, from the body surface. Held in contact with the skin by an adhesive or a strap mounting, they are largely insensitive to airborne sounds.

The speech signal is badly degraded by transmission through the tissues of the body (Figure 4–16), but vocal fundamental frequency is unaltered. Koike (1973) found that the improvement of signal-to-noise ratio afforded by a contact microphone in the pretracheal region made it preferable to a standard microphone for

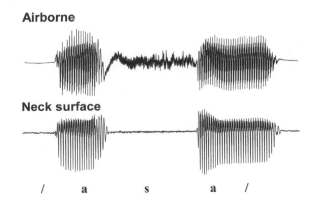

Airborne

Neck surface

/   a   s   a   /

Figure 4–16. Airborne (top) and neck-surface (bottom) pickup of speech signals.

analysis of fundamental frequency perturbation. While neck placement is usual, more esoteric locations (forehead, ear canal, mastoid, nose) have been evaluated by Snidecor, Rehman, and Washburn (1959).

TAPE RECORDERS

The tape recorder may be the one item of technical electronics with which absolutely every speech pathologist is familiar. It has become an indispensable tool in therapy and an invaluable aid in the maintenance of adequate patient records. Yet the way in which the ordinary tape recorder works remains a mystery to many, which often prevents them from gaining maximal advantage from it.

When asked what a tape recorder does, most users are likely to answer that it stores speech or music on a magnetic tape and allows it to be played back to reproduce the original material with high fidelity. For the general public, this is a perfectly adequate view, but for the speech professional it is far too narrow a formulation. What a tape recorder *really* does is to store *information* on a magnetic tape. That information might be (and most commonly is) speech or music, but it could just as easily be voltages representing intraoral pressure, jaw position, nasalization ratio, or any of the many measurements that a speech pathologist might make on a patient. Almost any kind of information can be stored on magnetic tape with just a little ingenuity and a bit of knowledge about the recording process.

Basic Principles of Tape Recording

Magnetic tape recording depends on the fact that an electric current causes a magnetic field to be produced around a conducting element. Conversely, movement of a magnetic field near a conductor causes an electric current to flow in it. Magnetic fields can be "frozen" and stored by allowing them to magnetize a susceptible material. A tape deck does all this with (1) a record system that generates magnetic fields; (2) a transport system that moves magnetically-sensitive material (the tape) into those magnetic fields in order to "capture" them; and (3) a playback system that detects the currents generated when the magnetic fields that have been captured on the tape are moved past a transducer (Figure 4–17).

RECORD TRANSDUCERS (RECORD HEADS)

The flow of current through a wire generates a magnetic field around the wire; the strength of that field is

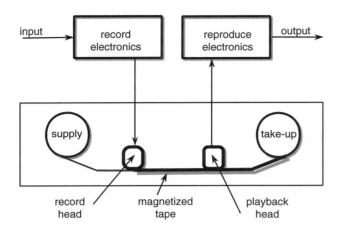

Figure 4–17. The functional components of a tape recorder.

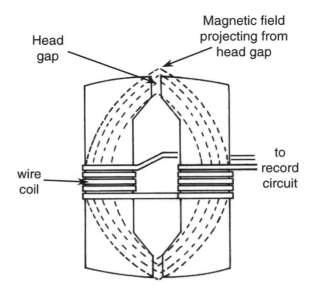

Figure 4–18. A tape-recorder head. A wire coil is wound on a core of magnetically permeable material. When current flows through the coil, a magnetic field is generated in the core and projects into the space at the head gap. Tape passing near the gap is magnetized.

proportional to the magnitude of the current. The magnetic field can be concentrated by winding the wire into a coil. Given these facts, it is easy to see how transduction of a tape-deck's input to a magnetic field is accomplished. This signal (a varying voltage that represents sound pressure, or pressure, or air flow, or whatever) is fed to an amplifier whose variable-current output is connected to a recording head, which is constructed as shown in Figure 4–18. The wire coils in the head generate a magnetic field that is further concentrated and directed by the metal core on which the coils are wound and by a set of "pole pieces." The net result is that a magnetic field whose strength is proportional to the current appears in the gap at the top of the head. (The gap itself is very narrow—on the order of 0.0005 cm.) The entire head is really nothing more than a specially-shaped electromagnet. One side of the gap is the magnet's north pole, the other side the south pole. Not only does the magnetic strength change with the magnitude of the current, but magnetic polarity reverses when current flow changes direction, as it periodically does in most AC signals.

RECORDING TAPE: THE STORAGE MEDIUM

Recording tape consists of a very thin plastic film backing on which is deposited an even thinner layer of microscopic crystals of an easily-magnetized material embedded in a binder. Each particle of magnetic material can be individually magnetized. In the recording process the gap of the record head is brought into intimate contact with the surface of the tape. As they travel past the record head each of the particles is magnetized to a degree proportional to the strength of the

head's magnetic field and with a polarity that matches it. Each particle therefore serves as a permanent record of the record-head's magnetic status at the time it passed by. From one end to the other, the tape preserves a record of the magnetic characteristics of the record head over time, which in turn represents the input signal over time.

The original magnetic material for tape recording was ferric oxide (Fe_2O_3), but special low-noise and high-output oxides have been developed in recent years. They have smaller, more densely packed magnetic particles, and so can provide an output up to 8 dB greater than older formulations. The increased output capability allows faithful reproduction of a wider range of signal intensities—a factor that is important to the speech pathologist because of the wide dynamic range of speech. Another development that has increased recording quality is the use of non-ferrous magnetic materials as the storage medium. Chromium dioxide (CrO_2) provides very high output levels, low signal distortion, and excellent frequency response. Tapes that use metal particles rather than an oxide are also available. They offer extremely high output levels and have a particularly good response at high frequencies, an important characteristic that can help overcome a major limitation of cassette tape decks. Furthermore, they tend to be less prone to saturation at high signal levels, thus offering greater protection from distortion. While the performance of metal tape is significantly better than that of metal-oxide tapes, it is considerably more expensive. Metal tape also needs stronger biasing than is provided for on some cassette tape units. More important than the specific material, however, may be the formulation and manufacturing technique used to produce a given tape: the binders and finish significantly affect a tape's performance. Fortunately, the quality of the major brands of recording tape is uniformly quite high. Differences in their ability to reproduce sound are likely to be small. More important, for most clinics, is the quality of the tape deck itself.

Recording tape can be made of any number of backing materials, but over the years acetate and polyester (Mylar®) have proven most useful. Acetate, however, turns brittle with age and is less dimensionally stable in the face of temperature and humidity changes. Polyester, which is much stronger and thereby better able to withstand the forces of tape starts and stops without parting, is considered superior for routine work, and has come to be the standard material. While polyester tape will not tear, it may stretch very badly when subjected to excessive tensile force. Acetate, in contrast, tends to snap fairly cleanly when it separates. A badly-stretched segment of a tape represents a significant length of recording forever destroyed. A clean break, on the other hand, can often be spliced, keeping the loss to a small fraction of a second. Under some very special circumstances, then, a recording is better protected when done on acetate tape. It is, unfortunately, difficult if not impossible to find.

Thickness of the backing material is also important; it varies from 0.5 mil (thousandths of an inch) to over 2 mils. (The thinner the tape the greater the length of tape that can be wound on a reel.) Very thin tapes—that is long tapes with extended recording time—should be avoided for two reasons. First, they are weaker and therefore more likely to tear or deform. Second, as the backing is made thinner the magnetized coatings on the tape surface lie much closer to each other when the tape is wound on the reel. In storage the magnetic fields in one layer can magnetize the coating in the next layer. On playback, one hears the original recording and a pre-echo of the material on the next tape layer. Aside from being distracting and disturbing to a listener, this "print-through" can interfere with analysis of the stored information. Print-

through is minimized by using thicker tape (1½ mils is adequate)—which translates in practice to using cassettes with shorter recording time. Tight winding of the tape is also to be avoided. Because fast-forward and rewind cause tight tape packing, recorded tapes are often stored on the take-up reel and rewound only before being played.[3]

REPRODUCE TRANSDUCERS (PLAYBACK HEADS)

Recall that moving a magnetic field near a wire causes a current to flow in it. Therefore, to reconvert the information stored in the tape's magnetic domains back to electrical signals, the tape need only be moved past the very same sort of coil-on-a-metal-core assembly that produced magnetic fields originally. As the magnetic domains on the tape pass the playback head they induce currents that are sensed by the output amplifiers, and the original signal is recreated.

It turns out that the current induced by the magnetic domains is proportional to their strength and to *the rate of change* of magnetization as the domains move along. This implies that signals of similar amplitudes but different frequencies (that is, signals whose rates of change are different) will induce very different currents in the playback head. In fact, the amplitude of the output of an ideal playback head increases with frequency at the rate of 6 dB per octave. Tape decks have "equalization" circuits that compensate for this distortion of AC signals. It should be clear that when the rate of change (that is, the frequency) of the stored signal drops to very low levels, the current induced in the playback head will ultimately become less than the random noise inherent in the system, and hence the signal will be irrecoverable. This is a formal way of saying that the ordinary tape system cannot record signals that approach DC.

Recording and Playback

MULTICHANNEL RECORDING AND PLAYBACK

It is possible to construct a composite head that contains two (or more) record- or reproduce-transducers in a stack. If each head in the stack is associated with its own circuitry, then different signals can be simultaneously recorded as magnetized stripes, or *tracks* on

---

[3]It is worth noting that print-through is also a threat to the long-term storage of videotapes. The same considerations and cautions prevail.

the tape, with each track separated from its neighbors by a *guard track* of unrecorded tape surface. While some specialized tape systems can record up to 14 tracks on a single (1 inch) tape, clinicians are most likely to encounter 2-channel tape decks. These are usually called *stereophonic*, but this term tends to obscure their real value to the speech pathologist: each channel can be used to store completely different information. Stimuli, for instance, can be put on one channel, while patient responses are recorded on the other. (This arrangement makes it much easier to extract patient data for analysis later.) With an appropriate adapter (see "FM Tape Recording," later) it is even possible to store physiological data (such as air flow or intraoral pressure) on one of the channels, while the speech signal is laid down in the usual way on the other.

BIASING

There is a problem in the storage, or tape magnetizing process, that has thus far been ignored: The degree of magnetization attained by the tape particles is by no means a linear function of the strength of the magnetic field produced by the record head. A typical relationship between the strength of the head's magnetizing force and the strength of the magnetization produced on the tape (called the *remanent magnetic flux*) is shown in Figure 4–19A. The "bent" transfer function has dire consequences for the accuracy of the representation of the stored signal (Figure 4–19B). Clearly, unless some corrective steps are taken, the magnetic representation on the tape may bear little resemblance to the original input signal, and the ultimate reproduction at the output will be a badly distorted version of what the record head laid down. A corrective measure has, in fact, been developed empirically. It is called *AC bias* and, as shown in Figure 4–19C, it involves adding a high-frequency complex waveform to the signal sent to the record head. When affected by the nonlinear transfer function, the composite signal produces a magnetic representation that is a much closer approximation of the original wave. The optimal frequency and amplitude of the bias signal depend on the range of frequencies to be recorded, on the characteristics of the record head, and on the material of which the recording medium is made. Generally, a bias signal of 100 kHz is used for audio recording, but the various magnetic materials (ferric oxide, chromium compounds, metallic particles) all require different bias currents. Manufacturers of tape decks usually provide a way to change the bias level to suit the kind of tape the user has selected. (It is unwise to buy a tape deck that does not offer this option.)

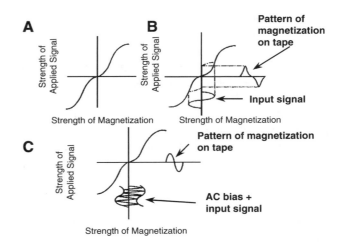

Figure 4–19. Recording-head AC bias. **A.** Magnetization of the tape is not a linear function of the magnetizing field. Hence, as shown in **B**, a recorded signal will be severely distorted. Linearization is achieved by adding a high-frequency wave to the signal to be recorded (**C**), causing it to be stored in an undistorted form. The high-frequency signal is called an "AC bias."

THREE-HEAD TAPE RECORDERS

In order to optimize performance, the record, reproduce, and erase heads should be designed differently. While it is perfectly possible to get acceptable recordings from a head that serves both record and reproduce functions, audio quality is significantly improved if separate, specially designed heads are used for the two functions. Accordingly, better-quality tape decks are usually "three-head" machines. This feature should be considered essential when selecting a tape deck for purchase, for two reasons. The first, of course, is the increased audio fidelity that separate heads provide. The second reason relates to the way in which the recording is monitored for quality. A combined record-reproduce head can only perform one function at a time. When it is recording it cannot, at the same time, reproduce what is on the tape. Therefore, when listening to the tape to check for quality during actual recording, what the listener hears is not the recording itself: the single head is operating in its record mode, and so is not available to transduce what has been put onto the tape. Rather, what the listener is hearing is the signal that is coming in to the recorder's amplifier. If there is any problem in the way in which the signal is laid down on the tape (including, for instance, incorrect bias or tape damage) it will not become apparent until later, when the tape is played back. On the other hand, a separate reproduce head can function while the recording is being made by the record head, so it is possible to monitor what has actually been put onto the tape. (In fact, three-head tape decks allow the user the choose between listening to the input amplifier or to the tape itself.)

ERASURE

One of the advantages of tape storage of information is the ease with which the magnetic domains on the tape can be eliminated and the recorded information expunged. Erasure is achieved by exposing the tape to a slowly diminishing cyclic magnetic field. While this sounds complex, it is actually quite easy to achieve: the tape is passed across a record head producing strong and rapidly alternating magnetic fields. As a given point on the tape moves further from the head, the effect of the head's magnetic field weakens, satisfying the "slowly diminishing" requirement. After this treatment the magnetic domains on the tape are left randomly magnetized (*"degaussed"*). Tape decks have a separate degaussing, or erase, head built into them. It is energized in the record mode and erases the tape just before it reaches the record head. Separate *bulk erasers* are also available: they can erase an entire reel or cassette of tape to a level at least 60 dB below that of a recorded signal.

EQUALIZATION

It was said earlier that the playback head inherently boosts the amplitude of signals of different frequencies at a rate of about 6 dB per octave. There are also non-linearities in the frequency-versus-amplitude curve due to inevitable losses produced by a number of physical phenomena. When these effects are taken together, the record-to-reproduce signal relationship is likely to resemble the one shown in Figure 4–20. Without correction a reproduced signal will be very different from the signal originally applied to the input.

The correction for these effects is called *equalization*. Basically it simply involves tailoring both the record and reproduce amplifiers' frequency responses to compensate for the inherent distortions of the tape recording process. Tape decks designed to handle instrumentation signals (as opposed to audio signals) exclusively achieve equalization by making the frequency response curve of the recorder's electronics the inverse of the record and reproduce curves, as in Figure 4–20B. The result, on playback, is a faithful reproduction of the original input.

Audio signals, however, present a greater challenge because the perceived loudness of equal-amplitude signals varies with frequency (see Chapter 5,

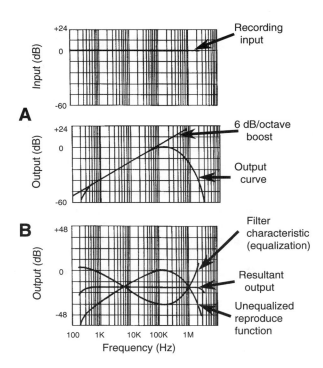

Figure 4–20. Equalization. **A**. Because of electrical and physical phenomena, equal amplitude recordings at different frequencies will be reproduced with different amplitudes. Applying a special filtering function (**B**) results in a linearized signal.

"Speech Intensity"). The equalization characteristics of audio tape decks compensate for these effects as well, and therefore are more complex. Furthermore, the different magnetic properties of the various kinds of tape now available call for different equalization curves. Fortunately, industry-wide standardization of equalization characteristics ensures that audio recordings made on one tape deck can be played back with equal fidelity on another. The U.S. standard equalization curve for consumer audio recorders is the National Association of Broadcasters (NAB) curve.

NOISE REDUCTION

Recording tapes have inherent random magnetic fluctuations that reproduce as tape hiss (high-frequency noise). Tape-deck electronics also contribute unwanted background noise. Optimizing the signal-to-noise ratio of recorded material is therefore important. One way to do this is to produce strong magnetic fields by recording at high signal levels. Sometimes, particularly with the thinner and narrower tape used in cassettes, this is of limited effectiveness, especially if it increases print-through. Ways have been sought to improve the signal-to-noise ratio by electronic manipulation of the signal.

The most widely used noise reduction method is the Dolby system. It provides a pre-recording emphasis of low-level input signals in the mid- and high-frequency ranges, where tape noise is most objectionable. On the tape, then, the amplitude of the higher frequencies is exaggerated. On playback, however, a matching de-emphasis is applied, so that the signal is restored to its original spectral characteristics. While the playback de-emphasis restores the recorded material to original levels, it also reduces objectionable hiss and noise in the frequency range of the de-emphasis. Since the noise signals were not boosted originally (because they were not part of the input, but rather came from the tape itself) they are attenuated in the final output. Recorded signals are reproduced at their real amplitudes. The net effect is that the signal-to-noise ratio is improved by several dB. It is this noise reduction, as much as any other factor, that makes a cassette recorder capable of high-fidelity recording.

AUTOMATIC GAIN CONTROL

Many tape recorders incorporate a special circuit that works to keep the signal at a constant level by increasing amplification when signal strength diminishes, and by reducing amplification when it increases. Known as an *automatic gain control* (AGC), this circuitry helps ensure that the signal strength remains optimal. It can be a very useful feature in circumstances where, for instance, the speaker-microphone distance cannot be kept constant (and signal strength therefore varies). On the other hand, the constant changes of amplification created by the AGC circuit may invalidate later measurements of speech intensity, and thus special caution needs to be exercised in using an AGC-equipped tape recorder. Speech clinicians, when selecting recording equipment, are best advised to purchase units in which the AGC circuit can be disabled.

Digital Tape Recording

Although there are several ways of reducing the noise in analog recordings, there is no way to eliminate it entirely. There is always at least a small amount of random magnetization on the tape. An analog signal itself, the random magnetization becomes part of the material that has been recorded and is heard as noise on playback. An important way around this problem is to store the input signal in *digital* form (after analog-to-digital conversion) on the tape, and to reconstruct it as part of the playback process.

The *digital audio tape* (DAT) recorder does exactly this.[4] What is laid down on tape is not an analog representation of the input, but rather a series of *bits* (see Chapter 3 and the section on analog-to-digital converters later in this chapter) organized into data "words." The advantage of doing this is that the bits (1s and 0s) are represented by regions of very strong and very weak (or absent) magnetization. The vast difference between the two levels of magnetization ensures that small background variations of magnetic flux (random noise on the tape) will not contaminate the data. Except in the most extreme situations, a "1" will always be read as a "1" and a "0" will always be retrieved as a "0." In short, noise on the tape plays essentially no role in the signal. Furthermore, there are mathematical techniques that can reconstruct a digital "word" even if part of it has been damaged. Thus, "error-correcting codes" can correct for tape imperfections that, in an analog recording, would interfere with accurate reproduction. The A/D converter that creates the data words operates at a constant (and very high) rate, and during playback a D/A converter translates them back to analog values at exactly the same rate. Therefore, unlike analog recorders, the sound reproduction process is essentially unaffected by minor variations in tape speed.

Because, in the DAT, the signal is not represented by analog changes in magnetization, the limitations on frequency and dynamic (intensity) range of magnetic tape are circumvented. Digital audio tape recording therefore provides reproduction that is much more faithful to the original input than any analog tape recording could hope to be.

Beyond the issue of greater recording fidelity, the DAT recorder offers certain conveniences beyond those available on analog tape decks. The digital values that represent the original audio signal can usually be retrieved (via a special digital connector), allowing them to be transferred directly to a computer for analytic processing. Given that the DAT is really a computer system, each location on the tape is associated with an "address" making it possible to go to it directly and automatically, exactly as on a compact disk. Clearly, DAT offers significant advantages to the speech clinician.

---

[4]A digital audio tape recording is, in essence, a compact-disk recording on tape.

Recording Technique

Ideally, a microphone would produce a perfectly accurate electrical analog of a single acoustic signal (for instance, a patient's speech) while disregarding all irrelevant sounds in the immediate environment. Ideally, that electrical analog would be precisely stored on the tape and would later be reproduced without any distortion. In a perfect world, an exact acoustic duplicate of the original sound waves would be generated by a speaker system. Perfection is not achieved in the real world, but with a little care it can be approached. What is required is a high-quality microphone, an excellent tape deck, and a well-designed speaker system. Clearly, given the nature of the work that they do, all speech pathologists should be equipped with the best audio system possible. A large proportion of everyday clinical work is founded on very careful listening. It is foolish to focus the finely honed perceptual skills of a first-rate therapist on a noisy, distorted, second-rate recording. First, then, clinicians will want to purchase the best possible recording instrument. The specifications of Table 4–1 serve as a basic selection guide.

At least as important as the quality of the equipment is adherence to a few basic and commonsense recording principles.

■ **Record in quiet surroundings.** Unlike the human auditory system, a microphone cannot be selectively attentive. That is, it cannot "focus in" on a single sound source and suppress all others. Except for directionality effects, a microphone transduces equally all sounds that reach it: the patient's speech, the clanking of a radiator, the rumble of passing trucks, and noises in the next room. It follows that the environment must be as quiet as possible. Excessively "live" or reverberant spaces should also be avoided: acoustic reflections may produce significant distortion of the audio signal. The sound-isolated rooms used for audiometric work serve quite well for recording and should be used whenever possible. The advantages outweigh the inconvenience of juggling of schedules that may be necessary.

■ **Isolate the microphone from vibration.** A microphone must be supported on (or from) something. The choice of support is far from trivial, since vibration of the microphone support will be transduced along with the sound input. A number of relatively simple steps can, and should, be taken to minimize this problem. The microphone should never be placed on the same surface as a tape recorder: the vibration of the recorder's motors is likely to produce background noise in the recording. Whenever possible, mount the microphone on a boom or other hanging support rather than on a desk-top microphone stand. This keeps it isolated from the noises produced when the patient or therapist

Table 4–1. Suggested minimal specifications for tape decks

Specification	Minimum Quality
Frequency response*	30 Hz – 15,000 Hz ± 3 dB
Signal / Noise ratio	
without Dolby®	55 dB or better
with Dolby®	60 dB or better
Wow and Flutter	
unweighted	0.15% or less
weighted˙	0.10% or less
Stereo separation	
(signal leakage between left and right channels)	40 dB or better
Cross-talk	
(signal leakage between adjacent tracks on multi-channel decks)	60 dB or better

˙Different frequency components in the signal are given different prominences in the mathematical computation. *Caution*: There are a number of different weighting systems in use, and they produce slightly different values for the same quality of performance.

drops something on the table, kick its leg, and so on. The boom stand can be positioned to the side of the speaker (out of the way of inadvertent kicks and knocks) while allowing great flexibility of placement of the microphone itself.

■ Manufacturers can usually provide **shock mounts** for their microphones, which cushion them and provide isolation from floor and building vibration. They are commonly worth their moderate cost.

■ Another excellent option is a high-quality head-mounted microphone. **Head-mounting** has the advantage of keeping a fixed position of the microphone with respect to the speaker, irrespective of the latter's movements. This can be particularly useful when dealing with restless patients (especially children) or when long-term intensity measurements (that require an invariant mouth-to-microphone distance) are to be made (See Chapter 5, "Speech Intensity").

■ **Place the microphone correctly in relation to the speaker.** "Correct" is determined by the directionality characteristics of the microphone being used. In general, the microphone should be pointed toward the speaker, slighly below and about 30 cm from the mouth. Closer placement may be useful, but it tends to subject the microphone to the puffs of air accompanying plosives and strong fricatives, which result in loud noise bursts in the recording. This problem can be mitigated by the use of a windscreen, a plastic-foam hood that fits over the microphone head. Note also that special microphone placements are recommended for measurements of speech intensity (see Chapter 5, "Speech Intensity").

■ Recording is much more of an art than a science. Clinicians should experiment with different locations, microphone placements, and mounting techniques to optimize results in their own settings. The time spent doing so is very likely to pay off in higher-quality and more useful patient recordings.

FM Tape Recording

The analog recording process discussed thus far, in which the instantaneous amplitude of the input signal is encoded in the strength of the stored magnetic field, is called *direct* or *amplitude modulated* recording. Recall that the voltage produced by the reproduce head of a tape deck is proportional to the *rate of change* of the magnetic field that it senses. Now, as the frequency of a recorded signal falls, the rate of change of the magnetic strength of the domains on the tape is reduced. Therefore, as frequency diminishes, the amplitude of

the reproduced signal gets smaller. An attempt to record DC by direct recording is doomed to total failure: since the rate of change of a DC signal is zero, the reproduce head will be unaffected by it.

Many physiological signals (airflow and air pressure, for instance) characteristically have very low rates of change, and some come close to being DC. The direct recording techniques discussed thus far will not work for them. They could, of course, be recorded by digital techniques (which can encode the magnitude of *any* voltage, changing or not). But the significant expense of these instruments may be difficult to justify in many clinical settings.

There is another option: the data signal can be encoded in a different analog form that is compatible with the direct recording system. There are many ways of doing this, but the most widely used method is *frequency modulation* (FM).

In frequency modulation, a waveform (called the *carrier*) is made to vary in frequency in proportion to the amplitude of some other signal. An example is shown in Figure 4–21. A sine-wave *carrier* (upper trace) changes frequency as the voltage of a *modulating signal* (lower trace) rises and falls. Note how, in the figure, the frequency of the modulated carrier is proportional to the instantaneous voltage of the modulating signal. When the modulating sine wave is at minimal voltage, the frequency of the modulated carrier signal is only a fraction of the frequency it has when the modulating signal is at a maximum. The amount of variation of the carrier frequency for a given change in the modulating voltage is an important parameter of frequency modulation, and is expressed as the amount of

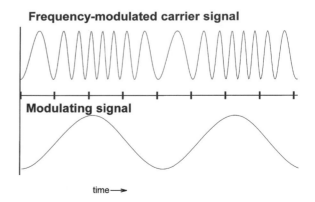

Frequency-modulated carrier signal

Modulating signal

time⟶

Figure 4–21. The frequency of a sine-wave *carrier* (upper trace) changes with changes in the voltage of a *modulating signal* (lower trace). Note how the frequency of the modulated carrier is proportional to the instantaneous voltage of the modulating signal.

frequency change of the carrier for a unit change in modulating-signal voltage. If, for example, the carrier frequency changed by 125 Hz as the modulating signal varied from zero to 5 volts, then the *frequency deviation* of the carrier would be said to be 25 Hz/V.

In frequency modulation, then, the *frequency* of a carrier waveform (usually a square wave) represents the *amplitude* of some other signal. Since the carrier is an AC wave it can be tape recorded, allowing a coded representation of a DC signal to be stored on magnetic tape. The only restriction (from the tape recorder's point of view) is that the highest and lowest frequency that the *carrier* might assume must lie in the range of the tape deck. Information theory also indicates that the carrier frequency limits the frequency of the data that can be coded. It is not possible, for instance, to obtain an accurate representation of a 100 Hz sine wave with a 150 Hz carrier frequency. In fact, for accurate data representation, the carrier frequency should be much higher than the highest frequency component in the modulating signal. For example, the instrumentation standards currently in effect call for a center frequency of 54 kHz to encode signals from DC to 10 kHz. It also turns out that the maximal deviation (produced by the maximal voltage change from 0 volts) must not be too great, or nonlinearities will occur. Industry standardization of FM tape decks permits a maximal deviation of ±40% about the center frequency. For a DC-to-10-kHz system, then, the center frequency of 54 kHz would vary from a minimum of 32.4 kHz to a maximum of 75.6 kHz.

FM tape decks contain all the necessary electronics for encoding an input into a frequency-modulated signal, storing it on the tape, and decoding it on playback. Usually these machines are multichannel, to provide for simultaneous recording of different data, and there is often at least one direct-recording channel for audio signals or experimenter "banter."

FM tape recorders are moderately expensive and are, in any case, less readily available than they were in the predigital world of a few years ago. Few clinics, moreover, are likely to be enthusiastic about investing in a tape deck that is of very limited value for audio work. Fortunately, there is a relatively low-cost alternative to buying an FM tape system. The frequency modulation and demodulation can be done by an external system which is then connected to a direct-recording tape deck. Multichannel *FM adapters* are commercially available and their characteristics are optimized to

work with ordinary audio tape decks. Alternatively, integrated circuits that perform voltage-to-frequency (frequency modulation) and frequency-to-voltage (frequency demodulation) conversion are also widely available (for about $1.00 each!). Any technician—and a great many amateurs—should have very little trouble designing an acceptable FM adapter with them.

ANALOG-TO-DIGITAL (A/D) CONVERTERS

If computers are to evaluate them, the acoustic and physiologic events of speech and voice must be converted from their naturally analog to a computer-compatible numerical form. This task is accomplished by an analog-to-digital (A/D) converter. The basic principles of A/D conversion were considered in Chapter 3; in this section we consider several aspects of A/D operation that are important to their everyday clinical utility.

Quantization Level

Conceptually, A/D conversion is the process of taking a ruler to a signal and measuring its size: A continuously varying function (perhaps a microphone signal) is thereby transformed to a set of discrete measurements. It is obvious that, the finer the gradations of the ruler, the more precise the measurements will be. Clearly, one can measure more precisely with a ruler on which tenths of a millimeter are marked than on one on which only millimeter lines are scribed. The minimal space between the ruler's markings is called its **resolution**, and it defines the precision of measurement that the ruler offers.

The effect of increasingly poor measurement precision is illustrated in Figure 4–22. At the top is a waveform, such as might be associated with one cycle of an acoustic signal. The y-axis of the data plot runs from -128 to $+127$, and the amplitude of the signal varies from about -80 to about $+90$.[5] Now suppose that the signal amplitude is measured at regular intervals by an instrument that can measure to the nearest ("quantizing step size") 4 units. When plotted, the results of that measurement yield the curve labeled "4." Some of the smoothness of the original curve has been lost because the data plot's amplitude changes in abrupt jumps of 4 units. Four units is about 1.5% of the

---

[5]In arbitrary units, which are used here to underscore the fact that the problem being discussed is unrelated to the units of measurement chosen.

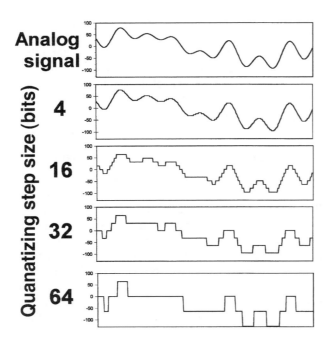

Figure 4–22. The effect of increasingly poor measurement precision. As the quantization step size becomes larger more and more details of the signal are lost.

total range of the graph, and about 2.4% of the peak-to-peak amplitude of the signal itself. The resolution of the measurement system can be expressed as 4 units, or approximately 2.3% of full scale, or about 2.4% of the signal amplitude. At least to the eye, this resolution seems to be acceptable: the details of the original data curve are well represented, but the signal curve has become a bit "choppy."

With a quantizing step size of 16 units (6.25% of full scale and about 9.50% of maximal signal amplitude), its is clear that, although the general waveshape is preserved, some detail of the original signal is lost. When the quantizing step size is 32 units (12.5% full scale, about 19% of signal amplitude) only the grossest features of the original signal are present. No one would consider this a good representation of the original signal. Finally, with a very coarse step size of 64 units (25% of full scale, about 38% of signal amplitude), the representation of the original signal is very poor indeed.

The degradation of the measured version of the original signal is due to *quantization*. If, for example, the recording system can measure the signal with a resolution of 4 units, and if the measurement system has a maximum range of 256 units, then the original signal must be represented by 256 / 4 = 64 *quantiza-*

tion levels, each of which is 4 units. In other words, the amplitude of original signal has to be squeezed into the range of 0 to 63 (and only whole-number values are available). If the measurement resolution is 8 units, then—for a maximal input range of 256 units, there will be 32 quantization levels available, and the original signal's amplitudes will be transformed to whole numbers in the range 0 to 31.

The number of quantization levels available is expressed as the number of bits (see Chapter 3, "Digital Systems") required to express the largest number the measurement system can produce. If, for example, there are 64 available quantization levels, then the magnitude of an input signal will be expressed as a number between 0 and 63. The base-two representation of 63_{10} is 111111_2, which is 6 bits long. An A/D converter with 6-bit resolution transforms analog signals into numbers in the range of 0 to 63. An 8-bit A/D converter produces numbers in the range 0 to 255, and so on. If one knows the bit resolution and the input voltage range over which an A/D converter is set to function, then the resolution of the A/D converter in volts can easily be calculated. Consider, for instance a 10 bit A/D system that can digitize inputs in the range of −5 to +5 volts (a range of 10 V). The range of numbers expressible with 10 bits is from 0 to 1111111111_2 = 1023_{10}, which provides for 1024 quantization levels. Each quantization level thus represents

$$\frac{10 \text{ volts}}{1024 \text{ levels}} = 0.00977 \text{ V},$$

or 9.77 mV per 1-digit increase in the A/D's output. More generally stated, the voltage increment, V, represented by each 1-digit increase in A/D output is:

$$V = \frac{\text{Input range}}{2^N},$$

where N is the number of bits available.

While it is obvious that quantization necessarily coarsens the appearance of the signal that has been converted, there is another effect that is not so immediately apparent. The original analog signal varies smoothly and continuously with time, whereas the digitized signal has very abrupt (in principal, instantaneous) shifts from one quantization state to another. Very rapid changes of state are associated with energetic high-frequency components in the signal's spectrum (see Chapter 7, "Sound Spectrography"). So, to convert a signal from a smoothly-varying (analog) form to a discontinuous discrete-valued (digital) form, is to *add* high-frequency spectral components to the original signal. These spurious components are called *quantization noise*. While unavoidable, quantization noise is minimized by using the greatest number of quantization levels possible.

The details of an input signal are best preserved, and the amount of quantization noise minimized, by using the best bit resolution possible. There are, however, two significant costs of increased resolution. First, a greater number of bits requires more complex circuitry. Fortunately, this is not a problem because, within the limits with which speech pathologists need be concerned, the complexity is easily handled by modern circuit-making methods. More important is that, in general, A/D speed (the number of conversions that can be performed per unit time) decreases as bit resolution increases, and adequate conversion speed is extremely important. On the whole, 12 bits of resolution will meet clinical needs, and A/D boards that provide this level of precision at acceptable speeds (see next section) are widely available at reasonable prices.

There is one final issue—too often overlooked—that is of critical importance. To get the best results from an A/D converter one must actually use all of the bits available. Consider, for instance, a 10-bit A/D with an input range of 0 to 5 volts. Each one-digital increment of the A/D's output is equivalent to

$$\frac{\text{Range}}{2^{10}} = \frac{5}{1024} = 4.88 \text{ mV}.$$

This is about 0.001 of the total range, so the precision of the A/D converter could be said to be 0.1%.

Now let us assume that a signal being converted ranges from a minimum of 0 V to a maximum of 2 V in amplitude. Each count of the A/D converter still represents 4.88 mV, but this is

$$\frac{0.00488}{2 \text{ V}} = .0024\%.$$

So, for this particular input, the precision achieved is 0.24%, less than half as good as what the A/D converter is capable of. The reason is not hard to understand. If 5 V into the system is converted to the output value 1023, then 2 V—the maximum amplitude of the input—will be represented by the number 410, which

is 110011010_2. In short, the largest voltage value going into the A/D converter requires only 9 bits of the 10 available for its quantification. One bit is completely "unused" by this input. For the signal in question, the A/D converter has effectively been converted to a 9-bit converter. The potential precision of an A/D converter is obtained only if all of its available bits are actually used. Ensuring this is relatively easy: ***an input signal should be amplified so that its amplitude range approximates that of the A/D converter to which it is applied.*** Before computer data-gathering is started, the signal should be monitored (perhaps with an oscilloscope) and the amplifier gain adjusted to ensure that the largest signal peaks (positive or negative) are just slightly less than the maximal voltages (positive or negative) that the A/D converter is set to handle.[6]

Sampling Rate

A/D converters examine an analog input every so often and convert the observed voltage to a number. "Every so often" is expressed as the ***sampling rate***, stated in samples per second (samples/s). While most clinical users of computer systems will never need to be concerned about such A/D characteristics as the input voltage range or the numerical encoding system, even those who use only commercially-available computer software will commonly be required to make decisions about the sampling rate. Intuitively, and correctly, one feels that the higher it is the more the digital output will capture all of the information in the analog input. But higher sampling rates result in more data, which take up more room in computer memory, occupy more space on computer disks, and require more time to process during data analysis. The idea, then, is to sample the input as slowly as possible, but fast enough to preserve data fidelity. When a data-acquisition program asks the user to specify a sampling rate, the question that must be answered is "How fast is fast enough?"

THE NYQUIST SAMPLING THEOREM

It turns out that, for everyday purposes, there is a quick and (relatively) easy answer to that question, but it is important to understand the reasoning behind

---

[6] An impediment to doing this might be that changing the amplifier gain would invalidate signal calibration. The solution is simple: Calibration is best done *after* data gathering. The recommended procedure, in short, is to gather the "cleanest," and highest-precision data possible and then, after the fact, to establish what it "meant"—in the sense of its calibration factors. It is almost always possible to proceed in this "reverse" manner, and it is not one whit less valid.

it. Therefore, we will defer the final answer until we have explored a bit of its logic.[7] The consideration that follows is by no means rigorous, and, in order to develop an intuitive sense of what is at issue, many simplifying assumptions have been made. To clarify the discussion issues of information preservation (with which the sampling considerations are really concerned) are combined with problems of signal reconstruction (which is really a separate issue). Those who need to understand the theory underlying signal reconstruction should consult a text on digital signal processing, such as Rabiner and Schafer (1978), Orfanidis (1995), Lyons (1996), and Proakis and Manolakis (1996).

In Figure 4–23 a 100-Hz sine wave (top trace) is sampled at several different rates. The results are illustrated in the lower four traces, in which the sample values are shown by large dots. (The sample values, unlike the original signal, are discrete and discontinuous, but they have been connected in the figure for illustrative purposes.) At a sampling rate of 1000 samples per second (1K/s) there are 10 sample points for every period of the 100 Hz wave, and it is clear that the frequency of the original signal is well represented: There are 10 cycles of the original signal in the time interval depicted, and the sample values clearly also alternate about the center line 10 times.

When the sampling rate is reduced to 500 samples per second the visual impression suggests significant distortion of the original waveform. But the data series of sample points still alternates about the center line 10 times during the sampling period, and so the frequency of the original signal remains discernible.

At a sampling rate as low as 250 samples per second there are only 2.5 samples (on average) per period of the original waveform. But there are still 10 maxima and 10 minima in 100 milliseconds, so the F_0 of the reconstructed series remains correct at 100 Hz.

When the sampling rate is only 160 samples per second, however, the situation changes. On average there are now only 1.6 sample points per period of the original signal. The maxima and minima now demarcate fewer than 10 cycles in the 100 milliseconds of the sampled signal. When reconstructing on the basis of the sampled data points, the original signal is now represented by a signal of much lower frequency. The reason for this state of affairs is that it takes at least two data points (of different values) to define a cycle, and,

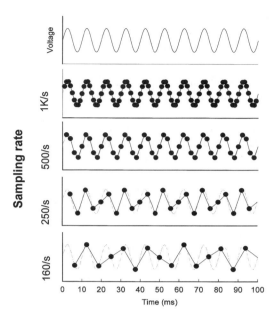

Figure 4–23. Aliasing: Lowering the sampling rate below a critical value causes extra (aliased) frequencies to be added.

at a sampling rate of 160 samples per second, sampling is not fast enough to allow every cycle to be sampled twice. As a result, the original 100-Hz waveform is now represented by a much lower frequency. *Aliasing*—the representation of one frequency by a different frequency—has occurred.

Now, if two data points are required to define a cycle, the question "How fast is fast enough" almost answers itself. Clearly, we must sample at a frequency (sampling rate) that is *at least* twice as high as the frequency of the waveform being converted. This is more formally stated as the *Nyquist sampling theorem*, which says that, if x(t) is a signal with no frequency components higher than f_n, then x(t) is uniquely determined by its samples x[nT] , n = 0, 1, 2, . . . , if and only if the sampling frequency is greater than $2f_n$. The value f_n is referred to as the *Nyquist frequency* and a sampling rate equal to twice this, $2f_n$, is called the *Nyquist rate*. Therefore, if we wish to sample in a way that will preserve all the information in a periodic signal with a frequency of say, 5000 Hz, we will have to sample at a rate of *no less than* 10,000 samples/s, which is the Nyquist rate.

---

[7] The discussion that follows assumes that sampling is periodic. That is, that the samples are equally spaced in time. It is possible to use a variable sampling interval, but the mathematics of the situation is very sticky indeed. It is unlikely that—outside of the most unusual and exotic circumstances—anything other than periodic sampling will ever be encountered.

The Frequency of the Signal

Suppose that we wish to analyze spectrographically a prolonged vowel by a young female patient. Her comfortable vocal F_0, we know from previous testing, is about 240 Hz. The first step, obviously, is to capture her production and save it as a computer file, using an A/D converter. What is the minimal sampling rate we can use?

At first glance, it might seem that, taking account of the Nyquist sampling theorem, we could sample at as little as 480 samples/s and still preserve all of the information in the original vocalization. But that ignores the fact that the vocal signal is rich in harmonics, and that it is the harmonics that define its waveshape. Furthermore, there may be a great deal of noise (for example, breathiness) in her voice, and we have to capture that, too, if we are going obtain a spectral analysis that will have any clinical use. A sampling rate of 480 samples/s will capture the F_0, but it will produce aliasing of all frequencies higher than that basal frequency. The resulting digital representation will contain a vast amount of erroneous information. In short, we need a much higher sampling rate—one which is at least twice the highest frequency *that is to be included* in the spectral analysis that is to be performed.

What frequency is that? How does one decide what the highest frequency of interest is? There are a couple of guidelines available. The easier one is "the highest frequency of interest is the highest frequency that the analysis ought to include." Spectral analyses, for example, traditionally extend to 8000 Hz. If that is the contemplated limit for the spectrogram's frequency scale, then—in principle—the signal to be analyzed should be sampled at 16,000 samples/s. If the spectrogram is to be limited to a display of up to only 4000 Hz, then sampling could be as slow as 8000 samples/s. On the other hand, if the spectrogram needs to extend to 16,000 Hz, the A/D converter needs to be set for no less than 32,000 samples/s.

The problem with the first guideline is that it may limit analysis options. It is not hard to imagine, for example, that a spectrogram with a 4000 Hz scale might show an interesting noise component extending from 3000 to 4000 Hz—the upper limit of the display. It would be useful to know to what upper frequency limit that noise component really extends. But if, in anticipation of an analysis only up to 4000 Hz, the voice signal had been sampled at only 8000 Hz, spectral analysis of higher frequencies would be impossible. Generally, for speech signals that are to be analyzed for spectral content, the sampling rate should not be less than 20K samples/s.

With respect to periodic physiologic (for example, airflow) signals, a good rule of thumb is that essentially all of the energy lies below the tenth harmonic. Therefore, if one has captured the tenth harmonic, one has probably preserved essentially all of the meaningful information in the original signal. Since (for a periodic signal) harmonics are integer multiples of the fundamental frequency, the highest frequency of interest for the patient in question is 2400 Hz, which is thus the Nyquist frequency. The *minimal* sampling rate (the Nyquist rate) then needs to be 4800 Hz. The word *minimal* is emphasized because real signals will include low levels of added noise—even after being "cleaned up"— and that noise is likely to raise the upper frequency limit of the signal. Therefore, one is advised to sample at a rate higher (perhaps by about 20%) than the Nyquist rate.

In summary,

- speech signals are best sampled at not less than 20K samples/s
- in *periodic* physiologic signals, the highest frequency of interest is usually $10F_0$, and thus the minimum sampling (Nyquist) rate is $20F_0$, plus a bit more for insurance.
- aperiodic signals, or signals that contain significant aperiodic components (such as turbulence noise) are almost certain to have significant high-frequency energy, and should (depending on the kinds of analysis to be done) be sampled at no less than 20K samples/s.

Anti-Aliasing Filtering

A moment's reflection shows that it is not enough to choose an apparently-adequate sampling rate. If the Nyquist frequency is the highest frequency that will be preserved in the digitized version of the signal, the implication is that frequencies higher than the Nyquist frequency will be aliased. That is, they will appear in the digitized version as lower, spurious frequencies. Therefore, the signal to be analyzed must be band limited; that is, it must have a known frequency limit. And the Nyquist frequency must, in fact, be the highest frequency in the signal that is to be digitized. To assure this most signals must be modified by a low-pass **"anti-aliasing filter"** before being processed by the A/D converter.

Ordinary low-pass filters are generally inadequate for anti-aliasing purposes. They usually have relatively gentle roll-off characteristics (see Chapter 2, "Analog Electronics"). A frequency component that is, for example, one octave higher than the filter's cutoff frequency may be attenuated by as little as 12 dB or so. That hardly qualifies as being eliminated from the signal. Therefore, anti-aliasing filters must have extremely steep roll-offs: they must come as close as possible to infinite attenuation of any frequency component in the signal that is even marginally greater than the cutoff frequency. In the real world perfection is not to be attained. And, for a variety of technical reasons, even coming close presents a significant challenge. Nonetheless, anti-aliasing filters that achieve a reasonable approximation to the ideal are commercially available at reasonable cost.

Except in very special circumstances, anti-alias filtering is essential to valid A/D conversion. Aliasing can distort the digital representation of a signal very badly indeed and, for all practical purposes, there is no way to correct the problem once it has occurred. An investment in good anti-aliasing filters is just as important as an investment in a good computer system.

OSCILLOSCOPES

An oscilloscope makes electrical waveforms and voltage conditions visible on a screen (Figure 4–24). It allows us to "see" speech signals and physiological variables, such as air flow rate, movement patterns, or pressures. It can also show stimulus characteristics and provide information on the calibration status of other instruments. Although it is almost a symbol of the research laboratory, the oscilloscope should also be considered an absolutely indispensable item of equipment for any clinician who routinely performs any kind of objective measurement. It will be used for checking the performance of almost every other electronic device, for obtaining basic measurements, and even for visual feedback to a patient during the course of therapy.

Basic Principles and Oscilloscope Design

CATHODE RAY TUBES

The heart of an oscilloscope is the *cathode ray tube* (CRT, Figure 4–25A), which looks very much like a TV picture tube, of which it is, in fact, the forerunner. The visual display appears on the front surface; the long neck contains most of the electronic elements. The tube is evacuated to a very high vacuum.

It has been known since the 19th century that electrons can be made to travel in straight lines in a vacuum if they are subjected to an accelerating force. The CRT elements that accomplish this are in the elec-

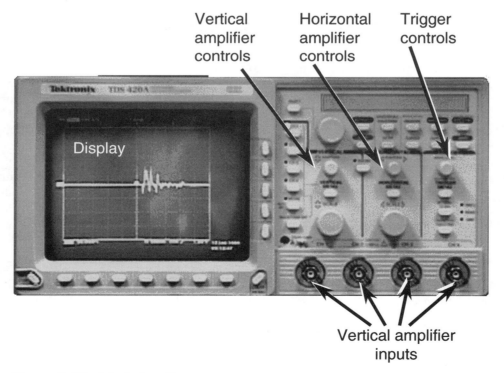

Figure 4–24. A typical oscilloscope.

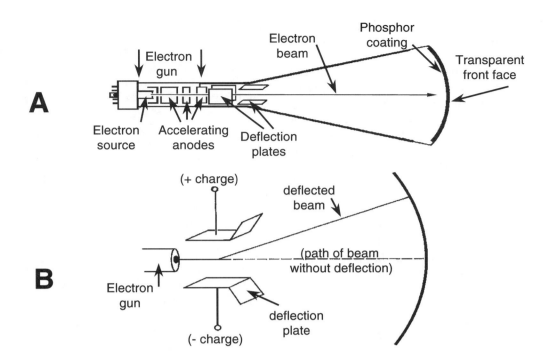

Figure 4–25. The cathode-ray tube (CRT). **A.** Internal organization. **B.** Generation and focusing of the electron beam. Deflection of the electron beam (dotted line) by the plates. Equal charge on opposing plates allows the beam to pass undeflected; positive charge on the upper plate deflects the beam upward. (From Figures 1–1, 1–2, and 1–3, pp. 3, 5, and 7. *Understanding oscilloscopes and display waveforms,* by K. W. Sessions and W. A. Fisher, 1978, New York: John Wiley and Sons, Inc. © 1978 John Wiley and Sons, Inc. Reprinted by permission.)

tron gun. Here, electrons are "boiled off" a metal surface that is kept very hot by a heater wire. A cloud of electrons forms near the heated plate. Electrons are negatively charged, implying that they will be repelled by other negatively-charged bodies and attracted to positively charged ones. The electron gun uses this fact. The metal plate from which the electrons are emitted is connected to the negative terminal of a voltage source, whose positive terminal is connected to a metal cylinder just in front of the emitting surface. The electrons are attracted out of the electron cloud toward and into the positively charged tube. The negative, or electron-producing, pole of the system is called a ***cathode***; the positive pole is the ***anode***. The stream of electrons drawn out of the electron cloud at the negative pole is therefore called a ***cathode ray***.

The speed at which the electrons move toward the anode is proportional to the voltage difference between the cathode and the anode. In the CRT very large voltages (perhaps 3000 V or more) are used.[8] The speed attained by the electrons will be so great that most of them will fly right on through the accelerating anode tube, to encounter and be stopped by a plate that closes its far end. The plate, however, does have a small hole in its center, and the path of a few of the electrons will carry them right through the hole and out of the electron gun. What has been created is a very thin beam (called a "pencil") of electrons traveling along the central axis of the CRT toward its face. Generally, the thin beam is made to pass through another anode at even higher voltage, to speed up the electrons still more. Along the path there will also be a special anode designed to compress the beam and to focus it. (Other control elements may be included in the gun assembly, but they need not concern us here.) The high-speed electrons now race the

---

[8] The oscilloscope is one of the few instruments in the clinical setting that uses genuinely high voltages. The implication is that, unless very certain of what they are doing, untrained personnel should not attempt internal adjustments of these devices. Servicing is best left to a qualified technician.

length of the tube until, if they are properly focused, they all crash into a single point on the inner surface of its flat screen.

Unfortunately, the human eye is not sensitive to electron radiation: we cannot see the electron beam. However, there are a number of substances that give off visible light when they are excited by electrons. The inside of the screen is coated with these *phosphors*, and the coating gives off light wherever the beam strikes it. The electron beam's impact is thus made visible.[9] The brightness of the phosphor's glow depends on the number of electrons striking it. A front-panel control on the oscilloscope allows the brightness level to be varied. Other controls adjust beam focus and astigmatism (directional inequality of focusing). A grid pattern, or *graticule*, etched onto a plastic covering or onto the glass of the screen itself, divides the usable screen area into squares on the order of 1 cm on a side for easy measurement of beam position.

The method by which the beam, and hence the spot of phosphorescent light, is moved around in conformity with an input signal also depends on the attraction of electrons to (relatively) positively-charged bodies. Figure 4–25B shows how deflection of the beam is achieved in most oscilloscopes. The speeding electrons pass between a pair of metal plates. If the two are at the same voltage the beam is unaffected. But if one of the plates is more positively charged than the other, the electrons will be attracted toward it. Therefore, as the electrons whiz by, they are diverted somewhat from their straight-line path and the beam as a whole is deflected a bit. The result is that the spot of light moves toward the edge of the screen that corresponds to the position of the positively charged plate. The more positive that plate is, the more strongly the electrons are attracted to it and the greater the deflection of the beam. If the charge on the plate is controlled by the input signal to the oscilloscope, the location of the spot of light on the screen will represent the signal voltage. Oscilloscopes have two pairs of **deflection plates**. The *vertical plates* are oriented horizontally and deflect the beam vertically; the *horizontal plates*, oriented vertically, control side-to-side positioning. Neither set of plates is connected directly the oscilloscope inputs, of course. Instead, they are controlled by amplifiers and other circuitry.

OSCILLOSCOPE ELECTRONICS

Oscilloscopes are available with a very wide range of features that are designed to facilitate different kinds of displays or signal analyses. Certain functions, however, are fundamental and are included in all oscilloscopes. Some oscilloscopes are "dedicated" instruments: They are designed to perform one task and are permanently adjusted to optimize for that task alone. (A television set is an extreme example of just such a specialized oscilloscope.) In these instruments there is relatively little the user need do beyond turning the instrument on. But most oscilloscopes are built to be as versatile as possible, which implies that adjustment and "tuning" of the instrument must be done by the user for each task. Doing this is not difficult if the oscilloscope's functional components are well understood. Therefore, this section will provide an introduction to the oscilloscope's functional blocks, those that are common to all oscilloscopes and a few that are optional but likely to be of special value to the speech clinician. Details of the specific electron circuits that perform the various functions will not be explored, but more information along these lines is available in many books at all levels of sophistication at most technical bookshops.

Basic Functional Units

Figure 4–26 shows the organization of a minimal, "barebones" oscilloscope. Controlling the CRT deflection plates are vertical and horizontal amplifiers, a sweep generator, and a trigger circuit.

Vertical and Horizontal Amplifiers

The basic function of the vertical and horizontal amplifiers is obvious: They modify the voltage of the input signal to a level that is adequate for the deflection plates (perhaps 25 V or so). In keeping with the objective of maximal versatility, the gain of these amplifiers can be varied by front-panel controls to accommodate inputs from just a few millivolts to over 100 V. (For very large signals the amplifier has fractional gain, and therefore acts as an attenuator.) Calibration of the amplifier is not in terms of gain, but rather is expressed as **sensitivity**—the input voltage required to deflect the beam 1 grid division on the screen's graticule. One

---

[9] The phosphor coating cannot tolerate heavy electron bombardment for very long. Light is not the only result of electron radiation: significant heat is also produced. If the beam is focused on a single spot for a long time, enough heat may be generated to burn away the phosphor, permanently damaging the CRT.

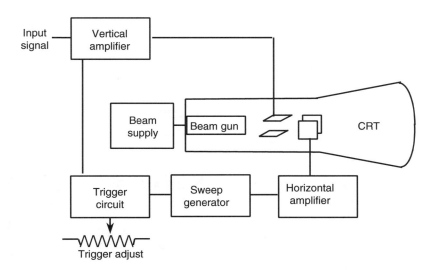

Figure 4–26. Organization of an oscilloscope.

gain setting of the amplifier, for example, might read "5 mV/division," indicating that the gain is set to cause the deflection plates to move the beam exactly 1 screen division for each 5 mV of signal strength. (If the screen is 10 divisions high—or wide—then a change in input up to 50 mV could be displayed.) Another setting might be labeled "1 V/div," another "5 V/div," and so on. Expressing the amplifier gain in this way makes the oscilloscope a kind of graphical voltmeter.

The input amplifiers are almost always of the DC-coupled type, meaning that they will amplify unchanging or extremely low frequency inputs. This is generally advantageous, since physiological signals, for instance, are very often quasi-DC. However, as mentioned previously, it is often desirable to eliminate a DC "bias" signal in order to be able maximally to boost a small AC component of interest riding on it. For example, in some types of dysphonia there is an uninterrupted flow of air during phonation, with only a small periodic fluctuation that represents the vocal signal. If a flow signal is being monitored on the oscilloscope most of the beam deflection will be produced by the constant flow (DC signal) with the phonation being shown as small ripples (AC signal) in the displayed trace. Amplification will enlarge the small AC ripple, but it will increase the DC level by an equal enlargement, perhaps driving the entire display off the screen. Here is a case in which elimination of the DC signal would make it easier to see the AC ripple that might of interest. To meet this need, the amplifier has a front-panel switch that allows the user to block DC and convert the circuit to an AC amplifier.

Usually the AC/DC amplifier switch has a third setting marked "ground." When the switch is in this position the amplifier input is disconnected from the front-panel connections and is instead connected to ground. The amplifier then has a 0 V input, and the position of the beam on the screen represents the zero baseline, from which voltages are measured. The baseline itself can be changed by means of a control marked "position" or "center" on the front panel. It changes the no-signal voltage relationship of the deflection plates.

Sweep Circuits (Time Base)

Although all oscilloscopes have vertical and horizontal amplifiers, most of the controls just described are provided only for the vertical one. While it is always possible to connect an external signal to it, the horizontal amplifier is really designed to handle internally generated voltages that will make the electron beam sweep from left to right at a known speed across the screen, establishing a *time base* for the display. If the beam is moving horizontally at a constant speed, then the horizontal axis of the screen is a *time* axis: Successive vertical deflections will occur further and further to the right in the display. The distance between any two points will be a measure of the amount of time that separates them. An oscilloscope whose vertical deflection is produced by an input signal and whose horizontal deflection represents a time base generates a graph of the input over time—a very useful form of data display.

The timebase is established by a circuit called a *sweep generator*, which is an oscillator that produces a "sawtooth wave" similar to the one in Figure 4–27. The voltage rises steadily from negative to positive, and then rapidly returns to the original negative level. If this voltage pattern is applied to one of the CRT's horizontal plates the beam will be deflected from left to right in a pattern that matches the waveform.

At the start of the cycle, the plate has a large negative charge, which deflects the beam maximally to the left. As the plate's charge becomes increasingly less negative, and ultimately more and more positive, the beam moves to the right. Since the charge on the deflection plate varies in a smooth and linear manner with time, the beam moves from left to right at a constant speed during the period of time, t_s, that the plate voltage is rising. At the end of the t_s interval the plate voltage drops rapidly to its original negative voltage. This interval is the *retrace period*, t_r, during which the beam will quickly return to its original, far-left, position. As the cycle repeats, the beam moves relatively slowly from left to right and then very quickly retraces its path back to the left, ready to sweep across the screen again. (Most oscilloscopes have a *blanking circuit* that dims the beam during the retrace portion of the cycles, so that the return stroke does not appear in the display.) While the beam is being moved across the screen the vertical input signal is also producing vertical beam deflection. Thus, the input voltage produces a graph of its magnitude over time.

In Figure 4–27 the rising portion of the sawtooth wave takes 100 ms, so this is the time required for the beam to cross the screen. If the graticule on the oscilloscope in question has, for example, ten divisions horizontally, the beam would traverse each division in 10 ms. The sweep time can be varied by changing the repetition rate of the sawtooth: the higher its frequency, the less time required for a complete transit of the beam from left to right and the less time each graticule-division on the screen will represent. The time-base control on the oscilloscope's front panel is calibrated in "sweep time per screen division": available settings commonly range from 1 μs/division to 5 s/division. The higher sweep speeds spread out vertical deflections so that closely spaced (that is, high frequency) events can be seen clearly. Very high sweep rates are of little use in clinical practice, since signals associated with speech production rarely have components exceeding a few thousand hertz. But increased time sensitivity is likely to be advantageous if the oscilloscope is also used for maintenance and adjustment of other clinical instruments.

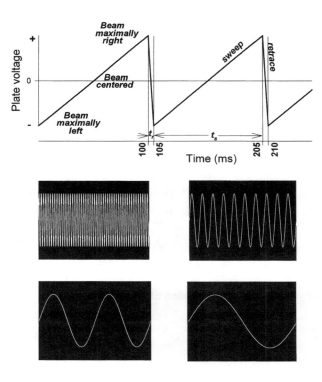

Figure 4–27. The time-base generator sweep signal.

Trigger Circuit

Although a usable oscilloscope could be built with only the functional elements discussed so far, the addition of another component will overcome one remaining inconvenience that results from the independence of the input and sweep signals. To appreciate the problem, consider the situation depicted in Figure 4–28. The sine-wave input (top) has a period just slightly longer than the time base sweep-retrace cycle (middle). Therefore, each sweep of the beam across the screen begins a bit earlier in the input wave's cycle than the previous sweep, with successive representations of the waveform as shown at the bottom of the figure. Because the sweep repetition rate is very high, the display takes on the characteristics of a motion picture, and the waveform seems to drift across the screen. Of course, this problem could be overcome by adjusting the sweep repetition rate to precisely match the frequency of the input signal, but such a solution has a number of inadequacies. Most signals that the speech clinician will want to see are not perfectly periodic—their repetition rate varies slightly from cycle to cycle. In order to get a stable display the sweep rate would have to be continually adjusted. Not only is this a practical

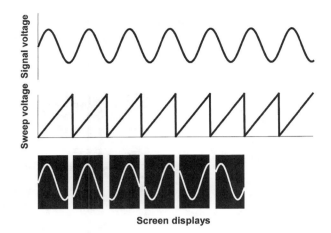

Screen displays

Figure 4–28. When the input signal and sweep signal are not synchronized, each sweep starts at a different point in the input wave. The result is a display that seems to drift across the screen. (From *Understanding oscilloscopes and display waveforms*, by K. W. Sessions and W. A. Fisher, 1978, Figure 2–14, p. 36, New York: John Wiley and Sons, Inc. © 1978 John Wiley and Sons, Inc. Reprinted by permission.)

impossibility but, even if it could be achieved, it would mean that the time axis of the display would be constantly changing, frustrating any attempt to derive time-based data. And even if these limitations were not objectionable, there would remain the problem of how nonrepetitive signals appear on the screen. If the sweep circuit is *free running*, an isolated event could appear at any point in the sweep. Thus, it might show up anywhere from left to right on the screen, and it might even run off the right edge. It would then be continued by the next sweep, meaning that it would "wrap around" to continue on the left edge of the screen.

The solution to all these problems is called a *trigger circuit*. A trigger is a pulse that initiates the function of another circuit. In the case of triggered oscilloscopes, the trigger generator produces a pulse that lets the sweep generator produce a single sawtooth wave. The trigger circuit itself can be controlled by an external signal that the user supplies (via a front-panel connection) so that the beam will be swept across the screen once every time an external pulse is delivered to the scope. This is useful for synchronizing the display to some external event. For instance, a pressure probe in the mouth, connected to appropriate interface circuitry, can cause the oscilloscope to trigger a sweep every time there is a pressure release for /p/, perhaps to show the sound pressure waveform (transduced by a microphone) applied to the vertical input.

The voice onset time for /p/ would then be easily determinable.

But there is an even more helpful, and more common, use to which the trigger circuit is put. In almost all oscilloscopes it can be set to monitor the vertical input signal itself and to produce a trigger pulse only when the amplitude and polarity of the input have certain values. In short, this means that the oscilloscope sweep can be started at the same point in each of a series of repetitive input waves, as shown in Figure 4–29. This holds the display stable on the screen. Note that the sweep rate (the speed of the beam's travel across the screen) is not altered by the trigger: each pulse allows one sweep at whatever speed has been preselected. The time base calibration remains valid. But each sweep starts at the same point in the waveform (which point depends on the front-panel, trigger-control setting) and, when sweeps are retriggered in rapid sequence, a steady display is perceived.

X-Y Display: Lissajous Figures

Almost all oscilloscopes allow the user to disable the sweep and to apply a signal directly to the X-axis circuitry. This allows one variable to be plotted as a function of the other. If both inputs are periodic (or nearly so) the result is a handy display called a *Lissajous figure* that can be of use for visual feedback in frequency- or amplitude-matching tasks. Figure 4–30 demonstrates how Lissajous figures can be generated and put to therapeutic use. In the case illustrated, the problem was to assist a patient in matching the F_0 of his phonation to that of a stimulus tone in order to obtain a voice range profile (see Chapter 6, "Vocal Fundamental Frequency"). The stimulus tone was produced by a tone generator that provided both triangle and sine waves. The triangle wave was used as the stimulus, while the sine wave (at the same frequency as the triangle wave) was applied to the X-axis (horizontal) input of the oscilloscope. The EGG waveform of the patient's phonation was fed to the oscilloscope's Y (vertical) input. When the F_0 of the patient's voice *exactly* matches that of the stimulus tone the Lissajous figure is a single loop. When the patient's F_0 is twice the stimulus frequency (that is, there is a one-octave frequency error), the Lissajous figure has two loops, showing that the X and Y input frequencies are in the ratio of 1 to 2. Finally, when the stimulus and phonatory F_0s are close (but not exactly equal) to each other a complex loop structure fills the screen. The visual information provides the tester with easily perceived information about the quality of the F_0 match, and the patient with guidance for controlling his or her vocal production.

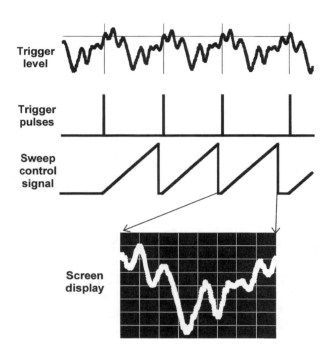

Figure 4–29. Action of the sweep triggering system. An input signal (top) is monitored by the trigger circuitry, which is set to react whenever the signal exceeds a user-set "trigger level" (represented by the thin horizontal line). The trigger circuit produces a pulse (second from top) whenever the trigger level is reached. The trigger pulses, in turn, turn on the sweep circuit, which generates a saw-tooth wave (third from top) of fixed characteristics. The oscilloscope beam is thus made to sweep from left to right at a steady and predetermined rate. The trace that would appear on the oscilloscope screen during the last of the sweep intervals is shown at the bottom.

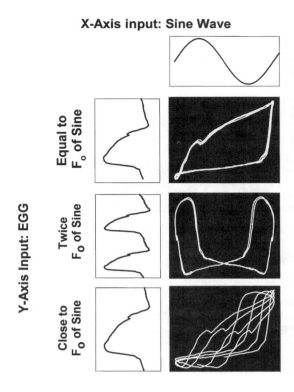

Figure 4–30. A sine wave, at the same frequency as a stimulus tone, is applied to the X-axis (horizontal) input of the oscilloscope, while an EGG waveform of a patient's phonation is applied to the oscilloscope's Y (vertical) input. When the patient's F_0 *exactly* matches that of the stimulus tone, the Lissajous figure appearing on the oscilloscope will form a single loop.

Special Oscilloscope Features

The utility of the ordinary oscilloscope can be greatly enhanced by a number of optional features that are offered by almost all manufacturers. Those that are most helpful to the speech clinician are considered here.

Dual Trace

Oscilloscopes are widely available that will allow two different input signals (such as the speech signal and oral airflow) to be shown on the screen at the same time. These *dual trace* or *dual channel* instruments use a single electron gun and one set of deflection plates that are shared by two separate vertical amplifiers. A switching circuit (called a *chopper*) alternately connects channel 1 and channel 2 to the deflection plates, so that a single beam is deflected for both of them. If each is associated with a different DC voltage (supplied by the oscilloscope circuitry) the segments representing channel 1 will appear at one level on the screen, and those representing channel 2 will appear at a different level.

Since a single deflection system is serving both signals, it is clear that both cannot be shown on the screen at exactly the same instant. Most dual-channel oscilloscopes offer a choice of methods for displaying the input signals in some sort of "time-sharing" fashion. In the *alternate* mode the chopper first connects channel 1 to the deflection plates for an entire sweep, and then connects channel 2 for the next sweep. The first-one-then-the-other pattern continues. When the sweep time is long, the user sees first the upper trace (channel 1) and then the lower one (channel 2). But for fast sweeps, persistence of phosphoresence and of vision combine to produce the *illusion* that both traces are on the screen at the same time. Therein lies a problem that grows more serious as the sweep time grows longer. It is possible that something of interest might happen on one channel while the other is being displayed. If the event is short enough it might be over by the time its channel is shown.

To counter this possibility a different form of alternation is provided. In the *chopped* mode the signals from the two channels are applied to the deflection plates for very brief periods in rapid succession during each sweep of the beam. The result is that a very short segment of the channel 1 signal is shown, then a very short segment of the channel 2 signal, and so on. Each trace is really a dashed line, with the dashes of one alternating with the dashes of the other. (Unless the sweep rate is extraordinarily high the individual dashes cannot be seen, and each line looks solid.) The two lines are, of course, separated on the screen by the different DC level applied to each to accomplish just that. In this mode not all of each trace is really present, but the pieces that are missing are extremely brief, and it is unlikely that any meaningful event will be missed—especially at the frequencies characteristic of speech events.

Display Storage

The trace on the oscilloscope screen is very temporary, lasting only as long as the phosphor continues to glow after it has been excited. In the case of the most popular phosphor, the glow persists only for about 30 ms. If the waveform being observed is repetitive or continuous (for example, a sustained speech sound) there is no problem. By the time one sweep's trace has disappeared another, identical, one is written. Imagine, for instance, that the therapist wants his client to see the noise component in her dysphonic voice. For this purpose the sweep rate of the oscilloscope can be quite fast, and there will always be a waveform to observe. Suppose, however, that the objective is to provide feedback of intraoral air pressure to a patient with velopharyngeal inadequacy. In this case the beam will have to move slowly across the screen (because speech events are relatively slow) and the patient has to observe the pattern of air pressure change during an entire utterance. There is no difficulty in getting the beam to sweep slowly, but since the phosphor only glows for a small fraction of a second no trace is produced. All that appears on the screen is a dot, moving up and down according to the air pressure, leaving no trail to show what the pattern of change has been. Transient events, such as a plosive, present a similar problem. Their trace is gone from the screen far too fast

for the clinician to clearly perceive, much less evaluate, them.

Storage oscilloscopes have modifications of the CRT which "freeze" a trace on the screen for a long period of time—typically, up to an hour. The effect is achieved by a special second screen inside the CRT made of a material that serves as a charge-storage device. The second screen is essentially analogous to a standard projection slide. It retains the pattern laid down by the original sweep of the CRT beam, and thereafter allows electrons (which are allowed to flood the inside of the tube) to pass to the viewing screen only in areas where the storage screen has previously been exposed. Thus, an image is projected on the display screen. Special electrical pulses can neutralize the storage screen, thereby erasing and preparing it for the next image.

A modification of the storage principle allows for *variable persistence* displays, in which the path that the beam has taken keeps glowing for an amount of time selected by the user. Slowly changing phenomena can be displayed with slow sweeps, and the trace persistence can be adjusted so that the trace remains visible for the duration of the entire sweep. The advantage of variable persistence over simple storage is that the display can be slow and *continuous* instead of intermittent, as with ordinary image storage.

Oscilloscope Cameras

A permanent record of the oscilloscope trace requires that the display be photographed. Special cameras make this fairly easy to do. Typically, such a camera has a hood that attaches to a mounting in front of the screen. The hood excludes ambient light and keeps the lens a fixed distance from the screen surface. (The camera is permanently focussed at this distance.) The back of the camera holds standard Polaroid™ film, providing instant copies of the trace at reasonable expense. Oscilloscope cameras are available for almost any type of instrument at very moderate cost. Although the need for them has lessened (because data can now also be easily stored in and displayed by computers and "hard copied" by the computer's printer), clinicians may find it convenient to have an oscilloscope camera on hand for making permanent records of oscilloscopic observations.

Digital Oscilloscopes

Digital oscilloscopes are not really oscilloscopes (in the traditional sense) at all. They are really very highly specialized microcomputers that, by using digital signal processing techniques, can perform all of the functions of their analog counterparts, and much more.

A typical digital oscilloscope can display several input channels simultaneously. Each can be sampled at very high rates (100 megasamples per second is a typical maximum) and converted to numeric values. These are then stored in memory and displayed on a screen using a format defined by the user. Because the system is really a computer, labels and informational text can be added to the screen display and because the data are resident in memory ("record lengths" of over 100,000 samples are commonly possible) they are available for any form of numeric analysis. Thus, the digital computer can show not only data traces, but, for example, the F_0 and rms amplitude associated with each can also be shown on the screen. Options are usually available for more advanced signal processing, such as Fourier analysis (see Chapter 7, "Sound Spectrography").

Beyond these capabilities, however, are two others that make the digital oscilloscope infinitely more useful than analog instruments. First, because data are stored to memory as they come in, it is possible to trigger the "sweep" when a defined event occurs, and to display not only the data following the trigger (as an analog oscilloscope would do), but to show the data *before* the trigger as well. Thus, data characteristics leading up to the triggering events—that would be lost in the case of an analog oscilloscope—can easily be explored. This capability can be of enormous value to the clinician. Suppose, for instance, that the vocal tract behavior of a stutterer is being evaluated. It is known, from previous observations, that stuttered events are characterized by plosive-like releases of high intraoral pressure. If the oscilloscope is displaying intraoral pressure, the trigger could be set to initiate a "sweep" only when the intraoral pressure dropped very rapidly (plosive release), and the display could show the pressure events for a short time before the sudden decrease. From the pressure record before the stuttered event it might well be possible to infer abnormal behaviors of the vocal tract that characterized the patient's dysfluent episodes. To be sure, the same observations might be possible by making a continuous record of the aerodynamics of the patient's speech and then searching out dysfluent events and analyzing the data record around them. But such an undertaking is time-consuming and tedious. The special capabilities of the digital oscilloscope isolate the events of interest and display the data most relevant to the clinician's assessment needs.

Second, because the digital oscilloscope is really a computer, it can communicate with other microcomputer systems. This is usually achieved via the medium of the GPIB (General Purpose Instrumentation Bus) interface, which is internationally standardized. (Software for implementing this function is provided by the oscilloscope's maker.) Through it the oscilloscope's operating and display characteristics can be modified by the microcomputer system to which it is attached, and, even more usefully, the data in the oscilloscope's memory can be transferred to the computer (or elsewhere!) for permanent storage (as on computer diskettes), more elaborate analysis, or specialized graphical display, and the screen display can be transferred for printing by an ordinary computer printer, thereby creating—more conveniently and less expensively than an oscilloscope camera—a permanent record of the observational data.

Digital oscilloscopes thus offer enormous advantages over the more "traditional" analog devices, and, almost always, are a better choice when deciding on the purchase of a new instrument.

REFERENCES

Barlow, S. M., Suing, G., Grossman, A., Bodmer, P., & Colbert, R. (1989). A high-speed data acquisition and protocol control system for vocal tract physiology. *Journal of Voice, 3,* 283–293.

Coughlin, R. F., Driscoll, F. F., & Driscoll, F. F. (1997). *Operational amplifiers and linear integrated circuits.* Englewood Cliffs, NJ: Prentice-Hall.

Franco, S. (1998). *Design with operational amplifiers and analog integrated circuits.* New York: McGraw-Hill.

Harford, E. R. (1980). The use of a miniature microphone in the ear canal for the verification of hearing aid performance. *Ear and Hearing, 1,* 329–337.

Harford, E. R. (1981). A new clinical technique for verification of hearing aid response. *Archives of Otolaryngology, 107,* 461–468.

Jamieson, D. G., Nearey, T. M., & Ramji, K. (1989). CSRE: A speech research environment. *Canadian Acoustics/Acoustique Canadienne, 17,* 236–25.

Koike, Y. (1973). Application of some acoustic measures for the evaluation of laryngeal dysfunction. *Studia Phonologica, 7,* 17–23.

Lyons, R. G. (1996). *Understanding digital signal processing.* New York: Addison-Wesley.

Orfanidis, S. J. (1995). *Introduction to signal processing.* Englewood Cliffs, NJ: Prentice-Hall.

Proakis, J. G., & Manolakis, D. G. (1996). *Digital signal processing: Principles, algorithms, and applications.* Englewood Cliffs, NJ: Prentice-Hall.

Rabiner, L. R., & Schafer, R. W. (1978). *Digital processing of speech signals.* Englewood Cliffs, NJ: Prentice-Hall.

Roark, R. M., Schaefer, S. D., Kondraske, G. V., Watson, B. C., Freeman, F. J., Butsch, R. W., & Dembowski, J. (1990). Systems architecture for quantification of dynamic myoelectric and kinematic activity of the human vocal tract. *Annals of Otology, Rhinology, and Laryngology, 99,* 902–910.

Rossiter, D., & Howard, D. M. (1996). ALBERT: A real-time visual feedback computer tool for professional vocal development. *Journal of Voice, 10,* 321–336.

Sessions, K. W., & Fischer, W. A. (1978). *Understanding oscilloscopes and display waveforms*. New York: John Wiley.

Snidecor, J. C., Rehman, I., & Washburn, D. D. (1959). Speech pickup by contact microphone at head and neck positions. *Journal of Speech and Hearing Research, 2*, 277–281.

Stout, D. F., & Kaufman, M. (1976). *Handbook of operational amplifier circuit design*. New York: McGraw-Hill.

Villchur, E. and Killion, M. C. (1975). Probe-tube microphone assembly. *Journal of the Acoustical Society of America, 57*, 238–240.

Walsh, V., Peyton, A. J., & Walsh, Y. (1993). *Analog electronics with op amps: A source book of practical circuits*. New York: Cambridge.

5

Speech Intensity

BACKGROUND
    Intensity and Intensity Level (IL)
    Sound Pressure Level (SPL)
    IL and SPL
INSTRUMENTATION
    Sound Level Meter
    Level Recorder
    VU Meters
INTENSITY MEASUREMENTS
    General Procedure
    Speech Intensity
    Vocal Intensity
    Amplitude Variability
REFERENCES

BACKGROUND

Sound is the perception of changes in air pressure. The variations to which the human is sensitive are very rapid and exceptionally small, but they are conceptually no different from the slow fluctuations in air pressure measured by a weather barometer. The "amount" of sound is referred to by the terms acoustic power, intensity, sound pressure, loudness, or volume. Although frequently used synonymously in casual discourse, these terms are not equivalent and cannot be interchanged in technical contexts.[1]

Acoustic power describes the amount of energy per second radiated by a sound source. Like other forms (such as electrical, steam, or mechanical) of power, acoustic power is measured in *watts*. (The acoustic power of speech, however, is millions of times less than the mechanical power of even a small household appliance.)

Intensity is the description of *power per unit area*. (The standard area is one square meter, m^2.) It differs from acoustic power in that sound is propagated as an ever-expanding sphere of energy with the source at its center. The further from the source, the greater the radius of the sphere. The surface area of a sphere is given by $A = 4\pi r^2$, so the surface area of a sphere of acoustic energy is proportional to the square of the distance from the source (the radius): $\pi \propto 1/d^2$. This is referred to as the *inverse square law*. Since, as one moves away from the sound source, the sphere is ever enlarging, the radiated sound energy is spread over a greater and greater area. And because the increase in area is proportional to the square of the radius, the sound power per unit area diminishes in proportion to the square of the distance. Therefore, intensity, *I*, is

$$I = P/(4\pi r^2),$$

where P is the total power emitted by the source. Intensity is almost always expressed not absolutely, but rather in comparison to some standard reference power. This relative measure (in dB) is called the *intensity level*.

Sound pressure refers to the average pressure (force of the moving air molecules acting on a unit surface area) of the sound wave. Like intensity, the sound pressure is almost never expressed directly, but rather is stated in relationship to a standard reference pressure, when the measurement is referred to as the *sound pressure level* (SPL).

Loudness is a *perceptual* attribute that cannot be measured instrumentally; it can only be assessed by a listener. The psychophysical scaling of loudness is very complex. In addition to the sound power, loudness is strongly influenced by the fundamental frequency and the spectral properties of the stimulus. Figure 5–1, taken from Fletcher (1934), shows this quite clearly: For all of the different tones considered loudness does not grow linearly with intensity, and different tones (human voice, violin, clarinet) are perceived to have different loudnesses at any given power level.

Volume is an undefined term, commonly used on audio amplifiers. It expresses in some unspecified way a relative "quantity" of sound. It is perhaps equivalent to the dynamical notation (*forte, fortissimo, piano,* and so on) used in musical scoring.

Intensity and Intensity Level (IL)

The *intensity* (I) of an acoustic signal is its *power* per unit area in watts (W). It turns out, however, that

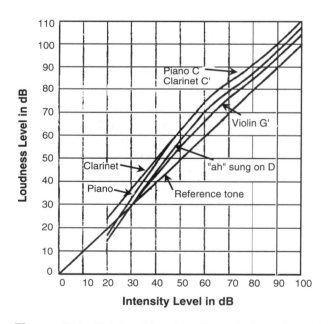

Figure 5–1. Relationship of loudness to intensity and timbre. (From "Loudness, Pitch, and the Timbre of Musical Tones and Their Relation to the Intensity, the Frequency, and the Overtone Structure," by H. Fletcher, 1934. *Journal of the Acoustical Society of America, 6,* 59–69. Reprinted by permission.)

---

[1] The basic theory of sound intensity and its measurement is concisely summarized in Gade (1982a, 1982b). A good introduction is also provided by Speaks (1996), Chapter 4. For an overview of speech intensity control see Titze (1994), Chapter 9.

using a simple power designation is inconvenient in a number of important ways. First, the human auditory system is sensitive to a vast range of acoustic power, from a barely audible 1×10^{-16} W/cm2 (0.0000000000000001 W/cm^2) to a very painful 1×10^{-3} W/cm^2 (0.001 W/cm^2). This is a range of about 1 to 10 trillion. Describing sound intensities in terms of power values would require the use of very cumbersome numbers indeed.

Second, the relationship between intensity and loudness is by no means a linear one (neither, of course, is the association between frequency and pitch). It was discovered long ago that all sensory perception tends to be exponentially related to stimulus magnitude. Loudness grows irregularly with intensity, and it is strongly influenced by frequency (Fletcher & Munson, 1933), but the underlying exponential relationship is well documented. It is more useful to have a measurement of sound intensity that grows in a way that parallels, at least crudely, increases in perceived loudness. Finally, we are usually interested in one sound only in terms of its relationship to another. For instance, in assessing hearing we are generally more concerned with how much greater the minimum power required for perception is than what the absolute power of the sound may be. On the productive side, to cite another example, we are often concerned with a speaker's intensity range, that is, with how great the spread is from minimal to maximal sound intensity.

The need for intensity *comparison* provides a useful starting point for exploring the standard scaling system that has been universally adopted. Suppose that a given speaker can phonate /ɑ/ at a minimal intensity of 3.5×10^{-9} W/cm^2 and at a maximum intensity of 1×10^{-7} W/cm^2. His vocal intensity range is therefore $(1 \times 10^{-7}$ W/cm$^2) - (3.5 \times 10^{-9}$ W/cm$^2)$, which is 9.65×10^{-8} W/cm^2 (or 0.0000000965 W/cm^2).

But this number is not only less than optimally useful, it is downright confusing. A better approach might be to generate a ratio of the speaker's two intensities. For the speaker in question, maximal intensity relative to minimal intensity would be expressed as $(3.5 \times 10^{-9}$ W/cm$^2 / 1 \times 10^{-7}$ W/cm$^2) = 28.57$. This is a more useful and comprehensible number, but the problems of the range over which such ratios might extend and the nonlinearity of loudness perception have not been dealt with.

To express the total possible range of intensities and, at the same time, to scale intensity in keeping with the underlying principle of nonlinear loudness growth, relative intensity is quantified as the ***logarithm*** of the ratio of one sound power (W_1) to a reference power (W_r). When the procedure is applied, the resultant measure is called the ***intensity level***—designated ***IL***. (The word *level* is an indicator of this sort of *relative* measure.) The unit of IL is the ***bel*** (B). In standard notation,

$$IL = \log 10 (W_1 / W_r). \tag{1}$$

For the example under consideration,

$$\begin{aligned} IL &= \log_{10} (3.5 \times 10^{-9} \text{ W/cm}^2 / 1 \times 10^{-7} \text{ W/cm}^2) \\ &= \log_{10} 28.57 \\ &= 1.46 \text{ bel.} \end{aligned}$$

In practice, it turns out that the bel is a little too coarse. The one-to-ten trillion range of normal hearing, for example, is covered by only 13 bels. Therefore, intensity level is more commonly expressed in tenths of a bel, or ***decibels*** (dB).[2] The decibel value is derived by multiplying bels by 10, and thus intensity level in dB equals

$$IL_{dB} = 10 \log_{10}(W_1 / W_r). \tag{2}$$

A few examples will serve to demonstrate some of the important characteristics of the decibel scale. Given that the threshold of hearing at 1 kHz is about 1×10^{-16} W/cm^2, what is the intensity level re: threshold of a stimulus having a power of 2×10^{-16} W/cm^2? We are comparing the power of a stimulus (W_1) to a threshold power of 1×10^{-16} W/cm^2 as the reference (W_r). Therefore,

$$\begin{aligned} IL_{dB} &= 10 \log_{10}(W_1 / W_r) \\ &= 10 \log_{10} (2 \times 10^{-16} / 1 \times 10^{-16}) \\ &= 10 \log_{10} 2 \\ &= 10 (.3010) \\ &= 3.01 \text{ dB.} \end{aligned}$$

Consider another case. A researcher measures the acoustic power of various phonemes, and determines that the average intensity of /m/ is 15 mW while /l/ has

---

[2] Following standard conventions, the "d," which symbolizes 1/10, is written in lower case; the unit symbol, "B," is upper case. The whole is a symbol, not an abbreviation, and therefore is not terminated with a period.

an average intensity of 7.5 mW. What is the intensity level of /m/ with respect to /l/? Clearly,

$$IL = 10 \log_{10} (\text{power}_{/m/} / \text{power}_{/l/})$$
$$= 10 \log_{10}(15 \text{ mW} / 7.5 \text{ mW})$$
$$= 10 \log_{10} 2$$
$$= 10 \, (.3010)$$
$$= 3.01 \text{ dB.}$$

Note that whenever the power doubles there is an increase in intensity level of just about 3 dB. (In general, we are willing to ignore the ".01" as too small to be meaningful.) It does not matter if the doubling is from 1×10^{-16} to 2×10^{-16} or from 7.5 mW to 15 mW: the IL increase will always be about 3 dB. Conversely, of course, halving the sound power results in a change of -3 dB.

It is important to understand that the addition (or loss) of 3 dB for a doubling (or halving) of the sound power works anywhere on the dB scale. The following example may help clarify this point. Suppose that a patient with a serious problem initially produces /m/ at an intensity of 3×10^{-9} W/cm². This vocal power is taken as a reference against which any therapeutic progress will be judged. After a couple of weeks of therapy the patient produces /m/ at 9×10^{-9} W/cm². The intensity level of this new /m/ with respect to his original /m/ is

$$IL_{\text{new }/m/} = 10 \log_{10} (W_{\text{new }/m/} / W_{\text{original }/m/})$$
$$= 10 \log_{10} (9 \times 10^{-9} / 3 \times 10^{-9})$$
$$= 10 \log_{10} 3$$
$$= 4.8 \text{ dB.}$$

After more therapy the patient manages to produce a maximally loud /m/ at 18×10^{-9} W /cm². What is the intensity of this better /m/ compared to the power of /m/ with which he entered therapy? By the same calculation:

$$IL = 10 \log_{10} (W_{\text{better }/m/} / W_{\text{original }/m/})$$
$$= 10 \log_{10} (18 \times 10^{-9} / 3 \times 10^{-9})$$
$$= 10 \log_{10} 6$$
$$= 7.8 \text{ dB.}$$

Note that the doubling of sound power (from 9 to 18 nanowatts) has moved the intensity level up 3 dB—from about 4.8 to 7.8 dB.

Summary: If a power of x represents intensity level y dB, then a power of $2x$ repre-sents an intensity level of $y + 3$ dB, and a power of $x/2$ is equal to an intensity level of -3 dB.

By a similar process we could show that a tenfold increase (or decrease) in power raises (or lowers) the intensity by 10 dB, since

$$IL = 10 \log_{10} (10 / 1) = 10(1) = 10.$$

Therefore:

If a power of x represents intensity level y dB, then a power of $10x$ represents $y + 10$ dB. A power of $x/10$ represents an intensity of $y - 10$ dB.

Intensity level, then, is a ratio of acoustic powers expressed on a logarithmic scale. By convention, unless otherwise stated, the reference level is assumed to be 1×10^{-12} W/m² (in the MKS system) or 1×10^{-16} watts/cm² (in the cgs system) which is approximately the threshold of normal hearing.

Sound Pressure Level (SPL)

In actual practice, sound intensities are usually measured in terms of sound pressures as transduced by a very precise microphone. These pressures are converted to electrical voltages that are conditioned by the measurement circuitry and output as dB. Now, it happens that sound intensity (I)

$$I = P^2 / Z_{\text{air}} \tag{3}$$

where P is pressure and Z_{air} represents the impedance of air as a transmission medium. Under ordinary circumstances the air's transmissive characteristics are constant. Therefore

$$I \propto P^2.$$

That is, intensity is directly proportional to the *square* of the sound pressure. If we let P^2 substitute for power, we can express intensity level in dB as

$$dB = 10 \log_{10} (W_1 / W_r) \tag{4}$$
$$= 10 \log_{10} (P_1^2 / P_r^2). \tag{5}$$

Recalling that

$$P_1^2 / P_r^2 = (P_1 / P_r)^2$$

and that

$$10 \log_{10} (P_1 / P_2)^2 = 2 (10 \log_{10}(P_1 / P_r)),$$

we have derived an expression for dB based on sound pressure:

$$dB_{SPL} = 20 \log_{10}(P_1 / P_r).$$

The sound pressure *level* (where the term "level" continues to signify a relative measure), denoted **SPL**, is a logarithmic transform of the ratio of two sound pressures.

Because the logarithm of the pressure ratio is multiplied by 20 (rather than by 10, as was the case for sound power) doubling a pressure raises the SPL by 6 dB (rather than by 3 dB). Similarly, increasing pressure by a factor of 10 increases SPL by 20 dB.

> **Summary: Doubling sound pressure raises SPL by 6 dB; halving sound pressure lowers SPL by 6 dB. Increasing pressure tenfold raises SPL by 20 dB; dividing pressure by 10 lowers SPL by 20 dB.**

The standard reference pressure for SPL, to be assumed if no other pressure reference is stated, is 20 micropascals (μPa), which, under specified standard conditions, is the pressure produced in air by a sound wave having a power of 1×10^{-12} W/m^2 (MKS) or 1×10^{-16} W/cm^2 (cgs). (This, incidentally, is equivalent to a pressure of 0.000000204 cmH$_2$O, which is a striking illustration of the sensitivity of the human auditory system.) Before the relatively recent acceptance of the MKS system as the norm for scientific reporting, the standard pressure was usually stated as 0.0002 dyne per square centimeter (d/cm^2). This is the same as 0.0002 microbar, a unit that also had some currency. All of these represent the same pressure, however, so the reference pressure has not changed despite the updating of the units used.

IL and SPL

The fact that doubling sound *power* raises IL by 3 dB but SPL by 6 dB often leads to significant, but needless, confusion. It is almost as if there are different dB scales for quantifying different sound signals.[3] This is simply not the case. Any acoustic signal can be measured in terms of either IL or SPL and the resultant dB values will be the same, assuming that equivalent power- or pressure-reference values have been used.

The confusion seems to stem from a failure to recall that power is proportional to the *square* of the pressure. Therefore, if pressure, P, is doubled (multiplied by 2), the power, W, is increased by 2^2, that is, by 4. So 2P = 4W in our equations. Therefore,

$$dB_{SPL} = 20 \log_{10}(2P / P) = 20 \log_{10}2$$
$$= 20 (.3010)$$
$$= 6.02 \ dB_{SPL},$$

and, equivalently,

$$dB_{IL} = 10 \log_{10}(4W / W) = 10 \log_{10}4$$
$$= 10(.6020)$$
$$= 6.02 \ dB_{IL}.$$

Conversely, pressure increases as the square root of the increase in power. So if the power of a signal doubles, the pressure must have been multiplied by $\sqrt{2} = 1.414$. Therefore

$$dB_{IL} = 10 \log_{10}(2W / W)$$
$$= 3.01 \ dB_{IL}$$

while

$$dB_{SPL} = 20 \log_{10}\sqrt{2P/P}$$
$$= 20 \log_{10} 1.414$$
$$= 20(.1505)$$
$$= 3.01 \ dB_{SPL}.$$

It is clear that, if a signal is increased or diminished in strength, its magnitude changes by the same number of dB on either the IL or SPL scales.

INSTRUMENTATION

Determination of sound pressure level is, at least in principle, a relatively easy and straightforward undertaking. It is only necessary to obtain a voltage proportional to the sound pressure and then to implement the necessary equations, either numerically with a computer or electronically with an appropriate analog circuit. The latter might seem a formidable task, but in

---

[3] A good example of the confusion is shown in the letter by Kallstrom (1976), and responses to it by Kramer (1977), Feth (1977), and Ward (1977).

practice it is not difficult. The block diagram of Figure 5–2 conceptualizes the requisite instrumentation.

The acoustic pressure is transduced to a voltage by a microphone. It should be obvious that the validity of the final SPL value depends very heavily on the accuracy of the initial sound pressure-to-voltage conversion, and therefore on the quality of the input transducer. For this reason SPL measurements are almost always done with a condenser microphone (see Chapter 4, "General-Purpose Tools"), since this type has the best linearity and stability. A precision low-noise amplifier boosts the microphone signal up to a usable level. The output of the amplifier is a voltage analog of the acoustic pressure.

Since it is the overall magnitude of the signal in which we are interested, rather than the size of a local maximum (or peak), the next step is to derive the root-mean-square (RMS) voltage of the waveform. This is accomplished by a special circuit whose output is proportional to the integral of the voltage. For the present purposes this can be considered to be a special "average" of the wave's amplitude. Because power is proportional to the square of the pressure (or, as in this case, of the equivalent voltage) the next circuit element multiplies the rms voltage by itself. A final set of circuit components derives the equivalent of the logarithm of the squared rms voltage, which represents R_{RMS}^2.

The process of comparing the signal to a reference pressure (in order to obtain sound pressure *level*) is neatly accomplished by adjusting all of the circuitry to produce an output reading of 0 whenever the reference signal is applied to the input. Once the instrument is

adjusted in this way the output will always indicate the number of dB above or below that reference. In fact, it is not even necessary to derive the logarithm of the pressure-squared signal. It is just as valid (and a lot easier) to mark the face of the output meter with a logarithmic, rather than a linear, scale. Commercially-available sound level devices often use just this strategy.

Fortunately, there is no need to construct one's own speech intensity instrument, since accurate and reliable devices have been readily available for a long time. While they are designed mainly for the engineer and the audiologist, they are very versatile and are likely to serve the needs of the speech pathologist quite well.

Sound Level Meter

The sound level meter (Figure 5–3) is a portable, self-contained precision instrument system for determination of the SPL. It consists of several specially-matched and sequentially arranged elements that transduce the acoustic signal and perform the necessary mathematical operations on the resultant voltages. The output is shown on a meter; no permanent record is generated by the instrument itself.

Input to the sound level meter is from a high-precision condenser microphone (see Chapter 4, "General-Purpose Tools"). An input amplifier boosts the microphone signal (which is only a few millivolts), and its output is fed to a variable attenuator that is adjusted by the user. The attenuator divides the voltage by an adjustable amount to ensure that the rest of the circuitry is not overwhelmed by too strong a signal. In so doing, it subtracts a certain number of decibels from the signal,[4] and the attenuator setting is therefore calibrated in dB.

Following the attenuator is a set of standardized filter networks that can be selected by the user. These adjust the relative amplitudes of frequency components in the input signal in different ways. The "A" scale (which is the most commonly used), for instance, weights component frequencies according to their approximate contributions to the perception of loudness. Intensities measured using the "A" weighting scale would be indicated in "dB(A)." Provision is also made for connecting external filters to the meter to allow the intensity evaluation of selected frequency

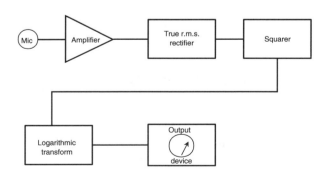

Figure 5–2. General scheme for measuring sound pressure level.

---

[4] Remember that the decibel is a logarithmic unit. Dividing one number by another is the same as subtracting the logarithm of one from the logarithm of the other. Therefore, to divide a number by some amount is to subtract a number of decibels from it.

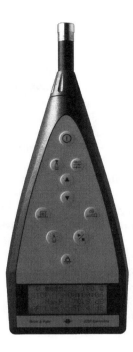

Figure 5–3. Sound level meters. (Courtesy of Bruel and Kjäer Instruments, Inc., Marlborough, MA.)

bands—for example, to include only a speaker's fundamental frequency. Finally, a special rectifying circuit produces an output proportional to the rms voltage (see Chapter 2, "Analog Electronics") of the filtered signal. This voltage drives a meter whose logarithmic scale runs from −10 to +10 dB.

For use, the sound level meter is first adjusted so that the meter reads 0 dB for a standard signal. This reference can be anything the user chooses—a 1 kHz sine wave at 0.0002 d/cm2, for instance, or a patient's phonation of /ɑ/—but until it is readjusted the meter will indicate dB re: this reference. The microphone is pointed at the sound source and the variable attenuator is adjusted so that the meter pointer is somewhere on the scale. The SPL of the signal is then equal to the attenuator setting plus the meter reading.

In many modern sound level meters the input signal is converted to numerical form by an analog-to-digital converter (see Chapters 3 and 4), and further processing is done by a microprocessor. This offers

numerous advantages: no attenuator settings are needed, intensity can be shown on a numeric display (usually to the nearest 0.1 dB), and the display can also show the maximum, minimum, and average SPL of a sample.

The sound level meter has the advantages of simplicity, ease of operation, and portability. But the inherently sluggish action of the display[5] and the absence of a graphic record of the data[6] make it best suited to the measurement of steady-state sounds, such as prolonged vowels.

Level Recorder

The sound level recorder, first described by Wente, Bedell, and Swartzel, (1935), produces a strip-chart record of sound pressure level. While it is an extremely versatile instrument whose characteristics can be adjusted to meet almost any intensity-measurement

[5] Determination of an rms amplitude inherently requires averaging signal strength over time. The *averaging time* involved, selectable by the user, is an important consideration in interpreting the output. It is discussed in the following discussion of sound level recorders.

[6] Note, however, that many sound level meters provide an output whose voltage is proportional to the SPL in dB. This output might, in turn, be fed to a computer or a graphic device to produce a permanent record.

need, it is not a complete system for sound measurement, nor is it self-contained or easily portable. It also requires more than minimal expertise and planning on the part of user. For these reasons, except for evaluating extremely long samples, most of its functions are probably more conveniently performed by a microcomputer. Still, sound level recorders are often available in settings where hearing research is performed, and thus may be readily accessible to the speech pathologist.

The function of the level recorder is quite different from that of the sound level meter. In order precisely to control the position of a pen on writing a strip chart, it contains what is technically known as an "automatic null balancing bridge." Because this application of cybernetic theory is an excellent example of important instrumentation principles, and because the validity of the data generated by the instrument depends quite heavily on the user's intelligent application of a basic understanding of how the instrument works, the operative principles of this device are worth exploring.

FUNCTIONAL ELEMENTS

The block diagram of Figure 5–4 shows the basic function units of a typical sound level recorder. Attenuation (set by a calibrated dial on the instrument by the user) is used to force the input signal to "fit" the analysis range of the instrument. (As in the case of the sound level meter, the user is subtracting a known number of dB from the input.) The attenuated signal is then amplified, rectified, and fed to a comparator, which is really the heart of the instrument. Here, the amplitude of the input is compared to a stable reference voltage. The comparator produces a voltage that is proportional to the *discrepancy* between the reference and the (attenuated) input. It Is known, therefore, as an *error*

voltage, and it is used to power a magnetic drive mechanism that moves a mechanical linkage to both the recording pen and the attenuator control. The error voltage thereby adjusts a yet another attenuating potentiometer and continues to do so until the (rectified) input to the comparator equals the reference voltage. When it does, of course, the error voltage disappears. If the input amplitude changes, the comparator will again see a difference between the reference and input, and the new error voltage that results causes the mechanical drive to readjust the potentiometer so that the input is again attenuated just enough to exactly match the internal reference voltage of the instrument. In short, the entire system functions automatically to maintain a *null balance* condition in which the error voltage is forced to zero.

The position of the potentiometer control is always proportional to the discrepancy between the input and the internal reference seen by the comparator. Since the pen is attached to the same mechanical linkage that controls the potentiometer, the record it produces on the strip-chart is an accurate reflection of this discrepancy over time, which is, in turn, a permanent record of the changes in sound intensity produced. Logarithmic scaling, which is needed for an output in dB, results from the fact that the potentiometer is itself designed with a logarithmic characteristic. That is, the position of the potentiometer's control rod and the degree of attenuation produced by that position are logarithmically related. Because of the pen–to–potentiometer linkage, this means that the pen's position on the paper is logarithmically related to the amplitude of the input signal. Hence, the written record has a dB scale, with linearly-spaced intervals. The setting of the (user-controlled) input potentiometer determines the baseline level to which the dB values of the strip-chart record are added.

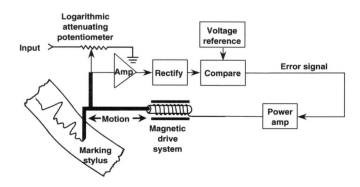

Figure 5–4. Simplified block diagram of the Bruel and Kjäer sound level recorder.

Averaging Time

There is one other feature of the level recorder (and indeed, of all intensity measurement systems, whether analog or digital) that must be understood if valid use of the instrument is to be made. This is the variable averaging time of the system, which is controlled primarily by the writing speed, a term which indicates the maximum speed at which the recording pen can move.[7] It is not hard to visualize the effect of writing speed on averaging time. Imagine an input signal, such as running speech, with very rapid changes in instantaneous amplitude. An oscillogram of such a signal is shown in Figure 5–5A. Now suppose that the SPL of the signal is analyzed with the level recorder set for a very high writing speed, perhaps 1000 mm/s, as in Figure 5–5B. The pen moves quickly enough to follow the peaks associated with the different syllables fairly accurately, and this readout has a strong resemblance to the oscillogram. Now suppose that the writing speed is reduced significantly, say to 500 mm/s. At this speed the pen cannot move quite fast enough to keep up with the rapid changes in the signal. Before it can get to the "target" position on the paper that actually represents the SPL of a peak, the event to which it is responding is over and the pen is being influenced by the level of the signal at a later point in time. Figure 5–5C shows that the peaks in the record are lowered and the troughs are raised because the pen is always responding to events over a moderately broad time interval. In fact, the write-out no longer represents the actual acoustic events, but rather a moving average of them over an averaging time of about 0.02 s. When the writing speed is lowered to an even slower 160 mm/s (Figure 5–5D) the pen is quite sluggish. Before it can fully respond to any given major change in SPL several other changes have taken place in the speech signal. At this writing speed its position at any one time represents an average of what has been going on in the past 0.075 s. At an extremely slow writing speed of 25 mm/s or so, all rapid fluctuations are lost in the written trace (Figure 5–5E). With an averaging time of about 0.5 s what is produced in an indication of the overall average SPL of the entire utterance.

The user must decide what averaging time best meets the measurement needs of the moment. If, for example, the intensity level of a given phoneme as it occurs in context is needed, then the averaging time will have to be sufficiently short (that is, writing time must be adequately fast) to capture a transient event.

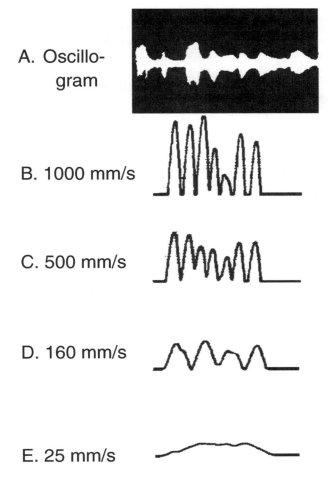

A. Oscillo-gram

B. 1000 mm/s

C. 500 mm/s

D. 160 mm/s

E. 25 mm/s

Figure 5–5. A. Oscillogram of the utterance "Joe took father's shoe bench out." **B—E.** Sound level recorder analysis at successively slower writing speeds.

But if the average SPL of, let's say, sustained /ɑ/ is wanted, a long averaging time that will smooth out minor intensity fluctuations is probably more useful. Then again, if the degree of *instability* of a patient's intensity is to be observed, a fast writing speed that will show small but relatively brief intensity variations is in order. There are few absolute and universal rules.

VU Meters

At least in theory almost any meter or chart recorder could be used to measure IL or SPL. If a standardized

---

[7] The exact relationship between writing speed and averaging time has been investigated by Broch and Wahrman (1961).

measure that is comparable to data gathered by others is needed, however, the acoustic signal will have to be conditioned as shown in the sound level meter. But if an "in-house" comparison of the intensity of two comparable samples is all that is required, then much simpler means are suitable. A clinician might, for instance, want to establish that a given intervention immediately results in increased speech intensity. For this, a simple pre–post comparison is adequate. Similarly, elaborate signal processing is rarely important in the provision of visual feedback of patient "loudness."[8] In short, in everyday clinical practice situations often arise in which an informal measure of intensity suffices quite well. In these circumstances the equipment to be found in most clinics can be pressed into service, provided that its limitations are clearly understood and respected.

Many recording devices—especially older ones—have a level indicator called a *VU meter* that is marked in decibels. "VU" stands for "volume unit," whose zero reference is a steady-state power of 1 mW into a circuit of 600 W impedance. The meter itself has certain specified dynamic characteristics. It was developed to provide a useful measure of the average power of music and speech signals that typically have very rapid and large sound pressure fluctuations.

The complexity of the relationship between dB VU and dB SPL makes conversion from one to the other impractical. The readings of VU meters are, however, comparable to each other if test conditions are the same and if the same trained observer reads the meter. Special procedures have been proposed to meet the need for high reliability (Levitt & Bricker, 1970; Brady, 1971). Therefore, while not the method of choice, VU meters can be used quite successfully in clinical practice, and even, with a little ingenuity, in some relatively simple in-the-field research (Fisichelli, Karelitz, Eichnauer, & Rosenfeld, 1961).

INTENSITY MEASUREMENTS

General Procedure

No matter the means by which intensity is to be evaluated, there are certain general procedural rules that must be observed. The choice of a microphone is very important, since much depends on the accuracy of the sound pressure-to-voltage conversion that it performs.

To the extent that the microphone response is not linear or deviates from acceptable flatness (see Chapter 4, "General-Purpose Tools") the final measures will be less that valid. For this reason, a condenser microphone should be used if at all possible. In its absence, the best quality microphone available should be selected. Microphone unidirectionality will help eliminate background noise.

Another fact that is often overlooked is the microphone amplifier, which might be part of a recording system if the speech sample is being saved for later evaluation. It is obvious that it must be a high-quality unit—a requirement met at very reasonable expense by equipment that is available commercially. Perhaps less apparent is the importance of matching the amplifier input characteristics to the microphone in order to preserve the fidelity and noise-free characteristics of the microphone signal. Some tape recorders have automatic level control circuits that adjust their gain to compensate for changes in signal strength. Such a circuit directly alters the intensity variable that is being evaluated, and so it must be turned off. Finally, it is very important that the amplifier never be overloaded by the signal. This means that some metering device should be available to check that the amplifier is functioning in its linear region over the entire range of sound intensities to be measured.

Special precautions must be taken to assure that the distance between the speaker's mouth and the microphone remains constant. The intensity of sound diminishes in proportion to the square of the distance from the source ($I \infty 1/d^2$). A relatively small change in position of the microphone can therefore have a significant effect on the intensity level. (Zaveri, 1971, presents a good summary of how to measure sound in a free field.) There are a number of common techniques that help assure mic–to–mouth constancy. A rod may be fixed to the microphone, its free end placed in contact with some stable area (perhaps the forehead) of the speaker's face. Alternatively, the speaker's head can be held against a stable support (such as the headrest of an examining chair) and the microphone set on a stand at a convenient distance in front of him or her. Typically, a mouth-to-microphone distance of about 30 cm is used.

If the microphone is sufficiently small it may be mounted on a short boom that is attached to a headband fitted on the patient. Such microphone headsets are widely available, and, if one is selective about the

---

[8]A simple device that provides an acoustic cue of excessive loudness has been described by Holbrook, Rolnick, and Bailey (1974).

quality of the microphone, the signals they provide can be just as useful as those derived from the larger microphones that have more typically been used (Winholtz & Titze, 1997a). Headband-mounted microphones eliminate the problem of variations in mouth-to-microphone distance caused by head movement, an advantage that is particularly important with children, who often cannot be induced to sit still. Headband-mounted microphones also have the advantage of being close to the mouth, maximizing the strength of the direct signal in relationship to the echoes in an inevitably reverberant environment and to extraneous noises.

Finally, there are extremely small but very accurate microphones (Villchur & Killion, 1975) that can simply be taped to the upper lip. These provide an excellent solution to the distance-variation problem. Although contact microphones might seem an obvious choice for intensity measurement, one can never be certain about how transmission through soft tissue—which is the route by which sound signals reach these microphones—influences sound amplitude (Horii, 1982), especially in situations involving speech, where F_0 changes.

CALIBRATED SPL MEASUREMENT

At first glance, it might appear that calibrating sound pressure measurements to a known reference is a fairly straightforward undertaking. In principle, one need only adjust the sound level meter to a signal of known intensity, emitted from a speaker in the same position that will be occupied by the test subject. If the sound level meter is set to read zero when the calibrating tone is produced all further readings will be in dB re: the calibrating tone.

In practice, however, a number of complications enter into the picture. First, when the test subject is producing the signals there are echoes from the face and body that add to the signal "heard" by the sound level meter. Then, too, the test room is usually somewhat reverberant, and the acoustic reflections can create standing waves in the environment. If, for instance, the sound level meter happens to be located where a standing wave peaks its readings will be inflated. Finally, almost all recording environments—frequently including sound-isolated rooms—are contaminated by low frequency sounds (traffic vibrations, machinery noises, and the like) that the meter includes in its reading.

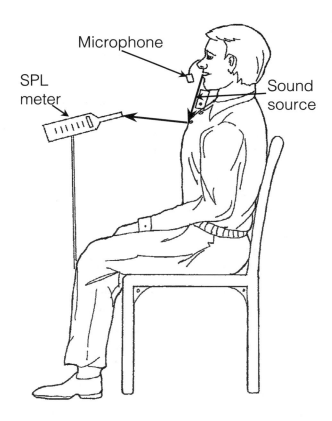

Figure 5–6. Arrangement of subject and instrumentation for calibrated sound level measurement. (From "Conversion of a Head-mounted Microphone Signal into Calibrated SPL Units," by W. S. Winholtz and I. R. Titze, 1997. *Journal of Voice, 11*, 417–421. Figure 1, p. 418. Used by permission.)

Winholtz and Titze (1997b) have proposed a relatively simple procedure, which requires subject positioning and instrumentation as shown in Figure 5–6, to compensate for these deleterious influences in order to obtain a much more valid estimate of speech sound pressure level. At some time during the session at which the speech sample is taken a sound generator capable of producing a stable sound is placed close to the patient's mouth and at least 1 second of its output is entered into the computer in exactly the same way that the speech sample is gathered. This calibrating sample provides a reference that is then used to correct the actual speech samples. After all the recordings have been done, the data from the calibration and speech

---

[9]If the data were sampled at, for example, 10,000 samples/s, then the rms value would be computed with a window size of 1,250 data points. (Window size = time constant × sampling rate.)

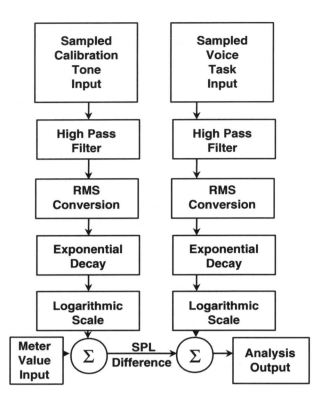

Figure 5–7. Data processing scheme for calibrated sound pressure level measurement. (Adapted from "Conversion of a Head-mounted Microphone Signal into Calibrated SPL Units," by S. Winholtz and I.R. Titze, 1997. *Journal of Voice*, *11*, 417–421. Figure 2, p. 419. Used by permission.)

samples are both processed according to the schema of Figure 5–7, which essentially is a digital implementation of the processing done by a sound level meter.

The data are first filtered with a linear phase high-pass filter having a cutoff frequency of 60 Hz and a roll-off of 24 dB/octave (see Chapter 2, "Analog Electronics"). The root-mean-square (rms) value of the signal is then determined using a time constant of 125 ms.[9] Then, in accordance with ANSI standards, the data are subjected to an exponential decay of no more than 0.5 s per dB. The resulting data are then converted to a $\log_{10}$ scale. The correction factor for the speech data is determined by taking the difference between the level of the reference signal and the calibration reference of the meter. This factor is then applied to the speech data to yield a final calibrated SPL reading.[10]

Speech Intensity

Because speech contains periods of silence, because intensity is varied for syllable and word stress (Fry, 1955; Lieberman, 1960), and because different phonemes are characterized by very different acoustic powers, the intensity level of connected speech shows very large fluctuations over short time intervals. The comparability of intensity levels of different samples of connected speech therefore depends very heavily on the type of averaging used (for example, peak or rms), the averaging time of the measurement system, and the utterances being spoken. Speech intensity also changes according to the communicative ambiance: one presumably speaks more loudly to an audience of 50 people than to a single interlocutor across the table. Interestingly, while interspeaker distance does affect speech intensity, the magnitude of the change is not nearly as large as might be imagined (Markel, Prebor, & Brandt, 1972; Johnson, Pick, Siegel, Cicciarelli, & Gerber, 1981). These considerations are important factors in deciding how to evaluate a speech sample.

ACOUSTIC POWER OF PHONEMES

As part of his investigations of the acoustics of speech, Fletcher (1953) considered the absolute and relative acoustic power of the phonemes of English. In presenting data derived by Sacia and Beck (1926), Fletcher warns that "although sixteen people were used in obtaining these data [on] sounds made in various combinations, they are still insufficient to give average values which can be said to be typical" (p. 83). Nonetheless, the findings of Table 5–1 do provide a firm idea of the general orders of magnitude of the radiated power of the phonemic components of the speech signal.

Fletcher (1953) also did an analysis of the *phonetic power* of phonemes. He based his measure on two psychophysical determinations of power. *Threshold scores* represent the amount of attenuation required to render a sound inaudible to the listener. *Articulation scores*, on the other hand, give the average degree of attenuation required to reduce the sound to a level at which it is misunderstood some arbitrary percentage of the total number of presentations. A combination of these measures has been derived to represent the *phonetic power*. These data, indexed to the weakest phone (/θ/ = 1) are given in Table 5–2.

---

[10] Program source code (in Fortran) is available from The Wilbur James Gould Voice Research Center, 1245 Champa Street, Denver CO 80204.

Table 5–1. Acoustic Power of Phonemes Measured at the Mouth

Phone	Average Power		Maximum Power	
	µWatt	dB re: /u/	µWatt	dB re: /u/
/u/	235	0.0	700	0.0
/ʊ/	470	3.01	890	1.04
/o/	435	2.67	1300	2.69
/ɔ/	615	4.18	1500	3.31
/ʌ/	450	2.82	1700	3.85
/ɑ/	700	4.74	1600	3.59
/æ/	650	4.42	1800	4.10
/ɛ/	500	3.28	1700	3.85
/e/	525	3.49	1700	3.85
/ɪ/	350	1.73	1300	2.69
/i/	310	1.20	1500	3.31
/m/	110	−3.30	200	−5.44
/n/	47	−6.99	70	−10.00
/ŋ/	97	−3.84	170	−6.15
/l/	130	−2.57	230	−4.83
/r/	200	−0.70	600	−0.67
/v/	25	−9.73	30	−13.68
/f/	3	−18.94	4	−22.43
/z/	30	−8.94	40	−12.43
/s/	30	−8.94	55	−11.05
/θ/	1	−23.71	1	−28.45
/ð/	9	−14.17	10	−18.45
/ʒ/	40	−7.69	55	−11.05
/ʃ/	110	−3.30	130	−7.31
/b/	7	−15.26	7	−20.00
/p/	6	−15.93	7	−20.00
/d/	4	−17.69	7	−20.00
/t/	16	−11.67	19	−15.66
/dʒ/	24	−9.91	36	−12.89
/tʃ/	52	−6.55	60	−10.67
/g/	8	−14.68	9	−18.91
/k/	6	−15.93	9	−18.91

Source: From *Speech and Hearing in Communication* by H. Fletcher, 1953, New York: Van Nostrand. Reprinted by permission. Decibel values have been calculated from the author's data, and do not appear in the original.

Table 5–2. Phonetic Power of Phonemes*

Phone	Relative Power	Phone	Relative Power
/ɔ/	680	/tʃ/	42
/ɑ/	600	/n/	36
/ʌ/	510	/dʒ/	23
/æ/	490	/ʒ/	20
/o/	470	/z/	16
/ʊ/	460	/s/	16
/e/	370	/t/	15
/ɛ/	350	/g/	15
/u/	310	/k/	13
/l/	260	/v/	12
/i/	220	/ð/	11
/r/	210	/b/	7
/l/	100	/d/	7
/ʃ/	80	/p/	6
/ŋ/	73	/f/	5
/m/	52	/θ/	Reference = 1

*Based on a combination of "threshold" and "articulation" scores. (See text.) Ratio of power of a given phone to that of the least powerful (= /θ/). "As produced by an average speaker."

Source: From Speech and Hearing in Communication. by H. Fletcher, 1953, New York: Van Nostrand. Reprinted by permission.

Tables 5–1 and 5–2 both show that the vowels are the most intense phonemes, but they are not equally powerful. The differences among them have been explored by Black (1949), by Fairbanks, House and Stevens (1950), and by Lehiste and Peterson (1959b). While specific intensity rank orders of the vowels differ somewhat among these several studies, all found that the intensities did, in fact, differ significantly. The important lesson for the clinician is that comparative measures must be based on the same utterance each time, even if the utterance is a monosyllable.

Within syllables the intensity of a phoneme is influenced by the context in which it is produced. This effect has been studied primarily for the syllables' vowel nuclei. Lehiste and Peterson (1959b) have determined that vowels are most strongly affected by neighboring semivowels and voiced plosives, next most strongly by glides, nasals, and voiced fricatives, and least strongly by voiceless fricatives and plosives. These findings generally support the earlier ones by House and Fairbanks (1953). Blood (1981) has examined the average SPL of 20 English vowels and diphthongs in the same CVC contexts used by Lehiste and Peterson (1959a). The average intensity of the (pooled) vowel nuclei is shown for different categories of surrounding consonants in Table 5–3. Very similar results were obtained by House and Fairbanks (1953).

Correlates of Phonemic Intensity

The intensity (or, perceptually, the loudness) of a phone is correlated to a number of variables. One of the clearest relationships is to intraoral pressure (P_{io}), as has been documented by Ringel, House, and Montgomery (1967), Malécot (1969), and Brown and McGlone (1974). Hixon, Minifie, and Tait (1967) have found that, for /s/ and /ʃ/ as produced by two speakers, SPL $\propto P_{io}^{1.2-1.4}$. Intraoral air pressure is itself correlated to speech effort (Hixon, 1966) or "force of articulation" (Malécot, 1966, 1969) and, therefore, it is not surprising that effort level is correlated to SPL. Leeper and Noll (1972) found that SPL for /t/ and /d/ increased logarithmically (power function = 0.56) with effort level on

Table 5–3. Average SPL of English Vowels in CVC Monosyllables.*

Consonant category**	Average SPL (dB)
Voicing:	
Voiced (13)	82.5
Voiceless (10)	78.8
Mode of Production:	
Plosive (6)	80.3
Fricative (8)	80.4
Affricate (2)	80.9
Glide (5)	81.5
Nasal (2)	82.7
Place of Production:	
Bilabial (5)	80.9
Labiodental (2)	81.8
Linguadental (2)	80.1
Alveolar (7)	81.6
Palatal (4)	80.3
Velar (2)	79.9
Glottal (1)	78.7

Source: From "The Interactions of Amplitude and Phonetic quality in Esophageal Speech," by G. Blood, 1981, *Journal of Speech and Hearing Research, 24* 308–312. © American Speech-Language-Hearing Association, Rockville, MD. Reprinted by permission.

*Three adult male speakers, 30-cm mouth-to-microphone distance. Utterance: "Say _____ again."

**Parenthetical data show number of consonants in each category.

a magnitude production task. It is possible, in fact, that the speaker's vocal effort plays a role in a listener's perception of loudness (Lehiste & Peterson, 1959b; Brandt, Ruder, & Shipp, 1969). Note also that changes in speech and singing SPL are also associated with alterations of vocal F_0, ventilatory movements, mean and instantaneous airflow, and vocal fold oscillatory movements (Sundberg, Titze, & Scherer, 1993; Holmberg, Hillman, Perkell, & Gress, 1994). These relationships are commonly different in adults and children (Stathopoulos & Sapienza, 1997).

The fact that measured sound pressure of the vowel during repetitions of /pɑ/ is not significantly affected by the presence of a face mask and oral pressure probe (Till, Jafari, Crumley, & Law-Till, 1992) suggests that valid assessment of the pressure/intensity relationship in the clinical setting (see Chapter 8, "Air Pressure") is entirely feasible. An estimate of normal sound pressure values measured with a pneumotachograph face mask in place is provided by Wilson and Leeper (1992), and is summarized in Table 5–4.

CONNECTED SPEECH

Speech intensity is significantly reduced in some speech and voice disorders, especially those involving CNS, laryngeal, or ventilatory pathology. Achieving adequate loudness is therefore a frequent therapeutic goal.

The intensity levels of connected speech are quite different from those of sustained phonations or of isolated monosyllables. The major cause of the difference lies in the significantly long pauses that are either physiologically required or linguistically prescribed in a complex utterance. To some extent they are bound to reduce

Table 5–4. Sound Pressure Level of /ɑ/ at Comfortable Pitch: Pneumotachograph Mask in Place*

Percentile of Intensity Range	Mean (and SD) dB SPL	
	Men	*Women*
25	65.6	69.3
	(3.2)	(8.1)
50	79	82
	(3.6)	(7.2)
75	92.2	94
	(4.3)	(6.9)

Source: From "Changes in Laryngeal Airway Resistance in Young Adult Men and Women as a Function of Vocal Sound Pressure Level and Syllable Context," by J. V. Wilson and H. A. Leeper, 1992, *Journal of Voice*, 6, 235–245.

*8 females, ages 22y 6m to 29y 8m (mean 25y 4m); 7 males, ages 23y 7m to 30y (mean 26y 1m)

15 cm mouth–microphone distance

Sound level meter, C (fast response) scale

Measured with subjects in pneumotachograph face mask.

the overall average intensity. Therefore, intensity measures of connected speech are probably best obtained together with an estimate of the proportion of the sample occupied by silent or quasi-silent intervals.

In the precomputer era, the task of isolating silent intervals was a daunting one. An ingenious electronic solution was proposed by Bricker (1965), who used a signal-driven electronic switch to toggle the output of a voltage-to-frequency converter to the input of an accumulator. (While the circuit he describes might seem very complex, it is, in fact, easily assembled from off-the-shelf integrated-circuit components.) Today, however, many of the microcomputer software systems marketed for speech analysis include some method for dealing with silent intervals. The problem is that the algorithm involved is frequently only poorly documented (if it is explained at all) by the vendor, with the result that the user is at a loss to evaluate critically the numeric results that result. It is impossible to know, therefore, whether data from one system are comparable to those from another, or whether, indeed, differences in the spoken material explain variations in measured intensity. The clinician thus needs to exercise extreme caution in interpreting computer-generated results.

Note also that, when measuring the range of speech intensities available to a speaker, the nature of the elicitation task and the instructions provided to the subject are likely to affect results significantly (Schmidt, Gelfer, & Andrews, 1990).

Expected Results

By and large, the data of Table 5–5 suggest that the SPL of connected speech lies in the general range of 70 dB. The mean SPLs reported in the literature obscure the normal sound pressure variations that are typical of running speech. Gelfer and Young (1997), however, examined the variability of their subjects' comfortable speech intensity (their means are included in Table 5–5) and found the mean SPL range associated with conversational-level reading of young adult subjects to be from 61.5 dB (SD = 3.1) to 80 dB (SD = 3.6) for men and from 60.4 dB (SD = 3.1) to 77.2 dB (SD = 2.8) for women. Recall, however, that communicative conditions—including personality traits of the speaker (Rekart & Begnal, 1989)—affect loudness and its physical correlate, intensity. Intuitively one expects more power from a speaker addressing an audience; less from a speaker in a one-to-one conversation. In the studies cited in Table 5–5, the speakers were asked to speak more or less naturally, as if to just a few people close by. Common experience suggests that a normal speaker's intensity will increase as the "audience" is perceived to be further away. The effect has been validated in a number of studies (Markel, Prebor, & Brandt, 1972; Johnson et al., 1981; Michael, Siegel, & Pick, 1995). Representative results (Healey, Jones, & Berky, 1997) when a speaker was asked to imagine a listener at given distances and when confronted with a

Table 5–5. SPL of Connected Speech: Normal Speakers, Reading

No./Sex	Mean Age	Material	Microphone Distance	dB Peak	dB Average	Source
10 M	21.3	Rainbow (2nd sent.)	12 in (30 cm)	73.65	71.36	f
10 F	21.3	Rainbow (2nd sent.)	12 in (30 cm)	68.70	67.14	f
20 M	24.5	Rainbow (2nd & 3rd sent)	12 in (30 cm)		70.4 (SD=3.10)	e
20 F	24.4	Rainbow (2nd & 3rd sent)	12 in (30 cm)		68.2 (SD=2.51)	e
1 F 7 M	23.2	Song lyrics	12 in (30 cm)	73.5	70.4	a
15	Adult	Rainbow (2nd sent.)	6 in (15 cm)		69.3	b
17 M	35–75	Rainbow (1st para)	8 in (20 cm)	78.5		c
7 M	40–65	Grandfather	6 in (15 cm)	79		d

Sources:

a. "Voicing Duration and Vocal SPL Changes Associated with Stuttering Reduction During Singing," by R. D. Colcord and M. R. Adams, 1979, *Journal of Speech and Hearing Research, 22,* 468–479.

b. "A Comparative Acoustic Analysis of Laryngeal Speech, Esophageal Speech, and Speech Production After Tracheoesophageal Puncture," by J. Robbins, H. B. Fisher, J. Logermann, J. Hillenbrand, and E. Blom, 1981, Paper presented at the annual convention of the American Speech and Hearing Association, Los Angeles, CA.

c. "Speech Characteristics of Patients with Parkinson's Disease. I. Intensity, Pitch, and Duration," by G. J. Canter, 1963, *Journal of Speech and Hearing Disorders, 28,* 221–229.

d. "An Experimental Study of Artificial Larynx and Esophageal Speech," by M. Hyman, 1955, *Journal of Speech and Hearing Disorders, 20,* 291–299.

e. "Comparisons of Intensity Measures and Their Stability in Male and Female Speakers," by M. P. Gelfer and S. R. Young, 1997, *Journal of Voice, 11,* 178–186.

f. "Superimposition of Speaking Voice Characteristics and Phonetograms in Untrained and Trained Vocal Groups," by S. N. Awan, 1993, *Journal of Voice, 7,* 30–37.

real listener at the same distances are summarized in Table 5–6. Note, however, that intensity changes observed in these studies do not compensate for the inverse-square decrease of sound power with distance, an effect that has been noted by others.

Vocal Disorder

Angerstein and Neuschaefer-Rube (1998) found that hyperfunctional voice disorder had little effect on the intensity of sustained vowels elicited at a loudness that was "comfortable for talking in everyday conversation." On the other hand, when individuals were asked to call "hello" as loudly as possible, a group of 72 male and female hyperfunctional dysphonics averaged only 99.5 dB(A) (SD = 10.3 dB), compared to 107.5 dB(A) (SD = 7.1 dB) for a comparable group of normal speakers. Furthermore, the decrease in the intensity of loudest speech was related to the severity of voice disorder.

The Effect of Delayed Auditory Feedback

It was recognized quite early that delayed auditory feedback (DAF) has a clear and consistent effect on speech intensity (Lee, 1950). Clinicians who use DAF as a diagnostic or treatment modality may find the data

Table 5–6. Mean (and SD) Speech Intensity in dB as a Function of Distance of Imaginary and Real Listeners.*

Distance	Men	Women
IMAGINARY LISTENER		
3 ft	69.0	65.8
0.9 m	(4.9)	(2.6)
15 ft	72.2	71.6
4.6 m	(4.3)	(1.4)
30 ft	77.6	76.2
9.2 m	(4.7)	(6.1)
REAL LISTENER		
3 ft	74.6	61.8
0.9 m	(8.0)	(2.1)
15 ft	78.5	72.8
4.6 m	(7.6)	(4.3)
30 ft	81.0	79.3
9.2 m	(7.4)	(4.7)

Source: "Effects of Perceived Listeners on Speakers' Vocal Intensity," by E. C. Healey, R. Jones, and R. Berky, 1997, *Journal of Voice*, 11, 67–73.

*12 men, age 20 to 52 y (mean 27.4 y); 12 women age 21 to 56 y (mean 30.5 y)

Mic–mouth distance 15 cm

Reading passage

Differences related to distance are significant, but there are also significant sex and real/imaginary interactions.

of Table 5–7 useful as a guide to interpreting a patient's response to this alteration of sidetone.

Alaryngeal Pseudophonation

Achieving adequate pseudovocal intensity is one of the specific objectives of the rehabilitation of the alaryngeal speaker. The intensity that can be produced will depend on many highly variable factors, including several, such as the type and extent of surgery performed, that are beyond the control of the therapist. In general, alaryngeal speakers will have noticeably lower SPLs (Blood, 1981), in large part because of the limited power supply (pressure in the esophageal reservoir)

driving the pseudoglottis (van den Berg & Moolenaar-Bijl, 1959; Snidecor & Isshiki, 1965; Diedrich, 1968). Table 5–8, which includes some findings for the Singer-Blom (1980) and Staffieri and Serafini (1976) modifications, can be used as a yardstick by which expectations may be scaled.

One note of caution is in order. Tracheostomized patients often produce significant "stoma noise." The microphone used for measurement of their vocal intensity should therefore be placed so as to maximize pickup of the oral signal and minimize the transduced level of the ventiatory turbulence. Furthermore, it should be remembered that the signal-to-noise ratio is a very important factor in alaryngeal speech (Horii & Weinberg, 1975).

Parkinson Disease

Reduced vocal loudness is a commonly-perceived feature of the speech of Parkinsonian patients (Logemann, Fisher, Boshes, & Blonsky, 1978). Illes, Metter, Hanson, and Iritani (1988) and Fox and Ramig (1997) have documented associated diminution of SPL compared to normal speakers, although earlier studies (Canter, 1963, 1965; Boshes 1966; Metter & Hanson, 1986) had not. Comparison of results is confounded in part by differences in test methodology. Although it has been shown that breathing and phonatory excercises can improve the vocal intensity of the Parkinson patient (Ramig, Bonitati, Lemi, & Horii, 1994; Ramig, Countryman, Thompson, & Hurii, 1995), it appears that the improvement is due not to an increase in subglottal pressure, but to better glottal function (Ramig & Dromey, 1996).

Vocal Intensity

Vocal intensity is dependent on the interaction of subglottal pressure (P_s), the biomechanics and aerodynamics at the level of the vocal folds, and the status of the vocal tract (Isshiki, 1964, 1965, 1969; Rubin, LeCover, & Vennard, 1967; Bernthal & Beukelman, 1977; for a general review see Titze, 1994, Chapter 9). Overall, sound power is roughly proportional to the cube of the subglottal pressure: $W \propto Ps^{3.18}$ (Tanaka & Gould, 1983) and to approximately the tenth power of the transglottal air flow ($W \propto Flow^{9.62}$). The range of powers at which voice can be produced is one indication of the limits of adjustment of the phonatory system and is therefore a potentially important measure in the assessment of vocal disorder (Michel & Wendahl, 1971; Hirano, 1989)

TABLE 5–7. Speech Intensity Increase Produced by Delayed Auditory Feedback.

Delay (seconds)	Mean SPL Increase (dB re: Simultaneous Feedback)			
	Adult		8 yr old	5 yr old
	(source a)	(source b)	(source b)	(source b)
0.0 (simultaneous)	0.0		0.0	0.0
0.03	2.4			
0.06	3.0			
0.09	5.2			
0.12	5.6			
0.15	5.7			
0.18	5.6			
0.21	5.7			
0.24	6.4			
0.25		5.4	7.71	6.1
0.27	6.9			
0.30	6.4			
0.375		4.7	6.0	5.6
0.500		4.0	8.0	3.9
0.625		4.1	5.8	4.5

Sources:

a. Adapted from "The Effect of Delayed Side-tone Upon Vocal Rate and Intensity," by J. W. Black, 1951, *Journal of Speech and Hearing Disorders, 16*, 56–60.

b. Adapted from "Delayed Auditory Feedback with Children," by G. M. Siegel, C. A. Fehst, S. R. Garber, and H. L. Pick, Jr., 1980, *Journal of Speech and Hearing Research, 23*, 802–813. 10 college undergraduates, 10 children age 7.1–8.8 y, 7 children 4.5–5.8 y, reading 30 simple sentences used by MacKay (1968). (Differences from simultaneous feedback have been computed from tabled data.) Differences due to age are not statistically significant.

VOCAL INTENSITY OF SUSTAINED VOWELS

When asked to prolong a vowel, the sound pressure level produced by normal speakers will vary as a function of the instructions given with respect to expected loudness and according to the pitch level used. Some slight variation in measured intensity of comfortably loud vowels may also be expected as a function of the vowel (Gelfer, Andrews, & Schmidt, 1991) because of acoustic phenomena in the vocal tract and because of changes in sound radiation patterns resulting from different lip openings. A sense of the variations to be expected is provided by the data of Tables 5–9 and 5–10. Note that, while many disorders result in a reduction of speech loudness, hearing impairment can cause comfortable vocal intensity to increase by a few decibels. Weatherley, Worrall, and Hickson (1997), for instance, found that older hearing impaired speakers sustained /ɑ/ at a mean of 72.6 dB, while their normal-hearing counterparts produced a significantly-different 70.4 dB.

MAXIMUM AND MINIMUM VOCAL INTENSITY: THE VOICE RANGE PROFILE (VRP)

Given the several interactions involved, it is not surprising that maximum and minimum vocal intensity vary with phonatory fundamental frequency (Finkelhor, Titze, & Durham, 1987; Gramming, 1988; Gramming, Sundberg, Ternström, Leanderson, & Perkins, 1988; Verdolini-Marston, Titze, & Druker, 1990; Titze, 1992b). Several studies have confirmed the tendency of both to increase as F_0 rises (Wolf & Sette, 1935; Wolf, Stanley, & Sette, 1935; Stout, 1938; Colton, 1973;

Table 5–8. Sound Pressure Level (SPL) of Speech of Alaryngeal Speakers

N	Mean Age	Material	Microphone Distance	SPL (dB)	Source
Esophageal					
15	48–80	Rainbow, 2nd sent.	15 cm	59.3	a,e
8	40–65	Grandfather, 1st sent.	6 in (15 cm)	73	b
22	36–81	Rainbow, 1st para.	12 in (30 cm)	62.4	d
10	61–67	Rainbow, 2nd sent.	30 cm	70	f
Singer-Blom					
15	53–65	Rainbow, 2nd sent.	15 cm	79.4	a,e
10	52–68	Rainbow, 2nd sent.	30 cm	82	f
Staffieri					
2	55–69	Rainbow, 1st para.	12 in (30 cm)	63.5	c

Sources: Adapted from:

a. "A Comparative Acoustic Analysis of Laryngeal Speech, Esophageal Speech, and Speech Production After Tracheoesophageal Puncture," by J. Robbins, H. B. Fisher, J. Logemann, J. Hillenbrand, and E. Blom, 1981, Paper presented at the annual convention of the American Speech and Hearing Association, Los Angeles, CA.

b. "An Experimental Study of Artificial Larynx and Esophageal Speech," by M. Hyman, 1955, *Journal of Speech and Hearing Disorders*, 20, 291–299.

c. "Acoustic characteristics of voice production after Staffieri's surgical reconstructive procedure," by J. Robbins, H. B. Fisher, and J. A. Logemann, 1982, *Journal of Speech and Hearing Disorders*, 47, 77–84.

d. "Relationship of Selected Acoustic Variables to Judgments of Esophageal Speech," by H. R. Hoops and J. D. Noll, 1969, *Journal of Communication Disorders*, 2, 1–13.

e. "A Comparative Acoustic Study of Normal, Esophageal, and Tracheoesophageal Speech Production," by J. Robbins, H. Fisher, E. Blom, and M. I. Singer, 1984, *Journal of Speech and Hearing Disorders*, 49, 202–210.

f. "Fundamental Frequency and Intensity Measurements in Laryngeal and Alaryngeal Speakers," by G. Blood, 1984, *Journal of Communication Disorders*, 17, 319–324.

Table 5–9. Mean (and SD) Sound Pressure Level (SPL) of Sustained Vowels by Normal Adults

Sex	No.	Frequency	Vowel	dB SPL
F	24	Comfortable	/i/	75.4 (4.4)
F	24	Comfortable	/a/	75.0 (4.5)
F	24	Comfortable	/u/	75.9 (4.5)

Source: "Effects of Prolonged Loud Reading on Selected Measures of Vocal Function in Trained and Untrained Singer," by M. P. Gelfer, M. L. Andrews, and C. P. Schmidt, 1991, *Journal of Voice*, 5, 158–167.

Coleman, Mabis, & Hinson, 1977). Stone and Krause (1980) have confirmed the effect on minimum vocal SPL and have shown that the increase with F_0 is approximately linear at a rate of between 7.5 and 12 dB/octave. It has also long been recognized that speakers raise their F_0 when asked to speak with greater effort (Black, 1961; Titze, Jiang, & Druker, 1988; Titze, 1989; Buekers & Kingma, 1997). (A simple instrumen-

Table 5–10. Sound Pressure Levels (SPL) of Sustained Vowels at Different Frequency and Intensity Levels in the Modal Register

Sex	F_o Level	Vowel	Intensity Level	dB SPL Mean (SD)	Source
M	25%	/a/	Minimal	66	a
			Comfortable	81	a
			Maximal	95	a
M	50%	/a/	Minimal	70	a
			Comfortable	84	a
			Maximal	101	a
M	75%	/a/	Minimal	72	a
			Comfortable	86	a
			Maximal	98	a
F	Comfortable	/i/	"relatively soft"	75.4 (4.4)	b
F	Comfortable	/ɑ/	"relatively soft"	75.0 (4.5)	b
F	Comfortable	/u/	"relatively soft"	75.9 (4.5)	b

a. "Vocal Intensity in the Modal and Loft Registers," by R. H. Colton, 1973, *Folia Phoniatrica, 25,* 62–70. 8 "young adult" males, vocally untrained. Frequency levels are percent of total phonational frequency range in the modal register. 9 inch ($\approx$ 23 cm) microphone-to-mouth distance. Compared to falsetto register and to trained singers.

b. "Effects of Prolonged Loud Reading on Selected Measures of Vocal Function in Trained and Untrained Singers," by M. P. Gelfer, M. L. Andrews, and C. P. Schmidt, 1991, *Journal of Voice, 5,* 158–167. 24 "Young adult" women without vocal training. 5 inch ($\approx$ 13 cm) microphone-to-mouth distance. Compared to performance after 1 hour of reading and to trained singers.

tation system to display vocal intensity as a function of vocal F_0 on an oscilloscope screen has been designed by Komiyama, Watanabe, Nishinow, and Yanai, 1977.)

The interrelationship of glottal adjustment and driving pressure underlies a graph showing a speaker's minimum and maximum measured phonatory intensity at frequencies that cover his F_0 range. Data plots of this type, introduced by Stout (1938) and explored early on by Calvet and Malhiac (1952) and Damsté (1970), have become very much more popular in recent years. An example is shown in Figure 5–8. A plot of this type has been referred to by several different names—including *fundamental frequency-sound pressure level profile* (Coleman, Mabis, & Hinson, 1977), *Stimmfeld* (Rauhut, Stürzbecher, Wagner, & Seidner, 1979; Klingholz & Martin, 1983; Klingholz, Martin, & Jolk, 1985; Seidner, Krüger, & Wernecke, 1985), *voice profile*

(Bloothooft, 1982), *phonogram* (Komiyama, Watanabe, & Ryu, 1984), and *phonetogram* (Damsté, 1970; Schutte & Seidner, 1983; Gramming & Sundberg, 1988). Those terms, for various reasons, have been felt to be less than optimal. In a report published in 1992, the Committee on Voice of the International Association of Logopedics and Phoniatrics recommended that they be replaced by the name *voice range profile* (VRP)—or its direct translation in other languages (Bless & Baken, 1992). That recommendation has been accepted for the discussion that follows.[11]

VRP Test Procedure

Despite its increasing popularity, there is effectively no standardization of either the method by which the data for the VRP are to be obtained or the manner in which

---

[11] An overall review of the voice range profile and various factors affecting is has been published by Gramming (1991).

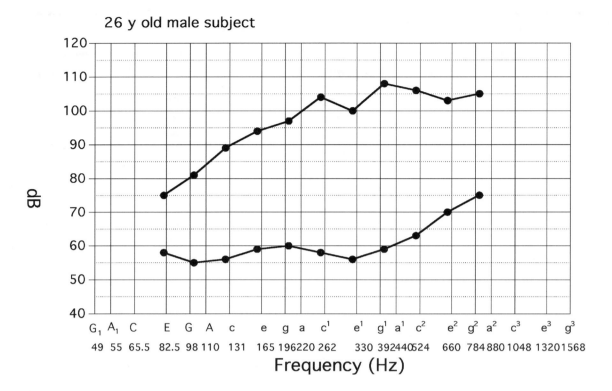

Figure 5–8. A typical voice range profile.

they are to be displayed. The literature thus presents a host of investigator-specific formats that, quite often, defy meaningful comparison in any but the broadest ways. The absence of consensus also means that the clinician is responsible for a number of crucial methodological decisions. In making them, however, the clinician is also free, within certain limits, to optimize the VRP to meet her preferred style of practice. It is also worth noting that automating the test procedure, using a computer and videotape presentation, produces quite acceptable results (Titze, Wong, Milder, Hensley, & Ramig, 1995).

There are, however, some elements of procedure that, while perhaps not universally agreed upon, approach what could be called "common usage" in obtaining VRPs:

Test setting. Although Schutte and Seidner (1983) recommend that testing be done in an acoustic envi-ronment that approximates a normal conversational setting, issues of noise and echoes are pertinent. A sound-isolated area (such as an audiometric test booth) is probably better, even if it proves to be some-what acoustically strange to the patient.

Mouth-to-microphone distance. The distance main-tained between the speaker's mouth and the micro-phone has varied widely—from as little as 3.8 cm (Stone, Bell, & Clack, 1978) to as much as 50 cm (Pabon & Plomp, 1988). The preferred distance, how-ever, seems to be approximately 30 cm.[12] On the other hand, headband-mounted microphones will necessar-ily be closer to the mouth, and a distance of approxi-mately 15 cm or less is more reasonable for them. Differences in measured intensity by the two methods can be resolved by application of the inverse square law. The vocal signal is not radiated uniformly in all directions, and early studies (Dunn & Farnsworth,

---

[12] The distance can be set and maintained by strapping a rod to a boom-mounted microphone, such that the tip of the rod extends 30 cm beyond the microphone. The apparatus is then positioned so that the rod just touches the patient's forehead or chin.

1939; Flanagan, 1960) suggest that the microphone should be positioned about 45° below the horizontal level of the mouth.

Stimulus tones. Stimulus tones are typically generated by a good-quality oscillator equipped with a "momentary on" switch. Triangle waves are probably the best choice for the stimulus waveform.

On the other hand, individual decisions will need to be made with respect to the following:

Vowel. The VRP is always based on a sustained vowel. Which vowel to use, however, remains an unresolved issue that may be of some import.[13] In particular, for acoustic reasons largely unrelated to the quality of glottal function, measured vocal intensity will be significantly greater for those productions for which the patient's F_0 lies at (or close to) a vowel formant frequency (Gramming & Sundberg, 1988). Schutte and Seidner (1983), writing on behalf of the Union of European Phoniatricians, recommend that the test vowels be /ɑ/, /i/, and /u/ and that the resulting data plots be color coded: /ɑ/—blue; /i/—red; /u/—green. On the basis of an experimental investigation of the issue, Gramming and Sundberg (1988) recommended the use of /ɑ/ because its relatively high first formant (F1) is likely, at least for male subjects, to lie outside of most of the vocal F_0 range. The lower F1s of /i/ and /u/, on the other hand, are likely especially to affect the lower (minimal intensity) boundary of the VRP. (Gauffin and Sundberg, 1980 have also noted that, at high vocal intensities, the strongest component of the signal may be a harmonic, rather than the fundamental, frequency.) "The ultimate goal of a clinical voice analysis is an efficient mapping of the physiology of *vocal fold vibration*. However, the relationship between the voice source and the SPL values shown in the [VRP] will be complicated as soon as the patient changes articulation" (Gramming, Gauffin, & Sundberg, 1986, p. 422; emphasis added). Unless articulatory influences are of interest—and they might be, particularly in singers—it is probably best to generate the VRP using only /ɑ/.

Stimulus frequencies. Although the VRP is intended to include phonations across the entire range of phonatory frequencies of which the patient is capable (but see the following section on vocal quality), pragmatic concerns demand that the vocal range be sampled at a limited number of frequencies. Intertest comparability requires that a general rule for selecting the test frequencies must therefore be established.

A common means of choosing the frequencies to be tested is to select equally-spaced frequencies in the patient's (previously determined) maximal phonational frequency range (MPFR).[14] If, as is usual, a 10% interval is chosen, there will thus be 11 stimulus frequencies—a reasonable number for everyday testing purposes. The question then arises about the meaning of "equally spaced." Two definitions are common. The simpler calculates the intervals in terms of absolute frequency. That is, if the patient's minimum and maximum F_0s are, for example, 75 Hz and 800 Hz respectively, then his maximum phonational frequency range of 725 Hz is divided into ten equal intervals of 72.5 Hz each. To generate the VRP he would be required to phonate at eleven frequencies: 75 Hz, 148 Hz, 220 Hz, and so on, up to 800 Hz. While this method offers the advantage of easy calculation of the stimulus frequencies, it does not take the generally-exponential nature of phonatory frequency control into account.

Better sampling is obtained by choosing the test frequencies in terms of semitones (see Chapter 6, "Vocal Fundamental Frequency"). Instead of dividing the patient's frequency range in hertz into equal intervals, the maximal phonational frequency range is expressed in semitones (ST) and then divided into an appropriate number of intervals. So, for the example just presented, the difference between 75 Hz and 800 Hz is 41 ST. If ten equal intervals are desired, they will each be 4.1 ST. The first sample frequency will be at minimal F_0 (75 Hz), the next 4.1 ST higher at 95 Hz, the third at 8.2 ST above 75 Hz, or at 120 Hz, the fourth at 12.3 ST above 75 Hz, or at 153 Hz, and so on to 800 Hz. In this way the spacing between the frequency samples is made logarithmic, with closer spacing at low frequencies and wider frequency intervals as one approaches the upper limits of the frequency range. Although the use of ST intervals involves somewhat greater computational effort, the extra requirements are easily met by a microcomputer or even a programmable hand calculator.

The "frequency resolution" of the VRP—the ability to discern closely-spaced changes along the frequency axis—is, of course, inversely related to the frequency-

---

[13] A fairly extensive examination of acoustic and physiologic factors that influence the VRP has been done by Titze (1992b).

[14] Note that there is a possibility that the measured maximal phonational frequency range may be influenced by factors of test method (Awan & Mueller, 1990; Reich, Frederickson, Mason, & Schlauch, 1990a, 1990b). See Chapter 6, "Vocal Fundamental Frequency".

sampling interval. A desire not to miss relatively small details (such as a fairly narrow notch) argues in favor of small frequency intervals and thus more test frequencies. But the exigencies of test efficiency urge wider intervals, fewer test frequencies, and a shorter test time. Clinicians will have to balance the opposing constraints according to their own best lights, but no fewer than ten frequency levels should be tested.

Intensity measurement. It is common to use a sound level meter to measure the intensity of the patient's vocal response. Two issues with respect to meter settings are relevant.

- The "A" weighting scale has commonly been used for VRP generation, but it discriminates against low frequencies, thus affecting readings at the lower end of the typical male range, especially at low phonatory intensities (Gramming & Sundberg, 1988). It is preferable to set the sound level meter for a flat response or to use "C" weighting (Coleman, Mabis, & Hinson, 1977; Coleman & Mott, 1978; Gramming, 1988, 1991; Pabon & Plomp, 1988).
- Fast meter response is important. At the extremes of vocal function phonation may be sustainable for only short periods of time. Accurate readings of intensity demand that the meter respond fast enough to have reached a final value before phonation ceases.

Vocal quality. It is common to limit the voice range profile to either the speaking or singing voice. In general, the esthetic quality of the vowel produced is not at issue. Hacki (1988, 1993, 1996) has made a case for the value of comparing the voice range profiles of a speaker's singing, speaking, and *shouting* productions. He has demonstrated, for instance, that the voice range profile of the speaking voice tends to be located in the lower frequency region of that of the singing voice, that intensity levels of the two are similar, and that the lower frequency boundary of the shouted voice tends to occur near the modal-falsetto register transition. It is his feeling that "irregularities in the relationship of voice range profiles of different voice modalities are evidence of voice disorders" (Hacki, 1996, p. 128).

Validity and reliability. To be useful, both from the research and from the clinical perspectives, steps must be taken to assure that the VRP is both valid (that is, that it measures what it purports to) and reliable (that is, that successive tests will yield at least closely com-

parable results).

- F_0 precision of patient productions. The most common way of eliciting phonations requires that the patient match the pitch of a stimulus tone. Unfortunately, many subjects (especially those without significant musical training) perform poorly at pitch-matching tasks. Errors ranging from several semitones to an entire octave are common (Schutte, 1980b, Chapter 2; Weiner, Lee, Cataland, & Stemple, 1996). The vowel intensities that the patient produces are usually plotted along the frequency axis at the *stimulus* frequency. The validity of doing this obviously depends on the accuracy of the patient's match to the stimulus frequency. Various methods, including visual feedback (Neuschaefer-Rube, 1997) can improve the accuracy of the patient's production, but no method can be relied on to assure precision matches. There must be some means for evaluating matching accuracy.
- Most commonly—and perhaps unfortunately—the accuracy of the frequency match is vouched for by the "trained ear" of the tester. The problem is that the ears of many (and perhaps most) clinicians are not nearly as trained or accurate as might be wished. Furthermore, the "trained ear" of the clinician is judging pitch, while the data axis is one of frequency. The two are not the same, and several well-known principles of psychoacoustics suggest that judgment errors are likely to be common. Assurance of test validity would therefore encourage instrumental assessment of the stimulus-response F_0 match. If specialized equipment is not available to do this, at least two easily-implemented techniques are available. Both are best accomplished using the EGG, rather than a microphone, signal,[15] whose utility for this purpose may be enhanced, where possible, by appropriate band-pass filtering.

The F_0 of the EGG signal can be measured directly by a frequency meter. (Digital oscilloscopes can usually measure F_0 as well.)

The EGG signal and the stimulus tone can be applied to the X and Y axes of an oscilloscope to generate a Lissajous figure (see Chapter 4, "General-Purpose Tools"). When the Lissajous figure has a *single* loop (irrespective of loop shape), the EGG and stimulus tones have the same F_0. (Judging the magnitude of the frequency mismatch will

---

[15] It must be recognized, however, that the EGG signal becomes very weak, and thus increasingly unreliable, at minimal vocal intensities. Low vocal intensity is also a problem for all other measurement methods, however.

require some familiarity—most easily gained by experience—with Lissajous figures.)

The objective is a frequency mismatch of no more than about 2–3%. Achieving this may require that the tester do some vocal training, for which the F_0 measurement system may be pressed into service. Alternatively, of course, the patient's response—if not too far from the intended frequency—might be plotted at its appropriate location along the frequency axis, rather than at the location of the stimulus frequency.

Vocal quality and duration. Although the subject has received some attention (Schutte, 1980b) there is no general agreement about the perceptual "quality" of phonations that may be accepted for VRP recording and, in fact, specifications in the literature tend to be very broad and general.[16] Schutte (1980b, p. 17) for instance, requires that the sample "not sound hoarse or breathy, or contain some other deviating quality" although this restriction cannot easily be imposed when testing a dysphonic patient. The question of vocal register (which, in the case of VRPs, is almost always perceptually defined) is also not formally resolved. In general, there is at least tacit agreement that both modal- and loft (falsetto)-register phonations are to be included, but that pulse (fry)-register phonations are not.

The presence of vibrato—which involves not only a controlled frequency variation but an associated intensity change as well—is a common feature of the musically trained voice. (Untrained subjects may produce uncontrolled vibrato-like modulations.) In the musical voice, vibrato may involve anywhere from 3 to perhaps 12 variations per second (Gemelli, Sacerdote, & Bellussi, 1954), although a rate betweem 4 and 7 per second seems more likely (Luchsinger & Arnold, 1965; Campbell & Michel, 1979; Shipp, Leanderson, & Sundberg 1979; Shipp, 1980). The extent of F_0 modulation may range from 0.5 to 2 ST (Winckel, 1953; Pommez, 1962; Mason & Zemlin, 1966; Shipp, Sundberg, & Doherty, 1988). Vibrato characteristics are apparently not consistently influenced by the baseline F_0 or intensity of phonation (Michel & Grashel, 1980; Shipp, Doherty, & Hakes, 1989). They may, however, be related to spectral characteristics of the vowel (Horii & Hata, 1988). The associated intensity change is generally in the range of 2 or 3 dB (Coleman, 1979;

Large, 1979; Shipp, Leanderson, & Sundberg, 1979, 1980). Clearly, vibrato introduces a complication in interpreting the VRP, which is, at least in part, founded on the assumption of a steady-state prolongation of a vowel. Unless the objective is specifically to assess selected aspects of the singing voice, it is best discouraged.

Minimal intensity. There is a general sense that reliable reproduction of minimal intensity is more difficult than reliable reproduction of maximal intensity. Stone and his coworkers have evaluated the reliability of measures of minimum SPL. They have found (Stone & Krause, 1980; Stone & Ferch, 1982) that subjects tended to come within 3 dB or their original mean measurements when retested after 1 day and after 13 days. (The perceptual insignificance of such a small difference is underscored by the fact that a perceived doubling of loudness requires an intensity increase on the order of 10 dB (Steinberg & Gardner, 1937). Generally, then, it is likely that testing of minimum vocal intensity is a reliable procedure.

Duration. Most investigators would agree that phonations need to be sustained for at least two seconds in order to be considered acceptable for the VRP.

Plotting the data. The shape and "smoothness" of the VRP is often at least as important to clinicians as the actual numerical values represented. Decisions about graph dimensions and axes may radically alter the appearance of the VRP. The geometric alterations effected by modification of the axes may easily engender varying interpretations of the data represented.

There is, unfortunately, no standard for plotting the VRP test data and, in fact, the style of VRP plots in the literature varies dramatically. The Union of European Phoniatricians (Schutte & Seidner, 1983) has recommended that the VRP's sound pressure scale (Y-axis) range from 40 to 120 dB(A)—with 10 dB occupying 15 mm of axis length. The frequency scale (X-axis) under this standard extends from 49 to 1568 Hz (five octaves, from G_1 to g^3), and 1 octave represented by a constant distance of 36 mm along the axis, implying a logarithmic scale. Gramming and her colleagues (Gramming, Gauffin, & Sundberg, 1986; Gramming & Åkerlund, 1988; Gramming & Sundberg, 1988; Gramming et al., 1988) have published VRPs in which the frequency (X) axis is either decile increments of the vocal range or vocal F_0 on a logarithmic scale. Pabon and Plomp (1988), Sulter, Wit, Schutte, and Miller (1994), and

---

[16] An automated VRP generator described by Pabon and Plomp (1988) includes selected vocal quality parameters in the data plot.

other producers of computer-automated VRPs (see below) use axes that are idiosyncratic, but perhaps optimized to the computer methodology involved.

The vertical axis of the VRP is always dB; the clinician need decide only the axis range. The horizontal, or frequency, axis is more problematic. Common options, and the resulting VRP geometry are illustrated in Figure 5–9. (VRPs on the left are for a typical male; those on the right for an average female.) Note how the plotting option selected influences the overall impression of the data. Clinicians should decide which representation is most consonant with their approach to evaluation of vocal capabilities and best meets the needs of their style of practice.

Automatic Generation of the VRP

Several computerized systems have been developed to automate the generation of the voice range profile. They offer convenience and greatly reduced testing time. The data they plot, however, are different in some important ways from those derived when testing is done "by hand." Specifically, computer systems generally work by marking a VRP form (which is likely to be different in style from those produced by other testers) at the F_0–dB locus of each cycle of the patient's phonation. The result is a "cloud" of markings, the limits of which, in principle, define the boundaries of the patient's VRP. The problem is that, especially for dysphonic individuals, there may be just a few cycles—in a burst or scattered throughout the trial—whose F_0 or intensity significantly exceeds the average for the phonation being measured. When these are marked on the VRP plot they extend the margins of the VRP, suggesting a greater range than is actually the case. (The problem is obviated when using a frequency intensity meter by the time-averaging that is built into these measuring systems.) Different software producers handle this situation in different ways. The clinician will need to take this situation into account when interpreting the VRPs that computerized systems generate.

VRP Measurement Method

While there is no standardized method for obtaining VRP data, Coleman (1993) has provided a moderately detailed description of a method that has proven successful in a large clinical practice. The recommendations that follow are based on his suggestions.

1. During a warm-up session the examiner demonstrates phonation at extremes of frequency and intensity, and the patient practices producing vowels of different frequency and intensity and musical

scales with both discrete and glissando tones. In addition to preparing the patient, this session also allows the examiner to assess the patient's ability to match tones, generate a maximal effort, and the like.

2. The patient's maximal phonational frequency range is then determined. Beginning at a comfortable pitch, the patient is instructed to produce ever lower pitches, first in discrete steps and then glissando. The reliability of this minimal F_0 is assessed by having the patient produce a vowel at it several times. The same procedure, but with ascending pitches, is used to determine the patient's maximal phonatory F_0.

The vowels produced need not be—and probably will not be—of acceptable quality from a musical point of view. The object of the test is to determine the frequency range of *any* phonation—what has sometimes been called the "physiological" range. If musical quality is at issue (as it may be in testing singers), the range may be retested with this restriction.

3. Stimulus frequencies are then selected according to the sampling system preferred by the examiner. Sample frequencies at intervals of one tenth of the frequency range (for a total of 11 test frequencies) are common, but a smaller interval may be desirable. (Steps larger than 1/10 of the F_0 range are not recommended.) Depending on examination objectives or tester predilection, intervals may be selected linearly (that is, in terms of a fraction of the *frequency* range) or logarithmically (in terms of the *semitone* range). The examples below show how this is done for 10% intervals.

- **Linear (frequency-based) intervals**: The patient's minimal F_0 is subtracted from his maximal F_0 to derive the maximum phonational frequency range. This value is then divided by ten to determine the frequency width (ΔF_0) of each interval. The sample frequencies are then minimal F_0, minimal $F_0 + \Delta F0$, minimal $F_0 + 2\Delta F_0$, minimal $F_0 + 3\Delta F_0$, ... minimal $F_0 + 10\Delta F_0$.

- **Logarithmic (semitone-scaled) intervals**: Maximal and minimal vocal F_0s are each converted to semitones (re: 16.35 Hz, see Chapter 6, "Vocal Fundamental Frequency"). The difference (in semitones) between the two is the maximal semitone range. This is then divided by 10 to determine the width (ΔST) of each 10% interval. The test stimuli in semitones will then be minimal ST, minimal ST + ΔST, minimal ST + 2ΔST, minimal ST + 3ΔST, ... minimal ST +

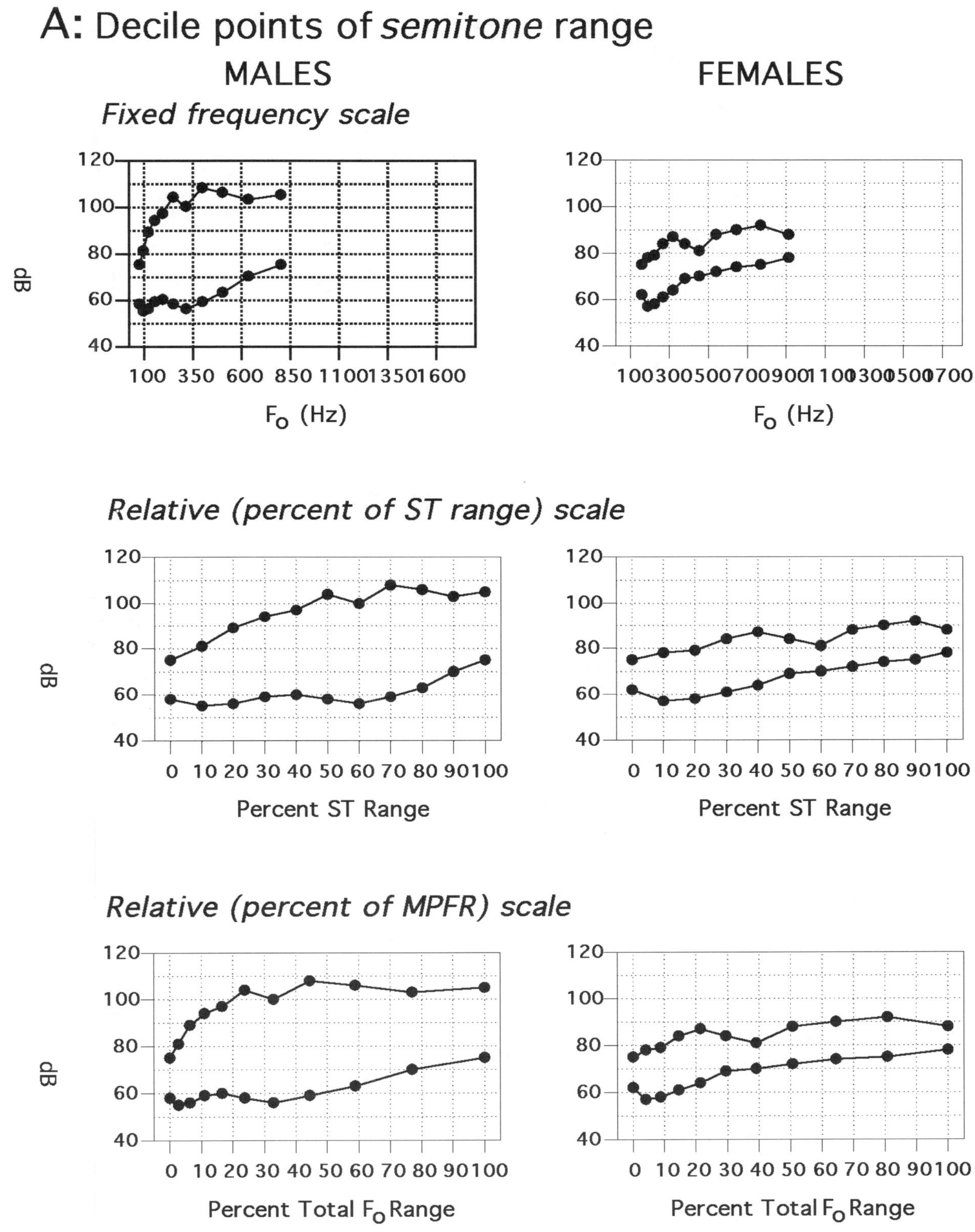

A: Decile points of *semitone* range

MALES

Fixed frequency scale

dB

100 350 600 850 1100 1350 1600

F_O (Hz)

FEMALES

100 300 500 700 900 1100 300 500 700

F_O (Hz)

Relative (percent of ST range) scale

dB

0 10 20 30 40 50 60 70 80 90 100

Percent ST Range

0 10 20 30 40 50 60 70 80 90 100

Percent ST Range

Relative (percent of MPFR) scale

dB

0 10 20 30 40 50 60 70 80 90 100

Percent Total F_O Range

0 10 20 30 40 50 60 70 80 90 100

Percent Total F_O Range

Figure 5–9. The effect of different plotting methods on the VRPs of men and women. **A.** Using decile points of the semi-tone phonational range.

B: Decile points of frequency range (MPFR)

MALES   FEMALES

Fixed frequency scale, LINEAR

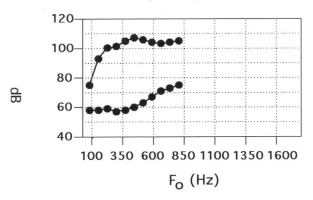
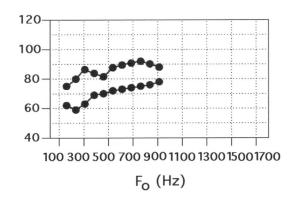

Fixed frequency scale, LOGARITHMIC

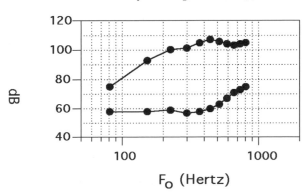
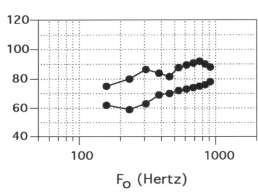

Relative (percent of MPFR) scale

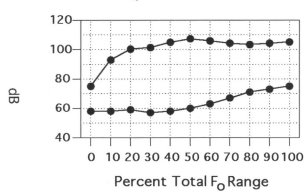
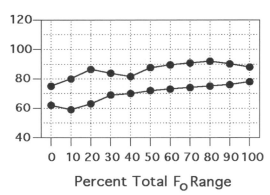

Figure 5–9 (continued). B. Using decile points of the maximum phonational frequency range.

$10\Delta ST$. Finally, the several semitone levels are converted back to frequencies.

4. Maximum and minimum vocal intensities are then determined at each of the stimulus frequencies. The first measurement is made at a frequency close to the center of the patient's vocal frequency range. The stimulus-generator is tuned to the appropriate frequency to produce a stimulus at about 75 dB SPL which the patient is asked to match. When an appropriate pitch match is attained the stimulus tone is turned off while the patient continues to phonate. The unaccompanied vowel production provides the VRP data.

At each frequency the patient is first asked to produce the softest tone he can, and then the loudest tone possible without straying from the target frequency. After the initial recording near midrange the lower levels of the pitch range are tested, and then, finally, the higher levels.

It is important to test both intensity limits several times at each frequency, since there may be significant inter-trial variability. Also, repeated trials over the course of the day may show an improvement in intensity limits (Sihvo & Sala, 1996).

5. Productions are acceptable if:

- the error of the patient's match to the stimulus frequency is no greater than about 3%;
- Minimum and maximum intensities on repeated trials differ by no more than 3 dB. Additional trials may have to be made until this criterion is met;
- The vowel is sustained for at least 3 seconds;
- Intensity limits at neighboring 10% frequency levels differ from each other by no more than 6 dB. A greater difference requires retesting of the frequencies in question to assure validity.

Expected Results

In general, intensity data are most widely available for the modal (chest) and loft (falsetto) vocal registers.

Intensity as a Function of F_0

Coleman, Mabis, and Hinson (1977) tested young men and women at 10% intervals of their maximum phonational frequency range. Sound pressure level (re: 0.0002 d/cm^2 was measured at 6 inches (15.24 cm) from the lips by a sound level meter set for a "fast" response. The data are summarized in Table 5–11. What the summary of values obscures, however, is the very

real difference in performance at different F_0 levels. Plots of the experimental data (Figure 5–10) show that both minimum and maximum SPL do indeed tend to increase as F_0 rises, and that the SPL range is greatly restricted at the extreme frequency levels. At the upper end of the range this might be due, at least in part, to the use of loft (falsetto) register, in which the intensity range is known to be smaller than in the modal (chest) register (Colton, 1973).

Greater detail is provided by Sulter, Schutte, and Miller (1995), who tested a large enough number of subjects that their data might tentatively be considered normative. A summary of these data is given in Table 5–12; plotting these data (Figure 5–11) provides a tentatively normative VRP shape.

Children

A number of studies demonstrate the possibility of successfully generating the VRP of relatively young children (Pedersen, Munk, Bennet, and Müller, 1983; Pedersen, Müller, Krabbe, Munk, Bennet, & Kitzing, 1984; Klingholz, Martin, & Jolk, 1985; Klingholz, Jolk, & Martin, 1989). McAllister, Sederholm, Sundberg, and Gramming (1994) suggest that an important difference between the VRPs of adults and children is the latter's compression along the dB axis, representing the somewhat more restricted intensity range of the children's voices. Böhme and Stuchlik (1995) have measured the VRP of 67 girls and 45 boys in the age range of 7 to 10

Table 5–11. Maximum, Minimum, and Range of Vocal Sound Pressure Level (SPL) in dB re: 0.0002 d/cm^2*

Measurement	*Men*	*Women*
Mean maximum SPL	117	113
Mean minimum SPL	58	55
Mean SPL range (at a single F_0)	54.8	51
Lowest single SPL	51	48
Greatest single SPL	126	122

Source: From "Fundamental Frequency—Sound—Pressure Level Profiles of Adult Male and Female Voices," by R. F. Coleman, J. H. Mabis, and J. K. Hinson, 1977, *Journal of Speech and Hearing Research*, *20*, 197–204. © American Speech-Language-Hearing Association, Rockville MD. Used by permission.

*Method: 10 men, age 21–.4 y; 12 women, age 20–39 y. Vowel sustained for at least 2 s; 10% intervals of F_0 range; 6" mouth-mic distance; means of 2 trials > 48 hours apart.

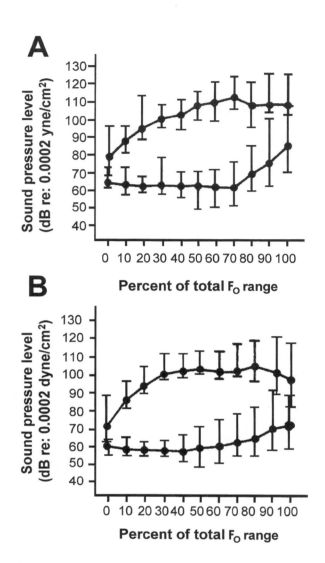

Figure 5–10. Range of sound pressure level as a function of fundamental frequency level for (A) men and (B) women. (From "Fundamental Frequency—Sound Pressure Level Profiles of Adult Male and Female Voices," by R. F. Coleman, J. H. Mabis, and J. K. Hinson, 1977, *Journal of Speech and Hearing Research, 20,* 97–204. © American Speech-Language-Hearing Association, Rockville, MD. Reprinted by permission.)

years, with results that are illustrated in Figures 5–12 and 5–13.

The Effect of Training

If the voice range profile depicts something real about the physiological capabilities of the larynx, and if vocal training has a beneficial effect on vocal function, one would expect that the area of the voice range profile

would expand as a result of vocal exercises. Whether this is so has been explored by Sulter, Schutte, and Miller (1995), who examined comparable groups of vocally-trained and -untrained men and women. A comparison of the (averaged) results at 10% intervals of the maximal phonational frequency range for the two sex groups is illustrated in Figure 5–14. Significant (p < .05) effects include a downward extension of the minimal frequency level and of the "soft" intensity contour at all frequencies below the 90th percentile. Awan (1991), however, using somewhat more restrictive acceptance criteria, found that the effect of (singing) training was to increase maximal intensity at frequencies above the zero percentile level and to decrease the minimal intensity at frequencies greater than the 20th percentile level. Gramming et al. (1988) found great inconsistency in the voice-range-profile differences between trained and untrained male speakers, while Åkerlund, Gramming, and Sundberg (1992) present voice range profiles for women that show an apparent improvement in both maximal and minimal intensity levels—associated with much greater subglottal pressure (Åkerlund and Gramming, 1994)—in trained speakers compared to their untrained counterparts. It is clear that, on the whole, vocal training is associated with an improvement in voice range profile, but not dramatically so, and with a consistency that has yet to be established.

In contrast to group effects, the change in an individual's voice range profile produced by voice training was assessed by Sulter and Meijer (1996), who examined a group of 25 young women (mean age = 18.4 years) before and after 2 1/2 years of several types of voice training (Coblenzer & Muhar, 1965, 1976; Veldkamp, 1965; Eldar, 1976; Smith, 1980; Pahn & Pahn, 1986). Results are illustrated in Figure 5–15. Although the subjects' frequency range showed no increase, the changes in both the maximum and minimum intensity contours are significant.

Measurement Variability

Vocal intensity does not remain absolutely stable, even over the short interval during which the intensity measurement is done. Gramming, Sundberg, and Åkerlund (1991) explored the extent to which SPL varies while a vowel is sustained by the speaker for VRP measurement. The *short term variation* that they observed in normal untrained speakers and in patients with "non-organic" dysphonia is summarized in Table 5–13. They also examined the variability over several test sessions, remeasuring the VRP of 1 normal male and 1 normal female 15 times over a 3-week period, with results that are tabulated in Table 5–14.

Table 5–12. Maximum and Minimum Vocal Intensities of Untrained Subjects at 10% Semitone-levels of the Maximum Phonational Frequency Range*

F_o Level (%)	FEMALES			MALES		
	Mean F_o (Hz)	Maximum Intensity (dB)	Minimum Intensity (dB)	Mean F_o (Hz)	Maximum Intensity (dB)	Minimum Intensity (dB)
0	157.3 (21.4)	63.1 (10.5)	53.9 (6.9)	86.1 (14.0)	59.2 (10.2)	52.0 (7.7)
10	192.6 (23.4)	82.4 (6.7)	51.4 (6.5)	107.1 (16.1)	77.2 (6.7)	46.9 (6.0)
20	235.9 (26.2)	90.0 (5.2)	53.4 (6.6)	133.3 (18.9)	85.7 (4.8)	46.6 (5.7)
30	289.3 (30.6)	94.5 (5.03)	56.1 (6.5)	166.0 (23.0)	90.7 (4.7)	48.7 (5.2)
40	354.7 (37.9)	97.4 (5.6)	58.4 (6.3)	206.9 (29.2)	94.8 (5.0)	52.0 (5.7)
50	435.2 (49.5)	97.3 (6.4)	61.0 (6.7)	258.1 (38.4)	97.9 (5.4)	56.9 (6.2)
60	534.5 (67.2)	97.5 (5.7)	65.2 (7.4)	322.0 (51.7)	100.3 (5.6)	61.5 (7.2)
70	656.9 (93.1)	99.6 (5.5)	70.6 (7.7)	401.9 (71.0)	98.0 (5.9)	65.3 (8.1)
80	807.8 (129.6)	102.0 (6.0)	76.8 (8.6)	502.4 (98.4)	97.3 (7.3)	71.2 (8.7)
90	993.8 (180.3)	103.8 (6.3)	83.6 (10.2)	628.0 (136.2)	99.7 (8.1)	77.9 (9.2)
100	1223.7 (249.4)	102.7 (8.7)	97.7 (11.5)	785.4 (188.4)	96.4 (11.2)	92.0 (12.2)

Italicized parenthetical data are standard deviations.

Source: Adapted and condensed from "Differences in Phonetogram Features Between Male and Female Subjects with and without Vocal Training" by A. M. Sulter, H.K. Schutte, and D. G. Miller, 1995, *Journal of Voice, 9*, 363–377.

Method: 92 women (age 17 to 44 y, mean 20.3 y) and 47 men (age 17 to 35 y, mean 25.0 y). Sustained /a/ of 1 s minimum duration, mouth-mic distance 30 cm. Measured frequencies were the musical pitches c, e, g, a in each octave of the subject's maximum phonational frequency range, and intensities at 10% ST levels of the range were determined by interpolation. "Fast" sound level meter setting, dB(A) weighting. Measurement was accomplished by a FST-II "phonetometer" augmented computer system.

Analysis and Extension of the VRP

Enhancement of the VRP

There is a strong sense that the utility of the voice range profile would be enhanced if it were to display other variables along with vocal frequency and intensity. Systems have accordingly been devised to evaluate and display maximal phonation time (Frank & Donner, 1983; Gross & Collo, 1983; Neuschaefer-Rube & Klajman, 1996; Neuschaefer-Rube, Sram, & Klajman, 1997), "comfortable" intensity (Awan, 1991, 1993), jitter, spectral slope, and noise (Pabon & Plomp, 1988) as part of the voice range profile. While intuitively appealing, the ultimate utility of these improvements of the standard voice range profile has not been clearly demonstrated, nor are the specialized measurement systems yet commercially available.

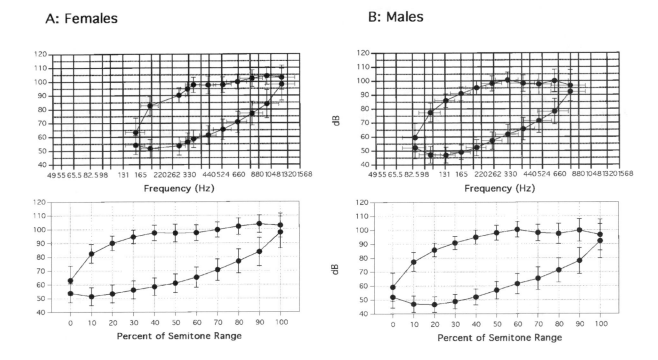

A: Females

B: Males

Figure 5–11. Tentative norms for the voice range profiles of normal men (A) and women (B), plotted by absolute frequency and at decile levels of the semitone vocal range. Error bars indicate ±1 SD. (Data are from Sulter, Schutte, and Miller, 1995).

Table 5–13. Intensity Variation of Sustained Vowels During VRP Measurement. (Averaged across F_0 levels; in dB SPL)*

Subject Group	Maximally Loud		Minimally Loud	
	Mean	Median	Mean	Median
Normal male	2.2	2.0	5.2	5.0
Normal female	2.1	2.0	4.7	4.0
Dysphonic females	1.7	1.0	4.0	3.5

Note: Data for dysphonic patients are significantly different from those of normal subjects. Intensity variability of dysphonic (but not of normal) subjects was less in the upper levels of their F_0 range.

Source: Adapted from "Variability of Phonetograms," by P. Gramming, J. Sundberg, and L. Åkerlund, 1991, *Folia Phoniatrica, 43*, 79–92.

Ten normal untrained females (age range 19–58 y, mean 39 y) ; 10 normal untrained males (age 25–44 y, mean 33 y); 10 dysphonic females (age range 20–56 y, mean 33 y) with no visible laryngeal pathology. Subjects sustained /a/ at maximal and minimal intensity at 4 pitches in each octave of the F_0 range.

Quantitative Description of VRP Characteristics

Attempts have been made to define and quantify the essential features of the voice range profile so as to improve its evaluative power and optimize its utility for differential diagnosis. Generally, these efforts have focused on the derivation of statistical descriptors or on the identification of characteristics related to diagnostic category or to rehabilitative or drug-treatment outcome (Pedersen, 1991, 1995; Behrman, Agresti, Blumstein, & Sharma, 1996; Heylen et al., 1998). Some, on the other hand, have attempted to capture the geometric charac-

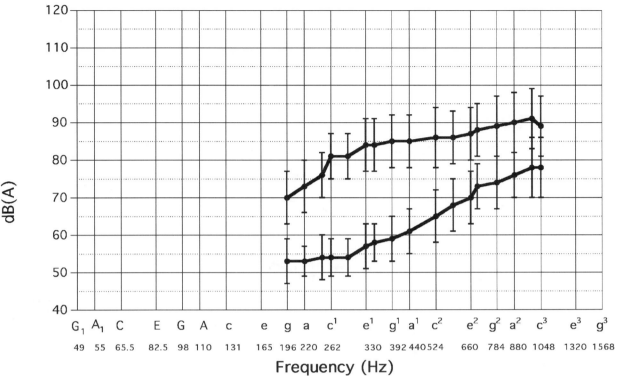

Figure 5–12. Average voice range profile of 45 boys, age 7 to 10 years. Error bars are ±1 SD. (Plotted from the data of Böhme and Stuchlik, 1995.)

Table 5–14. Long-term Variability of Vocal Intensity Across F_o Levels. (Mean of the Standard Deviations of Measured Intensity in dB SPL)*

Sex	Variation of:	
	Minimum Intensity	**Maximum Intensity**
Female	2.7	2.4
Male	3.0	3.4

Source: From "Variability of Phonetograms," by P. Gramming, J. Sundberg, and L. Åkerlund, 1991, *Folia Phoniatrica 43*, 79–92.

*One normal male, age 36 y and one normal female, age 50 y, retested on 15 different days over a 3-week period. "The standard deviation tended to increase towards the fundamental frequency extremes for both subjects" (p. 87).

teristics of the voice range profile plot (Klingholz & Martin, 1983; Airainer & Klingholz, 1993).

Perhaps the most extensive analytic method has been proposed by Sulter et al. (1994). Employing rather sophisticated mathematical techniques (some or which

were originally devised for automated handwriting analysis), the shape of a plot can be described by a series of Fourier descriptors. Enclosed area, contour regularity, and the slope of the data set are among the features considered and quantified. The method has the

Girls age 7-10

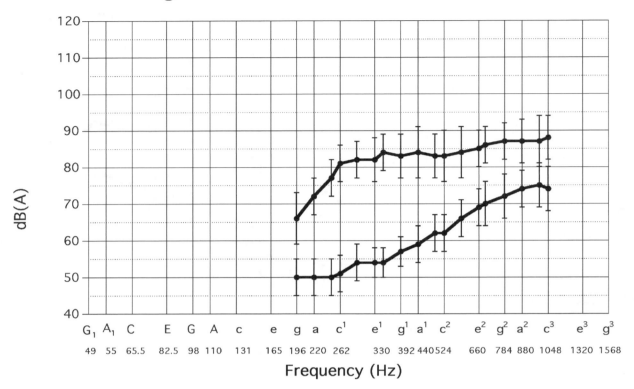

Figure 5–13. Average voice range profile of 67 girls, age 7 to 10 years. Error bars are ±1 SD. (Plotted from the data of Böhme and Stuchlik, 1995.)

distinct advantage of producing a quantitative description that is independent of the specific data values, thus making voice range profiles fully comparable across subjects and conditions. The ultimate diagnostic utility of the method has, however, yet to be determined.

THE EFFECT OF AGING ON VOCAL INTENSITY

Age seems to have a real, but not dramatic, effect on the maximum SPL of adults. Ptacek et al. (1966) had young and old adults shout /a/ as loudly as possible for at least 1 s at a self-selected pitch. SPL was measured 12 inches from the lips. The data, summarized in Table 5–15, show that maximum SPL falls off on the order of 6 dB (that is, sound pressure drops by half) between young adulthood and old age.

PULSE REGISTER

The limits of the vocal intensity range in pulse (vocal fry) register have not been adequately explored. A study by Murry and Brown (1971), however, provides some basis for initial and tentative conclusions. Five young adult men and five women were asked to sustain pulse register phonation for at least 4 s at the 25, 50, and 75 percentile levels of their pulse frequency range. The mean (self-selected) SPL used by the subjects was a bit more than 50 dB at the lowest frequency, rising to close to 60 dB at the highest frequency. When corrected for differences in microphone placement, these data are close to the mean *minimum* SPL for the modal and loft (falsetto) registers reported by Coleman, Mabis, and Hinson (1977). The conclusion, buttressed by everyday perceptual experience, that pulse register phonation is produced at a lower intensity seems reasonable.

More interesting, perhaps, is the fact that Murry and Brown's (1971) subjects not only changed intensity with F_0, but, when asked to change intensity by specific amounts, they did so by altering F_0. In the case of both F_0 matching and intensity matching, the correlation coefficient of F_0 with intensity level was about 0.85.

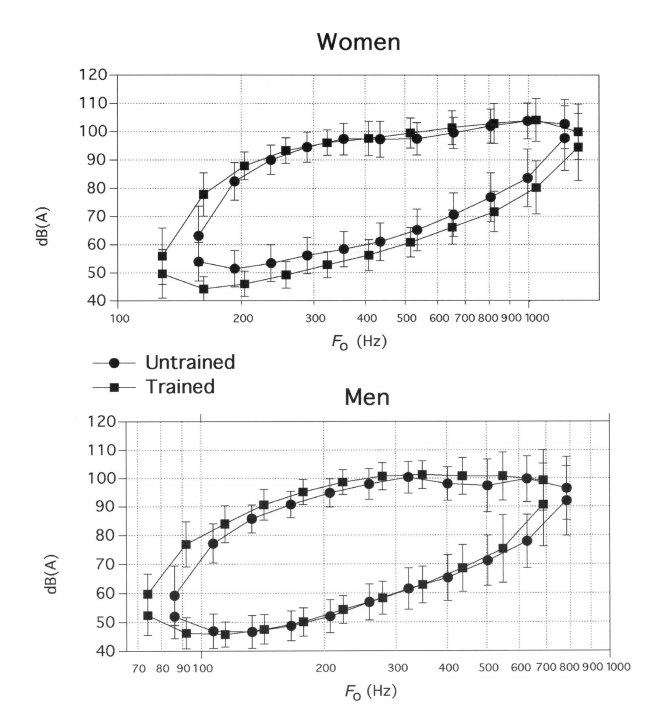

Figure 5–14. Comparison of voice range profiles of trained and untrained men and women. Men: 47 untrained (mean age 25.0 years, range 17—35 years); 43 trained (minimum of 2 years of singing experience, mean age 47.5 years, range 21—75 years). Women: 92 untrained (mean age 20.3 years, range 17—44 years); 42 trained (minimum 2 years of singing experience, mean age 35.1 years, range 18—59 years). Data gathered according to recommendations of European Union of Phoniatricians, but using the "FST-II phonetometer" computer system. Microphone distance 30 cm; dB(A) weighting, fast meter response. (Plotted from the data of Sulter, Schutte, and Miller, 1995.)

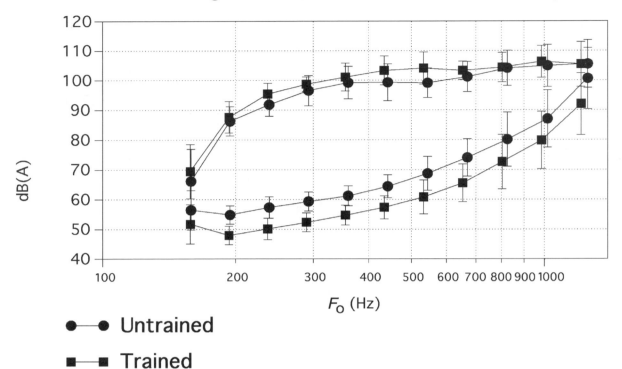

Figure 5–15. Effect of 2.5 years of voice training on the voice range profile of 25 females (mean age 18.4 years, range 17–21 years), speech therapy students in the Netherlands. VRP measurement according to the recommendations of the European Union of Phoniatricians, except data gathered by "FST-II phonetometer" computer system. Microphone distance 30 cm, vowel /ɑ/; dB(A) weighting, fast meter response. Error bars are ±1 SD. (Plotted from the data of Sulter and Meijer, 1996).

Table 5–15. Maximum Vocal Intensity: Effect of Aging

Subjects			Maximum SPL (dB re: 0.0002 d/cm²)		
Number	**Sex**	**Age range (yrs)**	**Mean**	**SD**	**Range**
31	M	18–39	105.8	5.1	92–116
27	M	66–89	100.5	5.9	88–110
30	F	18–38	106.2	3.0	99–112
34	F	66–93	98.6	4.5	90–104

Source: From "Phonatory and Related Changes with Advanced Age," by P. H. Ptacek, E. K. Sander, W. H. Maloney, and C. C. R. Jackson, 1966, *Journal of Speech and Hearing Research*, *9*, 353–360. © American Speech-Language-Hearing Association, Rockville, MD.

/ɑ/ sustained >1 s; self-selected pitch, 12" (≈30.5 cm) mouth-to-microphone distance; three trials each.

Vocal F_0 and intensity level seem very much more interdependent in pulse register than in other phonatory modes.

VOCAL RISE TIME

Acoustically, different types of vocal attack are discriminable by the vocal rise time, among other things. This is the duration of the interval between the onset of voice and the point at which amplitude reaches a stable value. Since vocal therapy may have modification of vocal onset characteristics as a goal, information concerning acoustic rise time is likely to be of clinical value. It is generally recognized that, perceptually, there are at least three broad categories of vocal attack: soft, breathy (or aspirate), and hard (or glottal). Research suggests that listeners judge "abruptness" of vocal onset on the basis of the logarithm of the slope of the voice amplitude envelope (Peters, Boves, & van Dielen, 1986). Oscilloscopic representations of the vowel /ɑ/ initiated with each of the attack types are shown in Figure 5–16. Note that the rise time is different in each case.

Koike, Hirano, and von Leden (1967) and Koike (1967) have studied vocal rise time together with F_0 and aerodynamic variables in normal subjects. They derived the data of Table 5–16 from measurement of oscillograms.

Koike (1967) has also measured the rise time associated with the softest vocal initiation that could be produced by patients with several different types of laryngeal pathology. These data are summarized in Table 5–17.

Table 5–16. Vocal Rise Time for Different Vocal Attacks

Attack Type	Rise Time (ms)*		
	Mean	SD	Range
Hard (glottal)	29	9.5	18–50
Soft	261	54.2	163–325
Breathy (aspirate)	148	66.6	65–243

Source: From Koike, Y., 1967, Experimental Studies on Vocal Attack. *Practica Otologica Kyoto, 60*, 663–688. Reprinted by permission.

10 normal males (Japanese speakers). Voluntary production of each type of attack. "Optimal pitch." Loudness and pitch constant.

*"The time duration from the onset of sound to the point at which the envelope of acoustic waves reached the mean amplitude of the steady portion of the phonation" (Koike, p. 664).

Amplitude Variability

The stability of the vocal signal can be assessed by measures of amplitude variability. There are a number of ways in which this can be done, depending on the intended purpose and on the nature of one's analytic model. Many proposed measures—such as the statistical distribution of wave amplitudes (Niederjohn & Haworth, 1983; Klingholz & Martin, 1989)—examine relatively long-term features of the speech signal. Very

Table 5–17. Vocal Rise Time of Softest Possible Initiation: Laryngeal Disorders

Diagnosis	No.	Sex of Subjects	Mean Age	Rise Time (ms)*		
				Mean	SD	Range
Cancer, glottic	5	M	60	50.8	48.9	25–138
Paralysis, unilateral	2	M	41.5	130.5	26.2	112–149
	2	F	35.5	120.5	19.1	107–134
Laryngitis, acute	2	F	34.5	62.0	19.8	48–76

Source: From "Experimental Studies on Vocal Attack," by Y. Koike, 1967, *Practica Otologica Kyoto, 60*, 663–688.

*Calculated from author's data.

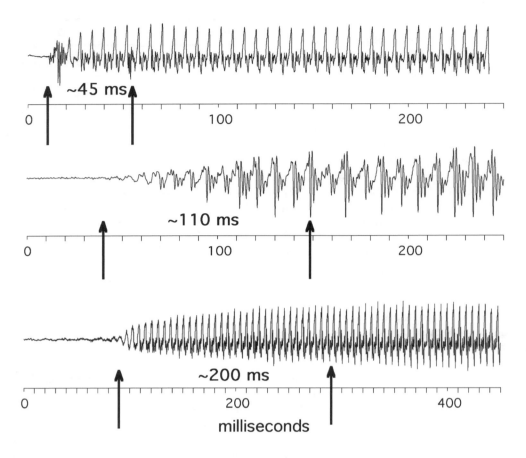

Figure 5–16. Sound pressure records of different vocal rise times. Vocal rise time (in ms) is measured from the onset of voice to the point at which the waveform achieves the mean amplitude of the steady portion of the vowel. Top: Hard attack; middle: breathy attack; bottom: soft attack. (The descriptive terms refer to Koike's 1967 categorization.)

few have had more than preliminary investigation in the clinical context. Much more popular, more thoroughly explored, and intuitively more closely connected to our understanding of vocal tract function have been the indices of short-term variation known as amplitude perturbation.

AMPLITUDE PERTURBATION (SHIMMER)

Measures of *amplitude perturbation*—generally called *shimmer*—are analogous to those of fundamental frequency perturbation discussed in Chapter 6. (Those unfamiliar with the concepts and terms related to perturbation should read that discussion first.) Like frequency-perturbation scores, shimmer values serve to quantify short-term amplitude instability that does not alter the qualitative features of the vocal waveform (Titze, 1995, p. 6). It is likely that shimmer is at least as

important as jitter (and perhaps more so) in its contribution to the perception of hoarseness, although there is no unanimity on this point (Wendahl, 1966a, 1966b; Hecker & Kreul, 1971; Takahashi & Koike, 1975; Klingholz & Martin, 1983; Eskenazi, Childers, & Hicks, 1990; Kempster, Kistler, & Hillenbrand, 1991; Wolfe & Martin, 1997; McAllister, Sundberg, & Hibi, 1998). The relationship of amplitude perturbation to specific abnormalities of glottal function—or of more global disorders of speech (see, for example, Hall and Yairi, 1992, and Gamboa et al., 1997)—remains, at the very best, extremely unclear (Hirano et al., 1988; Hirano, 1989; Feijoo & Hernández, 1990; Laver, Hiller, & Beck, 1992; Wolfe, Fitch, & Cornell, 1995). It seems clear, however, that shimmer values tend to normalize as laryngeal pathology abates (Verdolini-Marston, Sandage, & Titze, 1994; Shaw, Searl, Young, & Miner, 1996).[17]

---

[17]A review of issues related to vocal perturbation is provided by Laver, Hiller, and Beck, 1992.

Shimmer has not been as carefully studied as jitter. The effects of vocal fundamental frequency, frequency perturbation, and mean amplitude on amplitude perturbation remain incompletely characterized. Preliminary investigations suggest, however, that shimmer may be inversely (but nonlinearly) proportional to mean vocal intensity (Orlikoff & Kahane, 1991) and that shimmer and jitter (frequency perturbation) tend to covary (Heilberger & Horii, 1982). Possible differences due to age and sex also await clarification, as does the extent to which shimmer is independent of other acoustic characteristics of the vocal signal (Hillenbrand, 1987; Wong, Lange, Titze, & Guo, 1995). And, as is the case for frequency perturbation, the relationship of shimmer magnitude and vocal pathology is very murky. Still, shimmer measures remain popular among clinicians, perhaps, since they are included in most automated voice analysis systems (Read, Buder, & Kent, 1990), because computer-based systems make them easy to obtain.

Measurement Methods

The collection of a sample for shimmer analysis is simply a matter of capturing (with an adequate sampling rate) a sustained phonation of the type that requires evaluation. As is the case with any intensity measure, a constant mouth–to–microphone distance is very important. Also, the patient must be urged to produce the most stable phonation possible and the resulting phonation should, within reasonable limits, be classifiable as Type I: continuously periodic (Titze, 1995). The deleterious effect of occasional discontinuities on measured shimmer may, however, not be as serious as previously believed, at least for some computer software packages (Karnell et al., 1997).[18]

For frequency measurement a "clean" signal can be obtained by using an accelerometer, or contact microphone, but this is not advisable for amplitude studies. Horii (1982) has found that shimmer values of accelerometer signals may be lower than those derived from an air microphone for the same utterances. (This is presumably due to the fact that vocal tract phase-shifts affect the airborne wave but do not strongly influence the neck-wall vibrations that are sensed by a contact microphone.) Also, although it has been done for special purposes (Haji, Horiguchi, Baer, & Gould, 1986), amplitude variations of the EGG signal (see Chapter 10, "Laryngeal Function") cannot be substituted for acoustic variations. Shimmer measurement clearly requires a high-quality air microphone.

Amplitude perturbation is a measure based on the *peak* amplitude of the acoustic wave associated with each phonatory cycle. This is a different value from the rms or average amplitude (see Chapter 2, "Analog Electronics") that is typically used as the basis of sound pressure level (SPL), and the two must not be confused. The average peak amplitude that is derived for some of the shimmer measures is *not* the average that results from integration of the wave—which is the basis of rms amplitude. Without a very elaborate (and highly impractical) mathematical evaluation of the complex vowel waveform, there is no way to convert average peak amplitude to a different intensity measure.

Measurement Accuracy

Clearly, the accuracy of the amplitude perturbation measure can be no better than the precision of the peak amplitude values from which it is computed. The most important limiting factor is the bit resolution of the analog-to-digital converter (see Chapters 3 and 4). Titze, Horii, and Scherer (1987) have examined this issue in some detail. They point out that, under ideal circumstances, the system-dependent "maximum normalized theoretical shimmer"—that is, the magnitude of measurement error—is

$$\% \text{ shimmer} = \left(\frac{100}{A_0}\right)\left(\frac{1}{n}\right)\left| \sum_{i=1}^{n} \pm \left(\frac{1}{2}\frac{A}{2^N}\right) \right|$$

where A = the total amplitude range of the a/d converter

A_0 = the mean signal amplitude of the sample

n = the number of cycles in the sample

N = the number of bits used by the a/d converter (bit resolution).

If the full range of the converter's amplitude range is not used, then the reduction factor may be stated as

$$R = \frac{A}{A_0}$$

and the maximal relative error is

$$\% \text{ shimmer} = 50\left(\frac{R}{2^N}\right).$$

---

[18]A good summary of technical requirements for data-collection instruments is provided by Laver, Hiller, and Beck (1992). Refer also to the consideration of data precision and requisite sample characteristics for jitter measurements in Chapter 6, "Vocal Fundamental Frequency."

It is clear that measurement accuracy can be improved by using an a/d converter with the largest possible bit resolution (10 bits should be considered a minimum) and by using as much of the converter's input range as possible. That is, if the a/d converter has, for example, an input range of ±5 volts, then the voice signal should be amplified so that its maximum instantaneous amplitude is just slightly less than |5 V|.

Other factors also affect the accuracy of shimmer values. Low-pass filtering of the signal can alter the peak amplitudes, leading to measurable error. The filter cutoff frequency should be kept as high as possible, but in no case less than 1 octave above F_0. Sample size also matters, and at least 30 consecutive cycles should be included.

Finally, although some investigations have done so (Glaze, Bless, & Susser, 1990) it is generally not advisable to derive shimmer measures from samples taken with direct tape recorders (see Chapter 4, "General-Purpose Tools"), which can be expected to produce very significant errors into the shimmer estimate (Titze, Horii, & Scherer, 1987; Gelfer & Fendel, 1995; Perry, Ingrisano, & Blair, 1996; Jiang, Lin, & Hanson, 1998). Digital audio tape recordings are generally acceptable, however, as (to a lesser extent) are recordings made on an FM or pulse code modulation recording system (Doherty & Shipp, 1988; Bless & Baken, 1992).

Shimmer Measures

Today's computerized systems provide measures of intensity variability. But different systems commonly report differ shimmer values for the same signal (Karnell, Hall, and Landahl, 1995; Bielamowicz, Kreiman, Gerratt, Dauer, and Berke, 1996). Because of this, users must be certain that they understand the *exact* method by which the shimmer data are derived before making comparisons to published data. (Note that some systems employ algorithms (for example, Milenkovic, 1987) for which there are few, if any published results. It is also very important to be certain that the computer program does not automatically and surreptitiously eliminate what it deems to be "unacceptable" segments of the sample.

Even though, with today's technology, the clinician will almost never be called upon to calculate shimmer from a readout of successive cycle amplitudes, an understanding of the basis of each of the measures in common use is essential to intelligent interpretation and comparison of test results. The vari-

ous methods are therefore briefly discussed in the discussion that follows.[19]

Directional Perturbation Factor

Originated by Hecker and Kreul (1971) as a measure of period perturbation, the *directional perturbation factor* (DPF) can also be used to scale amplitude variation. The measure tallies the number of times that the amplitude difference between two successive waves shifts direction. Computation of the DPF sounds complex, but it is not really difficult in practice. The technique for calculating DPF for fundamental periods is described (together with a computational example) in Chapter 6. If "amplitude" is substituted for "period," that discussion is fully applicable to the amplitude DPF.

Sorenson and Horii (1984) have studied the amplitude DPF in normal men and women. Their data (Table 5–18) may be taken as tentative norms for this measure.

Table 5–18. Directional Perturbation Factor (% Sign Change) for Amplitude: Normal Men and Women*

	Vowel		
	/ɑ/	/u/	/i/
	Men		
Mean	59.47	58.91	61.13
Range	52.0–68.3	43.5–67.0	52.8–66.7
SD	3.89	5.40	3.91
	Women		
Mean	63.13	56.76	61.71
Range	52.3–69.4	51.3–70.9	57.5–72.6
SD	4.27	4.66	3.56

Source: From "Frequency and Amplitude Perturbation in the Voices of Female Speakers," by D. Sorensen and Y. Horii, 1983, *Journal of Communication Disorders, 16,*) 57–61. © 1983 by Elsevier Publishing Co., Inc. Reprinted by permission.

No correlation between DPF and actual shimmer magnitude values. Period perturbation (jitter) studied in the same group (see Chapter 6).

*20 men, 20 women (all nonsmokers) age 25–49 y (means: males 38.1 y; females 36.4 y); sustained vowels, 70–80 dB SPL for approximately 5 s.

---

[19] The mathematical relationships among many different shimmer measures have been explored by Pinto and Titze (1990).

Table 5–19. Amplitude Variability Index: Normal and Hoarse*

Vowel	NORMAL		HOARSE	
	Mean	SD	Mean	SD
/u/	−0.1287	0.2241	0.4142†	0.6497
/i/	−0.1330	0.4087	0.5706†	0.8831
/ʌ/	−0.0389	0.2432	0.5977†	0.8486
/a/	−0.0619	0.4036	0.2163	0.6389
/æ/	−0.0216	0.2557	0.1550	0.5876
Overall	−0.0768		0.3908†	

Source: From "Some Waveform and Spectral Features of Vowel Roughness," by R. E. Deal and F. W. Emanuel, 1978, *Journal of Speech and Hearing Research*, 21, 250–264. © American Speech-Language-Hearing Association, Rockville, MD. Reprinted by permission.

*Method: 20 normal males; 20 hoarse males with diagnosed laryngeal pathology. Analysis of 1 s portion of 7 s productions; vocal intensity 75 dB SPL; signal narrow-band filtered.

†All significantly different from $p < .05$.

Amplitude Variability Index

The *amplitude variability index* (AVI) of Deal and Emanuel (1978) resembles their period variability index (see Chapter 6). It is not an average of the cycle-to-cycle amplitude variation, but rather it represents the average degree of variation from the mean peak amplitude of the entire sample. In this respect it is unique among perturbation measures, and it is clearly not equivalent to the other amplitude variability indices that have been proposed.

The AVI is based on a *coefficient of variation* (CV) that can be applied to either periods or amplitudes. This is defined as

$$CV = \frac{\left[\frac{1}{n}\sum_{i=1}^{n}(x_i - \bar{x})^2\right]}{\bar{x}^{-2}}$$

where n = number of peaks measured

x_i = individual amplitude values

$\bar{x}$ = mean peak amplitude

The CV, then, is the average of the deviations from the mean peak amplitude ($[x_i - x]^2$) divided by the square of the mean amplitude. The AVI is then calculated as

$$AVI = \log_{10}(CV \times 1000).$$

Deal and Emanuel (1978) evaluated their index with samples (originally collected by Hanson, 1969, and by Sansone and Emanuel, 1970) of sustained vowels produced by normal adult males and by clinically hoarse men with confirmed laryngeal pathologies. AVI values for both groups are summarized in Table 5–19. A peculiarity of the analysis method, however, requires the use of caution in interpreting these data. Before oscillographic write out, all signals were conditioned by an extremely narrow (10 Hz) band-pass filter with its center frequency at the first harmonic of the voice signal. Such a filter smoothes out irregularities in the signal, but the exact extent to which it did so in the samples analyzed cannot be determined.

Shimmer in dB

Given that the dB scale is based on a ratio of amplitudes it is an easy matter to use it for quantifying shimmer. The ratio need only be that of two contiguous cycles (A_i and A_{i+1}) for which the amplitude difference in dB is

$$dB_{shimmer} = 20 \log^{10}(A_i/A_{i+1}).$$

The average shimmer for a sample of n cycles is then

$$dB_{shimmer} = \frac{\sum_{i=1}^{n-1}\left|20\log_{10}\left(\frac{A_i}{A_{i+1}}\right)\right|}{n-1}$$

This approach to the quantification of shimmer has the distinct advantage of freeing the measurement

Table 5–20. Shimmer in dB: Normal Adults*

Vowel	Men** Mean (SD)	Women† Mean (SD)
/ɑ/	0.47 (0.34)	0.33 (0.22)
/i/	0.37 (0.28)	0.23 (0.08)
/u/	0.33 (0.31)	0.19 (0.04)
Overall‡	0.39 (0.31)	0.25 (0.11)

Sources: Data for men from "Vocal Shimmer in Sustained Phonation," by Y. Horii, 1980, *Journal of Speech and Hearing Research, 23,* 202–209. © American Speech-Language-Hearing Association, Rockville, MD. Used by permission. Data for women from "Frequency and Amplitude Perturbation in the Voice of Female Speakers," by D. Sorensen and Y. Horii, 1983, *Journal of Communication Disorders, 16,* 56–61. © Elsevier Science Inc., New York. Used by permission.

*Method: 20 women, aged 25–49y (mean 36.8y); 31 men, aged 18–38y (mean 26.6y); sustained vowels of 5 s duration; 70–80 dB SPL; F_0 controlled ±10 Hz; 3 s segment of the least variable of 3 trials analyzed.

**Significant difference ($p < .05$) /ɑ/ > /i/ and /u/. 95% critical region: > 0.98 dB.

†Significant difference ($p < .05$) /ɑ/ > /i/ and /u/.

‡Male/female shimmer values are significantly different ($p < .05$) for /i/ and /u/ but not for /ɑ/. The overall mean shimmer values for men and women are not significantly different.

from the absolute amplitude. In this it is analogous to the F_0 compensation used for several jitter measures. It is the method used by Horii (1980) to generate the data of Table 5–20.

Orlikoff and Kahane (1991) have shown that $dB_{shimmer}$ tends to be inversely related to vocal SPL in normal men. Their findings are summarized in Table 5–21. $dB_{shimmer}$ increases significantly with age, and good physical condition (as measured by blood pressure, ventilatory capacity, weight, and blood cholesterol levels) or participation in vigorous physical activity is associated with lower $dB_{shimmer}$ scores, as shown by the data in Table 5–22.

Finally, Fuller and Horii (1986) have explored shimmer in the hunger, "fussing," pain, and "cooing" vocalizations of normal infants between the ages of 2 and 6 months. The mean shimmer values for these conditions

Table 5–21. Mean (and SD) Shimmer in dB as a Function of Baseline Vocal SPL

	Phonatory Condition		
	Soft	Moderate	Loud
Baseline level	63.32 (1.99)	74.30 (2.13)	84.80 (2.06)
Mean (SD) dB shimmer	0.37* (0.14)	0.31 (0.11)	0.21* (0.11)

*Difference between soft and loud conditions is significant ($p < .01$).

Source: R. F. Orlikoff and J. C. Kahane, 1991, Influence of mean sound pressure level on jitter and shimmer measures. *Journal of Voice, 5,* 113–119. 10 normal men, age 26–37y (mean 31.8y). Sustained /a/. Evaluation of at least 8 s, excluding first and last seconds.

ranged from 0.796 dB to 1.132 dB (grand mean = 1.002 dB) but did not differ significantly from each other.

Compensation for Long-term Changes: APQ

Long-term changes in vocal intensity are not the issue in evaluation of shimmer, but they are bound to increase its measured magnitude. Eliminating the effects of amplitude "drift" in order to get a truer index of the underlying shimmer itself has been attempted by the same kind of trend-line smoothing used for jitter analysis (see Chapter 6). Kitajima and Gould (1976) have proposed using deviation from a least-squares trend line, but that suggestion has not met with much acceptance.

Takahashi and Koike (1975) and Koike, Takahashi, and Calcaterra (1977) have suggested a measure that they call the *amplitude perturbation quotient (APQ)*, which is analogous to the relative average perturbation originally devised by Koike (1969). The function uses an 11-point average for smoothing and is defined as

$$APQ = \frac{\dfrac{1}{n-10}\sum\limits_{i=6}^{n-5}\left|\dfrac{A_{i-5}+A_{i-4}+...+A_i...A_{i+5}}{11}-A_i\right|}{\dfrac{1}{n}\sum\limits_{i=1}^{n}A_i}$$

where A_i = peak amplitude of each wave

n = number of waves measured.

Table 5–22. Shimmer in dB for Subjects with Different Levels of Physical Fitness

Mean Age	Age range or (SD)	Physical Condition or State	dB Shimmer and (SD)	Note
		Men		
29.5	26-35	Good	0.20 (0.05)	1
32.3	25-38	Poor	0.29 (0.33)	1
53.0	16-56	Good	0.28 (0.14)	1
52.6	42-59	Poor	0.34 (0.25)	1
67.5	62-75	Good	0.31 (0.11)	1
69.1	64-74	Poor	0.52 (0.23)	1
66.1	(2.2)	Active	0.34 (0.19)	2
67.4	(3.9)	Sedentary	0.42 (0.29)	2
73.3	68-80 (3.7)	Good cardiac health	0.39 (0.11)	3
70.3	60-79 (6.5)	Atherosclerotic	0.46 (0.12)	3
		Women		
66.4	(3.1)	Active	0.36 (0.19)	2
67.6	(3.8)	Sedentary	0.50 (0.49)	2

Sources:

1. Ringel and Chodzko-Zajko, 1987. "Physiological condition" defined on the basis of blood pressure, forced vital capacities, serum cholesterol and triglyceride levels, and percent body fat. See also Ramig and Ringel, 1983.

2. Xue and Mueller, 1997. "Physically active" defined as "regular and/or active participation in physical exercises, training programmes, and other physical activities." "Physically sedentary" defined as "rare or no participation" in any of these.

3. Orlikoff, 1990. Six men in each group. "Good cardiac health" indicated by absence of observable cardiovascular pathology and normal blood pressure. Atherosclerotic men had diagnosed chronic atherosclerosis with no bradycardia or respiratory problems. Cardiac patients were not taking medication likely to impair autonomic function.

Davis (1976, 1979, 1981) has evaluated the effect of window size (that is, of the number of waves in the running average) and has found that the APQ function is optimized at a window size of 5. He prefers, however, to evaluate the peaks of the residue signal after inverse filtering, which eliminates the effects of the acoustic characteristics of the vocal tract. Davis' data are not, therefore, directly comparable with those of Takahashi and Koike, but because they are reflective of the information derived by a commercially distributed system (ILS) that still has some currency, they are included in Table 5–23. Note also that Takahashi and Koike's samples were collected using a pretracheal contact microphone. Data for various pathologies are included in the table. Although not normative, they do provide an approximate indication of the shimmer increases that might be expected.

Serial Correlation Function

The serial correlation function is described more completely in connection with F_0 perturbation (see Chapter 6). It has been found (von Leden & Koike, 1970) that the same technique applied to amplitude measures can

Table 5–23. Amplitude Perturbation Quotients: Normal and Pathologic*

Number	Sex	Mean Age	Mean F_o	APQ Mean	APQ SD	Note
				Mean	*SD*	
Normal						
Acoustic signal:						
7	M	27.7	108.1	40.3×10^4	13.6×10^{-4}	a
2	F	29.5	206.0	32.9×10^{-4}	20.9×10^{-4}	a
Inverse-filtered residue signal:						
8	M	28.4	120.0	5.97%	3.10%	b
2	F	29.5	206.0	6.81%	3.15	b
Pathologic						
Chronic laryngitis:						
2	F	46.0	193.5	16.7×10^{-4}	8.3×10^{-4}	b
Unilateral paralysis:						
2	M	49.5	193.0	111.3×10^{-4}	0.64×10^{-4}	b
Nodules:						
2	M	54.5	118.5	41.0×10^{-4}	31.8×10^{-4}	b
1	M	11	271.	28.5×10^{-4}		b
1	F	33	205.	38.3×10^{-4}		b
Tumors:						
1	M	50	155	120.1×10^{-4}		b
1	F	61	149	137.3×10^{-4}		b
Partial laryngectomy:						
2	M	66	100.0	93.1×10^{-4}	4.1×10^{-4}	b

Source: Adapted from:

a. "Some Perceptual Dimensions and Acoustical Correlates of Pathologic Voices," by H. Takahashi and Y. Koike, 1975, *Acta Oto-Laryngologica, Suppl. 338*, 1–24. Eleven-point smoothing, pretracheal contact microphone.

b. "Acoustic Characteristics of Normal and Pathological Voices," by S. B. Davis,1979. In N. J. Lass (ed.), *Speech and language: Basic advances in research and practice*, (Vol. 1, pp. 271–335). New York: Academic Press. Five-point smoothing. Data based on samples collected by Y. Koike and J. Markel, 1975, "Application of Inverse Filtering for Detecting Laryngeal Pathology," A*nnals of Otology, Rhinology, and Laryngology, 84*, 117–124.

*Sustained /ɑ/, comfortable pitch and loudness. Analysis of steadiest 1.5 s.

be a very sensitive indicator of the presence of laryngeal pathology. Von Leden and Koike emphasize that, because cyclicity of perturbation tends to be a relatively short-term phenomenon, it is only necessary to use lags of 1 to 15 for analysis. They have categorized amplitude-perturbation correlograms into four basic types, schematized in Figure 5–17.

The type 1 correlogram is typical of a normal speaker. The very high correlation at lag = 1 is indicative of the similarity of successive waveforms. The correlation decreases smoothly as the comparison is made across a greater lag, and the negative peak between lag = 10 and lag = 15 tends to show a longer term periodicity of amplitude variation, perhaps like vibrato. The type 1 pattern is also seen in mild, transient, laryngeal involvements.

The type 2 correlogram is similar to the Type 1, but the irregularity of the correlation decrease points to

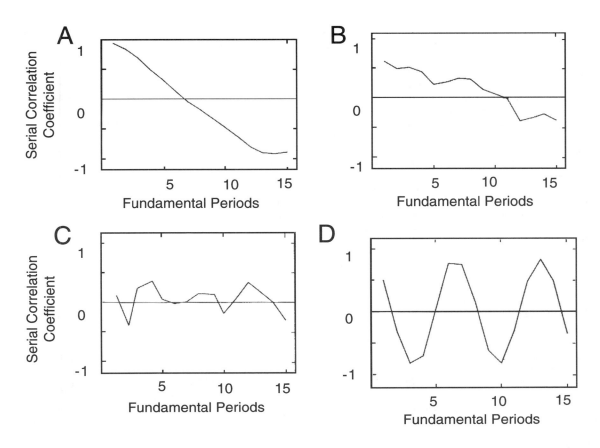

Figure 5–17. Amplitude perturbation correlogram categories. **A.** Type I: normal. **B.** Type 2: inflammation, small nodules. **C.** Type 3: incomplete closure, paralysis. **D.** Type 4: malignancy, papillomatosis. (Adapted from "Detection of Laryngeal Disease by Computer Technique," by H. von Leden and Y. Koike, 1970. *Archives of Otolaryngology, 91,* 3–10. Reprinted by permission.)

erratic, short-term amplitude perturbation. This pattern is commonly associated with benign changes of the vocal folds, such as fibrosis, inflammatory tumors, or severe inflammation.

An absence of correlational periodicity is characteristic of the Type 3 correlogram. It is a common concommittant of disorders that result in incomplete glottal closure, such as unilateral paralysis and benign neoplasms. Type 4 patterns are associated with serious laryngeal pathology, including malignant tumors of the vocal folds (Koike, 1969; Izdebski & Murry, 1980), and multiple papillomatosis. The clearly-marked positive and negative correlational peaks indicate fairly rapid and strongly periodic amplitude modulation.

The research concerning serial correlation functions is not sufficiently rigorous or extensive to permit firm diagnostic conclusions, but the promise of significant utility is clearly present. Further work may put this diagnostic technique on a firmer footing.

REFERENCES

Airainer, R., & Klingholz, F. (1993). Quantitative evaluation of phonetograms in the case of functional dysphonia. *Journal of Voice, 7,* 136–141.

Åkerlund, L., & Gramming, P. (1994). Average loudness level, mean fundamental frequency, and subglottal pressure: Comparison between female singers and nonsingers. *Journal of Voice, 8,* 263–270.

Åkerlund, L., Gramming, P., & Sundberg, J. (1992). Phonetogram and averages of sound pressure levels and fundamental frequencies of speech: Comparison between female singers and nonsingers. *Journal of Voice, 6,* 55–63.

Angerstein, W., & Neuschaefer-Rube, C. (1998). Sound pressure level examinations of the calling and speaking voice in healthy persons and in patients with hyperfunctional dysphonia. *Logopedics Phoniatrics Vocology, 23,* 23–25.

Awan, S. N. (1991). Phonetographic profiles and F_0-SPL characteristics of untrained versus trained vocal groups. *Journal of Voice, 5,* 41–50.

Awan, S. N. (1993). Superimposition of speaking voice characteristics and phonetograms in untrained and trained vocal groups. *Journal of Voice, 7,* 30–37.

Awan, S., & Mueller, P. B. (1990). Comment on "Methodological variables affecting phonational frequency range in adults." *Journal of Speech and Hearing Disorders, 55,* 804–805.

Behrman, A., Agresti, C., Blumstein, E., & Sharma, G. (1996). Meaningful features of voice range profiles from patients with organic vocal fold pathology: A preliminary study. *Journal of Voice, 10,* 269–283.

Bernthal, J. E., & Beukelman, D. R. (1977). The effect of changes in velopharyngeal orifice area on vowel intensity. *Cleft Palate Journal, 14,* 63–77.

Bielamowicz, S., Kreiman, J., Gerratt, B., Dauer, M., & Berke, G. (1996). Comparison of voice analysis systems for perturbation measurement. *Journal of Speech and Hearing Research, 39,* 126–134.

Black, J. W. (1949). Natural frequency, duration, and intensity of vowels in reading. *Journal of Speech and Hearing Disorders, 14,* 216–221.

Black, J. W. (1951). The effect of delayed side-tone upon vocal rate and intensity. *Journal of Speech and Hearing Disorders, 16,* 56–60.

Black, J. W. (1961). Relationships among fundamental frequency, vocal sound pressure, and rate of speaking. *Language and Speech, 4,* 196–199.

Bless, D. M., & Baken, R. J. (1992). International Association of Logopedics and Phoniatrics (IALP) Voice Committee discussion of assessment topics. *Journal of Voice, 6,* 194–210.

Blood, G. (1981). The interactions of amplitude and phonetic quality in esophageal speech. *Journal of Speech and Hearing Research, 24,* 308–312.

Blood, G. (1984). Fundamental frequency and intensity measurements in laryngeal and alaryngeal speakers. *Journal of Communication Disorders, 17,* 319–324.

Bloothooft, G. (1982). Nieuwe ontwikkelingen in de fonetografie. *Logopedie en Foniatrie, 54,* 78–90.

Böhme, G., & Stuchlik, G. (1995). Voice profiles and standard voice profile of untrained children. *Journal of Voice, 9,* 304–307.

Boshes, B. (1966). Voice changes in Parkinsonism. *Journal of Neurosurgery, 21,* 286–288.

Brady, P. T. (1971). Need for standardization in the measurement of speech level. *Journal of the Acoustical Society of America, 50,* 712–714.

Brandt, J. F., Ruder, K. F., & Shipp, T., Jr. (1969). Vocal loudness and effort in continuous speech. *Journal of the Acoustical Society of America, 46,* 1543–1548.

Bricker, P. D. (1965). Technique for objective measurement of speech levels. *Journal of the Acoustical Society of America, 38,* 361–362.

Broch, J. T., & Wahrman, C. G. (1961). Effective averaging time of the level recorder type 2305. *B & K Technical Review, 1,* 3–23.

Brown, W. S., Jr., & McGlone, R. E. (1974). Aerodynamic and acoustic study of stress in sentence productions. *Journal of the Acoustical Society of America, 56,* 971–974.

Buekers, R., & Kingma, H. (1997). Impact of phonation intensity upon pitch during speaking: A quantitative study in normal subjects. *Logopedics Phoniatrics Vocology, 22,* 71–77.

Calvet, J., & Malhiac, G. (1952). Courbes vocales et mue de la voix. *Journal Français d'Oto-Rhino-Laryngologie, 1,* 115–124.

Campbell, W. M., & Michel, J. F. (1979). The effects of auditory masking on vocal vibrato. In Lawrence, V. (Ed.), *Transcripts of the eighth symposium: Care of the professional voice* (pp. 50–56). New York: The Voice Foundation.

Canter, G. J. (1963). Speech characteristics of patients with Parkinson's disease. I. Intensity, pitch, and duration. *Journal of Speech and Hearing Disorders, 28,* 221–229.

Canter, G. J. (1965). Speech characteristics of patients with Parkinson's disease. II. Physiological support for speech. *Journal of Speech and Hearing Disorders, 31,* 44–49.

Coblenzer, H., & Muhar, F. (1965). Die Phonationsatmung. *Wiener Klinische Wochenschrift, 77,* 946–953.

Coblenzer, H., & Muhar, F. (1976). *Atem und Stimme.* Vienna: Gerin.

Colcord, R. D., & Adams, M. R. (1979). Voicing duration and vocal SPL changes associated with stuttering reduction during singing. *Journal of Speech and Hearing Research, 22,* 468–479.

Coleman, R. F. (1993). Sources of variation in phonetograms. *Journal of Voice, 7,* 1–14.

Coleman, R. F. (1979). Acoustic and perceptual factors in vibrato. In V. Lawrence (Ed.), *Transcripts of the eighth symposium: Care of the professional voice* (pp. 36–39). New York: The Voice Foundation.

Coleman, R. F., Mabis, J. H., & Hinson, J. K. (1977). Fundamental frequency-sound pressure level profiles of adult male and female voices. *Journal of Speech and Hearing Research, 20,* 197–204.

Coleman, R., & Mott, J. (1978). Fundamental frequency and sound pressure profiles of young female singers. *Folia Phoniatrica, 30,* 94–102.

Colton, R. H. (1973). Vocal intensity in the modal and loft registers. *Folia Phoniatrica, 25,* 62–70.

Damsté, P. H. (1970). The phonetogram. *Practica Oto-Rhino-Laryngologica, 32,* 185–187.

Davis, S. B. (1976). *Computer evaluation of laryngeal pathology based on inverse filtering of speech.* (SCRL Monograph No. 13). Santa Barbara, CA: Speech Communications Research Lab, Inc.

Davis, S. B. (1979). Acoustic characteristics of normal and pathological voices. In N. J. Lass (Ed.), *Speech and language: Basic advances in research and practice,* (Vol. 1, pp. 271–335). New York: Academic Press. (Reprinted in: *ASHA Reports* [1981], *11,* 97–115.)

Deal, R. E., & Emanuel, F. W. (1978). Some waveform and spectral features of vowel roughness. *Journal of Speech and Hearing Research, 21,* 250–264.

Diedrich, W. M. (1968). The mechanism of esophageal speech. *Annals of the New York Academy of Sciences, 155,* 303–317.

Doherty, E. T., & Shipp, T. (1988). Tape recorder effects on jitter and shimmer extraction. *Journal of Speech and Hearing Research, 31,* 485–490.

Dunn, H. K., & Farnsworth, D. W. (1939). Exploration of pressure field [sic] around the human head during speech. *Journal of the Acoustical Society of America, 10,* 184–199.

Eldar, A. (1976). *Spreken en zingen.* Assen, the Netherlands: Van Gorcum.

Eskenazi, L., Childers, D. G., & Hicks, D. M. (1990). Acoustic correlates of vocal quality. *Journal of Speech and Hearing Research, 33,* 298–306.

Fairbanks, G., House, A. S., & Stevens, E. L. (1950). An experimental study of vowel intensities. *Journal of the Acoustical Society of America, 22,* 457–459.

Feth, L. L. (1977). Letter to the editor. *Asha, 19,* 225–226.

Fisichelli, V. R., Karelitz, S., Eichbauer, J., & Rosenfeld, L. S. (1961). Volume-unit graphs: their production and applicability in studies of infants' cries. *Journal of Psychology, 52,* 423–427.

Feijoo, S., & Hernández, C. (1990). Short-term stability measures for the evaluation of vocal quality. *Journal of Speech and Hearing Research, 33,* 324–334.

Finkelhor, B. K., Titze, I. R., & Durham, P. L. (1987). The effect of viscosity changes in the vocal folds on the range of oscillation. *Journal of Voice, 1,* 320–325.

Flanagan, J. L. (1960). Analog measurements of sound radiation from the mouth. *Journal of the Acoustical Society of America, 32,* 1613–1620.

Fletcher, H. (1934). Loudness, pitch and the timbre of musical tones and their relation to the intensity, the frequency, and the overtone structure. *Journal of the Acoustical Society of America, 6,* 59–69.

Fletcher, H. (1953). *Speech and hearing in communication.* New York: Van Nostrand.

Fletcher, H., & Munson, W. A. (1933). Loudness, its definition, measurement, and calculation. *Journal of the Acoustical Society of America, 5,* 82–108.

Fox, C. M., & Ramig, L. O. (1997). Vocal sound pressure level and self-perception of speech and voice in men and women with idiopathic Parkinson disease. *American Journal of Speech-Language Pathology, 6*(2), 85–94.

Frank, F., & Donner, F. (1983). Stimmfeldmessungen unter besonderer Berücksichtigung der Tonhaltedauer bei Durchschnittsstimmen und Kunstgesangsstimmen. In L. Spitzer (Ed.), *Bericht über das 4. Gesangspädagogische Symposion* (pp. 65–75). Bad Ischl, Germany: Springer.

Fry, D. B. (1955). Duration and intensity as physical correlates of linguistic stress. *Journal of the Acoustical Society of America, 27,* 765–768.

Fuller, B. F., & Horii, Y. (1986). Differences in fundamental frequency, jitter, and shimmer among four types of infant vocalizations. *Journal of Communication Disorders, 19,* 441–447.

Gade, S. (1982a). Sound intensity (Part I: Theory). *B & K Technical Review, 3,* 3–39.

Gade, S. (1982b). Sound intensity (part II: Instrumentation and applications). *B & K Technical Review, 4,* 3–32.

Gamboa, J., Jiménez-Jiménez, F. J., Nieto, A., Montojo, J., Ortí-Pareja, M., Molina, J. A., García-Albea, E., and Cobeta, I. (1997). Acoustic voice analysis in patients with Parkinson's disease treated with dopaminergic drugs. *Journal of Voice, 11,* 314–320.

Gauffin, J., & Sundberg, J. (1980). Data on the glottal voice source behaviour in vowel production. *Speech Transmission Laboratory—Quarterly Progress and Status Report, 2–3,* 61–70.

Gelfer, M. P., Andrews, M. L., & Schmidt, C. P. (1991). Effects of prolonged loud reading on selected measures of vocal function in trained and untrained singers. *Journal of Voice, 5,* 158–167.

Gelfer, M. P., & Fendel, D. M. (1995). Comparisons of jitter, shimmer, and signal-to-noise ratio from directly digitized versus taped voice samples. *Journal of Voice, 9,* 378–382.

Gelfer, M. P., & Young, S. R. (1997). Comparisons of intensity measures and their stability in male and female speakers. *Journal of Voice, 11,* 178–186.

Gemelli, A., Sacerdote, G., & Bellussi, G. (1954). Analisi elettroacustica della voce cantata. *Bolletino della Società Italiana della Fonetica Sperimentale, 4,* 3–8.

Glaze, L. E., Bless, D. M., & Susser, R. D. (1990). Acoustic analysis of vowel and loudness differences in children's voice. *Journal of Voice, 4,* 37–44.

Gramming, P. (1988). Non-organic dysphonia. In P. Gramming, *The phonetogram: An experimental and clinical study* (pp. 133–141). Malmö, Sweden: University of Lund.

Gramming, P. (1991). Vocal loudness and frequency capabilities of the voice. *Journal of Voice, 5,* 144–157.

Gramming, P., & Åkerlund, L. (1988). Phonetograms for normal and pathological voices. In P. Gramming, *The phonetogram: An experimental and clinical study* (pp. 117–132). Malmö, Sweden: University of Lund.

Gramming, P., Gauffin, J., & Sundberg, J. (1986). An attempt to improve the clinical usefulness of phonetograms. *Journal of Phonetics, 14,* 421–427.

Gramming, P., & Sundberg, J. (1988). Spectrum factors relevant to phonetogram measurement. *Journal of the Acoustical Society of America, 83,* 2352–2360.

Gramming, P., Sundberg, J., & Åkerlund, L. (1991). Variability of phonetograms. *Folia Phoniatrica, 43,* 79–92.

Gramming, P., Sundberg, J., Ternström, S., Leanderson, R., & Perkins, W. (1988). Relationship between changes in voice pitch and loudness. *Journal of Voice, 2,* 118–124.

Gross, M., & Collo, D. (1983). Funktionelle Ergebnisse nach Larynxteilresektion mit kranial gestielter Halsfaszendeckung. *Archives of Oto-Rhino-Laryngology,* (Suppl. II), pp. 201–202.

Hacki, T. (1988). Die Beurteilung der quantitativen Sprechstimmleistungen. *Folia Phoniatrica, 40,* 190–196.

Hacki, T. (1993). Die Untersuchung und diagnostische Bedeutung der Rufstimmproduktion. In T. Hacki, (Ed.), *Aktuelle phoniatrisch-pädaudiologische Aspekte 1993* (Vol. 1, pp. 182–189). Berlin: Gross.

Hacki. T. (1996). Comparative speaking, shouting, and singing voice range profile measurement: physiological and pathological aspects. *Logopedics, Phoniatrics, and Vocology, 21,* 123–129.

Haji, T., Horiguchi, S., Baer, T., & Gould, W. J. (1986). Frequency and amplitude perturbation analysis of electroglottograph during sustained phonation. *Journal of the Acoustical Society of America, 80,* 58–62.

Hall, K. D., & Yairi, E. (1992). Fundamental frequency, jitter, and shimmer in preschoolers who stutter. *Journal of Speech and Hearing Research, 35,* 1002–1008.

Hanson, W. (1969). *Vowel spectral noise levels and roughness severity ratings for vowels and sentences produced by adult males presenting abnormally rough voice.* Unpublished doctoral dissertation, University of Oklahoma, Norman.

Healey, E. C., Jones, R., & Berky, R. (1997). Effects of perceived listeners on speakers' vocal intensity. *Journal of Voice, 11,* 67–73.

Hecker, M. H. L., & Kreul, E. J. (1971). Descriptions of the speech of patients with cancer of the vocal folds. Part I: Measures of fundamental frequency. *Journal of the Acoustical Society of America, 49,* 1275–1282.

Heilberger, V. L., & Horii, Y. (1982). Jitter and shimmer in sustained phonation. In N.J. Lass (Ed.), *Speech and language: Advances in basic research and practice,* (Vol. 7 pp. 299–332). New York: Academic Press.

Heylen, L., Wuyts, F. L., Mertens, F., De Bodt, M., Pattyn, J., Croux, C., & Van de Heyning, P. H. (1998). Evaluation of the vocal performance of children using a voice range profile index. *Journal of Speech, Language, and Hearing Research, 41,* 232–238.

Hillenbrand, J. (1987). A methodological study of perturbation and additive noise in synthetically generated voice signals. *Journal of Speech and Hearing Research, 30,* 448–461.

Hirano, M. (1989). Objective evaluation of the human voice: Clinical aspects. *Folia Phoniatrica, 41,* 89–144.

Hirano, M., Hibi, S., Yoshida, Y., Hirade, Y., Kasuya, H., & Kikuchi, Y. (1988). Acoustic analysis of pathological voice. *Acta Otolaryngologica, 105,* 432–438.

Hixon, T. J. (1966). Turbulent noise sources for speech. *Folia Phoniatrica, 18,* 168–182.

Hixon, T. J., Minifie, F. D., & Tait, C. A. (1967). Correlates of turbulent noise production for speech. *Journal of Speech and Hearing Research, 10,* 133–140.

Holbrook, A., Rolnick, M. I., & Bailey, C. W. (1974). Treatment of vocal abuse disorders using a vocal intensity controller. *Journal of Speech and Hearing Disorders, 39,* 298–303.

Holmberg, E., Hillman, R. E., Perkell, J. S., & Gress, C. (1994). Relationships between intra-speaker variation in aerodynamic measures of voice production and variation in SPL across repeated recordings. *Journal of Speech and Hearing Research, 37,* 484–495.

Hoops, H. R., & Noll, J. D. (1969). Relationship of selected acoustic variables to judgments of esophageal speech. *Journal of Communication Disorders, 2,* 1–13.

Horii, Y. (1980). Vocal shimmer in sustained phonation. *Journal of Speech and Hearing Research, 23,* 202–209.

Horii, Y. (1982). Jitter and shimmer differences among sustained vowel phonations. *Journal of Speech and Hearing Research, 25,* 12–14.

Horii, Y., & Hata, K. (1988). A note on phase relationships between frequency and amplitude modulations in vocal vibrato. *Folia Phoniatrica, 40,* 303–311.

Horii, Y., & Weinberg, B. (1975). Intelligibility characteristics of superior esophageal speech presented under various levels of masking noise. *Journal of Speech and Hearing Research, 18,* 413–419.

House, A. S., & Fairbanks, G. (1953). The influence of consonant environment upon the secondary acoustical characteristics of vowels. *Journal of the Acoustical Society of America, 25,* 105–113.

Hyman, M. (1955). An experimental study of artificial larynx and esophageal speech. *Journal of Speech and Hearing Disorders, 20,* 291–299.

Illes, J., Metter, E. J., Hanson, W. R., & Iritani, S. (1988). Language production in Parkinson's disease: Acoustic and linguistic considerations. *Brain and Language, 33,* 146–160.

Isshiki, N. (1964). Regulatory mechanism of voice intensity variation. *Journal of Speech and Hearing Research, 7,* 17–29.

Isshiki, N. (1965). Vocal intensity and air flow rate. *Folia Phoniatrica, 17,* 92–104.

Isshiki, N. (1969). Remarks on mechanism for vocal intensity variation. *Journal of Speech and Hearing Research, 12,* 665–672.

Izdebski, K., & Murry, T. (1980). Glottal waveform variability: A preliminary inquiry. In V. Lawrence and B. Weinberg (Eds.), *Transcripts of the ninth symposium: Care of the professional voice,* (Vol. I pp. 39–43). New York: The Voice Foundation.

Jiang, J., Lin, E., & Hanson, D. G. (1998). Effect of tape recording on perturbation measures. *Journal of Speech, Language, and Hearing Research, 41,* 1031–1041.

Johnson, C. J., Pick, H. L., Jr., Siegel, G. M., Cicciarelli, A. W., & Garber, S. R. (1981). Effects of interpersonal distance on children's vocal intensity. *Child Development, 52,* 721–723.

Kallstrom, L. A. (1976). A small portion falls short. (Letter to the Editor.) *Asha, 18,* 879–800.

Karnell, M. P., Chiang, A., Smith, A., & Hoffman, H. (1997). Impact of signal type of [sic] validity of voice perturbation measures. *NCVS Status and Progress Report, 11,* 91–94.

Karnell, M., Hall, K., & Landahl, K. (1995). Comparison of fundamental frequency and perturbation measurements among three analysis systems. *Journal of Voice, 9,* 383–393.

Kempster, G. B., Kistler, D. J., & Hillenbrand, J. (1991). Multidimensional scaling analysis of dysphonia in two speaker groups. *Journal of Speech and Hearing Research, 34,* 544–548.

Kitajima, K., & Gould, W. J. (1976). Vocal shimmer in sustained phonation of normal and pathological voice. *Annals of Otolaryngology, 85,* 377–381.

Klingholz, F., & Martin, F. (1983). Die quantitative Auswertung der Stimmfeldmessung. *Sprache-Stimme-Gehör, 7,* 106–110.

Klingholz, F., & Martin, F. (1989). Distribution of the amplitude in the pathologic voice signal. *Folia Phoniatrica, 41,* 23–29.

Klingholz, F., Jolk, A., & Martin, F. (1989). Stimmfelduntersuchungen bei Knabenstimmen (Toölzer Knabenchor). *Sprache Stimme Gehör, 13,* 107–111.

Klingholz, F., Martin, F., & Jolk, A. (1985). Die Bestimmung der Registerbrüche aus dem Stimmfeld. *Sprache–Stimme-Gehör, 9,* 109–111.

Koike, Y. (1967). Experimental studies on vocal attack. *Practica Otologica Kyoto, 60,* 663–688.

Koike, Y. (1969). Vowel amplitude modulations in patients with laryngeal diseases. *Journal of the Acoustical Society of America, 45,* 839–844.

Koike, Y., Hirano, M., & von Leden, H. (1967). Vocal initiation: acoustic and aerodynamic investigations of normal subjects. *Folia Phoniatrica, 19,* 173–182.

Koike, Y., & Markel, J. (1975). Application of inverse filtering for detecting laryngeal pathology. *Annals of Otology, Rhinology, and Laryngology, 84,* 117–124.

Koike, Y., Takahashi, H., & Calcaterra, T. C. (1977). Acoustic measures for detecting laryngeal pathology. *Acta Oto-Laryngologica, 84,* 105–117.

Komiyama, S., Watanabe, H., Nishinow, S., & Yanai, O. (1977). A new phonometer. *Otologia (Fukuoka), 23,* 105–110.

Komiyama, S., Watanabe, H., & Ryu, S. (1984). Phonographic relationship between pitch and intensity of the human voice. *Folia Phoniatrica, 36,* 1–7.

Kramer, M. B. (1977). Kallstrom creates concern from a doctoral candidate. (Letter to the Editor.) *Asha, 19,* 225.

Large, J. (1979). An air flow study of vocal vibrato. In V. Lawrence (Ed.), *Transcripts of the eighth symposium: Care of the professional voice* (pp. 39–45). New York: The Voice Foundation.

Laver, J., Hiller, S., & Beck, J. M. (1992). Acoustic waveform perturbations and voice disorders. *Journal of Voice, 6,* 115–126. (Reprinted in *The gift of speech* (pp. 328–349) by J. Laver, 1991. Edinburgh, UK: Edinburgh University.)

Lee, B. S. (1950). Some effects of side-tone delay. *Journal of the Acoustical Society of America, 22,* 639–640.

Leeper, H. A., & Noll, J. D. (1972). Pressure measurements of articulatory behavior during alterations of vocal effort. *Journal of the Acoustical Society of America, 51,* 1291–1295.

Lehiste, I., & Peterson, G. E. (1959a). Linguistic considerations in the study of speech intelligibility. *Journal of the Acoustical Society of America, 31,* 280–286.

Lehiste, I., & Peterson, G. E. (1959b). Vowel amplitude and phonemic stress in American English. *Journal of the Acoustical Society of America, 31,* 428–435.

Levitt, H., & Bricker, P. D. (1970). Reduction of observer bias in reading speech levels with a VU meter. *Journal of the Acoustical Society of America, 47,* 1583–1587.

Lieberman, P. (1960). Some acoustic correlates of word stress in American English. *Journal of the Acoustical Society of America, 32,* 451–454.

Logemann, J. A., Fisher, H. B., Boshes, B., & Blonsky, E. R. (1978). Frequency and cooccurrence of vocal tract dysfunctions in the speech of a large sample of Parkinson patients. *Journal of Speech and Hearing Disorders, 43,* 47–57.

Luchsinger, R., & Arnold, G. (1965). *Voice-speech-language: Clinical communicology, Its physiology and pathology,* (Chapter 6). Belmont, CA: Wadsworth Publishing.

MacKay, D. G. (1968). Metamorphosis of a critical interval: Age-linked changes in the delay in auditory feedback that produces maximal disruption of speech. *Journal of the Acoustical Society of America, 43,* 811–821.

Malécot, A. (1966). The effectiveness of intra-oral air-pressure-pulse parameters in distinguishing between stop cognates. *Phonetica, 14,* 65–81.

Malécot, A. (1969). The effect of syllabic rate and loudness on the force of articulation of American stops and fricatives. *Phonetica, 19,* 205–216.

Markel, N. N., Prebor, L. D., & Brandt, J. F. (1972). Biosocial factors in dyadic communication: Sex and speaking intensity. *Journal of Personality and Social Psychology, 23,* 11–13.

Mason, R., & Zemlin, W. (1966). The phenomenon of vocal vibrato. *NATS Bulletin, 22,* 12–17.

McAllister, A., Sederholm, E., Sundberg, J., & Gramming, P. (1994). Relations between voice range profiles and physiological and perceptual voice characteristics in ten-year-old children. *Journal of Voice, 8,* 230–239.

McAllister, A., Sundberg, J., & Hibi, S. R. (1998). Acoustic measurements and perceptual evaluation of hoarseness in children's voices. *Logopedics Phoniatrics Vocology, 23,* 27–38.

Metter, E. J., & Hanson, W. R. (1986). Clinical and acoustical variability in hypokinetic dysarthria. *Journal of Communication Disorders, 19,* 347–366.

Michael, D. D., Siegel, G. M., & Pick, H. L., Jr. (1995). Effects of distance on vocal intensity. *Journal of Speech and Hearing Research, 38,* 1176–1183.

Michel, J., & Grashel, J. (1980). Vocal vibrato as a function of frequency and intensity. In V. Lawrence (Ed.), *Transcripts of the ninth symposium: Care of the professional voice* (pp. 45–48). New York: The Voice Foundation.

Michel, J. F., & Wendahl, R. (1971). Correlates of voice production. In L. E. Travis (Ed.), *Handbook of speech pathology and audiology,* chapter 18 (pp. 465–480). Englewood Cliffs, NJ: Prentice-Hall.

Milenkovic, P. (1987). Least mean square measures of voice perturbation. *Journal of Speech and Hearing Research, 30,* 529–538.

Murry, T., & Brown, W. S., Jr. (1971) Regulation of vocal intensity during vocal fry phonation. *Journal of the Acoustical Society of America, 49,* 1905–1907.

Neuschaefer-Rube, C. (1997). Comparison of voice performance in auditory and visually assisted phonetography. *Logopedics Phoniatrics Vocology, 22,* 3–8.

Neuschaefer-Rube, C., & Klajman, S. (1996). Computergestüzte 3D-Phonetographie. *HNO, 44,* 585–589.

Neuschaefer-Rube, C., Šram, F., & Klajman, S. (1997). Three-dimensional phonetographic assessment of voice performance in professional and non-professional speakers. *Folia Phoniatrica et Logopaedica, 49,* 96–104.

Niederjohn, R. J., & Haworth, D. G. (1983). The relationship between rms level and the average absolute magnitude of long-time continuous speech. *Journal of the Acoustical Society of America, 74,* 444–446.

Orlikoff, R. F., & Kahane, J. C. (1991). Influence of mean sound pressure level on jitter and shimmer measures. *Journal of Voice, 5,* 113–119.

Pabon, J. P. H., & Plomp, R. (1988). Automatic phonetogram recording supplemented with acoustical voice-quality parameters. *Journal of Speech and Hearing Research, 31,* 710–722.

Pahn, J., & Pahn, E. (1986). Die Nasalierungsmethode. *Logopädie und Phoniatrie, 58,* 126–132.

Pedersen, M. F. (1991). Computed phonetograms in adult patients with benign voice disorders before and after treatment with a nonsedating antihistamine (Loratadine). *Folia Phoniatrica, 43,* 60–67.

Pedersen, M. F. (1995). Stimmfunktion vor und nach Behandlung von Hirngeschädigten. Mit Stroboskopie, Phonetographie und Luftstromanalyse durchgefürt. *Sprache Stimme Gehör, 19,* 84–89.

Pedersen, M. F., Müller, S., Krabbe, S., Munk, E., Bennet, P., & Kitzing, P. (1984). Change of voice in puberty in choir girls. *Acta Otolaryngologica, Suppl. 412,* 46–49.

Pedersen, M. F., Munk, E., Bennet, P., & Müller, S. (1983). The change of voice during puberty in choir singers measured with phonetograms and compared to androgen status together with other other phenomena of puberty. *Proceedings of the Tenth International Congress of Phonetic Sciences,* 604–608.

Perry, C. K., Ingrisano, D. R.-S., & Blair, W. B. (1996). The influence of recording systems on jitter and shimmer estimates. *American Journal of Speech-Language Pathology, 5*(2), 86–89.

Peters, H. F., Boves, L., & van Dielen, I. C. (1986). Perceptual judgment of abruptness of voice onset in vowels as a function of the amplitude envelope. *Journal of Speech and Hearing Disorders, 51,* 299–308.

Pinto, N. B., & Titze, I. R. (1990). Unification of perturbation measures in speech signals. *Journal of the Acoustical Society of America, 87,* 1278–1289.

Pommez, J. (1962). Étude acoustique du vibrato de la voix chantée. *Revue de Laryngologie (Bordeaux), 83,* 249–264.

Ptacek, P. H., Sander, E. K., Maloney, W. H., & Jackson, C. C. R. (1966). Phonatory and related changes with advanced age. *Journal of Speech and Hearing Research, 9,* 353–360.

Ramig, L. O., Bonitati, C. M., Lemke, J. H., & Horii, Y. (1994). Voice therapy for patients with Parkinson's disease: Development of an approach and preliminary efficacy data. *Journal of Medical Speech-Language Pathology, 2,* 191–210.

Ramig, L. O., Countryman, S., Thompson, L. L., & Horii, Y. (1995). A comparison of two forms of intensive speech treatment for Parkinson disease. *Journal of Speech and Hearing Research, 38,* 1232–1251.

Ramig, L. O., & Dromey, C. (1996). Aerodynamic mechanisms underlying treatment-related changes in vocal intensity in patients with Parkinson disease. *Journal of Speech and Hearing Research, 39,* 798–807.

Rauhut, A., Stürzbecher, E., Wagner, H., & Seidner, W. (1979). Messung des Stimmfeldes. *Folia Phoniatrica, 31,* 110–119.

Read, C., Buder, E. H., & Kent, R. D. (1990). Speech analysis systems: A survey. *Journal of Speech and Hearing Research, 33,* 363–374.

Reich, A. R., Frederickson, R. R., Mason, J. A., & Schlauch, R. S. (1990a). Methodological variables affecting phonational frequency range in adults. *Journal of Speech and Hearing Disorders, 55,* 124–131.

Reich, A. R., Frederickson, R. R., Mason, J. A., & Schlauch, R. S. (1990b). Phonational frequency range: Reply to Awan and Mueller. *Journal of Speech and Hearing Disorders, 55,* 805–806.

Rekart, D. M., & Begnal, C. F. (1989). Acoustic characteristics of reticent speech. *Journal of Voice, 3,* 324–336.

Ringel, R. L., & Chodzko-Zajko, W. J. (1987). Vocal indices of biological age. *Journal of Voice, 1,* 31–37.

Ringel, R. L., House, A. S., & Montgomery, A. H. (1967). Scaling articulatory behavior: Intraoral air pressure. *Journal of the Acoustical Society of America, 42,* 1209A.

Robbins, J., Fisher, H. B., & Logemann, J. A. (1982). Acoustic characteristics of voice production after Staffieri's surgical reconstructive procedure. *Journal of Speech and Hearing Disorders, 47,* 77–84.

Robbins, J., Fisher, H. B., Logemann, J., Hillenbrand, J., & Blom, E. (1981, November). *A comparative acoustic analysis of laryngeal speech, esophageal speech, and speech production after tracheoesophageal puncture.* Paper presented at the annual convention of the American Speech and Hearing Association, Los Angeles, CA.

Robbins, J., Fisher, H., Blom, E., & Singer, M. I. (1984). A comparative acoustic study of normal, esophageal, and tracheoesophageal speech production. *Journal of Speech and Hearing Disorders, 49,* 202–210.

Rubin, H. J., LeCover, M., & Vennard, W. (1967). Vocal intensity, subglottic pressure, and air flow relationships in singers. *Folia Phoniatrica, 19,* 393–413.

Sacia, C. F., & Beck, C. J. (1926). The power of fundamental speech sounds. *Bell System Technology Journal, 5,* 393–403.

Sansone, F. E., Jr., & Emanuel, F. (1970). Spectral noise levels and roughness severity ratings for normal and simulated rough vowels produced by adult males. *Journal of Speech and Hearing Research, 13,* 489–502.

Schmidt, C. P., Gelfer, M. P., & Andrews, M. L. (1990). Intensity range as a function of task and training. *Journal of Voice, 4,* 30–36.

Schutte, H. K. (1980a). *The efficiency of voice production.* Groningen, the Netherlands: Rijksuniversiteit te Groningen.

Schutte, H. K. (1980b). Untersuchungen von Stimmqualitäten durch Phonetographie. *HNO-Praxis, 5,* 132–139.

Schutte, H. K., & Seidner, W. (1983). Recommendation by the Union of European Phoniatricians (UEP): Standardizing voice area measurement/phonetography. *Folia Phoniatrica, 35,* 286–288.

Seidner, W., Krüger, H., and Wernecke, K. (1985). Numerische Auswertung Spektraler Stimmfelder. *Sprache, Stimme, Gehör, 9,* 10–13.

Shaw, G. Y., Searl, J. P., Young, J. L., & Miner, P. B. (1996). Subjective, laryngoscopic, and acoustic measurements of laryngeal reflux before and after treatment with omeprazole. *Journal of Voice, 10,* 410–418.

Shipp, T. (1980). Variability in vibrato rate: extent and regularity. In V. Lawrence (Ed.), *Transcripts of the ninth symposium: Care of the professional voice* (pp. 44–45). New York: The Voice Foundation.

Shipp, T., Doherty, E. T., & Hakes, J. (1989). Mean frequency of vocal vibrato relative to target frequency. *Journal of Voice, 3,* 32–35.

Shipp, T., Leanderson, R., & Sundberg, J. (1979). Vocal vibrato. In V. Lawrence (Ed.), *Transcripts of the eighth symposium: Care of the professional voice* (pp. 46–49). New York: The Voice Foundation.

Shipp, T., Leanderson, R., & Sundberg, J. (1980). Some acoustic characteristics of vibrato. *Journal of Research in Singing, 4,* 18–25.

Shipp, T., Sundberg, J., & Doherty, E. T. (1988). The effect of delayed auditory feedback on vocal vibrato. *Journal of Voice, 2,* 195–199.

Siegel, G. M., Fehst, C. A., Garber, S. R., & Pick, H. L., Jr. (1980). Delayed auditory feedback with children. *Journal of Speech and Hearing Research, 23,* 802–813.

Sihvo, M., & Sala, E. (1996). Sound level variation findings for pianissimo and fortissimo phonations in repeated measurements. *Journal of Voice, 10,* 263–268.

Singer, M., and Blom, E. (1980). An endoscopic technique for restoration of voice after laryngectomy. *Annals of Otology, Rhinology, and Laryngology, 89,* 529–533.

Smith, S. (1980). *Die Akzentmethode und ihre theoretische Voraussetzungen.* Flensburg, Germany: Spezial-Pädagogische Verlag.

Snidecor, J. C., and Isshiki, N. (1965). Air volume and air flow relationships of six male esophageal speakers. *Journal of Speech and Hearing Disorders, 30,* 205–216.

Sorensen, D., and Horii, Y. (1983). Frequency and amplitude perturbation in the voices of female speakers. *Journal of Communication Disorders, 16,* 56–61.

Sorenson, D., and Horii, Y. (1984). Directional perturbation factors for jitter and for shimmer. *Journal of Communication Disorders, 17,* 143–151.

Speaks, C. E. (1996). *Introduction to sound: Acoustics for the hearing and speech sciences,* 2nd ed. San Diego, CA: Singular Publishing Group.

Staffieri, M., and Serafini, I. (1976). La riabilitazione chirurgica della voce e della respirazaione dopo laryngectomia totale. *Atti del 29 Congresso nazionale.* Bologna, Italy.

Stathopoulos, E. T., and Sapienza, C. M. (1997). Developmental changes in laryngeal and respiratory function with variations in sound pressure level. *Journal of Speech, Language, and Hearing Research, 40,* 595–614.

Steinberg, J. C., and Gardner, M. B. (1937). The dependence of hearing impairment on sound intensity. *Journal of the Acoustical Society of America, 9,* 11–23.

Stone, R. E., Jr., Bell, C. J., and Clack, T. D. (1978). Minimum intensity of voice at selected levels within pitch range. *Folia Phoniatrica, 30,* 113–118

Stone, R. E., Jr., and Ferch, P. A. K. (1982). Intra-subject variability in F_0-SPL_{min} voice profiles. *Journal of Speech and Hearing Disorders, 47,* 134–137.

Stone, R. E., Jr., and Krause, P. (1980). Intra-subject variability in minimum SPL of voice at selected fundamental frequencies. Paper presented at the annual convention of the American Speech and Hearing Association.

Stout, B. (1938). The harmonic structure of vowels in singing in relation to pitch and intensity. *Journal of the Acoustical Society of America, 10,* 137–146.

Sulter, A. M., and Meijer, J. M. (1996). Effects of voice training on phonetograms and maximum phonation times in female speech therapy students. In A. M. Sulter, *Variation of voice quality features and aspects of voice training in males and females* (pp. 133–147). Groningen, the Netherlands: Rijkuniversiteit Groningen.

Sulter, A. M., Schutte, H. K., and Miller, D. G. (1995). Differences in phonetogram features between male and female subjects with and without vocal training. *Journal of Voice, 9,* 363–377.

Sulter, A. M., Wit, H. P., Schutte, H. K., and Miller, D. G. (1994). A structured approach to voice range profile (phonetogram) analysis. *Journal of Speech and Hearing Research, 37,* 1076–1085. (Reprinted in A. M. Sulter (1996). *Variation of voice quality features and effects of voice training in males and females* (Chapter 7). Groningen, the Netherlands: Rijksuniversiteit Groningen.)

Sundberg, J., Titze, I., and Scherer, R. (1993). Phonatory control in male singing: A study of the effects of subglottal pressure, fundamental frequency, and mode of phonation on the voice source. *Journal of Voice, 7,* 15–29.

Takahashi, H., and Koike, Y. (1975). Some perceptual dimensions and acoustical correlates of pathologic voices. *Acta Oto-Laryngologica, suppl. 338*, 1–24.

Tanaka, S., and Gould, W. J. (1983). Relationships between vocal intensity and noninvasively obtained aerodynamic parameters in normal subjects. *Journal of the Acoustical Society of America, 73*, 1316–1321.

Till, J. A., Jafari, M., Crumley, R. L., and Law-Till, C. B. (1992). Effects of initial consonant, pneumotachographic mask, and oral pressure tube on vocal perturbations, harmonics-to-noise, and intensity measurements. *Journal of Voice, 6*, 217–223.

Titze, I. R. (1984). Parameterization of the glottal area, glottal flow, and vocal fold contact area. *Journal of the Acoustical Society of America, 75*, 570–580.

Titze, I. R. (1989). On the relation between subglottal pressure and fundamental frequency in phonation. *Journal of the Acoustical Society of America, 85*, 901–906.

Titze, I. R. (1992a). Phonation threshold pressure: A missing link in glottal aerodynamics. *Journal of the Acoustical Society of America, 91*, 2926–2935.

Titze, I. R. (1992b). Acoustic interpretation of the voice range profile (phonetogram). *Journal of Speech and Hearing Research, 35*, 21–34.

Titze, I. R. (1994). *Principles of voice production*. Englewood Cliffs, NJ: Prentice-Hall.

Titze, I. R. (1995). *Workshop on acoustic voice analysis: Summary statement*. Iowa City, IA: National Center for Voice and Speech.

Titze, I. R., Horii, Y., and Scherer, R. C. (1987). Some technical considerations in voice perturbation measurements. *Journal of Speech and Hearing Research, 30*, 252–260.

Titze, I. R., Jiang, J. J, and Druker, D. (1988). Preliminaries to the body-cover theory of pitch control. *Journal of Voice, 1*, 314–319.

Titze, I. R., Wong, D., Milder, M. A., Hensley, S. R., and Ramig, L. O. (1995). Comparison between clinician-assisted and fully automated procedures for obtaining a voice range profile. *Journal of Speech and Hearing Research, 38*, 526–535.

van den Berg, J., and Moolenaar-Bijl, A. J. (1959). Cricopharyngeal sphincter, pitch, intensity, and fluency in oesophageal speech. *Practica Oto-Rhino-Laryngologica, 21*, 298–315.

Veldkamp, K. (1965). *De techniek van het spreken*. Groningen, the Netherlands: Wolters-Noordhoff.

Verdolini-Marston, K., Sandage, M., and Titze, I. R. (1994). Effect of hydration treatments on laryngeal nodules and polyps and related voice measures. *Journal of Voice, 8*, 30–47.

Verdolini-Marston, K., Titze, I. R., and Druker, D. G. (1990). Changes in phonation threshold pressure with induced conditions of hydration. *Journal of Voice, 4*, 142–151.

Villchur, E., and Killion, M. C. (1975). Probe-tube microphone assembly. *Journal of the Acoustical Society of America, 57*, 238–240.

von Leden, H., and Koike, Y. (1970). Detection of laryngeal disease by computer technique. *Archives of Otolaryngology, 91*, 3–10.

Ward, W. D. (1977). . . . from an acoustician. (Letter to the Editor.) *Asha, 19*, 226.

Weatherley, C. C., Worrall, L. E., and Hickson, L. M. H. (1997). The effect of hearing impairment on the vocal characteristics of older people. *Folia Phoniatrica et Logopaedica, 49*, 53–62.

Weiner, J. B., Lee, L., Cataland, J., and Stemple, J. C. (1996). An assessment of pitch-matching abilities among speech-language pathology graduate students. *American Journal of Speech-Language Pathology, 5*(2), 91–95.

Wendahl, R. W. (1966a). Some parameters of auditory roughness. *Folia Phoniatrica, 18*, 26–32.

Wendahl, R. W. (1966b). Laryngeal analog synthesis of jitter and shimmer auditory parameters of harshness. *Folia Phoniatrica, 18*, 98–108.

Wente, E. C., Bedell, E. H., and Swartzel, K. D., Jr. (1935). A high speed level recorder for acoustic measurements. *Journal of the Acoustical Society of America, 6*, 121–129.

Wilson, J. V., and Leeper, H. A. (1992). Changes in laryngeal airway resistance in young adult men and women as a function of vocal sound pressure level and syllable context. *Journal of Voice, 6*, 235–245.

Winholtz, W. S., and Titze, I. R. (1997a). Miniature head-mounted microphone for voice perturbation analysis. *Journal of Speech and Hearing Research, 40*, 894–899.

Winholtz, W. S. and Titze, I. R. (1997b). Conversion of a head-mounted microphone signal into calibrated SPL units. *Journal of Voice, 11*, 417–421.

Winckel, F. (1953). Physikalische Kriterien für objektive Stimmbeurteilung. *Folia Phoniatrica, 5*, 232–252.

Wolf, S. K., and Sette, W. J. (1935). Some applications of modern acoustic apparatus. *Journal of the Acoustical Society of America, 6*, 160–168.

Wolf, S. K., Stanley, D., and Sette, W. J. (1935). Quantitative studies on the singing voice. *Journal of the Acoustical Society of America, 6*, 255–266.

Wolfe, V., Fitch, J., and Cornell, R. (1995). Acoustic prediction of severity in commmonly occurring voice problems. *Journal of Speech and Hearing Research, 38*, 273–279.

Wolfe, V., and Martin, D. (1997). Acoustic correlates of dysphonia: Type and severity. *Journal of Communication Disorders, 30*, 403–416.

Wong, D., Lange, R., Titze, I., and Guo, C. G. (1995). Mechanisms of jitter-induced shimmer in a driven model of vocal fold vibration. *NCVS Status and Progress Report, 8*, 33–41.

Zaveri, K. (1971). Conventional and on-line methods of sound power measurements. *B & K Technical Review, 3*, 3–27.

Zue, A., and Mueller, P. B. (1997). Acoustic and perceptual characteristics of the voices of sedentary and physically active elderly speakers. *Logopedics Phoniatrics Vocology 22*, 51–60.

6

Vocal Fundamental Frequency

There is long-standing and widespread agreement that pitch is an important factor—perhaps etiologically and certainly symptomatically—in voice disorders (Fairbanks, 1940; Brodnitz, 1961; Luchsinger & Arnold, 1965; West & Ansberry, 1968; Boone, 1971; Cooper, 1971; Moore, 1971; Perkins, 1971a, 1971b; Stone & Sharf, 1973; Okamoto, Yoshida, Tanimoto, Takyu, & Inoue, 1984; Hirano, 1989; Andrews, 1991; Hirano, Tanaka, Fujita, & Terasawa, 1991, Harris, Harris, Rubin, & Howard, 1998). This vocal attribute has traditionally been evaluated solely according to the therapist's perception and estimate of magnitude, generally on a low-to-high continuum. The perception then formed the basis of a rather crude adequacy judgment: too high, normal, too low, erratic, and so on.

A purely perceptual assessment is likely to be inadequate. The descriptive terms are crude and unstandardized. They are also incapable of resolving moderately small differences. Listeners' judgments of pitch have been found to be unreliable (Laguaite & Waldrop, 1964; Montague, Hollien, Hollien, & Wold, 1978). As Brodnitz (1961, p. 51) has pointed out, conclusions about adequacy or acceptability are very likely to be influenced by "personal tastes, preferences of fashion in voices . . . and personal identifications." Beyond this lies the very important fact that pitch is not, by any means, the simple perception of fundamental frequency—the rate at which the vocal folds are oscillating, which is usually what needs to be known. Rather, the frequency, intensity, and spectral properties of a sound interact in very complex ways to lead to a pitch perception that may be a very poor reflection of the F_0 (Houtsma & Goldstein 1972; Goldstein, 1973). In a study of vocal change following treatment for myasthenia gravis, for example, Maxwell and Locke (1969, p. 1904) noted that "perception of pitch and measurement of fundamental frequency were in marked disagreement, not just in magnitude of discrepancy but also in direction of shift" between the pre- and post-treatment observations. Fletcher and Munson (1933), Fletcher (1934), Licklider (1951), and Pierce (1983) provide good elementary discussions of basic aspects of the phenomena of pitch perception, while the work of Shepard (1964) and Deutsch (1992) highlight some unsuspected and surprising oddities of pitch perception. The curves derived by Fletcher (1934) show the influence of intensity quite clearly. The perceived pitch of a tone changes as the loudness changes—and the effect is maximal in the expected range of human vocal pitch.

These considerations lead to two conclusions. First, perceptual judgments alone may well mislead the clinician. Perceived abnormality of pitch may, for instance, partly reflect the speaker's vocal intensity, and vice versa. The judgment of unacceptablility may betray clinicians' attitudes as well as patients' deviance. Comparison to a norm requires that both the norm and the behavior in question be based on unbiased and objective scales if the factors contributing to the final vocal product are to be understood and addressed in therapy. So, while it is likely to be important that the therapist judge vocal pitch acceptability, it is vital that the fundamental frequency be measured.

Second, the terms **pitch** and **frequency** should be kept separate and distinct. Even a casual survey of the literature of voice production shows that they are quite commonly interchanged.[1] The confusion that results may have meaningful clinical consequences. The terms will be differentiated in this chapter. Pitch will refer to a perceptual attribute of sound, generally scaled on a high-low continuum. Frequency, on the other hand, will always be used to refer to a physical attribute of certain signals: essentially, the repetition rate of a recurring waveshape.

It was not very long ago that fundamental frequency measurements were difficult, time consuming, and often quite expensive to obtain. The advent first of sophisticated analog instruments and then of computer technology has changed all of that. As long as the measurement technique and its limitations are well understood it is now simple to find a measurement method that will meet the needs of almost any clinical setting.

PERIODICITY

Measurement of fundamental frequency depends critically on the assumption that the signal is at least approximately **periodic**. A signal is said to be periodic if it is characterized by a recurring waveform that repeats itself *exactly* at a fixed and unvarying rate. Whether the recurring waveform is simple or complex is immaterial. What matters is that it repeats itself without variation, and that it does so at a constant rate. Each repetition of the waveform is referred to as a **cycle**. Given the requirement of invariance of waveshape and of repetition rate, it is clear that to see one cycle of a periodic signal is to see all cycles.

The shape of a waveform represents the variation of some property (voltage, pressure, or airflow, for example) as a function of time, *f(t)*. With this in mind Titze (1994, pp. 87–88, 1995, p. 8) offers a slightly more formal definition of periodicity. "A series of events is termed periodic if the events cannot be distinguished

---

[1] The confusion is perhaps encouraged by the standard use of "pitch" and "pitch period" for frequency and period in the electrical engineering literature.

from one another by shifting time forward or backward by a specific interval, nT_0,

$$f(t \pm nT_0) = f(t),$$

where n is any positive integer" and T_0 is the duration of a single repetition, or cycle.

Figure 6–1 illustrates periodic and non-periodic waveforms. Signal A satisfies Titze's definition, and is thus periodic. If any one of the cycles is slid left or right (earlier or later in time) by the proper distance it will *exactly* coincide with the cycle next to it. Sliding it again by the same distance will cause it to coincide exactly with the next cycle in the series, and so on. Hence, the original cycle is indistinguishable from any other cycle that is a multiple of a fixed distance (in time) away.

Signal B, however, is clearly radically different. No amplitude variation is exactly like any other in either amplitude or duration. It is said to be **aperiodic**. In fact,

it is stereotypically so in that it is the kind of signal one intuitively imagines when the term aperiodic is used.

Wavetrains C, D, and E have the appearance of periodicity because they appear quite regular. In each of them, however, there is a momentary deviation from perfect repetition. In C one of the cycles (beginning at 0.6 s) is shorter than the others. In D periodicity is violated by a cycle (at 0.3 s) whose amplitude is reduced. And in E the shape of the cycle beginning at 0.3 s is different from that of the others in the series.[2]

Technically, none of the signals represented by C, D, or E is periodic. One senses, however, that they are "almost" so. There is a feeling that, in the technical sense, these signals may not be periodic *but* . . . Signals that are almost periodic—that have only some slight deviation from perfect repetition—are often referred to as **quasiperiodic**. While the term literally translates as "almost periodic," the fact is that, strictly speaking, it is properly applied only to the situation in which a waveform represents a combination of two or more periodic signals whose frequency relationship to each other cannot be expressed by an integer ratio. (When this is the case the component frequencies are said to be **incommensurate**.) Titze (1995, p. 8), apparently sensing that there is already enough terminological confusion, suggests that the term quasiperiodic be avoided (except when it is strictly applicable) and that **nearly periodic** be used instead. That convention will be adopted in this text. The characteristics of some nearly-periodic signals will be discussed under the heading *Near-Periodicity*.

Units of Measurement

The fundamental frequency, denoted F_0, is the rate at which a waveform is repeated per unit time. Older literature measures frequency in **cycles per second** (cps), but a special frequency unit, the **hertz**, has since been universally adopted. One hertz (Hz) is equal to one cycle per second.[3] The **period** (denoted t) is the duration of a single cycle. Frequency and period are therefore mutually reciprocal:

$$t = 1/F_0$$
$$F_0 = 1/t.$$

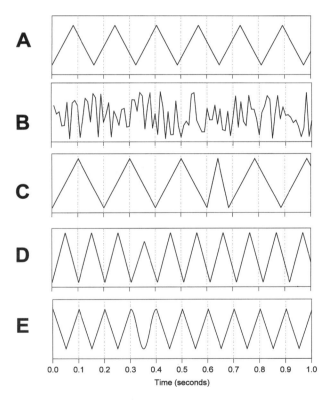

Figure 6–1. Periodicity and aperiodicity. While A is clearly periodic, and B is clearly aperiodic, C, D, and E, are "almost" periodic.

Some of the methods discussed in this chapter depend on counting the number of cycles per second—that is,

---

[2] Period (or frequency) and amplitude perturbation are known as *jitter* and *shimmer*, respectively, and are commonly measured for clinical purposes. Waveshape perturbation has no common name, and has only rarely been considered in the clinical literature. (But see Feijoo and Hernández, 1990.)

[3] Note that "Hz" is a *symbol*, not an abbreviation. It is therefore not followed by a period.

they measure frequency in Hz. Others determine the length of the period (generally given in milliseconds). To know one value is to know the other.

FUNDAMENTAL FREQUENCY AND PITCH

In general, pitch (a perceptual attribute of sound) increases with fundamental frequency (a physical parameter of vibration). But the relationship is not linear. The auditory system is more sensitive to some frequency changes than to others (Stevens, Volkmann, & Newman, 1937; Stevens & Volkmann, 1940). In particular, the average listener is more sensitive to changes at lower frequencies. Raising F_0 from 100 Hz to 200 Hz results in a much greater change in perceived pitch than going from 3000 Hz to 3100 Hz. The standard musical scale reflects this fact. For example the frequency of C below middle C is 65.41 Hz, while the D below middle C, perceived to be one note higher, is 73.42 Hz. A change of one note requires an increase of a bit more than 8 Hz. But going from the C *above* middle C to the D *above* middle C entails a frequency shift from 261.6 Hz to 293.7 Hz, four times as much. The semitone scale reflects this situation by an exponential growth function.[4] That is, the difference in semitones between two frequencies grows more slowly as frequency increases. The relationship is graphically illustrated in Figure 6–2.

SEMITONE SCALING

On the semitone scale, raising a frequency, f_1, by n semitones (ST) results in a higher frequency, f_2, according to the relationship

$$f_2 = (12\sqrt{2})^n f_1.$$

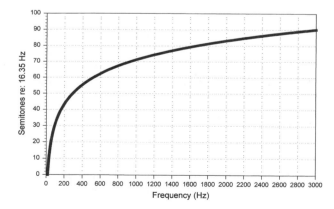

Figure 6–2. Relationship of semitones to frequency.

For example, the frequency ($n =$) 6 semitones above ($f1 =$) 100 Hz is

$$f_2 = (12\sqrt{2})^6 f_1$$
$$f_2 = (1.059463)^6 \, (100)$$
$$f_2 = 1.414(100)$$
$$f_2 = 141.4 \text{ Hz}$$

The semitone difference, n, between two frequencies, f_1 and f_2, is given by

$$n = \frac{12(\log_{10} f_2 - \log_{10} f_1)}{\log_{10} 2}$$

A mathematically equivalent form is

$$n = \frac{12\log_{10}(f_2/f_1)}{\log_{10} 2}$$

This formula can be made somewhat less intimidating by reducing the constants:

$$\log_{10} 2 = 0.30103 \text{ and}$$
$$12/\log_{10} 2 = 39.86.$$

Therefore we have

$$n = 39.86 \, (\log_{10} f_2 - \log_{10} f_1) \text{ or}$$
$$n = 39.86 \, \log_{10}(f_2/f_1).$$

So, for example, the semitone difference between ($f_1 =$) 200 Hz and ($f_2 =$) 400 Hz is

$$n = \frac{12(\log_{10} 400 - \log_{10} 200)}{\log_{10} 2)}$$
$$n = \frac{12(2.6020 - 2.3010)}{0.3010}$$
$$n = \frac{12(0.3010)}{0.3010}$$
$$n = 12 \text{ semitones.}$$

That is, 400 Hz is 12 semitones higher than 200 Hz. This is, of course, the expected answer: doubling a frequency is equivalent to raising the tone one octave. There are 12 semitones in an octave.

---

[4] This is **not** to say that semitone values actually scale perceived pitch. The perceptual "mel" scale values can only be derived by asking listeners to assign pitch values to tones. The underlying perceptual processes are too irregular to be expressed in any simple mathematical formula.

If the semitone scale is to be used for more than frequency comparisons, some frequency must be assigned a semitone value of 0. This done, the scale becomes definite and absolute. Fletcher (1934) proposed that zero semitones be set at 16.35 Hz, which has the effect of making all musical Cs integral multiples of 12 semitones. Also, 16.35 Hz is representative of the lower frequency limit of human hearing.

The semitone scale, then, was devised for much the same reasons as the dB scale, to which it is obviously analogous. Its ability to simplify inter-subject comparisons and its utility in quantifying frequency variations, coupled with its foundations in the familiar Western musical scale, have made it quite popular among phonatory researchers. It is encountered often in the literature of voice production.

NEAR-PERIODICITY

Natural sounds (including, and more to the point, vocal sounds) are never strictly periodic. More than 70 years ago Simon (1927, p. 83) noted that "there are no tones of constant pitch in either vocal or instrumental sounds." There is always at least some minimal cycle-to-cycle variation. Therefore, clinical evaluation of fundamental frequency is at best a matter of dealing with a nearly-periodic signal. There are many ways in which signals can deviate from periodicity, and several are of particular concern to clinicians.

Random Variation

Figure 6–3 shows the sound pressure (top trace) and EGG (middle trace) records of a normal middle-aged male sustaining the vowel /ɑ/ at comfortable pitch and loudness. The duration of each phonatory cycle has been measured, converted to F_0 and plotted at the bottom. Two features of this F_0 record are typical of normal phonation. First, while the fundamental frequency is relatively stable, it is not completely so: there is slight variation from one cycle to the next. Second, the cycle-to-cycle variations show no evident pattern; they appear to be random. Because of this, the F_0 of this sample is well described by its mean (which happens to be 112.6 Hz, and is represented as a dotted line) and its standard deviation (which is 1.4 Hz).

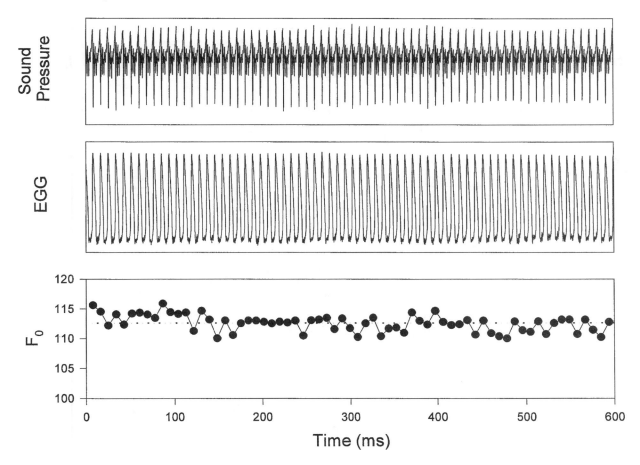

Figure 6–3. Normal phonation, exemplified by the sound pressure and electroglottographic records, is characterized by slight random variation of fundamental frequency.

Modulation of F₀

A signal is said to be *modulated* when one of its properties (most commonly its frequency or its amplitude) changes in proportion to the magnitude of some controlling variable. The fundamental frequency of the voice, for example, might be altered by changing the tension applied to the vocal folds. The controlled signal is called the *carrier* signal, while the controlling phenomenon is the *modulating* signal. The voice is subject to modulation for communicative purposes (such as lexical stress or intonation contouring), but may also show modulation that is not intentional.

The vocal sample evaluated in Figure 6–4 shows a relatively constant fall of F_0. While not usually thought of as such, this represents a special case of vocal modulation: there is a steady change of some controlling variable (perhaps the contractile state of the cricothyroid muscle) over the duration of the sample. Although the mean (dotted line, 139.2 Hz) and standard deviation (9.84) are valid descriptors of this sample, they do not convey its essential characteristic of steady change. For that the slope of the regression line (plotted here as

a line among the F_0 data points) is required. (For this sample it is about 0.165 Hz/ms.)

A different, more complex pattern of modulation (and one that is likely to be more clinically significant) is shown in Figure 6–5, where the F_0 varies in a fairly regular cyclic (essentially sinusoidal) way, perhaps resulting from tremor of one or more of the laryngeal muscles. At a minimum, what is needed to describe this F_0 record is its mean (which is an estimate of the "baseline" frequency about which the variations occur —in this case it is about 122.5 Hz), the extent of the F_0 variations about the mean (here on the order of ±10 Hz which, in a way, is a measure of the magnitude of the underlying causative phenomenon), and the cycle length (about 203 ms, or about 5 per second).

Subharmonic (Period Doubling) Oscillation

Under some circumstances (which, at present, remain only poorly understood) phonation is characterized by cycles that show a regular alternation of two periods or amplitudes (or of both). This pattern results from the

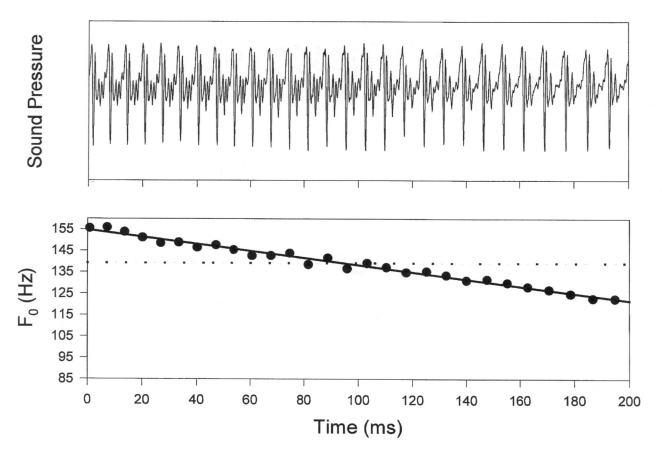

Figure 6–4. The lower trace shows the fundamental frequency of each period in the sound pressure record at the top. The normal random variation of fundamental frequency are superimposed on a falling F_0 contour.

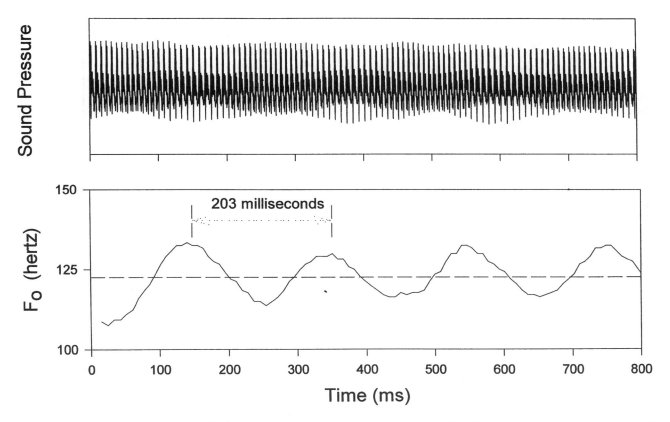

Figure 6–5. Upper trace: sustained vowel by a dysphonic male. Lower trace: plotting the fundamental frequency of each glottal cycle shows a cyclic variation of F_0. The extent of the frequency modulation is on the order of ± 10 Hz, and the rate of modulation is about 5 per second.

presence of a frequency of one half the fundamental ($F_0/2$) in the spectrum of the signal, and is thus called a **subharmonic** oscillation. Alternatively, of course, one could say that there is a component of the signal with a period that is twice the fundamental period ($2T_0$), which explains the alternate name, **period doubling**, for this phenomenon.

Viewed from a different perspective, it is clear that there are two ways of measuring the period of this waveform. Either each component oscillation could be seen as a cycle, or each pair of oscillations can be considered a single repetition of the waveform. In the first case the F_0 is the number of oscillations, but the alternation of two different oscillatory varieties creates a one-for-two component, which obviously occurs at half the rate of the oscillations, and hence has a frequency of $F_0/2$.

In the clinical literature vocal periodicity of this sort has been called **diplophonia, dichrotic phonation** or, occasionally, **biphonation**. However, it is probably better to adopt the terminology that is current in the science of nonlinear dynamics and refer to this phenomenon as a **period−2** sequence. The basis for this terminological choice is explored more completely in the next section.

Period-n and Chaotic Oscillation

In recent years the insights and analytical methods of the science of nonlinear dynamics have increasingly been applied to the study of voice production (Awrejcewicz, 1990; Baken, 1990, 1991, 1994a, 1994b, 1995a, 1995b; Herzel, Steinecke, Mende, & Wermke, 1991; Herzel, Berry, Titze, & Saleh, 1994; Herzel, 1993, 1996; Wong, Ito, Cox, & Titze, 1991; Titze, Baken, & Herzel, 1993; Kakita & Olkamoto, 1994; Steincke & Herzel, 1995; Behrman & Baken, 1997). That application has resulted in new ways of looking at many of the features of vocal signals and, in particular, has generated an appreciation of some of the complex patterning that may be buried in apparently-random F_0 contours.

A close look at the periodicity of abnormal phonation often reveals that period-2 oscillations are not the only pattern of regular irregularity to be found. Figure 6–6, for instance, plots the fundamental frequencies of successive cycles in the phonation of three individuals with spasmodic dysphonia, all of whom show brief bursts of period-n phenomena (circled). Sample A shows two different patterns of period-3 oscillation, while samples B and C demonstrate two different pat-

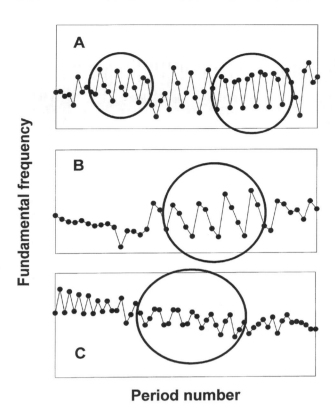

Figure 6–6. Patterned, and very rapid, variation of F_0, exemplifying period–3 and period–4 oscillation.

terns of period-4 oscillation. Much more complex period-n behavior is often found intermittently in disordered phonation.

It is very unlikely that the F_0 patterns of these samples are produced by contractions (voluntary or otherwise) of the laryngeal musculature or by shifts in driving pressures. They are simply too rapid to be accounted for by the ordinary physiological processes that control phonation. Rather, it is now widely accepted that these sudden changes in the qualitative characteristics of the phonatory system's behavior are **bifurcations**, and are evidence of **chaos** in the phonatory system. Note that the term *chaos* is strictly defined in the science of nonlinear dynamical systems, and must not be taken in its colloquial sense of "completely without order." Although they may superficially appear

to function randomly, chaotic systems are, in fact, organized, but the underlying deterministic principle is often deeply hidden.[5] The implication is that, in many cases, vocal irregularity may ultimately be found to have an identifiable basis in the dynamics of the phonatory system. (In fact, even some normal phenomena of vocal production, such as register transitions [Lucero, 1996], may well turn out to have their explanations in chaos theory.) This, in turn, may open the way to controlling deviant oscillatory behavior. Some elementary means of probing for chaotic characteristics of phonatory signals will be considered later in this chapter.

Signal Types

If acoustic analysis of vocal signals—including estimation of fundamental frequency—is to be meaningful it is important that the vocal signal have characteristics adequate for the analysis to be performed. (It is not possible, for instance, to measure the F_0 of an aperiodic signal. F_0, after all, specifies the rate at which a cyclic waveform repeats; aperiodic signals have no repetitive waveform and hence can have no F_0.[6])

It is important, therefore, to recognize that there are qualitatively different kinds of vocal signals and to deal with each appropriately. Along these lines Titze (1995) has proposed that vocal signals be grouped into three major categories. In addition, it seems reasonable to recognize subtypes within each of Titze's groups, and these have been added in italics.

Type 1: Nearly periodic (or, in the ideal case, periodic) waveforms that do not undergo qualitative changes during the time interval to be analyzed. Any modulating or subharmonic frequencies that may be present have an energy that is at least one order of magnitude less than that of the fundamental frequency.

Subtype A: minor random variation of F_0 *or waveshape;*

Subtype B: minor monotonic modulation (that is, F_0 *or amplitude steadily increasing or decreasing);*

Subtype C: minor cyclic variation (modulation) of F_0 *or amplitude.*

---

[5] The science of nonlinear dynamics ("chaos theory") is likely to have a very powerful influence on the development of our understanding of abnormal laryngeal function. It is, however, a very complex subject. Because it has recently been a "hot" topic, the recent past has seen the proliferation of books and articles on the subject. Among the better general sources for those wishing to explore more deeply are Holden (1986), Thompson and Stewart (1986), Moon (1987), Cvitanovic (1989), Baker and Gollub (1990), and Krasner (1990). Gleick (1987) is the classic (and entertaining) text for those wanting a nonmathematical overview of the area.

[6] A computer-based speech analysis system might, in fact, calculate the putative "F_0" of *any* signal—even if it is aperiodic! That does not mean that the number displayed is actually a F_0 value or that it has any meaning at all. It simply underscores the importance of the user's attention to, responsibility for, and evaluation of, the system's functioning.

Type 2: Signals that have sudden qualitative changes (that is, bifurcations) in the interval to be analyzed, or that have modulating or subharmonic frequencies whose energy is comparable to that of the fundamental frequency. Although Type 2 signals are clearly ordered and organized, there is no single F_0 value that validly characterizes the entire segment analyzed.

Subtype A: signal bifurcation(s) present;

Subtype B: F_0 or amplitude discontinuity;

Subtype C: large-scale modulation of F_0.

Type 3: Without apparent periodicity, and hence not validly susceptible to F_0 measurement. Type 3 signals may, however, be chaotic, implying that there is a covert organizing principle that might be discoverable through the techniques of dynamical systems theory.

Subtype A: no observable structure;

Subtype B: deep-level (chaotic) organization.

Evaluation of a signal's fundamental frequency necessarily presupposes that it should, within reasonable limits, be classifiable as Type I, subtype A. However, occasional discontinuities may not have as seriously deleterious an effect on the quantification of variability, at least as achieved by some software packages, as was previously generally believed (Karnell, Chang, Smith, & Hoffman, 1997).

MEASURING FUNDAMENTAL FREQUENCY

In the "old days" there were a limited number of options available for measuring F_0. An absence of sophisticated equipment led to a number of approaches to the problem, some of them quite ingenious. Even those with no measurement instruments at all, for instance, were able to visualize and count magnetic regions on recording tape (Black, 1949; Leeper & Leeper, 1976; Mueller, Adams, Baehr-Rouse, & Boos, 1979) and thereby to obtain an estimate of F_0. Thanks to the digital computer, there are now a very large number of ways of measuring the duration of vocal periods, and hence of evaluating F_0. The implementation of different measurement methods is likely to account for the variation in values returned by different measuring systems (Read, Buder, & Kent, 1990; Read, Buder, and Kent, 1992; Hakel, Healey, & Sullivan, 1994; Morris & Brown, 1996). While it is impossible to discuss them all in detail, this section will consider the basic principles of several different approaches to the problem.

Estimating F_0 from an Oscilloscope Trace

It is not unusual to need an approximate value of F_0, rather than a precise measurement of it. When this is the case there is no need to resort to an elaborate analytic program: an adequate estimate can usually be obtained from an oscilloscopic display of the vocal waveform (or of one of its correlates). The method is simple and fast, and commonly serves clinical purposes quite well. Figure 6–7 illustrates what is required.

The signal whose frequency is to be estimated is displayed on the screen. (In Figure 6–7 the electroglottographic waveform has been used, since its relatively simple shape makes the task easier.) An oscilloscope screen is partitioned into divisions, each representing an amount of time, according to the sweep-speed chosen by the user. In the figure each vertical division represents 10 milliseconds. Since there are 8 vertical divisions in the display, the screen shows a total of 80 ms of the vocalization that is to be evaluated.

The task now is to count the number of cycles shown. Note that, in the figure, the first wave on the left begins at what appears to be the very start of its rising portion. Reading the display to the right, the start of the next rising excursion signals the end of the first cycle and the start of the second. Repeating the processes eventually brings us near the right edge of the display, at which point 10 complete cycles will have been counted. There still remains a part of a cycle, and we may estimate by eye that it is approximately ¼ of a wave.

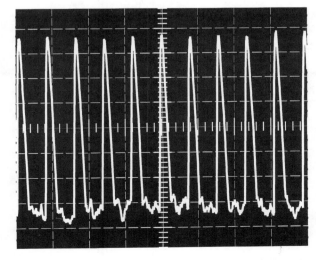

10 mS / div

Figure 6–7. Electroglottographic waveform as shown on an oscilloscope screen.

There are thus about 10¼ cycles in a display that covers 80 ms of time. On average, then, each cycle has a duration, or period, of 80/10.25 ≈ 7.8 ms. The frequency is the reciprocal of the period, so the average F_0 of this sample is 1/0.0078 s ≈ 128 Hz. This estimate is within one or two hertz of the true average value, which is certainly good enough for everyday clinical purposes.

Strategies for Measuring F_0

Whether implemented with analog instrumentation or (as is more common today) by means of digital computation, there are certain broad categories of approach to the problem of F_0 measurement. A number of these classes are considered here in terms of analog processing (where appropriate) and their equivalent digital algorithms.[7]

ZERO-CROSS DETECTION

A sine- or other simple wave crosses the zero axis twice during every cycle: once in a positive-going and once in a negative-going direction. The simplest way to measure its frequency is to count the number of zero crossings in one direction or the other per second. It happens that this is very easy to accomplish with analog circuitry. The basic plan is schematized in Figure 6–8. The signal to be evaluated is applied to one input of a circuit that converts it, by using great amplification and signal clipping, to a series of square pulses. A high-pass filter (see Chapter 2, "Analog Electronics") is then used to isolate the square-wave transition regions, producing a series of negative- and positive-going spikes that represent the "upward" and "downward" zero crosses of the input. A rectifier selects spikes of one direction or the other (positive-going in the figure) and these are passed to a

counter which tallies the number of spikes per second. The fundamental frequency of the input wave is shown by the counter's output.

The practical problem, of course, is that most signals—and especially speech signals—are not simple waves. They usually cross the zero axis several times in each cycle. This situation is shown in Figure 6–9, which plots the sound pressure record of a vowel sustained by a dysphonic female. Approximately one cycle is shown in the upper record, where the zero-volt level is indicated by the dotted line. Counting the number of zero crosses for this wave would result in a grossly invalid measure of F_0, since there are, in fact, more than one zero-axis crossings in the cycle. But we can take advantage of the fact that this particular wave has a single,

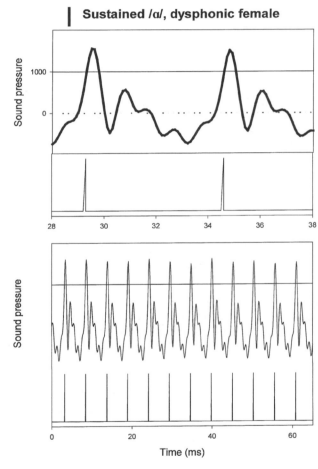

Figure 6–9. Top: A speech waveform and, below it, the signal from a circuit that produces a pulse whenever the waveform crosses the 1000 (A/D units) line. Bottom: A longer segment of the same phonation, demonstrating the demarcation of vocal periods by the "zero–cross" detector.

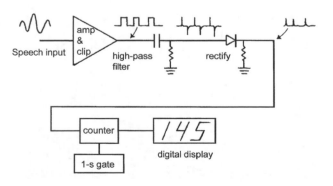

Figure 6–8. Scheme for measuring F_0 by counting zero crossings.

---

[7] Despite the ascendancy of the digital computer, there are probably a meaningful number of analog systems still in daily use. It is usually possible to interface them to a computer. See Horii (1983a) for an example.

relatively distinct, major peak in each cycle. All we need to do to get a valid "zero-cross" detection of each period is to use a value other than zero. Inspection of the original data suggests that, in this case, finding the points at which the waveform crosses the 1000 point[8] (for the case shown, in the positive-going direction) would result in a valid marking of each cycle. The resulting "1000-cross" markers are illustrated underneath the top graph. The result of applying a "1000-cross" rule to a longer segment of the vowel production is shown in the bottom half of the figure.

This solution does not always work, however. Figure 6–10 shows another major problem that is not so easily resolved. In this case a momentary baseline shift of the electroglottogram causes a major problem. Choosing a threshold level of about 650 (arbitrary units) is required in order to "capture" the smallest peak present (at about 75 ms). Unfortunately, a threshold of 650 is below the minimum value of two other peaks in the record (between about 55 and 65 ms) and, to make matters worse, it is just below the maximal value of one of the small oscillations that characterize the "trough" of each EGG wave. The comparator record shows the result: the peaks in the 55–65 ms region are detected as one very long waveform maximum, and the small trough oscillation results in a brief compara-

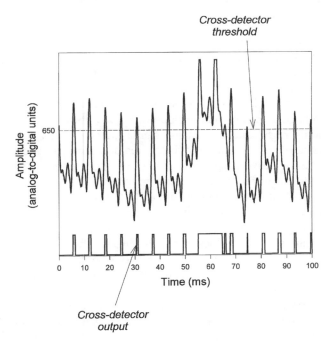

Figure 6–10. Failure of zero–cross detection. The shifting baseline of the signal causes inevitable errors in period detection.

tor output of its own. The comparator record is seriously flawed. What is worse, the flaw might not be detectable if one were to use a counter to find the number of comparator peaks during a one-second sample. That's because, through pure coincidence, the number of comparator peaks—sixteen—is the same as the number of waveform peaks. Although the total count is correct in this particular situation, the intervals that separate them are not. Evaluation of frequency perturbation (see later section, this chapter) based on this detection would have very poor validity.

The problem of "baseline shift," illustrated in Figure 6–10, is not completely insoluble. One approach to its solution is to obtain the derivative of the EGG signal, and use the peaks of the differentiated waveform to demarcate cycles (Schoentgen & Guchteneere, 1991). Another approach is to use band-pass filtering (Vieira, McInnes, & Jack, 1996), discussed in Chapter 2.

PEAK-PICKING

Many signals have a single peak of maximal amplitude (of either positive or negative polarity) in each cycle. A simple way to determine the fundamental frequency, then, is to count the number of peaks of one polarity (either positive or negative) that occur in every second. Alternatively, with a bit more difficulty, one can locate the exact temporal location of each peak, and thus measure the interval (period) from one peak to the next. These tasks may be accomplished electronically with clever use of a combination of analog circuits known as **comparators** and **slope detectors**.

The comparator produces one of two different outputs depending on whether the signal at its input does or does not exceed a pre-set threshold. When, as in Figure 6–11A, the input signal is greater than the threshold value the comparator output voltage is high. When the input is less than the threshold value, the comparator's output voltage is low. There are no intermediate output states. The use of a comparator is schematized in Figure 6–11B. It has two inputs; the threshold voltage is applied to one of them, while the signal to be evaluated is applied to the other. Whenever the input signal has a voltage greater than the threshold, the output of the comparator is at a maximum, often referred to as the "high" state. When the signal amplitude is less than the threshold voltage the output is minimal, or "low." (Since most sound pressure waveforms have more than one "peak" in each cycle, using the comparator assures that only one—the highest—is evaluated.) The comparator's "high" output is used to enable a **slope detector**, a circuit that indicates the direction of change of its input by

---

[8] Not 1000 volts, but rather an analog-to-digital conversion value of 1000.

A

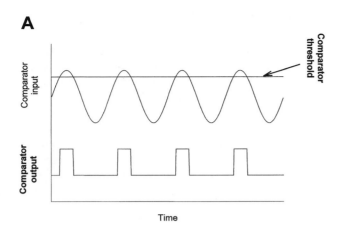

B

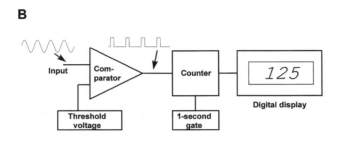

Figure 6–11. **A**. The output of a comparator (lower trace) is maximal whenever the magnitude of an input signal exceeds its threshold. The comparator output is minimal at all other times. **B**. Simple scheme for measuring F_0 by counting the number of comparator pulses per second.

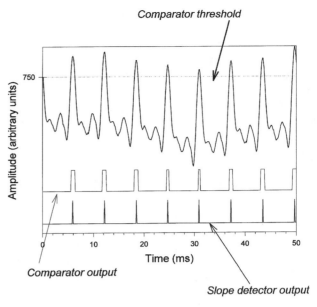

Figure 6–12. The comparator output signals the presence of the highest peak of the waveform (in this case, an electroglottogram). The comparator outputs (lower trace) can be used to enable a slope–detector, whose output is compared to the input voltage in order to determine when the signal is decreasing from a maximum. When it just begins to do, so a peak in the input voltage has occurred.

producing, like a comparator does, an output that has only two states. When the comparator enables it, the slope detector begins to keep track of the direction of change of the input signal. When the slope detector output changes from an indication of positive-going slope to one of negative-going, a peak must have occurred. That change of slope-detector output can be used to generate a brief pulse. The interval between pulses can be measured by a timer to provide the period, or the number of pulses per second can be tallied to measure the frequency.

Figure 6–12 shows the result of using a comparator and slope detector to find the peaks of an electroglottographic signal, which normally has only one maximal peak per cycle. Examination of the signal shows that the smallest value of any maximal peak is somewhat greater than 750 (arbitrary units). The comparator threshold was therefore set to 750 to ensure that every cycle would exceed the comparator threshold voltage at some time. Note how, in the lower trace, the comparator output does in fact "go high" whenever the threshold is passed. The

result is that there is one comparator pulse for each electroglottogram cycle. During the time that the comparator output is high the slope detector examines the rate of change of the signal voltage, producing a "low" output whenever signal voltage is increasing. When the input voltage begins to fall the slope-detector voltage changes to its "high" state. This change signals that a peak has just occurred. The instant that the comparator changes state a pulse is delivered either to a timer (for period detection) or to a counting circuit (for determining the F_0).[9]

Digital implementation of the peak-picking technique can be accomplished in a manner that emulates the analog approach. (The Alamed Corporation's Voice+ analysis software does this quite directly and, uniquely, produces screen graphics of the ongoing analytic process.) Suppose, for instance, that a threshold value is initially chosen. Clearly it should be somewhat lower than the lowest peak height. The places at which the signal begin to exceed the threshold value can be taken as the locations at which the program begins to examine the data list for a local maximum—that is, for a peak.

The problem with the peak-picking scheme, whether implemented by analog or digital means, is illustrated in

---

[9] Visual inspection of the data shows eight cycles in the 50 ms displayed; The mean period is therefore 6.25 ms, and the mean F_0 is $1/.00625 = 160$ Hz.)

Figure 6–13. It is not uncommon, as in this signal, for each cycle to have more than one peak, and, unfortunately, the multiple peaks may be of similar size. Under these circumstances, of course, the peak-picking method may fail badly.

WAVEFORM MATCHING

Another approach to the problems of F_0 extraction is to use a number of criteria to identify a cycle, and then to adjust them so as to minimize the difference between the cycle currently being evaluated and its neighbors. Various peaks—both positive and negative—can be detected and used as waveform-delineating criteria, for instance. When carefully applied, the waveform-matching method can produce very precise estimates of periods (although rapid frequency change seriously limits accuracy). Waveform matching, in a number of different forms, is considered by Gold (1962), Gold and Rabiner (1969), Hillenbrand (1987), Milenkovic (1987), and Titze and Liang (1993).

Optimizing Signals for F_0 Extraction

There are a number of techniques that often help to make F_0 detection by peak-picking and zero-crossing easier and more valid. Among the easiest to apply are filtering, substitution of correlate waveforms, and prior estimation of the fundamental period.

FILTERING

The "extra" peaks in each cycle of a complex waveform represent the harmonic frequencies in the signal. *Low-pass* filtering can be used to attenuate these higher frequencies, creating a much simpler waveform with the

same F_0 as the original. The filter should be set for a cutoff frequency (see Chapter 2, "Analog Electronics") just above the estimated fundamental frequency, and the filter roll-off should be as steep as possible. In Figure 6–14 a sound pressure signal was filtered using a low-pass cutoff frequency of $1.2F_0$, and a roll-off of approximately 42 dB/octave. (Any relatively slow baseline changes in the signal can be removed by *high-pass* filtering. The filter cutoff frequency should be somewhat below the estimated F_0—perhaps at 0.7 F_0—and a steep filter roll-off should be used.

In fact, an analog instrument known as the Fundamental Frequency Indicator (FFI) that depends on relatively sophisticated filtering was described in an unpublished paper by Hollien and Tamburrino in 1965. They fed tape-recorded voice signals to eight low-pass filters, arranged in parallel. Each had a cutoff frequency ½ octave higher than the one below it. The filter outputs were all connected to a special logic unit that identified the filter with the lowest cutoff frequency that was producing an output. Given the spacing of the cutoff frequencies, this output was essentially sinusoidal; that is, it had no harmonics. It was converted to a square wave and tape recorded on the second channel of the tape

Sound Pressure

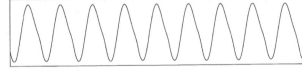

Filtered sound pressure

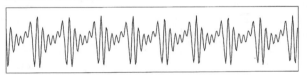

EGG

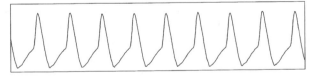

Accelerometer

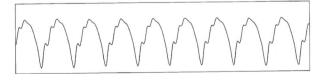

Figure 6–14. Four recordings of the same sustained vowel. The filtered sound pressure, electroglottographic (EGG) and accelerometer signals, which are correlates of the vocal signal, have a much weaker harmonic structure, making them simpler and easier to use for F_0 detection.

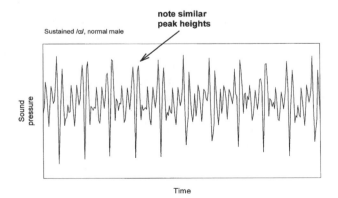

Figure 6–13. Peak detection is likely to fail when two or more peaks within a single period have similar amplitudes, as in this example of a sustained vowel.

deck. When the recording was played again (at half speed) the number of square wave pulses per second—that is, the fundamental frequency—was determined by a counter circuit. Although the system may seem crude by today's standard, it was, in fact, quite reliable and found considerable use in studies of F_0 in the modal and loft registers (Saxman & Burk, 1967; Weinberg & Zlatin, 1970; Hollien & Shipp, 1972; Hollien & Jackson, 1973). The low-frequency limitation of the tape recorder, however, was a significant impediment to the exploration of pulse register (Michel, 1968).

Most of the instrumentation commercially available today includes some form of filtering to facilitate the extraction of F_0 and a choice of filter characteristics is sometimes required of the user. The basis for that choice is the examiner's estimate of the patient's probable F_0. The consequences of the selection made by the examiner with respect to resultant measurement errors are not completely clear (Karnell, Scherer, & Fischer, 1991; Perry, Ingrisano, & Scott, 1996).

CORRELATE WAVEFORMS

Another way of dealing with the problem of complex waveforms is to ignore the sound pressure signal and to analyze instead a correlate of vocal fold activity that has a weak harmonic structure. There are two correlate signals—electroglottographic and accelerometric—that are easily available and well-suited for this purpose, and a third—photoglottographic—that, while mildly invasive, is nonetheless easily obtained during endoscopic examination.

Contact microphones and **accelerometers** are primarily sensitive to body-surface vibrations. When placed on the pretracheal surface of the neck their output reflects vocal fold movement and the response of the body wall to the acoustic wave in the trachea. Figure 6–14 shows how much "cleaner" than the radiated sound pressure signal the accelerometer wave is. Its harmonic content is obviously much weaker, and it is also relatively free of articulatory influences, making it much more suitable for F_0 extraction (Sugimoto & Hiki, 1962; Koike, 1973; Hencke, 1974a, 1974b; Stevens, Kalikow, & Willemain, 1975; Askenfelt, Gauffin, Sundberg, & Kitzing, 1980).

The **electroglottograph** (Fourcin & Abberton, 1971, 1976; Fourcin, 1974; Lecluse, Brocaar & Verschuure, 1975; Croatto & Ferrero, 1979) provides another alternative. The output of this device (discussed more fully in Chapter 10, "Laryngeal Function") represents the electrical resistance across the laryngeal region, a variable that changes in a highly predictable way during the phonatory cycle. While there remains debate about the precise relationship between the electroglottographic signal and the details of vocal fold behavior, it is nonetheless true that the periodicity of the electroglottographic waveform is an accurate

reflection of that of the vocal folds. Although it may be difficult to get a clear electroglottographic trace in some subjects (particularly those with a thick fatty layer over the neck), if a signal can be obtained it represents an excellent choice for F_0 measurement: EGG- and acoustic-derived estimates of F_0 show an almost perfect correlation (Verdonck-de Leeuw, 1998). Some electroglottographs therefore include circuitry that produces a voltage analog of the vocal F_0, and may also provide some form of readout of the instantaneous F_0.) It is not perfect, however, and EGG-based jitter can differ somewhat from acoustic-based jitter (Haji, Horiguchi, Baer, & Gould, 1986; Horiguchi, Haji, Baer, & Gould, 1987; Orlikoff, 1995; Vieira, et al., 1997).

Guidelines for choosing between accelerometry and electroglottography have been provided by Askenfelt and his colleagues (1980), who compared the two methods in normal adults. They suggest that

1. If a clear electroglottographic signal can be obtained from a patient this method should be used. The electroglottograph is less influenced by articulatory activity than the accelerometer, but the anatomy of the patient's neck may preclude a clear signal. Furthermore, the electroglottograph output may not accurately reflect F_0 if the vocal folds do not contact each other during the glottal cycle (as, for instance, in cases of paralysis).

2. The accelerometer works on all subjects, but its output is occasionally confounded by articulatory events. It is also more sensitive to changes in vocal intensity than the electroglottograph is.

In summary, Askenfelt et al. recommend that "for practical use in the phoniatric clinic, it seems that the [electroglottograph] should be preferred as long as it works well, and it should be replaced by the contact microphone for remaining patients. If . . . it is considered important that the same method be used on a great number of subjects, the contact microphone would represent the best choice." (p. 272)

Clinicians might also want to consider that accelerometers are very much less expensive than electroglottographs. On the other hand, of course, electroglottographs are needed for other aspects of vocal evaluation.

Photoglottography, (see Chapter 10, "Laryngeal Function") in which the opening and closing of the glottis modulates a beam of light (Sonesson, 1960; Kitzing & Sonesson, 1974) also provides an electrical signal that is usually simple enough for reliable F_0 determination (Lisker, Abramson, Cooper, & Schvey, 1966; Coleman & Wendahl, 1968; Vallancien, Gautheron, Pasternak, Guisez, & Paley, 1971; Kitzing & Sonesson, 1974). Since the larynx is brightly illuminated during endoscopic examination, all that is required to obtain a photoglottogram is the placement of a photodetector over the upper trachea.

PRIOR ESTIMATION OF THE FUNDAMENTAL PERIOD

Another way of dealing with the problem of multiple peaks in a signal is to give the analysis program an a priori estimate of the length of the period. Assume, for example, that the signal whose F_0 is to be determined is the one shown in Figure 6–15. Inspection of the sound pressure record (which might, in the clinical setting, be done on an oscilloscope) shows that the fundamental period is on the order of 10 ms. (The arrow above the data trace has a length of that duration.) The computer program doing the F_0 evaluation can be told to search for the largest value in a 10 ms window. Having found this first peak, the program can then search for the highest point that is about 10 ms later, and so on. It is also possible to build some simple logical rules into the software so that the estimate of the period is updated every time a new period is delineated. In many circumstances the "search-within-an-interval-approximately-equal-to-the-period" method prevents confounding by the presence of secondary peaks. It assumes, of course, that the fundamental period does not change radically over a short time span and that there really is only one maximal peak in each cycle.

INTERPOLATION

One problem with computer implementation of both peak-picking and zero-cross detection of fundamental periods stems from the discrete nature of the digital data that they work on. Recall that, before computer

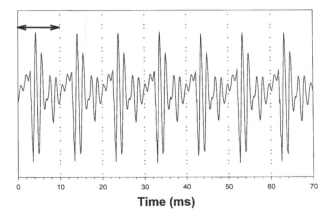

Figure 6–15. Examination of this sound pressure signal shows that it has a period of approximately 10 ms (demarcated by the arrow). An F_0 extraction system could therefore be instructed to search for a single major sound pressure peak in each 10 ms segment, minimizing the possibility of error.

processing, the (analog) signal must be converted to digital form by being sampled a fixed number of times per second. We cannot know the time at which a peak lies or a zero-cross occurs with greater precision than the sampling interval. That is, if we have sampled the original waveform at, let us say, 1000 times per second, then, using a simple examination of the data, the best we can do is locate the peak or the zero-cross to the nearest 1/1000 second. While this might seem sufficiently accurate it is, in fact, not nearly good enough for many clinical purposes, such as the computation of jitter indices. Fortunately, *interpolation* methods make it relatively easy to estimate the location of a peak or a zero-cross with much greater precision.

Interpolation is the process of estimating the unknown location of a data point (in this case, the point at which the zero-cross or peak occurs) on the basis of the known data points that surround it. There are many ways of doing this, but what is involved in all of them is the generation of an equation that describes the data curve and then applying that equation to obtain the coordinate of a point that is not already a part of the data set. The accuracy of the interpolation can be enhanced by use of a number of sophisticated techniques, discussed in many introductory texts of mathematics (for example, Hildebrand, 1956; Tuma, 1989; or Killingbeck, 1991). For almost all clinical purposes, however, the improvement in the precision of F_0 measurement that is gained by a simple linear method is likely to be more than adequate.

What is involved in linear interpolation is illustrated in Figure 6–16. The plot at the top shows the data points resulting from sampling a vocalic sound pressure waveform at a rate of 10,000 samples/s. A zero-cross level of −1500 mV has been chosen. The vertical lines on the plot show where each (negative-going) zero-cross has occurred. If the region of the third zero-cross (around 15 ms) is enlarged, as in the center graph, it becomes clear that the zero-cross did not occur exactly at one of the sample points. Instead, it lies somewhere between the samples at 14.2 ms and 14.3 ms. The ultimate estimate of the fundamental period or F_0 would be greatly improved if we were to interpolate so as to find out *where* between the two samples the cross is estimated to have actually occurred.

Further enlargement of the area around the zero-cross (bottom plot) shows how we can do this. Examination of the values of the data points in the computer file (which the computer can do quite easily!) shows that the point just before the zero-cross has a value of −1146 mV; the one just after is −1645 mV. The points are therefore separated by 499 mV. This separation is divisible into two parts. The pre-cross point is 354 mV higher than the zero-cross threshold of −1500 mV. This distance is labeled Y_1. The postcross point is 145 mV below the threshold. It is labeled Y_2. The time difference between the pre − and

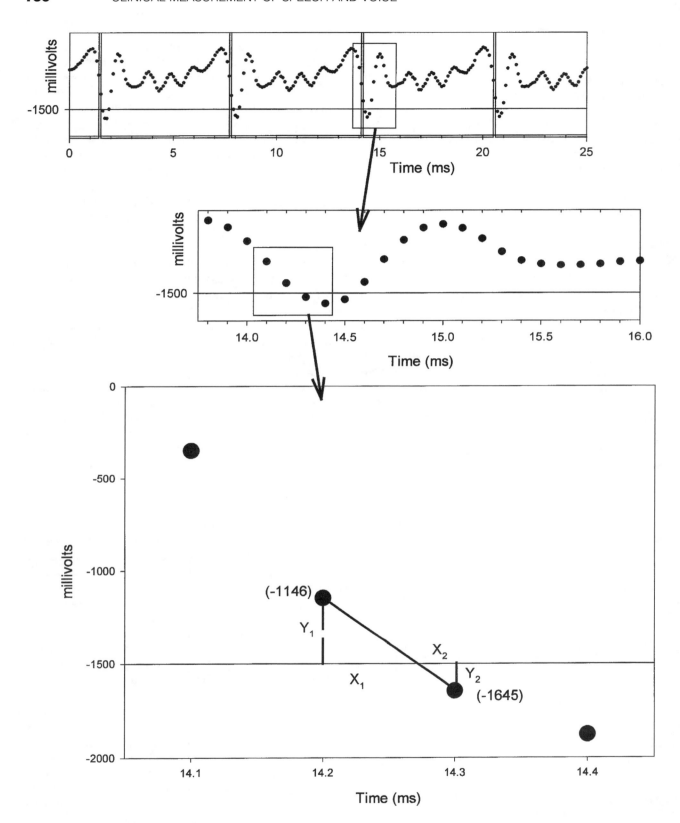

Figure 6–16. Linear interpolation. The task is to estimate where on the time axis the crossing of the threshold voltage (−1500 mV) actually occurs. See text.

postcross samples must be 0.1 ms. (We know this because the sampling rate was 10,000 samples/s; the interval between samples must therefore be 1/10,000 second.) This interval is also divisible into two parts: X_1 is the part before the zero-crossing occurred; X_2 is the part after it.

Now, it is clear from the principles of Euclidean geometry that

$$\frac{Y_1}{Y_1 + Y_2} = \frac{X_1}{X_1 + X_2}$$

We solve for X_1, the interval between the precross sample and the time that (according to a linear estimate) the threshold-crossing actually occurred. Therefore:

$$\frac{354}{499} = \frac{X_1}{.0001}$$

$$X_1 = 0.0001 \left(\frac{354}{499}\right)$$

$$X_1 = .00007094 \text{ s}$$

$$X_1 \approx .071 \text{ millisecond.}$$

The threshold crossing is thus estimated to be 0.071 ms after the pre-crossing sample, so it may be said to occur at $14.2 + .071 = 14.271$ ms. This represents a considerable improvement in the accuracy of the data from which the F_0 is calculated.

Computational Approaches to F_0 Estimation

The methods for estimating F_0 discussed so far depend on detecting a recurring feature (threshold-crossing or peak amplitude) in a periodic signal. The detection can be achieved by analog instrumentation or by digital processing. There are also methods that do not simply measure the temporal distance from one recurring event to the next, but rather explore more subtle features of the signal. These approaches are more mathematical and hence, while it is possible to implement some of them using analog instrumentation, it is much easier, faster, and convenient to have digital computers do the analytic work. Scientists and engineers have developed a very large number of such methods; it is not possible to discuss them all in detail. But most are variations and refinements of two basic (and related) techniques: *autocorrelation* and *spectral analysis*. The conceptual bases of these methods are described in the following sections.

AUTOCORRELATION

Autocorrelation methods represent a rather direct application of Titze's definition of periodicity (Titze, 1994, 1995) cited earlier: A series of events is considered to be periodic if they cannot be distinguished from each other by shifting forward or backward in time by an appropriate amount, nT_0. That is, $f(t \pm nT_0) = f(t)$. It turns out that, if the signal is at least nearly periodic, there is a relatively easy method to determine what an "appropriate amount" of shifting is. That method involves assessing the strength of the relationship of the signal's magnitude at a given point in time to its magnitude a bit later. If we keep increasing the time difference between the points whose relationship is being examined we should ultimately find a time difference that shows an optimal relationship. That time difference equals the period. The relationship between points can be quantified by the correlation coefficient. Since the signal is being correlated to (a later part of) itself, the procedure is called *autocorrelation*.[10]

To see how autocorrelation is used to detect fundamental periods we can examine another sound pressure signal, shown in Figure 6–17. When the signal is acquired by the computer it is digitized. Therefore, the appearance of the plot notwithstanding, it is not in the

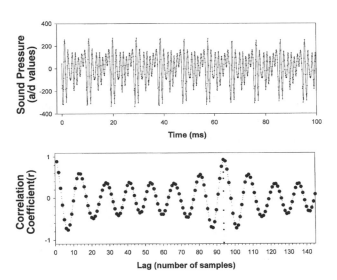

Figure 6–17. Autocorrelation analysis of the sound pressure waveform at the top results in the autorcorrelation function shown at the bottom. It peaks at 94 samples —which is the number of samples in one fundamental period. Since the sampling rate is known, it is a simple matter to find the fundamental period.

---

[10]An interesting, and clearly explained, example of the use of autocorrelation (together with a pre-estimation of the probable period value) is available in Feijoo and Hernández (1990).

form of a continuous line, but rather consists of a series of discrete points. Each point is a number that specifies the magnitude of the signal at the instant that the sample was taken. In the computer, then, the signal of Figure 6–17 has the form

43
−174
−147
−315
−282
−318
−181
−82
61
214
245
259
227
68
−47
−181
−245
−297
−255
−171
−73
28
108
148
168
129
95

. . . and so on, for a thousand values.

Now, suppose we were to correlate each value in this list with the value that follows it. In other words, we find the association between the list and itself, with a *lag* of 1:

43 ↔ −174
−174 ↔ −147
−147 ↔ −315
−315 ↔ −282
−282 ↔ −318
−318 ↔ −181
−181 ↔ −82
−82 ↔ 61
61 ↔ 214
214 ↔ 245

. . . and so on.

The correlation coefficient that results is 0.888. (The strong relationship is not surprising: In most signals, values are strongly correlated with the values that immediately follow them.)

We can now correlate each value with the value that is two samples later. That is, we change the lag to 2:

43 ↔ −147
−174 ↔ −315
−147 ↔ −282
−315 ↔ −318
−282 ↔ −181
−318 ↔ −82
−181 ↔ −61
−82 ↔ 214
61 ↔ 245
214 ↔ 245

. . . and so on.

With a lag of 2, the correlation coefficient drops to 0.627.

The correlation coefficient, r, can be recalculated as the lag is steadily increased: when the lag is 3, $r = 0.24$, when it is 4, $r = -0.16$, and so on. Plotting r against the lag results in the lower plot, the *correlogram*, of Figure 6–17. Note that, in the range of lags from 1 to 145, the highest measured correlation coefficient is .925, and it occurs at a lag of 94 samples. Since the sampling rate is 10,000 samples/s, this lag corresponds to a time lag of 9.4 ms. What this signifies is that the strongest relationship is found when a point in the wave is compared to a point 9.4 ms later. In other words, shifting ahead (or backward) 9.4 ms brings us to a point that is extremely similar to the point we were at. Hence, by the definition of periodicity that we have been using, we have not only established a very close approximation to periodicity, but we have measured the duration of the repetition interval, or period. (The regular oscillation of r reflects the presence of harmonics in the sound pressure waveform; their frequencies are reflected in the spacing of the local maxima of r.)

The sound pressure record of Figure 6–17—which is obviously nearly-periodic and quite free of noise—does not show the true utility of an autocorrelation method. Sound pressure signals are often not quite so neat and clean. Figure 6–18 shows a much less ideal sound pressure record: it is, in fact, exactly the same signal that we have already analyzed, but with a considerable amount of random noise added. The result of the autocorrelation analysis, shown in the lower graph, reveals a maximal correlation coefficient, r, that is a very modest 0.322. This reduction of the maximal r is due to the presence of significant noise. But the maximal r occurs at the same lag—94—as it did for the cleaner version of the waveform. The autocorrelation has "seen through" the noise to uncover the underlying 9.4-ms period.

SPECTROGRAPHY

Although usually generated to examine characteristics of the supraglottal vocal tract (that is, "filter" functions) the sound spectrogram does, of course, include information about the signal's fundamental frequency.

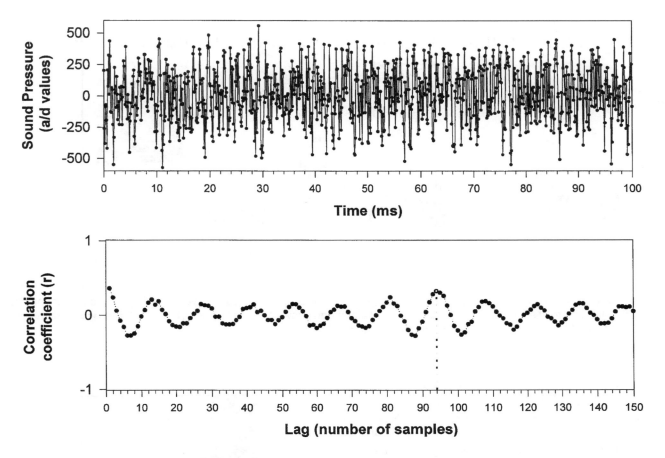

Figure 6–18. Autocorrelation analysis of a very noisy signal (upper). The plot of the autocorrelation function (lower) shows a peak, demonstrating that there is a periodic signal with a period of 94 samples obscured by the noise.

Depending on the type of spectrographic display, the information appears in different forms. It is, however, always moderately easy to derive. (Sound spectrography is considered in detail in Chapter 7.)

When the bandwidth of the spectrum-analyzing filter is large compared to the fundamental frequency, a "wide-band" spectrogram, like the one shown in Figure 6–19 results. Each of the vertical striations is produced by a single closure of the glottis. All that need be done to find the F_0 is to count the number of vertical striations between two points along the time axis, and then divide the number of glottal pulses thus represented by the time-equivalent of the horizontal distance. That is

$$F_0 = \frac{\text{Number of striations}}{\text{Duration of interval}}.$$

This procedure has been applied to the spectrogram of Figure 6–19. In the marked-off interval (the diphthong /ou/) there are 15 vertical striations. The interval has a

duration of 0.115 s. Therefore, $F_0 = 15/0.115 \approx 130$ Hz. (The same counting procedure can be applied to every voiced segment.) With a computer-based spectrograph it is generally possible to place cursors at the boundaries of the interval in which striation-counting is done, and their location in time is almost always indicated in the display. With less sophisticated—usually analog—analysis systems an accurate timing signal is needed to determine the distance-to-time equivalence. Often, as was the case for Figure 6–19, the spectrograph can produce those timing marks.

There is one important caution that must be kept in mind when determining F_0 in this way: The F_0 value obtained is the average F_0 for the time interval in question. Short-term changes in F_0 are not detected. An *average* F_0 is perfectly acceptable if the assumption can be validly made that the F_0 is constant during the measurement period or if any shift of F_0 is of no interest.

An analyzing filter with a bandwidth that is narrow compared to the F_0 of the signal being analyzed generates a spectrogram that resolves the vocal harmonics. Since

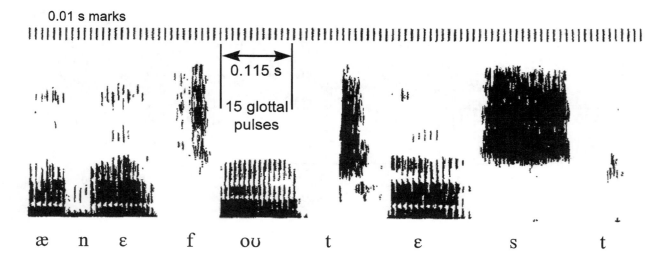

Figure 6–19. Wide-band sound spectrogram of the utterance "an eff-oh test." Fundamental frequency can be determined by counting the number of vertical striations, generated by glottal closures, in a voiced segment and comparing the count to the segment's duration. In this case, the /oʊ/ diphthong shows 15 striations in 0.115 s. The average fundamental frequency for this interval must therefore be 15/0.0115 = 130.4 Hz.

they are at integral multiples of the fundamental frequency, change in the vocal F_0 will always produce proportional change in the harmonics, making it very easy to see the F_0 contour. This can be particularly useful in detecting tremulous voice, which has cyclic variations of the fundamental frequency (Lebrun et al., 1982).

If the vertical scale of the spectrograph display can be expanded the fundamental frequency might be directly read from the spectrogram, as in Figure 6–20. But, because the harmonics bear a simple mathematical relationship to F_0, the fundamental frequency can almost always be determined easily. One need only find the frequency of the nth harmonic and divide it by n. Thus, if the sixth harmonic is at 650 Hz, the fundamental frequency must be about 108 Hz.

Cepstrum

A very powerful means of extracting the fundamental frequency of a speech signal was originally described by Noll (1964). Relying on Fourier analysis, it represented a departure from the evolutionary line of analog methods that would not have been possible without the high-speed digital processor. This method, referred to as ***cepstrum analysis***, has seen only occasional application in the clinical realm, but its unexploited potential makes it a good candidate for more widespread use in the medium-term future, the more so in that, while it isolates the fundamental frequency, it simultaneously reveals important characteristics of the vocal tract filter function. While the mathematical

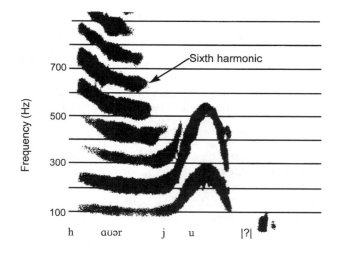

Figure 6–20. Narrow band (45 Hz) spectrogram, with an expanded frequency scale, of the utterance "How're you?" The frequency of any harmonic is an integer multiple of the fundamental frequency.

bases of this technique are, as might be expected, extraordinarily complex, the basic conceptualization is not overly difficult, and thus merits at least an overview here. More complete consideration can be found in Wakita (1976, 1977), Randall and Hee (1981), and in a very clear presentation by Noll (1967).

The vocal signal radiated at the lips is shaped by both the characteristics of the glottal source and the action of the vocal tract resonances on the laryngeal pulsations. More formally stated, the voiced speech sound, denoted *f(t)*, is the convolution of a source signal, *s(t)*, and a tract response, *h(t)*. Symbolically,

$$f(t) = s(t) * h(t)$$

"Convolution" (designated by the *) implies an interaction of two sets of spectral properties. The spectrum is represented by the Fourier transform, denoted $\mathscr{F}$. Therefore

$$\mathscr{F}[f(t)] = \mathscr{F}[s(t)] \times \mathscr{F}[h(t)].$$

That is, the spectrum of the voiced speech signal is the complex product[11] of the glottal source spectrum and the vocal tract transfer function.

The main problem is finding an efficient way of separating the source and transfer-function characteristics. Now, it is clear from elementary algebra that $\log(x \cdot y) = \log x + \log y$. Therefore, the logarithm of the spectrum of the vocal signal is equal to the sum of the logarithm of the source spectrum and the logarithm of the transfer function:

$$\log \mathscr{F}[f(t)] = \log \mathscr{F}[s(t)] + \log \mathscr{F}[h(t)].$$

The complex multiplication function is thereby replaced by a simpler additive one, greatly facilitating the ultimate separation of the two spectral responses.

The cepstrum method, flow-charted in Figure 6–21, begins by filtering out the highest-frequency components of the speech signal before converting the signal to digital form. The next step is to derive the spectrum of

the waveform, that is, to discover its frequency components and their amplitudes. Here a problem arises. Clearly to do the necessary computation one needs to take a string of numbers that represents at least one complete cycle of the speech waveform. But it is not known how long a cycle is. (If the length of the cycle were known, then the frequency would be known, and the analysis would be a pointless exercise.) One can be certain of getting at least one full vocal cycle if a long enough string of numbers is considered. To be absolutely certain, it might be decided to deal with a digital string representing, say, 40 ms of time. (A period of 40 ms is equivalent to a frequency of 25 Hz. Any voiced signal is almost certain to have a higher fundamental frequency—and therefore a shorter period—than that.)

The long sample duration solves one problem but introduces a somewhat more subtle difficulty of its own, illustrated in Figure 6–22. At the top is a vowel waveform with an F_0 of roughly 90 Hz. When a 40-ms sample of this wave is taken, the computer is left with the wavetrain shown in the lower plot. The fact that there is more than one complete cycle is no problem at all: the Fourier analysis takes account of that possibility. The "tags" of partial waves at either end of the sample, however, are a thornier issue. We know that they

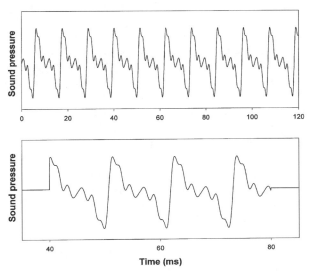

Figure 6–22. Speech signal (top) with a F_0 of approximately 90 Hz. A 40–ms extract of the speech wave (bottom) will have sharp discontinuities at either end. These appear to be impulse-like onset and offset phenomena to the computer, which does not "know" that they are a sampling artifact. (In actual practice, of course, the waves are represented by strings of numbers.)

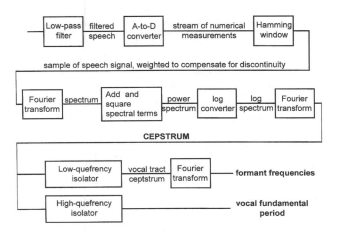

Figure 6–21. Schema of F_0 extraction using cepstrum analysis.

---

[11] The term "complex" is used here in its mathematical sense of having both real and imaginary parts.

are parts of waves; the computer does not. It "thinks" that the wave begins and ends at the baseline. The tags are seen as impulse-like onset and offset components. If the Fourier analysis is done using such a wave the spectrum of an impulse (an infinite series of lines spaced across the frequency axis) will be inextricably mixed into the actual spectrum of the wave that has been sampled. To prevent this artifact the sample of the digitized wave is put through the digital equivalent of a special filter called a "window" that adjusts the relative importance of data points so that the two ends contribute relatively little to the final analysis.

The result of processing to this point is a set of weighted measurements of the speech wave. These are now subjected to the Fourier transform to produce a series of real and imaginary terms that represent the frequency, amplitude, and phase relationships of the components of the original wave. In other words, the frequency spectrum is derived. These real and imaginary terms are squared and added to generate what is known as the "power spectrum." Finally, the logarithm of each of the power-spectrum terms is taken to derive the "logarithm power spectrum" upon which the result of the analysis is based.

The usefulness of all of this processing becomes more intuitively clear when a logarithm power spectrum, such as the one in Figure 6–23, is examined. Notice that the spectrum is formed of a series of regularly spaced lobes. That is, the spectrum itself shows periodicity, and it turns out that the "period" of this pronounced "ripple" is the same as the period of the glottal pulses. The spectrum also has a lower-frequency (and less regular) undulation to it, emphasized in Figure 6–23 by the dashed line. This feature is due to the vocal tract resonances.

How can the two features of the logarithm power spectrum be separated? Since they represent the simple sum of two functions (rather than the complex convolution) the matter is fairly easy. All that is necessary is to handle the logarithm power spectrum as if it were itself a waveform and apply a Fourier analysis to *it*. The Fourier transform of the logarithm power spectrum (formally known as the *inverse Fourier transform*) is a new quantity that has been named the **cepstrum** (a partial reversal of the word "spectrum").[12] The horizontal scale has been assigned the designation **quefrency** to distinguish it from the "frequency" of a real time function. Quefrency is measured in seconds and is therefore equivalent to period. Figure 6–23 (*bottom*) is the cepstrum that results from a Fourier analysis of the logarithm power spectrum shown in Figure 6–23 (*top*).

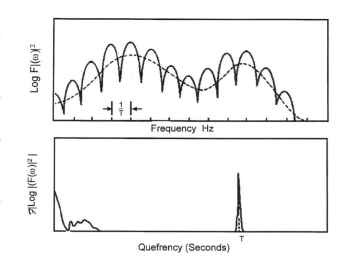

Figure 6–23. Top: The logarithm power spectrum of a voiced speech segment. Bottom: Cepstrum of the power spectrum. (From "Cepstrum Pitch Determination," by A. M. Noll, 1967, Figure 3, p. 296. *Journal of the Acoustical Society of America, 41,* 293–309. Reprinted by permission.)

The sharp, high-quefrency peak represents the period of the logarithm power spectrum, while the broad, low-quefrency peak represents the factors (vocal tract resonances) that produce the undulations. The fundamental period of the vocal signal is the quefrency peak in the cepstrum; the fundamental frequency is the reciprocal of this quefrency. Once the peak's location is determined (and the fundamental frequency thereby found) the computer can call for another sample of the speech input and repeat the process. The output of the computer is then a data series that shows the fundamental frequency of the speech signal over time.

(Although not directly relevant to the problem of F_0 extraction, it is worth noting that the vocal tract resonance peaks (formants) can be derived from the broad, low-quefrency peaks of the cepstrum. One simply treats the cepstrum as an ordinary waveform and subjects it to yet another Fourier analysis. The output of this third spectrum derivation has the unit "frequency" and the curve that results is essentially that of the vocal tract transfer function.)

The cepstrum method, then, provides a very effective way of deriving vocal F_0 and evaluating vocal tract characteristics in a totally noninvasive way (Schafer & Rabiner, 1970). Originally difficult to implement, today's powerful desktop computers and the development of the Fast Fourier Transform (Cooley & Tukey, 1965) have made it a very practical tool.

---

[12] Technically, the cepstrum results when the inverse Fourier transform is squared, an operation which serves to sharpen the cepstral peaks.

INVERSE FILTERING

While the cepstrum procedure essentially sidesteps the problems caused by convolution of the glottal source and vocal tract transfer characteristics, inverse filtering (first proposed by Miller, 1959) attacks them head on. It is possible, by very sophisticated techniques, to determine several properties of the vocal tract by mathematical analysis. Fundamental frequency extraction by inverse filtering takes advantage of these techniques in the way schematized in Figure 6–24.

As with cepstrum analysis, the assumption is made that the sound pressure signal represents the product of the glottal resonances, vocal tract resonances, and lip radiation characteristics acting on the glottal wave (the pulsatile flow of air through the glottis). If the effect of the nonlaryngeal acoustics could be determined, it would be possible to subtract them from the radiated acoustic signal, restoring it to a "purer" or simpler form that is more representative of what the larynx itself produced. This, in fact, is what is done in inverse filtering.

The sound pressure signal is analyzed to determine the effects of the lip-radiation and vocal tract acoustics. In other words, the speaker's nonglottal resonance properties are determined and expressed as a transfer function (of the kind that speech pathologists typically study in their beginning courses in acoustic phonetics). The reciprocal of this transfer function is calculated and used as a filter through which the speech signal is passed. The result of this inverse-filtering is a relatively simple waveform—the remainder after after the vocal tract and lip radiation influences are removed from the sound pressure signal. If the process has been done correctly, that remainder could only be the glottal volume velocity waveform. This form of inverse filtering is therefore called **glottal inverse filtering**.

It is possible to carry the process one step further. The glottal volume velocity wave (which is the acoustical excitation of the vocal tract) derives its form from the acoustic characteristics of the glottal space as they interact with pulsatile air bursts. It is possible to estimate the acoustic properties of the glottis and to compensate for them as well as for the vocal tract and lip radiation characteristics. The sound pressure signal can then be filtered to remove essentially everything except for the abrupt pulses of air that are the purest form of vocal system excitation. This more complete filtering process is called **residue inverse filtering**. The residue is, in a sense, the very essence of voice—*raw* puffs of air with all of the influences of the vocal tract removed. (This is the form of inverse filtering schematized in Figure 6–24.) The residue signal has a very sharp pulse at the beginning of every fundamental period. It is a fairly simple matter to measure the spacing of the pulses and thereby to determine the fundamental frequency of the original signal.

The conceptual simplicity of inverse filtering obscures the enormous complexity of implementation. More detailed descriptions of the inverse-filtering process, the principles on which it rests, and its utility in detecting laryngeal dysfunction are available in Miller (1959), Miller and Mathews (1963), Koike and Markel (1975), Davis (1976, 1979), and Wakita (1976, 1977).

FUNDAMENTAL FREQUENCY MEASUREMENTS

A Note on Vocal Registers

Over the years, few issues have been quite so liable to provoke (often acrimonious) debate among the many kinds of vocal specialists as that of vocal registers. Disagreement has characterized almost every aspect of the discussion, and true consensus still has yet to be achieved on most basic points. What is a register? Is it an acoustic attribute of voice? A purely perceptual phenomenon? A product of laryngeal function or of vocal tract characteristics? How many registers are there, and what should they be called? A measure of the confusion was presented by Mörner, Fransson, and Fant (1963), who managed to compile a list of more than 100 terms used to describe vocal registers. McGlone and Brown (1969) showed that the cross-over point between different registers is not reliably perceived, a fact that adds to the confusion of categorization.

In a cogent discussion of the register problem, Hollien (1974) attempted to bring a degree of order to the prevailing conceptual and terminological morass by proposing that a register be defined as a "totally laryngeal unit." That is, in his view a register is the reflection of a

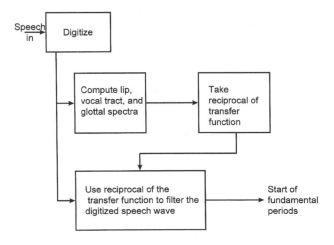

Figure 6–24. General scheme of residue inverse filtering.

specific mode of laryngeal action, rather than of supraglottal resonances. Each register consists of "a series or range of consecutively phonated frequencies which can be produced with nearly identical *vocal* quality" (pp. 125–126). Ordinarily, adjacent registers have little F_0 overlap. While it is apparently possible to identify a host of different registers on the basis of perceptual attributes[13] Hollien's insistence on the "laryngeality" of vocal registers seems most relevant to addressing the problems of vocal assessment and rehabilitation. It is therefore the approach to categorization that has been accepted for the present purposes.

The three registers that can be identified by Hollien's criteria have purposely been given new names in order to avoid confusion due to prior—sometimes fanciful and often confusing—usage. Hollien's recommended terminology is summarized below[14]:

Modal register designates the range of fundamental frequencies and vocal quality most commonly used in speaking and singing. The name is derived from the statistical "mode," signifying the most common value in a set. It may include the musical "chest" and "head" or "low," "mid," and "high" registers, depending on how these are defined.

Pulse register applies to the phonatory range at the low end of the frequency scale in which the laryngeal output is perceived as pulsatile. (The pulse register has been described more fully in Hollien, Moore, Wendahl, and Michel, 1966; Hollien and Michel, 1968; and Hollien and Wendahl, 1968.) The term is essentially synonymous with "vocal fry," "glottal fry," and perhaps the musical "strohbass."

Loft register refers to those frequencies at the upper end of the vocal continuum. It generally corresponds to the older musical term "falsetto."

"Pulse" and "modal" have attained considerable, although certainly not universal, acceptance as register descriptors. Perhaps because—unlike other musical terms like "head" and "chest"—the term "falsetto" is not prone to cause misunderstanding, there has been little motivation to abandon it.

General Considerations

Vocal fundamental frequency is reflective of the biomechanical characteristics of the vocal folds as they interact with the translaryngeal airflow. The biomechanical properties are determined by laryngeal structure and by applied muscle forces. Adjustment of the latter, in turn, is a function of reflexive, affective, and learned voluntary behaviors.

The vocal fundamental frequency provides insight into the adequacy of the interaction of all of those variables that influence the vocal fold status.[15] The ability to vary F_0 demonstrates a great deal about the mechanical adequacy of laryngeal structures and about the precision and extent of laryngeal control. The stability of phonatory adjustment is reflected in the amount of short-term variability (perturbation) of the voice signal. The speech pathologist may therefore be interested in any of several aspects of vocal F_0. A number of different measurements that are likely to be useful are presented in this section.

SPEAKING FUNDAMENTAL FREQUENCY (SF$_0$)

There has been a longstanding interest in the F_0 characteristics of speech, and the period of modern research dates from at least the first third of the twentieth century (for example, Weaver, 1924). A significant database, however, did not develop until measurement of F_0 was made easier by the development of appropriate electronic instrumentation in the 1950s and later.

There is an expectation that vocal pitch will be appropriate in some ill-defined way to a speaker's age and sex (Michel & Wendahl, 1971; Wolfe, Ratusnik, Smith, & Northrop, 1990) and perhaps to body type, social situation, emotional state, and other factors as well (Hecker, Stevens, von Bismarck, & Williams, 1968; Williams & Stevens, 1972, 1981; Griffin & Williams, 1987; Ruiz, Legros, & Guell, 1990; Przybyla, Horii, & Crawford, 1992). When that expectation is not realized further investigation may be warranted. Evaluation of the fundamental frequencies actually used during speech will show whether a given speaker's voice is really different in frequency from that of comparable speakers or whether the listener's perception of abnormality is based on other aspects of voicing.

Finally, there is a clinical expectation that the speaking fundamental frequency (SF$_0$, sometimes also abbreviated SFF) will fall at a roughly predictable point in a speaker's total F_0 range. The "normal" level is as yet not empirically well-established, and the effects of training are not certain, nor are the possible implications or consequences of deviation from the norm clear (Gramming,

---

[13] Titze (1994, Chapter 10) provides a summary of the essentials of register perception.

[14] Note that other vocal adjustments can be imposed on the basic register configurations to produce more complex vocal qualities. An overview is provided by Laver and Hanson (1981).

[15] The importance of subglottal pressure change in the regulation of vocal F_0 has been the subject of some debate (Ladefoged & McKinney, 1963; Lieberman, Knudson, & Mead, 1969) but it is not generally held to be a major contributor in normal speakers (Hixon, Klatt, & Mead, 1971; Shipp, Doherty, & Morrissey, 1979; Baken & Orlikoff, 1987a, 1987b, 1988).

1991; Awan, 1993; Drew and Sapir, 1995; Morris, Brown, Hicks, and Howell, 1995; Rossiter & Howard, 1997).

Speech is not usually monotonous: the normal speaker uses a range of fundamental frequencies in linguistically prescribed patterns to indicate word and sentence stress, statement form, and affective content. Given this fact, two basic and general properties of the SF_0 are of interest: the frequency average and variability.

Average SF_0 denotes the "average" fundamental frequency value. It seems to be a clear enough term. But there are three different common measures that can, in different senses, be considered to be "averages." They will be discussed with reference to the sample set of waveforms shown in Figure 6–25 and tabulated in Table 6–1. The speaker who provided the sample prolonged /ɑ/ at comfortable pitch and loudness.

1. *Mean* SF_0 is the sum of the frequency measurements divided by the number of waves measured. That is

$$\text{Mean } F_0 = \frac{\sum_{i=1}^{n} F_{Oi}}{n}.$$

In other words, it is the parameter that most people associate with the term "average." For the sample shown, the mean is

$$\text{Mean } F_0 = \frac{(f_1 + f_2 + \ldots + f_{25})}{25}$$

$$= \frac{106.05 + 108.17 + \ldots + 106.04}{25}$$

$$= 106.32 \text{ Hz}$$

There is a problem with computation of the mean that is subtle, and hence commonly overlooked. Suppose that, in a 3-s sample of a sustained vowel, there are 2 seconds of phonation at 100 Hz and 1 second at 200 Hz. Since there are as many 200 Hz cycles in 1 second as there are 100 Hz cycles in 2 seconds, the arithmetic of

$$\frac{\sum F_0}{n}$$

biases the mean in favor of high frequency. A way around this is to calculate the mean F_0 not for the entire sample, but for successive time frames (perhaps 50 ms long). The mean of these time-frame means then serves as an estimate of the mean F_0 of the entire sample.

Which is the "real" mean: the average for the entire sample, or the average of the time-frame averages? It depends on one's viewpoint and needs. If, for example, one is interested in exploring

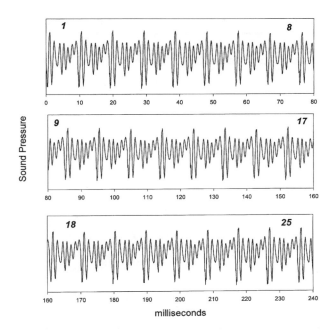

Figure 6–25. Sound pressure record of a sustained vowel by a normal male speaker. The periods have been numbered from 1 to 25.

certain aspects of vocal physiology, then one might be interested in the "average" cycle, and

$$\frac{\sum F_0}{n}$$

might well be the best choice. ***But if one wants to answer the question, "If I choose an arbitrary point in the time course of phonation, what is the F_0 likely to be?" a time-frame approach might well be better.***

2. The *median* SF_0 is the fundamental frequency value that marks the 50th percentile of the distribution. That is, half of all the values in the set are greater than the median, and half are smaller. To find the median fundamental frequency for the sample the individual wave measurements are listed in increasing (or decreasing) order. The number at the middle of the list is the median. (If there is an even number of entries the median can be taken as the mean of the two center values.) For the sample of Figure 6–25/Table 6–1 the median is 106.25 Hz.

3. The *modal* SF_0 is the value that occurs most frequently in the list. It is, in other words, the most common entry. For the sample, the model SF_0 is 106.25 Hz.

At this point the logical question is: If there are three different measures that can be considered to be "averages," which one should be used? The answer, of

Table 6–1. Period and F_0 Data Derived from Figure 6–25

Period No.	Period (ms)	F_0	Period No.	Period (ms)	F_0
1	9.43	106.05	13	9.51	105.13
2	9.24	108.17	14	9.52	105.06
3	9.35	106.97	15	9.39	106.47
4	9.50	105.22	16	9.40	106.43
5	9.36	106.89	17	9.42	106.17
6	9.33	107.12	18	9.25	108.06
7	9.48	105.52	19	9.37	106.75
8	9.52	105.03	20	9.41	106.25
9	9.37	106.67	21	9.25	108.16
10	9.46	105.68	22	9.41	106.25
11	9.64	103.73	23	9.30	107.53
12	9.51	105.09	24	9.31	107.43
25	9.43	106.04			

course, is "That depends ... " First, on the way in which the values are spread out and second, on what one wants to know.

Irrespective of any other factors, the modal frequency has a certain advantage. By virtue of the fact that it is the most common frequency value in the sample, it is the closest objective approximation of "habitual pitch," considered to be an important speech characteristic by many voice therapists. On the other hand, if the objective is, let us say, to identify a representative vocal fundamental frequency, a value that might represent a "basal" F_0 level from which intonational pitch changes are launched, the choice is more difficult.

Whether the median or the mean is more representative depends on the distribution characteristics. Suppose that the frequency of occurrence for two different samples is as shown in Figures 6–26 and 6–27. In Figure 6–26 all of the values are arranged with a fair amount of symmetry about a central, quite clearly modal, value. Visual inspection of this graph makes it clear that the median is likely to be close to the mode. In this instance, where the distribution approaches what the statistician refers to as "normality," the mean is the best measure of the "average."

The situation is very different for the sample shown in Figure 6–27, which is said to be "skewed." The long "tail" to the right of the mode influences the mean and inflates its value. In this case, the median is more representative of a typical value, and hence might be considered a better "average."

As a general rule, all other things being equal, the mean is a good average value if the distribution is more or less symmetrical; the median is preferable if the distribution is markedly skewed. But in clinical work all other things are rarely equal, especially with respect to the all-important question of what the therapist needs to know. As in so many aspects of therapeutics, the decision will have to be made on the basis of the facts of the individual case.

SF$_0$ Variability

Normal speech requires variation of fundamental frequency, but too little or too much is undesirable. How may the degree of F_0 variation be expressed? One simple way is to state the SF$_0$ range, which in simply the difference between the highest and lowest F_0 found in a sample. (It is common to express the range in semitones.) This gives some idea of variability, but it is based on the extreme values found in the sample and therefore may provide a distorted picture of what is happening. Suppose, for instance, that the F_0s of cycles in a sample are

105.6   105.9   104.8   105.7   106.1   105.9

106.2   121.3   104.9   105.5   106.0   105.8.

The mean F_0 of the sample is 107.1 Hz. The range is (121.3 − 104.8 =) 16.5 Hz, which is 2.5 semitones. But the range is enlarged by a single, obviously unrepresentative, reading of 121.3 Hz, which may well have been an accident, a momentary "slip of the larynx" or a transient failure of the analysis software. It seems

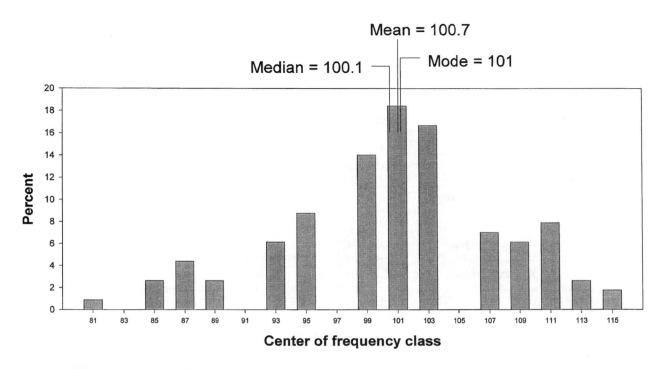

Figure 6–26. Distribution of fundamental frequencies in a sample for which the mean is likely to be the best "average."

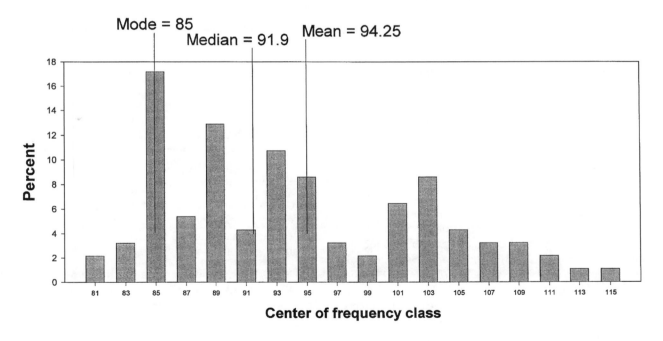

Figure 6–27. Distribution of fundamental frequencies in a sample for which the median is likely to be the "best" average.

unfair to include it in an estimate of variability, because it distorts the picture of vocal function. If it is omitted from the sample the variability drops to (106.2 − 104.8 =) 1.4 Hz, or a mere 0.2 ST.

A better approach to the description of variability is to measure the average distance of values from the mean. Such a measure, called the "standard deviation" (SD) is defined as the square root of the sum of the squares of the deviations from the mean.[16] Algebraically,

$$SD = \sqrt{\frac{1}{n}\sum_{i=1}^{n}(\bar{x} - x_i)^2}.$$

The standard deviation is a measure of dispersion that has been quite popular as an index of F_0 variability. The symbol for the standard deviation is the lower-case Greek letter sigma (σ), and so the standard deviation of the fundamental frequency (often expressed in semitones) has often been called *pitch sigma*.

By its very nature, pitch sigma is associated with the mean F_0. Particularly in cases where the median is used as the average, different measures of variability are needed. In these instances it is common to employ the 90% (sometimes 95%) range, which is defined as the frequency values above and below the average between which 90% (or 95%) of the observed frequencies fall. Curry (1940) called the 90% range the *effective range*.

Measuring SF$_0$

Determination of the speaking fundamental frequency requires an adequate speech sample. Two basic decisions about the speech task must be made: Should the patient read a standard test passage or speak spontaneously?[17] How much material must be analyzed to assure a valid measure?

Reading Versus Spontaneous Speech

Using a reading task rather than spontaneous speech has a definite advantage: If the same material is always used it is possible to do comparisons—patient-to-patient or session-to-session. On the other hand, reading ability and style may affect the results, especially in the case of children (Fairbanks, Herbert, & Hammond, 1949; Fairbanks, Wiley, & Lassman, 1949).

The question of whether the SF_0 characteristics of material that is read are different from those of spontaneous speech is pivotal in selecting a sample method (Ramig & Ringel, 1983). Snidecor (1943), Mysak (1959), Saxman and Burk (1968), Hollien and Jackson (1973), and Hollien, Hollien, and de Jong (1997) and have done studies in which the same research subjects

both read and spoke spontaneously. (Snidecor's subjects actually read verbatim transcripts of the extemporaneous speech that they had delivered a week earlier.) All found that the mean SF_0 during reading was slightly higher than the mean for spontaneous speech. The average differences ranged from 1.78 to 0.47 ST. No large differences were found in F_0 variability. Given the small difference between the two tasks, it would seem more efficient to use a reading passage in instances where there is no clinical requirement for a special type of sample and where reading ability is not at issue. Since a great deal of research has been done with Fairbank's (1960) "Rainbow Passage," it is the material that clinicians will probably prefer to use.

Sample Size

There is a tradeoff between the length of the sample analyzed and the accuracy of the SF_0 estimate obtained. Shorter samples are perhaps more convenient, but they reflect the actual values of the larger body of speech that they are intended to represent less accurately. The problem is to find the shortest possible sample that yields an acceptably accurate measure.

Shipp (1967) cited an unpublished study by the Stanford Speech Research Laboratory that showed that SF_0 measures of the second sentence of the Rainbow Passage correlated almost perfectly ($r = .99$) with the same measures of the entire first paragraph. Horii (1975) has done a more extensive investigation of the sampling problem and has come to the following conclusions:

1. For determination of the mean SF_0 use of the second or fourth sentences extracted from a reading of the entire first paragraph of the Rainbow Passage is acceptable. This avoids any special effects associated with initial and final sentences and yields an estimate of tolerable accuracy;

2. If analysis of a fixed amount of time (rather than a certain number of linguistic units) is preferred, an accuracy of about ±3 Hz will require analysis of about 14 s of speech;

3. Using the same sentence, rather than voice sample of equivalent duration, without respect to content, significantly reduces errors of mean SF_0 estimates;

---

[16] The complication in getting the average distance is necessary, and is not due to the whim of statisticians. The square-root-of-the-squares overcomes the problem that the simple sum of the distances of all values <u>from the</u> mean must be zero. If the square root is not taken, the result is SD², which is known as the "variance." Therefore, $SD = \sqrt{\text{Variance}}$. Textbooks of statistics give more efficient ways of calculating the standard deviation than the one described here.

[17] The temptation to use a sustained vowel or a syllable rather than a spoken passage to estimate SF_0 is best resisted. To be sure, the examination task is made considerably easier, analysis is somewhat simplified, and the resulting number somewhat less ambiguous. Unfortunately, the relationship of the F_0 of a sustained vowel to actual SF_0 is, at the very best, unclear and probably unstable (Black, 1940; Fitch, 1990; Higgins, Nelson, & Schulte, 1994; Murry, Brown, & Morris, 1995).

4. The low correlation between the SF_0 variability of a single sentence and that of the entire passage indicates that significantly longer samples are needed to evaluate this parameter.

The length of the test session, and the presumptive vocal fatigue induced by repetition of many test tokens, might reasonably be feared to alter vocal performance. Yet the results of research studies are equivocal in this regard, at least for normal speakers (Neils & Yairi, 1987; Gelfer, Andrews, & Schmidt 1991; Verstraete, Forrez, Mertens, & Debruyne, 1993; Vilkman, Sihvo, Alku, Laukkanen, & Pekkarinen,1993; Brenner, Doherty, & Shipp, 1994; Stemple, Stanley, & Lee, 1995; Rantala, Määttä, & Vilkman, 1997). Common sense would suggest, however, that patients with voice disorders might be less immune to vocal "load." It is prudent, therefore, to limit the strenuousness of testing.

Finally, it is well documented that speakers' F_0 varies from trial to trial, on the same day or across longer time intervals. There is some evidence that this normal variability is greater in some groups than others, but the research to date does not provide unequivocal guidance (Brown, Murry, & Hughes, 1976; Garrett & Healey, 1987; Higgins & Saxman, 1989; Fitch, 1990; Nittrouer, McGowan, Milenkovic, & Beehler, 1990; Coleman & Markham, 1991; Higgins, et al., 1994; Murry et al., 1995). Clinicians should therefore exercise appropriate caution in interpreting changes of measured F_0.

It is well known that vocal F_0 varies as a function of subglottal pressure, which, in turn, is a major physiologic determinant of vocal intensity. More intense speech is likely to be speech at a higher F_0. Buekers and Kingma (1997) have, in fact, confirmed a real and sizable relationship between vocal intensity increase and elevation of SF_0. As far as possible, therefore, testing should be done at a standard intensity level.

Expected Values of SF_0

The literature on SF_0 is quite extensive. Vocal pitch is a very prominent feature of speech and has been explored in terms of emotion (Fairbanks, 1940; Huttar, 1968), mental disorder (Saxman & Burk, 1968; Chevrie-Muller, Dodart, Sequier-Dermer, & Salmon, 1971), overall voice quality (Snidecor, 1943, 1951;

Michel, 1968), intellectual deficit (Michel & Carney, 1964; Montague, Brown, & Hollien, 1974, Montague et al.,1978), laryngeal pathology (Murry, 1978), general systemic, neurologic, and endocrine disorders (Canter, 1965a; Weinberg, Dexter & Horii, 1975; Vuorenkoski, Perheentupa, Vuorenkoski, Lenko, & Tjernlund, 1978; Strand, Buder, Yorkston, & Ramig, 1994), hearing impairment (Martony, 1968; Boothroyd & Decker, 1972; Gilbert & Campbell, 1980), and even sudden infant death syndrome (Colton & Steinschneider, 1980, 1981). It has also been the subject of numerous studies of average normal speakers from birth to old age. Comparability of these studies is often problematic because of differences in sample analysis methods, criteria for subject selection, and the like. This section presents summaries of findings in several categories that are likely to be useful to speech clinicians. Caution in drawing inferences from comparisons of the results of different studies is extremely important.[18]

Life-span Changes of SF_0: An Overview

It is a matter of common observation, confirmed by numerous research studies, that SF_0 changes in a broadly predictable way across the life span. Figure 6–28, an overall summary of the results of several widely-accepted investigations, demonstrates the pattern to be expected.[19]

In early childhood the SF_0s of males and females are comparable. But, because the human larynx is sexually dimorphic, adult women generally have a higher SF_0 than men. In both men and women SF_0 tends to decrease with increasing maturity until, as old age advances, it is likely to rise again. The effect is greater in men and occurs at an earlier age than in women. There is some dispute in the literature about whether the elevation of SF_0 is, in fact, characteristic of aged women's voices. A review of several investigations that used age-stratified samples suggests that SF_0 does, in fact, decline in older women until advanced old age, when it begins to increase. (See, for example, Dordain, Chevrie-Muller, and Grémy [1967] or Charlip [1968]. It is possible, therefore, that increased SF_0 is a characteristic of aged voices that appears considerably later in women than in men. It has been suggested by Baken (1994a) that this effect, among others, is due to increased nonlinearity of laryngeal properties associated with geriatric tissue changes. Other views of the

---

[18] The impact of several factors that may have affected the normative data available in the literature is assessed by Hollien, Hollien, and de Jong (1997).

[19] The figure is a synthesis of the findings of Pronovost (1942), Pilhour (1948), Fairbanks, Herbert, and Hammond (1949), Hanley (1951), Mysak and Hanley (1958, 1959), McGlone and Hollien (1963), Canter (1965a), Michel, Hollien, and Moore (1966), Saxman and Burk (1967), Hollien and Paul (1969), Fitch and Holbrook (1970), Chevrie-Muller, Salmon, and Ferrer (1971), Hollien and Shipp (1972), Hollien and Jackson (1973), Stoicheff (1981), Ramig and Ringel (1983), Chevrie-Muller, Perbos, and Guidet (1983), Morris and Brown (1988), Krook (1988), Linville, Skarin, and Fornatto (1989), Higgins and Saxman, (1991), and Hollien, Hollien, and de Jong (1997).

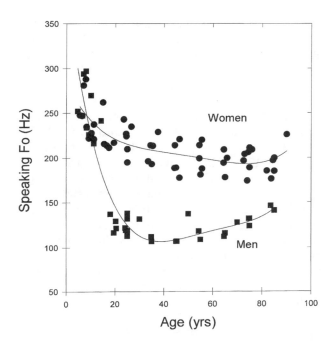

Figure 6–28. Overview of the general trend of SF_0 across the life span. The data points are taken from many different studies; see text.

elderly have also been advanced (see, for example, Hollien, 1987; Ringel and Chodzko-Zajko, 1987; Chodzko-Zajko, Ringel, and Vaca, 1995).

Average SF_0: Normal Adults

Table 6–2 summarizes the findings of several studies that have explored the speaking fundamental frequency level of normal adults. Fitch and Holbrook (1970) have provided good data on *modal* SF_0. They evaluated the "middle 55 words of the Rainbow Passage" as read by 100 men (ages 18 to 25.2 years) and 100 women (ages 17.75 to 23.5 years). Modal SF_0 was determined with a special electronic device, the Florida 1. The resultant data, which may be considered normative for this age group, are given in Table 6–3.

Race. The question of possible racial differences in SF_0 has been addressed by several investigators. Hollien and Malcik (1962, 1967) and Hollien, Malcik, and Hollien (1965) have found a slightly lower SF_0 in young African-American males as compared to their Euro-

pean-American counterparts. Hudson and Holbrook (1981, 1982) found that modal SF_0 was somewhat lower for male and female African-Americans than for European-Americans, and the former also had a somewhat greater mean SF_0 range. Morris (1997), in a study of African-American and European-American boys age 8 through 10 years, found no significant difference in SF_0 (although pitch sigma was greater for the older African-American boys). None of these differences, however, was large enough to be clinically meaningful.[20]

Average SF_0: Normal Aged Adults

Although there is considerable debate about the specific details, it is generally accepted that the voices of aged individuals are different from those of younger adults. Whether there is a specific pattern to the change of SF_0 with advancing old age remains a debated issue. The effect of professional voice training and use also remains to be definitively characterized (Morris, Brown, Hicks, and Howell, 1995). The results of several studies are summarized in Table 6–4.[21]

Average SF_0: Normal Children

There have been a number of studies of the SF_0 of children, the results of which are summarized in Table 6–5. Hollien and Malcik (1967) and Hollien, Malcik, and Hollien (1965) matched the experimental procedure of Curry (1940) in an attempt to determine the age of vocal maturation in boys. On the basis of their own data and those of comparable studies by others they concluded that vocal mutation

1. appears to occur at less than 14 years of age;

2. occurs at about the same age in Caucasian and black males;

3. is unrelated to climatic differences;

4. may be occurring earlier than in the past.

The relationship of SF_0 to hormonal levels and somatic signs of puberty has been carefully studies in boys and girls by Pedersen and her colleagues (Pedersen, Kitzing, Krabbe, & Heramb, 1982; Pedersen et al., 1985, 1986, 1990; Pedersen, 1993).

Cross-sectional studies are unfortunately inadequate for assessing vocal maturation. Addressing this

---

[20] The findings for SF_0 mirror those for the F_0 of sustained vowels. See, for instance, Mayo (1990), Walton and Orlikoff (1994), Mayo and Grant (1995), and Sapienza (1997).

[21] The table includes primarily studies of English speakers, for which the database is most extensive. Information for speakers of other languages may be found in Dordain, Chevrie-Muller, and Grémy (1967), Chevrie-Muller (1971), and Boë, Contini, and Rakotofiringa (1975) for French; Rappaport (1958) and Arndt and Leithäuser (1968) for German; and Krook (1988) for Swedish.

Table 6–2. Speaking Fundamental Frequency of Normal Adults*

Mean	Age Range	No. of Subj.	Mean SF$_0$ Hz	Mean SF$_0$ ST	Mean SF$_0$ Range	Median F$_0$ Hz	SD† ST	Range (ST)	Total Range (ST)	90% Range	Source
						Males					
Spontaneous Speech											
Adult		25	120	34.6				2.64	16.84		1
21–26		6	109.1	32.9							17
20.3	17.9–25.8	157	123.3		90.5–165.2			3.2			2
20.5	18–25	142	116	33.8				3.4			14
47.9	32–62	15	100.0	33.0		107.9	32.6		16.6	9.4	3
73.3	65–79	12	119.3	34.4		120.1	34.3		17.0	9.6	3
85.0	80–92	12	136.2	36.7		136.2	36.7		19.4	11.4	3
Reading											
Adult		25	132	36.3		129	36.0	3.3	19.78		1
Adult		6				132	36.5				6
> 18		10	110.3	33.0				3.1			5
21–26		6	112.9	33.4							17
20.3	18–26	157	129.4	35.7	92.6–178.1						14
20.5	18–25	142	121.5	34.6	95.0–159.4						14
21.3	SD = 1.5	10	123.0	34.9	102–137						15
47.9	32–62	15	113.2	33.4		110.3	32.9		16.79	9.5	3
54.1	26–79	65	112.5	33.4	84–151	110.7	33.1	2.41		7.95	8
18.1	17.8–18.5	6				137.1	36.8	3.58			4
20.3	17.9–25.8	157	129.4	35.8				3.2			2
24.4	20–29	25	119.5	34.4							7
34.9	30–39	25	112.2	33.3							7
45.4	40–49	25	107.1	32.5							7
54.3	50–59	25	118.4	34.3							7
34.6	60–69	25	112.2	33.3							7
74.7	70–79	25	132.1	36.2							7
85.0	80–92	12	141.0	37.2		142.6	37.4		19.6	11.2	3
83.6	80–89	25	146.3	37.9							7

Females

Reading

Mean	Age Range	No. of Subj.	Mean SF$_0$ Hz	Mean SF$_0$ ST	Mean SF$_0$ Range	Median F$_0$ Hz	SD† ST	Range (ST)	Total Range (ST)	90% Range	Source
15.5		89	215.7	44.6	158.6–259.6			3.06			12
16.5		185	213.9	44.5	153.7–256.4			2.96			12
17.5		193	211.5	44.3	127.3–263.1			3.34			12
Adult		6				212	44.4				5
Univ students		27	199.8	43.3		201.0	43.4		23.3	9.32	10
21–26		6	206.4	43.9	93–146						17
21.3	SD = 1.5	10	206.6	43.9	186–230						15
24.6	20–29	21	224.3	45.3	192.2–275.4			3.78			13
27.5	20–32	21	192.4	42.8	175.8–210.2						16
33.5	30–40	9	196.3	43.0	171.4–221.7			2.46			11
35.4		193	211.5	44.3	127.3–263.1			3.34			12

(*Continued*)

Table 6–2: (*continued*)

Mean	Age Range	No. of Subj.	Mean SF₀ Hz	Mean SF₀ ST	Mean SF₀ Range	Median F₀ Hz	SD† ST	Range (ST)	Total Range (ST)	90% Range	Source
44.4	40–50	9	188.6	42.3	168.5–208.3			2.76			11
46.4	40–49	21	220.8	45.1	189.8–272..9			4.00			13
54.4		17	199.3	43.3	176.4–241.2			4.33			13
65.8	60–69	15	199.7	43.3	142.8–234.9			4.25			13
72.6	65–79	10	196.6	43.0	154.5–264.6			2.96	19.1	9.42	9
75.4	τ70	19	202.2	43.5	170.0–248.6			4.70			13
85.0	80–94	19	199.8	43.3	182.9–225.3			2.7	17.7	8.56	9

Spontaneous Speech

21–26		6	210.3	44.2	179–256						17

*Data in the original sources presented in ST or in Hz. Necessary conversions have been done to present the authors' data in both scales for the purposes of this table.

†"Pitch sigma"

Sources:

1. Snidecor, 1943. Impromptu speech followed one week later by reading of verbatim transcript of earlier impromptu statement. Subjects were classed as "superior" talkers by a panel of judges. Hand measurement of mid 23–27 s of samples. Data represent the mean of successive 0.038-s segments.

2. Hollien and Jackson, 1973. Reading of a passage by R. L. Stevenson, as well as extemporaneous speech—about three minutes of each. Analysis by the Fundamental Frequency Indicator (see text).

3. Mysak, 1959. Youngest group are sons of the other two groups. Reading first paragraph of the Rainbow Passage. Analysis by special F₀ analyzer (Dempsey et al., 1950).

4. Curry, 1940. Reading of a 52-word passage. Hand measurement of output. Data represent means of successive 0.038 s segments.

5. Michel, 1968. Reading of Rainbow Passage. Analysis by the Fundamental Frequency Indicator (see text).

6. Pronovost, 1942 and Snidecor, 1951. Reading of sentences 2–5 of the Rainbow Passage. Speakers were judged "superior" by a panel of judges. Hand measurement of output. Data represent means of successive 0.038 s intervals. Estimated error about 0.5%.

7. Hollien and Shipp, 1972, and Shipp and Hollien, 1969. Reading first paragraph of the Rainbow Passage. Analysis by the Fundamental Frequency Indicator (see text).

8. Horii, 1975. Reading of first paragraph of the Rainbow Passage. Analysis by a special computer program.

9. McGlone and Hollien, 1963. Reading of first paragraph of the Rainbow Passage, rehearsed. Hand measurement of oscillographic output.

10. Linke, 1973. Test passage unspecified. Subjects represented a range of speaker "effectiveness." Phonellographic analysis.

11. Saxman and Burk, 1967. Reading of the Rainbow Passage, rehearsed. Analysis by the Fundamental Frequency Analyzer (see text).

12. Hollien and Paul, 1969, and Michel, Hollien, and Moore, 1966. Reading of the Rainbow Passage. Analysis by the Fundamental Frequency Indicator (see text). Note that 307 of the total of 467 subjects were high school cheerleaders, a fact that may have influenced the results.

13. Stoicheff, 1981. Reading of the first paragraph of the Rainbow Passage. Analysis by the Fundamental Frequency Indicator (see text). All subjects were nonsmokers. Older three age groups had significantly lower SF₀s than the younger three groups.

14. Hollien, Hollien, and de Jong, 1997. Two groups: Male university students and military personnel, closely matched in age. Reading material—a passage from R. L. Stevenson—was the same for both groups.

15. Awan (1993). Based on Visi-Pitch® analysis of tape recordings of second sentence of the first paragraph of the Rainbow Passage. Compared to trained singers.

16. Brown, Morris, and Michel (1989). Second sentence of Rainbow Passage, read at conversational loudness. Analysis of tape recordings. Compared to aged women.

17. Fitch, 1990. Middle 55 words of the Rainbow Passage. Spontaneous speech was in response to "common questions that required extended answers," 3 minutes of which was analyzed.

Table 6–3. Modal Speaking Fundamental Frequency (SF_0) of Normal Adults

Sex	Mean age	SF_o Average (Hz)	SF_o Modal (ST*)	S.D. (ST)	Range of Modes (Hz)	Range of Modes (ST)
Male	19.5	116.65	34.0	2.11	85–155	28.5–38.9
Female	19.5	217.00	44.8	1.70	165–255	40.0–47.5

*Computed from authors' data

Source: From "Modal Fundamental Frequency of Young Adults," by J. L. Fitch and A. Holbrook, 1970, Archives of Otolaryngology, 92, 379–382. Table 2, p. 381. Reprinted by permission.

problem, Bennett (1983) has undertaken a longitudinal study of a group of normal boys and girls, and has published SF_0 data for them for ages 8–11 years. Her findings, summarized in Table 6–5B, show that SF_0 is the same for boys and girls over the age range in question and that SF_0 declines across the period. Bennett's study underscores the inadequacy of cross-sectional data for describing age-related changes in children's fundamental frequency.

The subject of racial and/or ethnic influences on children's SF_0 has been addressed in a small number of studies. Awan and Mueller (1996), for instance, have found that African-American kindergartners had a lower mean SF_0 than their Hispanic age-mates, but that neither group was significantly different from kindergartners of European descent. Their data, and those of Wheat and Hudson (1988) for African-American youngsters, are included in Table 6–5A.

The import or implication of any observed differences among racial or ethnic groups (despite statistical significance) is obscured by the virtually universal absence of a definition of the classifying characteristics as well as by a general failure to control for linguistic and social variables.

Normal Infant Cry

The cry of the infant has been the object of considerable research attention for some time (Flatau & Gutzmann, 1906). Two basic interests have motivated this work. First, there has been a persistent conviction that the infant's cry can provide the basis for very early diagnosis of abnormality. This rationale was perhaps best exemplified in the work of Karelitz and his associates (Karelitz & Fisichelli, 1962, 1969; Fisichelli, Karelitz, Eichbauer, & Rosenfeld, 1961; Fisichelli, Haber,

Davis, & Karelitz, 1966) and in that of Michelsson and Wasz-Höckert (1980). Second, developmental specialists have been concerned with the way in which cry changes with maturation and with its relationship to the ultimate acquisition of speech (Prescott, 1975). A number of findings in this general area may be of interest to speech clinicians.[22]

The question of whether the infant's cry varies as a function of the provoking stimulus and whether listeners can categorize cries accordingly is a very old one. As opposed to some earlier work (Wasz-Höckert, Partanen, Vuorenkoski, Valanne, & Michelsson, 1964a, 1964b) recent research has tended to cast doubt on the ability of adult listeners to differentiate types of infant cries with certainty, although mothers apparently can reliably judge whether an infant vocalization is a true cry or just "fussing" (Petrovich-Bartell, Cowan, & Morse, 1982). Nor, it seems, can adults reliably identify infant sex on the basis of the fundamental frequency of the cry (Muller, Hollien, & Murry, 1974; Murry, Hollien, & Muller, 1975). The data of Table 6–6, taken from a study by Murry, Amundson, and Hollien (1977), were derived by hand measurement of oscillographic read-outs of the first and third 15-s intervals of cry samples of at least 90-s duration. The "pain" stimulus was a rubber band snapped against the baby's foot, while startle was the result of a loud noise. Vocal response to withholding of food was labeled a "hunger" cry.

There is, in these data, a clear tendency for males to cry with a higher mean F_0 than females, a finding in agreement with the results of Sheppard and Lane (1968) who studied two children, but not with those of Colton and Steinschneider (1980) who measured the cries of 66 normal infants. Pain also seems to elicit cries with higher F_0 than other stimuli do. There is considerable overlap in the data, however. Some females had

---

[22] Extensive consideration of many aspects of infant cry is provided by Lind (1965) and by Wasz-Höckert, Lind, Vuorenkoski, Partanen, and Valanne (1968).

Table 6–4. Mean Phonational F_o of Normal Aged Speakers

Age Range	Mean Age	No. of Subj.	Mean SF$_o$ (Hz)	SD (Hz)	Sustained /ɑ/ mean F$_o$ (Hz)	SD or range of sustained /ɑ/ (Hz)	Source
				Men			
60–69		21			118	15.8	2
69–85	75	20	162	30.7	162	32.4	1
60–92	ca. 73	6	126.2	25.8			8
> 65		18	130.1	16.7			9
65–85	75	15	127	3.1			11
70–79		27			121	26.9	2
80–92		22			127	22.7	2
	75.3	10			132*	20.2	5
	88	7			126	110–142	3
				Women			
60–69		36			179	27.7	2
60–77	69	20			191.8†	155–215 (SD = 13.9)	7
60–92	ca. 73	15	172.65	13.6			8
69–85	75	20	177	26.7	165	32.5	1
65–85	79	19	175	2.4			11
70–79		54			186	29.4	2
	74.6	11			211*	31.5	5
75–90	79.4	17	175.3	13.4	176.7	19.04	6
80–96		67			178	30.7	2
	88	18			181	131–228	3
100–107	102	5			140†	19.5†	4
	105	1	219	78			10

* Vowel /æ/

† Vowel /i/

Sources:

1. Honjo and Isshiki, 1980. F_o by spectrum analysis. F_o data gathered with perceptual ratings of voice quality.

2. Mueller, Sweeney, and Baribeau, 1984. Subjects "free of major medical problems, particularly those affecting the pulmonary-laryngeal system, as well as communication disorder of significant hearing loss." F_o readout by Visi-Pitch® 6087A system.

3. Mueller, 1982. "Only persons who were free of major medical problems, particularly those affecting the larynx or tracheobronchial system were included. Subjects who exhibited speech, voice, language and/or significant hearing difficulties were excluded." Maximally sustained /a/ in "normal speaking voice." Maximum phonation time also assessed.

4. Mueller, 1989. Subjects were "able to hear speech at normal conversational levels, were free of speech or language defects, were lucid and oriented to the task and did not suffer from dementia. . . . None . . . were afflicted with neurological disease and/or distress of the upper respiratory tract." 9-second sample of extemporaneous speech, evaluated by Visi-Pitch® system.

5. Higgins, M. B., and Saxman, J. H. A comparison of selected phonatory behaviors of healthy aged and young adults. *Journal of Speech and Hearing Research, 34* (1991) 1000–1010.

6. Brown, Morris, and Michel, 1989. Subjects had no history of neurological or respiratory disease and had no hearing loss > 35 dB at 500, 1K, and 2K Hz in at least one ear. Sustained /a/ and second sentence of Rainbow Passage at conversational loudness. Analysis from tape recordings. Compared to young women, see Table 6–2.

7. Biever and Bless, 1989. Subjects were free of neurological disease, no history of laryngeal surgery or disorder, nonsmokers, vocally untrained, hearing threshold better than 35 dB at octave frequencies 500 to 4K Hz in better ear, between 62 and 68 inches (139 cm and 152 cm). Analysis of tape recorded samples.

8. Weatherley, Worrall, and Hickson, 1997. SF_o calculated from spoken phrases consisting exclusively of voiced phones. Compared to hearing-impaired aged subjects.

9. Morris, Brown, Hicks, and Howell, 1995. Combined reading (Rainbow Passage) and spontaneous speech (picture description). Compared to younger men and to professional singers.

10. Max and Mueller, 1996. Conversational speech (radio interview) of an independently-living woman.

11. Brown, Morris, Hollien, and Howell, 1991. Reading of first paragraph of Rainbow Passage. Comparison to professional singers.

Table 6–5A. Speaking Fundamental Frequency of Normal Children

Age (y) Mean	Age (y) Range	No. of Subj.	Mean F_o* (Hz)	Mean F_o* (ST)	Range	SD (ST)	Sources
				Boys			
Spontaneous Speech							
3.8	3.2–4.6	10	283	49.4	241–322		10
4.6		15	252.4	47.4	217.2–292.7		4
‡‡5.4	5.1–6.0	16	249.0		218.2–287.5	5.39	8
††5.5	5.0–6.0	18	241.3		204.9–274.3	5.26	8
5.6	5.1–6.3	15	240.1	46.5	211.9–263.1	4.38	8
††	6.0–6.9	50	219.5	44.9	134.8–298.7		9
6.5		14	247.3	47.0	204.1–274.4		4
††8.3		15	230	45.8		2.1	11
8.4		15	213	44.4		2.5	11
††9.5		15	217	44.8		2.5	11
9.4		15	219	44.9		1.9	11
††10.6		15	204	43.7		3.2	11
10.5		15	220	45.0		2.3	11
Reading							
7.0	6.8–7.2	15	294	50.0		2.2	2
8.0	7.8–8.1	15	297	50.2		2.0	2
††8.3		15	233	46.0		2.1	11
8.4		15	220	45.0		2.1	11
††9.5		15	232	45.9		2.6	11
9.4		15	232	45.9		1.9	11
††10.6		15	215	44.6		3.4	11
10.5		15	225	45.4		2.5	11
10.0	9.8–10.2	6	269.7	48.7		2.38	3
	8.7–12.9	19	273	48.7			7
11.2	10–12	18	226.5	45.5	192.1–268.5	1.51	5
14.2	13.9–14.3	6	241.5	46.8		3.4	3
	13–15.9	15	184	41.9			7
	16–19.5	14	125	35.2			7
				Girls			
Spontaneous Speech							
5.5		18	247.6	47.0	211.9–295.2		4
5.6	5.1–6.1	20	243.4	46.7	195.2–291.1	5.59	8
††5.6	5.1–6.3	17	231.5	45.9	208.1–261.7	5.03	8
‡‡5.6	5.1–5.9	19	248.0	47.1	217.6–274.0	4.64	8
††	6.0–6.9	50	211.3		137.6–297.5		9
6.4		19	247.0	47.0	217.7–274.1		4
Reading							
7.0	6.8–7.2	15	281	49.2		2.0	1
7.9	7.8–8.1	15	288	49.6		2.8	1
	8.6–12.9		256	47.6			6
11.2	10–12	18	237.5	46.32	198.1–271.1	1.51	5
	13–15.9		248	47.1			6
	16—19.8		241	46.6			6

(Continued)

Table 6–5A. (continued)

*Data in original sources is given in either Hz or ST. Conversions have been done so as to present all data in both scales for purposes of this table.

† "Pitch sigma"

†† African-American

‡‡ Hispanic

Sources and notes:

1. Fairbanks, Herbert, and Hammond, 1949. Simple 52-word passage embedded in a longer reading selection. Hand measurement of oscillographic readout.

2. Fairbanks, Wiley, and Lassman, 1949. Same procedure as (1), above.

3. Curry, 1940. Same procedure as (1), above.

4. Weinberg and Zlatin, 1970. Thirty-second sample of elicited spontaneous speech. Compared to Down syndrome children.

5. Horii, 1983b. Normal 5th and 6th grade children reading the Rainbow Passage and the Zoo Passage of Fletcher (1971). Computer derivation of data.

6. Pedersen, Møller, Krabbe, Bennett, and Svenstrup, 1990. Three age groups, 8.6–19.8 ys. 47 subjects; number in each age group not specified. All subjects were students in a music school. Reading of Danish translation of a standard passage: "The North Wind and the Sun." Measurement of 2000 consecutive EGG cycles by special computer program. Relationship to hormonal levels and somatic signs of puberty examined.

7. Pedersen, Møller, Krabbe, S., and Bennett, 1986. All subjects were students at the Copenhagen Singing School. Reading of Danish translation of a standard passage: "The North Wind and the Sun." Measurement of 2000 consecutive EGG cycles by a special computer program. Relationship to hormonal levels and somatic signs of puberty examined. Data also evaluated in Pedersen, Møller, Krabbe, Munk, and Bennett, 1985.

8. Awan and Mueller, 1996. Description of picture. Analysis by Kay Elemetrics CSL system.

9. Wheat and Hudson, 1988. Conversational speech. Analysis by Florida I analyzer (Fitch & Holbrook, 1970).

10. Hall and Yairi, 1992. Spontaneous speech. Analyzed by Cspeech. Compared to age-matched stutterers.

11. Morris, 1997. Same children produced spontaneous speech and reading (second grade level) samples. Analysis by Kay Elemetrics MDVP. software. SF_0 did not differ significantly by race, but pitch sigma was significantly greater for 9- and 10-year-old African-American boys than for their European-American counterparts.

considerably higher cry F_0s than some males, and no stimulus condition produced consistently higher or lower F_0s. The result of the data dispersion is that none of the observed tendencies is statistically significant.

Exploration of developmental changes in cry has been even less complete. Fairbanks (1942) did hand measurement of cry tracings of a single male infant over a period of nine months, but his finding of a mean F_0 as high as 814 Hz casts doubt on the validity of his methods. More recently, Murry, Gracco, and Gracco (1979) have studied the cries of a single female infant from age 2 to 12 weeks. Their data for distress cries are summarized in Table 6–7, while similar data from Prescott (1975) are given in Table 6–8. Hunger cries consistently had a higher mean F_0 than discomfort cries, but no clear developmental trend is apparent.

Spontaneous (nondistress) vocalizations may be more analogous to adult speech than crying is and are of potentially greater interest. They are also harder to study, since they are produced largely at the infant's whim and hence cannot be reliably elicited (Keating & Buhr, 1978). Murry, Gracco, and Gracco (1979) evaluated the nondistress (pleasure) vocalizations of the same infant evaluated in Table 6–6 from the age of 8 to 12 weeks. Mean F_0 for these sounds was 355.8 Hz— almost exactly the same as that of the child's discomfort cries at the same ages. The average F_0 range was considerably smaller, however.

Laufer and Horii (1977) have done a somewhat more extensive exploration of nondistress vocalizations. In a longitudinal study of normal infants (2 boys and 2 girls) they measured the F_0 of utterances of more than 200 ms duration, often resulting from interactions with adults, produced under quasi-naturalistic conditions. Table 6–9 summarizes their findings. There is little variation in average F_0 during the period of the study. On the other hand, the average standard deviation of the F_0 (that is, pitch sigma) dropped to a low in the 5- to 8-week interval and then tended to increase with age. The mean data obscure individual variations in development that may well be meaningful: different infants did, in fact, show different patterns of age-related change. This fact underscores the need for caution in dealing with developmental data on young infants. Each one tends to be unique in many ways, and meaningful differences in vocalization can be observed as early as the perinatal period (Ringel & Kluppel, 1964).

Table 6–5B. Average SF_0 from Ages 8 to 11 (Longitudinal Study)*

Sex	Mean SF_0	SD	Range
Mean Age: 8y 2m			
Boys	234	19.76	204–270
Girls	235	12.31	221–258
Combined	234	16.88	204–270
Mean Age: 9y 2m			
Boys	226	16.42	198–263
Girls	228	9.37	215–239
Combined	226	13.65	198–263
Mean Age: 10y 2m			
Boys	224	14.68	208–259
Girls	228	9.37	215–239
Combined	226	12.76	208–259
Mean Age: 11y 2m			
Boys	216	15.04	195–259
Girls	221	13.43	200–244
Combined	218	14.57	195–259

Source: From "A 3-year Longitudinal Study of School-aged Children's Fundamental Frequencies," by S. Bennett, 1983, *Journal of Speech and Hearing Research, 26*, Table 1, p.138. (c) American Speech-Language-Hearing Association, Rockville, MD. Reprinted by permission.

*15 boys, mean age 8y 3m (SD = 0.48y) at start; 10 girls, mean age 8y 1m (SD = 0.41 y) at start. Repetition of "There is a sheet of paper in my coat pocket." Hand measurement of *all* voiced segments on oscillographic readout. Data for each subject is the average of mean frequencies in 50-ms segments.

Table 6–6. Fundamental Frequency of Infant Distress Cries*

Subjects	Fundamental Frequency (Hz)		
	Pain	Hunger[†]	Startle[†]
Males			
Mean	457.4	451.4	442.2
SD of means**	(59.2)	(47.4)	(41.1)
Females			
Mean	424.7	425.7	400.3
SD of means**	(47.1)	(52.6)	(24.5)
Overall	441.0	438.5	421.3

Source: From "Acoustical Characteristics of Infant Cries: Fundamental Frequency," by T. Murry, P. Amundson, and H. Hollien, 1977, *Journal of Child Language, 4*, Table 1, p. 323. Reprinted by permission.

*Four male and 4 female infants. Age 3 months to 6 months. Method: see text.

[†]See definitions in text.

**Calculated from authors' data.

Information about the fundamental frequency of utterances during the early stages of language development is provided by the results of Robb and Saxman (1985). They used narrow-band spectrograms (see Chapter 7, "Sound Spectrography") to determine the F_0 of the vowel segments of at least 70 utterances (spontaneously produced during play with the parents and with an examiner) by each child. The data are tabulated in Table 6–10. There clearly seems to be a tendency for F_0 to lower with age, although the large intersubject variability prevented this trend from reaching statistical significance. The age-related decrease in F_0 variability, however, was statistically significant.

Average SF_0: Abnormal Speakers

Mental Retardation. There is a considerable body of opinion to the effect that retarded individuals have unusual voices, but there is only a little evidence to support the conclusion that F_0 is a distinguishing feature. Neelley, Edison, and Carlile (1968) found that, on the average, a mixed group of retarded young adults had average SF_0s 2.7 ST higher than a comparable group of normal speakers, but this small difference is unlikely to be the basis of a perceptual difference between groups.

The vocal characteristics of children with Down syndrome have perhaps been investigated more fully than those of any other form of mental retardation. Although Benda (1949), for instance, claimed that the lower-pitch voices of these children were so typical as to permit diagnosis of the disorder, more recent research has clearly indicated that the perceived low pitch is not likely to be due to differences in SF_0. Weinberg and Zlatin (1970) found that higher SF_0 and somewhat greater F_0 variability characterized the spontaneous speech of trisomy-21 boys and girls (age 5.5 to 6.5 years). Michel and Carney (1964), Hollien and Copeland (1965), and Pentz and Gilbert (1983) all failed to find any meaningful differences between the SF_0s of Down syndrome boys and girls and normal children. Montague, Brown, and Hollien (1974) and Montague et al. (1978) have determined that, although the perceived pitch of Down syndrome children is lower than that of normal children, the actual F_0s of the two groups are not meaningfully different. The perception, it was felt, may be due to vocal resonance phenomena. This contention has some support in the research literature (Fisichelli & Karelitz, 1966).

Table 6–7. Fundamental Frequency of Infant Distress Cries: Development in a Single Child*

| Age (wks) | Hunger[†] | | | | Discomfort** | | | |
	Mean F_o (Hz)	F_o Range (Hz)	(ST)	Pitch Sigma (Hz)	Mean F_o (Hz)	F_o Range (Hz)	(ST)	Pitch Sigma (Hz)
2	396.5	110–700	32.0	79.9	372.6	80–620	35.5	74.1
4	403.8	80–700	37.6	107.7	341.9	80–680	37.0	115.7
6	449.1	180–740	24.5	80.2	346.7	60–600	39.9	93.1
8	341.3	80–740	38.5	106.9	340.4	40–620	47.4	104.7
10	417.8	100–680	33.2	90.8	380.6	110–560	2802	88.0
12	427.9	90–680	35.0	93.4				
Mean	406.1	106.7–706.7	33.5		356.5	74.0–616.0	37.6	
SD (Hz)	36.8	37.8–27.3			18.8	26.1–43.4		

Source: From *Infant vocalization during the first twelve weeks* by T. Murry, V. L. Gracco, and L. C. Gracco, 1979. Paper presented at the Annual Convention of the American Speech and Hearing Association. Also from "Infant vocalization: A longitudinal study of acoustic and temporal parameters," by T. Murry, J. Hoit-Dalgaard, and V. Gracco, 1983, *Folia Phoniatrica 35*, 245–253. Reprinted by permission.

*One female infant. Measurement of oscillographic output.

[†]Food withheld after feeding begun.

**Soiled diaper.

Table 6–8. Fundamental Frequency of Infant Distress Cries: Development*

| Age | F_o (Hz) | | Pitch Sigma (Hz) |
	Mean	SD	
1–10 days	384	38	32
4–6 weeks	453	67	30[†]
6–8 weeks	495	53	53[†]
6–9 months	415	39	53

*Normal infants, sex unspecified. Spontaneous cries, cause undetermined. Recording in the child's normal environment.

[†]Significantly different (p<.05) and not related to cry duration.

Source: From "Infant cry sound: developmental features," by R. Prescott, 1975, *Journal of the Acoustical Society of America*, *57*, 1186–1191. Data extracted from Table 1, p. 1189. Reprinted by permission.

Laryngeal Pathology. Most disorders of the larynx do not, in and of themselves, appear to have a consistent influence on the mean SF_0. (Ng et al. [1997], for instance, have documented a decrease of SF_0 in acute laryngitis in men, but a laryngitic increase of SF_0 in women.) Some representative data are included in Table 6–11. F_0 variability and range do seem to reflect tissue changes more consistently, at least in the case of some pathologies. Hecker and Kreul (1971), for example, found that patients with laryngeal cancer had a restricted SF_0 range during reading of the second sentence of the Rainbow Passage. They also showed a smaller rate of change of the fundamental frequency.

Orlikoff et al. (1997) observed a slightly lower-than-normal pitch sigma (1.89 ST) in 19 male patients with advanced laryngeal cancer, and they found that it rose slightly (to an average of 2.28 ST) after a strongly positive response to chemotherapy. Murry (1978) studied patients with different laryngeal disorders. His data (summarized in Table 6–11) showed that only the standard deviation and range of the SF_0 of men with unilateral vocal fold paralysis were different from normal. (His data tend to support Hecker and Kreul's [1971] finding of reduced SF_0 range in cases of cancer, however.) Murry was led to conclude that "organically based voice disorders are not characterized by a [SF_0] that is lower than that found in normal voices" (p. 378). Laguaite and Waldrop (1964) and Hufnagle and Hufnagle (1984) have observed that the fundamental frequency of dysphonic patients does not change significantly as a result of therapy. Vocal fold edema may represent an exception to the general rule. Fritzell, Sundberg, and Strange-Ebbesen (1982) discovered that some women with confirmed vocal fold edema have SF_0s considerably lower than expected. Further, the SF_0 of all of their patients rose significantly following surgical stripping of the vocal folds.

It appears that SF_0 may also be influenced by extralaryngeal problems in the neck. Debruyne et al. (1997), for instance, studied the SF_0 of women who underwent thyroidectomy (for a variety of reasons) but who suffered no apparent injury to the laryngeal innervations pre- or post-operatively. Their results, summarized in Table 6–12, are generally consistent with those of similar studies (Kark, Kissin, Auerbach, & Meikle, 1984; Keilmann & Hülse, 1992), and suggest the pos-

Table 6–9. Fundamental Frequency of Nondistress Vocalizations by Normal Infants (1–2 weeks)*

Age (weeks)		Mean F_o (Hz)	Median F_o (Hz)	Modal F_o (Hz)	SD Hz	SD ST
1–4	Mean	317	319	329	38.8	2.24
	SD	328.2	38.2	48.0	15.2	0.95
5–8	Mean	338	338	344	27.7	1.40
	SD	40.8	39.9	43.3	13.5	0.66
9–12	Mean	338	337	346	31.2	1.63
	SD	40.1	10.9	43.6	15.2	0.79
13–16	Mean	339	341	346	30.4	1.57
	SD	41.7	41.6	44.8	15.5	0.71
17–20	Mean	337	339	349	33.3	1.74
	SD	43.3	43.8	50.4	14.5	0.75
21–24	Mean	342	341	356	37.8	1.94
	SD	51.5	53.8	62.5	18.0	0.84

Mean Lowest, Mean Highest, and Mean Range of Fundamental Frequencies within Utterances

Age (weeks)		Mean Lowest (Hz)	Mean Highest (Hz)	Mean 5th %ile (Hz)	Mean 95th %ile (Hz)	Mean 5–95th %ile (Range in ST)
1–4	Mean	217	412	251	372	6.89
	SD	62.2	75.9	49.0	54.0	3.15
5–8	Mean	268	408	294	381	4.34
	SD	50.0	69.8	40.5	58.5	2.15
9–12	Mean	247	410	285	382	5.07
	SD	52.7	63.3	43.6	53.7	2.58
13–16	Mean	252	413	286	283	4.94
	SD	48.4	72.9	41.4	56.7	2.34
17–20	Mean	239	423	281	383	5.33
	SD	49.7	76.2	44.5	55.8	2.45

*Longitudinal study, 2 male and 2 female normal infants. Spontaneous (sometimes elicited) vocalizations in a quasi-normal environment. Analysis by special computer program.

Source: From "Fundamental frequency characteristics of infant non-distress vocalizations during the first 24 weeks," by M. Z. Laufer and Y. Horii, 1977, *Journal of Child Language, 4*, 171–184. Table 1 p. 175. Reprinted by permission.

Authors caution that "individual variation in each of the measures was obscured when averaged as mean data."

sibility that SF_0 might serve to gauge the status of post-surgical recovery.

Stutterers. It has become fairly clear that the fluent speech of stutterers differs from that of normal speakers. An investigation by Healey (1982) measured the F_0 characteristics of declarative and interrogative sentences as spoken by adult stutterers and nonstutterers (Table 6–13). Stutterers had a significantly lower pitch sigma and used a more restricted pitch range. This finding is consistent with the results of earlier work by Travis (1927), Bryngelson (1932), and Schilling and Göler (1961), and argues for that view of stuttering that extends beyond simple dysfluency. On the other hand, Hall and Yairi (1992) failed to find a statistically significant difference between the SF_0s of fluent and stuttering children in the age range of 3 to 4 years.

Esophageal Pseudophonation. Unusual vocal pitch is a common hallmark of esophageal voice and is often the object of attempts at therapeutic modification. The data summarized in Table 6–14 provide guidelines of what can be expected of the laryngectomized speaker.[23]

---

[23] Some data for patients with surgically constructed neoglottises are available. See, for example, Robbins, Fisher, and Logemann (1982).

The relationship between the SF_0 of esophageal pseudophonation and voice acceptability has been explored by Shipp (1967) who had a very large group of naïve listeners rate tape recordings of 33 male esophageal speakers for general speech acceptability. He then compared those with above-average ratings to those who were deemed less adequate, and he contrasted the six best speakers to the rest. SF_0 data were generated by wave-by-wave analysis of the second sentence of the Rainbow Passage. Pitch sigma and the 90% SF_0 data were generated by wave-by-wave analysis of the second sentence of the Rainbow Passage. Pitch sigma and the 90% SF_0 range had no significant correlation with rated speech acceptability. The relationship of mean SF_0 was significant ($p < .05$) but the correlation, at $r = -.35$ was not very strong. It was clear from Shipp's analysis that respiratory noise, duration of the sentence, and percent periodic phonation were more important to the judges.

Esophageal speakers, then, can be expected to have an SF_0 about one octave below that of normal speakers (Kyttä, 1964) with variability (in ST) comparable to normal adults. The perceived lack of variability of esophageal pitch probably lies in the nonlinearity of pitch perception at very low frequencies (Stevens & Volkmann, 1940), which has the effect of requiring more F_0 change per unit change in pitch. (Clinically significant aspects of the physiology of esophageal pitch variation are considered by van den Berg and Moolenaar-Bijl, 1959.)

Table 6–10. Fundamental Frequency of Nondistress Vocalizations by Normal Infants (11–25 Months)*

Age (months)	No. in Group	Mean (Hz)	Range (Hz)	SD (Hz)
11–13	2	400	366–435	187
14–16	4	378	305–537	154
17–19	3	363	320–407	38
20–22	2	328	310–362	50
23–25	3	314	269–364	60

*Seven boys, 7 girls. Spontaneous utterances during play. Narrow-band spectrographic measurement. >70 utterances per child.

Source: From "Developmental trends in vocal fundamental frequency of young children," by M. P. Bobb and J. H. Saxman, 1985, *Journal of Speech and Hearing Research, 28*, 421–427. Table 4, p. 425. (c) American Speech-Language-Hearing Association, Rockville, MD. Reprinted by permission.

Table 6–11 Speaking Fundamental Frequency: Laryngeal Pathology

Group	Mean SF_0 (Hz)	SD of SF_0	Range of SF_0	Sources
Normal (Men)	121.9	4.63 ST	10.60 ST	1
Paralysis (Men)	127.0	3.64 ST[†]	7.55 ST[†]	1
Benign mass (Men)	133.0	4.34 ST	10.55 ST	1
Cancer (Men)	133.3	3.89 ST	9.04 ST	1
Normal (Men)	129.0			2
Laryngitis (Men)	97.8			2
Normal (Women)	204.9			2
Laryngitis (Women)	223.8			2
Normal (Men)	137	6 Hz	106–190 Hz	3
Radiation (Men)	194[†]	14 Hz	132–326 Hz	3
Normal (Women)	186	13 Hz	162–214 Hz	3
Radiation (Women)	271[†]	25 Hz	228–336 Hz	3

[†]Significantly different from normals.

Sources:

1. Murry, T., 1978. 80 males: 20 normal (mean age 52.5 y, SD 11.9); 20 unilateral paralysis (mean age 53.0y, SD 11.35); 20 benign mass (mean age 57.6y, SD 10.05); 20 laryngeal cancer (mean age 60.7y, SD 8.74). Measurement of oscillographic readout of third sentence of the Rainbow Passage, extracted from a reading of the entire selection.

2. Ng and Lerman, 1997. 8 women, 3 men. "Normal" voices are those of the same speakers after recovery from acute laryngitis. Nature of recorded material unspecified.

3. Dagli, Mahieu, and Festen, 1997. 16 men (mean age 63.3 y, range 43–86 y) and 4 women (mean age 71.5 y, range 57–87 y) who had been treated with radiation for T1a or T1b glottic carcinoma no less than 1 y before data collection. None had observable recurrence of tumor at time of testing. Normal subjects matched to cancer group by age and sex.

Table 6-12. Speaking Fundamental Frequency of Women Before and After Thyroidectomy

Thyroidectomy	N	SF$_o$		
		Preoperative	4th Day Post-op	15th Day Post-op
Bilateral	32	207.8	194.3	202.2
Unilateral	15	216.0	208.3	212.5
Overall	47	210.4	198.8	205.4

*Thyroidectomy was performed for goiter or hyperthyroidism. No malignant tumors were present.

Source: Debruyne, Ostyn, Delaere, and Wellens (1997).

Table 6-13. Variability of the Speaking Fundamental Frequency: Stutterers

Statistic	Declarative		Interrogative	
	Stutterers	Normals	Stutterers	Normals
Mean SF$_0$ (Hz)	105.65	107.69	113.79	119.25
SD of SF$_0$ (ST) (pitch sigma)	1.35	1.74	1.59	3.19
Range of SF$_0$ (ST)	5.24	7.28	4.88	8.80

*10 male stutterers, age 16–52 (mean 29) and 10 normal males matched to stutterers for age and mean SF$_0$. Two all-voiced phrases (declarative and interrogative) embedded in a carrier. Hand measurement of oscillographic readout. Only fluent portions analyzed.

Source: From "Speaking fundamental frequency characteristics of stutterers and nonstutterers," by E. C. Healey, 1982, *Journal of Communication Disorders*, *15*, 21–29. Table 1, p. 27. Copyright 1982 by Elsevier Science Publishing Co., Inc. Reprinted by permission.

Pitch sigma and SF$_0$ range differences between normals and stutterers are significant ($p < .05$).

Pulse Register Versus "Harsh" Voice. It has been shown (Michel & Hollien, 1968) that the "harsh" quality that characterizes some vocal disorders is perceptually distinct from pulse register (vocal fry). The basis for the perception was explored by Michel (1968). Ten normal adult male speakers read the Rainbow Passage using their customary voices and then using continuous pulse register. Another group of 10 men whose voices had been judged clinically "harsh" read the same material. SF$_0$ was measured with a phonellograph (pulse register samples) or with the Fundamental Frequency Indicator (normal and harsh voices). Results are summarized in Table 6–15.

It is obvious that pulse register had a much lower mean SF$_0$ than did harsh voice. The measures of variability failed to discriminate between harsh and pulse register voice, although there was considerably greater heterogeneity of the total range of harsh-voice speakers than of pulse-register users. It seems clear that perceptual differentiation of harsh vocal quality from normal pulse register phonation depends heavily on an SF$_0$ discrimination.

MAXIMUM PHONATIONAL FREQUENCY RANGE

Measures of SF$_0$ provide information about how a speaker uses her voice. The *maximum phonational frequency range* (MPFR) says something about her basic vocal ability. It is also likely that the MPFR reflects the physical condition of the phonatory mechanism. Michel and Wendahl (1971 p. 470) are of the opinion that "during speech utilizing a normal phonational mechanism, a certain degree of variability in frequency is expected and indeed deemed necessary. The extent to which the mechanism does not or cannot produce a range of frequencies may be the first indication of non-normal function." "*Does not*" is in the province of the SF$_0$; "*cannot*" may be assessed by the MPFR.

The MPFR is also the starting point in generating the voice range profile (formerly called the *phonetogram*, see Chapter 5, "Speech Intensity"). It is defined (Hollien, Dew, & Philips, 1971) as "that range of vocal frequencies encompassing both the modal and falsetto registers; its

Table 6–14. Speaking Fundamental Frequency: Esophageal Pseudophonation

Number	Mean SF$_o$ Hz (ST)	Mean SF$_o$ (Range)	Mean Hz (ST)	SD of SF$_o$ (Range)	Mean Highest SF$_o$ Hz (ST)	Mean Highest SF$_o$ Range	Mean Lowest SF$_o$ Hz (ST)	Mean Lowest SF$_o$ Range	Sources
Men									
22	65.59 (24.0)	42.92–85.81 16.7–28.7	14.66	7.79–25.00					1
18	57.4 (21.74)			(4.15)					2
6	63.0 (23.2)	50.9–76.7 (19.4–26.8)			115.3 (33.7)	95.2–135.5 (30.4–36.6)	25.3 (8.3)	17.2–32.2 (8.0–11.8)	3
15	65.7 (24.1)			(4.12)					4
10	64.6	56.0–104.0							5
15	77.1		22.5	range = 118.1Hz					6
Women									
15	86.65 (28.87)			(3.94)					2

Sources:

1. Hoops and Noll, 1969. First paragraph of the Rainbow Passage. Measurement of oscillogram.

2. Weinberg and Bennett, 1971, 1972. Second sentence of the Rainbow Passage. Measurement of oscillogram. Poor speakers excluded. Male / female differences were significant ($p < .01$).

3. Curry and Snidecor, 1961; Snidecor and Curry, 1959; Curry, 1962. Six superior speakers. Rainbow Passage. Measurement of oscillogram.

4. Torgerson and Martin, 1980. Second sentence of Rainbow Passage. Poor speakers excluded. Measurement of oscillogram. Data are derived from averages of successive 50-ms intervals. Comparison to nonlaryngectomee esophageal speakers.

5. Blood, 1984. Second sentence of Rainbow Passage. SF$_0$ derived from contiguous samples by then-current model of Kay Visi-Pitch.

6. Robbins, Fisher, Blom, and Singer, 1984. Second sentence of Rainbow Passage. Wave-by-wave measurement by means of an interactive computer system

Table 6–15. Speaking Fundamental Frequency: Pulse Register and "Harsh" Voices*

Sample	Mean SF$_0$ (Hz)	SD of SF$_0$ (ST)	Total Range (ST)	90% Range (ST)
"Normal" mean	110.6	3.1		
Pulse mean SD	36.4†	4.4 (0.81)	25.6 (2.1)	13.5 (2.2)
"Harsh" mean SD	122.1	3.3 (0.86)	25.6 (6.4)	11.8 (3.9)

*See text for method.

†Mean SF$_0$ of pulse register is significantly different ($p < .01$) from harsh or normal. Normal and harsh SF$_0$s are not significantly different from each other.

Source: From "Fundamental frequency investigation of vocal fry and harshness," by J. F. Michel, 1968, *Journal of Speech and Hearing Research, 11,* 590–594. Table 1, p. 593. © American Speech-Language-Hearing Association, Rockville, MD. Reprinted by permission.

extent is from the lowest tone sustainable in the modal register to the highest in falsetto, inclusive" (p. 755). Modal and loft (falsetto) are both included in the range because of the difficulty of reliably differentiating them perceptually. Pulse register ("vocal fry") is excluded because it is not normally used continuously for running speech, and the very concept of fundamental frequency is of dubious validity for phonation that is characteristically highly irregular in repetition rate.

Measurement Technique

The MPFR has typically been determined using a pitch-matching procedure. The patient is asked to sustain a vowel (usually /ɑ/) at the same pitch as a stimulus tone presented through an earphone. (A triangle- or saw-tooth-wave oscillator is commonly used to generate the stimuli.) Beginning at a comfortable fundamental frequency the stimuli are lowered in pitch (perhaps in 2-ST steps) until the patient can no longer sustain modal-register phonation. Stimulus frequency then ascends from the comfortable level until loft register phonation becomes unsustainable. The F_0 actually achieved by the patient in response to the highest- and lowest-frequency stimuli is determined by instrumental analysis of the vocal signal, using any of the techniques discussed earlier. Neither the musical quality of the phonation nor the accuracy of the match to the stimulus is a criterion for trial acceptability.

However, Reich, Frederikson, Mason, & Schlauch (1990) have shown that, in modal register, the maximal phonatory F_0 is increased, and hence MPFR is expanded, by having adult subjects follow glissando stimuli whose frequency sweeps two octaves above and two octaves below starting points of 277 Hz for men and 392 Hz for women. (The effect of the glissando elicitation method on minimal F_0 was small.) The effect of glissando stimuli on measured MPFR was similar in children (Reich, Mason, Frederikson, and Schlauch, 1989). Having patients produce a "sweep" across their vocal frequency range is likely to produce a better estimate of MPFR and may therefore be preferred to eliciting discrete F_0 increments.

The reliability of measurements of lowest sustainable vocal F_0 has been addressed by Cooper and Yanagihara (1971) in adults and by Austin and Leeper (1975) in children. Both studies found significant variation as a function of time of day. Gelfer (1989) has evaluated the MPFR of each of 10 men and 10 women at several times during a single day and at similar times during a day 1 to 2 months later. She concluded that men's MPFR is significantly greater in the morning than in the late afternoon / early evening. Women's MPFR did not show significant diurnal change. The measured MPFR of neither sex showed significant variation as a function of the 1- to 2-month sampling interval.

Expected Results

Normal Speakers

Table 6–16 summarizes the findings of several comparable studies of the MPFR of normal adults. While men do not differ from women in the extent of their ranges, it is clear that the older speakers' ranges are restricted by reduced ability to achieve high vocal F_0. Ramig and Ringel (1983) have studied men in three age groups 25 to 35, 45 to 55, and 65 to 78 years. Eight members of each group were in good physical condition, as estimated by resting heart rate, diastolic and systolic blood pressure, and forced vital capacity. The other eight men in each group were in relatively poor physical condition, as judged by the same measures. The groups were not significantly different in terms of highest or lowest sustainable F_0. Age did not significantly affect MPFR

(which was measured somewhat differently from the other studies summarized in Table 6–16) but physical condition *was* a significant factor. Subjects in good physical condition had larger phonational ranges than those in poor condition. It is therefore conceivable (but not yet proven) that biological aging (as reflected in physical condition) is a much more powerful restrictor of MPFR than simple chronological age.

An interesting study by Fishman and Shipp (1970) evaluated the effect of subject posture on MPFR, which was determined for each of fifteen males, ages 21 to 33 years, in standing and supine positions. Data were derived from a 10-ms segment of each vowel prolongation. The results (Table 6–17) showed that both upper and lower fundamental frequency limits are reduced in the supine position, with a consequent reduction in the MPFR. Although the difference in the two ranges was statistically significant ($p < .05$) it was quite small, suggesting that "unless the absolute limits of the frequency range are of critical importance, valid vocal range data can be obtained from untrained naïve subjects in the supine position" (Fishman & Shipp, 1970, p. 432). The clinician need not be overly concerned about patient posture during testing.

MPFR is commonly determined as part of a larger, more complete vocal evaluation that includes laryngeal endoscopy. In this regard, it is worth noting that the anesthesia of the pharyngeal region, induced as a standard part of the endoscopic examination technique, has an adverse effect on MPFR (Kim et al., 1998). Although it might seem unnecessary to point out, examination of vocal characteristics should be done before administration of drugs or invasive devices.

Abnormal Speakers

Amyotrophic Lateral Sclerosis (ALS). Silbergleit et al. (1997) have examined a number of vocal characteristics of men and women with ALS who had perceptually normal speech. Among the factors that differentiated these patients from comparable normal speakers was a restricted MPFR. A summary of their findings is given in Table 6–18.

Parkinson Disease. Canter's (1965a, 1965b) study of the speech of Parkinsonian patients demonstrates the effect that neuropathology may have on laryngeal adjustment capabilities. The data of Table 6–19 show a highly noticeable and statistically significant ($p < .01$) difference in the median lowest frequency attainable by the two groups. Highest F_0s do not differ significantly, however. The MPFR is accordingly reduced in Parkinson's patients. The data of Gamboa et al. (1997), also included in Table 6–19, confirm a reduced MPFR, even in patients who are in active drug therapy for the disorder. The inability to achieve a very low F_0 is consistent with the increased muscle tone that is characteristic of Parkinson disease. Other neuropathologies may well influence the MPFR in ways that are consistent with their particular effects on the neuromotor system.

Pulse and Loft Registers.   Pulse register is, by definition, excluded in the determination of the MPFR[24]; loft register is considered, however. The limits of F_0 adjustment of these registers have been determined separately, however. The data are summarized in Table 6–20, along with findings for the modal register alone.

Table 6–16. Maximal Phonational Frequency Range

Age Mean	Age Range	No. of Subj	Lowest F_0* Mean	Lowest F_0* Range	Highest F_0* Mean	Highest F_0* Range	MPFR* Mean	MPFR* Range	Sources
					Men				
20.3	17.9–25.8	157	79.5	62.0–110.0	763.6	292.0–1568.0	864.1		3
			/27.4/	/23.1–33.0/	/66.5/	/55.0–79.0/	/38.8/	/29–54/	3
21.4	18–36	332	80.1	61.7–123.5	674.6	220.0–1567.8	594.5		1
			/27.5/	/23–35/	/64.4/	/45–79/	/37.9/	/13–55/	1
	young adult	14	87	69–110	571	440–698	484		4
			/28.9/	/24.9–33.0/	/61.5/	/57.0–65.0/	/32.4/	/29–36/	4
27.1	23–33	10	84.8	61.7–123.5	752.8	493.8–932.2			7
			/28.5/	/23–35/	/66.3/	/59–70/	/37.8/	/30–45/	7
27.6	18–39	31	77.3		567.3		490		2
			/26.9/		/61.4/		/34.5/		2
76.9	68–89	27	85.3		394.2		308.9		2
			/28.6/		/55.1/		/26.5/		2
56.8[†]	35.5–75.0	17	80[†]	40–120	260.0[†]	190–440			5
			/27.5[†]/	/15.5–34.5/	/47.9[†]/	/42.5–57.0/	/22.1[†]/	/8–36/	5
					Women				
21	18–33	44	141.4	93.8–190.1	884.1	334.1–1917.4	743.4	199.6–1816.0	6
			/37.3/	/30.2–45.2/	/85.4/	/52.2–82.5/	/30.3/		6
22.8	18–36	202	140.2	98–196	1121.5	587.3–2092.8	981.3		1
			/37.2/	/31–43/	/73.2/	/62.0–84.0/	/37.0/	/23–50/	1
23.5	18–38	31	134.6		895.3		760.7		1
			/36.5/		/69.3/		/32.8/		2
27.1	23–33	10	127.1	98.0–164.8	1102.2	830.5–1666.1			7
			/35.5/	/31–40/	/72.9/	/68–80/			7
76.9	66–93	36	133.8		570.6		436.8		2
			/36.4/		/61.5/		/25.1/		2

Data have been converted from Hz to ST, or vice versa, as required.

*Data within slashes (/ /) are in ST, others in Hz.

[†]Median

Sources:

1. Hollien, Dew, and Phillips, 1971.

2. Ptacek, Sander, Maloney, and Jackson, 1966.

3. Hollien and Jackson, 1973. "Extreme intersubject variability." SF0 data are also available for these subjectcs.

4. Shipp and McGlone, 1971.

5. Canter, 1965a. Research compared normals and parkinsonian patients.

6. Kim, Oates, Phyland, and Campbell, 1998. Compared to performance after pharyngeal anesthesia.

7. Gelfer, 1989. Data are means of three trials on each of two days, 1 to 2 months apart.

---

[24] A word of caution is in order, however. It has repeatedly been noted that a hallmark of pulse register phonation is the alternation of long and short periods (Moore & von Leden, 1958; Timcke, von Leden, & Moore, 1959; Wendahl, Moore, & Hollien, 1963; Hollien, Girard, & Coleman, 1977; Cavallo, Baken, & Shaiman, 1984). The exact meaning of "fundamental frequency" in such a circumstance may be debatable.

Table 6-17. Maximal Phonational Frequency Range: Effect of Posture

	Standing		Supine	
	Mean Hz	Mean ST*	Mean Hz	Mean ST*
Highest F_o	639.8	63.5	629.1	63.2
Lowest F_o	81.1	27.7	84.2	28.4
MPFR	558.7	35.7	544.9	34.8

*Computed from authors' data.

Source: From "Subject positioning and phonation range measures," by B. Fishman and T. Shipp, 1970, Journal of the Acoustical Society of America, 48, 431–432. Table 1, p. 432. Reprinted by permission.

Table 6-18. Maximum Phonational Frequency Range: Amyotrophic Lateral Sclerosis

		Age		
Group	N/Sex	Mean	Range	MPFR
Normal	13 M	56.1	34–77	22.7*
	13 F	56.5	37–72	
ALS	15 M	57.2	31–88	16.4*
	5 F	63.2	37–79	

*Groups are significantly different, $p = .0025$

Sustained /a/ and /i/. Analysis by Cspeech.

Source: Silbergleit, Johnson, and Jacobson (1997).

Table 6-19. Maximum Phonational Frequency Range: Parkinson Disease*

		Lowest F_0		Highest F_0		Range in ST[†]		
Group	Unit	Median	Range	Median	Range	Median or Mean and (SD)	Range	Sources
Normal Men	Hz	80**	40–120	260	190–440			1
	ST‡	27.5	15.5–34.5	47.9	42.5–57.0	22.1**	8.0–36.4	1
Normal Men	ST					20.9 (4.84)		2
Normal Women	ST					19.9 (3.92)		2
Parkinson Men: Untreated	Hz	100**	80–130	220	140–330			1
	ST‡	31.4	27.5–35.9	45.0	37.2–52.0	15.0**	4.0–22.0	1
Parkinson Men: treated	ST					18.4 (3.68)		2
Parkinson Women: treated	ST					17.3 (4.96)		2

*17 subjects in each group. Age 35.5–75 years; median 56.8; groups matched. Hand measurement of oscillograms.

[†]Original data in octaves

**Significant differences: median lowest ($p < .01$), median range ($p < 0.5$)

‡Computed from author's data.

Parkinson patients: 24 males, 17 females. Mean subject age 69.8 y (SD = 6.8 y); Mean age at disease onset 65.0 y (SD = 7.8y). All subjects in drug treatment, 37 with levodopa or levodopa in combination with other drugs.

1. Canter, G. J., 1965b, Speech characteristics of patients with Parkinson's disease: II. Physiological support for speech. Journal of Speech and Hearing Disorders, 30, 44–49. Table 1,p. 46. © American Speech-Language-Hearing Association, Rockville MD. Reprinted by permission.

2. Gamboa, Jiménez-Jiménez, Nieto, Montojo, Orti-Pareja, Molina, Garcia-Albea, and Cobeta, 1997.

Table 6–20. Maximum Phonational Frequency Range: Pulse and Loft Registers (Young Adults)

No. of Subjects	Units	Lowest F_o Mean	Lowest F_o Range	Highest F_o Mean	Highest F_o Range	MPFR	Source
				Pulse			
Men							
5	Hz	26.8	22–32	80.0	62–92	53.2	1
	ST	8.4	5.1–11.6	27.3	23.1–29.9	18.9	1
12	Hz	24		52		28	2
	ST	6.6		20.0		13.4	2
Women							
11	Hz	18		46		28	2
	ST	1.7		17.9		16.2	2
				Modal			
Men							
5	Hz	78.2	65–98	462	330–523	383.8	1
	ST	26.9	23.9–31.0	57.6	52–60	30.7	1
12	Hz	94		287		193	2
	ST	30.3		49.6		19.4	2
Women							
11	Hz	144		538		394	2
	ST	37.7		60.5		22.8	2
				Loft			
Men							
12	Hz	275		634		359	2
	ST	48.9		63.3		14.4	2
Women							
11	Hz	495		1131		636	2
	ST	59.0		73.3		14.3	2

Sources:

1. Murry, 1971

2. Hollien and Michel, 1968

Note: Data have been converted to ST if not so given in original source

FREQUENCY PERTURBATION (JITTER)

Definition and Significance

While MPFR assesses certain aspects of the limits of laryngeal adjustment, and SF_0 measures how those adjustments are used in running speech, the degree of frequency perturbation is intended to provide an index of the stability of the phonatory system.

Frequency (or *period*) *perturbation*—commonly called *jitter*—is the variability of the fundamental frequency (or, reciprocally, of the fundamental period) from one cycle to the next. When measured during running speech, variability is reflected in pitch sigma.

Jitter measurements, however, are concerned with short-term variation. That is, jitter is a measurement of how much a given period differs from the period that immediately follows it, and not how much it differs from a cycle at the other end of the utterance. Jitter, then, is a measure of the frequency variability not accounted for by voluntary changes in F_0. If the phonatory system were an ideal and perfectly stable mechanism, there would be absolutely no difference in fundamental periods except when a speaker purposely changed pitch; frequency perturbation would be zero. To the extent that jitter is not zero, "perturbation is an acoustic correlate of erratic vibratory patterns" (Beckett, 1969, p. 418) that result from diminished neuromotor and aerodynamic control, altered tissue rheology (Hemler, Wieneke, & Dejonkere, 1997) and presumably even modified auditory-feedback control over the phonatory system (Elliott & Niemoller, 1970; Sorenson, Horii, & Leonard, 1980; Ternström, Sundberg, & Colldén, 1988; Burnett, Senner, & Larson, 1997).

More than seventy years ago Simon (1927, p. 83) concluded that "there are no tones of constant pitch in either vocal or instrumental sounds." The phonatory system is in no way a perfect machine and every speaker's vibratory cycles are erratic to some extent. But, on the face of it, one would guess that an abnormal larynx should produce a more erratic voice than a healthy one. On the whole this turns out to be the case.[25] There is by now a considerable body of literature that asserts the validity, in many and varied situations, of frequency perturbation measures for the evaluation or categorization of laryngeal and vocal pathology and for the validation of perceptual attributes of the disordered voice (Kitajima, Tanabe, & Isshiki, 1975; Davis, 1976; Horii, 1979; Lieberman, 1961, 1963; Hecker & Kreul, 1971; Klingholz & Martin, 1983; Hartmann & von Cramon, 1984; Zyski, Bull, McDonald, & Johns, 1984; Haji et al., 1986; Ramig, Scherer, Titze, & Ringel, 1988; Scherer, Gould, Titze, Meyers, & Sataloff, 1988; Ramig et al., 1990; Wolfe, Cornell, & Palmer, 1991; Kempster, Kistler, & Hillenbrand, 1991; Baker, Ramig, Johnson, & Freed, 1997; Wolfe & Martin, 1997; McAllister, Sundberg, & Hibi, 1998).[26] This should not be taken to imply that jitter can be used as the sole diagnostic criterion, or that it accounts for all of what the listener perceives in the disordered voice. Far from it: factors such as amplitude perturbation (Wendahl et al., 1963; Wendahl, 1966a, 1966b; Takahashi & Koike, 1975; Horii, 1980), spectral noise (Emanuel, Lively, & McCoy, 1973; Emanuel & Scarinzi, 1979, 1980; Emanuel & Austin, 1981) and glottal waveform changes (Coleman, 1971) account for a great deal, probably most, of what is heard as abnormality. But frequency perturbation is sufficiently sensitive to pathological changes in the phonatory process, and perhaps even to severe respiratory insufficiency (Gilbert, 1975) to warrant careful consideration.

Still, a major caveat is in order. Although, as the data tables that follow make clear, increased vocal jitter is clearly associated with voice disorder, the magnitude of jitter—no matter how measured—is not a guide to the cause of the dysphonia. In this respect jitter measures have proven to be a major disappointment to the vocal diagnostician. For better or worse, however, computer analysis systems make the evaluation of jitter extremely—maybe even overly—easy, with the result that jitter indices are perhaps overused. Furthermore,

there is a large number of different measures, all of which can legitimately be called indices of jitter. The plethora of measurement methods and the perils of interpretation call for careful exploration and judicious —**very** judicious—application of jitter measures.

Sources of Perturbation

Although the term *jitter* is generally accepted as a designation of the *random* variations in vocal F_0, one should not by any means assume that the randomness is real (because there may be underlying, but undetected, regularity) or that it is necessarily without identifiable causes. In fact, a number of factors are felt, or have been demonstrated, to contribute to vocal perturbation. While some, in fact, seem to result in random variation, others are more deterministic. Clinicians might want to keep the following potential sources of jitter in mind as they evaluate test results.

1. *Neurogenic*. The contractile status of muscles is controlled by discharges of motoneurones exciting the muscles' motor units. The individual muscle excitations last only a very small fraction of a second; the tonus of the muscle reflects the averaging of the contributing muscle "twitches" over space and time. That averaging, or integration, is necessarily imperfect, with the result that there are very small, apparently-random deviations from a steady-state muscle tension. These variations are likely to be an important contributor to frequency and amplitude perturbation (Baer, 1980; Larson, Kempster, & Kistler, 1987; Titze, 1991).

2. *Aerodynamic*. The pulses of air emerging from the glottis are injected into the supraglottic space as concentrated jets, much like the thin stream of fluid leaving the tip of a hypodermic needle. Under some (often very subtle) conditions these jets of gas may, quite unpredictably, attach to (or separate from) the surrounding walls of the lower airway and they may generate different degrees of air turbulence. This erratic aerodynamic behavior may contribute significantly to the vocal signal and is possibly a significant source of vocal perturbation (Kaiser, 1983; Teager & Teager, 1983; Liljencrants, 1991; Shadle, Barney, & Thomas, 1991).

3. *Mechanical*. Alteration of the biomechanical properties of the vocal fold, including changes in mass

---

[25] There are, however, clear exceptions and serious limitations. See Wolfe, Fitch, and Cornell (1995) or Ross, Noordzji, and Woo (1998) for examples.

[26] Frequency perturbation may show promise as a means of assessing the effects of drugs. See, for example, Nevlud, Fann, and Falck (1983).

and tissue structure associated with pathology, appear to be a major cause of increased vocal perturbation (Jiang, Titze, Wexler, & Gray, 1994). But other mechanical phenomena—sometimes distant from the vocal tract—are capable of causing short-term alterations of the vocal signal. For example, relatively rapid changes in airway impedance (most commonly associated with consonant production) can significantly alter vocal F_0 (Baken & Orlikoff, 1987a, 1987b, 1988; Kitajima & Tanaka, 1995). F_0 is also affected by the heartbeat, probably because of varying stiffness of the vascular bed of the vocal folds as a function of the cyclic change of blood pressure (Orlikoff & Baken, 1989a, 1989b; Orlikoff, 1989; Orlikoff, 1990a, 1990b, 1990c, 1990d).

4. *Stylistics.* Particularly in the performing arts, variation of F_0 is used to adorn the vocal output. Vibrato is probably the most common of the artistic alterations of F_0, and may be defined as a periodic variation of vocal F_0 of up to about 3% or about 1.4 ST at a rate of from about 4 to about 7 cycles per second (Hakes, Shipp, & Doherty, 1987; Ramig & Shipp, 1987). The regular variation of frequency is commonly accompanied by comparable variability of amplitude. Variational characteristics, however, are modified by the physiological context and by cultural preferences (Rothman & Arroyo, 1987; Michel & Myers, 1991; Schutte & Miller, 1991; Horii, 1989; Keidar, Hurtig, & Titze, 1987).

5. *Chaotic oscillation.* Chaotic behavior appears random, but is the product of a deterministic system and has deeper-level structure that can often be described and characterized. It is, most emphatically, not simply disorganized or unpredictable activity. There are a number of behavioral features that are typical of a chaotic system, including the sudden qualitative changes described as "bifurcations." A growing corpus of work suggests that the vocal apparatus is a chaotic system and that the methods of nonlinear dynamics (the parent science of which chaos theory is a part) may have much to offer to our understanding of abnormal vocal production (Awrejcewicz, 1990; Baken, 1990, 1991, 1995a, 1995b; Mende, Herzel, & Wermke, 1990; Herzel et al., 1991; Titze et al., 1993; Berry, Herzel, Titze, & Story, 1996; Behrman & Baken, 1997; Behrman, 1999).

Another caution is the fact that medium-term events, such as the "spasms" of spasmodic dysphonia

may inflate jitter measures. (See, for example, Crevier-Buchman, Laccourreye, Papon, Nurit, and Brasnu, 1997.) While one might quite obviously want to assess such transient shifts of F_0 (as, for example, in Ramig, 1986), they are not what is usually meant by "jitter" and can be assessed by more telling means.

These considerations strongly underscore the need to examine the F_0 data to be analyzed, preferably in graphic form. That is, undertaking a numerical analysis of vocal frequency perturbation without checking for signs of patterns of F_0 variation is very poor practice indeed. Figure 6–29 demonstrates why. This 81-year-old woman was diagnosed as spasmodic dysphonic, and indeed there were occasional spasmodic vocal episodes. But looking at the record of her F_0 over time shows a slow ($\approx$ 3/min) frequency tremor, which is often overlaid with a higher-frequency tremor and, most unusually, intervals of "diplophonia" whose onset occurs as she approaches the low point of each major F_0 swing. Simply obtaining a jitter index for this patient would have missed the most salient features of her vocal frequency problem.

Measurement Methods

In principle, frequency perturbation can be measured from either running speech or from sustained phonation of a vowel. But, by common understanding, jitter is concerned with unintentional changes in F_0: its *raison d'être* is the assessment of the stability of phonational frequency. In normal speech, F_0 is volitionally made to vary for purposes of stress, intonation, and the like. These purposive variations confound the quantification of the involuntary frequency variability that is of interest. "Sustained vowel phonations," suggests Horii (1979, p. 5) "would seem to be an appropriate phonatory task when more or less random perturbations caused by mechanophysiologic conditions of the vocal folds are in question." The sustained vowel in question, of course, might be released by a plosive, so that simultaneous assessment of associated physiological variables such as subglottal pressure (see Chapter 8, "Air Pressure") and glottal resistance can be done.[27] On the other hand, there are occasionally situations—such as assessing the effect of consonants on vowel stability (Nittrouer et al.,1990)—when measurement of jitter in running speech might be appropriate. It is likely that the measured perturbation of spoken material will be very much higher than that of a sustained vowel (McAllister, Sederholm, Ternström, and Sundberg,

---

[27] The presence of a face mask and intraoral pressure-sensing tube does not seem to have an adverse effect on perturbation measurement (Till et al., 1992).

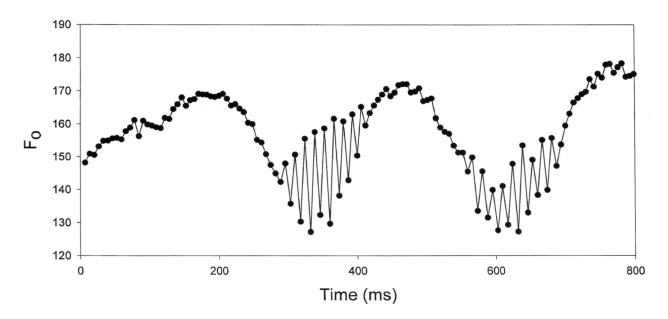

Figure 6–29. Frequency of successive vocal periods during a sustained vowel by an 81–year-old female with a diagnosis of spasmodic dysphonia. Among the features of the very complex patterning of her F_0 variability are a low-frequency tremor with evidence of a superimposed tremor of higher rate (evident at the upper limits of her F_0 swings) and, quite prominently, the development of "diplophonia" as she approaches the low limit of each regular alternation of F_0. None of these features would be evident in a single perturbation index of this patient's voice.

1966) although, under some circumstances, preliminary investigation suggests that jitter estimated from short vowel segments extracted from running speech may not be meaningfully different from the jitter measured from a longer sustained vowel (Leddy & Bless, 1989).

There is a very large number of ways in which an index of frequency perturbation might be calculated, and each has different advantages and drawbacks. In the days before personal computers ease of calculation was an issue in selecting a measurement method. (Troughear and Davis [1979] even described a "home-built" computer system to deal with the problem.) The ubiquity of desktop computers has eliminated that problem, but at a cost: In the "old days" one was exposed to the raw data from which the jitter measure was to be derived. One thus had a sense of the quality of the vocal sample. And, since the calculations had to be done at least partly by hand, one also had a good sense of what a given jitter measurement actually represented. Today's computers, of course, usually take care of data acquisition and take care of all of the computation "out of sight." The quality of the data and the mathematical reality of the resultant measure are largely hidden.[28]

Measurement Precision

The measurement of frequency perturbation can obviously be no more accurate than the measurement of the periods (or, equivalently, of the frequencies) from which it is calculated. The accuracy of those period- (or frequency-) determinations is limited, in turn, by the sampling frequency (see Chapters 3 and 4) and the accuracy of the specific F_0-extraction method used. In fact, if the sampling frequency is Fs, then the samples are spaced $\dfrac{1}{F_s}$ seconds apart. The location of any event (including the beginning or end of a vocal cycle) can only be directly determined with an accuracy of $\pm \dfrac{1}{2}\left(\dfrac{1}{F_s}\right)$ seconds.

As F_0 increases the duration of each cycle decreases, and so the number of samples that represent each cycle grows smaller. But the measurement error remains the same. Thus, the *relative* magnitude of the error grows in proportion to the vocal fundamental frequency. Titze, Horii, and Scherer (1987) point out

---

[28] A brief useful review of conceptual and technical issues relevant to the assessment and interpretation of perturbation is available in Laver, Hiller, and Black (1992).

that, under ideal conditions, the maximal error due to sampling rate is

$$\% \, \text{Error}_{\text{Jitter}} = \left(\frac{100F_0}{n}\right) \sum_{i=1}^{n} \left| \pm \frac{1}{2} F_s^{-1} \right|,$$

where F_0 = the mean fundamental frequency of the sample;
  n = the number of vocal cycles in the sample and
  F_s = the sampling frequency.

Some algebraic manipulation of this relationship shows that the maximal error is

$$\% \, \text{error}_{\text{Jitter}} = 50 \frac{F_0}{F_s}.$$

Thus, if the sampling rate (Fs) is 25000 / s, the relative maximum jitter error for a voice whose F_0 averages 100 Hz would be

$$\pm 50 \left(\frac{100}{25000}\right) = 0.2\%.$$

But if the mean F_0 were 300 Hz (as a child's might well be), the relative maximum error rises to

$$\pm 50 \left(\frac{100}{25000}\right) = 0.6\%.$$

In fact, compared to the expected jitter of a normal voice, the error in both cases is quite large. While, in principle, the error could be reduced to acceptable levels by raising the sampling rate, the fact is that this is not likely to be feasible: very few facilities are equipped with analog-to-digital converters that are fast enough to do the job. The limitations of sampling rate can be greatly lessened by the use of interpolation (discussed earlier in this chapter) to provide data adequate to the needs of everyday practice (Titze et al., 1987).

The choice of F_0-extraction method can also limit the precision of F_0 determination and hence of jitter measurement.[29] There are basically three choices of algorithm: zero crossing, peak picking, and waveform matching (Milenkovic, 1987). Their adequacy to the needs of perturbation analysis has been analyzed by Titze and Liang (1993). Their overall conclusions are that:

1. Waveform-matching best meets the need for precision F_0 extraction if the signal-to-noise ratio is favorable and amplitude modulation is < 5%.

2. If frequency variations are large, however, the waveform-matching algorithm may suffer a serious loss of accuracy.

3. Peak-picking and zero-cross methods cannot be relied upon to provide adequately high precision, especially for perturbations characteristic of those of normal voices. They are seriously affected by additive noise.

4. While filtering the vocal signal can, in principle, improve the performance of peak-picking and zero-cross methods, it may also degrade the accuracy of the resulting jitter measure. It is important that filter characteristics be chosen in light of the specific perturbational pattern to be detected, but this is rarely known beforehand.

Hardware factors must also be considered. It is clear, from everyday clinical experience and from formal studies, that different analysis systems may produce dissimilar results when analyzing the same signal, and software characteristics do not account for all of the variability (Karnell, Scherer, & Fischer, 1991; Karnell, Hall, & Dahl, 1995). Until inter-laboratory standards are agreed upon, comparison of data sets must be undertaken with caution.

The choice of microphone may be meaningful. A preliminary study by Titze and Winholtz (1993) suggests that cardioid condenser microphones (see Chapter 4, "General-Purpose Tools") with a balanced output are to be preferred over other types and they should be set close to the speaker.

Minimal Sample Size

The minimal number of periods that must be evaluated to ensure a valid estimate of F_0 perturbation depends on a number of factors. For **normal** voices, with only minimal roughness, as few as 30 consecutive cycles may be adequate (Titze et al., 1987), although having more cycles tends to minimize the variability that may be produced by analyzing from different "starting points" (inplying different amounts of residual onset transition) in the sample (Jafari, Till, Truesdell, & Law-Till, 1993). **Clinically disordered** voices can be "graded" as to severity with only that many cycles, but more precise quantification of dysfunction will require larger samples. Karnell (1991) suggests that, for a high-quality recording, up to 190 cycles are necessary to achieve an estimate with a minimal value (which is taken to be optimally valid). On the other hand, 110

---

[29] An idea of the magnitude of the differences introduced by various F_0-extraction and analysis methods can be gotten from Deem, Manning, Knack, and Matesich (1989).

consecutive samples are likely to produce an estimate of jitter that is within 5% of a minimal value, and this may well be good enough for routine clinical use.

Tape Recording

Finally, analog tape recorders introduce considerable frequency and amplitude variations of their own (Doherty & Shipp, 1988). This tends to inflate perturbation measures, and so they should therefore not be used to acquire samples for jitter analysis unless absolutely necessary (Titze, Horii, & Scherer, 1987; Gelfer & Fendel, 1995; Jiang, Lin, & Hanson, 1998). Instead, recording should be done with a digital audio tape recorder, which introduces significantly less added perturbation (Doherty & Shipp, 1988) or the sample should be acquired via the A/D system directly into the computer.

Jitter Measures

On the assumption that a reasoned choice of a perturbation measure requires more familiarity with the measurement method than is provided simply by the computational formula, the actual computation of several types of perturbation index will be undertaken using the vocalic sample of Figure 6–30. (Note that, for the sake of illustration, a small sample is considered. Clinical evaluation would require a very much larger vocal sample.) Although casual inspection of the waveform record by eye might suggest that there is excellent uniformity of cycle duration, actual measurement of the duration of the several cycles shown (Table 6–21) reveals meaningful variability.

That variability is graphically illustrated by plotting the F_0 of each of the periods, as in Figure 6–31. It is the "scatter" of the data points in that plot that perturbation measures attempt to portray.[30]

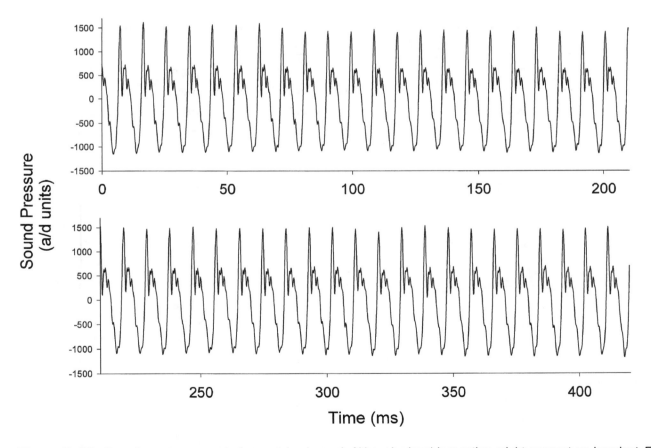

Figure 6–30. Sound pressure record of a sustained vowel. Although visual inspection might suggest an invariant F_0, measurement reveals that the periods do vary slightly.

---

[30] The various approaches to perturbation analysis represent different ways of portraying the vocal variability. The mathematical relationship of the various perturbation measures has been explored by Pinto and Titze (1990).

Distributions

Fundamental Frequency Histogram.   Perhaps the simplest way to analyze the F_0 data is to construct a F_0 *histogram*, which is nothing more than a bar graph of the occurrences of F_0s in the sample. For the example of Figure 6–30/Table 6–21 the distribution of F_0s can be tabled as shown in Table 6–22. The histogram that results from graphing these values is shown in Figure 6–32. (A larger sample would have resulted in a smoother graph.) Schultz-Coulon, Battner, and Fedders (1979) were of the opinion that this form of analysis provided the most useful information in voice evaluation, although it does not really measure jitter per se. While it is easy to construct, there is little information about the significance of the histogram's "shape." The method is not currently in general use,

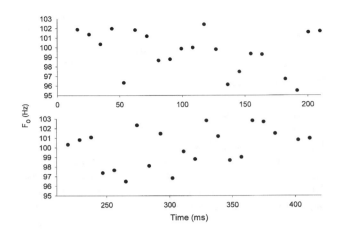

Figure 6–31. Plot of the F_0 of successive cycles of the sample shown in Figure 6–30.

Table 6–21. *F_0* and Period of Consecutive Cycles in Figure 6–30

Cycle No.	F_o (Hz)	Period (ms)	Cycle No.	F_o (Hz)	Period (ms)
1	101.88	9.81	23	100.33	9.96
2	101.37	9.86	24	100.82	9.91
3	100.35	9.96	25	101.08	9.89
4	101.97	9.80	26	97.37	10.26
5	96.32	10.38	27	97.65	10.23
6	101.82	9.82	28	96.48	10.36
7	101.18	9.88	29	102.34	9.77
8	98.64	10.13	30	98.11	10.19
9	98.77	10.12	31	101.46	9.85
10	99.87	10.01	32	96.82	10.32
11	99.98	10.00	33	99.60	10.03
12	102.40	9.76	34	98.80	10.12
13	99.80	10.01	35	102.82	9.72
14	96.12	10.40	36	101.18	9.88
15	97.46	10.25	37	98.68	10.13
16	99.33	10.06	38	99.01	10.09
17	99.26	10.07	39	102.80	9.72
18	103.30	9.67	40	102.68	9.73
19	96.70	10.34	41	101.47	9.85
20	95.48	10.47	42	103.54	9.65
21	101.57	9.84	43	100.80	9.92
22	101.68	9.83	44	100.96	9.90

Mean F_0 = 100.007 Hz

SD of F_0 = 2.155 Hz

Mean period = 10.004 ms

SD of period = 0.217 ms

although some attempts have been made to relate it to perceptual attributes of abnormal voices (Hammarberg, Fritzell, Gauffin, Sundberg, & Wedin, 1980).

Durational Differences Histogram. Lieberman (1961, 1963) and Iwata and von Leden (1970) demonstrated the usefulness of examining the distribution of the magnitude of the differences between adjacent periods. The method requires plotting the percent

Table 6–22. Distribution of Fundamental Frequencies in the Standard Sample of Table 6–21

Center of Interval	N	Center of Interval	N
95.25	1	99.75	4
95.75	0	100.25	2
96.25	3	100.75	3
96.75	2	101.25	6
97.25	2	101.75	5
97.75	1	102.25	2
98.25	1	102.75	3
98.75	4	103.25	1
99.25	3	103.75	1
		Total	44

occurrence (known in descriptive statistics as the relative frequency of the occurrences) of the function $\Delta t = \mid t_n - t_{n-1} \mid$. In descriptive terms, this is the absolute difference between a period, t, (or, equivalently, a frequency, f) and the period (or frequency) preceding it. The procedure for generating the distribution curve can be illustrated with the data of Table 6–21, as shown in Table 6–23.

First, the several Δts are found by subtracting the period of each cycle from the period of the cycle just before it. (One therefore begins with the second cycle, and the number of differences will be one less than the number of cycles in the sample.) Since only the absolute value of the difference is needed, the sign of the result is ignored. Now the number of occurrences in each value interval[31] is determined (Table 6–24), and the percentage of all observations found in each interval is calculated. In the example at hand, for instance, 4 of the differences had magnitudes between 0.16 and .020 millisecond. This interval, then, contained 4/43, or 9.3%, of all the differences. The percentages are then plotted, as in Figure 6–33.

The distribution shown in Figure 6–34 is taken from Lieberman (1961) and is based on more than 7,000 vocal periods produced by six normal male speakers. It shows that most of the period-to-period differences were quite small (< 0.4 ms); perturbations equal to or greater than 0.5 ms account for only about 20% of all observations. (In later work using more accurate measurement, Lieberman (1963) found that

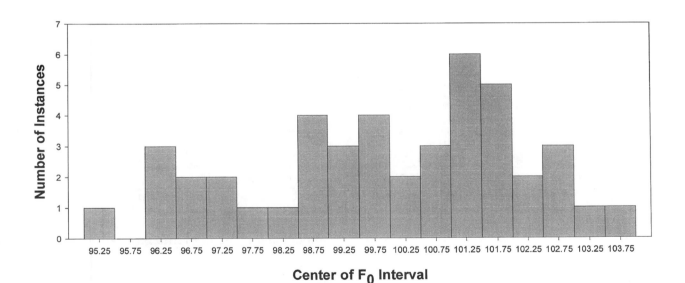

Figure 6–32. Frequency distribution of the fundamental frequencies of Table 6–22.

---

[31] The *minimum* size of the interval depends on the precision of the original period measurements.

Table 6–23. Durational Differences for the Standard Sample of Table 6–21

Cycle (n)	Period (ms)	$|t_n - t_{n-1}|$ (ms)	Cycle (n)	Period (ms)	$|t_n - t_{n-1}|$ (ms)
1	9.81	—	23	9.96	.13
2	9.86	.05	24	9.91	.05
3	9.96	.10	25	9.89	.02
4	9.80	.16	26	10.26	.37
5	10.38	.58	27	10.23	.03
6	9.82	.56	28	10.36	.13
7	9.88	.06	29	9.77	.59
8	10.13	.25	30	10.19	.42
9	10.12	.01	31	9.85	.34
10	10.01	.11	32	10.32	.47
11	10.00	.01	33	10.03	.29
12	9.76	.24	34	10.12	.09
13	10.01	.25	35	9.72	.40
14	10.40	.39	36	9.88	.16
15	10.25	.15	37	10.13	.25
16	10.06	.19	38	10.09	.04
17	10.07	.01	39	9.72	.37
18	9.67	.40	40	9.73	.01
19	10.34	.67	41	9.85	.12
20	10.47	.13	42	9.65	.20
21	9.84	.63	43	9.92	.27
22	9.83	.01	44	9.90	.02

Table 6–24. Distribution of the Period Differences

Δt Interval (ms)	No. of Occurrences	Relative Frequency (%)
.01–.05	11	25.6
.06–.10	3	7.0
.11–.15	6	13.9
.16–.20	4	9.3
.21–.25	4	9.3
.26–.30	2	4.7
.31–.35	2	4.7
.36–.40	4	9.3
.41–.45	1	2.3
.46–.50	1	2.3
.51–.55	0	0.0
.56–.60	3	7.0
.61–.65	1	2.3
.66–.70	1	2.3
.71–.75	0	0.0
.76–.80	0	0.0
.81–.85	0	0.0
.86–.90	0	0.0
.91–.95	0	0.0
Total:	43	100

interperiod differences >0.5 ms constituted only about 15% of the total number.) For normal speakers the overall shape of the distribution was always the same, although the emotional content of the spoken material did affect the height of the right-hand "shoulder" (Lieberman, 1961; Lieberman & Michaels, 1962). Hoarse speakers had a greater proportion of large differences and the "tail" of the curves was therefore elevated in such cases. This fact led to the creation of the "perturbation factor," discussed below. For those willing to go through the trouble of plotting the individual period values, the distribution of the relative frequency of occurrence can provide a "picture" of a patient's vocal perturbation that may prove useful.

Numerical Indices of Frequency Perturbation

In general one would prefer to generate not a curve, but a "score" that might serve as a perturbation rating. Hopefully, such an index would reflect different kinds of disorders and would be sensitive to either improvement or deterioration of the patient's vocal function. A host of approaches to the quantification of frequency perturbation has been created. The more

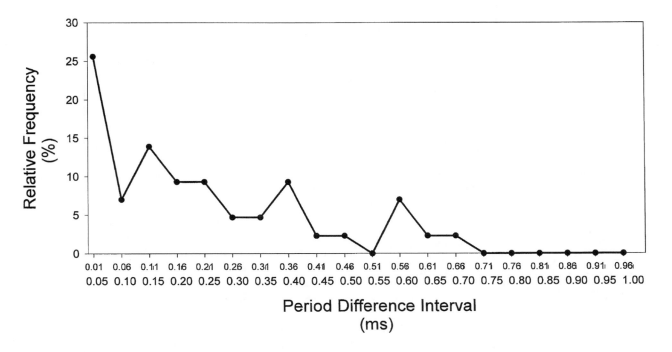

Figure 6–33. Distribution of the period-to-period differences for the specimen jitter sample.

useful—or at least the more widely accepted—are considered here.

Absolute Jitter Measures. Period perturbation measures that ignore the speaker's F_0 can be said to be "absolute." Several such indices have been devised, although none has proven very popular.

Perturbation Factor. Lieberman's (1961, 1963) research on the frequency perturbation of normal and pathological voices tended to confirm the observation of von Leden, Moore, and Timcke (1960) that the normal vibratory patterns of the vocal folds are disrupted in the presence of laryngeal pathology and, in particular, that there is a greatly increased tendency for rapid and frequent lapses of vibratory regularity. Specifically, Lieberman (1963) reasoned that frequency perturbations effect (1) changes in glottal periodicity; (2) alterations of the glottal waveform; and (3) variations of vocal tract configuration that result in phase shifts of the acoustic wave. The first of these (which was of prime interest) was considered to produce cycle-to-cycle period differences greater than 0.5 ms. Lieberman therefore proposed an index that he called the *perturbation factor*, defined as "the integral of the frequency distribution of $\Delta t > 0.5$ ms." More simply stated, the perturbation factor is the percentage of all perturbations equal to or greater than a half millisecond. In the data for the specimen sample of Table 5–18 there are 5 period differences greater than 0.5 ms. The perturbation factor for this sample is therefore 5/43 = 11.6%.

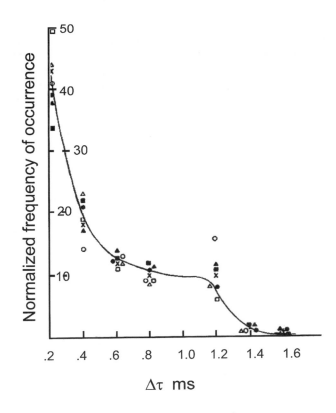

Figure 6–34. Distribution of the period-to-period differences in a large sample from 6 speakers. (From "Perturbations in Vocal Pitch," by P. Lieberman, 1961, Figure 4, p. 598. *Journal of the Acoustical Society of America, 33,* 597–603. Reprinted by permission.)

The perturbation factor may be useful as a screening measure for detection of laryngeal disorder. Lieberman (1963) was of the opinion that it

is sensitive to the size and location of pathologic growths in the speaker's larynx. When growths occur on the speaker's vocal cords the differences between the perturbation factors of the normal and pathologic larynges are proportional to the size of the pathologic growths as long as the growths do not interfere with normal closure of the vocal cords. ... Inflammatory conditions and very small nodules ... have, in general, comparatively small effect on either the perturbation factor or on the acoustic waveform (p. 353).

Some validation of these conclusions has been done (Iwata & von Leden, 1970), but more will be needed before one can feel comfortable about interpreting the perturbation factor in this way.

Directional Perturbation Factor.   A different kind of perturbation measure has been proposed by Hecker and Kreul (1971). Their *directional perturbation factor* (DPF) ignores the magnitude of period perturbations:

it is concerned only with the number of times that the frequency change shifts direction. The DPF

takes into account the algebraic sign rather than the magnitude of the difference between adjacent glottal pulse intervals. It was defined as the percentage of the total number of differences for which there is a change in algebraic sign [p. 1279].

While the definition might, at first blush, seem somewhat confusing, the calculation of DPF is easily demonstrated by example. Using the data of the specimen sample, Table 6–25 shows how it is done. The period of each cycle is determined, and the difference between the successive periods is found by subtraction. For the DPF, however, the sign of the difference is preserved. For example, the difference between cycles 11 and 12 of the sample is −0.24, but between cycles 12 and 13 it is +0.25. Now the tabulation of period differences is scanned, and the number of times that the sign of the difference *changes* is counted. The DPF is this sign-change count divided by the total number of differences in the tabulation. In Table 6–25 there are 29 changes of sign among a total of 43 period differences. Therefore, DPF = 29/43 = 67%.

Table 6–25. Computation of the Directional Perturbation Factor for the Specimen Sample of Table 6–21

Cycle (n)	Period (ms)	$\|t_n - t_{n-1}\|$ (ms)	Sign-change Count	Cycle (n)	Period (ms)	$\|t_n - t_{n-1}\|$ (ms)	Sign-change Count
1	9.81	—		23	9.96	+.13	12
2	9.86	+.05		24	9.91	−.05	13
3	9.96	+.10		25	9.89	−.02	
4	9.80	−.16	1	26	10.26	+.37	14
5	10.38	+.58	2	27	10.23	−.03	15
6	9.82	−.56	3	28	10.36	+.13	16
7	9.88	+.06	4	29	9.77	−.59	17
8	10.13	+.25		30	10.19	+.42	18
9	10.12	−.01	5	31	9.85	−.34	19
10	10.01	−.11		32	10.32	+.47	20
11	10.00	−.01		33	10.03	−.29	21
12	9.76	-.24		34	10.12	+.09	22
13	10.01	+.25	6	35	9.72	-.40	23
14	10.40	+.39		36	9.88	+.16	24
15	10.25	−.15	7	37	10.13	+.25	
16	10.06	−.19		38	10.09	−.04	25
17	10.07	+.01	8	39	9.72	-.37	
18	9.67	−.40	9	40	9.73	+.01	26
19	10.34	+.67	10	41	9.85	+.12	
20	10.47	+.13		42	9.65	−.20	27
21	9.84	−.63	11	43	9.92	+.27	28
22	9.83	−.01		44	9.90	−.02	29

Mean directional perturbation factor for older men (age 42 to 75 years, mean = 63.2 years) has been measured at 33.3% (SD = 4.2) during reading of a sentence of the Rainbow Passage (Hecker & Kreul, 1971). Izdebski and Murry (1980) found a somewhat higher mean DPF of 58.4% (SD = 7.54) for productions of /ɑ/ at comfortable pitch and loudness by 5 normal adults.

Sorensen and Horii (1984) have determined the DPF for 20 men and 20 women. Their data (Table 6–26) are so far the most complete available, and may be considered tentative norms for this measure.

TABLE 6–26. Directional Perturbation Factor: Normal Adults (Percent Sign Change)*†

Vowel	/ɑ/	/u/	/i/
Men			
Mean	46.24	49.26	46.37
Range	39.0–52.1	41.0–61.1	34.6–60.3
SD	3.59	5.54	6.32
Women			
Mean	48.79	52.77	52.04
Range	39.3–60.0	40.6–62.7	44.7–61.1
SD	4.78	6.69	5.23

*20 men, 20 women (all nonsmokers). Age 25–49 y (mean: males 38.1 y; females 36.4 y). Sustained vowels at 70–80 dB SPL for approx. 5 s.

†Amplitude perturbation factor also assessed for this group. See Chapter 5.

Source: From: "Directional perturbation factors for jitter and for shimmer," by D. Sorensen and Y. Horii, 1984, *Journal of Communication Disorders*, 16, 143–151. Table 1, p. 147. © 1984 by Elsevier Science Publishing Co., Inc. Reprinted by permission of the publisher.

F_0-Related Jitter Measures. The magnitude of frequency perturbation shows considerable correlation with mean fundamental frequency. A number of researchers (Lieberman, 1963; Beckett, 1969; Koike, 1973; Horii, 1979, 1980; Orlikoff & Baken, 1990) have noted that larger cycle-to-cycle period differences are associated with longer fundamental periods. (Reciprocally, higher fundamental frequencies tend to have less perturbation.) Horii (1979) had each of six men sustain tones at approximately 2 ST intervals from 98 to 298 Hz and measured the frequency perturbation of each production. The averages for the group are shown in Table 6–27. It is clear that the mean perturbation decreases as F_0 increases (the correlation is $-.95$) but the relationship is not monotonic or even invariable.

Analyses by Horii (1979) and by Hollien, Michel, and Doherty (1973) tend to demonstrate that there is no way to compensate exactly for the effect of mean F_0 in order to achieve an "uninfluenced" jitter index. The best compromise is to generate a ratio of some form of mean perturbation to mean period. It is this tack that most jitter indices take. (Honjo and Isshiki (1980) have expressed jitter in semitones, which does make for a frequency-compensated measure. The effectiveness of the correction has not been assessed, however.)

Jitter Ratio and Jitter Factor. The simplest form of F_0-adjusted perturbation index is the mean perturbation divided by the mean waveform duration. When done in terms of period, the measure is called the *jitter ratio* (Horii, 1979). By definition:

$$\text{Jitter Ratio} = \frac{\frac{1}{n-1}\left[\sum_{i=1}^{n-1}|P_i - P_{i+1}|\right]}{\frac{1}{n}\sum_{i=1}^{n}P_i} \times 1000$$

where P_i = the period of the ith cycle in ms, and

n = the number of periods in the sample.

Table 6–27. Mean Jitter at Different Fundamental Frequencies*

	Semitones above 98 Hz										
	2	**4**	**6**	**8**	**10**	**12**	**14**	**16**	**18**	**20**	**22**
MeanJitter (μs)	51	52	45	41	44	35	30	26	28	28	24
SD†	13.7	14.8	14.2	13.1	17.8	10.2	11.9	5.9	9.1	9.0	4.6
Range	38–89	32–79	23–69	24–65	21–77	22–57	17–54	16–38	17–45	16–51	17–32

*Six men, age 28–43. Sustained /i/, pitch matching, two trials each.

†Computed from author's data.

Source: From "Fundamental frequency perturbation observed in sustained phonation," by Y. Horii, 1979, *Journal of Speech and Hearing Research*, 22, 5–19. Table 2, p. 11. © American Speech-Language-Hearing Association, Rockville, MD. Reprinted by permission.

For those with little experience in this form of algebraic notation, the mathematics might seem complex. In fact, this is not the case. Put discursively, the numerator is the sum of the absolute values of the differences between successive periods, divided by the number of differences measured (n − 1). In short, it is the average magnitude of perturbation. The denominator is the sum of the periods divided by the number of periods—that is, it is the mean period. Multiplication by 1000 serves only to make the resultant ratio larger as a matter of convenience.

Table 6–28 uses the specimen sample of Table 6–21 again for the purpose of illustration. The individual periods have been tabulated and summed to give

$$\sum_{i=1}^{n} P_i.$$

The absolute value of the difference between each period and its successor ($|P_i - P_{i+1}|$) is then determined, and the sum of these values,

$$\sum_{i=1}^{n} |P_i - P_{i+1}|,$$

is also taken. The sums are inserted into the formula to find the jitter ratio which, for the specimen sample, turns out to be 22.62.

The frequency-based equivalent of jitter ratio is known as **jitter factor** (Hollien, Michel, & Doherty,

Table 6–28. Computation of the Jitter Ratio (JR) for the Standard Sample of Table 6–21

Cycle (n)	P_i (ms)	$|P_n - P_{n+1}|$ (ms)	Cycle (n)	P_i (ms)	$|P_n - P_{n+1}|$ (ms)
1	9.81	.05	23	9.96	.02
2	9.86	.10	24	9.91	.02
3	9.96	.16	25	9.89	.37
4	9.80	.58	26	10.26	.03
5	10.38	.56	27	10.23	.13
6	9.82	.06	28	10.36	.59
7	9.88	.25	29	9.77	.42
8	10.13	.01	30	10.19	.34
9	10.12	.11	31	9.85	.47
10	10.01	.01	32	10.32	.29
11	10.00	.24	33	10.03	.09
12	9.76	.25	34	10.12	.40
13	10.01	.39	35	9.72	.16
14	10.40	.15	36	9.88	.25
15	10.25	.19	37	10.13	.04
16	10.06	.01	38	10.09	.37
17	10.07	.40	39	9.72	.01
18	9.67	.67	40	9.73	.12
19	10.34	.13	41	9.85	.20
20	10.47	.63	42	9.65	.27
21	9.84	.01	43	9.92	.02
22	9.83	.13	44	9.90	
			Total:	439.95	9.73

Computation:

$$JR = \frac{\frac{1}{n-1}\left[\sum_{i=1}^{n-1} |P_i - P_{i+1}|\right]}{\frac{1}{n}\sum_{i=1}^{n}P_i} \times 1000$$

$$= \frac{\frac{1}{44-1}[9.73]}{\frac{1}{44}(439.95)} \times 1000$$

$$= \frac{0.226}{9.99} \times 1000 = 22.62$$

1973). That is, jitter factor is the mean difference between the *frequencies* of adjacent cycles divided by the mean frequency, multiplied by 100. Formally stated

$$\text{Jitter Factor} = \frac{\frac{1}{n-1}\left[\sum_{i=1}^{n-1}|F_i - F_{i-1}|\right]}{\frac{1}{n}\sum_{i=1}^{n}F_i} \times 100.$$

The jitter factor for the specimen sample of Table 6–21, computed in Table 6–29, is 2.24. Typical values of jitter ratio and jitter factor for normal men are shown in Table 6–30.

Period Variability Index. Deal and Emanuel (1978) adopted an approach to the quantification of period perturbation that derives from descriptive statistics. Termed the *period variability index* (PVI) it requires the computation of a coefficient of variation (CV), defined as

$$CV = \frac{\frac{1}{n}\sum_{i=1}^{n}[(P_i - \overline{P})^2]}{\overline{P}^2},$$

where P_i = period of the ith cycle and the bar signifies "mean."

The term $(P_i - \overline{P})$ represents the difference between the ith period and the mean of the periods in the sample. In descriptive terms, then, the coefficient of variation is the mean of the squares of the deviations from the mean divided by the square of the mean. It is akin to the standard deviation of the period, and is not, in actual fact, a true measure of cycle-to-cycle variability per se. The PVI is the CV times 1000.

In Table 6–31 the PVI is computed for the specimen sample. First, the sum of the periods is divided by the number of periods to find the mean period, $\overline{P}$. Next, the mean period is subtracted from each period value and the result is squared to provide the series of $(P_i - \overline{P})^2$ s in the third column. These values are added to give

$$\sum_{i=1}^{n}(P_i - \overline{P})^2.$$

The results of these arithmetic processes are then used according to the formula to derive the coefficient of variation, which is multiplied by 1000 to give the PVI.

The PVI values for normal adult males, shown in Table 6–32, may be used as a basis for comparison with clinical cases seen in everyday practice.

Relative Average Perturbation. Changes of fundamental frequency are of two types: relatively slow and steady increases or decreases and abrupt, rapid, apparently-random shifts. The first are, in most cases, related to

Table 6–29. Computation of Jitter Factor (JF) for the Sample of Table 6–21

1 Cycle (i)	2 Freq (F_i) (Hz)	3 $|F_i - F_{i+1}|$ (Hz)
1	101.88	0.51
2	101.37	1.02
3	100.35	1.63
4	101.97	5.65
5	96.325	5.50
6	101.82	.643
7	101.18	2.54
8	98.64	0.12
9	98.77	1.10
10	99.87	0.11
11	99.98	2.42
12	102.40	2.60
13	99.80	3.67
14	96.12	1.34
15	97.46	1.86
16	99.33	.066
17	99.26	4.04
18	103.31	6.60
19	96.71	1.22
20	95.49	6.09
21	101.58	.106
22	101.68	1.34
23	100.34	0.49
24	100.83	0.26
25	101.09	3.71
26	97.38	0.28
27	97.66	1.17
28	96.49	5.85
29	102.34	4.23
30	98.11	3.35
31	101.46	4.63
32	96.83	2.78
33	99.61	0.80
34	98.80	4.02
35	102.82	1.64
36	101.18	2.50
37	98.69	0.33
38	99.02	3.79
39	102.81	0.12
40	102.69	1.21
41	101.48	2.06
42	103.54	2.74
43	100.80	0.16
44	100.96	—
Sum	4400.29	96.33

$$JF = \frac{\frac{1}{n-1}\left[\sum_{i=1}^{n-1}|F_i - F_{i+1}|\right]}{\frac{1}{n}\sum_{i=1}^{n}F_i} \times 100$$

$$= \frac{\frac{1}{44-1}[96.33]}{\frac{1}{44}(4400.29)} \times 100$$

$$= \frac{2.24}{100.01} \times 100$$

$$JF = 2.24$$

Table 6–30. Jitter Ratio and Jitter Factor Values for Normal Subjects

Age (y)	Subjects Sex	N	F_0 (Hz)	Absolute Jitter	Relative Perturbation Mean	Range	Sources
				Jitter Ratio			
28–43	M	6	98–298			5.3–7.6	1
23–38	F	24	210.3		2.96		4
26–33	M	6	109.8	0.042 ms	0.461	0.408–0.590	5
68–80	M	6	120.1	0.053 ms	0.625	0.468–0.740	5
				Jitter Factor			
21–37	M	4	102	0.48	0.47	0.39–0.54	2
			142	0.76	0.53	0.33–0.86	
			198	0.85	0.43	0.36–0.52	
			275	2.67	0.97	0.77–1.34	
55–71 (mean 63.8)	M	5	115.3		0.99	0.76–1.49	3

Sources:

1. Horii, 1979

2. Hollien, Michel, and Doherty (1973)

3. Murry and Doherty (1980)

4. Gelfer, Andrews, and Schmidt (1991). Tabled data are means of values for three vowels (/ɪ,a,u/) given in authors' Table 2. Comparison to trained singers and to sung tones.

5. Orlikoff, 1990b. Compared to elderly atherosclerotic men.

linguistic variables and hence are volitional. They are best evaluated by measures such as pitch sigma. The sudden, involuntary changes are those that are usually classed as perturbational. In running speech the two types of fundamental frequency modulation occur simultaneously. Any measure that evaluates one inevitably includes the effects of the other. Even during sustained vowels, F_0 may undergo slow changes that are not of interest but that may inflate the jitter measure. All of the frequency perturbation indices discussed so far, therefore, suffer from a potential problem.

Relative average perturbation (Koike, 1973), also called the *frequency perturbation quotient* (Takahashi & Koike, 1975) attempts to mitigate the difficulty by using a form of straightline averaging that greatly reduces the effect of relatively slow changes in F_0. The way it works can be explained with the help of Figure 6–35, in which the periods of successive cycles in a hypothetical sample are plotted (filled circles) in the upper graph. It is obvious that the length of the period is increasing, but the vocal jitter makes the increase erratic. What we want to know is how much each period differs from the period before it, *after correcting for the general tendency for periods to increase*. In other words, we want to know by how much the value of a period differs from what it would be if periods were increasing in a perfectly regular fashion.

We can achieve an estimate of the "expected" ("overall-increase-free") value of a given period by taking the average of its value together with the values of the periods that precede and follow it. For example, periods 4, 5, and 6 have values of 7.2, 7.6, and 7.3 ms, respectively. The best estimate of the "overall-increase-free" value of period number 5 is therefore

$$\frac{P_4 + P_5 + P_6}{3} = \frac{7.2 + 7.6 + 7.3}{3} = 7.37 \text{ ms.}$$

An estimate of the "overall-increase-free" value of each period in the data set (except, of course, for the first and last periods in the sample) can be obtained in this way. These estimates are plotted with crosses in the upper graph of Figure 6–35.

To estimate the size of the period-to-period variations that are not accounted for by the increasing trend of the period values we can subtract the actual value from the estimated value of each period. Since the direction of the deviation is of no interest to us, we take the absolute value of this difference. That is, for any given period, P_i, we can compute

$$\left| \frac{P_{i-1} + P_i + P_{i+1}}{3} - P_i \right|.$$

Table 6–31. Computation of the Period Variability Index (PVI) for the Sample of Table 6–21

Cycle	P_i sec $\times 10^{-3}$	$(P_i - \bar{P})^2$ sec $\times 10^{-3}$
1	9.81	.032
2	9.86	.017
3	9.96	.0009
4	9.81	.032
5	10.38	.152
6	9.82	.029
7	9.88	.012
8	10.14	.022
9	10.12	.017
10	10.01	.0004
11	10.00	.0001
12	9.76	.053
13	10.02	.0009
14	10.40	.250
15	10.26	.073
16	10.07	.029
17	10.07	.029
18	9.68	.048
19	10.34	.194
20	10.47	.325
21	9.845	.004
22	9.83	.005
23	9.97	.005
24	9.92	.0004
25	9.89	.0001
26	10.27	.137
27	10.24	.116
28	10.36	.212
29	9.77	.017
30	10.19	.084
31	9.86	.002
32	10.33	.185
33	10.04	.020
34	10.12	.048
35	9.73	.029
36	9.88	.0004
37	10.13	.053
38	10.10	.040
39	9.73	.029
40	9.74	.026
41	9.85	.003
42	9.66	.058
43	9.92	.0004
44	9.90	.000
Sum	439.95×10^{-3}	2.391×10^{-3}

$$\bar{P} = 9.99 \times 10^{-3}$$

$$\sum_{i=1}^{n} (P_i - \bar{P})^2 = 5.717 \times 10^{-6}$$

$$CV = \frac{\dfrac{1}{n}\left[\sum_{i=1}^{n} (P_i - \bar{P})^2\right]}{\bar{P}^2}$$

$$= \frac{\dfrac{1}{44}(5.717 \times 10^{-6})}{(9.99 \times 10^{-3})^2}$$

$$= \frac{1.299 \times 10^{-7}}{9.980 \times 10^{-5}}$$

$$CV = 1.302 \times 10^{-3}$$

$$PVI = CV \times 1000$$

$$PVI = 1.302$$

Table 6–32. Period Variability Index Values for Normal Males*[†]

| Vowel | Period Variability Index | |
	Mean	S.D.
/u/	0.4451	.01051
/i/	0.4898	0.1288
/ʊ/	0.4196	0.0979
/a/	0.4412	0.1595
/æ/	0.4951	0.1167

*20 normal adult males. 7 s of phonation at 75 dB SPL. Signal narrow band filtered, analysis of first harmonic.

[†]Samples originally collected by Sansone and Emanuel, 1970.

Source: From "Some waveform and spectral features of vowel roughness," by R. E. Deal and F. W. Emanuel, 1978, *Journal of Speech and Hearing Research*, *21*, 250–264, Table 1. P. 256. © American Speech-Language-Hearing Association, Rockville MD. Reprinted by permission.

Doing this (as shown in the lower graph of Figure 6–35) gives us deviation values of 0.03, 0.23, and 0.20 ms for period numbers 4, 5, and 6.

We have, in short, defined average trend-line-corrected jitter as the average difference between period values and their estimates. The relative average perturbation (RAP) performs exactly this process (but without the graphs, of course). The RAP function is defined as

$$RAP = \frac{\dfrac{1}{n-2}\sum_{i=2}^{n-1}\left| \dfrac{P_{i-1} + P_i + P_{i+1}}{3} - P_i \right|}{\dfrac{1}{n}\sum_{i=1}^{n} P_i}.$$

The numerator, called the **average absolute perturbation**, should be recognizable as the average difference between actual periods and their three-point estimates.[32] The denominator, of course, is the mean period, which is included to normalize the jitter measurement by expressing it as a proportion of the mean period.

Table 6–33 generates the RAP for the specimen sample that has served as the example for all the other measures of jitter. Koike (1973) originally found that the mean frequency for RAP for 30 adult speakers of both sexes and various ages was about 0.0046 for the midsection of a sustained /a/. The results of some further studies of normal individuals are summarized in Table 6–34. While attempts have been made to establish a mathematical basis for discriminating the data of patients with

---

[32]A similar technique that allows any number of periods to be averaged is discussed by Davis (1976, 1979, 1981).

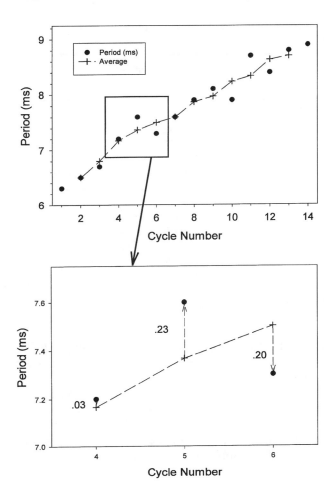

Figure 6–35. Top: Plot of the period values of successive cycles in a hypothetical sample. Filled circles are the actual period durations, while crosses show the averages of cycles n − 1, n, and n + 1. **Bottom:** enlargement of a portion of the upper graph, showing the deviation of the actual period values from their average-estimates.

vocal pathologies from normals on the basis of their RAP, success has been highly elusive (Koike, Takahashi, & Calcaterra, 1977; Davis, 1979, 1981).

Factors Influencing Frequency Perturbation

Whichever perturbation measure is chosen, it is likely to be sensitive to a number of jitter-producing variables. Some of these are normal phenomena of voice production, while others are of pathologic origin.

Normal Phonation

Voice onset and termination typically have much greater frequency perturbation than the steady-state midportion of a sustained vowel (Lieberman, 1961; Horii, 1979). Koike (1973), in his study of normal men and women found that, whereas steady-state phonation had a mean relative average perturbation of 0.0046, the first 17 glottal cycles of a normal (soft) vocal initiation had a frequency perturbation of 0.0276 when measured the same way. The rating for a breathy voice onset was 0.0123. Unless voice onset itself is the phonatory feature being examined, clinicians will want to evaluate sustained vowels no less than a half-second or so after voice initiation.

Horii's (1979) data show that dividing absolute frequency perturbation by the mean fundamental frequency tends to overcompensate for the change in jitter that is attributable to F_0 level. This is shown in Figure 6–36, in which the positive slope of the regression line for jitter ratio is a measure of the inadequacy of the compensation. Hollien, Michel, and Doherty (1973) have observed the same phenomenon when using their jitter factor and Verstraete et al. (1993) found an increase of RAP at high frequencies in female voices. There is no reason to believe that it is not the case for other relative measures. Clinicians should therefore expect *relative* perturbation to be somewhat higher in high-frequency voices, while *absolute* jitter magnitude should decrease with increasing F_0.

Vocal intensity is also a factor to consider. An unpublished study (Jacob, 1968) suggested that jitter ratio tended to decrease with increasing vocal intensity. That effect was confirmed in men by Orlikoff and Kahane (1991). It would seem prudent to do all measurements at a standard intensity level.

The question of whether jitter varies systematically across different vowels is as yet not fully resolved. Wilcox and Horii (1980) and Horii (1980) found that /ɑ/ and /i/ had significantly greater jitter than /u/, whereas Johnson and Michel (1969) observed a tendency for high vowels to show greater jitter than low ones. Further work by Horii (1982) failed to validate any significant difference in mean jitter across ten English vowels, while Sorensen and Horii (1983) found significantly more jitter for /i/ than for /u/ or /ɑ/ in productions at comfortable pitch and loudness by women. On the other hand, this pattern was not observed in the data of Gelfer et al. (1991) or of Orlikoff (1995), whose results supported those of Horii (1982). Nonetheless, pending further clarification of the issue, it seems obvious that comparisons of jitter values are most safely done only for measurement of the same vowel.

Finally, preliminary evidence (Sorensen & Horii, 1983) points to the possibility that adult females might normally have more vocal jitter than men, at least for some vowels. Fortunately, the observed sex difference is not great enough to lead to diagnostic error, especially if several different vowels are tested.

Table 6–33. Computation of the Relative Average Perturbation (RAP) for the Sample of Table 6–21

Cycle No. (i)	Period (P_i)	$\dfrac{P_{i-1} + P_i + P_{i+1}}{3}$	$\dfrac{P_{i-1} + P_i + P_{i+1}}{3} - P_i$
1	9.81		
2	9.86	9.88	.017
3	9.96	9.88	.087
4	9.80	10.05	.247
5	10.38	10.00	.380
6	9.82	10.03	.207
7	9.88	9.94	.063
8	10.13	10.04	.087
9	10.12	10.09	.033
10	10.01	10.04	.033
11	10.00	9.92	.077
12	9.76	9.92	.163
13	10.01	10.06	.047
14	10.40	10.22	.180
15	10.25	10.24	.011
16	10.06	10.13	.067
17	10.07	9.933	.137
18	9.67	10.03	.357
19	10.34	10.16	.180
20	10.47	10.22	.253
21	9.84	10.05	.207
22	9.83	9.88	.047
23	9.96	9.90	.060
24	9.91	9.92	.010
25	9.89	10.02	.130
26	10.26	10.13	.133
27	10.23	10.28	.053
28	10.36	10.12	.240
29	9.77	10.11	.337
30	10.19	9.94	.253
31	9.85	10.12	.270
32	10.32	10.07	.253
33	10.03	10.16	.127
34	10.12	9.96	.163
35	9.72	9.91	.187
36	9.88	9.91	.030
37	10.13	10.03	.097
38	10.09	9.98	.110
39	9.72	9.85	.127
40	9.73	9.77	.037
41	9.85	9.74	.107
42	9.65	9.81	.157
43	9.92	9.82	.097
44	9.90		
Σ	439.95		5.857

$$RAP = \frac{\dfrac{1}{n-2} \displaystyle\sum_{i=2}^{n-1} \left| \dfrac{P_{i-1}+P_i+P_{i+1}}{3} - P_i \right|}{\dfrac{1}{n} \displaystyle\sum_{i=1}^{n} P}$$

$$= \frac{\dfrac{1}{42}(5.857)}{\dfrac{1}{44}(439.95)}$$

$$RAP = \frac{.1395}{9.999} = 0.01395$$

Table 6–34. Relative Average Perturbation* (RAP) Values for Normal Adults

Group	Age (y)	N	Vowel	Mean F_o (Hz)	RAP × 100 Mean	RAP × 100 SD	Sources
Men							
Japanese	27.7	7	/a/	108.1	0.57	0.134	1
European- American	30	50	/a/	107.5	0.28	0.12	2
American	18–25	24	/a/	117.8	0.38	0.169	3
"	"	"	/i/	128.1	0.42	0.565	3
"	"	"	/u/	137.2	0.58	0.877	3
"	30	5	/a/	112.1	0.21	0.058	4
"	"	"	/pa/	112.1	0.25	0.072	4
African -American	29	50		108.8	0.40	0.36	2
Women							
American	18–25	25	/a/	222.9	0.89	0.622	3
"	"	"	/i/	234.7	0.54	0.463	3
"	"	"	/u/	241.8	0.84	0.976	3
"	27.4	5	/a/	221.2	0.28	0.061	4
"	"	"	/pa/	221.2	0.303	0.080	4
Japanese	29.5	2	/a/	206	0.61	0.056	1

*Also called Frequency Perturbation Quotient

1. Takahashi and Koike (1975). Japanese subjects, sustained /a/.

2. Walton and Orlikoff (1994). Male prisoners, sustained /a/.

3. Dwire and McCauley (1995). Data are means of 2 test sessions, separated by 1 to 2 weeks. Measurement by Kay Elemetrics "Visi-Pitch."

4. Till, Jafari, Crumley, and Law-Till, 1992. Comparison of vocal perturbation for a sustained /a/ and for the sustained vowel in /pa/. No significant effect of syllable type, but a significant sex difference was observed. Presence of a face mask and intraoral pressure probe (data not included above) did not significantly affect jitter values.

Aging. An extensive literature documents the anatomic and physiologic changes of the larynx and vocal tract as a function of aging (Hommerich, 1972; Honjo & Isshiki, 1980; Kahane, 1983, 1987; Hirano, Kurita, & Nakashima, 1983). Still, Brown and his colleagues (1989) found no significant difference between the jitter ratio of sustained /ɑ/ at comfortable loudness produced by young and old women (Table 6–35). Recent insights, however, confirm that aging is not merely a matter of the passage of time: people of the same chronological age can have very different "biological" ages. Table 6–36 suggests the magnitude of jitter—which seems strongly to influence the perception of aging (Ringel & Chodzko-Zajko, 1987) —that may be expected in aged subjects, in particular as it relates to their overall physical condition.

Vocal Pathology

Studies by a variety of means have shown that frequency perturbation is one of the physical correlates of perceived "hoarseness" or "harshness" (von Leden et al., 1960; Dunker & Schlosshauer, 1961; Lieberman, 1963; Bowler, 1964; Moore & Thompson, 1965; Isshiki, Yanagihara, & Morimoto, 1966; Deal & Emanuel, 1978). Wendahl (1966b), using synthetic stimuli, found that jitter of as little as ± 1 Hz around a 100 Hz median F_0 was perceived as rough, while increased jitter magnitude was associated with increased perceived roughness.

Although frequency perturbation is not the only—and perhaps not even the most important—correlate of hoarseness, it nonetheless seems to be an important concomitant of the laryngeal pathologies that produce the hoarse voice. In this regard it is worth repeating, for instance, that Lieberman (1963) found that while inflammatory and very small growths on the vocal folds only minimally influenced the perturbation factor, larger masses produced increased perturbation in proportion to their size. Koike (1967) has confirmed these findings, and Orlikoff et al. (1997) have documented that jitter decreased as chemotherapy reduced the size of malignant lesions of the vocal folds.

Interestingly, Beckett (1969) reported that there was a very significant relationship between the degree of F_0 perturbation and subjective *vocal constriction*, defined as "the sensation of tightness and/or squeezing in and around the throat that a speaker experiences during phonation." There is also some preliminary basis for believing that jitter values might differentiate hyper- and hypofunctional voice disorders (Klingholz & Martin, 1985).

The data of Table 6–37 provide some idea of the perturbation values that might be expected in various disorders. (Values characteristic of normal speakers are included for comparison.) In general, too little work has been done to consider these results as normative. Caution must be exercised in using any of them as a criterion for diagnosis. Because there is significant overlap between perturbation scores of normal and disordered groups (Zyski et al., 1984) it is unwise to use perturbation assessment as a screening tool.

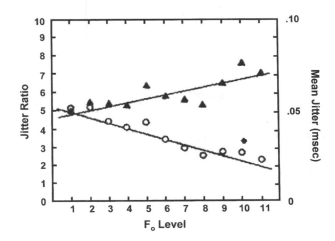

Figure 6–36. Mean absolute jitter in milliseconds (circles) and mean jitter ratios (triangles) for six subjects at various frequency levels. For each set of data a straight line approximation (regression line) has been generated. Mean absolute jitter falls with increasing fundamental frequency, as expected, but mean jitter ratio increases. This indicates that jitter ratio tends to overcorrect for the effect of fundamental frequency. (From "Fundamental Frequency Perturbation Observed in Sustained Phonation," by Y. Horii, 1979, *Journal of Speech and Hearing Research, 22*, 5–19. Figure 3, p. 12. © American Speech-Language-Hearing Association, Rockville MD. Reprinted by permission.)

Periodicity of Frequency Perturbation

Indices of jitter express *average* perturbation. The implication that the period-to-period variability is random is not necessarily valid. Various factors could cause the jitter to be regularly altered, resulting in a cyclic variation of F_0. An example is shown in Figure 6–37. At the top is a short segment piece of the electroglottogram of a late middle-aged male. Although casual inspection may not readily reveal anything unusual, a plot of the F_0 of each of 121 successive cycles of the man's phonation (middle plot) shows that his F_0 varies in a fairly regular way. That is, his F_0 is *frequency modulated*. It would clearly be useful to be able to detect such "periodicity of perturbation" in the jitter data. Obviously, plotting the F_0 of the individual periods, as was done for the center plot of Figure 6–37 is one way to do this. But the availability of digital computers

Table 6–35. Jitter Ratio of Sustained Vowels by Women of Different Ages at Three Loudness Levels.

| Loudness | Young | | Middle Aged | | Aged | | Sources |
	Mean	SD	Mean	SD	Mean	SD	
Soft	1.413(10)	0.309			1.285(13)	0.524	1
Conversational	0.782(21)	0.211			0.748(17)	0.333	1
Comfortable	0.523	0.181	0.550	.0298	0.913	1.309	2
Loud	1.181(14)	0.293			1.060(20)	0.408	1

Sources:

1. Brown, Morris and Michel (1989). 25 young women, age 20–32 y (mean 27.5 y); 25 old women, age 75–90 y (mean 79.4 y). No history of respiratory or neurologic disease. Hearing loss not greater than 35 dB SPL at 500, 1K and 2K Hz in at least one ear. **Measurements made on tape-recorded samples** of sustained /a/ at different subject-determined loudness levels. Tale entries are calculated from the authors' Table 1, p. 115. Subscripted parenthetical data are number of recorded samples contributing to the mean shown.

2. Linville and Fisher, 1985. 25 women in each age group. Free of visible laryngeal abnormality and having normal perceived voice quality, no neurologic or respiratory disease, no professional voice-use experience. Hearing at least 30 dB at 125, 250, 500, and 1K Hz. Sustained /æ/.

Table 6–36. Jitter Values for Sustained Vowels by Older Speakers with Different Levels of Overall Fitness

Mean Age	Age Range or (SD)	N	Physical Condition or State	Mean Jitter (SD)	Note Sources
			Men		
67.5	62–75	15	Good*	0.59% (0.11%)	1
69.1	64–74	15	Poor*	0.69% (0.26%)	1
66.1	(2.23)	8	Active†	0.47% (0.21%)	2
67.4	3.87	7	Sedentary†	1.30% (0.83%)	2
73.3	68–80	6	Good‡	0.625% (0.102)	3
			Atherosclerotic‡	0.831 (0.229)	3
			Women		
66.4	3.11	8	Active†	0.66% (0.43%)	2
67.6	3.81	8	Sedentary	2.23 2.38%)	2

*Difference between "good" and "poor" groups is significant.

†Difference between "active" and "sedentary" groups is significant.

‡Difference betweeen "good" and atherosclerotic groups is significant.

Sources:

1. Ringel and Chodzko-Zajko, 1987. "Physiological condition" defined on the basis of blood pressure, forced vital capacities, serum cholesterol and triglyceride levels, and percent body fat. See also Ramig and Ringel, 1983.

2. Xue and Mueller, 1997. "Physically active" defined as "regular and/or active participation in physical exercises, training programmes, and other physical activities." "Physically sedentary" defined as "rare or no participation" in any of these.

3. Orlikoff, 1990b. Aged normotensives with no clinical cardiac disease and atherosclerotic subjects with no other significant chronic disorders. Six subjects in each group.

offers a better way that depends solely on a mathematical analysis.

Correlation Coefficients

The *correlation coefficient* is a measure of the extent to which the change in one variable reflects the change in another. A correlation coefficient of 1.00 indicates a perfect relationship, implying that if one factor increases, the other must increase by an exactly proportional amount. If, on the other hand, the correlation coefficient is 0 there is no relationship at all between the two sets of numbers. The correlation coefficient, symbolized *r*, can be positive, indicating direct proportionality (x ∝ y) or negative, indicating inverse proportionality (x ∝ 1/y).

Some feel for the meaning of the correlation coefficient can be gotten by examining Table 6–38, in which various data about six hypothetical individuals are cor-

related. In A, age in years is matched with age in months. Obviously, these two data sets must be perfectly correlated, since age in months is a simple linear transform of age in years. That the relationship is perfect is shown by the correlation coefficient of +1.00. Data set B compares heights and weights. One would expect a relationship between the two, but not a perfect one. (Tall people can be very thin and weigh less than their short, fat fellows.) The correlation coefficient of +.90 reflects this. It can be taken to mean that weight is closely, but not perfectly, related to height; other variables enter into the relationship between the two. Lastly, mean SF_0 is correlated to bank balance in data set C. The correlation coefficient of 0.00 demonstrates a total absence of relationship here.

Another look at the center plot of Figure 6–37 shows how the correlation coefficient can be of help in finding perturbational periodicity. Because the pattern

Table 6–37. Frequency Perturbation for Normal and Disordered Voices

Disorder	Measure	Sex	No. of Subjects	Age Mean	Age SD or Range	Normal Mean	Normal SD of Range	Disordered Mean	Disordered SD of Range	Sources
Hoarse	PVI	M	20 + 20	Adult		0.4807	0.1216	0.8295	0.4783	1
Tumor	DPF	M	5	63.8	55–71	58.5%	45.8–65.3			3
	DPF	M	5	65.2	61–69			64.5%	55.4–76.7	3
	DPF	M	5	63.2	42–75	33.3%	4.2			2
	JF	M	5	65.8	55–71	0.55%	0.76–1.49			3
	JF	M	5	65.2	61–69			3.79%	0.77–9.71	3
	RAP	M	7	27.7		0.0057	0.00134			4
	RAP	M	1	50				0.00687		4
	RAP	F	2	29.5		0.0061	0.00056			4
	RAP	F	1	61				0.2022%		4
	RAP	M/F	15?	Adult				0.0176		5
	RAP	M	19	57.9	(7.7)			4.34%	(1.42%)	9
Paralysis	RAP	M/F	15?	Adult				0.0125		5
	RAP	M	2	49.5				0.0452	0.0537	4
Nodules	RAP	M/F	10	10	8.5			0.0123	0.0023–0.0472	8
	RAP	M	2	54.5				0.0084	0.00049	4
	Absolute	F	6	22	18–33			0.016	(0.008)	10
Inflammation	RAP	F	2	36				0.0074	0.00064	4
Esophageal	PF	F	2	36				0.0074	0.00064	6
	JR	M	22	58	36–81			41.1%	8.9–66.8	7
Parkinson (drug treated)	RAP	M	24	(70				0.90%	(0.47%)	11
	RAP	F	17	(70				1.10%	(0.78%)	11
Amyotrophic Lat. Sclerosis (Early)	RAP-M	M	1	69				0.39%	(0.07%)	13
Amyotrophic Lat. Sclerosis (Late)	RAP-M	M	1	69				0.33%	(0.15%)	13
Hearing Impaired aged	RAP	M&F	19	76.6	9.5			/a/ = 1.21% /i/ = 1.73% /u/ = 1.42%	(1.57%) (2.87%) (1.42%)	12
	RAP	M&F	21	72.9	8.1			/a/ = 0.75% /i/ = 0.63% /u/ = 0.77%	(0.88%) (0.63%) (0.91%)	12

PVI = period variability index; DPF = directional perturbation factor; JF = jitter factor; RAP = relative average perturbation; PF = perturbation factor; JR = jitter ratio. RAP-M = modified RAP: Jitter values vased on deviation from mean of preceding and following cycles.

*Sources:

1. Deal and Emmanuel, 1978. Based on samples collected by Sansone and Emanuel (1970) from normal, and by Hanson (1969) from hoarse, speakers. Analysis of narrow-band (10 Hz) filtered first harmonic. Normal and hoarse speakers were significantly different, except for /a/.

2. Hecker and Kreul,. 1971. **One sentence of the Rainbow Passage**. Tumors were malignant.

3. Murry and Doherty, 1980. At least 2 s of sustained /a/. DPF was a better discriminator of cancer cases than JF, but the authors caution about generalizing the data.

4. Takahashi and Koike, 1975. Sample of 1.5 s from the most stable portion of sustained /a/ at comfortable pitch and loudness. Mean computed from data processed in article; categories of disorder given here are not the same as is the original publication.

5. Koike, 1973. Thirty-two cycles of steady-state portion of sustained /a/.

6. Hoops and Noll, 1969. Special form of perturbation factor: percentage of observed perturbations greater than 1.o ms. **First paragraph of the Rainbow Passage.**

7. Smith, Weinberg, Feth, and Horii, 1978. 1-s segment of least variable production of /a/ for each subject.

8. Kane and Wellen, 1985. School children. 5-s production of /a/ following two practice trials. Analyzed by protocol of Davis, 1976.

9. Orlikoff, Kraus, Harrison, Ho, and Gartner, 1997. Sustained /a/. Compared to RAP values at later stages of successful chemotherapy for advanced laryngeal cancer.

10. Verdolini-Marston, Sandage, and Titze, 1994. Sustained /a/. Compared to jitter values after a regimen to improve laryngeal hydration.

11. Gamboa, Jiménez-Jiménez, Nieto, Montojo, Ortí-Pareja, Molina, García-Albea, and Cobeta, 1997. All patients were taking dopaminergic medications.

12. Weatherley, Worrall, and Hickson, 1997. Hearing impaired had mild/moderate sensorineural losses with mean PTA of 39.2 dB (SD = 9.6 dB) in the better ear. Four subjects had bilateral hearing aids and 2 were unilaterally aided. Difference between normal and hearing impaired subjects is not significant.

13. Ramig, Scherer, Klasner, Titze, and Horii, 1990. Single male ALS patient, followed over a 6-month period.

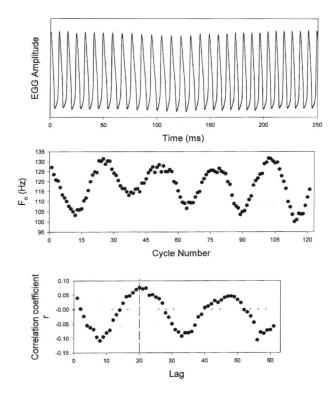

Figure 6–37. EGG record (top) of phonation by a middle-aged male. Plotting the F_0s of successive periods (middle) shows cyclic frequency variation. Autocorrelation analysis (bottom) demonstrates that the frequency variation occurs over a span of about 20 glottal cycles.

of F_0 repeats roughly every 20 cycles, the period of any given cycle should most closely match that of a cycle about 20 cycles away. That is, cycles should be most strongly correlated with those at a distance of about 20 cycles. Therefore, one could determine the correlation of the frequency of waves with those following them (F_i with $F_i + 1$), then with those that are two cycles away (F_i with $F_i + 2$), then those three cycles away (F_i with $F_i + 3$), and so on, trying to find the distance at which the correlation coefficient is maximal. The distance between the cycles being correlated is called the *lag*. The lag at which a maximum (positive) r is found indicates the number of cycles of the perturbational periodicity. The magnitude of the maximal r shows how much of the perturbation the cyclic variation accounts for.

Serial Correlation

The process that has just been described is known as *serial correlation*, and the way in which r varies as a function of the lag is the *serial correlation function*.

Table 6–38. Relationships Among Various Sets of Data for a Hypothetical Adult

A. Age in years compared to age in months

Subj. No.	Age (yr)	Age (mo)
1	21.3	255.6
2	37.1	445.2
3	19.8	237.6
4	47.0	564.0
5	33.5	402.0
6	25.8	309.6

Correlation coefficient: $r = +1.00$

B. Height compared to weight

Subj. No.	Height (cm)	Weight (kg)
1	172.7	71.4
2	177.8	70.5
3	165.1	61.4
4	188.0	75.9
5	175.3	68.6
6	177.8	73.2

Correlation coefficient: $r = +0.90$

C. SF_0 compared to bank balance

Subj. No.	SF_0 (Hz)	Bank Balance in Toogriks*
1	120	1133
2	111	1279
3	106	981
4	115	109
5	98	401
6	107	2521

Correlation coefficient $r = 0.00$

*The national currency of Mongolia

The serial correlation technique has been applied to the signal of which the topmost plot of Figure 6–37 is a sample, and the results are shown in the bottom plot. Note how the serial correlation function peaks at a lag of 20 (dashed line).

The calculation of the serial correlation function is relatively straightforward (Koike, 1969; Iwata, 1972), and is easily programmed:

$$r_k = \frac{1}{n-k} \sum_{i=1}^{n-k} \frac{P_i P_{i+k} - \overline{P}_1 \overline{P}_2}{S_1 S_2}$$

where:

$P_1, P_2, \ldots, P_i$ are successive frequency or period values;

n = number of values in the series

k = lag (distance between the cycles being correlated):

$$\overline{P}_1 = \sum_{i=1}^{n-k} \frac{P_i}{n-k}$$

$$\overline{P}_2 = \sum_{i=k+1}^{n-k} \frac{P_i}{n-k}$$

$$S_1 = \sqrt{\sum_{i=1}^{n-k} \frac{(P_i - \overline{P}_i)^2}{n-k}}$$

$$S_2 = \sqrt{\sum_{i=k+1}^{n-k} \frac{(P_i - \overline{P}_i)^2}{n-k}}.$$

Iwata and von Leden (1970) and Iwata (1972) have presented evidence that different serial correlation functions may be associated with different kinds of laryngeal pathologies, although there has been no definitive confirmation of that since. Koike (1969) also found intensity modulation in pathologic voices.

REFERENCES

Andrews, M. L. (1991). *Voice therapy for children: The elementary school years*. San Diego, CA: Singular Publishing Group.

Arndt, H., J., & Leithäuser, H. (1968). Die mittlere Sprechtonhöhe bein jungen und alten Menschen. *HNO, 16*, 114–116.

Askenfelt, A., Gauffin, J., Sundberg, J., & Kitzing, P. (1980). A comparison of contact microphone and electroglottograph for the measurement of vocal fundamental frequency. *Journal of Speech and Hearing Research, 23*, 258–273.

Austin, M. D., & Leeper, H. A. (1975). Basal pitch and frequency level variation in male and female children: A preliminary investigation. *Journal of Communication Disorders, 8*, 309–316.

Awan, S. N. (1993). Superimposition of speaking voice characteristics and phonetograms in untrained and trained vocal groups. *Journal of Voice, 7*, 30–37.

Awan, S. N., & Mueller, P. B. (1996). Speaking fundamental frequency characteristics of White, African American, and Hispanic kindergartners. *Journal of Speech and Hearing Research, 39*, 573–577.

Awrejcewicz, J. (1990). Bifurcation portrait of the human vocal cord oscillations. *Journal of Sound and Vibration, 136*, 151–156.

Baer, T. (1980). Vocal jitter: A neuromuscular explanation. In V. Lawrence & B. Weinberg (Eds.), *Transcripts of the eighth symposium: Care of the professional voice* (pp. 19–24). New York: Voice Foundation.

Baken, R. J. (1990). Irregularity of vocal period and amplitude: A first approach to the fractal analysis of voice. *Journal of Voice, 4*, 185–197.

Baken, R. J. (1991). Géométrie fractale et évaluation de la voix: Application préliminaire à la dysphonie. *Bulletin d'Audiophonologie: Annales Scientifique de L'Université de Franche-Comté*, VII N.S. (nos. 5 & 6), 731–749.

Baken, R. J. (1994a). The aged voice: A new hypothesis. *Voice (Journal of the British Voice Association), 3*, 57–73.

Baken, R. J. (1994b). L'analyse de la voix: Présent et avenir. *Bulletin d'Audiophonologie: Annales Scientifiques de l'Université de Franche-Comté (Médicine et Pharmacie)*, X (nos. 1 & 2), 38–55.

Baken, R. J. (1995a). Into a chaotic future. In W. J. Gould, J. S. Rubin, & R. Sataloff (Eds.), *Diagnosis and treatment of voice disorders* (pp. 502–509). New York: Raven.

Baken, R. J. (1995b). Between organization and chaos: A different view of the human voice. In F. Bell-Berti & L. J. Raphael (Eds.). *Producing speech: Contemporary issues. For Katherine Safford Harris* (pp. 233–245). New York: American Institute of Physics.

Baken, R. J., & Orlikoff, R. F. (1987a). Phonatory response to step-function changes in supraglottal pressure. In T. Baer, C. Sasaki, & K. S. Harris (Eds.), *Laryngeal function in phonation and respiration* (pp. 273–290). Boston, MA: Little, Brown.

Baken, R. J., & Orlikoff, R. F. (1987b). The effect of articulation on fundamental frequency in singers and speakers. *Journal of Voice, 1*, 68–76.

Baken, R. J., & Orlikoff, R. F. (1988). Changes in vocal fundamental frequency at the segmental level: Control during voiced fricatives. *Journal of Speech and Hearing Research, 31*, 207–211.

Baker, G. L., & Gollub, J. P. (1990). *Chaotic dynamics: An introduction*. New York: Cambridge University Press.

Baker, K. K., Ramig, L. O., Johnson, A. B., & Freed, C. R. (1997). Preliminary voice and speech analysis following fetal dopamine transplants in 5 individuals with Parkinson disease. *Journal of Speech, Language, and Hearing Research, 40*, 615–626.

Beckett, R. L. (1969). Pitch perturbation as a function of subjective vocal constriction. *Folia Phoniatrica, 21*, 416–425.

Behrman, A. (1999). Global and local dimensions of vocal dynamics. *Journal of the Acoustical Society of America, 106*, 432–443.

Behrman, A., & Baken, R. J. (1997). Correlation dimension of electroglottographic data from healthy and pathologic subjects. *Journal of the Acoustical Society of America, 102*, 2371–2379.

Benda, C. (1949). *Mongolism and cretinism*. New York: Grune and Stratton.

Bennett, S. (1983). A 3–year longitudinal study of school-aged children's fundamental frequencies. *Journal of Speech and Hearing Research, 26*, 137–142.

Berry, D. A., Herzel, H., Titze, I. R., & Story, B. H. (1996). Bifurcations in excised larynx experiments. *Journal of Voice, 10*, 129–138.

Biever, D. M., & Bless, D. M. (1989). Vibratory characteristics of the vocal folds in young adult and geriatric women. *Journal of Voice, 3*, 120–131.

Black, J. W. (1940). Natural frequency, duration and intensity of vowels in reading. *Journal of Speech and Hearing Disorders, 14*, 216–221.

Black, J. W. (1949). Natural frequency, duration, and intensity of vowels in reading. *Journal of Speech and Hearing Disorders, 14*, 216–221.

Blood, G. W. (1984). Fundamental frequency and intensity measurements in laryngeal and alaryngeal speakers. *Journal of Communication Disorders, 17*, 319–324.

Boë, L.-J., Contini, M., & Rakotofiringa, H. (1975). Etude statistique de la fréquence laryngienne. *Phonetica, 32*, 1–23.

Boone, D. R. (1971). *The voice and voice therapy*. Englewood Cliffs, NJ: Prentice-Hall.

Boothroyd, A., & Decker, M. (1972). Control of voice pitch by the deaf: An experiment using a visible speech device. *Audiology, 11*, 343–353.

Bowler, N. W. (1964). A fundamental frequency analysis of harsh vocal quality. *Speech Monographs, 31,* 128–134.

Brenner, M., Doherty, E. T., & Shipp, T. (1994). Speech measures indicating workload demand. *Aviation, Space and Environmental Medicine, 65,* 21–26.

Brodnitz, F. S. (1961). *Vocal rehabilitation.* Rochester, MN: American Academy of Ophthalmology and Otolaryngology.

Brown, W. S., Jr., Morris, R. J., Hollien, H., & Howell, E. (1991). Speaking fundamental frequency characteristics as a function of age and professional singing. *Journal of Voice, 5,* 310–315.

Brown, W. S., Jr., Morris, R. J., & Michel, J. F. (1989). Vocal jitter in young adult and aged female voices. *Journal of Voice, 3,* 113–119.

Brown, W. S., Jr., Murry, T., & Hughes, D. (1976). Comfortable effort levels: An experimental variable. *Journal of the Acoustical Society of America, 60,* 696–699.

Bryngelson, B. (1932). A phonophotographic analysis of the vocal disturbances in stuttering. *Psychological Monographs, 43,* 1–30.

Buekers, R., & Kingma, H. (1997). Impact of phonation intensity upon pitch during speaking: A quantitative study in normal subjects. *Logopedics Phoniatrics Vocology, 22,* 71–77.

Burnett, T. A., Senner, J. E., & Larson, C. R. (1997). Voice F_0 responses to pitch-shifted auditory feedback: A preliminary study. *Journal of Voice, 11,* 202–211.

Canter, G. J. (1965a). Speech characteristics of patients with Parkinson's disease: II. Physiological support for speech. *Journal of Speech and Hearing Disorders, 30,* 44–49.

Canter, G. J. (1965b). Speech characteristics of patients with Parkinson's disease: III. Articulation, diadochokinesis, and overall speech adequacy. *Journal of Speech and Hearing Disorders, 30,* 217–224.

Cavallo, S. A., Baken, R. J., & Shaiman, S. (1984). Frequency perturbation characteristics of pulse-register phonation. *Journal of Communication Disorders, 17,* 231–243.

Charlip, W. S. (1968). *The aging female voice: Selected fundamental frequency characteristics and listener judgments.* Unpublished thesis, Purdue University, West Lafayette, IN.

Chevrie-Muller, C. (1971). Etude du fondamental de la voix parlée sur des groupes d'enfants de 3 ans à 5 ans et demi. *Journal Français d'Oto-Rhino-Laryngologie, 20,* 451–455.

Chevrie-Muller, C., Dodart, F., Sequier-Dermer, N., & Salmon, D. (1971). Etudes des paramètres acoustiques de la parole au cours de la schizophrénie de l'adolescent. *Folia Phoniatrica, 23,* 401–428.

Chevrie-Muller, C., Perbos, J., & Guidet, C. (1983). Automated analysis of the electroglottographic signal: Application to the study of phonation of the elderly. *Bulletin d'Audiophonologie, 16,* 121–144.

Chevrie-Muller, C., Salmon, D., & Ferrer, G. (1971). Contribution à l'établissement de constantes acoustiques de la voix parlée chez la femme adolescente, adulte, âgée. *Bulletin d'Audiophonologie, 1,* 33–55.

Chodzko-Zajko, W., Ringel, R., & Vaca, V. (1995). Biogerontology implications for the communication sciences. In R. A. Huntley & K. S. Helfer (Eds.), *Communication in later life* (pp. 3–21). Boston, MA: Butterworth-Heinemann.

Coleman, R. F. (1971). Effect of waveform changes upon roughness perception. *Folia Phoniatrica, 23,* 314–322.

Coleman, R., & Markham, I. (1991). Normal variations of habitual pitch. *Journal of Voice, 5,* 173–177.

Coleman, R. F., & Wendahl, R. W. (1968). On the validity of laryngeal photosensor monitoring. *Journal of the Acoustical Society of America, 44,* 1733–1735.

Colton, R. H., & Steinschneider, A. (1980). Acoustic relationships of infant cries to the Sudden Infant Death syndrome. In T. Murry & J. Murry (Eds.), *Infant communication: Cry and early speech* (pp. 183–208). Houston, TX: College-Hill Press.

Colton, R. H., & Steinschneider, A. (1981). The cry characteristics of an infant who died of the Sudden Infant Death syndrome. *Journal of Speech and Hearing Disorders, 46,* 359–363.

Cooley, J. W., & Tukey, J. W. (1965). An algorithm for the machine calculation of complex Fourier series. *Mathematics of Computation, 19,* 297–301.

Cooper, M. (1971). Modern techniques of vocal rehabilitation for functional and organic dysphonias. In L. E. Travis (Ed.), *Handbook of speech pathology and audiology* (Chapter 23, pp. 585–616). Englewood Cliffs, NJ: Prentice-Hall.

Cooper, M., & Yanagihara, N. (1971). A study of the basal pitch level variations found in the normal speaking voices of males and females. *Journal of Communication Disorders, 3,* 261–266.

Crevier-Buchman, L., Laccourreye, O., Papon, J.-F., Nurit, D., & Brasnu, D. (1997). Adductor spasmodic dysphonia: Case reports with acoustic analysis following botulinum injection and acupuncture. *Journal of Voice, 11,* 232–237.

Croatto, L., & Ferrero, F. (1979). L'esame elettroglottografico applicato ad alcuni case di disodia. *Acta Phoniatrica Latina, 1,* 247–258.

Curry, E. T. (1940). The pitch characteristics of the adolescent male voice. *Speech Monographs, 7,* 48–62.

Curry, E. T. (1962). Frequency measurement and pitch perception in esophageal speech. In J. C. Snidecor (Ed.), *Speech rehabilitation of the laryngectomized* (Chapter 5, pp. 85–93). Springfield, IL: Charles C. Thomas.

Curry, E. T., & Snidecor, J. C. (1961). Physical measurement and pitch perception in esophageal speech. *Laryngoscope, 71,* 415–423.

Cvitanovic, P. (Ed.). (1989). *Universality in chaos* (2nd ed). Bristol, UK: Adam Hilger (IOP Publishing Ltd.).

Dagli, A. S., Mahieu, H. F., & Festen, J. M. (1997). Quantitative analysis of voice quality in early glottic laryngeal carcinomas treated with radiotherapy. *European Archives of Otorhinolaryngology, 254,* 78–80.

Davis, S. B. (1976). Computer evaluation of laryngeal pathology based on inverse filtering of speech. *SCRL Monograph number 13.* Santa Barbara, CA: Speech Communications Research Lab.

Davis, S. B. (1979). Acoustic characteristics of normal and pathological voices. In N. J. Lass (Ed.), *Speech and language: Advances in basic research and practice* (Vol. 1, pp. 271–235). New York: Academic Press.

Davis, S. B. (1981). Acoustic characteristics of normal and pathological voices. *ASHA Reports, 11,* 97–115.

Deal, R. E., & Emanuel, F. W. (1978). Some waveform and spectral features of vowel roughness. *Journal of Speech and Hearing Research, 21,* 250–264.

Debruyne, F., Ostyn, F., Delaere, P., & Wellens, W. (1997). Acoustic analysis of the speaking voice after thyroidectomy. *Journal of Voice, 11,* 479–482.

Deem, J. F., Manning, W. H., Knack, J. V., & Matesich, J. S. (1989). The automatic extraction of pitch perturbation using microcomputers: Some methodological considerations. *Journal of Speech and Hearing Research, 32,* 689–697.

Dempsey, M. E., Draegert, G. L., Siskind, R. P., & Steer, M. D. (1950). The Purdue pitch meter—a direct-reading fundamental frequency analyzer. *Journal of Speech and Hearing Disorders, 15,* 135–141.

Deutsch, D. (1992). Paradoxes of musical pitch. *Scientific American, 267*(2), 88–95.

Doherty, T. E., & Shipp, T. (1988). Tape recorder effects on jitter and shimmer extraction. *Journal of Speech and Hearing Research, 31,* 485–490.

Dordain, M., Chevrie-Muller, C., & Grémy, F. E. (1967). Etude clinique et instrumentale de la voix et de la parole des femmes âgées. *Revue Française de Gérontologie, 13,* 1–8.

Drew, R., & Sapir, S. (1995). Average speaking fundamental frequency in soprano singers with and without symptoms of vocal attrition. *Journal of Voice, 9,* 134–141.

Dunker, E., & Schlosshaier, B. (1961). Unregelmässige Stimmlippenschwingungen bei funktionellen Stimmstörungen. *Zeitschrift für Laryngologie und Rhinologie, 40,* 919–934.

Dwire, A., & McCauley, R. (1995). Repeated measures of vocal fundamental frequency perturbations obtained using the Visi-Pitch. *Journal of Voice, 9,* 156–162.

Elliott, L., & Niemoeller, A. (1970). The role of hearing in controlling voice fundamental frequency. *International Audiology, 9,* 47–52.

Emanuel, F. W. & Austin, D. (1981). Identification of normal and abnormally rough vowels by spectral noise level measurements. *Journal of Communication Disorders, 14,* 75–85.

Emanuel, F. W., Lively, M. A., & McCoy, J. F. (1973). Spectral noise levels and roughness ratings for vowels produced by males and females. *Folia Phoniatrica, 25,* 110–120.

Emanuel, F., & Scarinzi, A. (1979). Vocal register effects on vowel spectral noise and roughness: findings for adult females. *Journal of Communication Disorders, 12,* 263–272.

Emanuel, F., & Scarinzi, A. (1980). Vocal register effects on vowel spectral noise and roughness: Findings for adult males. *Journal of Communication Disorders, 13,* 121–131.

Fairbanks, G. (1940). Recent experimental investigations of vocal pitch in speech. *Journal of the Acoustical Society of America, 11,* 457–466.

Fairbanks, G. (1942). An acoustical study of the pitch of infant hunger wails. *Child Development, 13,* 227–232.

Fairbanks, G. (1960). *Voice and articulation drill book.* New York: Harper.

Fairbanks, G., Herbert, E. L., & Hammond, J. M. (1949). An acoustical study of vocal pitch in seven- and eight-year-old girls. *Child Development, 20,* 71–78.

Fairbanks, G., Wiley, J. H., & Lassman, F. M. (1949). An acoustical study of vocal pitch in seven and eight-year-old boys. *Child Development, 20,* 63–69.

Feijoo, S., & Hernández, C. (1990). Short-term stability measures for the evaluation of vocal quality. *Journal of Speech and Hearing Research, 33,* 324–334.

Fishman, B., & Shipp, T. (1970). Subject positioning and phonation range measures. *Journal of the Acoustical Society of America, 48,* 431–432.

Fisichelli, V. R., Haber, A., Davis, J., & Karelitz, S. (1966). Audible characteristics of the cries of normal infants and those with Down's syndrome. *Perceptual and Motor Skills, 23,* 744.

Fisichelli, V. R., & Karelitz, S. (1966). Frequency spectra of the cries of normal infants and those with Down's syndrome. *Psychometric Science, 6,* 195–196.

Fisichelli, V. R., Karelitz, S., Eichbauer, J., & Rosenfeld, L. S. (1961). Volume-unit graphs: Their production and applicability in studies of infants' cries. *Journal of Psychology, 52,* 423–427.

Fitch, J. (1990). Consistency of fundamental frequency and perturbation in repeated phonations of sustained vowels, reading, and connected speech. *Journal of Speech and Hearing Disorders, 55,* 360–363.

Fitch, J. L., & Holbrook, A. (1970). Modal fundamental frequency of young adults. *Archives of Otolaryngology, 92,* 379–382.

Flatau, T. S., & Gutzmann, H. (1906). Die Stimme des Säuglings. *Archiv für Laryngologie und Rhinologie, 18,* 139–151.

Fletcher, H. (1934). Loudness, pitch, and the timbre of musical tones and their relation to the intensity, the frequency, and the overtone structure. *Journal of the Acoustical Society of America, 6,* 59–69.

Fletcher, S. G. (1971). *Diagnosing speech disorders from cleft palate.* New York: Grune and Stratton.

Fletcher, H., & Munson, W. A. (1933). Loudness, its definition, measurement, and calculation. *Journal of the Acoustical Society of America, 5,* 82–108.

Fourcin, A. J. (1974). Laryngographic examination of vocal fold vibration. In B. Wyke (Ed.), *Ventilatory and phonatory control systems* (pp. 315–333). New York: Oxford University Press.

Fourcin, A. J., & Abberton, E. (1971). First applications of a new laryngograph. *Medical and Biological Illustration, 21,* 172–182. [Reprinted in: *Volta Review* (1972), *74,* 161–176.]

Fourcin, A. J., & Abberton, E. (1976). The laryngograph and the voiscope in speech therapy. *Proceedings of the XVI International Congress of Logopedics and Phoniatrics,* 116–122.

Fritzell, B., Sundberg, J., & Strange-Ebbesen, A. (1982). Pitch change after stripping oedematous vocal folds. *Folia Phoniatrica, 34,* 29–32.

Gamboa, J., Jiménez-Jiménez, F. J., Nieto, A., Montojo, J., Ortí-Pareja, M., Molina, J. A., García-Albea, E., & Cobeta, I. (1997). Acoustic voice analysis in patients with Parkinson's disease treated with dopaminergic drugs. *Journal of Voice, 11,* 314–320.

Garrett, K. L., & Healey, E. C. (1987). An acoustic analysis of fluctuations in the voices of normal adult speakers across three times of day. *Journal of the Acoustical Society of America, 82,* 58–62.

Gelfer, M. P. (1989). Stability in phonational frequency range. *Journal of Communication Disorders, 22,* 181–192.

Gelfer, M. P., Andrews, M. L., & Schmidt, C. P. (1991). Effects of prolonged loud reading on selected measures of vocal function in trained and untrained singers. *Journal of Voice, 5,* 158–167.

Gelfer, M. P., & Fendel, D. M. (1995). Comparisons of jitter, shimmer, and signal-to-noise ratio from directly digitized versus taped voice samples. *Journal of Voice, 9,* 378–382.

Gilbert, H. R. (1975). Speech characteristics of miners with black lung disease (pneumoconiosis). *Journal of Communication Disorders, 8,* 129–140.

Gilbert, H. R., & Campbell, M. I. (1980). Speaking fundamental frequency in three groups of hearing-impaired individuals. *Journal of Communication Disorders, 13,* 195–205.

Gleick, J. (1987). *Chaos: Making a new science.* New York: Viking Penguin.

Gold, B. (1962). Computer program for pitch extraction. *Journal of the Acoustical Society of America, 34,* 916–921.

Gold, B., & Rabiner, L. (1969). Parallel processing techniques for estimating pitch periods of speech in the time domain. *Journal of the Acoustical Society of America, 46,* 442–448.

Goldstein, J. L. (1973). An optimum processor for the central formation of pitch of complex tones. *Journal of the Acoustical Society of America, 54,* 1496–1516.

Gramming, P. (1991). Vocal loudness and frequency capabilities of the voice. *Journal of Voice, 5,* 144–157.

Griffin, G. R., & Williams, C. E. (1987). The effects of different levels of task complexity on three vocal measures. *Aviation, Space, and Environmental Medicine, 58,* 1165–1170.

Haji, T., Horiguchi, S., Baer, T., & Gould, W. J. (1986). Frequency and amplitude perturbation analysis of electroglottograph during sustained phonation. *Journal of the Acoustical Society of America, 80,* 58–62.

Hakel, M. E., Healey, E. C., & Sullivan, M. (1994). Comparisons of fundamental frequency measures of speakers with dysarthria and hyperfunctional voice disorders. In J. A. Till, K. M. Yorkston, & D. R. Beukelman (Eds.), *Motor speech disorders: Advances in assessment and treatment* (pp. 193–203). Baltimore, MD: Paul H. Brookes.

Hakes, J., Shipp, T., & Doherty, E. (1987). Acoustic properties of straight tone, vibrato, trill, and trillo. *Journal of Voice, 1,* 148–156.

Hall, K. D., & Yairi, E. (1992). Fundamental frequency, jitter, and shimmer in preschoolers who stutter. *Journal of Speech and Hearing Research, 35,* 1002–1008.

Hammarberg, B., Fritzell, B., Gauffin, J., Sundberg, J., & Wedin, L. (1980). Perceptual and acoustic correlates of abnormal voice qualities. *Acta Otolaryngologica, 90,* 441–451.

Hanley, T. D. (1951). An analysis of vocal frequency and duration characteristics of selected samples of speech from General American, Eastern American, and Southern American dialect regions. *Speech Monographs, 18,* 78–93.

Hanson, W. (1969). *Vowel spectral noise levels and roughness severity ratings for vowels and sentences produced by adult males presenting abnormally rough voice.* Unpublished doctoral dissertation, University of Oklahoma, Norman.

Harris, T., Harris, S., Rubin, J. S., & Howard, D. M. (1998). *The voice clinic handbook.* London, UK: Whurr.

Hartmann, E., & von Cramon, D. (1984). Acoustic measurement of voice quality in central dysphonia. *Journal of Communication Disorders, 17,* 425–440.

Healey, E. C. (1982). Speaking fundamental frequency characteristics of stutterers and nonstutterers. *Journal of Communication Disorders, 15,* 21–29.

Hecker, M. H. L., & Kreul, E. J. (1971). Description of the speech of patients with cancer of the vocal folds. Part I: Measures of fundamental frequency. *Journal of the Acoustical Society of America, 49,* 1275–1282.

Hecker, M. H. L., Stevens, K. N., von Bismarck, G., & Williams, C. E. (1968). Manifestations of task-induced stress in the acoustic speech signal. *Journal of the Acoustical Society of America, 44,* 993–1001.

Hemler, R. J. B., Wieneke, G. H., & Dejonckere, H. (1997). The effect of relative humidity of inhaled air on acoustic parameters of voice in normal subjects. *Journal of Voice, 11,* 295–300.

Hencke, W. L. (1974a). Signals from external accelerometers during phonation: Attributes and their internal physical correlates. *MIT Research Laboratory of Electronics Quarterly Progress Report, 114,* 224–231.

Hencke, W. L. (1974b). Display and interpretation of glottal activity as transduced by external accelerometers. *Journal of the Acoustical Society of America, 55,* S79A.

Herzel, H. (1993). Bifurcations and chaos in voice signals. *Applied Mechanics Review, 46,* 399–413.

Herzel, H. (1996). Possible mechanisms of vocal instabilities. In P. M. Davis & N. H. Fletcher (Eds.), *Vocal fold physiology: Controlling complexity and chaos* (pp. 63–75). San Diego, CA: Singular Publishing Group.

Herzel, H., Berry, D., Titze, I. R., & Saleh, M. (1994). Analysis of vocal disorders with methods from nonlinear dynamics. *Journal of Speech and Hearing Research, 37,* 1008–1019.

Herzel, H., Steinecke, I., Mende, W., & Wermke, K. (1991). Chaos and bifurcations during voiced speech. In E. Moselkilde (Ed.), *Complexity, chaos, and biological evolution* (pp. 41–50). New York: Plenum.

Higgins, M. B., Netsell, R., & Schulte, L. (1994). Aerodynamic and electroglottographic measures of normal voice production: Intrasubject variability within and across sessions. *Journal of Speech and Hearing Research, 37,* 38–45.

Higgins, M. B., & Saxman, J. H. (1989). A comparison of intrasubject variation across sessions of three vocal frequency perturbation indices. *Journal of the Acoustical Society of America, 86,* 911–916.

Higgins, M. B., & Saxman, J. H. (1991). A comparison of selected phonatory behaviors of healthy aged and young adults. *Journal of Speech and Hearing Research, 34,* 1000–1010.

Hildebrand, F. B. (1956). *Introduction to numerical analysis* (2nd ed.). New York: Dover.

Hillenbrand, J. (1987). A methodological study of perturbation and additive noise in synthetically generated voice signals. *Journal of Speech and Hearing Research, 30,* 448–461.

Hirano, M. (1989). Objective evaluation of the human voice: clinical aspects. *Folia Phoniatrica, 41,* 89–144.

Hirano, M., Kurita, S., & Nakashima, T. (1983). Growth, development, and aging of human vocal folds. In D. M. Bless & J. H. Abbs (Eds.), *Vocal fold physiology: Contemporary research and clinical issues* (pp. 22–43). San Diego, CA: College-Hill Press.

Hirano, M., Tanaka, S., Fujita, M., & Terasawa, R. (1991). Fundamental frequency and sound pressure level of phonation in pathological states. *Journal of Voice, 5,* 120–127.

Hixon, T. J., Klatt, D. H., & Mead, J. (1971). Influence of forced transglottal pressure changes on vocal fundamental frequency. *Journal of the Acoustical Society of America, 49,* 105.

Holden A. V. (Ed.). (1986). *Chaos.* Princeton, NJ: Princeton University Press.

Hollien, H. (1974). On vocal registers. *Journal of Phonetics, 2,* 125–143.

Hollien, H., & Copeland, R. H. (1965). Speaking fundamental frequency (SFF) characteristics of mongoloid girls. *Journal of Speech and Hearing Disorders, 30,* 344–349.

Hollien, H., Dew, D., & Philips, P. (1971). Phonation frequency ranges of adults. *Journal of Speech and Hearing Research, 14,* 755–760.

Hollien, H., Girard, G. T., & Coleman, R. (1977). Vocal fold vibratory patterns of pulse register phonation. *Folia Phoniatrica, 29,* 200–205.

Hollien, H., Hollien, P. A., & de Jong, G. (1997). Effects of three parameters on speaking fundamental frequency. *Journal of the Acoustical Society of America, 102,* 2984–2992.

Hollien, H., & Jackson, B. (1973). Normative data on the speaking fundamental characteristics of young adult males. *Journal of Phonetics, 1,* 117–120.

Hollien, H., & Malcik, E. (1962). Adolescent voice change in southern Negro males. *Speech Monographs, 29,* 53–58.

Hollien, H., & Malcik, E. (1967). Evaluation of cross-sectional studies of adolescent voice change in males. *Speech Monographs, 34,* 80–84.

Hollien, H., Malcik, E., & Hollien, B. (1965). Adolescent voice change in southern white males. *Speech Monographs, 32,* 87–90

Hollien, H., & Michel, J. F. (1968). Vocal fry as phonational register. *Journal of Speech and Hearing Research, 11,* 600–604.

Hollien, H., Michel. J., & Doherty, E. T. (1973). A method for analyzing vocal jitter in sustained phonation. *Journal of Phonetics, 1,* 85–91.

Hollien, H., Moore, P., Wendahl, R. W., & Michel, J. F. (1966). On the nature of vocal fry. *Journal of Speech and Hearing Research, 9,* 245–247.

Hollien, H., & Paul, P. (1969). A second evaluation of the speaking fundamental frequency characteristics of post-adolescent girls. *Language and Speech, 12,* 119–124.

Hollien, H., & Shipp, T. (1972). Speaking fundamental frequency and chronologic age in males. *Journal of Speech and Hearing Research, 15,* 155–159.

Hollien, H., & Wendahl, R. W. (1968). A perceptual study of vocal fry. *Journal of the Acoustical Society of America, 43,* 506–509.

Hommerich, K. W. (1972). Der alternde Larynx: Morphologische Aspekt. *Hals- Nasen- Ohrenaerzte, 20,* 115–120.

Honjo, I., & Isshiki, N. (1980). Laryngoscopic and voice characteristics of aged persons. *Archives of Otolaryngology, 106,* 149–150.

Hoops, H. R., & Noll, J. D. (1969). Relationship of selected acoustic variables to judgments of esophageal speech. *Journal of Communication Disorders, 2,* 1–13.

Horiguchi, S., Haji, T., Baer, T., & Gould, W. J. (1987). Comparison of electroglottographic and acoustic waveform perturbation measures. In T. Baer, C. Sasaki, & K. S. Harris (Eds.), *Laryngeal function in phonation and respiration* (pp. 509–518). San Diego, CA: College-Hill Press.

Horii, Y. (1975). Some statistical characteristics of voice fundamental frequency. *Journal of Speech and Hearing Research, 18,* 192–201.

Horii, Y. (1979). Fundamental frequency perturbation observed in sustained phonation. *Journal of Speech and Hearing Research, 22,* 5–19.

Horii, Y. (1980). Vocal shimmer in sustained phonation. *Journal of Speech and Hearing Research, 23,* 202–209.

Horii, Y. (1982). Jitter and shimmer differences among sustained vowel phonations. *Journal of Speech and Hearing Research, 25,* 12–14.

Horii, Y. (1983a). Automatic analysis of voice fundamental frequency and intensity using a Visipitch. *Journal of Speech and Hearing Research, 26,* 467–471.

Horii, Y. (1983b). Some acoustic characteristics of oral reading by ten- to twelve-year-old children. *Journal of Communication Disorders, 16,* 257–267.

Horii, Y. (1989). Acoustic analysis of vocal vibrato: A theoretical interpretation of data. *Journal of Voice, 3,* 36–43.

Houtsma, A. J., & Goldstein, J. L. (1972). The central origin of the pitch of complex tones: evidence from musical interval recognition. *Journal of the Acoustical Society of America, 51,* 520–529.

Hudson, A., & Holbrook, A. (1981). A study of the reading fundamental vocal frequency of young adult males. *Journal of Speech and Hearing Research, 24,* 197–201.

Hudson, A., & Holbrook, A. (1982). Fundamental frequency characteristics of young Black adults: spontaneous speech and oral reading. *Journal of Speech and Hearing Research, 25,* 25–28.

Hufnagle, J., & Hufnagle, K. (1984). An investigation of the relationship between speaking fundamental frequency and vocal quality improvement. *Journal of Communication Disorders, 17,* 95–100.

Huttar, G. L. (1968). Relations between prosodic variables and emotions in normal American English utterances. *Journal of Speech and Hearing Research, 11,* 481–487.

Isshiki, N., Yanagihara, N., & Morimoto, M. (1966). Approach to the objective diagnosis of hoarseness. *Folia Phoniatrica, 18,* 393–400.

Iwata, S. (1972). Periodicities of pitch perturbations in normal and pathological larynges. *Laryngoscope, 82,* 87–95.

Iwata, S., & von Leden, H. (1970). Pitch perturbations in normal and pathological voices. *Folia Phoniatrica, 22,* 413–424.

Izdebski, K., & Murry, T. (1980). Glottal waveform variability: A preliminary inquiry. In V. Lawrence & B. Weinberg (Eds.). *Transcripts of the ninth symposium: Care of the professional voice, Vol. 1,* pp. 39–43. New York: The Voice Foundation.

Jacob, L. (1968). *A normative study of laryngeal jitter.* Unpublished master's thesis, University of Kansas.

Jafari, M., Till, J. A., Truesdell, L. F., & Law-Till, C. B. (1993). Time-shift, trial, and gender effects on vocal perturbation measures. *Journal of Voice, 7,* 326–336.

Jiang, J., Lin, E., & Hanson, D. G. (1998). Effect of tape recording on perturbation measures. *Journal of Speech, Language, and Hearing Research, 41,* 1031–1041.

Jiang, J. J., Titze, I. R., Wexler, D. B., & Gray, S. D. (1994). Fundamental frequency and amplitude perturbation in reconstructed canine vocal folds. *Annals of Otology, Rhinology, and Laryngology, 103,* 145–148.

Johnson, K. W., & Michel, J. F. (1969). The effect of selected vowels on laryngeal jitter. *Asha, 11,* 96.

Kahane, J. C. (1983). A survey of age-related changes in the connective tissues of the adult human larynx. In D. M. Bless & J. H. Abbs (Eds.), *Vocal fold physiology: Contemporary research and clinical issues* (pp. 44–49). San Diego, CA: College-Hill Press.

Kahane, J. C. (1987). Connective tissue changes in the larynx and their effects on voice. *Journal of Voice, 1,* 27–30.

Kaiser, J. F. (1983). Some observations on vocal tract operation from a fluid flow point of view. In I. R. Titze & R. C. Scherer (Eds.), *Vocal fold physiology: Biomechanics, acoustics, and phonatory control* (pp. 359–386). Denver, CO: Denver Center for the Performing Arts.

Kakita, Y., & Okamoto, H. (1996). Visualizing the characteristics of vocal fluctuation from the viewpoint of chaos: An attempt toward qualitative quantification. In P. J. Davis & N. H. Fletcher (Eds.), *Vocal fold physiology: Controlling complexity and chaos* (pp. 79–95). San Diego, CA: Singular Publishing Group.

Kane, M., & Wellen, C. J. (1985). Acoustical measurements and clinical judgments of vocal quality in children with vocal nodules. *Folia Phoniatrica, 37,* 53–57.

Karelitz, S., & Fisichelli, V. R. (1962). The cry thresholds of normal infants and those with brain damage. *Journal of Pediatrics, 61,* 679–685.

Karelitz, S., & Fisichelli, V. R. (1969). Infants' vocalizations and their significance. *Clinical Proceedings of the Children's Hospital, 25,* 345–361.

Karelitz, S., Fisichelli, V. R., Costa, J., Karelitz, R., & Rosenfeld, L. (1964). Relation of crying activity in early infancy to speech and intellectual development at age three years. *Child Development, 35,* 469–777.

Kark, A. E., Kissin, M. W., Auerbach, R., & Meikle, M. (1984). Voice changes after thyroidectomy: role of the external laryngeal nerve. *British Medical Journal, 289,* 1412–1415.

Karnell, M. P. (1991). Laryngeal perturbation analysis: Minimum length of analysis window. *Journal of Speech and Hearing Research, 34,* 544–548.

Karnell, M. P., Chang, A., Smith, A., & Hoffman, H. (1997). Impact of signal type of validity of voice perturbation measures [sic]. *NCVS Status and Progress Report, 11,* 91–94.

Karnell, M. P., Hall, K. D., & Landahl, K. L. (1995). Comparison of fundamental frequency and perturbation measurements among three analysis systems. *Journal of Voice, 9,* 383–393.

Karnell, M. P., Scherer, R. S., & Fischer, L. B. (1991). Comparison of acoustic voice perturbation measures among three independent voice laboratories. *Journal of Speech and Hearing Research, 34,* 781–790.

Keating, P., & Buhr, R. (1978). Fundamental frequency in the speech of infants and children. *Journal of the Acoustical Society of America, 63,* 567–571.

Keidar, A., Hurtig, R., & Titze, I. R. (1987). The perceptual nature of vocal register change. *Journal of Voice, 1,* 223–233.

Keilmann, A., & Hülse, M. (1992). Dysphonie nach Strumektomie bei ungestörter respiratorischer Beweglichkeit der Stimmlippen. *Folia Phoniatrica, 44,* 261–268.

Kempster, G. B., Kistler, D. J., & Hillenbrand, J. (1991). Multidimensional scaling analysis of dysphonia in two speaker groups. *Journal of Speech and Hearing Research, 34,* 534–543.

Killingbeck, J. P. (1991). *Microcomputer algorithms: Action from algebra.* New York: Adam Hilger.

Kim, V. P. C., Oates, J. M., Phyland, D. J., & Campbell, M. J. (1998). Effects of laryngeal endoscopy on the vocal performance of young adult females with normal voices. *Journal of Voice, 12,* 68–77.

Kitajima, K., Tanabe, M., & Isshiki, N. (1975). Pitch perturbation in normal and pathological voice. *Studia Phonologica, 9,* 25–32.

Kitajima, K., & Tanaka, K. (1995). The effects of intraoral pressure change on F_0 regulation—Preliminary study for the evaluation of vocal fold stiffness. *Journal of Voice, 9,* 424–428.

Kitzing, P., & Sonesson, B. (1974). A photoglottographical study of the female vocal folds during phonation. *Folia Phoniatrica, 26,* 138–149.

Klingholz, F., & Martin, F. (1983). Speech wave aperiodicities at sustained phonation in functional dysphonia. *Folia Phoniatrica, 35,* 322–327.

Klingholz, F., & Martin, F. (1985). Quantitative spectral evaluation of shimmer and jitter. *Journal of Speech and Hearing Research, 28,* 169–174.

Koike, Y. (1967). Application of some acoustic measures for the evaluation of laryngeal dysfunction. *Journal of the Acoustical Society of America, 42,* 1209.

Koike, Y. (1969). Vowel amplitude modulations in patients with laryngeal diseases. *Journal of the Acoustical Society of America, 45,* 839–844.

Koike, Y. (1973). Application of some acoustic measures for the evaluation of laryngeal dysfunction. *Studia Phonologica, 7,* 17–23.

Koike, Y., & Markel, J. (1975). Application of inverse filtering for detecting laryngeal pathology. *Annals of Otology, Rhinology, and Laryngology, 84,* 117–124.

Koike, Y., Takahashi, H., & Calcaterra, T. C. (1977). Acoustic measures for detecting laryngeal pathology. *Acta Otolaryngologica, 84,* 105–117.

Krasner, S. (Ed.). (1990). *The ubiquity of chaos.* Washington, DC: American Association for the Advancement of Science.

Krook, M. I. P. (1988). Speaking fundamental frequency characteristics of normal Swedish subjects obtained by glottal frequency analysis. *Folia Phoniatrica, 40,* 82–90.

Kyttä, J. (1964). Spectrographic studies of the sound quality of oesophageal speech. *Acta Otolaryngologica, Suppl. 188,* 371–377.

Ladefoged, P., & McKinney, N. P. (1963). Loudness, sound pressure, and subglottal pressure in speech. *Journal of the Acoustical Society of America, 35,* 454–160.

Laguaite, J. K., & Waldrop, W. F. (1964). Acoustic analysis of fundamental frequency of voices before and after therapy. *Folia Phoniatrica, 16,* 183–192.

Larson, C. R., Kempster, G. B., & Kistler, M. K. (1987). Changes in voice fundamental frequency following discharge of single motor units in cricothyroid muscles. *Journal of Speech and Hearing Research, 30,* 552–558.

Laufer, M. Z., & Horii, Y. (1977). Fundamental frequency characteristics of infant non-distress vocalizations during the first 24 weeks. *Journal of Child Language, 4,* 171–184.

Laver, J., Hiller, S., & Beck, J. M. (1992). Acoustic waveform perturbations and voice disorders. *Journal of Voice, 6,* 115–126.

Laver, J., & Hanson, R. J. (1981). Describing the normal voice. In J. K. Darby (Ed.), *Speech evaluation in psychiatry* (pp. 57–78). New York: Grune and Stratton. [Reprinted in: Laver, J. (1991). *The gift of speech* (pp. 209–234). Edinburgh, UK: Edinburgh University Press.]

Lebrun, Y. Devreux, F., Rousseau, J.-J., & Darimont, P. (1982). Tremulous speech: A case report. *Folia Phoniatrica, 34,* 134–142.

Lecluse, F. L. E., Brocaar, P. M., & Verschuure, J. (1975). The electroglottography [sic] and its relation to glottal activity. *Folia Phoniatrica, 27,* 215–224.

Leddy, M., & Bless, D. M. (1989, November). *Normal jitter in sustained vowels and connected speech.* Presentation at the annual meeting of the American Speech-Language-Hearing Association.

Leeper, H., & Leeper, G. (1976). *Clinical evaluation of the fundamental frequency of normal children and children with vocal nodules employing a striation counting procedure.* Paper presented at the annual convention of the American Speech-Language-Hearing Association.

Licklider, J. C. R. (1951). Basic correlates of the auditory stimulus. In S. S. Stevens (Ed.), *Handbook of experimental psychology* (pp. 985–1039). New York: John Wiley.

Lieberman, P. (1961). Perturbations in vocal pitch. *Journal of the Acoustical Society of America, 33,* 597–603.

Lieberman, P. (1963). Some acoustic measures of the fundamental periodicity of normal and pathologic larynges. *Journal of the Acoustical Society of America, 35,* 344–353.

Lieberman, P., Knudson, R., & Mead, J. (1969). Determination of the rate of change of fundamental frequency with respect to subglottal pressure during sustained phonation. *Journal of the Acoustical Society of America, 45,* 1537–1543.

Lieberman, P., & Michaels, S. B. (1962). Some aspects of fundamental frequency and envelope amplitude as related to the emotional content of speech. *Journal of the Acoustical Society of America, 34,* 922–927.

Liljencrants, J. (1991). Numerical simulations of glottal flow. In J. Gauffin & B. Hammarberg (Eds.), *Vocal fold physiology: Acoustic, perceptual, and physiological aspects of voice mechanisms* (pp. 98–112). San Diego, CA: Singular Publishing Group.

Lind, J. (Ed.), (1965). *Newborn infant cry.* Uppsala, Sweden: Almqvist and Wiksells.

Linke, C. E. (1973). A study of pitch characteristics of female voices and their relationship to vocal effectiveness. *Folia Phoniatrica, 25,* 173–185.

Linville, S. E., & Fisher, H. B. (1985). Acoustic characteristics of women's voices with advancing age. *Journal of Gerontology, 40,* 324–330.

Linville, S. E., Skarin, B. D., & Fornatto, E. (1989). The interrelationship of measures related to vocal function, speech rate, and laryngeal appearance in elderly women. *Journal of Speech and Hearing Research, 32,* 323–330.

Lisker, L., Abramson, A. S., Cooper, F. S., & Schvey, M. H. (1966). Transillumination of the larynx in running speech. *Journal of the Acoustical Society of America, 45,* 1544–1546.

Lucero, J. C. (1996). Chest- and falsetto-like oscillations in a two-mass model of the vocal folds. *Journal of the Acoustical Society of America, 100,* 3355–3359.

Luchsinger, R., & Arnold, G. (1965). *Voice-speech-language.* Belmont, CA: Wadsworth Publishing.

Martony, J. (1968). On the correction of voice pitch level for severely hard of hearing subjects. *American Annals of the Deaf, 113,* 195–202.

Max, L., & Mueller, P. B. (1996). Speaking F_0 and cepstral periodicity analysis of conversational speech in a 105–year-old woman: Variability of aging effects. *Journal of Voice, 10,* 245–251.

Maxwell, S., & Locke, J. L. (1969). Voice in myasthenia gravis. *Laryngoscope, 79,* 1902–1905.

Mayo, R. (1990). *Fundamental frequency and vowel formant frequency characteristics of normal African-American and European-American adults.* Unpublished doctoral dissertation, Memphis State University, Memphis TN.

Mayo, R., & Grant, W. C. II. (1995). Fundamental frequency, perturbation, and vocal tract resonance characteristics of African-American and White American males. *Echo, 17,* 32–38.

McAllister, A., Sederholm, E., Ternström, S., & Sundberg, J. (1996). Perturbation and hoarseness: A pilot study of six children's voices. *Journal of Voice, 10,* 252–261.

McAllister, A., Sundberg, J., & Hibi, S. R. (1998). Acoustic measurements and perceptual evaluation of hoarseness in children's voices. *Logopedics Phoniatrics Vocology, 23,* 27–38.

McGlone, R. E. and Brown, W. S., Jr. (1969). Identification of the "shift" between vocal registers. *Journal of the Acoustical Society of America, 4,* 1033–1036.

McGlone, R. E., & Hollien, H. (1963). Vocal pitch characteristics of aged women. *Journal of Speech and Hearing Research, 6,* 164–170.

Mende, W., Herzel, H., & Wermke, K. (1990). Bifurcations and chaos in newborn cries. *Physics Letters, 145A*, 418–424.

Michel, J. F. (1968). Fundamental frequency investigation of vocal fry and harshness. *Journal of Speech and Hearing Research, 11*, 590–594.

Michel, J. F., & Carney, R. J. (1964). Pitch characteristics of mongoloid boys. *Journal of Speech and Hearing Disorders, 29*, 121–125.

Michel, J., & Hollien, H. (1968). Perceptual differentiation in vocal fry and harshness. *Journal of Speech and Hearing Research, 11*, 439–443.

Michel, J. F., Hollien, H., & Moore, P. (1966). Speaking fundamental frequency characteristics of 15, 16, and 17 year-old girls. *Language and Speech, 9*, 46–51.

Michel, J. F., & Myers, R. D. (1991). The effects of crescendo on vocal vibrato. *Journal of Voice, 5*, 293–298.

Michel, J. F., & Wendahl, R. (1971). Correlates of voice production. In L. E. Travis (Ed.), *Handbook of speech pathology and audiology* (pp. 465–480). Englewood Cliffs, NJ: Prentice-Hall.

Michelsson, K., & Wasz-Höckert, O. (1980). The value of cry analysis in neonatology and eary infancy. In T. Murry, & J. Murry (Eds.), *Infant communication: Cry and early speech* (pp. 152–182). Houston, TX: College-Hill Press.

Milenkovic, P. (1987). Least mean square measures of voice perturbation. *Journal of Speech and Hearing Research, 30*, 529–538.

Miller, R. L. (1959). Nature of the vocal cord wave. *Journal of the Acoustical Society of America, 31*, 667–677.

Miller, J. E., & Mathews, M. V. (1963). Investigation of the glottal waveshape by automatic inverse filtering. *Journal of the Acoustical Society of America, 35*, 1876.

Montague, J. C., Jr., Brown, W. J., Jr., & Hollien, H. (1974). Vocal fundamental frequency characteristics of institutionalized Down's syndrome children. *American Journal of Mental Deficiency, 78*, 414–418.

Montague, J. C., Jr., Hollien, H., Hollien, P. A., & Wold, D. C. (1978). Perceived pitch and fundamental frequency comparisons of institutionalized Down's syndrome children. *Folia Phoniatrica, 30*, 245–256.

Moon, F. C. (1987). *Chaotic vibrations: An introduction for applied scientists and engineers.* New York: John Wiley.

Moore, G. P. (1971). Voice disorders organically based. In L. E. Travis (Ed.), *Handbook of speech pathology and audiology* (pp. 535–569). Englewood Cliffs, NJ: Prentice-Hall.

Moore, P., & Thompson, C. L. (1965). Comments on physiology of hoarseness. *Archives of Otolaryngology, 81*, 97–102.

Moore, P., & von Leden, H. (1958). Dynamic variations of the vibratory pattern in the normal larynx. *Folia Phoniatrica, 10*, 205–238.

Mörner, M., Fransson, F., & Fant, G. (1963). Voice register terminology and standard pitch. *Speech Transmission Laboratory, Quarterly Status and Progress Report, 4/1963*, 17–23.

Morris, R. J. (1997). Speaking fundamental frequency characteristics of 8– through 10–year-old white- and African-American boys. *Journal of Communication Disorders, 30*, 101–116.

Morris, R. J., & Brown, W. S., Jr. (1988). Age-related differences in F_0 and pitch sigma among females. *IASCP Bulletin, 2*, 36–40.

Morris, R. J., & Brown, W. S., Jr. (1996). Comparison of various automatic means for measuring mean fundamental frequency. *Journal of Voice, 10*, 159–165.

Morris, R. J., Brown, W. S., Jr., Hicks, D. M., & Howell, E. (1995). Phonational profiles of male trained singers and nonsingers. *Journal of Voice*, 142–148.

Mueller, P. B. (1982). Voice characteristics of octogenarian and nonagenarian persons. *Ear, Nose and Throat Journal, 61*, 204–207.

Mueller, P. B. (1989). *Voice characteristics of centenarian subjects.* Presentation at the XXIst Congress of the International Association of Logopedics and Phoniatrics, Prague, Czechoslovakia.

Mueller, P. B., Adams, M., Baehr-Rouse, J., & Boos, D. A. (1979). A tape striation counting method for determining fundamental frequency. *Language, Speech, and Hearing Services in Schools, 10*, 246–248.

Mueller, P. B., Sweeney, R. J., & Baribeau, L. J. (1984). Acoustic and morphologic study of the senescent voice. *Ear, Nose and Throat Journal, 63*, 292–295.

Muller, E., Hollien, H., & Murry, T. (1974). Perceptual responses to infant crying: identification of cry types. *Journal of Child Language, 1*, 89–95.

Murry, T. (1971). Subglottal pressure and airflow measures during vocal fry phonation. *Journal of Speech and Hearing Research, 14*, 544–551.

Murry, T. (1978). Speaking fundamental frequency characteristics associated with voice pathologies. *Journal of Speech and Hearing Disorders, 43*, 374–379.

Murry, T., Amundson, P., & Hollien, H. (1977). Acoustical characteristics of infant cries: fundamental frequency. *Journal of Child Language, 4*, 321–328.

Murry, T., Brown, W. S., Jr., & Morris, R. J. (1995). Patterns of fundamental frequency for three types of voice samples. *Journal of Voice, 9*, 282–289.

Murry, T., & Doherty, E. T. (1980). Selected acoustic characteristics of pathological and normal speakers. *Journal of Speech and Hearing Research, 23*, 361–369.

Murry, T., Gracco, V. L., & Gracco, L. C. (1979). *Infant vocalization during the first twelve weeks.* Paper presented at the Annual Convention of the American Speech and Hearing Association.

Murry, T., Hoit-Dalgaard, J., & Gracco, V. (1983). Infant vocalization: A longitudinal study of acoustic and temporal parameters. *Folia Phoniatrica, 35*, 245–253.

Murry, T., Hollien, H., & Muller, E. (1975). Perceptual responses to infant crying: Maternal recognition and sex judgments. *Journal of Child Language, 2*, 199–204.

Mysak, E. D. (1959). Pitch and duration characteristics of older males. *Journal of Speech and Hearing Research, 2*, 46–54.

Mysak, E. D., & Hanley, T. D. (1958). Aging process in speech: Pitch and duration characteristics. *Journal of Gerontology, 13*, 309–313.

Mysak, E. D., & Hanley, T. D. (1959). Vocal aging. *Geriatrics, 14*, 652–656.

Neelley, J., Edison, S., & Carlile, L. (1968). Speaking voice fundamental frequency of mentally retarded adults and normal adults. *American Journal of Mental Deficiency, 72*, 944–947.

Neils, L. R., & Yairi, E. (1987). Effects of speaking in noise on vocal fatigue and vocal recovery. *Folia Phoniatrica, 39*, 104–112.

Nevlud, G. N., Fann, W. E., & Falck, F. (1983). Acoustic parameters of voice and neuroleptic medication. *Biological Psychiatry, 18*, 1081–1084.

Ng, M. L., Gilbert, H. R., & Lerman, J. W. (1997). Some aerodynamic and acoustic characteristics of acute laryngitis. *Journal of Voice, 11*, 356–363.

Nittrouer, S., McGowan, R. S., Milenkovic, P. H., & Beehler, D. (1990). Acoustic measurements of men's and women's voices: A study of context effects and covariation. *Journal of Speech and Hearing Research, 33*, 761–775.

Noll, A. M. (1964). Short-term spectrum and "cepstrum" techniques for vocal pitch detection. *Journal of the Acoustical Society of America, 36*, 296–302.

Noll, A. M. (1967). Cepstrum pitch determination. *Journal of the Acoustical Society of America, 41*, 293–309.

Okamoto, K., Yoshida, A., Tanimoto, C., Takyu, H., & Inoue, J. (1984). A clinical study of speaking fundamental frequency. *Otologia (Fukuoka), 30*, 33–39.

Orlikoff, R. F. (1989). Vocal jitter at different fundamental frequencies: A cardiovascular-neuromuscular explanation. *Journal of Voice, 3*, 104–112.

Orlikoff, R. F. (1990a). Vowel amplitude variation associated with the heart cycle. *Journal of the Acoustical Society of America, 33,* 2091–2097.

Orlikoff, R. F. (1990b). Heartbeat-related fundamental frequency and amplitude variations in healthy young and elderly male voices. *Journal of Voice, 4,* 322–328.

Orlikoff, R. F. (1990c). The relationship of age and cardiovascular health to certain acoustic characteristics of male voices. *Journal of Speech and Hearing Research, 33,* 450–457.

Orlikoff, R. F. (1990d). The atherosclerotic voice. *Ear, Nose, and Throat Journal, 69,* 833–837.

Orlikoff, R. F. (1995). Vocal stability and vocal tract configuration: An acoustic and electroglottographic investigation. *Journal of Voice, 9,* 173–181.

Orlikoff, R. F., & Baken, R. J. (1989a). The effect of the heartbeat on fundamental frequency perturbation. *Journal of Speech and Hearing Research, 35,* 576–583.

Orlikoff, R. F., & Baken, R. J. (1989b). Fundamental frequency modulation of the human voice by the heartbeat: Preliminary results and possible mechanisms. *Journal of the Acoustical Society of America, 85,* 888–893.

Orlikoff, R. F., & Baken, R. J. (1990). Consideration of the relationship between the fundamental frequency of phonation and vocal jitter. *Folia Phoniatrica, 42,* 31–40.

Orlikoff, R. F., & Kahane, J. C. (1991). Influence of mean sound pressure level on jitter and shimmer measures. *Journal of Voice, 5,* 113–119.

Orlikoff, R. F., Kraus, D. H., Harrison, L. B., Ho, M. L., & Gartner, C. J. (1997). Vocal fundamental frequency measures as a reflection of tumor response to chemotherapy in patients with advanced laryngeal cancer. *Journal of Voice, 11,* 33–39.

Pedersen, M. F. (1993). A longitudinal pilot study on [*sic*] phonetograms/voice profiles in pre-pubertal choir boys. *Clinical Otolaryngology, 18,* 488–491.

Pedersen, M. (1997). Biological development and the normal voice in puberty. *Acta Universitatis Ouluensis (Finland), D Medica 401,* 15–51.

Pedersen, M. F., Kitzing, P., Krabbe, S., & Heramb, S. (1982). The change of voice during puberty in 11 to 16 years [*sic*] old choir singers meaured with electroglottographic fundamental frequency analysis and compared to other phenomena of puberty. *Acta Otolarynologica, Suppl. 386,* 189–192.

Pedersen, M. F., Møller, S., Krabbe, S., & Bennett, P. (1986). Fundamental voice frequency measured by electroglottography during continuous speech. An new exact secondary sex characteristic in boys in puberty. *International Journal of Pediatric Otolaryngology, 11,* 21–27.

Pedersen, M. R., Møller, S., Krabbe, S., Bennett, P., & Svenstrup, B. (1990). Fundamental voice frequency in female puberty measured with electroglottography during continuous speech as a secondary sex caracteristic [*sic*]. A comparison between voice, pubertal stages, oestrogrens and androgens. *International Journal of Pediatric Otolaryngology, 20,* 17–24.

Pedersen, M. F., Møller, S., Krabbe, S., Munk, E., & Bennett, P. (1985). A multivariate statistical analysis of voice phenomena related to puberty in choir boys. *Folia Phoniatrica, 37,* 271–278.

Pentz, A. L., Jr., & Gilbert, H. R. (1983). Relation of selected acoustic parameters and perceptual ratings to voice quality of Down syndrome children. *American Journal of Mental Deficiency, 88,* 203–210.

Perkins, W. H. (1971a). Vocal function: Assessment and therapy. In L. E. Travis (Ed.), *Handbook of speech pathology and audiology* (pp. 505–534). Englewood Cliffs, NJ: Prentice-Hall.

Perkins, W. H. (1971b). *Speech pathology.* St. Louis, MO: Mosby.

Perry, C. K., Ingrisano, K. R.-S., & Scott, S. R. G. (1996). Accuracy of jitter estimates using different filter settings on Visi-Pitch: A preliminary report. *Journal of Voice, 10,* 337–341.

Petrovich-Bartell, N., Cowan, N., & Morse, P. A. (1982). Mothers' perception of infant distress vocalizations. *Journal of Speech and Hearing Research, 25,* 371–376.

Pierce, J. R. (1983). *The science of musical sound.* New York: Scientific American Books.

Pilhour, C. W. (1948). *An experimental study of the relationships between perception of vocal pitch in connected speech and certain measures of vocal frequency.* Unpublished doctoral dissertation, University of Iowa, Iowa City.

Pinto, N. B., & Titze, I. R. (1990). Unification of perturbation measures in speech signals. *Journal of the Acoustical Society of America, 87,* 1278–1289.

Prescott, R. (1975). Infant cry sound: Developmental features. *Journal of the Acoustical Society of America, 57,* 1186–1191.

Pronovost, W. (1942). An experimental study of methods for determining the natural and habitual pitch. *Speech Monographs, 9,* 111–123.

Przybyla, B. D., Horii, Y., & Crawford, M. H. (1992). Vocal fundamental frequency in a twin sample: Looking for a genetic effect. *Journal of Voice, 6,* 261–266.

Ptacek, P. H., Sander, E. K., Maloney, W. H., & Jackson, C. C. R. (1966). Phonatory and related changes with advanced age. *Journal of Speech and Hearing Research, 9,* 353–360.

Ramig, L. O. (1986). Acoustic analysis of phonation in patients with Huntington's disease. *Annals of Otology, Rhinology, and Laryngology, 95,* 288–293.

Ramig, L. O., & Ringel, R. L. (1983). Effects of physiological aging on selected acoustic characteristics of voice. *Journal of Speech and Hearing Research, 26,* 22–30.

Ramig, L. O., Scherer, R. C., Klasner, E. R., Titze, I. R., & Horii, Y. (1990). Acoustic analysis of voice in amyotrophic lateral sclerosis: A longitudinal study. *Journal of Speech and Hearing Disorders, 55,* 2–14.

Ramig, L., Scherer, R., Titze, I., & Ringel, R. (1988). Acoustic analysis of voices of patients with neurological disease: A rationale and preliminary data. *Annals of Otology, Rhinology and Laryngology, 97,* 164–172.

Ramig, L. A., & Shipp, T. (1987). Comparative measures of vocal tremor and vocal vibrato. *Journal of Voice, 1,* 162–167.

Randall, R. B., & Hee, J. (1981). Ceptstrum analysis. *Brüel and Kjær Technical Review, 3,* 3–40.

Rantala, L., Määttä, T., & Vilkman, E. (1997). Measuring voice under teachers' working circumstances: F_0 and perturbation features in maximally sustained phonation. *Folia Phoniatrica et Logopedica, 49,* 281–291.

Rappaport, W. (1958). Über Messungen der Tonhöhenverteilung in der deutschen Sprache. *Acustica, 8,* 220–225.

Read, C., Buder, E., & Kent, R. (1990). Speech analysis systems: A survey. *Journal of Speech and Hearing Research, 33,* 363–374.

Read, C., Buder, E., & Kent, R. (1992). Speech analysis systems: An evaluation. *Journal of Speech and Hearing Research, 35,* 314–332.

Reich, A. R., Frederickson, R. R., Mason, J. A., & Schlauch, R. S. (1990). Methodological variables affecting phonational frequency range in adults. *Journal of Speech and Hearing Disorders, 55,* 124–131.

Reich, A. R., Mason, J. A., Frederickson, R. R., & Schlauch, R. S. (1989). Factors influencing fundamental frequency range estimates in children. *Journal of Speech and Hearing Disorders, 54,* 429–438.

Ringel, R. L., & Chodzko-Zajko, W. (1987). Vocal indices of biological age. *Journal of Voice, 1,* 31–37.

Ringel, R. L., & Kluppel, D. D. (1964). Neonatal crying: A normative study. *Folia Phoniatrica, 16,* 1–9.

Robb, M. P., & Saxman, J. H. (1985). Developmental trends in vocal fundamental frequency of young children. *Journal of Speech and Hearing Research, 28,* 421–427.

Robbins, J., Fisher, H., Blom, E., & Singer, M. I. (1984). A comparative acoustic study of normal, esophageal, and tracheoesophageal speech production. *Journal of Speech and Hearing Disorders, 49,* 202–210.

Robbins, J., Fisher, H. B., & Logemann, J. A. (1982). Acoustic characteristics of voice production after Staffieri's surgical reconstructive procedure. *Journal of Speech and Hearing Disorders, 47,* 77–84.

Ross, J.-A., Noordzji, J. P., & Woo, P. (1998). Voice disorders in patients with suspected laryngo-pharyngeal reflux disease. *Journal of Voice, 12,* 84–88.

Rossiter, D., & Howard, D. (1997). Observed change in mean speaking voice fundamental frequency of two subjects undergoing voice training. *Logopedics, Phoniatrics, Vocology, 22,* 187–189.

Ruiz, R., Legros, C., & Guell, A. (1990). Voice analysis to predict the psychological or physical state of a speaker. *Aviation, Space, and Environmental Medicine, 61,* 266–271.

Rothman, H. B., & Arroyo, A. A. (1987). Acoustic variability in vibrato and its perceptual significance. *Journal of Voice, 1,* 123–141.

Sansone, F. E., Jr., & Emanuel, F. (1970). Spectral noise levels and roughness severity ratings for normal and simulated rough vowels produced by adult males. *Journal of Speech and Hearing Research, 13,* 489–502.

Sapienza, C. M. (1997). Aerodynamic and acoustic characteristics of the adult African American voice. *Journal of Voice, 11,* 410–416.

Saxman, J. H., & Burk, K. W. (1967). Speaking fundamental frequency characteristics of middle-aged females. *Folia Phoniatrica, 19,* 167–172.

Saxman, J. H., & Burk, K. W. (1968). Speaking fundamental frequency and rate characteristics of adult female schizophrenics. *Journal of Speech and Hearing Research, 11,* 194–203.

Schafer, R., & Rabiner, L. R. (1970). System for the automatic formant analysis of voiced speech. *Journal of the Acoustical Society of America, 47,* 634–648.

Scherer, R., Gould, W., Titze, I., Meyers, A., & Sataloff, R. (1988). Preliminary evaluation of selected acoustic and glottographic measures for clinical phonatory function analysis. *Journal of Voice, 2,* 230–244.

Schilling, von A., & Göler, D. V. (1961). Zur Frage der Monotonie —Untersuchung beim Stottern. *Folia Phoniatrica, 13,* 202–218.

Schoentgen, J., & Guchteneere, R. (1991). An algorithm for the measurement of jitter. *Speech Communication, 10,* 533–538.

Schultz-Coulon, H.-J., Battmer, R.-D., & Fedders, B. (1979). Zur quantitativen Bewertung der Tonhöhenschwankungen Rahmen der Stimmfunktionsprüfung. *Folia Phoniatrica, 69,* 56–69.

Schutte, H. K., & Miller, D. G. (1991). Acoustic details of vibrato cycle in tenor high voice. *Journal of Voice, 5,* 217–233.

Shadle, C. H., Barney, A. M., & Thomas, D. W. (1991). An investigation into the acoustics and aerodynamics of the larynx. In J. Gauffin & B. Hammarberg (Eds.), *Vocal fold physiology: Acoustic, perceptual, and physiological aspects of voice mechanisms* (pp. 73–82). San Diego, CA: Singular Publishing Group.

Shepard, R. N. (1964). Circularity in judgments of relative pitch. *Journal of the Acoustical Society of America, 36,* 2346–2353.

Sheppard, W. C., & Lane, H. L. (1968). Development of the prosodic features of infant vocalizing. *Journal of Speech and Hearing Research, 11,* 94–108.

Shipp, T. (1967). Frequency, duration, and perceptual measures in relation to judgments of alaryngeal speech acceptability. *Journal of Speech and Hearing Research, 10,* 417–427.

Shipp, T., Doherty, E. T., & Morrissey, P. (1979). Predicting vocal frequency from selected physiologic measures. *Journal of the Acoustical Society of America, 66,* 678–684.

Shipp, T., & Hollien, H. (1969). Perception of the aging male voice. *Journal of Speech and Hearing Research, 12,* 703–710.

Shipp, T., & McGlone, R. E. (1971). Laryngeal dynamics associated with voice frequency change. *Journal of Speech and Hearing Research, 12,* 761–768.

Silbergleit, A. K., Johnson, A. F., & Jacobson, B. H. (1997). Acoustic analysis of voice in individuals with amyotrophic lateral scleroris and perceptually normal voice quality. *Journal of Voice, 11,* 222–231.

Simon, C. (1927). The variability of consecutive wavelengths in vocal and instrumental sounds. *Psychological Monographs, 36,* 41–83.

Sorensen, D., & Horii, Y. (1983). Frequency and amplitude perturbation in the voices of female speakers. *Journal of Communication Disorders, 16,* 57–61.

Sorensen, D., & Horii, Y. (1984). Directional perturbation factors for jitter and for shimmer. *Journal of Communication Disorders, 17,* 143–151.

Smith, B. E., Weinberg, B., Feth, L., & Horii, Y. (1978). Vocal roughness and jitter characteristics of vowels produced by esophageal speakers. *Journal of Speech and Hearing Research, 21,* 240–249.

Snidecor, J. C. (1943). A comparative study of the pitch and duration characteristics of impromptu speaking and oral reading. *Speech Monographs, 10,* 50–57.

Snidecor, J. C. (1951). The pitch and duration characteristics of superior female speakers during oral reading. *Journal of Speech and Hearing Disorders, 16,* 44–52.

Snidecor, J. C., & Curry, E. T. (1959). Temporal and pitch aspects of superior esophageal speech. *Annals of Otology, Rhinology, and Laryngology, 68,* 623–629.

Sonesson, B. (1960). On the anatomy and vibratory pattern of the human vocal folds. *Acta Otolaryngologica, Suppl. 156.*

Sorenson, D., & Horii, Y. (1983) Frequency and amplitude perturbation in the voices of female speakers. *Journal of Communication Disorders, 16,* 57–61.

Sorenson, D., & Horii, Y. (1984). Directional perturbation factors for jitter and for shimmer. *Journal of Communication Disorders, 17,* 143–151.

Sorenson, D., Horii, Y., & Leonard, R. (1980). Effects of laryngeal topical anesthesia on voice fundamental frequency perturbation. *Journal of Speech and Hearing Research, 23,* 274–283.

Steincke, I., & Herzel, H. (1995). Bifurcations in an asymmetrical vocal fold model. *Journal of the Acoustical Society of America, 97,* 1874–1884.

Stemple, J. C., Stanley, J., & Lee, L. (1995). Objective measures of voice production in normal subjects following prolonged voice use. *Journal of Voice, 9,* 127–133.

Stevens, K. N., Kalikow, D. N., & Willemain, T. R. (1975). A miniature accelerometer for detecting glottal waveforms and nasalization. *Journal of Speech and Hearing Research, 18,* 594–599.

Stevens, S. S., & Volkmann, J. (1940). The relation of pitch to frequency: A revised scale. *American Journal of Psychology, 53,* 329–353.

Stevens, S. S., Volkmann, J., & Newman, E. B. (1937). A scale for the measurement of the psychological magnitude pitch. *Journal of the Acoustical Society of America, 8,* 185–190.

Stoicheff, M. L. (1981). Speaking fundamental frequency characteristics of nonsmoking female adults. *Journal of Speech and Hearing Research, 24,* 437–441.

Stone, R. E., Jr., & Sharf, D. J. (1973). Vocal change associated with the use of atypical pitch and intensity levels. *Folia Phoniatrica, 25,* 91–103.

Strand, E. A., Buder, E. H., Yorkston, K. M., & Ramig, L. O. (1994). Differential phonatory characteristics of four women with amyotrophic lateral sclerosis. *Journal of Voice, 8,* 327–339.

Sugimoto, T., & Hiki, S. (1962). On the extraction of the pitch signal using the body wall vibration at the throat of the talker. *Proceedings of the Fourth International Congress on Acoustics.*

Takahashi, H., & Koike, Y. (1975). Some perceptual dimensions and acoustical correlates of pathologic voices. *Acta Otolaryngologica, Suppl. 338,* 1–24.

Teager, H. M., & Teager, S. M. (1983). Active fluid dynamic voice production models, or There is a unicorn in the garden. In I. R. Titze & R. C. Scherer (Eds.), *Vocal fold physiology: Biomechanics, acoustics, and phonatory control* (pp. 386–401). Denver, CO: Denver Center for the Performing Arts.

Ternström, S., Sundberg, J., & Colldén, A. (1988). Articulatory F_0 perturbations and auditory feedback. *Journal of Speech and Hearing Research, 31,* 187–192.

Thompson, J. M. T., & Stewart, H. B. (1986). *Nonlinear dynamics and chaos.* New York: John Wiley.

Till, J. A., Jafari, M., Crumley, R. L., & Law-Till, C. B. (1992). Effects of initial consonant, pneumotachographic mask, and oral pressure tube on vocal perturbation, harmonics-to-noise, and intensity measurements. *Journal of Voice, 6,* 217–223.

Timcke, R., von Leden, H., & Moore, P. (1959). Laryngeal vibrations: measurements of the glottic wave. Part II: Physiologic variations. *Archives of Otolaryngology, 69,* 438–444.

Titze, I. R. (1991). A model for neurologic sources of aperiodicity in vocal fold vibration. *Journal of Speech and Hearing Research, 34,* 460–472.

Titze, I. R. (1994). *Principles of voice production.* Englewood Cliffs, NJ: Prentice-Hall.

Titze, I. R. (1995). *Workshop on acoustic voice analysis: Summary Statement.* Iowa City, IA: National Center for Voice and Speech.

Titze, I. R., Baken, R. J., & Herzel, H. (1993). Evidence of chaos in vocal fold vibration. In I. R. Titze (Ed.), *Vocal fold physiology: Frontiers in basic science* (pp. 143–182). San Diego, CA: Singular Publishing Group.

Titze, I. R., Horii, Y., & Scherer, R. C. (1987). Some technical considerations in voice perturbation measurements. *Journal of Speech and Hearing Research, 30,* 252–260.

Titze, I. R., & Liang, H. (1993). Comparison of F_0 extraction methods for high-precision voice perturbation measurements. *Journal of Speech and Hearing Research, 36,* 1120–1133.

Titze, I. R., & Winholtz, W. S. (1993). Effect of microphone type and placement on voice perturbation. *Journal of Speech and Hearing Research, 36,* 1177–1190.

Torgerson, J. K., & Martin, D. E. (1980). Acoustic and temporal analysis of esophageal speech produced by alaryngeal and laryngeal talkers. *Folia Phoniatrica, 32,* 315–322.

Travis, L. E. (1927). A phono-photographic study of the stutterer's voice and speech. *Psychological Monographs, 36,* 109–141.

Troughear, R., & Davis, P. (1979). Real-time, micro-computer based voice feature extraction in a speech pathology clinic. *Australian Journal of Human Communication Disorders, 7,* 4–21.

Tuma, J. J. (1989). *Handbook of numerical calculations in engineering.* New York: McGraw-Hill.

Vallancien, B., Bautheron, B., Pasternak, L., Guisez, D., & Paley, B. (1971). Comparaison des signaux microphoniques, diaphanographiques, et glottographiques avec application au laryngographe. *Folia Phoniatrica, 23,* 371–380.

Van den Berg, J., & Moolenaar-Bijl, A. J. (1959). Cricopharyngeal sphincter, pitch, intensity, and fluency in oesophageal speech. *Practica Oto-Rhino-Laryngologica, 21,* 298–315.

Verdonck-de Leeuw, I. M. (1998). Voice characteristics following radiotherapy: *The development of a protocol* (chap. 5). Unpublished doctoral dissertation, University of Amsterdam, the Netherlands.

Verdolini-Marston, K., Sandage, M., & Titze, I. R. (1994). Effect of hydration treatments on laryngeal nodules and polyps and related voice measures. *Journal of Voice, 8,* 30–47.

Verstraete, J., Forrez, G., Mertens, P., & Debruyne, F. (1993). The effect of sustained phonation at high and low pitch on vocal jitter and shimmer. *Folia Phoniatrica, 45,* 223–228.

Vieira, M. N., McInnes, F. R., & Jack, M. A. (1996). Analysis of the effects of electroglottographic baseline fluctuation on the F_0 estimation in pathological voices. *Journal of the Acoustical Society of America, 99,* 3171–3178.

Vieira, M. N., McInnes, F. R., & Jack, M. A. (1997). Comparative assessment of electroglottographic and acoustic measures of jitter in pathological voices. *Journal of Speech and Hearing Research, 40,* 170–182.

Vilkman, E., Sihvo, M., Alku, P., Laukkanen, A.-M., & Pekkarinen, E. (1993). Objective analysis of speech profile phonations of normal female subjects in a vocally-loading task. In T. Hacki (Ed.), *Aktuelle phoniatrisch-pädaudiologische Aspekte* (pp. 174–181). Berlin, Germany: Gross.

von Leden, H., Moore, P., & Timcke, R. (1960). Laryngeal vibrations: measurements of the glottic wave. Part III: The pathologic larynx. *Archives of Otolaryngology, 71,* 16–35.

Vuorenkoski, L., Perheentupa, J., Vuorenkoski, V., Lenko, H. L., & Tjernlund, P. (1978). Fundamental voice frequency during normal and abnormal growth and after androgen treatment. *Archives of Disease in Childhood, 53,* 201–209.

Wakita, H. (1976). Instrumentation for the study of speech acoustics. In N. J. Lass (Ed.), *Contemporary issues in experimental phonetics* (pp. 3–40). New York: Academic Press.

Wakita, H. (1977). Speech analysis and synthesis. In D. Broad (Ed.), *Topics in speech science* (pp. 69–157). Los Angeles, CA: Speech Research Laboratory.

Walton, J. H., & Orlikoff, R. F. (1994). Speaker race identification from acoustic cues in the vocal signal. *Journal of Speech and Hearing Research, 37,* 738–745.

Wasz-Höckert, O., Lind, J., Vuorenkoski, V., Partanen, T., & Valanne, E. (1968). *The infant cry: A spectrographic and auditory analysis.* London, UK: Heinemann.

Wasz-Höckert, O., Partanen, T., Vuorenkoski, V., Valanne, E., & Michelsson, K. (1964a). Effect of training on the ability to identify specific meanings in newborn and infant vocalizations. *Developmental Medicine and Child Neurology, 6,* 393–396.

Wasz-Höckert, O., Partanen, T., Vuorenkoski, V., Valanne, E., & Michelsson, K. (1964b). The identification of some specific meanings in newborn and infant vocalisation. *Experientia, 20,* 154.

Weatherley, C. C., Worrall, L. E., & Hickson, L. M. H. (1997). The effect of hearing impairment on the vocal characteristics of older people. *Folia Phoniatrica et Logopaedica, 49,* 53–62.

Weaver, A. T. (1924). Experimental studies in vocal expression. *Journal of Applied Psychology, 8,* 23–56.

Weinberg, B. and Bennett, S. (1971). A comparison of the fundamental frequency characteristics of esophageal speech measured on a wave-by-wave and averaging basis. *Journal of Speech and Hearing Research, 14,* 351–355.

Weinberg, B., & Bennett, S. (1972). Selected acoustic characteristics of esophageal speech produced by female laryngectomees. *Journal of Speech and Hearing Research, 15,* 211–216.

Weinberg, B., Dexter, R., & Horii, Y. (1975). Selected speech and fundamental frequency characteristics of patients with acromegaly. *Journal of Speech and Hearing Disorders, 40,* 253–259.

Weinberg, B., & Zlatin, M. (1970). Speaking fundamental frequency characteristics of five- and six-year old children with mongolism. *Journal of Speech and Hearing Research, 13,* 418–425.

Wendahl, R. W. (1966a). Some parameters of auditory roughness. *Folia Phoniatrica, 18,* 26–32.

Wendahl, R. W. (1966b). Laryngeal analog synthesis of jitter and shimmer auditory parameters of harshness. *Folia Phoniatrica, 18,* 98–108.

Wendahl, R. W., Moore, P., & Hollien, H. (1963). Comments on vocal fry. *Folia Phoniatrica, 15,* 251–255.

West, R. W., & Ansberry, M. (1968). *The rehabilitation of speech* (4th ed.). New York: Harper and Row.

Wheat, M. C., & Hudson, A. I. (1988). Spontaneous speaking fundamental frequency of 6–year-old Black children. *Journal of Speech and Hearing Research, 31,* 723–725.

Wilcox, K., & Horii, K. (1980). Age and changes in vocal jitter. *Journal of Gerontology, 35,* 194–198.

Williams, C. E., & Stevens, K. N. (1972). Emotions and speech: Some acoustical correlates. *Journal of the Acoustical Society of America, 52,* 1238–1250.

Williams, C. E., & Stevens, K. N. (1981). Vocal correlates of emotional states. In J. K. Darby, Jr. (Ed.), *Speech evaluation in psychiatry.* New York: Grune and Stratton.

Wolfe, V., Cornell, R., & Palmer, C. (1991). Acoustic correlates of pathologic voice types. *Journal of Speech and Hearing Research, 34,* 509–516.

Wolfe, V., Fitch, J., & Cornell, R. (1995). Acoustic prediction of severity in commonly occurring voice problems. *Journal of Speech and Hearing Research, 38,* 273–279.

Wolfe, V., & Martin, D. (1997). Acoustic correlates of dysphonia: Type and severity. *Journal of Communication Disorders, 30,* 403–416.

Wolfe, V. I., Ratusnik, D. L., Smith, F. H., & Northrop, G. (1990). Intonation and fundamental frequency in male-to-female transsexuals. *Journal of Speech and Hearing Disorders, 55,* 43–50.

Wong, D., Ito, M. R., Cox, N. B., & Titze, I. R. (1991). Observation of perturbation in a lumped-element model of the vocal folds with application to some pathological cases. *Journal of the Acoustical Society of America, 89,* 383–394.

Xue, A., & Mueller, P. B. (1997). Acoustic and perceptual characteristics of the voices of sedentary and physically active elderly speakers. *Logopedics Phoniatrics Vocology, 22,* 51–60.

Zyski, B. J., Bull, G. L., McDonald, W. E., & Johns, M. E. (1984). Perturbation analysis of normal and pathologic larynges. *Folia Phoniatrica, 36,* 190–198

7

Sound Spectrography

Speech, said Stetson (1928), is "movement made audible." The sounds of speech are the product of actions of the complex acoustic system called the vocal tract. Any change in the acoustic characteristics of the speech signal must, of necessity, represent movement of the organs of speech production.

If the physiology and acoustics of speech production were completely understood, it might be possible to evaluate a speech signal and to determine from its waveform exactly what the speaker's vocal tract was doing.[1] Our understanding remains far from perfect, and so it is frequently impossible to draw unequivocal conclusions about specific motor events on the basis of acoustic analysis alone. Furthermore, in most cases there is unlikely to be a strict one-to-one correspondence between individual motor acts and specific acoustic events. The entire speech system is characterized by many degrees of freedom, and so a given acoustic result might be produced by different combinations of vocal tract actions.

Still, acoustic analysis provides an extraordinarily potent tool for assessing speech system functioning, especially when combined with observation of appropriate physiological parameters, such as air pressure or flow. Doing so increases certainty about vocal tract behavior in a given situation. One of the most powerful acoustic analytic techniques, and one for which the requisite instrumentation is widely available, is **sound spectrography**—the dissection of an acoustic wave into its most basic components.

The amount of information displayed in a spectrogram—even one of a simple utterance—can be enormous. A lot of research involving spectrography has tried to clarify which features are clinically most meaningful and which may be ignored in drawing conclusions about speech production or perception. Every aspect of speech motor behavior contributes to the final acoustic product and, therefore, the spectrogram is likely to tell the clinician more than he wants to know about any given utterance. In consequence, the spectral features that are to be "read" and evaluated must be chosen according to the speech behaviors being examined, the nature of the dysfunction being characterized, and the objectives of clinical intervention.

The interpretation of sound spectrograms rests on a thorough knowledge of the acoustics and physiology of speech, on familiarity with the way in which spectrograms are generated, on experience, and on a practiced eye. The richness of the technique has been explored in a vast and ever-expanding body of literature. Many excellent volumes have been written about its methodology and about the relationship of spectral features to various aspects of speech physiology, auditory perception, or basic acoustic processes. Hundreds and hundreds of research articles deal with spectrographic observations of just about every aspect of human sound production and linguistic organization. It is not possible, by any stretch of the imagination, to summarize even a fraction of this information here. Accordingly, the intent of this chapter is to introduce the newcomer to the principles underlying sound spectrography, to the methods by which it is accomplished, and to some salient quantified results of spectrographic analysis.

Most sound spectrographic systems require that the user specify certain analysis parameters and choose among several options that determine how a sample is to be analyzed. The parameters specified and the options selected can change the appearance of the resulting spectrogram a great deal, highlighting or obscuring various features. The choices made by the user thereby constrain the ways in which the results are interpreted. Because of this, and because the user's decisions must be based on knowledge of how spectrography works, some of the functional details of the process will be considered in this chapter.

BASIC PRINCIPLES

Sound spectrography is a mathematical process, a fact that may intimidate the novice and, all too often, confound even the adventurous. While it is inescapably true that mastering the mathematics is essential for some purposes, it is fortunately possible to make valid use of spectrography based on an understanding of principles, leaving the computational details aside. The purpose of this section is to elucidate those principles in a discursive manner. To be sure, some rigor will be

---

[1]Over the years significant research effort has been devoted to the creation of ways of plotting the shape of the vocal tract from an acoustic analysis of the speech signal (Dunn, 1950; Stevens, Kasowski, & Fant, 1953; Stevens & House, 1955, 1961; Fant, 1962, 1980; Mermelstein, 1967; Schroeder, 1967; Paige & Zue, 1970a, b; Lindblom & Sundberg, 1971; Sondhi & Gopinath, 1971; Nakajima, 1977; Strube, 1977; Atal, Matthews, & Tukey, 1978; Ladefoged, Harshman, Goldstein, & Rice, 1978; Charpentier, 1984; Boë, Perrier & Bailly, 1992). Although the digital computer has moved us much closer to that goal, a truly practical, valid, and reliable means has yet to be perfected.

lost, but, it is hoped, better comprehension of crucial concepts will be gained. Understanding sound spectrography does, however, demand a firm grounding in physical and psychological acoustics, at least at the elementary level. The physics of sound and the psychology of perception are both part of the required academic preparation of speech pathologists, and it is assumed that the reader has mastered the relevant basic concepts in these areas. They will not be reviewed in detail here, but several good summaries are available.[2]

Fourier Analysis: Periodic Signals

The basis of sound spectrography is the Fourier theorem.[3] Put into simple everyday terms (with only a little loss of precision) it states that any periodic wave can be expressed as the sum of an infinite series of sine (and cosine) waves of different amplitudes, whose frequencies are in integer ratio to each other, and which have different phase angles with respect to each other. The waves that are so summed are referred to as a *Fourier series*. The prime condition that must be met for the Fourier theorem to be valid is that the waveform **must be periodic**.[4] That is, it must repeat exactly in time for a Fourier series to exist for it.

Stated formally, a Fourier series is defined as

$$x(t) = a_0 + \sum_{n=1}^{\infty} (a_0 \cos n_0 \omega t + b_n \sin n\omega_0 t),$$

where $\omega_0 = 2\pi f_0$, which is a means of expressing the frequency of the wave in terms of the number of complete cycles per second.[5] However intimidating the mathematical expression may appear, it says nothing more than what was stated discursively earlier. The meaning and implications of this theorem are best examined by means of some examples.

ADDING SINE WAVES

The Fourier series states that a complex periodic wave is composed of a series of sine waves. Figure 7–1 shows how this can be so. The frequencies and amplitudes of the sinusoids are:

Frequency (Hz)	Amplitude (arbitrary units)
100	1
200	0.5
300	0.333
400	0.25
500	0.20

If the magnitudes of these waves at a given point in time are added together we derive the summed magnitude at that instant. If that sum is redone at every point in time, and the results plotted along the time axis, the bottom waveform of Figure 7–1 results. It clearly has the same fundamental frequency (or repetition rate) as the top sinusoid in the figure (that is, its frequency is 100 Hz), but it has a much different shape. Five sinusoids have been added to create a complex wave. We have performed a *Fourier synthesis* of a waveshape.

This synthesis is, in fact, summarized by the preceding small table that specified the frequencies and amplitudes of the component waves. In fact, this *Fourier series* can be put into graphic form, as in Figure 7–2. It is called the amplitude *spectrum* of the wave that is shown as the sum in the figure. It is the result of a *Fourier analysis* of that waveform (Kersta, 1948; Stuart, 1966; Ramirez, 1985).

The amplitude spectrum can be considered a "recipe" for the construction of the sum waveform of Figure 7–1. It says: "Take a sine wave with a peak

---

[2]See, for instance, Lieberman (1977), Fry (1979), Shoup, Lass, and Kuehn (1982), Fujimura and Erickson (1997), Speaks (1999), and Pickett (1999).

[3]Developed by Jean Baptiste Joseph Fourier (1768–1830), a French mathematical physicist, and published in 1822, to describe the flow of heat through a solid mass.

[4]There are other conditions, of less importance to the speech clinician. In principle, the periodicity must have existed for all time in the past and it must continue to exist for all time in the future. (That is, the waveform must extend from time $= -\infty$ to time $= +\infty$.) Clearly there exists no such waveform, but we are permitted to bend the rules a bit and state that the periodicity must extend over the period of observation. Further, as a matter of technical fact, the waveform must not have an infinite number of discontinuities in any period; it must have a finite number of maxima and minima in any period, and it must be integrable in any period. None of these restrictions is likely to trouble clinical users.

[5]In elementary courses one is usually taught that a complete cycle goes through 360°. But, for reasons which are mathematically cogent but need not be explored here, it is frequently more convenient to express "rotation" not in degrees, but in *radians*. A radian is an angle that intercepts a length of the circle's circumference equal to the circle's radius, r. Since the circumference of the circle, c, has a length of $2\pi r$, an angle of 1 radian must intercept an arc of length $c/2\pi$, and the total angular displacement of a rotation that goes through a complete cycle (that is, describes a circle) must be 2π radians. Therefore, 360° $= 2\pi$ radians.

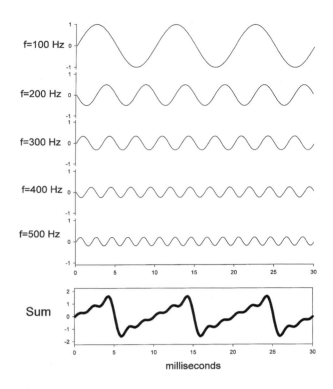

Figure 7–1. Addition of sine waves of different frequencies to produce a complex wave by Fourier synthesis.

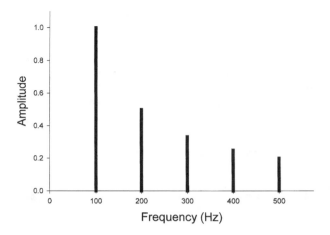

Figure 7–2. Amplitude spectrum of the complex wave generated in Figure 7–1.

amplitude of 1.00 and a frequency of 100 Hz, a sine wave of 200 Hz whose peak amplitude is 0.50, a sine wave of 300 Hz with a peak amplitude of 0.33, and so on. Add the magnitudes of these waves at every point in time and plot the results of all the additions to form this particular complex waveform."

TIME AND FREQUENCY DOMAINS

A moment's reflection reveals that the waveform and its spectrum contain exactly the same information, but represented differently. This must be so, since the spectrum can be followed as an exact guide to the construction of the waveform, and the waveform can be broken down into components that are represented as the spectrum. From the point of view of the information contained, we could therefore generate a sort of graphic equation:

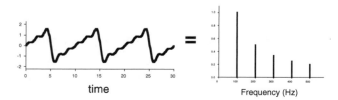

We say that the graph on the left, which is plotted as amplitude over time, is a representation of the complex waveform in the *time domain*. The representation on the right, where amplitude is plotted as a function of frequency, represents the wave in the *frequency domain*. The two representations are exactly equivalent: they contain the same information. The *Fourier transform* is a means of converting from the time to the frequency domains. (Going back again, from frequency domain to time domain, is achieved by the *inverse Fourier transform*.)

Actually, a careful inspection of Figure 7–1 shows a feature that we have thus far overlooked. The several sinusoids that make up the summed wave are not all "in synch." That is, while the 100, 300, and 500 Hz waves "begin" at the left axis with their amplitudes increasing from 0, the 200 and 400 Hz waves start out in just the opposite direction. The 200 and 400 Hz waves have a phase angle of 180° with respect to the 100 Hz wave, while the 300 and 500 Hz waves have a phase angle of 0° re: the 100 Hz wave. The fact is that the phase angle of each of the component sinusoids makes a difference in the shape of the summed waveform. In Figure 7–3 the frequencies and amplitudes of the component sinusoids are the same, but their phase relationship to the 100 Hz wave is different. The 200 Hz wave leads by 90°, 300 Hz lags by 90°, 400 Hz leads by 45°, and 500 Hz leads (or lags!) by 180°. The summation of these waves leads to a waveshape which is quite different from that of Figure 7–1, although the sinusoids are the same.

The phase relationships of Figure 7–3 can be summarized by plotting the phase angle as a function of frequency, as in Figure 7–4. This representation is

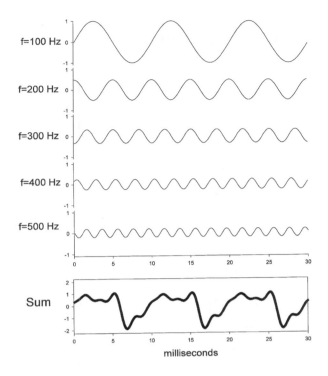

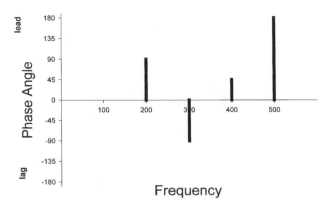

Figure 7–4. The *phase spectrum* shows the phase relationships of the component frequencies of Figure 7–3.

Figure 7–3. Adding the same frequency components as in Figure 7–1, but with different phase relationships, produces a different waveshape.

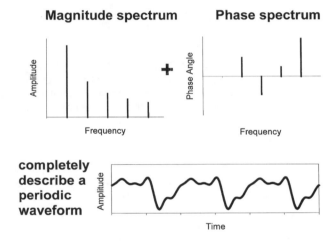

Figure 7–5. The magnitude and phase spectra together completely describe a periodic wave.

known as the **phase spectrum** of the signal. As emphasized in Figure 7–5, the amplitude spectrum together with the phase spectrum constitute a complete description of the waveform.

THE SPECTRUM OF A PERIODIC SIGNAL

We can now summarize a number of characteristics of the spectrum (the frequency-domain representation of the Fourier series) of a periodic waveform:

1. If a signal is periodic, it can be decomposed into a Fourier series: A set of sinusoids of differing frequencies, amplitudes, and phase relationships. The components of the series can be determined by application of the Fourier transform. Conversely, any periodic signal can be synthesized from a set of sinusoids by use of the inverse Fourier transform.

2. **The amplitude spectrum of a periodic waveform is its representation in the frequency domain**. It consists of a set of discrete lines arranged along a frequency axis. The lines represent the frequencies of the component sinusoids and their respective

amplitudes. There are no components between these lines. **The amplitude spectrum of a periodic wave is therefore known as a** *line spectrum.*

3. **The sinusoidal components of a periodic signal**, each of which is represented as a line in its amplitude spectrum, **are referred to as** *harmonics.*

4. **The spacing on the frequency axis between the harmonics is equal to the fundamental frequency**. (The amplitude of a harmonic may, however, be zero. In this case, the spacing between harmonics will be equal to an integer multiple of the fundamental frequency.)

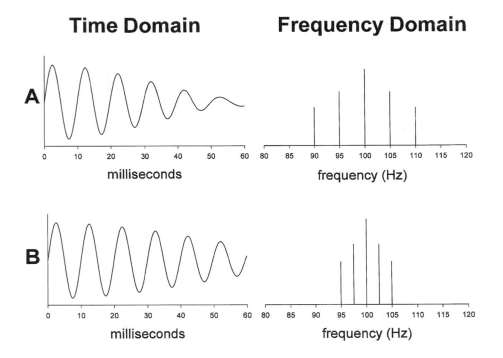

Figure 7–6. Examples of two damped sinusoids, represented in the time and frequency domains. Note that the frequency components of the signals are not integer multiples of the 100 Hz fundamental frequency. Signal A has greater damping than signal B, and its component frequencies are more widely spaced.

5. A complete description of a waveform also requires a description of the phase relationship of the harmonics. This is represented by the phase spectrum. Because phase information is of little importance or interest in speech analysis, it is rarely calculated and, for everyday clinical purposes, may be ignored.

6. Particularly with respect to speech analysis, it is useful to think of a complex waveform not as a single signal, but rather as an ordered bundle of different frequencies having greater or lesser amplitudes.

Fourier Analysis: Damped Signals

Damping refers to loss of energy over time. The laws of thermodynamics tell us that all oscillating systems are damped. That is, they will lose energy and the amplitude of their oscillations will diminish. A child on a playground swing offers a familiar example. Once started, the swing's arcs grow smaller and smaller. Energy is steadily lost to air resistance and to the frictional elements in the swing's setup. To maintain a constant arc something must be done to replace the energy that is constantly being bled away.

The acoustic oscillations in the vocal tract are also subject to damping because sound energy is absorbed by the tissues of the vocal tract or is radiated away to the surrounding environment. In some cases, such as pulse-register phonation (Coleman, 1963; Wendahl, Moore, & Hollien, 1963; Cavallo, Baken, & Shaiman, 1984), the damping is responsible for a distinctive vocal feature.

Figure 7–6 shows two damped sinusoids in both the time and frequency domains. Signal A dies away relatively rapidly: it has moderately strong damping. Signal B, on the other hand, loses energy more slowly, and thus has weaker damping. The frequency domain representations of both are line spectra: the signals are made up of discrete frequency components. But, in contrast to the case of periodic signals, the frequency components are not integer multiples of the fundamental frequency (which in the present case is 100 Hz). They are not, therefore, harmonics. Further, it is clear that A, the more strongly damped signal, has frequency components (90, 95, 100, 105, and 110 Hz) that are more widely spaced than the frequency components (95, 97.5, 100, 102.5, and 105 Hz) of the less-damped signal B. This illustrates a basic rule: increased damping (more rapid decrease of signal amplitude) is associated with wider spacing of the lines in the amplitude spectrum.[6]

Because systems with little damping lose energy slowly, they tend to respond for a long time after an initial excitation. A good example is a church bell, which is designed to have exceptionally low damping. Once excited by the blow of the clapper it oscillates for a very long time. On the other hand, a table top is an example of a system with very strong damping. After being rapped by one's knuckles it does not oscillate for an appreciable period of time. The sound emitted by the two structures—bell and table top—suggests another important difference between lightly damped and strongly damped systems, a difference which is also indicated in the line spectra of Figure 7–6. The sound of the bell has a very distinct pitch. In other words, the bell is frequency selective or sharply tuned. Its spectrum covers a narrow range of frequencies. The table top, however, produces a dull thud that lacks definite pitch when it is struck. Its spectrum is much broader (it includes a much wider range of frequencies) and so the table top is not tuned.

In summary:

- The oscillation of a strongly damped system is characterized by rapid loss of oscillatory amplitude; widely spaced components in the frequency domain; a wide-band spectrum.
- The oscillation of a weakly damped system, on the other hand, is characterized by slow loss of oscillatory amplitude; closely spaced components in the frequency domain; a narrow-band spectrum; relatively sharp tuning to a specific frequency.

Figure 7–6 illustrates one more interesting phenomenon. Wave A will clearly die away to zero amplitude long before wave B does. That is, it has a short duration. On the other hand, its spectrum is much wider than that of wave B. There is a reciprocity of time and frequency: greater extent in the time domain results in less extent in the frequency domain, and vice versa. This reciprocal relationship of time and frequency is universal—it is not merely a characteristic of damping. And it will be important in the interpretation of sound spectrograms.

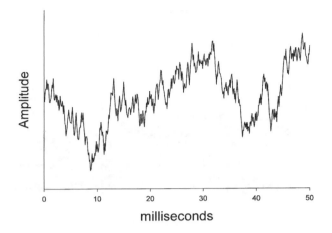

Figure 7–7. An aperiodic signal.

Fourier Analysis: Aperiodic Signals

Natural signals, and, in particular, speech signals, are not by any means exclusively periodic. Aperiodic waveforms can also be decomposed into component sinusoids, but the situation is considerably more complex.

Consider the aperiodic signal plotted in the time domain in Figure 7–7. As depicted, it has no discernible periodic structure. But suppose that the plot depicts only a portion—50 milliseconds in duration—of a very much longer waveform. It is possible that, if we could see more of it, we would find that this signal is, in fact, repetitive. That is, it might be periodic, but with a period very much longer than our viewing window. Now, in principle, an aperiodic signal does not repeat. But it might be considered to be part of a periodic wave whose period, T, is *infinite*.

With this perspective, if we recall that the spacing between the harmonic lines in the spectrum of a periodic wave is equal to the fundamental frequency, we can conceptually derive the form of the spectrum of an aperiodic wave. Give that the frequency is the reciprocal of the period, $f = 1/T$, then the "frequency" of the aperiodic signal must be $f = 1/\infty$. That is, the frequency is infinitesimally small. Now, if the space between the harmonic lines in the amplitude spectrum

---

[6]As the amplitude decrease becomes more and more gradual, the spectral lines get closer. Conceptually it is easy to see that, when the decrease becomes zero—and thus there is no damping—the spectral lines will have become so closely spaced that they will merge into the line of the fundamental frequency. In other words, the signal will have become periodic.

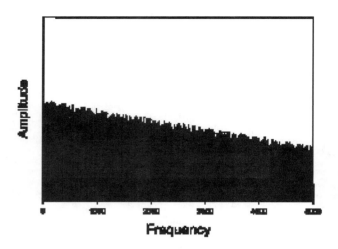

Figure 7–8. In a *continuous spectrum*, such as this, the space between the harmonic lines is zero. Therefore, the spectrum is filled with lines.

is equal to the frequency, then the space that separates the lines of the spectrum of the aperiodic wave must be equal to 1/ ∞, which is equal to 0. That is, there is *no space* between the harmonic lines: they are jammed up against each other, completely filling in the space along the frequency axis. The amplitude of the aperiodic wave might therefore look like Figure 7–8. (In principle, the spectrum extends to infinite frequency. Only the 0–5000 Hz portion is shown in the figure.) Because the spectrum fills the space along the frequency axis, it is called a *continuous spectrum*.

The infinitesimal spacing of the component frequencies of an aperiodic wave means that it cannot be expanded by the Fourier transform into a Fourier series. Rather, analysis of aperiodic signals requires the methods of the calculus. In particular, their frequency domain representations are accomplished by the *Fourier integral*.[7] Specifically, the frequency function, X(f) is derived from the time-domain values by

$$X(f) = \int_{-\infty}^{\infty} x(t)e^{-j\pi 2ft}\, dt,$$

where x(t) represents the time-domain function.[8] This calculation, of course, does not produce an infinite number of lines, so the plot of the function consists solely of the "tops" of the vertical frequency lines that were conceptualized above: the space below is not filled in. The continuous spectrum of Figure 7–8 would therefore look like Figure 7–9.

Fourier Analysis: The Real World

Acoustic signals in the real world are different in some important ways from the synthetic signals that are created by formula. A time-domain example (a few cycles of a sustained /ɑ/) is provided at the top of Figure 7–10. Below it is its digitally-created amplitude spectrum. One would expect that this waveform—which certainly appears periodic—would have a line spectrum, and yet clearly that expectation is not fulfilled. The problem is that, strictly speaking, "periodic" means repeated *exactly, precisely, and with no variation*, in time. No natural speech generator can achieve this. There is always added aperiodic background noise, there is noise added by the process of digitizing (see Chapter 3, "Digital Systems"), and, most of all, there is

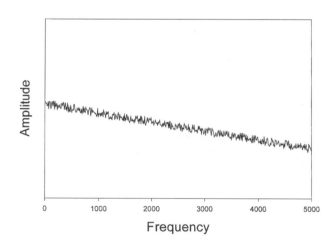

Figure 7–9. A truer rendering of the continuous spectrum of Figure 7–8. Only the "tops" of the "harmonic lines" are plotted.

---

[7]Essentially the same limitations as applied to the analysis of periodic signals pertain: there must be a finite number of maxima and minima, the number of discontinuities must be finite, and the function must be integrable. These considerations are not a problem in speech analysis.

[8]Transforming the frequency-domain function to the time domain is done with the inverse transform:

$$x(t) = \int_{-\infty}^{\infty} X(f)e^{j2\pi ft}\, df$$

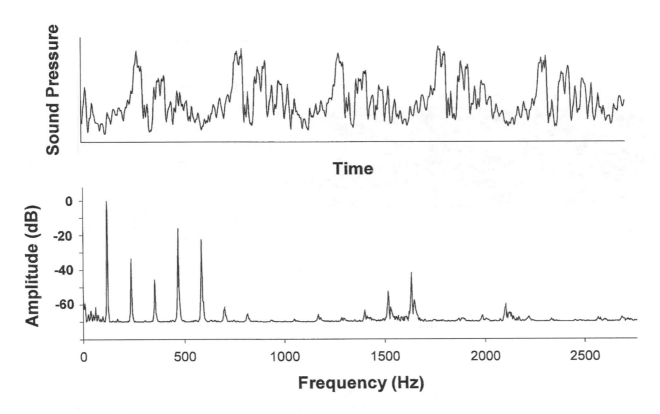

Figure 7–10. Top: Time-domain representation of sustained /ɑ/. Bottom: Computed amplitude spectrum of the sound

the irregularity of fundamental frequency known as jitter and the tiny instabilities of vocal tract posture that result in microvariations in vowel "quality." So the /ɑ/ waveform varies slightly from cycle to cycle. Which is to say that it is not periodic. But one would hardly label it aperiodic, either. Although, somewhat colloquially it would be called *quasiperiodic*,[9] we might better call it, as Titze (1995) suggests, *nearly periodic*. It contains both periodic and aperiodic elements.

The amplitude spectrum shows this in the frequency domain. While there are not discrete lines (which would characterize the spectrum of a periodic waveform) there are clearly distinct peaks in a continuous spectrum (which is characteristic of an aperiodic waveform). Each peak can be considered to be a "smeared" line. (Its smearing represents the variability of successive periods in the signal.) Also, the random-noise components add a little energy at every frequency, and thus tend to fill in the spaces between the "lines" of the amplitude spectrum. The peaks do have different heights, reflecting the fact that the

"smeared lines" of the spectrum have different amplitudes, just as they would in a line spectrum. Note also that the amplitude of the peaks does not vary randomly as a function of frequency: there are regions of strong harmonics, and regions of weak harmonics. The strong harmonics are in the neighborhood of resonant frequencies of the vocal tract, which are called *formants*. This subject will be considered in more detail later.

GENERATING THE SPEECH SPECTROGRAM: ANALOG AND DIGITAL APPROACHES

The Fourier transform is valid for analog signals, that is, signals that are continuous in time (see Chapter 2). The only practical way to accomplish analog processing is with (analog) electronic circuits. While today almost completely superseded by digital methods, essentially all of the research of the initial period of

---

[9]The term *quasiperiodic* has, in fact, the rather precise meaning of the superposition of two incommensurate frequencies.

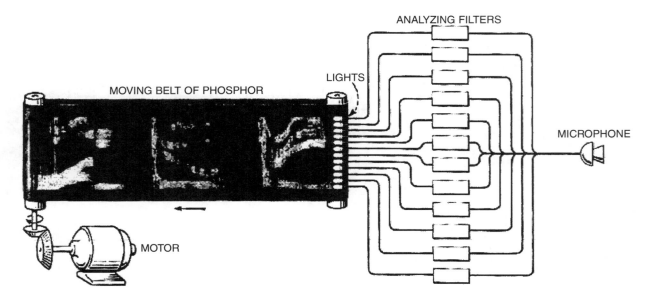

Figure 7–11. The *Visible Speech Translator* of Dudley and Gruenz, 1946. From *Visible Speech*, by R. K. Potter, G. A. Kopp, and H. Green, 1947, New York: Van Nostrand. Figure 1, p. 17. Reprinted by permission.

spectrographic investigation was accomplished by analog instruments, which handled the analog signals of the day.

Analog Methods

A conceptually simple analog method of visualizing the ever-changing spectrum of a speech signal was exemplified by the ***visible speech translator*** of Dudley and Gruenz (1946) as depicted in Figure 7–11. The speech input from a microphone was fed to a bank of bandpass filters (see Chapter 2, "Analog Electronics"). When there is a harmonic whose frequency falls within the band of one of the filters it is passed to that filter's output with an amplitude proportional to its strength. This output was used to light a miniature lamp associated with the responding filter. The lamp shone on a moving belt of phosphorescent material, which glowed with a brightness related to the brightness of the bulb. As the belt moved it displayed the recent history of the brightness of each of the lamps. The result was a three-dimensional record that showed the changes in frequency components and their amplitude (shown as brightness variations) over time. The phosphorescent screen thus displayed a sound spectrogram of the type that is still prevalent. This primitive system was improved upon by substitution of a cathode ray tube (oscilloscope) for the phosphorescent screen (Riesz & Schott, 1946) and by improvement of frequency resolution through the addition of special circuitry (Wood & Hewitt, 1963). Despite these improvements, this particular analog approach to Fourier analysis has very serious limitations.

A different approach was taken by the developers of the sound spectrograph (Koenig, Dunn, & Lacy, 1946). Marketed as the "Sonagraph" by the company now known as Kay Elemetrics, Inc. (Lincoln Park, NJ), it quickly became, and remained for several decades, the preferred tool for Fourier analysis of speech signals.[10]

THE SONAGRAPH®

Illustrated in Figure 7–12A, the Kay Sonagraph® was an electromechanical system in which a the signal to be evaluated was first recorded on the magnetized edge of a large revolving platter, which could store about 2.2 seconds of material. Mechanically coupled to the recording platter was a cylinder that was wrapped with a specially-coated paper that could be etched by an electric current. Because the recording platter and the cylinder were linked, each point in the recording (location on the edge of the platter) was associated with a

---

[10]Another instrument, which worked on very similar principles, was produced by Voice Identification using a recording system designed by Prestigiacomo (1957). It also enjoyed considerable popularity.

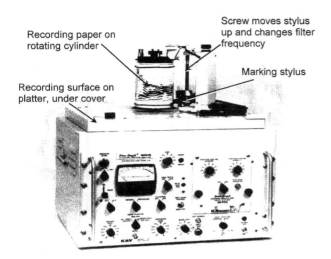
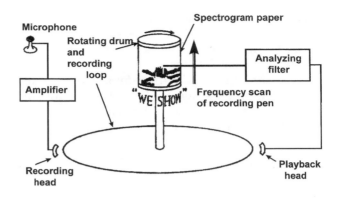

Figure 7–12. A. The Kay Elemetrics Sonagraph®, an analog spectrograph. Courtesy of Kay Elemetrics Corp., Lincoln Park, NJ. **B.** the general schema of its recording, playback and writing system from *The Sounds of Speech Communication: A Primer of Acoustic Phonetics and Speech Perception*, by J. M. Pickett, 1980, Baltimore, MD: University Park Press. Figure 15, p. 36. Reprinted by permission.

point on the circumference of the cylinder. To analyze the recording a playback head transduced the magnetic recording back into an electrical current, which was passed through a filter. If a frequency component of the signal fell within the filter's pass band it would appear at the filter output. This was amplified and was fed to a stylus in contact with the paper. The greater the amplitude of the frequency component that passed through the filter, the larger the stylus current would be, and the darker the mark made on the paper. In the course of one revolution of the platter the entire duration of the recorded signal would have been scanned for a narrow range of frequencies and—the cylinder rotating with the recording platter—marks would have been made on the paper around the cylinder wherever those frequencies were found. At the end of one rotation, therefore, the paper (when later unwound from the cylinder) would bear a permanent record of when (in terms of location along the paper) those frequencies were present as components of the signal.

Revolution of the platter not only turned the cylinder, it also turned a screw that was attached to a variable resistor in the filter circuit. The turning of the screw caused the filter's "center frequency" (the frequency in the middle of the pass band) to increase. Thus, with every revolution of the platter, and hence with every repetition of the signal, the filter frequency increased a bit. Furthermore, the marking stylus rode on the adjustment screw, so that the vertical position of the stylus was directly related to the frequency being detected. After many repetitions (done at much greater than the original recording speed) all frequencies

between (usually) 50 and 8000 Hz had been scanned and marks had been made on the paper at positions that indicated the temporal location (distance from left end of the paper) of any given component and the frequency (distance from bottom edge of the paper) of the component. Since the strength of the signal coming out of the filter controlled the magnitude of the stylus current, the marks on the page varied in darkness according to the magnitude of the frequency component being passed by the filter. In this way a three-dimensional (time, frequency, amplitude) *spectrogram* was built up.

The controls on the face of the Sonagraph® not only governed the way in which the signal to be analyzed was recorded, they also determined important parameters of the analysis process, including the frequency range of the analysis and the frequency resolution of the bandpass filter. Certain enhancement features—such as pre-emphasis—were also selectable. The user thus had to make quite a few adjustments and decisions. But exactly the same adjustments and decisions need to be made by users of today's digital systems.

Digital Methods

THE DISCRETE FOURIER TRANSFORM

Digital Fourier analysis is performed on discrete data-points, equally spaced in time, that are samples of the waveshape to be evaluated. Real-world signals are analog and therefore must first be sampled and digitized. The resulting analysis can be no better than the analog-to-digital conversion used to obtain them (see Chapter 3, "Digital Systems").

The **discrete Fourier transform** (DFT) is the process that converts digitized (discrete) data from the time domain to the frequency domain. It is the sampled-data equivalent of the Fourier integral:

$$X_d(k\Delta f) = \Delta t \sum_{n=0}^{N-1} x(N\Delta t)e^{-j2\pi\Delta f\Delta t}$$

where N = number of samples entering the analysis
Δt = the time between samples, or *sampling interval*[11]
Δf = the sample interval in the frequency domain, so that $\Delta f = 1/N\Delta t$
n = the sample number, which ranges from $n = 0, 1, 2, \ldots N-1$
k = the number of each of the computed frequency components
$x(n\Delta t)$ = the set of samples that describes the waveform being transformed
$X(k\Delta f)$ = the set of Fourier coefficients obtained by the analysis
e = the base of the natural logarithms
j = the imaginary number, $\sqrt{-1}$

Similarly, the **inverse discrete Fourier transform**, which converts from the frequency domain to the sampled time domain, is

$$X(n\Delta t) = \Delta f \sum_{k=0}^{N-1} X_d(k\Delta f)e^{j2\pi k\Delta f\Delta t}.$$

In the days before digital computers the DFT was an interesting, but little used, tool. The burden of computation by hand was simply too great.[12] It is, however, primarily a question of repeating a given set of operations over and over again. This makes it wonderfully suited to, and relatively easy to program for, a digital computer. There is, however, a problem: the DFT requires a very large number of computations. In fact, the required number of major computing operations is proportional to the square of the number of samples. This is not so bad if a signal is represented by, let us say, 30 or so sample points: only $30^2 = 900$ operations are needed. Today's computers can handle this very quickly. But suppose a sustained vowel were sampled

and digitized at the rate of 20,000 samples per second (which is a reasonable and common sampling rate). If the speaker's fundamental frequency is 100 Hz, then just a few vocal periods would be represented by perhaps 500 or so samples. The number of computer operations required for a Fourier transform of this interval is on the order of $500^2 = 250,000$ operations. This would take a computer a significant amount of time—not so long that Fourier analysis of reasonably long signals would be impossible, but certainly too long for it to be convenient.

Fourier analysis became very much more practical in the early 1960s with the invention of a highly efficient computational algorithm known as the **fast Fourier transform**, or **FFT** (Cooley & Tukey, 1965; Ramirez, 1985). The FFT is not different from the DFT—it is simply a way of computing the DFT that takes advantage of certain potential efficiencies when there are 2^N samples, where N is an integer. Using this procedure a Fourier transform on 2^N sample points can be accomplished with only $N \log_2 N$ operations. Thus an analysis of 512 ($= 2^9$) samples requires only $512(\log_2 512) = 4,608$ major computational operations. The FFT—usually in the form of one of its many improved offspring—lies behind almost all of today's digital speech spectrography.

Windows

Up to this point, the discussion of the Fourier transform and its use in deriving amplitude spectra has been theoretical. The formal requirement that a periodic signal must have existed for all past time, and must continue for all future time, has been somewhat casually dismissed by saying that we are entitled to bend the rules a bit. But that flexibility comes at a real price. The fact is that, when a signal is gathered for Fourier analysis it is grabbed from its context, and thus it begins abruptly at some point in time and ends just as abruptly some time later.

Imagine a sine wave that, in satisfaction of the formal requirements for a periodic wave, has been going on for all past time, and will continue to do so into the future. It is shown as the upper trace in Figure 7–13. We sample the waveform for some interval of time in order to have a representative segment on which we can do a Fourier analysis, and we choose a sampling rate of 10,000 samples/s. The FFT requires that we take 2^N

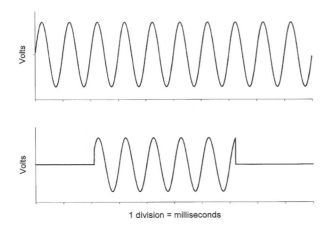

Figure 7–13. A sample (bottom), taken from a longer signal (top), is likely to have abrupt discontinuities at its ends.

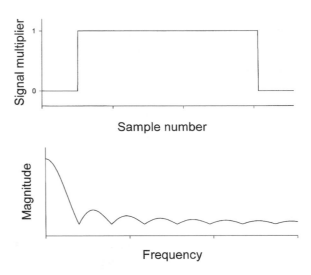

Figure 7–14. A square window (top) and the mathematical function that describes it (below).

samples, and we choose therefore to take 512 (2^9) samples. At the sampling rate that we are using this means that we extract a segment that is 512/10,000 = 0.0512 second in length. The analysis instrument or program that we will use will therefore apply the FFT to the segment shown as the lower trace in Figure 7–13. In essence, the analysis system is looking at the original signal through a window that is 512 samples wide. It cannot see anything beyond the limits of the window frame, and therefore makes the assumption that all values before the first sample and after the last sample are zero.

This may not seem like a problem until one compares the "real" signal to its windowed sample. The two have an important dissimilarity. Because of the arbitrary start and stop of the sampled interval, the segment to be analyzed has a very abrupt onset and offset. People may know that the sharp rise and fall at the beginning and end of the segment are artifacts created by looking at the waveform through a window, but the mathematics of the Fourier transform doesn't know that. Therefore, the analysis will be accomplished not on a sine wave, but on a peculiar wavetrain.

A sine wave such as that from which we've taken a segment has a line spectrum that consists of a single line at the frequency of the sine wave. But the abrupt rise and fall of the sample segment means that, from the analysis system's point of view, there is something other than a series of sine waves present. Furthermore, the extracted segment, seen as a whole, is a non-recurring complex wave. Therefore its spectrum is not a line spectrum, but a continuous spectrum with a major peak at the frequency of the sine wave and several minor peaks, or lobes.

This transformation of the spectrum from an isolated single line on the frequency axis to a continuous and complicated spectrum is easily understood by considering the window through which the sine wave was seen as itself a mathematical function. Basically, what it does is to multiply the amplitude of all parts of the periodic signal that fall *outside* of the window frame by zero, and to multiply all amplitudes *within* the window frame by 1. So the window function could be plotted as shown in the upper trace of Figure 7–14. This square pulse, of course, has a Fourier spectrum, which is shown in the lower trace. The spectrum of the extracted segment of the sine wave will therefore be a combination of the single-line sine-wave spectrum and the continuous multi-lobed spectrum of the window function. (Technically, the two "signals" are *convolved*.)

The presence of side lobes in the spectrum of the rectangular window is not a trivial matter. They imply that the window function is adding frequency components of meaningful amplitude to the signal that we are interested in analyzing. Since the problem is caused by the abrupt onset and offset transitions that the rectangular window introduces into the sampled segment, a fairly obvious approach to a solution presents itself: smudge the edges of the window. That is, choose a window function such that the closer a sample value is to the window's edge the more attenuated it is. There are many ways of doing this; three of the more popular are described in Figure 7–15, which can serve as a guide to users of software systems that offer a choice of window functions, as most do.

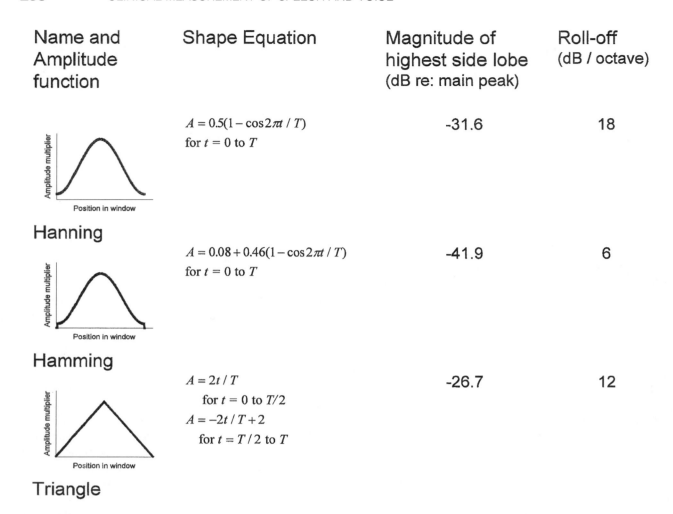

Name and Amplitude function	Shape Equation	Magnitude of highest side lobe (dB re: main peak)	Roll-off (dB / octave)
Hanning	$A = 0.5(1 - \cos 2\pi t\,/\,T)$ for $t = 0$ to T	-31.6	18
Hamming	$A = 0.08 + 0.46(1 - \cos 2\pi t\,/\,T)$ for $t = 0$ to T	-41.9	6
Triangle	$A = 2t\,/\,T$ for $t = 0$ to $T/2$ $A = -2t\,/\,T + 2$ for $t = T/2$ to T	-26.7	12

Figure 7–15. Some widely-used window functions. The shape equation states the function applied to the samples in the segment to be analyzed. (t is the sampling interval, and T is the length of the segment.) Magnitude of the highest side lobe is the greatest amplitude of any of the frequency components "added" to the spectrum by the window function. The roll-off specifies how the amplitude of "added" frequency components diminishes.

The Transfer Function and Resonance

Conceptually similar to an audiogram, the frequency response specifies how much attenuation a system—a microphone, an ear, or an electronic circuit, for example—imposes on its input as a function of frequency. The frequency response is not random: it is the manifestation of some underlying property. This property governs the way signals are transmitted from input to output, and it is known as the ***transfer function***. Figure 7–16 shows a simple transfer function. Although, when plotted on a linear frequency scale, it may not seem to be easily described, when redrawn on a logarithmic frequency axis, as in the lower right, it is clear that there is a very simple relationship between input and output amplitudes. Sinusoids at a frequency of

1000 Hz undergo no (0 dB) attenuation. But the attenuation increases by 6 dB for every octave higher or lower than this 1000 Hz "center frequency." So, for instance, a sinusoid at 500 Hz would be attenuated by 6 dB, and a sinusoid of 4000 Hz would be attenuated by 12 dB. In short, the transfer function of Figure 7–16 is the description of a filter. Essentially that is what a transfer function is: a statement of filtering characteristics. For complex systems, such as the vocal tract, the transfer function (filter characteristics) can be very complex indeed.

Figure 7–16, however, describes a simple system that can be said to be ***resonant***. A resonance is simply a frequency or band of frequencies to which a filter responds with less attenuation than it does to surrounding frequencies. The resonant frequency in Figure 7–16 is clearly 1000 Hz, but it is common also to

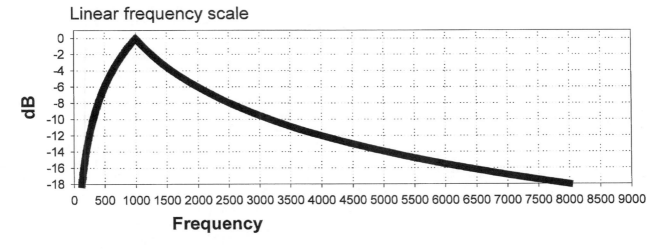

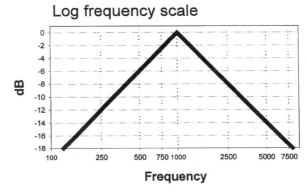

Figure 7–16. The transfer function of a system with a resonant peak at 1000 Hz, plotted with linear (top) and logarithmic (bottom) frequency axes.

describe the resonant peak in terms of its width, that is, the distance between those frequencies on either side of the "peak" at which the output is attenuated by 3 dB. The transfer function of Figure 7–16 might therefore be said to have a resonant peak with a width extending from about 700 Hz (attenuation ≈ 3 dB) to about 1400 Hz (attenuation ≈ 3 dB). Very narrow resonant peaks indicate precise frequency tuning and very little damping (see previous discussion). Broader peaks are obviously less discriminating of frequency and have greater damping. There is quite commonly more than one resonant peak in a transfer function; the vocal tract transfer function has several.

THE SOURCE SIGNAL

If a transfer function is a description of a filter, then the *source signal* is the waveform that will be subjected to filtering. A sample waveform with a fundamental frequency of 200 Hz is shown (in the time domain) at the top of Figure 7–17. We will subject this wave to the filtering described by the transfer function of Figure 7–

16. In the frequency domain (line spectrum, bottom of Figure 7–17) we are reminded that the wave is really a collection of discrete frequencies, each an integer multiple of 200 Hz, whose amplitudes diminish in a regular way as their frequency increases.

Now imagine that this bundle of frequencies (that constitute the wave) is subjected to the filter whose transfer function (filtering characteristic) is plotted in Figure 7–16. What will the result look like? Figure 7–18 suggests two possible output spectra (whose time-domain representations are shown in the insets). The envelope of spectrum A reproduces the shape of the transfer function, and thus might seem like a good candidate. But a moment's reflection shows why it is not. The transfer function specifies how much any given frequency component of the source signal is attenuated. So, the transfer function of Figure 7–16 specifies that a 400 Hz harmonic, for instance, would be attenuated by about 7.5 dB, while a 2200 Hz component would lose roughly 6.5 dB. And Figure 7–18A suggests just this. But the output's perfect mimicry of the transfer function could only occur if each harmonic

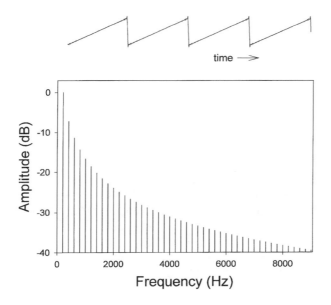

Figure 7–17. A complex wave, in the time and frequency domains, that will be subjected to filtering. It has a fundamental frequency of 200 Hz.

had an amplitude of 0 dB to begin with, which would make its final size dependent solely on the amount of attenuation imposed by the transfer function.

On the other hand, our source signal has a steady rolloff of harmonic amplitude. That means that each harmonic has already been attenuated by some amount before the transfer function acts on it. The transfer function's attenuation is imposed on the actual amplitude of the transfer function. When this is done by the transfer function of Figure 7–16 on the source signal of Figure 7–17 the harmonics are attenuated to the values shown in Figure 7–18B.

Figure 7–19 summarizes the principles just described. **The output of a system depends on the *interaction* of the source spectrum and the transfer function.** The output, therefore, looks like a combination of both, and is never simply a copy of either.

Probably the most common reason for doing speech sound spectrography is to obtain an estimate of the transfer function of the vocal tract system. (The importance of this will be discussed later.) But, especially with respect to speech signals, we are confronted with at least two major problems.

The transfer function, after all, specifies the frequency response of a system. That is, it describes how signal attenuation changes as a function of frequency. So, for instance, a transfer function might be such that a 100 Hz component of the signal is passed without loss (attenuation = 0 dB), a 190 Hz component suffers 5 dB of attenuation, 270 Hz undergoes an attenuation of 11 dB, and so on. How can we get an estimate of the characteristics of an unknown transfer function? Simply by putting known energies at various frequencies into the system and observing the output to determine how much attenuation each input has undergone. If enough different frequencies are tried a fairly good picture of the transfer function can be generated.

One major problem for speech analysis immediately becomes clear (and is suggested by Figure 7–18). Knowing the magnitude of a frequency component at the output of a system does no good unless its original (input) amplitude is known, at least in a relative sense. That is, one is trying to measure attenuation, and attenuation is a measure of *change*. To assess change one needs to know both before and after values. But the amplitudes of the various frequencies that are the natural (voice) input to the vocal tract are not known, except in a rather vague way. How can one tell, then, how much each has been attenuated? If one cannot determine the attenuation, one's conclusions about the transfer function will be limited indeed.[13]

To characterize the transfer function completely one needs to "probe" it at every frequency (at least in the range of frequencies that are of importance to a given purpose). But a periodic signal has energy only at its harmonic frequencies. So, for instance, if the fundamental frequency (F_0) is 100 Hz, there is energy in the signal only at 100, 200, 300, 400 Hz, and so on. If a periodic signal is used as the input, estimates of a system's frequency response (that is, of its transfer function) can be obtained only at the harmonic frequencies. Figure 7–20 shows what the problem is. At the top is a plot of the transfer function of a system. If the input signal used to evaluate this transfer function has a fundamental frequency of 10 Hz, then there is a harmonic frequency every 10 Hz. (We assume, for the sake of the example, that the harmonics of the input signal all have the same amplitude.) A line connecting the "tops" of the harmonics of the output signal, shown in the figure, is the best estimate of shape of the transfer function. When the harmonics are only 10 Hz apart, that

[13]Fortunately the general spectral characteristics of the vocal signal that is acted upon by the vocal tract are not completely unknown, which allows for reasonable assumptions, that lead to generally useful conclusions. The characteristics and assumptions are discussed more fully later.

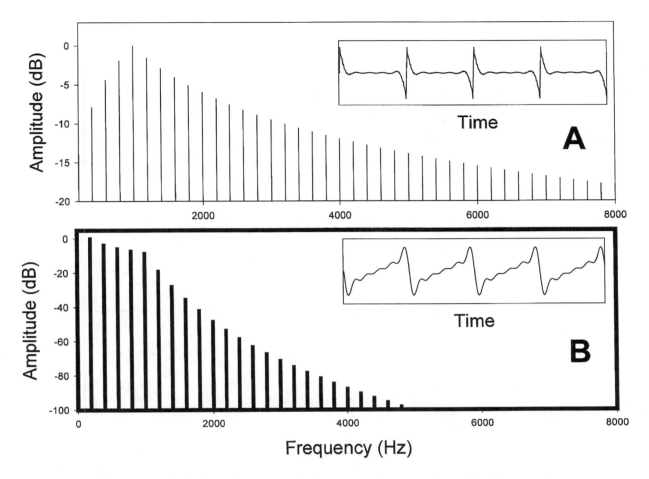

Figure 7–18. Two hypothetically possible outputs after the transfer function of Figure 7–16 has acted on the complex wave of Figure 7–17.

representation is very good. (It is unlikely, after all, that a major feature would occur in the narrow 10 Hz space between any two harmonics.)

When the input signal has an F_0 of 100 Hz there are fewer, more widely spaced harmonics, and thus the recreation of the transfer function formed by connecting their tops is cruder. Still, it is not too bad. Both peaks of the transfer function are represented, and the location of the center frequency of each is at least approximately correct. When, however, the F_0 rises to 200 Hz the wide spacing of the harmonic becomes a real problem. The "probes" of the transfer function are now so far apart that the "connect-the-tops" recon-

struction of the transfer function is quite poor. And when the F_0 is 300 Hz, the reconstruction is essentially useless. Fundamental frequencies of 100, 200, and 300 Hz are representative of the voices of men, women, and children.[14]

The 3-Dimensional Speech Spectrogram

Figure 7–21 is an example of a classical "3-dimensional" speech spectrogram, sometimes called a *sonagram*, of the utterance "Joe took father's shoe bench

---

[14]Young children commonly use F_0s that are significantly higher still (see Chapter 6, "Vocal Fundamental Frequency"), which makes the problem even worse.

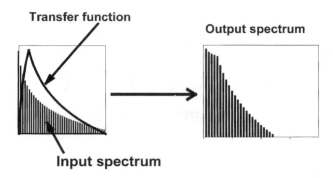

Figure 7–19. The output of a system is never a copy of either the source or the transfer functions, but rather is created by the source-transfer function interaction.

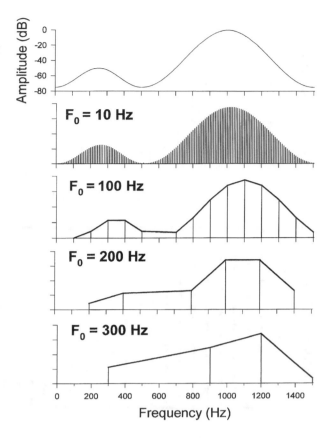

Figure 7–20. The characteristics of the transfer function are revealed only at those points where there is a "stimulus." As the harmonics of the source signal become more widely spaced, the "stimuli" are more separated, and the characterization of the transfer function becomes less exact.

out."[15] The top trace shows the signal in the time domain (that is, the sound pressure waveform), while the larger display shows the frequency domain representation over time. At first glance this analysis does not seem to have much in common with the spectrum displays that have been considered thus far. But that's because there is so much information condensed into it, and because some special tricks have been used so that changes in the spectrum over time can be shown. (After all, the speech signal is variable, and it is its variability which allows it to convey information. Therefore, it is not only the spectral properties of speech at a point in time that interest the clinician, but also—and perhaps even more—the ways in which the spectral properties change.) Just a casual glance at Figure 7–21 shows even a naïve viewer that there are regular features in it. The interpretation of those features is largely what evaluation of speech sound spectrograms is about. But in order to do so it is crucial to understand how the display is generated.

LINEAR PREDICTIVE CODING

Although the discussion thus far has related the concept of "spectrum" only to Fourier analysis, there are, in fact, many different ways in the content of a signal may be evaluated in the frequency domain. Most of these methods are primarily of use for specialized tasks, such as efficient data transmission. One, however, is of particular use in speech sound spectrography (Atal & Hanauer, 1971; Flanagan, 1972), and, in fact, is included in several commercial analysis packages. *Lin-*

ear predictive coding (*LPC*), as it is known, therefore warrants at least a brief description.

The basis for linear predictive coding is the fact the signals are, in fact, significantly predictable. That is, if a series of samples has been obtained, it constitutes a "history" about the waveform from which one might guess, with a fair degree of accuracy, what the value of the next sample will be. While there are a large number of ways in which such a guess might be made, one of the easiest (and computationally simplest) is to use a linear model. The predicted next value of the waveform can be formed by taking a kind of average of the previous values. In forming the average some previous samples are made more important than others by

---

[15]This sentence was chosen in honor of Harvey Fletcher, who used it in his pioneering early work of the acoustics and perception of speech at Bell Telephone Laboratories (Fletcher, 1929, 1953).

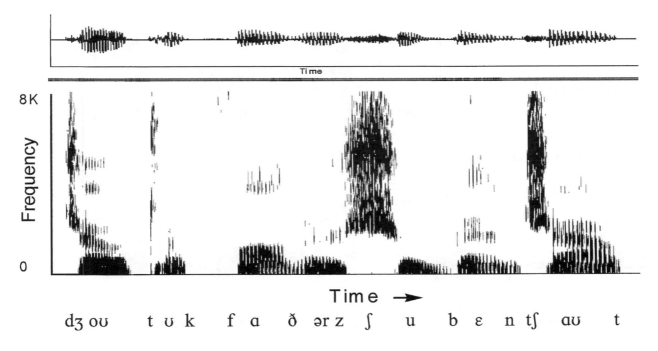

Figure 7–21. The standard "3-dimensional" sound spectrogram, which shows frequency and the amplitude of frequency components along the vertical axis against time on the horizontal axis. The time-domain representation (sound pressure signal) is shown at the top.

assigning them greater weights (that is, by multiplying them by larger coefficients). So, if s_i represents the ith consecutive sample of a waveform, then an estimate, $\hat{s}_{i+1}$, of what the next sample is, s_{i+1}, can be obtained from

$$\hat{s} = \sum_{j=1}^{N} a_j s_{i-j},$$

where a_j are the coefficients (weighting factors) assigned to each of the prior samples being used to make the prediction.

It is almost certain that this technique will not achieve a perfect estimate of the value of the next sample. There is bound to be some degree of error. Its magnitude, e_{i+1}, will be known as soon as the next sample is actually obtained. The error is equal to the difference between the prediction and the reality: $e_{i+1} = (s_{i+1} - \hat{s}_{i+1})$. Therefore, an accurate expression for the value of the ith sample of a speech wave is

$$\hat{s} = \left(\sum_{j=1}^{N} a_j s_{i-j} \right) - e.$$

It may seem that this is a very complex—and useless—way of going about things. The logical question is

"Why undertake this highly complicated business of making a prediction of the next value and then figuring out how much it is in error, when the next sample will actually be obtained, and its value will therefore be known precisely?" There are two answers: the first focuses on the needs of data compression (for example, to speed information transfer in communication systems), whereas the second is of particular import for speech synthesis and, what is more germane, to the needs of speech sound spectrography.

First, on the whole, speech signals do not change very abruptly and (on the time scale of electronic phenomena) they do not change very often. Therefore, if a signal is periodic, one set of predictive coefficients is likely to be valid for quite a long time. Therefore, the prediction equation does not have to be updated very often. So, instead of transmitting a waveform at a rate of, let us say, 10,000 samples per second, each sample having perhaps 10 bits of resolution, linear predictive coding might offer the advantage of sending the signal as a series of 20 or 30 coefficients and an error term, updated only 100 times per second. That's a very much more efficient way of transmitting the signal, with only a little loss of quality.

The second reason is more interesting to the speech specialist. Suppose, for the sake of example, the estimate of the value of the next sample is to be

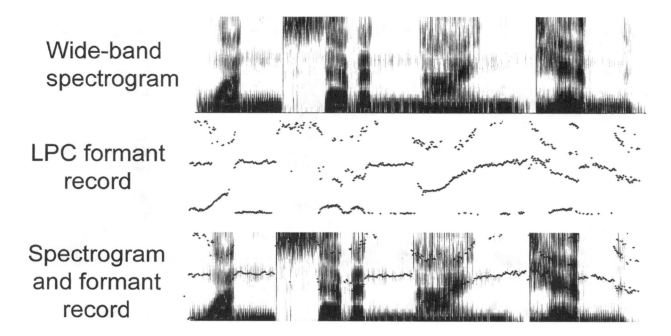

Figure 7–22. Top: A standard wide-band spectrogram of the utterance /wʊnsɛv̄n naɪn tɛn/. Center: Formant frequencies have been marked using linear predictive coding. Bottom: Overprint of "formant history" on original spectrogram.

determined on the basis of only the five preceding samples. Then the expression for the value of a single sample,

$$\hat{s} = \left(\sum_{j=1}^{N} a_j s_{i-j}\right) - e_i,$$

may be expanded to

$$\hat{s}_i = a_1 s_{i-5} + a_2 s_{i-4} + a_3 s_{i-3} + a_4 s_{i-2} + a_5 s_{i-1} - e_i.$$

A whole series of samples, then, can be expressed as

$$\hat{s}_1 = a_{11}s_{-5} + a_{12}s_{-4} + a_{13}s_{-3} + a_{14}s_{-2} + a_{15}s_{-1} - e_i$$
$$\hat{s}_2 = a_{21}s_{-4} + a_{22}s_{-3} + a_{23}s_{-2} + a_{24}s_{-1} + a_{25}s - e_i$$
$$\hat{s}_3 = a_{31}s_{-3} + a_{32}s_{-2} + a_{33}s_{-1} + a_{34}s + a_{35}s_1 - e_i,$$

and so on. In short, the signal is represented by a matrix of coefficients and error terms:

$$a_{11} + a_{12} + a_{13} + a_{14} + a_{15} - e_1$$
$$a_{21} + a_{22} + a_{23} + a_{24} + a_{25} - e_2$$
$$a_{31} + a_{32} + a_{33} + a_{34} + a_{35} - e_3$$

This series of numbers in the time domain, it turns out, represents a spectral plot in the frequency domain. But the spectrum is shows does not include the harmonics and other content of the source signal. Rather, it is a spectrum that shows the resonances of the system. In other words, *linear predictive coding provides a spectral representation of the formants of the speech signal.*

Linear predictive spectrography can be combined with Fourier spectrography to show the formant frequencies right on the spectrogram, as in Figure 7–22, saving a great deal of analysis time and effort. The upper record is a standard wide-band spectrogram of the utterance /wʊn sɛv̄n naɪn tɛn/. The display range is 0 to 4000 Hz. In the center, linear predictive coding techniques have been used to mark the formant frequencies. Finally, comparison to the spectrographic analysis is facilitated by overprinting the LPC formant history, as in the bottom record.

There are a few important limitations of LPC analysis. First, it may fail badly if the signal changes abruptly, as it well may do in some cases of speech disorder. Second, if the vocal F_0 is high (above, let us say, 350 Hz), estimating formants on the basis of LPC spectra may be less accurate than measuring the formant frequencies by hand (Monsen & Engebretson, 1983). Third, LPC analysis is not usually designed to take account of antiresonances (such as are often characteristic of nasalization (see Chapter 11, "Velopharyngeal Function"), which may cause results to be erroneous.

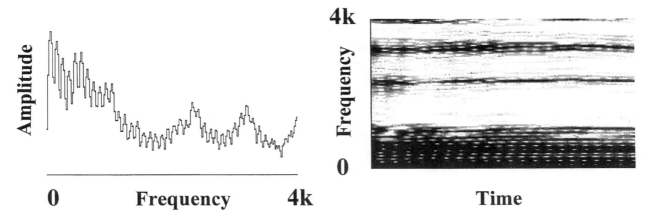

Figure 7–23. An amplitude spectrum (left) at one point in time during a sustained /ɑ/. A standard three-dimensional sound spectrogram (right) of a sustained /ɑ/ by the same speaker.

CREATING THE SPEECH SPECTROGRAM

Figure 7–23 shows, on the left, the amplitude spectrum of one instant during the production of the vowel /ɑ/. The evenly-spaced small peaks show the harmonic components, while the several regional maxima of harmonic amplitude are the result of resonances in the vocal tract. On the right is a standard 3-dimensional sound spectrogram—the workhorse display of speech evaluation—of a sustained /ɑ/ by the same speaker. It contains all of the same information as the amplitude spectrum on the left, but it also displays the time history of the amplitude spectrum. That is, it shows how the amplitude spectrum changes, or does not change, over time.

It may not be immediately obvious that the two displays are intimately related, and that is because the sound spectrogram displays its information, quite literally, from a different perspective. To understand what is involved, one first needs to consider that, in order to see how a signal's spectral characteristics change over time, one must first do a series of spectral analyses, each at a sequentially later point in the signal. Each analysis will require a short segment of the signal. (Since the acoustic signal will have been digitized, the length is specified as a number of samples. The segment length is thus the size of the window, discussed earlier. The significance of the number of samples entering into each analysis—and it is an important consideration—will be discussed later.) In general, the analysis segments will overlap. (For the sake of clarity, the overlap in Figure 7–24 has been greatly reduced.) A spectral analysis is done separately for each segment, and the process continues until the whole signal has been evaluated.

The resulting series of spectra can now be arranged, as shown in Figure 7–25, to form the spectrographic display. The several spectra (represented by the one in the lower left of the figure) are accumulated and arranged in a sequence, one next to the other, as shown.[16] The sequence is then rotated, so that the spectra run in a series from left to right. Since the spectra have been taken at regular time intervals, the horizontal axis really represents time. Finally, the entire plot is (at least conceptually) tilted up off the page. The result is that the viewer is seeing the spectra *from above*.

There is, however, something very wrong with this display: Each spectrum has become simply a vertical line on the page, extending from the lowest frequency detected in the analysis to the highest. Since we are looking from directly "overhead" the peaks and valleys are no longer discernible. The most critical result of the analysis has been hidden in the process of putting three information dimensions (frequency, amplitude, and time) onto a two-dimensional page. The solution to the problem is to use increasingly dark shades of gray to represent increasing energy. Doing this translates height into gray-scale levels that represent the otherwise-undetectable third dimension. Figure 7–26 shows the gray-scale relationship of a standard 3-dimensional spectrogram.

---

[16]Because, in actual practice, the spectra represent overlapping segments of the signal, the spectral traces also "overlap." There are no spaces between them. The separations in the figure have been included only for the sake of diagrammatic clarity.

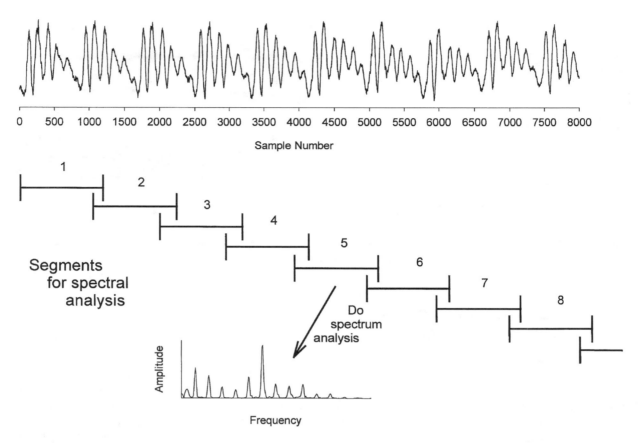

Figure 7–24. A long speech sample is divided into overlapping segments, for each one of which the amplitude spectrum is obtained.

Figure 7–27 shows an extract from a sound spectrogram of a prolonged vowel (on the right). The vertical axis represents frequency (from low to high), while the horizontal axis is time. To its left, plotted "on end," is the amplitude spectrum of the same utterance. Note how the height of the peaks in the amplitude spectrum (which, of course, represent the harmonic frequencies in the vocalic signal) corresponds to the darkness of the gray values in the spectrogram. (The fourth harmonic peak, for instance, has the greatest height of any point in the amplitude spectrum, and it is marked by the darkest of the gray "bars" in the spectrogram.)

Spectrogram Parameters

Although several sound spectrograms may be derived from the same spoken utterance, they may appear so different as to make it hard to imagine that they are all analyses of the very same recording. The differences among them, however, represent the state of several important analysis parameters that must be set by the user, no matter what analysis system is employed. The decision about any given setting is made on the basis of the nature of the signal to be analyzed and of the specific information that the analysis is intended to provide.

SAMPLING RATE / FREQUENCY RANGE

The frequency of the highest component that can be validly detected is limited by the Nyquist sampling theorem (see Chapter 3, "Digital Systems"). In the simplest terms, that theory states that one cannot capture frequencies that are greater than one half of the sampling rate. Thus, the maximum frequency range of the spectrogram is determined by the rate at which the speech sample has been digitized. Therefore, if one wanted, for instance, to observe relatively high-frequency components—let us say turbulence noise—in the neighborhood of 8000 Hz, one would have to digitize the speech signal at a minimum 16,000 samples

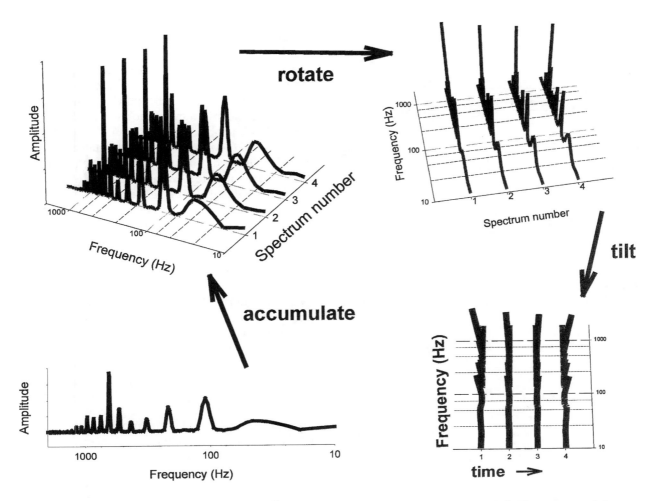

Figure 7–25. Generating a three-dimensional sound spectrogram. Clockwise from lower left: The spectra of the overlapping samples of the waveform are generated, and then are accumulated by being plotted "one behind the other." The plane holding the accumulated spectra is rotated, so that the frequency axis (on the left) becomes the y axis. Finally, the entire plane is "tilted" up off the background, so that the viewer is looking at the several spectra from above.

per second. That minimum assumes ideal conditions that are, in fact, never characteristic of the real world. Therefore, the sampling rate would need to be a bit higher, say 20 kHz. (As a rule of thumb, one is advised to sample at a rate equal to about 220% of the highest frequency to be observed.) One can, depending upon the options of one's analysis system, always limit the display's frequency range to less than the maximum frequency that the Nyquist sampling theorem allows. But, unfortunately, one cannot validly extend it beyond the Nyquist limit, and most analysis systems will not allow the user to try. There is no post-acquisition fix for too low a sampling rate, and so the user must judge wisely beforehand.

WINDOW SIZE: FREQUENCY AND TIME RESOLUTION

The ability to discriminate between two frequencies separated by an arbitrary distance on the frequency axis is called the *frequency resolution*. The frequency resolution, in turn, is governed by the size of the analysis window. That is, it is a function of the length of the signal segment that is analyzed. The effect on the amplitude spectrum is clearly shown in Figure 7–28, which plots several spectrum analyses of the same point during the production of a sustained /ɛ/. At the upper left the analysis window is 4096 samples (acquired at a rate of 44k samples per second). The

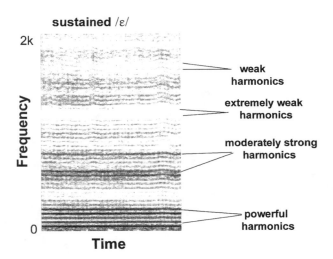

Figure 7–26. A standard three-dimensional spectrogram of a sustained /ɛ/. The darker grays indicate greater amplitude.

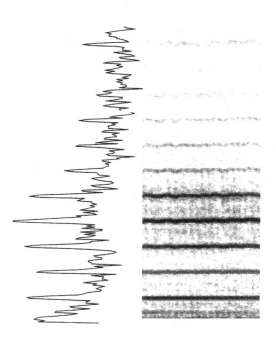

Figure 7–27. Shown at right is a three-dimensional sound spectrogram of a sustained vowel. Frequency increases along the vertical axis from about 10 to about 2000 Hz. The horizontal axis represents time. Depth of gray shading indicates the amplitude of the frequency components of the vowel signal. To the left is plotted (with frequency scaled from bottom to top) an amplitude spectrum of a point in the same utterance. Note how the magnitudes of the peaks of the amplitude spectrum coincide with the depth of gray shading in the spectrogram.

harmonics are clearly visible, and, given the frequency resolution of about 11 Hz, their actual values can be determined within 5 Hz or so. But if, as in the upper right, the window size is halved, so that only 2048 samples are used, resolution drops. At the resulting resolution of about 22 Hz the individual harmonics are still discernible, but they are not as sharply delimited. On the lower left the window size has once again been halved, to 1024 samples, and the frequency resolution has now dropped to about 43 Hz. Not all of the individual harmonics are now resolved. Finally, with a very small window size of only 512 samples, which provides a frequency resolution of 86 Hz, none of the harmonics is individually distinguishable. Instead, only the "envelope" of the spectrum can be read.

Since the three-dimensional sound spectrogram is composed of accumulated individual spectra, the loss of resolution naturally affects it as well. Figure 7–29 shows the result for the same sustained /ɛ/ whose amplitude spectra were examined. As the window becomes smaller, and frequency resolution decreases, the bars showing the harmonic energy become increasingly wider. Ultimately they merge together. The merging, however, confers an advantage that, depending on the purposes for which the spectrogram was generated, might constitute an advantage: in the merging of the individual harmonic lines, one is left with a more distinct impression of where, on the frequency scale, energy is locally concentrated. That is, in the darker broad bands one can more easily see the regions that are likely to constitute spectral peaks in the signal. In other words, resonances or—in the terminology of vocal tract acoustics, formants—are made more apparent.

There is another, very important, reason for sacrificing frequency resolution by selecting a smaller window size, and it is illustrated in Figure 7–30. It shows three spectrograms of the same production of the VCV disyllable /ɑtʰɑ/, produced by a normal man. The signal was digitized at a rate of 44k samples/s. At the top, the analysis window was 8192 samples wide. As expected, the component frequencies are well resolved, and the individual harmonics are identifiable. When the size of the analysis window is reduced to 2048 samples, the harmonic lines are much less distinct, a consequence of the reduced frequency resolution. Finally, with a window length of 1024 samples the harmonic lines have merged, and the regions of resonance that characterize the vowels are now more easily perceived as dark bands. At this window size, however, another feature has appeared: The spectrogram shows distinct *vertical* bands during the vowels.

These vertical striations are not an artifact, and their source is no mystery. Every time the glottis snaps shut, a sharp pulse of acoustic energy is created in the

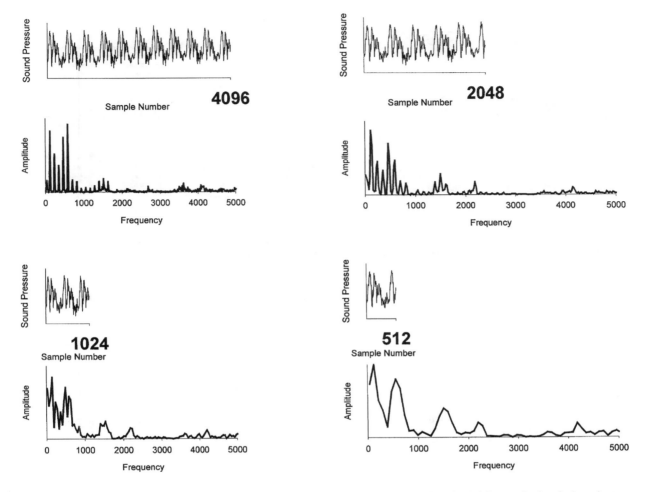

Figure 7–28. Frequency resolution of the amplitude spectrum decreases as the size of the analysis window decreases. Clockwise from upper left are results of spectral analyses of the same prolonged vowel, sampled at about 44k samples/s, using analysis-window sizes of 4096, 2048, 1024, and 512 samples.

vocal tract. (These pulses, to be discussed in more detail later, are, in fact, the vocal signal.) Each of these small bursts is subject to significant damping, and so its energy dies away rather quickly. No sooner has it significantly weakened, however, than another burst of acoustic energy is produced at the glottis. The vertical striations, then, represent this sudden onset and subsequent fading of the glottal acoustic excitation.

The appearance of these bursts in the short-window spectrogram results from the fact that it has much greater *time* resolution than the others. There is an inherent tradeoff between time and frequency resolution: the more one is improved the worse the other gets. Time and frequency resolution are, in other words, reciprocally related. (This fact was hinted at earlier, and, indeed, is foreshadowed by the simple state-

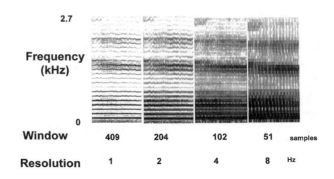

Figure 7–29. Four sound spectrograms of the same sustained vowel. As the analysis window becomes smaller (from left to right), the bars showing harmonic frequencies become wider, and ultimately merge. Smaller window size implies less resolution.

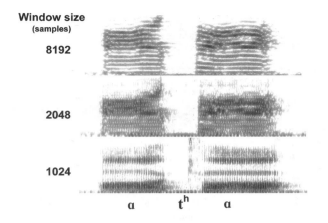

Window size
(samples)

8192

2048

1024

ɑ   tʰ   ɑ

time domain

600 samples / 49 Hz   100 samples / 293 Hz

↕ 391 Hz

256 samples / 114 Hz   75 samples / 391 Hz

125 samples / 229 Hz   50 samples / 586 Hz

Figure 7–30. Three sound spectrograms of the same production of /ɑtʰɑ/, using progressively shorter windows. Note that as the frequency resolution is lost there is a corresponding improvement in time resolution.

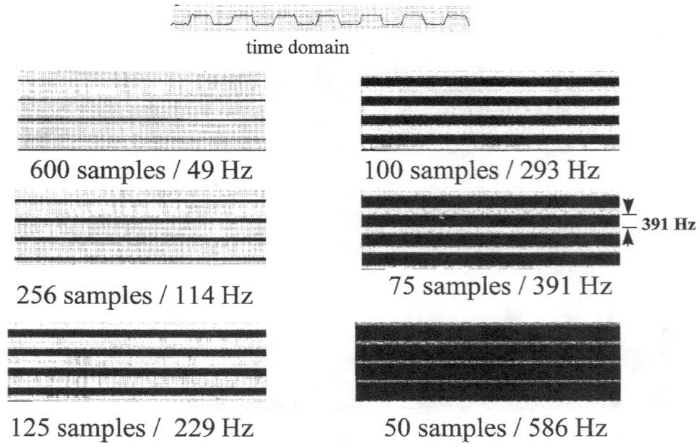

Figure 7–31. Spectrograms of a simple signal (shown at the top) that has harmonics about 1000 Hz apart using different window lengths/analyzing bandwidths. The horizontal bands show the presence of each harmonic over time. The thickness of each band is a function of the filter bandwidth.

ment that $f = 1/t$, that is, frequency is the reciprocal of period.)

In routine spectrographic work it is usual to refer not to the window size, but to the frequency resolution, which is a function of both window size and sampling rate. The frequency resolution is usually specified in terms of the *bandwidth*, because, in analog systems, it is represented by the bandwidth of the filter through which the signal is passed (see Chapter 2, "Analog Electronics"). Suppose a filter has a bandwidth of 100 Hz and a center frequency of 200 Hz. Now suppose that a signal is applied to the filter's input and is passed with minimal attenuation to its output. Without a frequency meter, what can we say about the frequency content of the input signal? Only that it had to lie in the range of 150 to 250 Hz—the range that is one-half of the bandwidth above and below the filter's center frequency. In a spectrogram, either digital or analog, the uncertainty produced by the bandwidth of the analyzer will appear in the output. A single sine wave will be represented not as a thin, precisely located line, but as a bar whose thickness (that is, its width on the frequency axis) is equal to the analyzer's bandwidth.

Figure 7–31 illustrates this fact. Sound spectrograms have been prepared of a relatively simple waveform that has harmonics about 1000 Hz apart. The window length has been shortened (and therefore the bandwidth of the analyzing filter increased) for each analysis. While the harmonics are well separated in the top left spectrogram—for which the bandwidth is 49

Hz—the harmonics are represented as bands 586 Hz wide at the bottom right. The top left illustration shows a *narrow-band* spectrogram; the one at the bottom right, a *wide-band* (or *broad-band*) spectrogram.

In summary, then:

- Window length (expressed as the number of samples in the analysis window) is inversely related to frequency resolution. The longer the window, the closer in frequency two signal components can be and still be identified as separate components.
- Time resolution is inversely related to frequency resolution. That is, the shorter the analysis window, the closer two events can be to each other in time and still be discriminated as separate events.
- The frequency resolution (and hence also the time resolution) is determined by both the sampling rate and the length of the analysis window.
- Frequency resolution (and hence also time resolution) can also be expressed as the bandwidth. The larger the bandwidth, the less the frequency resolution (and the greater the time resolution).
- For a periodic signal the terms "wide-band" and "narrow-band" have meaning only in terms of the fundamental frequency (which specifies the spacing of the harmonics). A 150 Hz bandwidth, for instance, is narrow-band with respect to a child's voice (whose F_0 might be 350 Hz) because it will

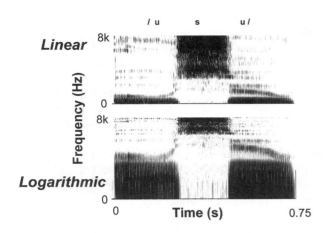

Figure 7–32. Appearance of sound spectrograms of /usu/ when generated with a linear (above) and a logarithmic (below) frequency scale.

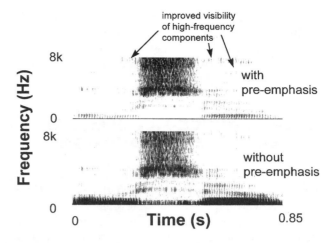

Figure 7–33. Appearance of sound spectrograms of /usu/ when generated with (above) and without (below) pre-emphasis. Pre-emphasis intensifies the higher-frequency components of the signal, making them more easily detectable in the spectrogram.

allow the harmonics to be individually represented. But the same bandwidth is wide-band when used with the average male voice, which has a F_0 of around 100 Hz. The 150 Hz filter will produce very broad bands on the frequency axis, each band containing more than one harmonic.

■ Although wide-band analyzers sacrifice resolution of individual harmonics, the resulting display may make identification of resonant (formant) frequencies easier.

LOG/LINEAR SCALING

Under most circumstances, spectrograms are created with a linear frequency scale. Since most of the acoustic energy of the speech signal is at relatively low frequencies, there may be circumstances in which there are significant details crowded into a narrow range at the lower end of the frequency axis. One way of expanding the lower portion of the frequency scale while preserving its full range is to use logarithmic scaling. (Figure 7–32 shows spectrograms with linear and logarithmic scaling of the same utterance.) Another virtue of logarithmic scaling, where equal distances on the axis represent equal ratios of values (as opposed to equal separation of values), is that some types of special measurement are made easier.

PRE-EMPHASIS

The spectral slope of the vocal source signal means that the higher harmonics of the speech output are generally very weak. As a result there may not be enough high-frequency energy present to make features at the upper end of the frequency range visible in the spectrographic display. To deal with this, many spectrographic analysis systems provide for "pre-emphasis." In essence, this means that the gain of the analysis system can be adjusted to be frequency dependent in some regular way, so that higher frequencies receive a boost. Pre-emphasis can be achieved by either analog or digital means. In an analog system, a simple high-pass filter is used. The most basic filter will provide a pre-emphasis of 6 dB / octave. (That is, for an input that has equal amplitude of all of its frequency components, output amplitude is doubled for every doubling of frequency.) Alternatively, digital pre-emphasis is achieved by subjecting the series of samples to a conversion formula of the form:

$$y_n = x_n - ax_{n-1,}$$

where a is a constant that determines the amount of pre-emphasis achieved.

The rolloff of the original signal's spectrum is thereby at least partially reversed, and more equal spectral strengths are created. Giving the higher frequencies greater emphasis makes them more visible in the spectrogram display. The effect of pre-emphasis is usually relatively subtle—so that the gross appearance of, and impression created by, the spectrogram is not seriously altered. An example, using the disyllable /usu/, is provided in Figure 7–33. Notice how, when pre-emphasis is used (upper spectrogram), the higher frequency range of the /s/ is more darkly marked than in the lower (without pre-emphasis) one and, more important, how very weak high frequency components in the vowels (perhaps turbulence noise) are now faintly, but distinctly, visible.

THE SOURCE-FILTER MODEL OF VOWEL PRODUCTION

A powerful theory that explains how the vocal tract generates different vowels is called the *source-filter model* of vowel production (Stevens, Kasowski, & Fant, 1953; Stevens & House, 1961). It describes the glottis as the source of a harmonic-rich signal that is applied to the complex filter of the vocal tract resonances. Some of the harmonics in the glottal signal fall at or near the resonance peaks in the vocal tract transfer function, and are therefore passed through the vocal tract with little attenuation. Other harmonics are more strongly attenuated because they lie beyond the cutoff frequencies of the resonance peaks. They therefore contribute much less to the shape of the final waveform at the mouth opening. As the vocal tract changes shape its resonant frequencies change, different acoustic products result, and the listener perceives different vowels.

The concepts of a source signal and a filter (or transfer) function were described earlier. Both contribute in important and identifiable ways to the characteristics of the product of any acoustic system. An important use of sound spectrography of speech signals is the identification of the contributions of the glottal sound source and the vocal tract filter, and, in any case, the two must frequently be disambiguated in order to interpret spectrographic features. It is profitable, therefore, to revisit those concepts here, in the context of the source-filter model and of sound spectrography of speech.

Glottal Sound Source Characteristics

A time-domain representation of a typical airflow signal (the *glottal volume velocity*) that is produced by the opening/closing action of the glottis is illustrated at the top of Figure 7–34. This airflow signal produces pressure changes—a complex acoustic wave—at the lower end of the vocal tract. This pressure signal is the source signal for any vocalic sound.

Since the source signal is (at least to a useful approximation) periodic, it must, according to the Fourier theorem, be composed of a series of sine waves —harmonics—that are separated along the frequency scale by a distance equal to the fundamental frequency. In fact, although it is rarely done, it is better to view the glottal sound source not as a pulse of airflow, but rather as an acoustic packet that is injected once every glottal cycle into the lower end of the vocal tract. That packet contains a bundle of frequencies that the vocal tract will shape into a vowel.

As is the case of most natural sounds, the strength of the harmonics in the glottal-source acoustic packet decreases as their frequency increases. That is, there is a *rolloff*. That rolloff is usually expressed as the *spectral slope*—the rate of amplitude decrease as a function of frequency. Usually the slope is stated in dB per octave: the number of decibels of attenuation associated with each doubling of harmonic frequency. Amplitude spectra of the bundle of frequencies that are the glottal source signal are also shown in Figure 7–33. (For the sake of generality, the horizontal axis represents the harmonic number: first, second, ... tenth, eleventh, and so on. The frequency of each harmonic is an integer multiple of the fundamental frequency. Thus, the frequency of a harmonic is its number times the F_0. If, for instance, $F_0 = 120$ Hz, then the 12th harmonic has a frequency of $12 \times 120 = 1440$ Hz.)

An important characteristic of normal vocal-fold oscillation is that glottal closure occurs much more rapidly than glottal opening. The airflow through the glottis therefore stops much more abruptly than it starts. This abrupt closure is responsible for most of the energy in the resulting acoustic wave and, in particular, it is responsible for the generation of the higher harmonics in the packet of frequencies that are the source signal. Figure 7–34 shows three different frequency domain (spectral) representations of the glottal source signal. The middle one has a spectral slope of -12 dB per octave. In other words, harmonic power is reduced by a factor of 16 for every doubling of harmonic frequency.[17] This rolloff is typical of normal, everyday, voice production.

If vocal intensity is raised, or if the speaker intentionally makes certain laryngeal adjustments, glottal closure becomes faster. The airflow is therefore

---

[17]Halving of power is equivalent to a drop of 3 dB. (See Chapter 5, "Speech Intensity".)

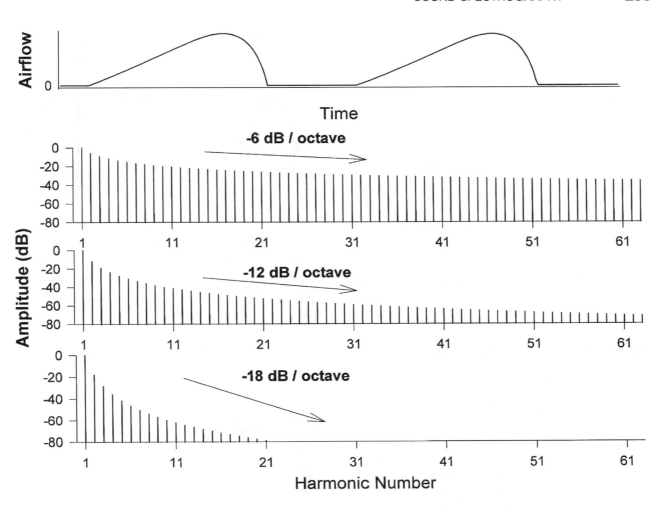

Figure 7–34. Top: Time domain representation of the glottal volume velocity signal. Bottom: Spectrum of that signal as vocal intensity goes from quite loud (upper spectrum) to very soft (lower spectrum). Note that the glottal volume velocity waveform also changes in the time domain as vocal intensity is modified.

pinched off even more quickly. Since rapid reduction of the glottal airflow is the major contributor to the strength of high-frequency components in the source signal, one would expect that, when viewed in the frequency domain, the higher harmonics of such phonation would have larger amplitude and the spectral slope would be reduced. This situation is depicted in the upper spectrum of Figure 7–34, where the spectral slope is −6 dB/octave. Perceptually, this source signal would produce a "brighter" or more "brassy" vocal quality.

In breathy phonation the glottal closing gesture is more sluggish. Since the airflow pinch-off is therefore slower, one would expect (by the logic just considered) that the higher harmonics of the source signal would be less powerful, and the spectral slope would be steeper, as is the case for the bottom spectrum of Fig-

ure 7–34, whose slope is −18 dB/octave. (Note also, however, that increased transglottal flow in general is associated with increased airflow turbulence. Turbulence is random and aperiodic, and so nonharmonic frequencies of significant strength will tend to fill in the interharmonic spaces of the spectrum.

Lest the impression be given that spectral slope changes are characteristic only in the ideal or synthetic case, Figure 7–35 presents amplitude spectra of the vowel /ɛ/ as produced at three levels of vocal loudness by a normal male. The arrows suggest the general trend of the spectral slope for each production, and each one is comparable to that which theory predicts. The amplitude spectrum of vowels produced by real speakers therefore contains information about the intensity of phonation or about the normality of phonatory adjustment.

/ɛ/

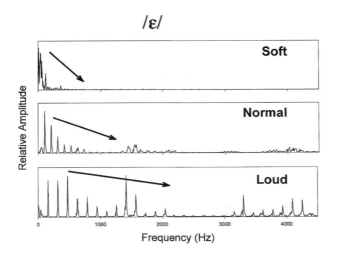

Figure 7–35. The amplitude spectra of vowel /ɛ/ produced at three levels of vocal intensity.

Vocal Tract Filter Characteristics

The supralaryngeal vocal tract behaves like a tube resonator, in many ways similar to an organ pipe. The specific details of vocal tract acoustics are moderately complex, and will not be discussed in detail here.[18] The principle most important to an understanding of speech production, however, is that the frequency response, or transfer function, of the vocal tract system is primarily dependent on vocal tract shape. Figure 7–36 shows some configurations of the vocal tract and the transfer functions associated with them. At the top is the relaxed shape of the tract, assumed for the neutral vowel 7/. This is the simplest shape of the tract, and it results in a simple transfer function. In fact, this transfer function is very similar to that of a straight tube. The peaks in the resultant transfer function show the frequencies at which the vocal tract is resonant. The resonance peaks of the vocal tract are called **formants**. There is a popular misconception that the formants are the emphasized frequencies in the final speech output. But this is most emphatically **not** the case. The distinction between vocal tract formants (resonances) and the amplitude of the spectral lines (emphasized frequencies) of the speech signal is an important one.

For a neutral vowel the formants are spaced at regular intervals across the frequency scale and have comparable, if not equal, amplitudes. Movements of

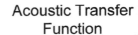
Vocal Tract Shape

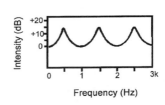
Acoustic Transfer Function

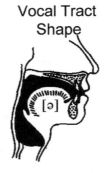

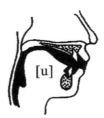

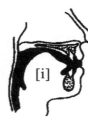

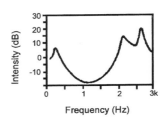

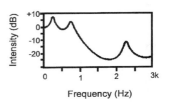

Figure 7–36. Configurations of the vocal tract and the acoustic transfer functions associated with them.

the articulators, especially of the tongue and lips, produce more complex vocal-tract configurations and hence much more complicated formant patterns. As the vocal tract assumes the postures required for different vowels, the formant peaks in the transfer function shift around and assume unequal heights. A large body of literature has shown that the perceptual classification of vocalic sounds (vowels, liquids, glides, and nasals) depends heavily on the formant characteristics as reflected in the final acoustic product radiated at the lips. These characteristics in turn depend on the location of constrictions in the vocal tract (Chiba & Kajiyama, 1941; Dunn, 1950; Stevens & House, 1955,

---

[18]Good reviews are available in Daniloff, Schuckers, and Feth (1980); Kent and Read (1992); Kent (1993, 1997); Titze (1994); Kent, Dembowski, and Lass (1996); Fujimura and Erickson (1997); and Pickett (1999).

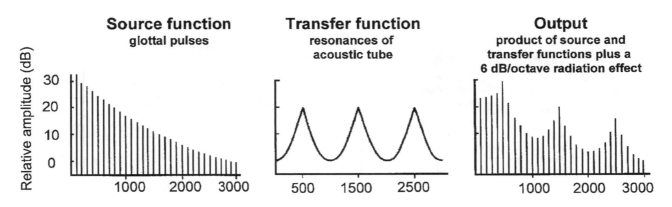

Figure 7–37. The spectral characteristics of the glottal source (left) interact with the resonant properties (or *transfer function*) of the vocal tract (center) to produce the spectral characteristics of the radiated sound wave. Reprinted from *Speech Science Primer: Physiology, Acoustics and Perception of Speech* (3rd ed.) by G. J. Borden, K. S. Harris, and L. J. Raphael, 1994, Baltimore, MD: Williams and Wilkins. Figure 5.13, p. 100. © 1994, The Williams and Wilkins Co., Baltimore, MD. Reprinted by permission.

1961; Fant, 1960, 1975). A good technical review of the relationships between vocal tract shape and the resultant acoustic signals has been published by Fant (1980).

Source-Filter Interaction

What we have for vowel production, then, is a glottal signal whose component harmonics progressively diminish in amplitude, and a vocal tract transfer function that has (usually) irregularly-spaced resonant peaks of differing heights and widths. The spectrum of the vowel that is ultimately produced is a function of both contributions, glottal and vocal tract. As shown in Figure 7–37, the two *interact*. Any acoustic analysis of the final product therefore evaluates both the glottal source and the supralaryngeal filter characteristics. One of the tasks of spectrographic analysis is to separate the two functions.

It should be noted in passing that the source-filter model assumes that the vocal tract acoustic characteristics have no significant effect on vocal-fold function. That is, the source is assumed to be independent of the filter. This is not really the case. For instance, constriction of the vocal tract (for example by linguapalatal contact) results in higher supraglottal air pressure. This alters the magnitude of the transglottal pressure drop, and thereby modifies the vocal signal (Baken & Orlikoff, 1987a; 1987b; 1988). Articulatory transitions between vocalic and voiceless segments can affect vocal-fold configuration and approximation in ways that may significantly alter glottal source characteristics (Löfqvist & McGowan, 1992). The influence of vocal

tract posture and movement on vocal-fold tension (via a mechanical and/or acoustic linkage) is commonly cited as the reason for the observation that high vowels (such as /i/ and /u/) tend to be associated with a higher mean vocal F_0 than low vowels (such as /æ/ and /ɑ/) produced within similar contexts (Black, 1949; House & Fairbanks, 1953; Lehiste & Peterson, 1961; Sonninen, 1968; Flanagan, Coker, Rabiner, Schafer, & Umeda, 1970; Honda, 1983, 1985; Sapir, 1989; Honda & Fujimura, 1991; Vilkman, Aaltonen, Raimo, Arajärvi, & Oksanen, 1989; Vilkman, Aaltonen, Laine, & Raimo, 1991; Vilkman, Laine, & Klojonen, 1991). From a clinical point of view, however, such "intrinsic vowel pitch" effects are like to be of negligible importance. Nonetheless, the clinician will want to bear in mind that consequential source-filter interactions are possible.

The frequency content of the vocalic signal is determined by the source signal, while the magnitude of each frequency component is determined by both the spectral slope of the source signal and the filter function of the vocal tract. Figures 7–38 and 7–39 illustrate how the source and filter functions appear in the sound spectrogram.

Figure 7–38 shows wide-band (top) and narrow-band (bottom) spectrograms of a prolongation of the vowel /ɛ/. The vocal F_0 during the middle third of the production is higher than at the beginning or at the end but, to the best of the speaker's ability, the vowel quality was held constant. The upper spectrogram was produced with a wide-band filter (short analysis window), and time resolution is quite good. Because of this, the vertical striations, each of which represents the burst of energy produced by a glottal closure, are easily visible. They are more widely spaced during the first and last

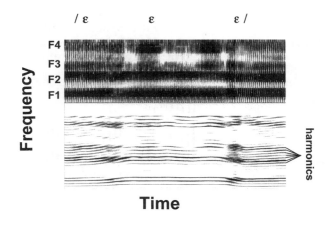

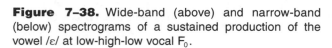

Time

Figure 7–38. Wide-band (above) and narrow-band (below) spectrograms of a sustained production of the vowel /ε/ at low-high-low vocal F_0.

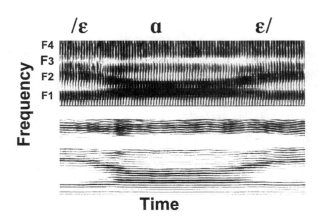

Time

Figure 7–39. Wide-band (above) and narrow-band (below) spectrograms of the utterance /εɑε/ produced with a relatively constant vocal fundamental frequency.

thirds of the record than during the middle third. This is evidence of a glottal source characteristic: Lower F_0 means a longer time between glottal pulses. When the F_0 rises, in the middle third of the vocalization, the period is shorter, and the pulses more closely spaced. The formant bands (labelled F1 through F4) in the wide-band analysis are constant throughout the production. The formants, then, are independent of F_0: They are a product of the vocal tract filter characteristics.

The lower spectrogram of the same production of /ε/ was done with a narrow-band (long analysis window) filter which has good frequency resolution. (The individual glottal pulses are not visible because, when the frequency resolution improves, the time resolution worsens.) The individual harmonics are well demonstrated, and it is clear that their separation is greater during the middle third of the production, when the F_0 is higher, than during the first and last third. This follows from the fact that the separation between the harmonics is equal to the fundamental frequency: The higher the F_0, the greater the spacing. The harmonics, then, are purely a function of the glottal source. In this spectrogram the formants are harder to see, but they can be discerned in darkening (intensification) of some harmonics. The frequency levels at which such intensifications occur are constant across the production, although, as the harmonics change frequency, different ones enter into and leave the zones of intensification (formant regions). The formant regions are vocal-tract dependent.

Figure 7–39, on the other hand, shows analyses of /εɑε/ at constant F_0, with a smooth transition between the vowels. In the upper, wide-band spectrogram the vertical striations are again visible, and they are of uni-

form spacing because F_0 does not change appreciably. The formant bands, however, do move as the vocal tract shape alters for the different vowels. Formant frequencies are characteristics of the vocal tract filter, not of the glottal source signal. The lower analysis shows that the harmonic frequencies are constant during this monopitch production. (Some of the harmonics are not visible because they are so weak.) As the resonant (formant) frequencies change, different harmonics are emphasized.

SPECTRAL CHARACTERISTICS OF SPEECH SOUNDS

The information displayed in the speech spectrogram is considered here under several broad headings. They have been assigned somewhat arbitrarily, but are likely to represent the spectrographic features of most interest to the practicing speech clinician.

Spectral Features: Vowels

Vowels are the nuclei around which syllables are built. They are characterized by pulsed glottal airflow that remains laminar as it traverses the open vocal tract. Aside from the spectral features of vowel sounds, considerable attention has been focused on their duration, which varies in a language- and dialect-specific way as a function of tense-lax distinction, consonant environment, position in the breath group, stress or prominence, speech rate, and even the information content of the word of which they are a part. All of these factors interact in very complex ways (House & Fairbanks, 1953; Fry, 1955; Fønagy & Magdics, 1960; Peterson & Lehiste, 1960; Lehiste & Peterson, 1961; Lindblom, 1963; Lindblom & Studdert-Kennedy, 1967; Bennett, 1968; Lehiste, 1972; Klatt, 1973, 1975b, 1976; DiSimoni, 1974b; Umeda, 1975; Allen, 1978; Kent, Netsell, & Abbs, 1979; Chollet, 1980; Kent & Forner, 1980; Prosek & Runyan, 1982; Crystal & House, 1988; Engstrand, 1988; Di Benedetto, 1989; Nearey, 1989; van Son & Pols, 1990; Fourakis, 1991; Moon & Lindblom, 1994; Deterding, 1997; Pickett, 1999). The discussion to follow, however, will be limited to the basic consideration of vowel spectral characteristics.

The vowel resonances are probably the most immediately obvious feature in the spectrogram of a speech utterance. While interest in them dates from the 19th century, the sound spectrograph, by making them readily observable, unleashed a flood of research into their characteristics and significance. As a result, formant patterns are understood better than most other spectral characteristics of speech. As in so many areas of scientific inquiry, the understanding achieved often points more to unresolved questions and the inability to formulate inviolable rules than to a complete and settled model. A number of significant caveats must therefore be kept in mind.

The formant pattern of a vocalic sound (and, in particular, the relationship of its first two formants) is crucial to its perceptual categorization by a listener (Potter et al., 1947; Potter & Peterson, 1948; Potter & Steinberg, 1950; Delattre et al., 1952; Fry, Abramson, Eimas, & Liberman, 1962; Carlson, Fant, & Granstrom, 1975). However, formant frequencies do not necessarily uniquely specify the vowel that is perceived. Some vowels share a common formant pattern yet are perceptually distinct (Peterson & Barney, 1952; Fairbanks & Grubb, 1961; Assmann, Nearey, & Hogan, 1982; Hillenbrand et al., 1995). Identification is influenced by the listener's linguistic experience, speaker fundamental frequency, voice quality, the vowel's phonetic context, stress or prominence, and formant amplitude (Ladefoged & Broadbent, 1957; Tiffany, 1959; Peterson, 1961; Öhman, 1966; Strange, Verbrugge, Shankweiler, & Edman, 1976; Verbrugge, Strange, Shankweiler, & Edman, 1976; Chistovich & Lublinskaya, 1979; Strange, Jenkins, & Johnson, 1983; Syrdal, 1984; Syrdal & Gopal, 1986; Assmann & Nearey, 1987; Assmann & Summerfield, 1989; Fox, 1989; Nearey, 1989; Strange, 1989; Hillenbrand & Gayvert, 1993; Hoemke & Diehl, 1994; Lotto, Holt, & Kluender, 1997).

Since formants reflect the size and shape of the vocal tract, there is no reason to expect that absolute formant frequencies should remain constant in the face of anatomical variation among speakers. What are important are the *relative* frequencies of the formant peaks, their positions with respect to each other, and to the formants of other vowels produced by the same speaker (Ladefoged & Broadbent, 1957; Nearey, 1980). However, even the relativity of formant frequencies may not be perfectly preserved across speakers. If it were, one would expect that, for a given vowel, the ratio of the frequencies of the first and second formants would remain stable across younger and older children, and across women and men, whose vocal tracts are all different in size and shape. Indeed, while there are linear trends in interpersonal formant scaling, the exact relationships are neither simple nor perfectly understood (Broadbent, Ladefoged, & Lawrence, 1956; Fant, 1966, 1975; Gerstman, 1968; Eguchi & Hirsch, 1969; Coleman, 1971; Kent, 1976, 1978, 1979; Kent & Forner, 1979; Nearey, 1980; Fox, 1983; Hillenbrand & Gayvert, 1993).

It is clear, then, that clinical use of formant data must be approached with due regard for constraints on their applicability and interpretation. For example, attempts to have a child exactly match the clinician's formant patterns would probably be futile—and almost certainly be pointless. Still, formant measures can have value in assessing developmental normality (Eguchi & Hirsh, 1969; Gilbert, 1970; Kent & Forner, 1979; Buhr, 1980; Kent & Murray, 1982; Kent, Osberger, Netsell, & Hustedde, 1987; Nittrouer, Studdert-Kennedy, & McGowan, 1989; Smith & Kenney, 1998) and a range of speech disorders, including dysfluency, dyslalia, apraxia, and dysarthria (Adams, 1978; Kahane, 1979; Kent, 1979; Kent, Netsell, & Abbs, 1979; Daniloff, Wilcox, & Stephens, 1980; Klich & May, 1982; Collins, Rosenbek, & Wertz, 1983; Gerratt, 1983; Kent & Rosenbek, 1983; Weismer, 1984a; Moran, 1986; Howell & Vause, 1986; Ziegler & von Cramon, 1986; Chaney, 1988; Huer, 1989; Kent, Kent, Weismer, Sufit, Brooks, & Rosenbek, 1989; Kent, Kent, Rosenbek, Weismer, Martin, Sufit, & Brooks, 1992; Keller, Vigneux, & Laframboise, 1991; Ansel & Kent, 1992; Howell & Williams, 1992; Weismer, Martin, Kent, & Kent, 1992; Walton & Pollock, 1993; Mulligan et al., 1994; Smith, Marquardt, Cannito, & Davis, 1994; Dromey, Ramig, & Johnson, 1995; Harteluis, Nord, & Buder, 1995; McLeod & Issac, 1995; Turner, Tjaden, & Weismer, 1995; Max & Caruso, 1998). Formant frequencies have also been used extensively to characterize the speech of the deaf and hearing-impaired (Angelocci, Kopp, & Holbrook, 1964; Monsen, 1976a, 1976b; Maki, Gustafson, Conklin, & Aumphrey-Whitehead, 1981; Simmons, 1983; Kent, Osberger, Netsell, & Austedde, 1987; Osberger, 1987; Lane & Webster, 1991; Economou, Tartter, Chute, & Hellman, 1992; Manning, Moore, Dunham, Lu, & Domico, 1992; Ryalls & Larouche, 1992).

FORMANT MEASUREMENT

Formants can be described in terms of three parameters: (1) frequency, (2) amplitude, and (3) bandwidth. The latter two are of limited interest to the speech clinician, and therefore will not be considered here. Good reviews of the problems of assessing them are provided by Dunn (1961) and by Fant, Fintoft, Liljencrantz, Lindblom, and Martony (1963).

Formant Frequencies

A formant is a local maximum in the vocal tract transfer function. It is a single frequency at which vocal tract transmission is more efficient than at nearby frequencies. The emphasis on transmission characteristics is important here: *The vocal tract system has formants even if no sound is being produced.* The fact is, however, that a formant frequency can be detected only when there is acoustic energy being transmitted. Therefore, a formant can be operationally defined as a peak in the displayed amplitude spectrum that is not due to source-spectrum properties.

This pragmatic definition raises a significant problem in that the vocal signal, which is the wave usually being transmitted, has a line spectrum. That is, it has significant energy only at discrete (harmonic) frequencies. So the formant becomes that point on the frequency scale where a harmonic has greater amplitude than its neighbors. It would be a fortunate coincidence if the frequency of a harmonic fell at exactly the true frequency of a formant peak: one could then be certain that the formant frequency had been precisely indicated. It is not surprising, given the essential independence of the glottal source and vocal-tract filter, that such a happy correspondence is likely to be rare and certainly not to be assumed.

Individual harmonics serve as "samples" of the vocal tract's resonant responses. The greater the space between harmonics, the larger the gaps between samples and the less certain the formant determination can be. Harmonic spacing is a direct correlate of fundamental frequency, and so formant frequency determination becomes less precise as vocal frequency rises (Cornut & Lafon, 1960; Bloothooft & Plomp, 1985; Maurer, Cook, Landis, & d'Heureuse, 1992; Maurer & Landis, 1996). As presented earlier, Figure 7–20 shows how serious the situation can become.

Obviously, the voices of women—and especially of children—are most likely to suffer this kind of estimation inaccuracy. Peterson (1959), after a lucid and concise review of the difficulty, found it to be essentially irresolvable. Even more recently developed mathematical analytic methods do not seem to hold the promise of a solution (Monsen & Engebretson, 1983). There are, however, a few tricks that circumvent the problem. One is to analyze whispered speech, since the broad-band noise signal of whispering will excite all the formants (Peterson, 1961; Watterson & Emanuel, 1981). Another is to substitute an external noise source or low-frequency signal for the patient's voice. A clever way of doing this is to have the speaker mouth the utterance while using an electrolarynx (Huggins, 1980).[19] The tricks do have their problems, however (Weiss, Yeni-Komshian, & Heinz, 1979). There is sound leakage from the electrolarynx directly to the microphone; the spectrum of the electrolaryngeal excitation is different from the natural voice spectrum, such that spurious peaks in the speech amplitude spectrum may result (Sáfrán, 1971); and speech rate tends to be slower both when using the electrolarynx and when whispering (Parnell, Amerman, & Wells, 1977). But, as shown in Figure 7–40, there is enormous improvement in formant resolution.

Expected Formant Values

If there is one thing that early spectrographic investigations of speech made clear, it is that there are no static signals. This holds true for vowels. The voluminous examples presented in the classic work of Potter, Kopp, and Green (1947) show that vowel formants change as they "grow" out of the preceding phoneme and merge into the following one. Not only do the formant transitions change as a function of the acoustic surroundings, but the formants of the vowel's *hub*, or midportion, show accommodative shifting as well. Therefore, studies designed to assess formant characteristics have usually used either a standard phonetic context or a simple prolongation of an isolated vowel.[20] Measurements are commonly made at the midportion of the vowel production. Assessment of a patient's speech should do the same if comparability with published data is to be preserved.

Table 7–1 summarizes formant frequency data from five research studies:

---

[19] An externally applied sine wave signal, rapidly swept through a wide frequency range, can provide an excellent delineation of formants (Fujimura & Lindqvist, 1971). However, it requires the speaker to maintain a static articulatory posture and entails more complexity than the clinical situation is likely to warrant.

[20] Some investigations of diphthongs have also been done: See Holbrook and Fairbanks (1962), for example.

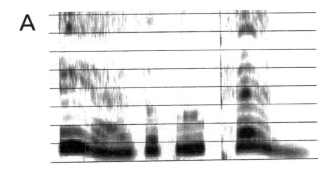

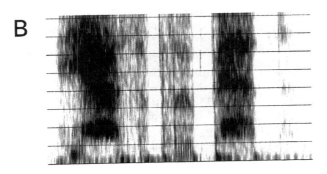

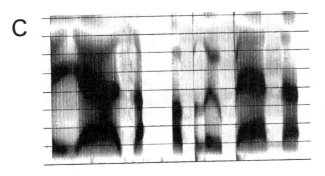

/hi hæz ə blu pɛn/

Figure 7–40. Three analyses of the utterance "He has a blue pen," each produced with a 293-Hz bandwidth. **A.** The speaker's relatively high vocal F_0 causes individual harmonics to be resolved. Determining accurate formant frequencies with such a display is difficult at best. **B.** Formant energy is more easily recognized when the utterance is whispered. **C.** Formants are particularly clear in this display where an electrolarynx has been used to provide the "source" signal.

1. Peterson and Barney (1952) evaluated a population of 33 men, 28 women, and 15 children (ages unspecified) that had been studied earlier by Potter and Steinberg (1950). Each speaker did two readings of a list of 10 words: *heed, hid, head, had, hod,*

hawed, who'd, hud, and *heard.* Formant frequencies were located in narrow-band sections taken at the midpoint of each vowel.

2. Angelocci, Kopp, and Holbrook (1964) studied two groups (normal and deaf speakers) of 18 boys each, age 11–14 years. (Only data for the normal boys are included in Table 7–1.) The same vowels as in the Peterson and Barney (1952) study (in a different phonetic context) were analyzed in very much the same way.

3. Eguchi and Hirsh (1969) explored developmental changes of a number of speech variables, including formant frequencies. The subject population included 5 children at each age from 3 to 10 years, 5 boys and 5 girls at each age from 11 to 13 years, and 5 men and 5 women. Each subject spoke two sentences: "He has a blue pen" and "I am tall." Narrow-band sections were used to locate the first two formants of each of the italicized vowels (/i/, /æ/, /u/, /ɛ/, /ɔ/) and the first vowel from the diphthong "I" (/ɑɪ/).

4. Hillenbrand, Getty, Clark, and Wheeler (1995) studied 45 men, 48 women, and 46 children (27 boys and 19 girls) ages 10–12 years. Each speaker read a list of 12 words that included those used by Peterson and Barney (1952), plus *hayed* and *hoed.* Formant frequencies were determined using LPC spectra at the "maximally steady" midpoint of each vowel.

5. Lee, Potamianos, and Narayanan (1999) studied 29 men, 27 women, and 436 children (229 boys and 207 girls) between the age of ages 5 and 18 years. Each speaker read or repeated the words *bead, bit, bet, bat, pot, ball, but, put, boot,* and *bird* in the carrier phrase "I say uh _____ again." Formant frequencies were determined using an automatic tracking LPC program supplemented by manual estimation based on visual inspection of spectral displays.

There is an orderly progression of formant frequencies in Table 7–1, a regularity that is made clearer in actual spectrograms of the same vowels (produced in the same /h—d/ contexts), as in Figure 7–41. There is a definite pattern of formant change across vowels. The pattern is most easily explored by preparing a graph, in which the second formant is plotted against the first formant. Figure 7–42A shows just such a plot, prepared by Peterson and Barney (1952) to demonstrate the formant positions of vowels spoken by all of their subjects. Note that there is considerable dispersion of the data points; the same vowel can have a very different F1/F2 relationship when produced by different speak-

Table 7–1. Mean Vocal Fundamental Frequency and Formant Frequencies (in Hz) for Vowels Produced by Normal Men, Women, and Children

	/i/	/ɪ/	/e/	/ɛ/	/æ/	/ɑ/	/ɔ/	/o/	/ʊ/	/u/	/ʌ/	/ɝ/	Source
					Vowels								
					Men								
F_0	136	135	—	130	127	124	129	—	137	141	130	133	a
	138	135	129	127	123	123	121	129	133	144	133	130	d
	132	136	—	129	123	135	127	—	149	144	130	134	e
F1	270	390	—	530	660	730	570	—	440	300	640	490	a
	288	—	—	555	645	—	653	—	—	344	—	—	c
	342	427	476	580	588	768	652	497	469	378	623	474	d
	292	458	—	590	669	723	601	—	501	342	610	471	e
F2	2290	1990	—	1840	1720	1090	840	—	1020	870	1190	1350	a
	2217	—	—	1726	1723	—	1048	—	1256	—	—		c
	2322	2034	2089	1799	1952	1333	997	910	1122	997	1200	1379	d
	2266	1851	—	1707	1725	1204	929	—	1269	1185	1288	1265	e
F3	3010	2550	—	480	2410	2440	2410	—	2240	2240	2390	1690	a
	3000	2684	2691	2605	2601	2522	2538	2459	2434	2343	2550	1710	d
	2930	2588	—	2549	2532	2496	2599	—	2466	2411	2557	1612	e
					Women								
F_0	235	232	—	223	210	212	216	—	232	231	221	218	a
	227	224	219	214	215	215	210	217	230	235	218	217	d
	228	235	—	219	215	231	213	—	246	243	218	222	e
F1	310	430	—	610	860	850	590	—	470	370	760	500	a
	338	—	—	589	761	—	666	—	—	356	—	—	c
	437	483	536	731	669	936	781	555	519	459	753	523	d
	360	532	—	694	787	894	726	—	595	412	740	543	e
F2	2790	2480	—	2330	2050	1220	920	—	1160	950	1400	1640	a
	2810	—	—	2111	2054	—	1135	—	—	1460	—	—	c
	2761	2365	2530	2058	2349	1551	1136	1035	1225	1105	1426	1588	d
	2757	2183	—	2057	2078	1459	1079	—	1522	1388	1609	1481	e
F3	3310	3070	—	2990	2850	2810	2710	—	2680	2670	2780	1960	a
	3372	3053	3047	2979	2972	2815	2824	2828	2827	2735	2933	1929	d
	3291	3064	—	3005	2916	2950	2986	—	2887	2804	2957	1884	e
					Children								
F_0	27	269	—	260	251	256	263	—	276	274	261	261	a
	246	241	237	230	228	229	225	236	243	249	236	237	d
F1	370	530	—	690	1010	1030	680	—	560	430	850	560	a
	452	511	564	749	717	1002	803	597	568	494	749	586	d
F2	3200	2730	—	2610	2320	1370	1060	—	1410	1170	1590	1820	a
	3081	2552	2656	2267	2501	1688	1210	1137	1490	1345	1546	1719	d
F3	3730	3600	—	3570	3320	3170	3180	—	3310	3260	3360	2160	a
	3702	3403	3323	3310	3289	2950	2982	2987	3072	2988	3145	2143	d
					(Boys)								
F_0	199	191	—	189	187	188	189	—	194	204	195	194	b
	212	211	—	206	203	210	202	—	221	218	206	204	e
F1	262	410	—	606	588	917	762	—	500	363	671	396	b
	370	—	—	652	645	—	724	—	—	427	—	—	c

(Continued)

Vowels

	/i/	/ɪ/	/e/	/ɛ/	/æ/	/ɑ/	/ɔ/	/o/	/ʊ/	/u/	/ʌ/	/ɝ/	Source
	367	520	—	692	798	857	700	—	568	430	696	550	e
F2	2776	2300	—	2079	2231	1376	1067	—		061	1427	1459	b
	2794	—	—	2047	1987	—	1193	—	—	1347	—	—	c
	2711	2217	—	2010	2050	1393	1063	—	1426	1559	1443	1486	e
F3	3251	2974	—	2908	2961	2705	2750	—	2791	2757	2813	1909	b
	3334	3095	—	3056	2954	2837	2970	—	2926	2765	2984	1955	e

(Girls)

	/i/	/ɪ/	/e/	/ɛ/	/æ/	/ɑ/	/ɔ/	/o/	/ʊ/	/u/	/ʌ/	/ɝ/	Source
F_0	240	244	—	234	231	239	232	—	261	246	236	234	e
F1	386	—	—	635	703	—	812	—	—	433	—	—	c
	437	573	—	748	840	943	763	—	628	462	760	628	e
F2	2994	—	—	2244	2188	—	1503	—	—	1443	—	—	c
	2852	2359	—	2166	2158	1567	1209	—	1571	1746	1672	1654	e
F3	3363	3255	—	3248	3100	3046	3139	—	3117	2922	3208	2172	e

Sources: (a) Peterson and Barney, 1952; (b) Angelocci, Kopp, and Holbrook, 1964; (c) Eguchi and Hirsh, 1969; (d) Hillenbrand, Getty, Clark, and Wheeler, 1995; and (e) Lee, Potamianos, and Narayanan, 1999. For sources c and e, data for boys and girls averaged over tabled values for 11–14 year olds. See text and original sources for details. (Sources a–c are reprinted, along with other classic papers in speech spectrography, in Baken and Daniloff, 1991.)

ers. Outlining the zone within which each vowel lies shows that the dispersion is great enough to produce overlap of vowel areas (for example, /ɝ/ and /ɛ/). What this indicates is that the formant pattern of, say, /ɔ/ for one speaker might be the same as a different speaker's pattern for /ɝ/. The formant similarity of two different vowels by two different speakers is a demonstration of the fact that formants do not uniquely specify the vowel category.[21]

Isovowel Lines and Formant Scaling

The F2/F1 graph can be simplified by plotting the mean formant values for each vowel. This has been done separately for the men, women, and children in Figure 7–42B. It now becomes even clearer that the orderly progression of formant changes across vowels is related in some way to the vocal tract configuration assumed for each one. Note how the mean relationships of the formants outline the classic vowel diagram. More important for the present purposes is the fact that there seems to be a regular relationship among the formant locations of men, women, and children. In Figure 7–42C, the F2/F1 loci of vowels as produced by the three groups are connected together

to demonstrate this. These so called *isovowel lines* (Broad, 1976) show that the progression is not fully regular, but there is a strong sense that the loci are "fleeing" from the origin of the graph.

What significance, validity, and applicability does this have? It helps, in answering these questions, to begin by considering how isovowel lines are generated. Suppose a group of speakers all produce several vowels. The formant frequencies of each production are determined and plotted, as in Figure 7–43A, forming "clouds" on the graph. Using a mathematical technique called regression analysis, two very important characteristics about each group of data points can be determined. One is the equation of a **best-fit** line (also called a **least squares** line) that can be drawn through each aggregation of points. (It is called "best fit" because the average distance of the data points from the line is minimized.) The equation of the line has the general form $F2 = bF1 + a$. The coefficient b is the slope of the isovowel line and represents the average F2/F1 ratio for the data points included in the analysis. Conceptually, the best-fit line depicts the locus of points along which all F2/F1 relationships would lie if the data were "pure," that is, uninfluenced by any external factor and not contaminated by error.

---

[21]See Miller (1989) and Nearey (1989) for detailed discussions of this issue. Also addressed are various attempts to improve acoustic vowel classification by "normalizing" formant frequencies using nonlinear semitone, mel, Koenig, and Bark scales.

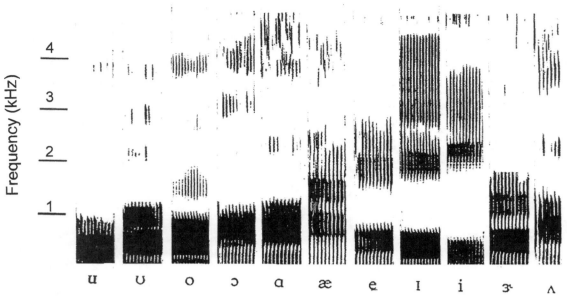

Figure 7–41. Formant patterns of the English vowels.

The extent to which this last concept holds is quantified in the **_correlation coefficient_**, which is the second important parameter determined by regression analysis. It specifies how spread out the data are, that is, how far on the average the data points lie from the idealization represented by the best-fit line. Obviously, the closer the points are to the line, the more likely it is that it does, in fact, represent some real underlying relationship and not just the meaningless product of a mathematical manipulation. Even better, the square of the correlation coefficient (called the **_coefficient of determination_**) is the proportion of F2/F1 position change that is attributable to the relationship represented by the best-fit line. (The rest of the data-point variability is attributable to other unknown influences and to error.) If, for example, the coefficient of determination is 0.5 or higher, we may conclude that there is a significant linear relationship among the points because at least 50% of the change in the F2/F1 position is accounted for by the equation of the best-fit line.

This kind of scaling has been explored by a number of acoustic phoneticians (see, for example, Peterson, 1961; Mol, 1963; Fant, 1973, 1975), but most relevantly by Kent (1978, 1979) and by Kent and Forner (1979), who studied the formants of /i, æ, ɑ, u, ɝ/ as produced by 4-, 5-, and 6-year-old boys and girls and by men and women. Regression analysis of the sort just described resulted in F2/F1 isovowel lines as shown in Figure 7–43B. As the coefficients of determination show, linear relationships are quite strong, except in the case of /æ/. If the "_a_" term is dropped from the best-fit equation, leaving only the "_b_" (slope) coefficient, extensions of the best-fit lines will all pass through the graph's origin, forming a set of radiating isovowel "rays."

Each of the rays represents the change in the F2/F1 ratio as the vocal tract increases in size. Data for the small vocal tracts of children lie more distant from the origin than those for men whose relatively large vocal tracts have lower formant frequencies. Also, in many ways the rays of the diagram represent the life history of the vocal tract. As an individual's vocal tract grows and changes, his vowel formants travel down the rays toward the graph's origin. Most of the movement will occur during childhood, but both anatomic (Israel, 1968, 1973) and acoustic (Endres, Bombach, & Flösser, 1971; Linville & Fisher, 1985; Rastatter & Jacques, 1990; Scukanec, Petrosino, & Squibb, 1991) studies provide ample reason to believe that vocal tract development extends across the life span.

Kent (1979) describes how the "universal" isovowel lines can be of use to the clinician. It is simply a matter of measuring a patient's formant frequencies and plotting them onto a graph with the appropriate isovowel lines (Figure 7–43C). The distance of the plotted data points from their respective isovowel lines is at least an approximate measure of deviance. Kent shows, for instance, how plotting the data of Angelocci, Kopp, and Holbrook (1964) for deaf boys on the isovowel lines results in a vowel triangle that is much smaller than normal (that is, its vertices do not extend to the isovowel lines), demonstrating severe vowel centralization in this population. (Similar data from Monsen, 1976b, also show this effect.) Using the same evaluation procedure, Kent, Netsell, and Abbs (1979) demonstrated that formant structure was largely undisturbed in cerebellar dysarthria, while Kent and Rosenbek (1983) have explored vowel errors in apraxics.

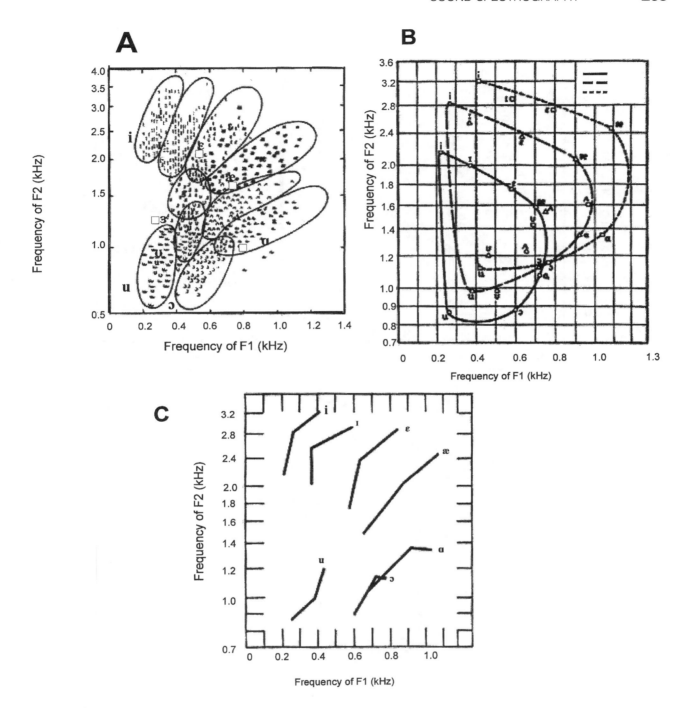

Figure 7–42. **A**. The frequency of the second formant plotted against the frequency of the first formant for vowels spoken by 76 speakers Adapted from Peterson and Barney (1952, p. 182). Reprinted by permission from *Speech Physiology and Acoustic Phonetics: An Introduction,* by P. Lieberman, 1977, New York: Macmillan, p. 68. **B**. F2/F1 relationships for vowels spoken by men, women, and children; and **C**. Isovowel lines created by connected the "man," "woman," and "child" loci of Figure 7–42B. (The "child" end of each line has been labeled by the IPA symbol for each vowel.)

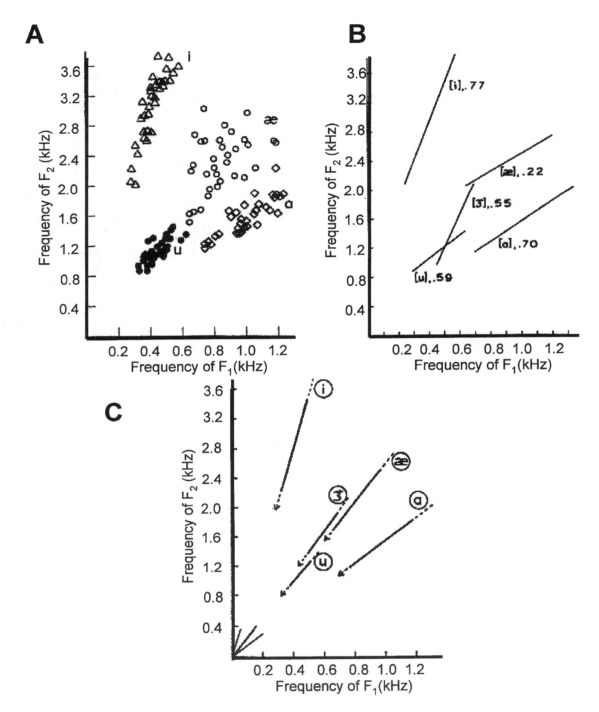

Figure 7–43. **A**. A scattergram of F2 and F1 frequencies of English vowels as spoken by 33 men, women, and children. Reprinted with permission from "Developmental Study of Vowel Formant Frequencies in an Imitation Task," by R. D. Kent and L. L. Forner, 1979, *Journal of the Acoustical Society of America, 65,* 208–217. Figure 2, p. 210. **B**. Isovowel lines (least-squares regression) for the data points of Figure 7–43A. The number associated with each line is its R² coefficient of determination, which indicates the proportion of variability accounted for by the F2/F1 relationship (Kent and Forner, 1979, Figure 3, p. 211. Reprinted with permission). **C**. Isovowel lines as determined by Kent (1979). The solid midportion of each line represents the region for which normative data were available; dashed segments were extrapolated. Each line can be described by an equation of the form F2 = *b*.F1, where *b* is the slope of the line. The coefficients for the lines shown are: /i/ = 7.11; /u/ = 2.48; /ɑ/ = 1.545; /ɑ/ = 2.65; and /ɜ/ = 2.79. Reprinted with permission from "Isovowel lines for the evaluation of formant structure in speech disorders," by R. D. Kent, 1979, *Journal of Speech and Hearing Disorders, 44,* 513–521. Figure 1, p. 515. © American Speech-Language-Hearing Association, Rockville, MD.

Kent (1979) suggests that F3/F2 plots can also be used to improve vowel-formant assessment. He also adds an important caution to the effect that the position of a patient's F2/F1 locus in relation to an isovowel line is not as important as its position with respect to the *age-appropriate segment* of the line. For example, an F2/F1 point for a man might fall directly on the isovowel line, but quite far from the origin. The distant (upper right) reaches of the line are normally the province of young children. As noted earlier, advancing age should move the F2/F1 points toward the lower left. Therefore, the hypothetical man in question has a highly abnormal set of formants, despite their exact coincidence with the isovowel norm.

While no exact age-division of the line can be done, Table 7–2 may help the clinician locate regions broadly associated with different ages. The data are taken from the Eguchi and Hirsh (1969) study described earlier. There are five children in each of the age or age-sex groups. In using these data, remember that the phonetic context of the vowels was very different from that of Kent's studies.

Plotting a patient's F2/F1"vowel space" and then comparing it with formant ratios obtained from normal speakers of similar age and sex can be another effective way to assess vocal tract function (see, for instance, Kahane, 1979, or Kamen and Watson, 1991). Figure 7–44 shows a similar representation for a child with a severe articulation disorder. Note that, in comparison with Eguchi and Hirsh's (1969) data for normal children, this patient's vowel space is greatly restricted and "centralized"—characteristics that are typical for speakers with reduced articulatory capabilities. Such vowel space representations thus may be used as an index of a speaker's articulatory posturing and flexibility.

Specific Influences on Vowel Spectra

Vocal tract shaping. From the studies cited at the opening of this chapter and others, it is possible to formulate a set of "rules" that relate specific changes in formant patterns to actions or shapes of the vocal tract. Caution is required in drawing inferences from them, since many were derived by changing a vocal tract analog (often an electrical circuit or computer model) and noting the effect on the resulting vowel formants. Reasoning in the other direction, from formant frequencies to vocal tract shape, is not necessarily valid, since there are many degrees of freedom. In theory, there are an infinite number of vocal tract shapes that could produce a given formant frequency. However, as a rough guide, the following relationships may prove useful. They are schematized in Figure 7–45.

1. *Vocal tract length*. The frequency of all formants lowers as the length of the vocal tract increases.

2. *Lip rounding*. Increasing the constriction of the labial port lowers all formant frequencies.

3. *Anterior oral constriction*. Elevation of the front of the tongue lowers F1 and raises F2.

4. *Posterior oral constriction*. Raising the posterior part of the tongue tends to lower F2.

5. *Pharyngeal constriction*. Narrowing the pharynx raises the frequence of F1.

6. *Nasalization*. The effects of coupling the nasal resonant space to the vocal tract are very complex. Not only are resonant frequencies altered, but anti-resonances are introduced. The overall result is highly variable. (Specific nasalization characteristics are summarized in Chapter 11, "Velopharyngeal Function.")

Vocal effort or intensity. A number of studies have shown that the glottal (source) wave changes with increasing vocal effort or intensity; that is, its rise and decay become steeper and its turning points become sharper and more abrupt (see Chapter 10, "Laryngeal Function"). Spectrally, these changes indicate more energy at high frequencies. In fact, the extended bandwidth of the vocal signal is one of the acoustical correlates of increased loudness (Zwicker, Flottorp, & Stevens, 1957; Brandt, Ruder, & Shipp, 1969). Therefore, as vocal intensity increases, the vocal source spectrum shows increased amplitude of high-frequency harmonics, which results in elevation of the amplitude of F2 and F3.

Speech rate. The effect of rate of syllable production on the formant frequencies is still a matter of some dispute. Lindblom (1963), Fourakis (1991), and Asano and Kiritani (1992) report that formants (and especially F2) change as speech rate increases (which causes vowel duration to decrease). In essence, these changes have been considered to represent an "undershoot" in the approximation of a target vocal-tract posture as increasing speed demands are placed on the system. On the other hand, studies by Gay (1978) and Engstrand (1988) have failed to detect a change in the formants of the vowel midpoint when speakers changed from a slow to a fast syllabic rate. Testing several vowels from written material recited at normal and fast rates, von Son and Pols (1990) also found little evidence of undershoot vowel reduction, but did note a systematic increase in F1 frequency across vowels when speech rate increased.

Table 7–2. Mean Formant Frequencies (in Hz) for Vowels Produced by Children at Different Ages

Age	/i/ F1	/i/ F2	/ɛ/ F1	/ɛ/ F2	/æ/ F1	/æ/ F2	/ɔ/ F1	/ɔ/ F2	/u/ F1	/u/ F2
					Boys and Girls					
3	484	3318	673	2683	786	2599	802	1485	578	1664
4	444	3050	566	2397	567	2281	762	1390	472	1528
5	408	3235	642	2418	643	2423	901	1513	452	1477
6	397	3108	512	2281	611	2238	689	1308	431	1385
7	411	3204	664	2280	736	2299	817	1398	481	1525
8	397	3104	585	2195	685	2222	743	1359	450	1437
9	403	3106	308	2296	647	2295	836	1352	469	1392
10	403	3028	645	2193	735	2255	814	1336	469	1351
					Boys					
11	397	2778	671	2109	620	2063	724	1284	448	1388
12	359	2877	618	2059	658	2012	705	1175	404	1253
13	355	2727	668	1974	658	1885	744	1120	428	1347
					Girls					
11	423	3134	628	2359	736	2266	799	1325	478	1474
12	358	2940	687	2169	700	2136	830	1382	422	1436
13	377	2907	590	2205	672	2161	806	1802	399	1420

Source: From "Development of Speech Sounds in Children," by S. Eguchi and I. J. Hirsh, 1969, *Acta Otolaryngologica, Suppl. 257*, 5–43. Table 1, pp. 9–13. Reprinted by permission. (Five children in each group; Analysis of the italicized vowels in "He has a blue pen" and "I am tall.")

Spectral Features: Consonants

Öhman (1967) has proposed that it is useful to view consonants as articulatory gestures superimposed on an underlying continuous variation of vowel productions. The consonants have several important characteristics that cause their spectra to differ in fundamental ways from those of the background vowels. Aside from the fact that consonants may include silent intervals, nasalizations, and aspirations, consonantal spectra are profoundly influenced by two critical facts:

1. While the sournd source for normal English vowels is always the periodic and harmonic-rich glottal pulse, consonants can be formed from the periodic glottal tone, aperiodic turbulence noise, or a combination of the two. The effects of this latitude on the spectrogram are obvious.

2. Consonants (even the relatively open /j/ and /w/) are produced with significantly more constriction of the vocal tract than vowels. Constriction, of course, reaches an extreme in the case of the plosives, for which there is a brief period of airway closure. The tighter constriction of consonants results in less radiated sound energy than vowels (see Chapter 5, "Speech Intensity").

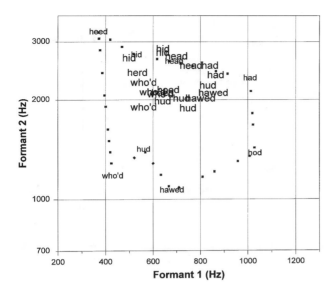

Figure 7–44. The reduced and centralized F2/F1 data of a child with a severe articulation disorder compared with the average "vowel space" determined by Eguchi and Hirsh (1969) for normal children (dotted line).

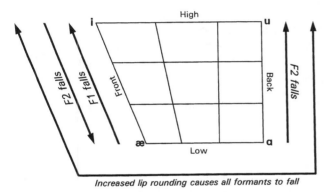

Increased lip rounding causes all formants to fall

Figure 7–45. Relationship between vowel position and formant values. Based on these changes, front vowels tend to have a relatively high separation between F1 and F2, whereas back vowels tend to have a relatively low F1–F2 separation.

In discussing vowels, the point was made that formant frequencies change during the transitions from the preceding, and to the following, sounds. Furthermore, it was said that, even in its stable midsection, the formant frequencies of a given vowel could be expected to be different as a function of the phonetic surroundings. The same effect is seen in consonants. Each begins with an onset transition period during which its acoustic characteristics are built upon the foundation of the preceding sound, and terminates as

an offset transition as its acoustic signal modifies toward that of the succeeding sound. And, as was the case for vowels, the acoustic midportion of the consonant can be expected to show substantial accommodation to its neighbors.

These effects, of course, are the acoustic manifestation of the constant motion of the articulators. Speech is not a sequence of static postures, each representing a discrete phoneme. Rather, the higher neurological control calls for, and the vocal tract biomechanics impose, an overlapping of sounds on the motor and acoustic level. In saying "spot," for example, lip closure for /p/ is occurring during /s/ production. The resonances of /s/ will reflect the ever-diminishing labial opening: Part of the /p/ "resides" in the /s/. In short, coarticulatory effects are significant.

Just as elementary courses in phonetics present a picture of rather idealized speech sounds, for the same reasons the following sections on the English consonants will deal with idealized spectral features. The physiological classification of speech sounds according to articulatory *manner* has its counterpart in spectral features and, thus, will be used to organize the discussion. It should be noted that temporal aspects of consonants are important to their perceptual differentiation but, with a few exceptions, durational aspects of consonant features will not be specifically addressed here. (More information on this subject is available in Liberman, Delattre, and Cooper, 1952; Denes, 1955; Liberman, Delattre, Gerstman, and Cooper, 1956; Liberman, Harris, Hoffman, & Griffith, 1957; Liberman, 1957; Hawkins, 1973; DiSimoni, 1974a, 1974b, 1974c; Klatt, 1974; Umeda, 1975, 1977; Parnell et al., 1977; Prosek and Runyan, 1982; Crystal and House, 1988; Weismer, 1984a; Jongman, 1989; and in Weismer and Liss, 1991).

SONORANTS

Phoneticians use the term *sonorant* in various ways. For the present discussion, it is considered to mean a voiced speech sound that is produced with airflow that is neither fully laminar (as for vowels) nor totally turbulent (as is the case with fricatives). There are two generally recognized classes of sonorant consonants: (1) The *approximants* (which can be further subdivided to include the *semivowels* or *glides*: /w/ and /j/; and the *liquids*: the *lateral* /l/ and the *retroflex* /r/), and (2) The *nasals* (which include /m/, /n/, and /ŋ/).

Semivowels

The semivowels /j/ and /w/ are aptly named. Although more constricted, they are physiologically and acoustically similar to /i/ and /u/, respectively. When combined with a vowel, these consonants produce a pattern of formant change that very much resembles a diphthong (Figure 7–46). The greater constriction of the consonants, however, results in lower F1 and F2 frequencies than is typical of these vowels. The third formant of /w/ is commonly weak or missing (weaker sound radiation for consonants), and the third formant of /j/ is often at a higher frequency than that of /i/.

An important difference between diphthongs and semivowel glides is the much briefer duration of the consonants, meaning the formant transitions are faster. Furthermore, the duration of these phonemes may be too short for the formants to stabilize at all. In that case, of course, /w/ and /j/ reduce to little more than a formant transition between two other sounds. This is not a problem since perceptual discrimination of different approximant consonants depends heavily on the transitional patterns of F2 and F3 (Lisker, 1957a; O'Connor, Gerstman, Liberman, Delattre, & Cooper, 1957; Lehiste & Peterson, 1961; Dalston, 1975; Sharf & Benson, 1982; Ohde & Sharf, 1992; Orlikoff & Baken, 1993; Pickett, 1999).

Liquids

The lateral consonant /l/ is characterized by great formant variability, particularly of F2, whose frequency is strongly influenced by the surrounding vowels. Syllabic /l/ is somewhat more stable (Tarnøczy, 1948; Lehiste, 1964). The syllable-final /ɫ/, however, tends to show a higher F1 and lower F2 than the more common /l/.

Despite the very great variety of articulator postures used for the retroflex /r/ (Delattre, 1965), the acoustic product is almost always characterized by extreme lowering of F3, bringing it close to F2. This phenomenon is the signature of /r/ in English (Lehiste, 1964; Klein, 1971; McGovern & Strange, 1977; Sharf & Benson, 1982; Hoffman, Schuckers, & Daniloff, 1989). On the other hand, the syllabic /ɝ/ and syllable-final /ɚ/ (typically referred to as "r-colored" vowels) have a higher F3. Acoustically, /r/ is influenced by its position in the utterance (initial, medial, etc.) more than by the physiological differences in production style (O'Connor et al., 1957; Hoffman, Schuckers, & Ratusnik, 1977). Initial /r/, for instance, has generally lower formants that other /r/s and, in general, is relatively immune to the influence of the following vowel. The formants of /ɝ/ or /ɚ/ are strongly influenced by the preceding vowel, however.

Dalston (1975) has studied word-initial /l, r, w/ as produced by normal children and adults. His data are comparable to those of the other investigators cited

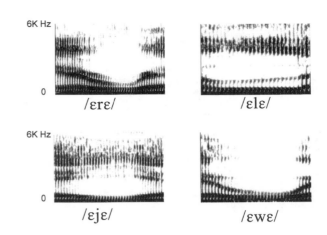

Figure 7–46. Wide-band spectrograms of intervocalic semivowel and liquid consonants.

above, and he confirmed that the formant transitions of the approximants are important to to their discrimination. Tables 7–3 and 7–4 summarize his findings of formant frequencies of the steady-state portions of the approximants and their formant transition characteristics. Shuster, Ruscello, and Smith (1992) report the successful use of spectrographic feedback to improve an 18-year-old patient's articulation of /r/ and //ɝ/. They also suggest that preliminary attempts to employ the technique with school-aged children who had been "resistant to [r] acquisition" are encouraging.

Nasals

The primary resonator for the nasal consonants is the pharynx and nasal cavity. The oral cavity serves as a dead-end (occluded) resonator that is coupled to the rest of the vocal tract approximately at its midpoint. (Because the oral cavity is occluded, this type of consonant is sometimes called a "stop-nasal.") The length of this side branch is longest for /m/ (labial occlusion) and shortest for /ŋ/ (linguavelar occlusion). Pharyngeal shape is essentially the same for all three nasal consonants, and the geometry of the nasal cavity itself cannot be voluntarily altered. It is, therefore, not surprising that the nasal consonants have similar formant peaks.

The addition of a side branch to the resonating system creates *antiresonances* in its transfer function. In contrast to formant peaks, that represent spectral maxima, antiresonances are valleys in the spectral envelope that represent spectral minima. Like formants, however, antiresonances are located at specific frequencies. It has been shown by Fant (1960, 1973)

Table 7–3. Steady-State Formant Frequencies (in Hz) of Word-Initial /w, r, l/ Produced by Normal Speakers of English*

	Men		Women		Children	
	Mean	(SD)	Mean	(SD)	Mean	(SD)
			/r/			
F1	348	(45.9)	350	(38.3)	431	(49.8)
F2	1061	(92.5)	1065	(85.4)	1503	(191.8)
F3	1546	(94.8)	2078	(346.1)	2491	(369.8)
			/w/			
F1	336	(39.2)	337	(30.4)	402	(59.7)
F2	732	(87.6)	799	(87.8)	1020	(148.8)
F3	2290	(335.8)	2768	(141.7)	3547	(223.7)
			/l/			
F1	344	(55.2)	365	(11.6)	412	(38.4)
F2	1179	(141.2)	1340	(96.8)	1384	(175.3)
F3	2523	(197.8)	2935	(174.4)	3541	(293.0)

*Subjects were 6 boys, age 3 years 3 months to 4 years 3 months (mean = 4 years 0 months); 4 girls, age 3 years 5 months to 4 years 3 months (mean = 3 years 11 months); 3 men (mean age 25 years); and 2 women (mean age 18 years). Word-initial /r, w, l/ combined with /(, ɑ, (/ in simple words; 5 repetitions of each word.

From "Acoustic characteristics of English /w, r, l/ spoken correctly by young children and adults," by R. M. Dalston, 1975, *Journal of the Acoustical Society of America*, *57*, 462–469. Table II, p. 464. Reprinted by permission.

that each antiresonance produced by coupling in a side-branch resonator is associated with an added resonance in the transfer function. Thus, the oral side branch produces resonance-antiresonance *pairs*. The frequency-separation between the added resonance peak and its counterpart antiresonance is a function of the amount of coupling between the side branch (oral cavity and the main resonator pharynx-nasal cavity). Strong coupling (that is, a large connecting orifice) results in wide separation between the resonance and antiresonance pair, whereas weak coupling causes the two to be closer together. In fact, with a very narrow communicating orifice between the two resonating chambers, the resonance and antiresonance may fall at essentially the same frequency. In this case, of course, they will cancel each other and produce no net change of the vocal tract transfer function. Specific spectral features of nasalization are considered in Chapter 11, to which the reader should refer for a more detailed listing of the effects of side-branch coupling on the speech signal.

The three nasal consonants of English (whose spectrograms are shown in Figure 7–47) are distinguished from each other by the frequency location of the resonance-antiresonances and by the formant transitions between the consonant and its surrounding sounds.

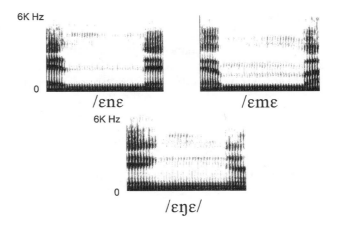

Figure 7–47. Wide-band spectrograms of intervocalic nasal consonants.

Table 7–4. Mean Formant Durations (in ms) and Transition Rates (in Hz/ms) of Word-Initial /w, r, l/ Produced by Normal Speakers of English

		Adults		Children	
		Mean	**(SD)**	**Mean**	**(SD)**
		$/r/$			
Steady-state portion	F1	39.2	(23.2)	40.3	(15.3)
	F2	35.5	(14.8)	41.2	(15.0)
Transition duration	F1	33.7	(20.4)	32.7	(19.2)
	F2	50.4	(17.3)	52.3	(21.5)
Transition rate	F1	3.9	(2.2)	8.0	(7.7)
	F2	10.5	(6.6)	11.7	(6.9)
		$/w/$			
Steady-state portion	F1	39.6	(16.1)	39.0	(23.1)
	F2	44.4	(20.2)	39.5	(21.9)
Transition duration	F1	32.7	(18.7)	36.9	(18.2)
	F2	58.3	(26.8)	55.0	(24.7)
Transition rate	F1	3.5	(3.5)	7.7	(7.5)
	F2	11.8	(6.9)	7.4	(9.5)
		$/l/$			
Steady-state portion	F1	67.0	(19.0)	56.7	(14.6)
	F2	57.0	(19.9)	55.4	(15.9)
Transition duration	F1	21.3	(15.7)	21.8	(14.1)
	F2	41.3	(26.7)	41.1	(28.1)
Transition rate	F1	8.5	(6.6)	11.2	(9.5)
	F2	11.4	(4.5)	19.0	(7.0)

Source: From "Acoustic Characteristics of English /w, r, l/ Spoken Correctly by Young Children and Adults," by R. M. Dalston, 1975, *Journal of the Acoustical Society of America, 57*, 462–469. Table II, p. 464. Reprinted by permission. (For method, see Table 7–3.)

Resonances and Antiresonances

The nasalization resonances and antiresonances are added to (or subtracted from) the transfer function of the major resonating tube. The antiresonance may be most easily detected in the spectral envelope. Its position depends on the length of the side branch: The longer it is, the lower the antiresonance frequency (House, 1957; Hattori, Yamamoto, & Fujimura, 1958). Typically, the major antiresonances are at about 1000 Hz for /m/, 3500 Hz for /n/, and above 5000 Hz for /ɰ/.

Second-Formant Frequency

The frequency of F2 also plays an important role in the perception of the place of articulation. Nakata (1959)

and Hecker (1962) have explored this parameter using synthetic speech signals. Their results indicate that second-formant frequencies in the range of 1200 Hz, 1800 Hz, and 2100 Hz are strong cues to /m/, /n/, and /ɰ/, respectively.

Formant Transitions

It is clear that formant transitions associated with oral occlusion and opening also play an important role in the discrimination of nasal consonants (Malécot, 1956; Fujimura, 1962; Larkey, Wald, & Strange, 1978; Recasens, 1983; Kurowski & Blumstein, 1984, 1987; Repp, 1986; Orlikoff & Baken, 1993; Pickett, 1999). The transition patterns are very complex and not yet completely characterized.

FRICATIVES

The aerodynamic feature that characterizes fricatives is airstream turbulence, generated by airflow through a tight constriction in the vocal tract (Stevens, 1971; Catford, 1977; Scully, Castelli, Brearley, & Shirt, 1992). The turbulence is random fluctuation of local air pressure, the acoustic correlate of which is aperiodic noise (Hughes & Halle, 1956; Strevens, 1960; Bauer & Kent, 1987; Behrens & Blumstein, 1988a, 1988b; Jongman, 1989). The vocal tract in which the noise is generated, however, is an active resonant space with a real transfer function that influences the radiated noise signal, limiting its bandwidth. Therefore, the spectra of fricatives contain a strong continuous-spectrum component extending over a frequency range that is broad but limited. This is clearly shown in Figure 7–48A. Note the ways in which /s/ differs from /i/: The absence of glottal pulses (voiceless), continuous spectrum (noise), and noise energy concentrated in the higher frequencies due to the influence of the vocal tract transfer function. When a voiced fricative is analyzed (Figure 7–48B) the spectrum shows the combined contributions of glottal pulsing and frication turbulence. Glottal pulsing continues throughout the fricative, although there is also a distinct high-frequency noise component. The amplitude spectrum shows the same evidence: During /ɑ/ the harmonics in the line spectrum are interspersed with random noise.

Although spectrally distinct as a group from other classes of speech sounds, the specific acoustic characteristics underlying the perceptual discrimination of individual fricative phones remain unclear. A number of listener identification criteria have been proposed, but none seems to completely separate a given fricative from all others (Hughes & Halle, 1956; Heinz & Stevens, 1961; Jassem, 1965). In fact, Harris (1954, 1958) has shown that discrimination of fricatives may depend heavily on the formant transitions of the post-fricative vowel rather than on the spectral properties of the consonant itself. Fricative formant transitions, particularly of F2, have since received a great deal of attention by investigators (Uldall, 1964; Soli, 1981; Nittrouer, Studdert-Kennedy, & McGowan, 1989)

Most attempts at characterizing the spectra of fricatives have centered on determination of the frequency limits of the noise band and on the location of any energy peaks within it. Differences in these parameters should, in theory, reflect changes in the length of the portion of the vocal tract anterior to the turbulence-producing constriction, since that is the effective resonating space. Several studies support that hypothesis (Heinz & Stevens, 1961; Pentz, Gilbert, & Zawadzki, 1979; Daniloff et al., 1980). Peak energy for /f/, which has an exceptionally short length of vocal

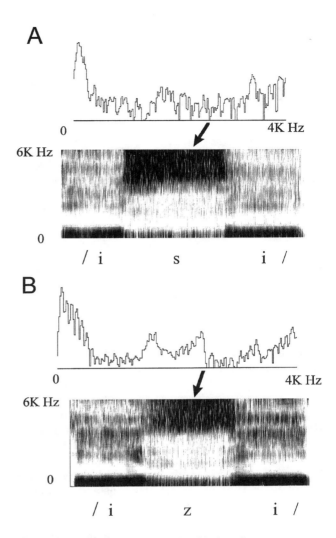

Figure 7–48. Spectrum and wide-band spectrograms for (**A**) /isi/ and (**B**) /izi/.

tract in front of the labiodental constriction, is at higher frequencies than peak energy for /ʃ/, whose constriction opens into a much larger resonating tube. The pattern of airflow and obstructions in the airstream also create acoustic differences by generating "spoiler" or "edge" noise that is added to the turbulence.

The formant peaks of the fricatives are not very strong, and they seem to show significant variation as a function of the vowel which follows them. Further complicating any attempt at a clear specification of the spectral properties is the fact that fricatives are prone to a great deal of allophonic modification and intersubject variability (Hughes & Halle, 1956; McGowan & Nittrouer, 1988; Nittrouer et al., 1989). All things considered, only a broad and general description of any given

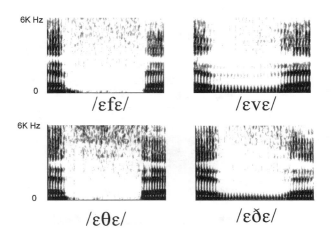

Figure 7–49. Wide-band spectrograms of intervocalic fricative consonants.

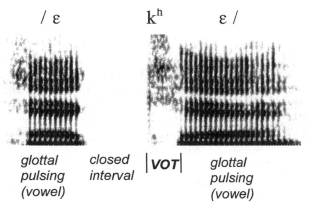

Figure 7–50. Wide-band spectrogram of an intervocalic plosive, delineating glottal pulsing, the closed interval (also called the "silent interval" or "stop gap"), and the voice onset time (VOT).

fricative can be offered. Figure 7–49 and Table 7–5 summarize their most salient features.

Given the fact that fricatives, and in particular /s/, are so often misarticulated in the school-age population, it is unfortunate that a firm grasp of the exact basis of their acoustic characteristics has been elusive. Both Mazza, Schuckers, and Daniloff (1979) and Daniloff, Wilcox, and Stephens (1980), for example, have studied the spectral features of children's /s/ misarticulations. While it was clear the listener's auditory impressions of abnormality had a basis in the acoustic signal, intersubject variability tends to be so high as to preclude a classification of more subtle /s/ distortions. Similar difficulties have been reported by Schäfersküpper, Amorosa, von Benda, and Dames (1986) and by Baum and McNutt (1990). However, the application of new analysis techniques, such as ***moment analysis***[22] (Forrest, Weismer, Milenkovic, & Dougall, 1988; McGowan & Nittrouer, 1988; Matthies, Svirsky, Lane, & Perkell, 1994; Buder, Kent, Kent, Milenkovic, & Workinger, 1996; Tjaden & Turner, 1997) and the ***self-organizing map*** (Mujunen, Leinonen, Kangas, & Torkkola, 1993), appear to hold promise as ways of discriminating the spectra of fricatives (and other obstruent consonants) judged to be acceptable from those perceived to be misarticulated.

PLOSIVES

The plosives (also called "stops" or "stop-plosives") are unique among the sounds of speech in that they include a variable period of total blockage of airflow during which sound output may cease. During this interval air pressure rises behind the point of closure to be released as a burst of acoustic energy. (The dynamics of airflow during stop consonants has been examined in detail by Rothenberg, 1968.) Plosive consonants are discriminated on the basis of three major parameters: (1) the characteristics of the burst (or impulse); (2) the nature of formant transitions before and after the silent (closure) period; and (3) the time required for reestablishment of glottal pulsing (voice onset time) following release of the closure. The appearance of these features in the spectrogram is illustrated in Figure 7–50.

Burst (Impulse) Characteristics

Release of the high back pressure associated with "voiceless" plosives gives rise to a more intense burst and often to significant aspiration. These are important cues to the voicing distinction in English. Intensity and aspiration aside, a number of studies have shown that the place of plosive articulation can be discriminated

---

[22] Briefly, moment analysis is a statistical approach used to assess the spectral *average* (that is, central tendency or "center of gravity"), the *diffuseness* of spectral energy, spectral *tilt*, and spectral *peakedness* (see Forrest et al., 1988, or Buder et al., 1996, for a detailed discussion of the analysis technique and the interpretation of moments).

Table 7–5. Spectral Characteristics of Fricatives Produced by Normal Speakers of English

Phone	Speaker	Noise Band Limits (Hz)	Energy Peak Locations (Hz)	Intensity	Source
f/v	Adults	1500–7000+	1900, 4000, 6800–8400	Low	a
			8200–12,000+		b
	Children		11,200–11,400		c
θ/ð	Adults	1400–7200+	2000	Low	a
s/z	Adults	>3500–8000+	Variable	Moderate	a
			3500–6400, 8000–8400		b
	Children		8300–8400		c
			6500, 10,000		d
ʃ/ʒ	Adults	1600–7000	Near Lower End	Moderate	a
			2200–2700, 4300—5400		b
	Children		5300		c

Sources: (*a*) Strevens, 1960; (*b*) Heinz and Stevens, 1961; (*c*) Pentz, Gilbert, and Zawadzki, 1979; and (*d*) Daniloff, Wilcox, and Stephens, 1980.

on the basis of the spectral characteriscs of the first 20 ms or so of the release burst (Halle, Hughes, & Radley, 1957; Liberman, 1957; Winitz, Scheib, & Reeds, 1972; Stevens & Blumstein, 1978; Blumstein & Stevens, 1979). In particular, the important features seem to be that:

1. The *labial* plosives /p, b/ have a primary energy concentration at low frequency (500–1500 Hz);

2. The *alveolar* plosives /t, d/ show either a flat burst spectrum or one in which energy is concentrated above 4000 Hz. There is also an energy peak at about 500 Hz; and

3. The *velar* plosives /k, g/ have their burst energy concentrated in the intermediate 1500–4000 Hz region.

These characteristics are by no means invariant and, in general, are subject to the following modifications:

1. Voiced plosives are likely to have continuous glottal pulsing that shows as a major concentration of energy below 300 Hz or so. (The burst interval will also have faint glottal striations in its spectrogram.)

2. The lower pressure of voiced plosives (see Chapter 8, "Air Pressure") results in less high-frequency energy in the burst. Hence, for example, /d/ would be expected to have less spectral amplitude above

4000 Hz than its voiceless cognate /t/.

3. The burst characteristics are modified by coarticulation of the following vowel (Fischer-Jørgensen, 1954). The velar plosives seem particularly susceptible to this effect. Their spectral peaks tend to shift toward the F2 of the vowel in which they are released.

Formant Transitions

A number of studies (most of them done at Haskins Laboratories) have demonstrated the extreme importance of the formant transitions of the following vowel to identification of a plosive's place of articulation (Cooper, Delattre, Liberman, Borst, & Gerstman, 1952; Delattre, Liberman, & Cooper, 1955; Malmberg, 1955; Liberman, 1957; Harris, Hoffman, Liberman, Delattre, & Cooper, 1958; Hoffman, 1958; Dorman, Studdert-Kennedy, & Raphael, 1977). While F3 transitions contribute to the discrimination, most of the necessary information is carried by F2.

The patterns of the formant transitions associated with different plosives do not show a strict one-to-one correspondence with perceived phonemic categories. Figure 7–51 illustrates the formant-transition patterns of synthetic stimuli that listeners identified as the syllables indicated. The first-formant movements are always the same and, therefore, can be presumed to play little if any role in the discrimination of specific

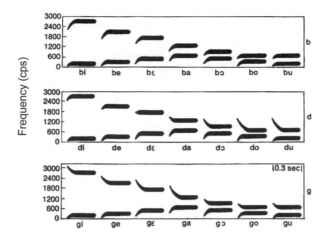

Figure 7–51. Formant transitions associated with the perception of specific plosive-vowel syllables. Adapted from "Acoustic Loci and Transitional Cues for Consonants," by P. C. Delattre, A. M. Lieberman, and F. S. Cooper, 1955, *Journal of the Acoustical Society of America, 27,* 769–773. Reprinted by permission from *Speech Physiology and Acoustic Phonetics: An Introduction,* by P. Lieberman, 1977, New York: Macmillan. Figure 7–3, p. 119.

plosives. For a given plosive, F2 can be assumed to originate at some frequency locus (that does not appear in the pattern) that is "pointed at" by the onset transition. Clearly, for /b/, for instance, the indicated F2 frequency-of-origin is very low, and the F2 of /b/ always "rises" from it. Hence, /b/ always has a rising F2 transition. By the same reasoning, it can be assumed that the origin of F2 of /g/ must be quite high, since all of /g/'s F2 transitions are falling. The locus for /d/ must be at some intermediate frequency: The transitions into the high F2s of /i, e, and ɛ/ rise, while the transitions into the lower F2s of the other vowels fall. That formant transitions should signal the place of stop production is not surprising, as they reflect movement of the articulators on release of the plosive.

Final plosives are often unreleased in English, so there are no burst and post-release formant transitions to identify them. It is clear in these cases that the formant transitions of the pre-plosive sound provide the basis for perceptual categorization. Wang (1959) showed that the greater these formant transitions were, the more certain a listener was of the plosive's identity. However, the reduction of information caused by the loss of the release phenomena was reflected in greater listener confusion than would be the case were the release burst available. English partially compen-

sates for the reduced acoustic cues of unreleased final plosives by requiring that the vowel preceding a voiced plosive have longer duration than a vowel preceding its voiceless cognate (House & Fairbanks, 1953; Denes, 1955; Peterson & Lehiste, 1960; Raphael, 1972; Krause, 1982).

Voice Onset Time

Voice onset time (VOT), an essential characteristic of plosive phones, is easily read from a wide-band spectrogram. It can be viewed as a variable that, in a sense, summarizes a very complex and extremely important aspect of articulator-laryngeal coordination. It can be measured from simple, easily elicited utterances that can be produced even by very young children. (Bond and Korte, 1983, have found that the VOT of spontaneous and imitative productions of 2- and 3-year-olds are not significantly different.) The pattern of VOT change during the period of speech acquisition is clear and relatively well-documented—and there is the possibility that it is sensitive to senescent involution as well. All of these facts point to VOT as a measure that is likely to be of use in describing or categorizing a range of developmental, neuromotor, or linguistic disorders (Farmer, 1977, 1980; Farmer & Lencione, 1977; Freeman, Sands, & Harris, 1978; Gilbert & Campbell, 1978; Weismer, 1979, 1984a, 1984b; Blumstein, Cooper, Goodglass, Statlender, & Gottleib, 1980; Itoh et al., 1982; Glasson, 1984; Healey & Gutkin, 1984; Shewan, Leeper, & Booth, 1984; Hardcastle, Barry, & Clark, 1985; Caruso & Burton, 1987; Young & Gilbert, 1988; Forrest, Weismer, & Turner, 1989; Morris, 1989; Baum, Blumstein, Naeser, & Palumbo, 1990; Waldstein, 1990; Seikel, Wilcox, & Davis, 1990, 1991; Keller et al., 1991; Ouellon, Ryalls, Lebeuf, & Joanette, 1991; Tyler & Saxman, 1991; Tyler & Watterson, 1991; Lieberman et al., 1992; Baum & Ryan, 1993). This potential utility to the speech pathologist may be one of the reasons for the heavy emphasis VOT has received in the research literature. It seems worthwhile, then, to consider it in some detail here.

The voice onset time is defined as the interval between the release of an oral constriction and the start of glottal pulsing (Lisker & Abramson, 1964). Although it is a temporal value that can be determined directly from the speech signal (Till & Stivers, 1981; Keller et al., 1991; Kent, 1993), it is more common to measure it from a wide-band spectrogram. In this context, VOT is defined as the time equivalent of the space from the onset of the plosive release-burst to the first vertical striation representing glottal pulsing (Liberman et al., 1952; Lisker & Abramson, 1964, 1967), as delineated in Figure 7–50.

Viewed solely from the perspective of physiological capability of glottal and supraglottal coordination, the VOT is free to vary over a wide and continuous range. However, most languages limit VOT to two or three relatively narrow and non-overlapping ranges (Ladefoged & Maddieson, 1996). For prevocalic plosives, the range into which a given VOT falls serves the listener as an important cue to the voicing category of the phone (Lisker & Abramson, 1964; Abramson & Lisker, 1965, 1968). The traditional distinction of phoneticians, based on a dichotomous presence or absence of voicing during plosive production, has been found inadequate to explain categorization along the voiced-voiceless dimension (Malécot, 1970; Ladefoged, 1971; Ohde, 1984; Kohler, 1982, 1985; Whalen, Abramson, Lisker, & Mody, 1993).

Interruption of glottal pulsing during plosives can be either passive or active. Passive unvoicing results when the air pressure behind an oral closure rises near the level of the subglottal pressure. With the effective elimination of a transglottal pressure drop, voicing must halt. On the other hand, voicing can be actively stopped by the simple expedient of abducting the vocal folds. Numerous studies have shown that the larynx commonly behaves as an active articulator in controlling unvoicing, although its function in this regard is complex and poorly understood (Haggard, Ambler, & Callow, 1970; Kim, 1970; Sawashima, 1970; Lisker & Abramson, 1971; Hirose & Gay, 1972; Warren & Hall, 1973; Summerfield & Haggard, 1977; Hirose & Ushijima, 1978; Löfqvist & Yoshioka, 1979, 1984; Murry & Brown, 1979; Haggard, Summerfield, & Roberts, 1981; Abramson & Lisker, 1985; Kohler, 1985; Goldstein & Browman, 1986; Löfqvist, Baer, McGarr, & Story, 1989; Hong & Kim, 1997). It is not yet clear whether variation of VOT is achieved by manipulation of glottal width during abduction for a plosive or by direct timing control by higher CNS centers (Kim, 1970; Benguerel, Hirose, Sawashima, & Ushijima, 1978; Benguerel & Bhatia, 1980). No matter what the control mechanism, it is widely recognized that the VOT is a reliable and easily measured correlate of an important and precisely regulated aspect of speech motor coordination. Furthermore, a moderately large body of work has confirmed a clear developmental pattern of VOT change that provides a basis for evaluation of one aspect of a patient's early developmental status.

Voice onset time in English. By convention, a VOT of 0 signals simultaneous onset of release-burst noise and glottal pulsing. Negative VOT values denote the time *before* burst noise that voice began (known as "prevoicing" or "voice lead"), while positive VOT values show the time of glottal striations *after* burst onset (known as "voice lag").

In their early studies of isolated words with initial plosives, Lisker and Abramson (1964, 1967) determined that VOT fell into three distinct ranges. Voiceless plosives had a relatively long VOT, ranging from +60 to +100 ms. On the other hand, VOTs associated with voiced plosives fell into two ranges: −75 to −25 ms (voicing lead) and 0 to +25 ms (short voicing lag). It has been demonstrated that perceptual categorization of English plosives along the voicing dimension requires only two categories (Lisker, 1957b; Lisker & Abramson, 1964; Abramson & Lisker, 1965; Zlatin, 1974). Listeners classify plosives with prevoicing or short voicing lags as voiced, while a long voicing lag underlies the perception of voiceless.[23] Therefore, the two "voiced" VOT ranges are generally collapsed into one category when discussing the English language.

The data in Table 7–6 are taken from a study by Zlatin (1974) in which normal English-speaking adults each produced 35 tokens of each of eight test words. There is very little overlap of the voiced and voiceless ranges. By and large the categories are quite distinct. The data also reveal that VOT tends to increase as the place of articulation is retracted. Labial plosives have the shortest VOTs, velars the longest. This effect was also noted by Lisker and Abramson (1964, 1967) and possible explanations for it, in terms of articulatory dynamics, have been proposed by Klatt (1975a). Thus, in stressed single-word utterances, a VOT less than 25 ms or so can be said to signal an English voiced plosive. Longer VOTs indicate a voiceless phoneme. Within the two ranges there are obviously overlapping subdivisions that offer some cue to place of articulation.

Contextual variability. The VOT of a given plosive varies as a function of the phonetic and suprasegmental characteristics of its environment. On the segmental level, the VOT of both voiced and voiceless plosives is significantly longer before sonorants. VOTs of voiceless plosives are lengthened by about 15% before the high vowels /i, u/ as compared with the low vowels /ɑ, æ/ (Klatt, 1975a, Port & Rotunno, 1979; Weismer, 1979). A similar effect can be seen in the data for "bees" and "bear" in Table 7–6. The addition of a second sylla-

---

[23] Other acoustic phenomena, including formant transition characteristics, burst intensity, fundamental frequency contour, and the like, play a role in real-life categorization (Slis & Cohen, 1969a, 1969b; Stevens, 1971; Stevens & Klatt, 1972, 1974; Summerfield & Haggard, 1977; Port & Dalby, 1982; Ohde, 1984; Revoile et al., 1987; Forrest & Rockman, 1988; Hayashi, Imiazumi, Harada, Seki, & Hosoi, 1992; Whalen et al., 1993).

Table 7–6. Voice Onset Time (in ms) for Word-Initial Plosives in Single-Word Utterances*

Word	Mean	(SD)	Mode	Median	Minimum	Maximum
bees	−23.17	(50.74)	10	5.79	−170	+30
bear	−12.02	(43.02)	10	7.54	−210	+50
dime	−5.20	(42.50)	10	10.30	−200	+50
goat	−0.08	(49.67)	20	19.75	−210	+50
bees	−23.17	(50.74)	10	5.79	−170	+30
VOICED	−10.12		10		−210	+50
peas	+79.17	(23.67)	70	74.05	+40	+220
pear	+83.77	(25.06)	70	.26	+10	+170
time	+87.12	(25.66)	70	82.52	+30	+180
coat	+90.73	(23.66)	70	86.93	+40	+170
VOICELESS	+85.15		70		+10	+220

*Subjects were 10 men and 10 women, age 23–40 years; General American dialect; 35 repetitions of each stimulus word, measured from wide-band spectrograms. [Note: The large differences among the mean, median, and mode in each class are indicative of the marked skewing of the distributions.]

Source: From "Voicing Contrast: Perceptual and Productive Voice Onset Time Characteristics of Adults," by M. A. Zlatin, 1974, *Journal of the Acoustical Society of America*, *56*, 981–994. Table 5, p. 989.

ble to a plosive-initial word shortens VOT only by about 8% (Klatt, 1975a).

The larger context, beyond the one or two syllables directly associated with the plosive, also influences its VOT. In particular, there is demonstrable sensitivity to such suprasegmental characteristics as speech rate, word stress, semantic importance, and utterance length (Lisker & Abramson, 1967; Umeda, 1977). Based on his own research findings, Klatt (1975a) has generated a series of rules for predicting VOT in sentence contexts. They are summarized in Table 7–7, along with his data for average VOT values for word-initial plosives and consonant clusters.

It is also important to realize that "citational" utterances of a single word for testing purposes may have VOTs that are significantly different from, and less variable than, the VOTs occurring in more naturalistic speech samples (Baran, Laufer, & Daniloff, 1977).

Developmental changes in VOT. Life-span changes in the VOT voicing contrast have been explored from the point of view of both perception and production. Most of the research has examined childhood development, but there are also indications that certain involutional changes might be associated with advanced age (Preston & Yeni-Komshian, 1967; Eguchi

& Hirsh, 1969; Preston & Port, 1969; Kewley-Port & Preston, 1974; Gilbert, 1975; Menyuk & Klatt, 1975; Zlatin & Koenigsnecht, 1975, 1976; Benjamin, 1982; Sweeting & Baken, 1982; Neiman, Klich, & Shuey, 1983; Forrest et al., 1989; Slawinski, 1994).

The picture of childhood development of VOT control that emerges indicates that infants produce plosives whose onset times fall rather uniformly along the VOT continuum. With further development, the VOTs of *all* plosives tend to cluster around the short-lead/short-lag (equivalent to the adult's "voiced") part of the range. As the child matures, the voiceless plosives are increasingly associated with greater voicing lag (that is, with a longer VOT).

Just around the time of speech onset, then, children's plosives have a unimodal distribution of VOTs; That is, the VOT ranges used by very young children to indicate the voiced-voiceless distinction tend to overlap almost completely, so that they are collapsed into a single productive category. This situation is readily apparent in the data of Kewley-Port and Preston (1974) and Zlatin and Koenigsknecht (1976). By the age of 6 years or so, the categories overlap very much less, thanks to the increased mean voicing lag that has come to the voiceless cognates. Somewhere past the age of 6, movement of voiceless plosives further into

Table 7–7A. Voice Onset Time (in ms): Average Values for Word-Initial Consonant Clusters*

Voiced		*Voiceless*		*/s/-Initial*	
/b/	11	/p/	47	/sp/	12
/d/	17	/t/	65	/st/	23
/g/	27	/k/	70	/sk/	30
/br/	14	/pr/	59	/spr/	18
/dr/	2	/tr/	93	/str/	37
/gr/	35	/kr/	84	/skr/	35
/bl/	13	/pl/	61	/spl/	16
/gl/	26	/kl/	77	/skw/	39
		/tw/	102		
		/kw/	94		

*Subjects were three normal men. Five words for each cluster, embedded in the carrier phrase "Say _____ again." Measured from wide-band spectrograms.

Source: From "Voice Onset Time, Frication, and Aspiration in Word-initial Consonant Clusters," by D. H. Klatt, 1975, *Journal of Speech and Hearing Research*, *18*, 686–706. Table 1, p. 689. © 1975, American Speech-Language-Hearing Association, Rockville, MD. Reprinted by permission.

Table 7–7B. Rules for Predicting VOT in Sentence Production*

Condition	*Multiply Table 7–7A Average Value by:*
VOICED PLOSIVES /b, d, g/	
—not in blend	1
—preceded by voiceless consonant	1.3
—preceded by nasal consonant	0.8
VOICELESS PLOSIVES /p, t, k/	
—in prestressed cluster	1
—not stressed, word-initial that is	
not in a blend	0.7
preceded by voiceless consonant (or silence)	0.9
—not stressed, word medial or final that is	
not in a blend	0.4
preceded by voiceless consonant	0.7

*Caution: "Individual VOT values may differ from the predictions due to unaccounted-for variability, especially in unstressed environments" (p. 706).

Source: From "Voice Onset Time, Frication, and Aspiration in Word-initial Consonant Clusters," by D. H. Klatt, 1975, *Journal of Speech and Hearing Research*, *18*, 686–706. Appendix, p. 706. © 1975, American Speech-Language-Hearing Association, Rockville, MD. Reprinted by permission.

the lag range results in complete separation of the two categories, with no overlap in the VOT ranges for isolated words. The skill that is acquired by children in controlling VOT is that of *delaying* voice onset a precise amount of time in order to mark a voiceless phoneme.[24]

An important index of a child's speech-motor development may be the restriction of VOTs for a given plosive to an acceptably narrow range that lies wholly to one side of the voiced-voiceless boundary (Macken & Barton, 1980). There is also evidence that VOT control may be slightly poorer in "language delayed" children compared with their peers (Bond & Wilson, 1980; Maxwell & Weismer, 1982; Catts & Jensen, 1983; Glasson, 1984; Forrest & Rockman, 1988; Tyler & Saxman, 1991). In the terminology of statistics, the mean VOTs of voiced and voiceless plosives should be widely separated, and the standard deviation associated with each should be small enough to prevent significant overlap of the distributions. On the motor-control level, what is implied is that a speaker should be able to attain a desired VOT target with minimal variation from trial to trial. Eguchi and Hirsh (1969) provide mean intraspeaker standard deviations that provide a useful gauge of the attainment of the required precision. Data for each of the age groups they studied are plotted in Figure 7–52. Note, in particular, the more adult-like precision attained by roughly 7 to 8 years of age.

AFFRICATES

Affricates are produced with a period of vocal-tract occlusion which is released, not into a relatively open vocal tract as is the case for plosives, but into a narrow constriction. This yields burst energy followed shortly by strong frication. There are two generally recognized affricate consonants in English, /tʃ/, and its voiced cognate /dʒ/. Both the occlusion and constriction occur at the same alveolar place of articulation.

Compared with fricative consonants, the frication associated with the affricates tends to be shorter in duration, but with a far more rapid onset and rise time (Gerstman, 1957; Cutting & Rosner, 1974; Howell & Rosen, 1983; Kent & Read, 1992) when produced in similar contexts, such as "chew" /tʃu/ vs. "shoe" /ʃu/. When occurring in a syllable-final context, the affricates are additionally distinguished by the closure interval, the presence of a release burst, and by formant

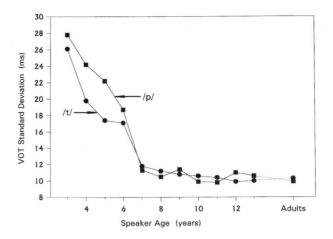

Figure 7–52. Average intra-subject VOT standard deviations associated with /p/ (in "pen") and /t/ (in "tall") from Eguchi and Hirsh's (1969) data by age group.

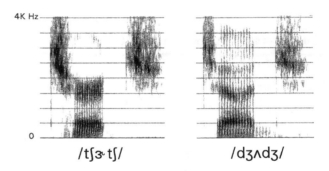

/tʃɝ·tʃ/   /dʒʌdʒ/

Figure 7–53. Wide-band spectrograms of the words "church" and "judge."

transitions associated with the preceding and following speech sounds (Raphael & Dorman, 1980). Figure 7–53 shows spectrograms of the words "church" and "judge" showing both English affricates in initial and word-final positions. Table 7–8 includes Howell and Rosen's (1983) data on /tʃ/ and /ʃ/ frication rise times, averaged across productions by two male and two female speakers of British English.

---

[24] It should be noted that acquisition of the voicing contrast does not seem to depend on learning to perceive the difference between long and short VOTs. Zlatin and Koenigsknecht (1975) have shown that 2-year-olds are capable of perceiving the VOT distinction, even though they may not be able to reproduce it. There is reason to believe that the perceptual ability is a function of inborn auditory feature detectors (Eimas, Siqueland, Jsczyk, & Vigorito, 1971; Kuhl, 1979) that are not unique to humans (Kuhl & Miller, 1975, 1978).

Table 7–8. Frication Rise Time (in ms): Average Values for /tʃ/ and /ʃ/ in Word- Initial, Medial, and Final Position*

Context	/tʃ/				/ʃ/			
	Initial	Medial	Final	All	Initial	Medial	Final	All
Nonsense Syllables*								
Mean	55.9	53.3	74.7	61.3	136.1	88.7	134.6	118.6
(SD)	(9.8)	(11.6)	(22.7)	(18.4)	(30.8)	(18.5)	(21.0)	(32.4)
Isolated Words†								
Mean	37.2	57.2	52.1	48.8	123.0	113.3	132.4	122.9
(SD)	(2.6)	(6.2)	(8.5)	(10.6)	(29.7)	(28.5)	(11.0)	(25.8)
Reading Passage††								
Mean	25.6	31.2	42.1	33.0	67.2	77.5	82.8	75.8
(SD)	(3.6)	(9.6)	(12.0)	(11.4)	(15.9)	(3.5)	(19.2)	(15.9)

*CV, VCV, and VC syllables; V = /i, u, æ, and ɑ/.

†Initial *choose/shoes*; Medial *matched/mashed*; and Final *ditch/dish*.

††Specially designed 4-sentence reading passage that included the following test words: Initial *childhood/shimmering*; Medial *catching/ocean*; and Final *beach/wash*.

Source: *Data derived from individual subject rise times reported by "Production and Perception of Rise Time in the Voiceless Affricate/Fricative Distinction," by P. Howell and S. Rosen, 1983, *Journal of the Acoustical Society of America, 73*, 976–984. Note: Rise times measured from sound pressure oscillograms and defined as duration of the time between "the onset of frication (i.e., ignoring the burst)" to the point when "the frication reached its maximum absolute level"; Authors' examination of spectrograms reportedly yielded no "spectral differences which might serve as a cue to the affricate/fricative distinction" [p. 977].

EVALUATION OF THE SOURCE SPECTRUM

Because the acoustic spectrum of speech is the product of the glottal source signal as well as the filter characteristics of the vocal tract, spectrum analysis provides a window on laryngeal function as well as on articulatory movements. Evaluative methods rely primarily on spectrograms of the types already discussed. Research has shown that analysis of the *long-term average spectrum* (*LTAS*), the mean of all sound spectra during a relatively long sample), in particular, holds great promise as an index of vocal quality (Carr & Trill, 1964; Tarnøczy & Fant, 1964; Schlorhaufer, Müller, Hussl, & Scharfetter, 1972; Frøkjaer-Jensen & Prytz, 1976; Wedin, Leanderson, & Wedin, 1978; Hammarberg, Fitzell, Gauffin, Sundberg, & Wedin, 1980; Izdebski, 1980; Weinberg, Horii, & Smith, 1980; Wendler, Doherty, & Hollein, 1980; Wedin & Ögren, 1982; Dejonckere, 1983; Löfqvist & Manderson, 1987; Novak, Dlouha, Capkova, & Vohradnick, 1991; Kitzing & Åkerlund, 1993; Mendoza, Valencia, Muñoz, & Trujillo, 1996). In addition to the LTAS, there are several other techniques of spectral analysis that have been found to be useful in the evaluation of vocal-fold pathology (Rontal, Rontal, & Rolnick, 1975a, 1975b;

Wolfe & Ratusnik, 1981; Pruszewicz, Obrebowski, Swindzinski, Demenko, Wika, & Wojciechowska, 1991; Remacle & Trigaux, 1991; Sasaki, Okamura, & Yumoto, 1991; Wolfe, Cornell, & Palmer, 1991; Leinonen et al., 1992; Rihkanen, Leinonen, Hitunen, & Kangas, 1994), esophageal voice (Tato, Mariani, DePicolli, & Mirasov, 1954), spasmodic dysphonia (Frint, 1974), metabolic disorder (Rontal, Rontal, Leuchter, & Rolnick, 1978), and vocal abnormalities associated with severe hearing impairment (Monsen, 1979; Wirz, Subtelny, & White-head, 1981).

The search for spectrographic methods of analyzing vocal quality has concentrated on characterizing or quantifying the acoustic energy that lies between the harmonic frequencies. The harmonic content of the vocal signal results from quasi-periodic interruption of airflow by the vocal folds. The interharmonic (noise) energy, however, is the acoustic correlate of an uninterrupted turbulent transglottal flow. By analogy with electrical signals, the "chopped" airflow is described as AC; the turbulent but continuous flow represents a DC component (Isshiki, Yanagihara, & Morimoto, 1966; Yanagihara, 1967a; Isshiki, 1981, 1985; Isshiki, Ohkawa, & Goto, 1985; see AC/DC Ratio, Chapter 10). As laryngeal function deteriorates and glottal efficiency declines, vocal-fold modulation of the airstream becomes less complete: The AC component weakens as the DC component grows. The spectral manifestation of this shift is progressive replacement of harmonic energy by aperiodic noise.[25]

Different aspects of glottal-source noise can be observed in wide- and narrow-band spectrograms (Nessel, 1962; Schönhärl, 1963; Cornut, 1971; Wolfe & Bacon, 1976; Kim, Kakita, & Hirano, 1982; Yoon, Kakita, & Hirano, 1984; Imaizumi, 1986; Keller et al., 1991; Dedo & Izdebski, 1999), such as those shown in Figure 7–54, in which normal and hoarse vowel productions are compared. Abnormality can be seen in the irregular spacing of the glottal striations and in the obvious high-noise background of the wide-band analyses. But the differences between the normal and hoarse voices are even more apparent in the narrow-band spectrograms because of the clear delineation of the voice harmonics. It is obvious why narrow-band analyses form the basis of spectrographic evaluation of voice.

Spectrographic Categories of Hoarse Voice

Yanagihara (1967a, 1967b) evaluated male and female speakers with varying degrees of hoarseness. Narrow-band spectrograms of their sustained /u, ɔ, ɑ, ɛ, i/ at "moderate loudness and medium pitch" could be categorized into four types that correlated well with hoarseness severity. Narrow-band spectrograms are assigned to the various classes according to the following criteria (Yanagihara, 1967b):

Type I. "The regular harmonic components are mixed with noise component chiefly in the formant region of the vowels."

Type II. "The noise components in the second formants of /ɛ/ and /i/ dominate over the harmonic components, and slight additional noise components appear in the high-frequency region above 3000 Hz in the vowels /ɛ/ and /i/."

Type III. "The second formants of /ɛ/ and /i/ are totally replaced by noise components, and the additional noise components above 3000 Hz further intensify their energy and expand their range."

Type IV. "The second formants of /ɑ/, /ɛ/, and /i/ are replaced by noise components, and even the first formants of all vowels often lose their periodic components. In addition, more intensified high frequency additional noise components are seen."

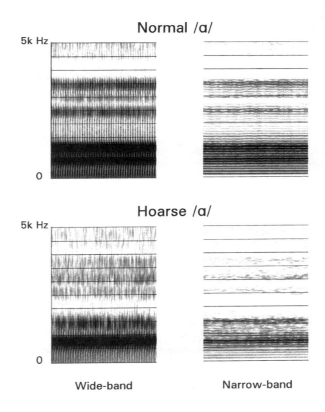

Figure 7–54. Wide-band (left) and narrow-band (right) spectrograms of normal (above) and hoarse (below) phonations of the vowel /ɑ/.

Measures of Spectral Noise

SPECTRAL NOISE LEVEL

Spectral noise and its relationship to vowel *roughness* (a term specially used to avoid the confusion associated with the term *hoarseness*) has been a particular interest of Emanuel and his coworkers (Emanuel & Sansone, 1969; Sansone & Emanuel, 1970; Lively & Emanuel, 1970; Emanuel, Lively, & McCoy, 1973; Emanuel & Smith, 1974; Whitehead & Emanuel, 1974; Arnold & Emanuel, 1979; Emanuel & Whitehead, 1979; Whitehead & Lieberth, 1979; Emanuel & Scarinzi, 1979, 1980; Emanuel & Austin, 1981; Trullinger, Emanuel, Skenes, & Malpass, 1988; Toner, Emanuel, & Parker, 1990; Emanuel, 1991; Newman & Emanuel,

---

[25]Another major contributor of noise, cycle-to-cyle period variability or "jitter," is discussed in Chapter 6, "Vocal Fundamental Frequency."

1991). Their method of analysis is best exemplified by the first of their reports (Emanuel & Sansone, 1969; Sansone & Emanuel, 1970). Speakers sustained each of several vowels for 7 s at a monitored intensity of 75 dB SPL. A 2-s tape segment of the vowel recording was formed into a loop and repeatedly scanned by a spectrum analyzer operated with a very narrow (3 Hz) bandwidth. The strip-chart output was an amplitude-by-frequency spectrum with very fine frequency resolution. From this record, the minimum noise value (in dB SPL) was measured for each 100-Hz segment of the spectrum from 200 to 8000 Hz. In this first study, normal men produced the vowels using their habitual voice and then using a "rough" voice. Findings were not always fully consistent across speakers, but several conclusions were justified:

1. All vowels—both normal and rough—have noise components over a broad spectral range. Rough vowels, however, have much more noise. This finding is consistent with the earlier work of Nessel (1962), Isshiki, Yanagihara, and Morimoto (1966), and Yanagihara (1967a, 1967b).

2. The noise level is related to the amount of frequency perturbation.

3. Spectral noise level varies with the height of the vowel. For both normal and rough productions, the high vowels /u/ and /i/ had the least, low vowel /æ/ had the most, and the vowels /ɑ/ and /ʊ/ had intermediate levels of spectral noise.

4. The correlation coefficients for overall spectral noise level and perceived vowel roughness were all significant ($p < .05$), ranging from .74 to .92. The correlations were even higher (.97–.98) when noise levels only in the range of 100 to 2600 Hz were considered. (Correlation coefficients resulting from several studies are summarized in Whitehead and Emanuel, 1974, and in Emanuel, 1991.)

Similar, and hence confirmatory, results have been obtained in studies of simulated rough vowels produced by women (Lively & Emanuel, 1970; Emanuel, Lively, & McCoy, 1973). Vocal effort (Thomas-Kersting & Casteel, 1989) and voice register also influence spectral noise levels. In normal speakers, pulse register is associated with more spectral noise, and loft (falsetto) register with less, than the modal register (Emanuel & Scarinzi, 1979, 1980).

The validity of spectral noise levels as a measure of roughness of genuinely (as opposed to simulated) dysphonic vowels has been assessed by Arnold and Emanuel (1979). They studied 10 normal boys and 10 boys with confirmed laryngeal lesions and rough voices. The analytic methods were the same as in the simulation studies, but two pitch levels were examined. Spectral noise was found to be higher in the voices of the dysphonic children. For all children, vowels differed in median noise level, generally following the order observed in adults. Among the normal children, high vocal fundamental frequency was associated with lower noise levels, but this effect did not hold for the dysphonic children. It has also been determined that spectral noise levels correlate moderately well with ratings of the "tension/harshness" of the voices of deaf speakers (Whitehead & Lieberth, 1979; Thomas-Kersting & Casteel, 1989; Wirz, Subtelny, & Whitehead, 1981). Unfortunately, spectral noise alone has been found to be only a fair differentiator of rough and abnormal voices (Emanuel & Austin, 1981).

Another important consideration is the harmonic amplitude level. As (interharmonic) spectral noise increases, it might be supposed that the energy at the harmonic frequencies would decrease. Emanuel and Whitehead (1979) found that this is indeed the case, but only up to a point. They reanalyzed the taped samples used by Sansone and Emanuel (1970) using the same spectrum analyzer. This time, however, the variable of interest was the amplitude of each of the first five harmonics and its relationship to perceived vowel roughness. Unfortunately, their results were not unequivocal. With a single exception (the third harmonic of /i/), the amplitude of the first three harmonics decreased as judged roughness increased. The correlation coefficients for the median of the judges' roughness ratings and harmonic amplitude level ranged from $-.32$ to $-.74$ (excluding the correlation for the third harmonic of /i/). Interestingly, the correlation coefficients for the second harmonic were considerably higher than those for the first and third, ranging from $-.70$ to $-.74$. These correlations are statistically significant ($p < .05$), but on the whole they are not impressive. A coefficient of $-.32$ indicates that the harmonic amplitude change accounts for a scant 10% of the change in perceived roughness. Even a coefficient of $-.74$ means that only 55% of the roughness variability is accounted for.

Confounding the harmonic-level interpretation even more is the fact that the fourth and fifth harmonics sometimes showed a significant *increase* in amplitude as roughness grew more severe. The authors hypothesized that this was due to high-frequency noise additively contributing to the energy of the upper formants. The supposition could not be tested, however.

THE HARMONICS-TO-NOISE RATIO

The major problem with Emanuel's approaches is that either the noise or the harmonic level is considered in isolation. However, the work of Isshiki, Yanagihara, and Morimoto (1966), Yanagihara (1967a, 1967b), and Kim, Kakita, and Hirano (1982) has shown that a characteristic feature of hoarseness is the replacement of harmonics by noise energy. That is, aperiodic sound intensifies at the expense of the periodic signal. It is reasonable to conclude that the best index of hoarseness might be the ratio of one to the other. This was the approach taken by Kojima, Gould, Lambiase, and Isshiki (1980) and Kitajima (1981). Their computational procedure, however, was complex and inconvenient. It was soon improved upon by Yumoto and his colleagues (Yumoto, Gould, & Baer, 1982; Yumoto, 1983; Yumoto, Sasaki, & Okamura, 1984; Yumoto, 1988), whose procedure was to objectify and quantify the features that appear in the spectrogram of the hoarse voice.

While the actual mathematical method is beyond the scope of the present discussion, the conceptual basis of Yumoto et al.'s measure is fairly simple and worth some consideration. The voice is considered to have two components: (1) Perfectly periodic waves, and (2) Random noise. Because the noise component represents random sound pressure variation about a zero value, summing the instantaneous noise amplitudes over a moderately long time interval will result in a net noise amplitude of zero. On the other hand, similarly adding the consecutive waves of the purely periodic component results in an ever-larger net-sum wave. Therefore, if the average amplitude of every point in a real vowel waveform is taken for a moderately large number of periods, the noise component should cancel out, leaving a pure periodic signal.

Now, it can be assumed that the pure (average) periodic wave is increasingly contaminated by random noise as hoarseness worsens. The degree of contamination can best be expressed as a period-to-noise amplitude ratio. It has just been shown that the periodic amplitude can be determined fairly easily by averaging waveforms. How can the noise level associated with each vocal period be determined?

It turns out that the answer is relatively simple. Since the averaged waveform represents a pure, noise-free vocal period, it suffices to subtract its value at every point in time from a real (noise-contaminated) vocal period. The remainder is the isolated noise content of the real waveform. The **harmonics-to-noise (H/N) ratio** is then just the mean amplitude of the average

wave divided by the mean amplitude of the isolated noise components for the train of waves.[26] For convenience, the H/N ratio is expressed in dB.

To test the utility of their index, Yumoto and his coworkers (1982) assessed the sustained /ɑ/ of 22 men and 20 women with no demonstrable vocal disorder. They were compared with the pre- and post-operative phonation of a roughly comparable group of 12 men and 8 women with various laryngeal pathologies and widely different degrees of hoarseness. The mean H/N ratio for the normal subjects was 11.9 dB (SD = 2.32; range 7.0–17.0 dB). Men and women were not significantly different. The 95% confidence limit was 7.4 dB. In contrast, the mean H/N ratio of the preoperative dysphonics was only 1.6 dB (range 15.2–9.6 dB). Three of the 20 preoperative subjects had H/N ratios greater than the 7.4 dB lower limit of normality, but they were the ones with very slight clinical hoarseness. Postoperatively, the patients' mean H/N ratio rose to 11.3 dB (SD = 3.13; range 5.9–17.6 dB) with about 95% achieving a ratio in the expected normal range. Equally interesting was the fact that the correlation between the H/N ratios and the spectrogram type (as determined by an experienced clinician) was an impressive .849. The pre- and postoperative change in H/N ratio was correlated with change in spectrogram type to the extent of a near-perfect coefficient of .944.

In a later study, Yumoto, Sasaki, and Okamura (1984) found that the correlation of the H/N ratio and psychophysical scaling of hoarseness was .809, although Wolfe, Fitch, and Cornell (1995) reported no significant correlation between the H/N ratio and the judged severity of dysphonia. Both Eskenazi, Childers, and Hicks (1990) and Ramig, Scherer, Klasner, Titze, and Horii (1990), however, found the H/N ratio to be a particularly potent index of overall severity of vocal disturbance and de Krom (1995) reported that the H/N ratio is an excellent predictor of perceived breathiness.

NORMALIZED NOISE ENERGY

Kasuya and his colleagues (Kasuya, Masubuchi, Ebihara, & Yoshida, 1986; Kasuya, Ogawa, Kikuchi, & Ebihara, 1986; Kasuya, Ogawa, Mashima, & Ebihara, 1986) have developed a measure they call the *normalized noise energy* (*NNE*), that, like the H/N ratio, assesses the relative level of vocal noise to that of the harmonics. One potential problem with the H/N ratio is that, should the speaker's vocal F_0 or SPL slowly vary

---

[26] Alternatively, the mean amplitude of the noise components can be divided by the mean amplitude of the average wave to yield a noise-to-harmonics (N/H) ratio. As yet, however, this measure has little currency in the voice literature.

over the course of the sampling interval, those regular changes will influence the assessment of noise. (This is analogous to the long-term voice "drift" problems that can plague "jitter" and "shimmer" measures, discussed in Chapters 5 and 6, respectively.) The NNE measure attempts to avoid this contaminating influence by basing its analysis on relatively few vocal periods while detecting the noise component of the spectrum by means of a specially designed adaptive comb filter. As with the H/N ratio, the NNE is expressed in dB.

Although published NNE data remain scarce, preliminary reports suggest that the measure performs well when discriminating abnormal voices (Kasuya, Masubuchi et al., 1986; Kasuya, Ogawa et al., 1986). In a study of normal and dysphonic 10-year-old children, McAllister, Sundberg, and Hibi (1998) reported a "reasonable correlation" between NNE and perceived breathiness, hoarseness, and roughness. For the 26 girls and 24 boys they tested, the correlation between NNE and hoarseness was .50 and .57, repectively. The correlation was higher between NNE and perceived breathiness (girls = .78; boys = .77) and far lower when NNE and roughness were compared (girls = .38; boys = .48).

Fex, Fex, Shiromoto, and Hirano (1994) attempted to use NNE to measure post-therapeutic voice improvement. For 10 adult patients they tested pre- and post-treatment, NNE values were found not be be significantly different despite a significant reduction in vocal jitter and shimmer and the patients' own claim "to be improved as voice users, with a general reduction of symptoms." However, when the NNE was based exclusively on energy between 1 and 4 kHz, there was a significant change following treatment. The clinical usefullness of NNE—or some modification of it—thus remains unclear.

Tracking Change in Source Characteristics

The most salient features of many vocal pathologies may be slow, sudden irregular, and rapid quasi-periodic alterations in glottal source characteristics. Wheras measures such as the H/N ratio and NNE attempt to assess interharmonic (noise) energy that is tied to the perception of hoarseness, breathiness, and the like, the narrow-band spectrogram can also be used quite fruitfully to assess the types of phonatory (harmonic) instability that are tied to, among other things, perceived tremulousness (Lebrun, Devreux, Rousseau, & Darimont, 1982; Horii & Hata, 1988; Aronson, Ramig, Winholtz, & Silber, 1992; Kent, Duffy, Vorperian, & Thomas, 1998), intermittent diplo-

phonia (Sirviö & Michelsson, 1976; Monsen, 1979; Michelsson, Raes, Thoden, & Wasz-Hockert, 1982; Robb & Saxman, 1988; Mende, Herzel, & Wermke, 1990; Wong, Ito, Cox, & Titze, 1991; Titze, Baken, & Herzel, 1993; Herzel, Berry, Titze, & Saleh, 1994; Švec, Schutte, & Miller, 1996), and pitch breaks (Ramig, 1986; Švec & Pešák, 1994). Several such features are shown in the narrow-band spectrograms displayed in Figure 7–55.

A comfortable sustained phonation produced by a women with vocal tremor is shown in Figure 7–55A. In the sound pressure waveform above it, the quasi-periodic changes in vocal intensity are quite clear. The associated spectrogram shows the coincident fluctuation of vocal frequency as reflected in the substantial oscillatory variation of the harmonics. Note, however, that the formant frequencies remain relatively stable throughout. Figure 7–55B, on the other hand, shows harmonics that are relatively stable, but change suddenly when the fundamental frequency drops in what is often referred to as a "pitch break." This is common in some vocal pathologies and is characteristic of male vocal mutation during puberty.

Transient *period-* or *harmonic-doubling* (also called a "double harmonic break"), as shown in Figure 7–55C, is a feature that occurs frequently in normal infant vocalization (see, for instance, Michelsson, 1980, Robb and Saxman, 1988, or Herzel and Reuter, 1997), but is often associated with a "creaky" or "diplophonic" dysphonia in older children and adults (Isshiki, Tanabe, Ishizaka, & Broad, 1977; Monsen, 1979; Keller et al., 1991; Orlikoff & Kraus, 1996). Harmonic doubling occurs when there are two glottal closing phases per vocal cycle as in, for instance, dichotic pulse register phonation (Orlikoff & Kahane, 1996), and is associated with low-amplitude *subharmonics* that fall between the regular harmonic components of the signal. These subharmonics are often an inconsistent feature when present in dysphonia, and are also evident in *biphonation,* a poorly understood phenomenon where harmonic and subharmonic components vary independently.

Lastly, Figure 7–55D show rapid F_0 shifts during syllable repetition as part of a "clonic" stuttering block. Spectrographic displays provided by Howell and Vause (1986), among others, suggest that both wide- and narrow-band analyses may help the clinician to differentiate between abnormal "source" and "filter" behavior during perceptually fluent and disfluent utterances. Spectrograms can be of similar assistance in the assessment of vocal and vocal-tract instability and discoordination that may be shown by dysarthric and apraxic speakers (Weismer, 1984a, 1984b).

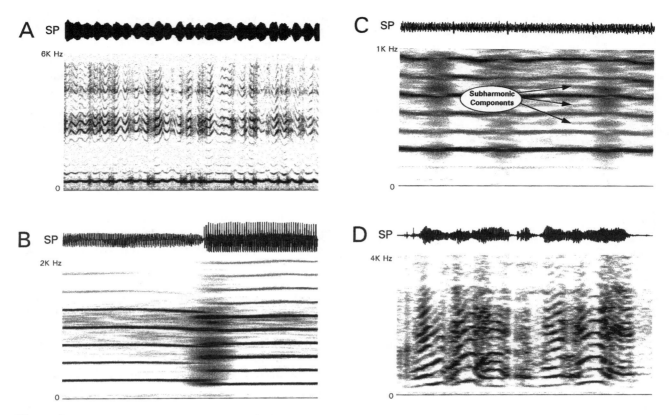

Figure 7–55. Narrow-band spectrograms of different vocal behaviors: **A.** Long-term harmonic instability associated with vocal tremor; **B.** Sudden shift in harmonic frequencies associated with a pitch break; **C.** The inconsistent appearance of subharmonic components; and **D.** F_0 shifts during stuttered /wʊ/-syllable repetition.

REFERENCES

Abramson, A. S., & Lisker, L. (1965). Voice onset time in stop consonants. *Haskins Laboratories Status Report on Speech Research, SR–3*, 1–17.

Abramson, A. S., & Lisker, L. (1968). Voice timing: Cross language experiments in identification and discrimination. *Haskins Laboratories Status Report on Speech Research, SR13/14*, 49–63.

Abramson, A. S., & Lisker, L. (1985). Relative power of cues: F_0 shift versus voice timing. In V. A. Fromkin (Ed.), *Phonetic linguistics: Essays in honor of Peter Ladefoged* (pp. 25–33). New York: Academic Press.

Adams, M. R. (1978). Further analysis of stuttering as a phonetic transition defect. *Journal of Fluency Disorders, 3*, 265–271.

Allen, G. D. (1978). Vowel duration measurement: A reliability study. *Journal of the Acoustical Society of America, 63*, 1176–1185.

Angelocci, A. A., Kopp, G. A., & Holbrook, A. (1964). The vowel formants of deaf and normal-hearing eleven- to fourteen-year-old boys. *Journal of Speech and Hearing Disorders, 29*, 156–170.

Ansel, B. M., & Kent, R. D. (1992). Acoustic-phonetic contrasts and intelligibility in the dysarthria associated with mixed cerebral palsy. *Journal of Speech and Hearing Research, 35*, 296–308.

Arnold, K. S., & Emanuel, F. W. (1979). Spectral noise levels and roughness severity ratings for vowels produced by male children. *Journal of Speech and Hearing Research, 22*, 613–626.

Aronson, A. E., Ramig, L. O., Winholtz, W. S., & Silber, S. R. (1992). Rapid voice tremor, or "flutter," in amyotrophic lateral sclerosis. *Annals of Otology, Rhinology, and Laryngology, 101*, 511–518.

Asano, K., & Kiritani, S. (1992). Phonetic characteristics of unstressed vowels in fast speech. *Annual Bulletin of the Research Institute of Logopedics and Phoniatrics, 26*, 45–50.

Assmann, P. F., & Nearey, T. M. (1987). Perception of front vowels: The role of harmonics in the first formant region. *Journal of the Acoustical Society of America, 81*, 520–534.

Assmann, P. F., Nearey, T. M., & Hogan, J. T. (1982). Vowel identification: Orthographic, perceptual, and acoustic aspects. *Journal of the Acoustical Society of America, 71*, 975–989.

Assmann, P. F., & Summerfield, Q. (1989). Modeling the perception of concurrent vowels: Vowels with the same fundamental frequency. *Journal of the Acoustical Society of America, 85*, 327–338.

Atal, B. S., Chang, J. J., Mathews, M. V., & Tukey, J. W. (1978). Inversion of articulatory-to-acoustic transformation in the vocal tract by a computer-sorting technique. *Journal of the Acoustical Society of America, 63*, 1535–1555.

Atal, B. S., & Hanauer, S. L. (1971). Speech analysis and synthesis by linear prediction of the speech wave. *Journal of the Acoustical Society of America, 50*, 637–655.

Baken, R. J., & Daniloff, R. G. (Eds.) (1991). *Readings in clinical spectrography of speech*. San Diego, CA: Singular Publishing Group and Kay Elemetrics Corp.

Baken, R. J., & Orlikoff, R. F. (1987a). Phonatory response to step-function changes in supraglottal pressure. In T. Baer,

C. Sasaki, & K. S. Harris (Eds.), *Laryngeal function in phonation and respiration* (pp. 273–290). Boston, MA: Little, Brown.

Baken, R. J., & Orlikoff, R. F. (1987b). The effect of articulation on fundamental frequency in singers and speakers. *Journal of Voice, 1,* 68–76.

Baken, R. J., & Orlikoff, R. F. (1988). Changes in vocal fundamental frequency at the segmental level: Control during voiced fricatives. *Journal of Speech and Hearing Research, 31,* 207–211.

Bauer, H. R., & Kent, R. D. (1987). Acoustic analyses of infant fricative and trill vocalization. *Journal of the Acoustical Society of America, 81,* 505–511.

Baran, J. A., Laufer, M. Z., & Daniloff, R. (1977). Phonological contrastivity in conversation: A comparative study of voice onset time. *Journal of Phonetics, 5,* 339–350.

Baum, S. R., Blumstein, S. E., Naeser, M. A., & Palumbo, C. L. (1990). Temporal dimensions of consonant and vowel production: An acoustic and CT scan analysis of aphasic speech. *Brain and Language, 39,* 33–56.

Baum, S. R., & Ryan, L. (1993). Rate of speech effects in aphasia: Voice onset time. *Brain and Language, 44,* 431–445.

Baum, S. R., & McNutt, J. C. (1990). An acoustic analysis of frontal misarticulation of /s/ in children. *Journal of Phonetics, 18,* 51–63.

Behrens, S. J., & Blumstein, S. E. (1988a). Acoustic characteristics of English voiceless fricatives: A descriptive study. *Journal of Phonetics, 16,* 295–298.

Behrens, S. J., & Blumstein, S. E. (1988b). On the role of the amplitude of the fricative noise in the perception of place of articulation in voiceless fricative consonants. *Journal of the Acoustical Society of America, 84,* 861–867.

Benguerel, A.-P., & Bhatia, T. K. (1980). Hindi stop consonants: An acoustic and fiberscopic study. *Phonetica, 37,* 134–148.

Benguerel, A.-P., Hirose, H., Sawashima, M., & Ushijima, T. (1978). Laryngeal control in French stop production: A fiberscopic, acoustic, and electromyographic study. *Folia Phoniatrica, 30,* 175–198.

Benjamin, B. J. (1982). Phonological performance in gerontological speech. *Journal of Psycholinguistic Research, 11,* 159–167.

Bennett, D. C. (1968). Spectral form and duration as cues in the recognition of English and German vowels. *Language and Speech, 11,* 65–85.

Black, J. W. (1949). Natural frequency, duration, and intensity of vowels in reading. *Journal of Speech and Hearing Disorders, 14,* 216–221.

Bloothooft, G., & Plomp, R. (1985). Spectral analysis of sung vowels. II: The effect of fundamental frequency on vowel spectra. *Journal of the Acoustical Society of America, 77,* 1580–1588.

Blumstein, S. E., Cooper, W. E., Goodglass, H., Statlender, S., & Gottlieb, J. (1980). Production deficits in aphasia: A voice-onset-time analysis. *Brain and Language, 9,* 153–170.

Blumstein, S. E., & Stevens, K. N. (1979). Acoustic invariance in speech production: Evidence from measurements of the spectral characteristics of stop consonants. *Journal of the Acoustical Society of America, 66,* 1001–1017.

Boë, L.-J., Perrier, P., & Bailly, G. (1992). The geometric vocal tract variables controlled for vowel production: Proposals for constraining acoustic-to-articulatory inversion. *Journal of Phonetics, 20,* 27–38.

Bond, Z. S., & Korte, S. S. (1983). Children's spontaneous and imitative speech: An acoustic-phonetic analysis. *Journal of Speech and Hearing Research, 26,* 464–467.

Bond, Z. S., & Wilson, H. F. (1980). Acquisition of the voicing contrast by language-delayed and normal-speaking children. *Journal of Speech and Hearing Research, 23,* 152–161.

Borden, G. J., Harris, K. S., & Raphael, L. J. (1994). *Speech science primer: Physiology, acoustics and perception of speech* (3rd ed.). Baltimore, MD: Williams and Wilkins.

Brandt, J. F., Ruder, K. F., & Shipp, T., Jr. (1969). Vocal loudness and effort in continuous speech. *Journal of the Acoustical Society of America, 46,* 1543–1548.

Broad, K. J. (1976). Toward defining acoustic phonetic equivalence for vowels. *Phonetica, 33,* 401–424.

Broadbent, D. E., Ladefoged, P., & Lawrence, W. (1956). Vowel sounds and perceptual constancy. *Nature, 178,* 815–816.

Buder, E. H., Kent, R. D., Kent, J. F., Milenkovic, P., & Workinger, M. (1996). FORMOFFA: An automated formant, moment, fundamental frequency, amplitude analysis of normal and disordered speech. *Clinical Linguistics and Phonetics, 10,* 31–54.

Buhr, R. D. (1980). The emergence of vowels in an infant. *Journal of Speech and Hearing Research, 23,* 73–94.

Carlson, R., Fant, G., & Granstrom, B. (1975). Two-formant models, pitch, and vowel perception. In G. Fant & M. A. A. Tatham (Eds.), *Auditory analysis and perception of speech* (pp. 55–82). New York: Academic Press.

Carr, P. B., & Trill, D. (1964). Long-term larynx-excitation spectral. *Journal of the Acoustical Society of America, 36,* 2033–2040.

Caruso, A. J., & Burton, E. K. (1987). Temporal acoustic measures of dysarthria associated with amyotrophic lateral sclerosis. *Journal of Speech and Hearing Research, 30,* 80–87.

Catford, J. C. (1977). *Fundamental problems in phonetics.* Bloomington, IN: Indiana University Press.

Catts, H. W., & Jensen, P. J. (1983). Speech timing of phonologically disordered children: Voicing contrast of initial and final stop consonants. *Journal of Speech and Hearing Research, 26,* 501–510.

Cavallo, S. A., Baken, R. J., & Shaiman, S. (1984). Frequency perturbation characteristics of pulse register phonation. *Journal of Communication Disorders, 17,* 231–243.

Chaney, C. (1988). Acoustic analysis of correct and misarticulated semivowels. *Journal of Speech and Hearing Research, 31,* 275–287.

Charpentier, F. (1984). Determination of the vocal tract shape from the formants by analysis of the articulatory-to-acoustic nonlinearities. *Speech Communication, 3,* 291–308.

Chiba, T., & Kajiyama, M. (1941). *The vowel: Its nature and structure.* Tokyo, Japan: Kaiseikan.

Chistovich, L. A., & Lublinskaya, V. V. (1979). The "center of gravity" effect in vowel spectra and critical distance between the formants: Psychoacoustical study of the perception of vowel-like stimuli. *Hearing Research, 1,* 185–195.

Chollet, G. (1980). Variability of vowel formant frequencies in different speech styles. In J. C. Simon (Ed.), *Spoken language generation and understanding* (pp. 293–308). Dordrecht, Germany: Reidel.

Coleman, R. F. (1963). Decay characteristics of vocal fry. *Folia Phoniatrica, 15,* 256–263.

Coleman, R. O. (1971). Male and female voice quality and its relationship to vowel formant frequencies. *Journal of Speech and Hearing Research, 14,* 565–577.

Collins, M., Rosenbek, J. C., & Wertz, R. T. (1983). Spectrographic analysis of vowel and word duration in apraxia of speech. *Journal of Speech and Hearing Research, 26,* 224–230.

Cooley, P. M., & Tukey, J. W. (1965). An algorithm for the machine computation of complex Fourier series. *Mathematics of Computation, 19,* 297–301.

Cooper, F. S., Delattre, P. C., Liberman, A. M., Borst, J. M., & Gerstman, L. J. (1952). Some experiments on the perception of synthetic speech sounds. *Journal of the Acoustical Society of America, 24,* 597–606.

Cornut, G. (1971). Vibrations normales et pathologiques des cordes vocales étudiées à l'aide du Sonagraph. *Folia Phoniatrica, 23,* 234–238.

Cornut, G., & Lafon, J.-C. (1960). Etude acoustique comparative des phonèmes vocaliques de la voix parlée et chantée. *Folia Phoniatrica, 12,* 188–196.

Crystal, T. H., & House, A. S. (1988). Segmental durations in connected-speech signals: Current results. *Journal of the Acoustical Society of America, 83,* 1553–1573.

Cutting, J., & Rosner, B. (1974). Categories and boundaries in speech and music. *Perception and Psychophysics, 16,* 564–570.

Dalston, R. M. (1975). Acoustic characteristics of English /w, r, l/ spoken correctly by young children and adults. *Journal of the Acoustical Society of America, 57,* 462–469.

Daniloff, R., Schuckers, G., & Feth, L. (1980). *The physiology of speech and hearing: An introduction.* Englewood Cliffs, NJ: Prentice-Hall.

Daniloff, R. G., Wilcox, K., & Stephens, M. I. (1980). An acoustic-articulatory description of children's defective /s/ productions. *Journal of Communication Disorders, 13,* 347–363.

de Krom, G. (1995). Some spectral correlates of pathological breathy and rough voice quality for different types of vowel fragments. *Journal of Speech and Hearing Research, 38,* 794–811.

Dedo, H. H., & Izdebski, K. (1999). Indirect teflon injection in unilateral vocal fold paralysis: A response to criticisms and discussion of essentials to successful outcomes. *Phonoscope, 2,* 15–22.

Dejonckere, P. H. (1983). Recognition of hoarseness by means of LTAS. *International Journal of Rehabilitation Research, 6,* 343–345.

Delattre, P. (1965). *Comparing the phonetic features of English, German, Spanish, and French: An interim report.* Heidelberg, Germany: Julius Groos Verlag.

Delattre, P. C., Lieberman, A. M., & Cooper, F. S. (1955). Acoustic loci and transitional cues for consonants. *Journal of the Acoustical Society of America, 27,* 769–773.

Delattre, P., Liberman, A. M., Cooper, F. S., & Gerstman, L. J. (1952). An experimental study of the acoustic determinants of vowel color. *Word, 8,* 195–210.

Denes, P. (1955). Effect of duration on the perception of voicing. *Journal of the Acoustical Society of America, 27,* 761–764.

Deterding, D. (1997). The formants of monophthong vowels in standard southern British English pronunciation. *Journal of the International Phonetic Association, 27,* 47–55.

Di Benedetto, M.-G. (1989). Vowel representation: Some observations on temporal and spectral properties of the first formant frequency. *Journal of the Acoustical Society of America, 86,* 55–66.

DiSimoni, F. G. (1974a). Effect of vowel environment on the duration of consonants in the speech of three-, six-, and nine-year-old children. *Journal of the Acoustical Society of America, 55,* 360–361.

DiSimoni, F. G. (1974b). Influence of consonant environment on duration of vowels in the speech of three-, six-, and nine-year-old children. *Journal of the Acoustical Society of America, 55,* 362–363.

DiSimoni, F. G. (1974c). Influence of utterance length upon bilabial closure duration of /p/ in three-, six-, and nine-year-old children. *Journal of the Acoustical Society of America, 55,* 1353–1354.

Dorman, M. F., Studdert-Kennedy, M., & Raphael, L. J. (1977). Stop consonant recognition: Release bursts and formant transitions as functionally equivalent, context-dependent cues. *Perception and Psychophysics, 22,* 109–122.

Dromey, C., Ramig, L. O., & Johnson, A. B. (1995). Phonatory and articulatory changes associated with increased vocal intensity in Parkinson disease: A case study. *Journal of Speech and Hearing Research, 38,* 751–764.

Dudley, H., & Gruenz, O., Jr. (1946). Visible speech translators with external phosphors. *Journal of the Acoustical Society of America, 18,* 62–73.

Dunn, H. K. (1950). The calculation of vowel resonances, and an electrical vocal tract. *Journal of the Acoustical Society of America, 22,* 740–753.

Dunn, H. K. (1961). Methods of measuring formant bandwidths. *Journal of the Acoustical Society of America, 33,* 1737–1746.

Economou, A., Tartter, V. C., Chute, P. M., & Hellman, S. A. (1992). Speech changes following reimplantation from a single-channel to a multichannel cochlear implant. *Journal of the Acoustical Society of America, 92,* 1310–1323.

Eguchi, S., & Hirsh, I. J. (1969). Development of speech sounds in children. *Acta Otolaryngologica, Suppl. 257,* 5–43.

Eimas, P. D., Siqueland, E. R., Jsczyk, P., & Vigorito, J. (1971). Speech perception in infants. *Science, 171,* 303–306.

Emanuel, F. W. (1991). Spectral noise. *Seminars in Speech and Language, 12,* 115–130.

Emanuel, F. W., & Austin, D. (1981). Identification of normal and abnormally rough vowels by spectral noise level measurements. *Journal of Communication Disorders, 14,* 75–85.

Emanuel, F. W., Lively, M. A., & McCoy, J. F. (1973). Spectral noise level and roughness rating for vowels produced by males and females. *Folia Phoniatrica, 25,* 110–120.

Emanuel, F. W., & Sansone, F. E., Jr. (1969). Some spectral features of "normal" and simulated "rough" vowels. *Folia Phoniatrica, 21,* 401–415.

Emanuel, F. W., & Scarinzi, A. (1979). Vocal register effects on vowel spectral noise and roughness: Findings for adult females. *Journal of Communication Disorders, 12,* 263–272.

Emanuel, F. W., & Scarinzi, A. (1980). Vocal register effects on vowel spectral noise and roughness: Findings for adult males. *Journal of Communication Disorders, 13,* 121–131.

Emanuel, F. W., & Smith, W. (1974). Pitch effects on vowel roughness and spectral noise. *Journal of Phonetics, 2,* 247–253.

Emanuel, F. W., & Whitehead, R. L. (1979). Harmonic levels and vowel roughness. *Journal of Speech and Hearing Research, 22,* 829–840.

Endres, W., Bombach, W., & Flösser, G. (1971). Voice spectrograms as a function of age, voice disguise, and voice imitation. *Journal of the Acoustical Society of America, 49,* 1842–1847.

Engstrand, O. (1988). Articulatory correlates of stress and speaking rate in Swedish VCV utterances. *Journal of the Acoustical Society of America, 83,* 1863–1875.

Eskenazi, L., Childers, D. G., & Hicks, D. M. (1990). Acoustic correlates of vocal quality. *Journal of Speech and Hearing Research, 33,* 298–306.

Fairbanks, G., & Grubb, P. (1961). A psychophysical investigation of vowel formants. *Journal of Speech and Hearing Research, 4,* 203–219.

Fant, G. (1960). *Acoustic theory of speech production.* The Hague: Mouton.

Fant, G. M. (1962). Descriptive analysis of the acoustic aspects of speech. *Logos, 5,* 3–17.

Fant, G. (1966). A note on vocal tract size and nonuniform F-pattern scalings. *Speech Transmission Laboratory Quarterly Progress and Status Report* (Royal Institute of Technology, Stockholm, Sweden), *4,* 22–30.

Fant, G. (1973). *Speech sounds and features.* Cambridge, MA: MIT Press.

Fant, G. (1975). Non-uniform vowel normalization. *Speech Transmission Laboratory Quarterly Progress and Status Report* (Royal Institute of Technology, Stockholm, Sweden), *2–3,* 1–19.

Fant, G. M. (1980). The relations between area functions and the acoustic signal. *Phonetica, 37,* 55–86.

Fant, G., Fintoft, K., Liljencrants, J., Lindblom, B., & Martony, J. (1963). Formant-amplitude measurements. *Journal of the Acoustical Society of America, 35,* 1753–1761.

Farmer, A. (1977). Stop cognate production patterns in adult athetotic cerebral palsied speakers. *Folia Phoniatrica, 29,* 154–162.

Farmer, A. (1980). Voice onset time production in cerebral palsied speakers. *Folia Phoniatrica, 32,* 267–273.

Farmer, A., & Lencione, R. M. (1977). An extraneous vocal behaviour in cerebral palsied speakers. *British Journal of Disorders of Communication, 12,* 109–118.

Fex, B., Fex, S., Shiromoto, O., & Hirano, M. (1994). Acoustic analysis of functional dysphonia: Before and after voice therapy (accent method). *Journal of Voice, 8,* 163–167.

Fischer-Jørgensen, E. (1954). Acoustic analysis of stop consonants. *Miscellanea Phonetica, 2,* 42–59.

Flanagan, J. L. (1972). *Speech analysis synthesis and perception* (2nd ed.). New York: Springer-Verlag.

Flanagan, J. L., Coker, C. H., Rabiner, L. R., Schafer, R. W., & Umeda, N. (1970). Synthetic voices for computers. *IEEE Spectrum, 7,* 22–45.

Fletcher, H. (1929). *Speech and hearing.* Princeton, NJ: Van Nostrand.

Fletcher, H. (1953). *Speech and hearing in communication.* Princeton, NJ: Van Nostrand.

Fónagy, I., & Magdics, K. (1960). Speed of utterance in phrases of different lengths. *Language and Speech, 3,* 179–192.

Forrest, K., & Rockman, B. K. (1988). Acoustic and perceptual analysis of word-initial stop consonants in phonologically disordered children. *Journal of Speech and Hearing Research, 31,* 449–459.

Forrest, K., Weismer, G., Milenkovic, P., & Dougall, R. (1988). Statistical analysis of word-initial voiceless obstruents: Preliminary data. *Journal of the Acoustical Society of America, 84,* 115–123.

Forrest, K., Weismer, G., & Turner, G. S. (1989). Kinematic, acoustic, and perceptual analyses of connected speech produced by Parkinsonian and normal geriatric adults. *Journal of the Acoustical Society of America, 85,* 2608–2622.

Fourakis, M. (1991). Tempo, stress, and vowel reduction in American English. *Journal of the Acoustical Society of America, 90,* 1816–1827.

Fox, R. A. (1983). Perceptual structure of monophthongs and diphthongs in English. *Language and Speech, 26,* 21–60.

Fox, R. A. (1989). Dynamic information in the identification and discrimination of vowels. *Phonetica, 46,* 97–116.

Freeman, F. J., Sands, E. S., & Harris, K. S. (1978). Temporal coordination of phonation and articulation in a case of verbal apraxia: A voice onset time study. *Brain and Language, 6,* 106–111.

Frint, T. (1974). Experimentelle Untersuchungen seltner Stimmphänomene bei einem Fall von spastischer Dysphonie. *Folia Phoniatrica, 26,* 422–427.

Frøkjaer-Jensen, B., & Prytz, S. (1976). Registration of voice quality. *B & K Technical Review, 3,* 3–17.

Fry, D. B. (1955). Duration and intensity as physical correlates of linguistic stress. *Journal of the Acoustical Society of America, 27,* 765–768.

Fry, D. B. (1979). *The physics of speech.* New York: Cambridge University Press.

Fry, D. B., Abramson, A. S., Eimas, P. D., & Liberman, A. M. (1962). The identification and discrimination of synthetic vowels. *Language and Speech, 5,* 171–189.

Fujimura, O. (1962). Analysis of nasal consonants. *Journal of the Acoustical Society of America, 34,* 1865–1875.

Fujimura, O., & Erickson, D. (1997). Acoustic phonetics. In W. Hardcastle & J. Laver (Eds.), *The handbook of phonetic sciences* (pp. 65–115). Oxford, UK: Blackwell.

Fujimura, O., & Lindqvist, J. (1971). Sweep-tone measurements of vocal-tract characteristics. *Journal of the Acoustical Society of America, 49,* 541–558.

Gay, T. (1978). Effect of speaking rate on vowel formant movements. *Journal of the Acoustical Society of America, 63,* 223–230.

Gerratt, B. R. (1983). Formant frequency fluctuation as an index of motor steadiness in the vocal tract. *Journal of Speech and Hearing Research, 26,* 297–304.

Gerstman, L. J. (1957). *Perceptual dimension for the friction portions of certain speech sounds.* Unpublished Ph.D. dissertation, New York University.

Gerstman, L. J. (1968). Classification of self-normalized vowels. *IEEE Transactions in Audio and Electroacoustics, AV–16,* 78–80.

Gilbert, H. R., & Campbell, M. I. (1978). Voice onset time in the speech of hearing impaired individuals. *Folia Phoniatrica, 30,* 67–81.

Gilbert, J. H. (1970). Formant concentration positions in the speech of children at two levels of linguistic development. *Journal of the Acoustical Society of America, 48,* 1404–1406.

Gilbert, J. H. V. (1975). A voice onset time analysis of apical stop production in 3–year-olds. *Journal of Child Language, 4,* 103–110.

Glasson, C. (1984). Speech timing in children with history of phonological-phonetic disorders. *Seminars in Speech and Language, 5,* 85–95.

Goldstein, L., & Browman, C. P. (1986). Representation of voicing contrasts using articulatory gestures. *Haskins Laboratories Status Report on Speech Research, SR − 85,* 251–254.

Haggard, M., Ambler, S., & Callow, M. (1970). Pitch as a voicing cue. *Journal of the Acoustical Society of America, 47,* 613–617.

Haggard, M., Summerfield, Q., & Roberts, M. (1981). Psychoacoustical and cultural determinants of phoneme boundaries: Evidence from trading F_0 cues in the voiced-voiceless distinction. *Journal of Phonetics, 9,* 49–62.

Halle, M., Hughes, G. W., & Radley, P. A. (1957). Acoustic properties of stop consonants. *Journal of the Acoustical Society of America, 29,* 107–116.

Hammarberg, B., Fritzell, B., Gauffin, J., Sundberg, J., & Wedin, L. (1980). Perceptual and acoustic correlates of abnormal voice qualities. *Acta Otolaryngologica, 90,* 442–451.

Hardcastle, W. J., Barry, R. A. M., & Clark, C. J. (1985). Articulatory and voicing characteristics of adult dysarthric and verbal dyspraxic speakers: An instrumental study. *British Journal of Disorders of Communication, 20,* 249–270.

Harris, K. S. (1954). Cues for the identification of the fricatives of American English. *Journal of the Acoustical Society of America, 26,* 952A.

Harris, K. S. (1958). Cues for the discrimination of American English fricatives in spoken syllables. *Language and Speech, 1,* 1–7.

Harris, K. S., Hoffman, H. S., Liberman, A. M., Delattre, P. C., & Cooper, F. S. (1958). Effect of third-formant transitions on the perception of voiced stop consonants. *Journal of the Acoustical Society of America, 30,* 122–126.

Harteluis, L., Nord, L., & Buder, E. H. (1995). Acoustic analysis of dysarthria associated with multiple sclerosis. *Clinical Linguistics and Phonetics, 9,* 95–120.

Hattori, S., Yamamoto, K., & Fujimura, O. (1958). Nasalization of vowels in relation to nasals. *Journal of the Acoustical Society of America, 30,* 122–126.

Hawkins, S. (1973). Temporal coordination of consonants in the speech of children: Preliminary data. *Journal of Phonetics, 1,* 181–217.

Hayashi, A., Imaizumi, S., Harada, T., Seki, H., & Hosoi, H. (1992). Effect of fundamental frequency and silent intervals on the voicing distinction for stop consonants in VCV contexts. *Annual Bulletin of the Research Institute of Logopedics and Phonatrics, 26,* 69–78.

Healey, E. C., & Gutkin, B. (1984). Analysis of stutterers' voice onset times and fundamental frequency contours during fluency. *Journal of Speech and Hearing Research, 27,* 219–225.

Hecker, M. H. L. (1962). Studies of nasal consonants with an articulatory speech synthesizer. *Journal of the Acoustical Society of America, 34,* 179–188.

Heinz, J. M., & Stevens, K. N. (1961). On the properties of voiceless fricative consonants. *Journal of the Acoustical Society of America, 33,* 589–596.

Herzel, H., Berry, D., Titze, I. R., & Saleh, M. (1994). Analysis of vocal disorders with methods from nonlinear dynamics. *Journal of Speech and Hearing Research, 37,* 1008–1019.

Herzel, H., & Reuter, R. (1997). Whistle register and biphonation in a child's voice. *Folia Phoniatrica, 49,* 216–224.

Hillenbrand, J., & Gayvert, R. T. (1993). Vowel classification based on fundamental frequency and formant frequencies. *Journal of Speech and Hearing Research, 36,* 694–700.

Hillenbrand, J., Getty, L. A., Clark, M. J., & Wheeler, K. (1995). Acoustic characteristics of American English vowels. *Journal of the Acoustical Society of America, 97,* 3099–3111.

Hirose, H., & Gay, T. (1972). The activity of the intrinsic laryngeal muscles in voicing control. *Phonetica, 25,* 140–164.

Hirose, H., & Ushijima, T. (1978). Laryngeal control for voicing distinction in Japanese consonant production. *Phonetica, 35,* 1–10.

Hoemke, K. A., & Diehl, R. L. (1994). Perception of vowel height: The role of F1–F0 distance, *Journal of the Acoustical Society of America, 96,* 661–674.

Hoffman, H. S. (1958). Study of some cues in the perception of the voiced stop consonants. *Journal of the Acoustical Society of America, 30,* 1035–1041.

Hoffman, P. R., Schuckers, G. H., & Daniloff, R. G. (1989). *Children's phonetic disorders: Theory and treatment.* Boston, MA: Little, Brown.

Hoffman, P. R., Schuckers, G. H., & Ratusnik, D. L. (1989). Contextual-coarticulatory inconsistency of /r/ misarticulation. *Journal of Speech and Hearing Research, 20,* 631–643.

Holbrook, A., & Fairbanks, G. (1962). Diphthong formants and their movements. *Journal of Speech and Hearing Research, 5,* 38–58.

Honda, K. (1983). Relationship between pitch control and vowel articulation. In D. M. Bless & J. H. Abbs (Eds.), *Vocal fold physiology: Contemporary research and clinical issues* (pp. 286–297). San Diego, CA: College-Hill Press.

Honda, K. (1985). Variability analysis of laryngeal muscle activities. In I. R. Titze & R. C. Scherer (Eds.), *Vocal fold physiology: Biomechanics, acoustics and phonatory control* (pp. 128–137). Denver, CO: The Denver Center for the Performing Arts.

Honda, K., & Fujimura, O. (1991). Intrinsic vowel F$_0$ and phrase-final F$_0$ lowering: Phonological vs. biological explanations. In J. Gauffin & B. Hammarberg (Eds.), *Vocal fold physiology: Acoustic, perceptual, and physiological aspects of voice mechanisms* (pp. 149–157). San Diego, CA: Singular Publishing Group.

Hong, K. H., & Kim, H. K. (1997). Electroglottography and laryngeal articulation in speech. *Folia Phoniatrica et Logopaedica, 49,* 225–233.

Horii, Y., & Hata, K. (1988). A note on phase relationships between frequency and amplitude modulations in vocal vibrato. *Folia Phoniatrica, 40,* 303–311.

House, A. S. (1957). Analog studies of nasal consonants. *Journal of Speech and Hearing Disorders, 22,* 190–204.

House, A. S., & Fairbanks, G. (1953). The influence of consonant environment upon the secondary characteristics of vowels. *Journal of the Acoustical Society of America, 25,* 105–113.

Howell, P., & Rosen, S. (1983). Production and perception of rise time in the voiceless affricate/fricative distinction. *Journal of the Acoustical Society of America, 73,* 976–984.

Howell, P., & Vause, L. (1986). Acoustic analysis and perception of vowels in stuttered speech. *Journal of the Acoustical Society of America, 79,* 1571–1579.

Howell, P., & Williams, M. (1992). Acoustic analysis and perception of vowels in children's and teenagers' stuttered speech. *Journal of the Acoustical Society of America, 91,* 1697–1706.

Huer, M. B. (1989). Acoustic tracking of articulation errors: [r]. *Journal of Speech and Hearing Disorders, 54,* 530–534.

Huggins, A. W. F. (1980). Better spectrograms from children's speech: A research note. *Journal of Speech and Hearing Research, 23,* 19–27.

Hughes, G. W., & Halle, M. (1956). Spectral properties of voiceless fricative consonants. *Journal of the Acoustical Society of America, 28,* 303–310.

Imaizumi, S. (1986). Spectrographic evaluation of laryngeal pathology. In C. W. Cummings & J. M. Fredrickson (Eds.), *Otolaryngology—Head and neck surgery* (Vol. 3, pp. 1838–1845). St. Louis, MO: Mosby.

Israel, H. (1968). Continuing growth in the human cranial skeleton. *Archives of Oral Biology, 13,* 133–137.

Israel, H. (1973). Age factor and the pattern of change in craniofacial structures. *American Journal of Physical Anthropology, 39,* 111–128.

Isshiki, N. (1981). Vocal efficiency index. In K. N. Stevens & M. Hirano (Eds.), *Vocal fold physiology* (pp. 193–207). Tokyo, Japan: University of Tokyo Press.

Isshiki, N. (1985). Clinical significance of a vocal efficiency index. In I. R. Titze & R. C. Scherer (Eds.), *Vocal fold physiology: Biomechanics, acoustics and phonatory control* (pp. 230–238). Denver, CO: The Denver Center for the Performing Arts.

Isshiki, N., Ohkawa, M., & Goto, M. (1985). Stiffness of the vocal cord in dysphonia—Its assessment and treatment. *Acta Otolaryngologica, Suppl. 419,* 167–174.

Isshiki, N., Tanabe, M., Ishizaka, K., & Broad, D. (1977). Clinical significance of asymmetrical vocal cord tension. *Annals of Otology, Rhinology, and Laryngology, 86,* 58–66.

Isshiki, N., Yanagihara, N., & Morimoto, M. (1966). Approach to the objective diagnosis of hoarseness. *Folia Phoniatrica, 18,* 393–400.

Izdebski, K. (1980). Long-time-average spectra (LTAS) applied to analysis of spastic dysphonia. In V. Lawrence & B. Weinberg (Eds.), *Transcripts of the Ninth Symposium: Care of the professional voice* (part I, pp. 89–94). New York: The Voice Foundation.

Itoh, M., Sasanuma, S., Tatsumi, I. F., Marakami, S., Fukusato, Y., & Suzuki, T. (1982). Voice onset time characteristics in apraxia of speech. *Brain and Language, 17,* 193–210.

Jassem, W. (1965). The formants of fricative consonants. *Language and Speech, 8,* 1–16.

Jongman, A. (1989). Duration of frication noise required for identification of English fricatives. *Journal of the Acoustical Society of America, 85,* 1718–1725.

Kahane, J. C. (1979). Pathophysiological effects of Möbius syndrome on speech and hearing. *Archives of Otolaryngology, 105,* 29–34.

Kamen, R. S., & Watson, B. C. (1991). Effects of long-term tracheostomy on spectral characteristics of vowel production. *Journal of Speech and Hearing Research, 34,* 1057–1065.

Kasuya, H., Masubuchi, K., Ebihara, S., & Yoshida, H. (1986). Preliminary experiments on voice screening. *Journal of Phonetics, 14,* 463–468.

Kasuya, H., Ogawa, S., Kikuchi, Y., & Ebihara, S. (1986). An acoustic analysis of pathological voice and its application to the evaluation of laryngeal pathology. *Speech Communication, 5,* 171–181.

Kasuya, H., Ogawa, S., Mashima, K., & Ebihara, S. (1986). Normalized noise energy as an acoustic measure to evaluate pathologic voice. *Journal of the Acoustical Society of America, 80,* 1329–1334.

Keller, E., Vigneux, P., & Laframboise, M. (1991). Acoustic analysis of neurologically impaired speech. *British Journal of Disorders of Communication, 26,* 75–94.

Kent, J. F., Kent, R. D., Rosenbek, J. C., Weismer, G., Martin, R. E., Sufit, R. L., & Brooks, B. R. (1992). Quantitative description of the dysarthria in women with amyotrophic lateral sclerosis. *Journal of Speech and Hearing Research, 35,* 723–733.

Kent, R. D. (1976). Anatomical and neuromuscular maturation of the speech mechanism: Evidence from acoustic studies. *Journal of Speech and Hearing Research, 18,* 421–447.

Kent, R. D. (1978). Imitation of synthesized vowels by preschool children. *Journal of the Acoustical Society of America, 63,* 1193–1198.

Kent, R. D. (1979). Isovowel lines for the evaluation of formant structure in speech disorders. *Journal of Speech and Hearing Disorders, 44,* 513–521.

Kent, R. D. (1993). Vocal tract acoustics. *Journal of Voice, 7,* 97–117.

Kent, R. D. (1997). *The speech sciences.* San Diego, CA: Singular Publishing Group.

Kent, R. D., Dembowski, J., & Lass, N. J. (1996). The acoustic characteristics of American English. In N. J. Lass (Ed.), *Principles of experimental phonetics* (pp. 185–225). St. Louis, MO: Mosby.

Kent, R. D., Duffy, J. R., Vorperian, H. K., & Thomas, J. E. (1998). Severe essential vocal tremor and oromandibular tremor: A case report. *Phonoscope, 1,* 237–253.

Kent, R. D., & Forner, L. L. (1979). Developmental study of vowel formant frequencies in an imitation task. *Journal of the Acoustical Society of America, 65,* 208–217.

Kent, R. D., & Forner, L. L. (1980). Speech segment durations in sentence recitations by children and adults. *Journal of Phonetics, 8,* 157–168.

Kent, R. D., Kent, J. F., Weismer, G., Sufit, R. L., Brooks, B. R., & Rosenbek, J. C. (1989). Relationships between speech intelligibility and the slope of second formant transitions in dysarthric subjects. *Clinical Linguistics and Phonetics, 3,* 347–358.

Kent, R. D., & Murray, A. D. (1982). Acoustic features of vocalic utterances at 3, 6, and 9 months. *Journal of the Acoustical Society of America, 72,* 353–365.

Kent, R. D., Netsell, R., & Abbs, J. H. (1979). Acoustic characteristics of dysarthria associated with cerebellar disease. *Journal of Speech and Hearing Research, 22,* 627–648.

Kent, R. D., Osberger, M. J., Netsell, R., & Hustedde, C. G. (1987). Phonetic development in identical twins differing in auditory function. *Journal of Speech and Hearing Disorders, 52,* 64–75.

Kent, R. D., & Read, C. (1992). *The acoustic analysis of speech.* San Diego, CA: Singular Publishing Group.

Kent, R. D., & Rosenbek, J. C. (1983). Acoustic patterns of apraxia of speech. *Journal of Speech and Hearing Research, 26,* 231–249.

Kersta, L. G. (1948). Amplitude cross-section representation with the sound spectrograph. *Journal of the Acoustical Society of America, 20,* 796–801.

Kewley-Port, D., & Preston, M. S. (1974). Early apical stop production: A voice onset time analysis. *Journal of Phonetics, 2,* 195–210.

Kim, C. W. (1970). A theory of aspiration. *Phonetica, 21,* 107–119.

Kim, K. M., Kakita, Y., & Hirano, M. (1982). Sound spectrographic analysis of the voice of patients with recurrent laryngeal nerve paralysis. *Folia Phoniatrica, 34,* 124–133.

Kitajima, K., (1981). Quantitative evaluation of the noise level in the pathologic voice. *Folia Phoniatrica, 33,* 115–124.

Kitzing, P., & Åkerlund, L. (1993). Long-time average spectrograms of dysphonic voices before and after therapy. *Folia Phoniatrica, 45,* 53–61.

Klatt, D. H. (1973). Interaction between two factors that influence vowel duration. *Journal of the Acoustical Society of America, 54,* 1102–1104.

Klatt, D. H. (1974). The duration of /s/ in English words. *Journal of Speech and Hearing Research, 17,* 51–63.

Klatt, D. H. (1975a). Voice onset time, frication, and aspiration in word-initial consonant clusters. *Journal of Speech and Hearing Research, 18,* 686–706.

Klatt, D. H. (1975b). Vowel lengthening is syntactically determined in a connected discourse. *Journal of Phonetics, 3,* 129–140.

Klatt, D. H. (1976). Linguistic uses of segmental duration in English: Acoustic and perceptual evidence. *Journal of the Acoustical Society of America, 59,* 1208–1221.

Klein, R. P. (1971). Acoustic analysis of the acquisition of acceptable *r* in American English. *Child Development, 42,* 543–550.

Klich, R. J., & May, G. M. (1982). Spectrographic study of vowels in stutterers' fluent speech. *Journal of Speech and Hearing Research, 25,* 364–370.

Koenig, W., Dunn, H. K., & Lacy, L. Y. (1946). The sound spectrograph. *Journal of the Acoustical Society of America, 18,* 19–49.

Kohler, K. J. (1982). F_0 in the production of lenis and fortis plosives. *Phonetica, 39,* 199–218.

Kohler, K. J. (1985). F_0 in the perception of lenis and fortis plosives. *Journal of the Acoustical Society of America, 78,* 21–32.

Kojima, H., Gould, W. J., Lambiase, A., & Isshiki, N. (1980). Computer analysis of hoarseness. *Acta Otolaryngologica, 89,* 547–554.

Krause, S. E. (1982). Vowel duration as a perceptual cue to postvocalic consonant voicing in young children and adults. *Journal of the Acoustical Society of America, 71,* 990–995.

Kuhl, P. K. (1979). The perception of speech in early infancy. In N. J. Lass (Ed.), *Speech and language* (Vol. I, pp. 1–47). New York: Academic Press.

Kuhl, P. K., & Miller, J. (1975). Speech perception by the chinchilla: Voiced-voiceless distinction in alveolar plosive consonants. *Science, 190,* 69–72.

Kuhl, P. K., & Miller, J. (1978). Speech perception by the chinchilla: Identification for synthetic VOT stimuli. *Journal of the Acoustical Society of America, 63,* 905–917.

Kurowski, K., & Blumstein, S. E. (1984). Perceptual integration of the murmur and formant transitions for place of articulation in nasal consonants. *Journal of the Acoustical Society of America, 76,* 383–390.

Kurowski, K., & Blumstein, S. E. (1987). Acoustic properties for place of articulation in nasal consonants. *Journal of the Acoustical Society of America, 81,* 1917–1927.

Ladefoged, P. (1971). *Preliminaries to linguistic phonetics.* Chicago, IL: University of Chicago Press.

Ladefoged, P., & Broadbent, D. E. (1957). Information conveyed by vowels. *Journal of the Acoustical Society of America, 29,* 98–104.

Ladefoged, P., Harshman, R., Goldstein, L., & Rice, L. (1978). Generating vocal tract shapes from formant frequencies. *Journal of the Acoustical Society of America, 64,* 1027–1035.

Ladefoged, P., & Maddieson, I. (1996). *The sounds of the world's languages.* Oxford, UK: Blackwell.

Lane, H., & Webster, J. W. (1991). Speech deterioration in postlingually deafened adults. *Journal of the Acoustical Society of America, 89,* 859–866.

Larkey, L., Wald, J., & Strange, W. (1978). Perception of synthetic nasal consonants in initial and final syllable position. *Perception and Psychophysics, 23,* 299–312.

Lebrun, Y., Devreux, F., Rousseau, J.-J., & Darimont, P. (1982). Tremulous speech: A case report. *Folia Phoniatrica, 34,* 134–142.

Lee, S., Potamianos, A., & Narayanan, S. (1999). Acoustics of children's speech: Developmental changes of temporal and spectral parameters. *Journal of the Acoustical Society of America, 105,* 1455–1468.

Lehiste, I. (1964). Acoustic characteristics of selected English consonants. *International Journal of American Linguistics, 30,* 1–197.

Lehiste, I. (1972). The timing of utterances and linguistic boundaries. *Journal of the Acoustical Society of America, 51,* 2018–2024.

Lehiste, I., & Peterson, G. E. (1961). Some basic considerations in the analysis of intonation. *Journal of the Acoustical Society of America, 33,* 419–425.

Leinonen, L., Kangas, J., Torkkola, K., & Juvas, A. (1992). Dysphonia detected by pattern recognition of spectral composition. *Journal of Speech and Hearing Research, 35,* 287–295.

Liberman, A. M. (1957). Some results of research on speech perception. *Journal of the Acoustical Society of America, 29,* 117–123.

Liberman, A. M., Delattre, P. C., & Cooper, F. S. (1952). The role of selected stimulus variables in the perception of the unvoiced stop consonants. *American Journal of Psychology, 65,* 497–516.

Liberman, A. M., Delattre, P. C., & Cooper, F. S. (1958). Some cues for the distinction between voiced and voiceless stops in initial position. *Language and Speech, 1,* 153–167.

Liberman, A. M., Delattre, P. C., Gerstman, L. J., & Cooper, F. S. (1956). Tempo of frequency change as a cue for distinguishing classes of speech sounds. *Journal of Experimental Psychology, 52,* 127–137.

Liberman, A. M., Harris, K. S., Hoffman, H. S., & Griffith, B. C. (1957). The discrimination of speech sounds within and across phoneme boundaries. *Journal of Experimental Psychology, 54,* 358–368.

Lieberman, P. (1977). *Speech physiology and acoustic phonetics: An introduction.* New York: Macmillan.

Lieberman, P., Kako, E., Friedman, J., Tajchman, G., Feldman, L. S., & Jimenez, E. B. (1992). Speech production, syntax comprehension, and cognitive deficits in Parkinson's disease. *Brain and Language, 43,* 169–189.

Lindblom, B. (1963). Spectrographic study of vowel reduction. *Journal of the Acoustical Society of America, 35,* 1773–1781.

Lindblom, B. E. F., & Studdert-Kennedy, M. (1967). On the rôle of formant transitions in vowel recognition. *Journal of the Acoustical Society of America, 42,* 830–843.

Lindblom, B. E. F., & Sundberg, J. E. F. (1971). Acoustical consequences of lip, tongue, jaw, and larynx movement. *Journal of the Acoustical Society of America, 50,* 1166–1179.

Linville, S. E., & Fisher, H. B. (1985). Acoustic characteristics of perceived versus actual vocal age in controlled phonation by adult females. *Journal of the Acoustical Society of America, 78,* 40–48.

Lisker, L. (1957a). Minimal cues for separating /w, j, r, l/ in intervocalic position. *Word, 13,* 256–267.

Lisker, L. (1957b). Closure duration and the intervocalic voiced—voiceless distinction in English. *Language, 33,* 42–47.

Lisker, L., & Abramson, A. S. (1964). A cross-language study of voicing in initial stops: Acoustic measurements. *Word, 20,* 384–442.

Lisker, L., & Abramson, A. S. (1967). Some effects of context on voice onset time in English stops. *Language and Speech, 10,* 1–28.

Lisker, L., & Abramson, A. S. (1971). Distinctive features and laryngeal control. *Language, 47,* 767–785.

Lively, M. A., & Emanuel, F. W. (1970). Spectral noise levels and roughness severity ratings for normal and simulated rough vowels produced by adult females. *Journal of Speech and Hearing Research, 13,* 503–517.

Löfqvist, A., & Manderson, B. (1987). Long-time average spectrum of speech and voice analysis. *Folia Phoniatrica, 39,* 221–229.

Löfqvist, A., & McGowan, R. S. (1992). Influence of consonantal environment on voice source aerodynamics. *Journal of Phonetics, 20,* 93–110.

Löfqvist, A., & Yoshioka, H. (1979). Laryngeal activity in Swedish voiceless obstruent clusters. *Haskins Laboratories Status Report on Speech Research, SR59/60,* 103–125.

Löfqvist, A., & Yoshioka, H. (1984). Intrasegmental timing: Laryngeal-oral coordination in voiceless consonant production. *Speech Communication, 3,* 279–289.

Löfqvist, A., Baer, T., McGarr, N. S., & Story, R. S. (1989). The cricothyroid muscle in voicing control. *Journal of the Acoustical Society of America, 85,* 1314–1321.

Lotto, A. J., Holt, L. L., & Kluender, K. R. (1997). Effect of voice quality on perceived height of English vowels. *Phonetica, 54,* 76–93.

Macken, M. A., & Barton, D. (1980). A longitudinal study of the voicing contrast in American English word-initial stops, as measured by voice onset time. *Journal of Child Language, 7,* 41–74.

Maki, J. E., Gustafson, M. S., Conklin, J. M., & Humphrey-Whitehead, B. K. (1981). The speech spectrographic display: Interpretation of visual patterns by hearing-impaired adults. *Journal of Speech and Hearing Disorders, 46,* 379–387.

Malécot, A. (1956). Acoustic cues for nasal consonants: An experimental study involving a tape-splicing technique. *Language, 32,* 274–284.

Malécot, A. (1970). The lenis-fortis opposition: Its physiological parameters. *Journal of the Acoustical Society of America, 47,* 1588–1592.

Malmberg, B. (1955). The phonetic basis for syllable division. *Studia Linguistica, 9,* 80–87.

Manning, W. H., Moore, J. N., Dunham, M. J., Lu, F. L., & Domico, E. (1992). Vowel production in a prelinguistic child following cochlear implantation. *Journal of the American Academy of Audiology, 3,* 16–21.

Matthies, M. L., Svirsky, M. A., Lane, H. L., & Perkell, J. S. (1994). A preliminary study of the effects of cochlear implants on the production of sibilants. *Journal of the Acoustical Society of America, 96,* 1367–1373.

Maurer, D., Cook, N., Landis, T., & d'Heureuse, C. (1992). Are measured differences between the formants of men, women and children due to F_0 differences? *Journal of the International Phonetic Association, 21,* 66–79.

Maurer, D., & Landis, T. (1996). Intelligibility and spectral differences in high-pitched vowels. *Folia Phoniatrica et Logopaedica, 48,* 1–10.

Max, L., & Caruso, A. J. (1998). Adaptation of stuttering frequency during repeated readings: Associated changes in acoustic parameters of perceptually fluent speech. *Journal of Speech, Language, and Hearing Research, 41,* 1265–1281.

Maxwell, E., & Weismer, G. (1982). The contribution of phonological, acoustic, and perceptual techniques to the characterization of a misarticulating child's voice onset time for stops. *Applied Psycholinguistics, 3,* 29–44.

Mazza, P. L., Schuckers, G. H., & Daniloff, R. G. (1979). Contextual-coarticulatory inconsistency of /s/ misarticulation. *Journal of Phonetics, 7*, 57–69.

McAllister, A., Sundberg, J., & Hibi, S. R. (1998). Acoustic measurements and perceptual evaluation of hoarseness in children's voices. *Logopedics Phoniatrics Vocology, 23*, 27–38.

McGovern, K., & Strange, W. (1977). The perception of /r/ and /l/ in syllable-initial and syllable-final position. *Perception and Psychophysics, 21*, 162–170.

McGowan, R. S., & Nittrouer, S. (1988). Differences in fricative production between children and adults: Evidence from an acoustic analysis of /ʃ/ and /s/. *Journal of the Acoustical Society of America, 83*, 229–236.

McLeod, S., & Issac, K. (1995). Use of spectrographic analyses to evaluate the efficacy of phonological intervention. *Clinical Linguistics and Phonetics, 9*, 229–234.

Mende, W., Herzel, H., & Wermke, K. (1990). Bifurcations and chaos in newborn infant cries. *Physics Letters A, 145*, 418–424.

Mendoza, E., Valencia, N., Muñoz, J., & Trujillo, H. (1996). Differences in voice quality between men and women: Use of the long-term average spectrum (LTAS). *Journal of Voice, 10*, 59–66.

Menyuk, P., & Klatt, M. (1975). Voice onset time in consonant cluster production by children and adults. *Journal of Child Language, 2*, 223–231.

Mermelstein, P. (1967). Determination of the vocal tract shape from measured formant frequencies. *Journal of the Acoustical Society of America, 41*, 1283–1294.

Michelsson, K. (1980). Cry characteristics in sound spectrographic cry analysis. In T. Murry & J. Murry (Eds.), *Infant communication: Cry and early speech* (pp. 85–105). San Diego, CA: College-Hill Press.

Michelsson, K., Raes, J., Thoden, C., & Wasz-Hockert, O. (1982). Sound spectrographic analysis in neonatal diagnostics. *Journal of Phonetics, 10*, 79–88.

Miller, J. D. (1989). Auditory-perceptual interpretation of the vowel. *Journal of the Acoustical Society of America, 85*, 2114–2134.

Mol, H. (1963). *Fundamentals of phonetics* (Janua Linguarum, no. 26). The Hague: Mouton.

Monsen, R. B. (1976a). Second formant transitions of selected consonant-vowel combinations in the speech of deaf and normal-hearing children. *Journal of Speech and Hearing Research, 19*, 279–289.

Monsen, R. B. (1976b). Normal and reduced phonological space: The production of English vowels by deaf adolescents. *Journal of Phonetics, 4*, 189–198.

Monsen, R. B. (1979). Acoustic qualities of phonation in young hearing-impaired children. *Journal of Speech and Hearing Research, 22*, 270–288.

Monsen, R. B., & Engebretson, A. M. (1983). The accuracy of formant frequency measurements: A comparison of spectrographic analysis and linear prediction. *Journal of Speech and Hearing Research, 26*, 89–97.

Moon, S.-J., & Lindblom, B. (1994). Interaction between duration, context, and speaking style in English stressed vowels. *Journal of the Acoustical Society of America, 96*, 40–55.

Moran, M. J. (1986). Identification of Down's syndrome adults from prolonged vowel samples. *Journal of Communication Disorders, 19*, 387–394.

Morris, R. J. (1989). VOT and dysarthria: A descriptive study. *Journal of Communication Disorders, 22*, 23–33.

Mujunen, R., Leinonen, L., Kangas, J., & Torkkola, K. (1993). Acoustic pattern recognition of /s/ misarticulation by the self-organizing map. *Folia Phoniatrica, 45*, 135–144.

Mulligan, M., Carpenter, J., Riddel, J., Delaney, M. K., Badger, G., Krusinski, P., & Tandan, R. (1994). Intelligibility and the acoustic characteristics of speech in amyotrophic lateral sclerosis. *Journal of Speech and Hearing Research, 37*, 496–503.

Murry, T., & Brown, W. S., Jr. (1979). Aerodynamic interactions associated with voiced-voiceless stop consonants. *Folia Phoniatrica, 31*, 82–88.

Nakajima, T. (1977). Identification of a dynamic articulatory model by acoustic analysis. In M. Sawashima & F. S. Cooper (Eds.), *Dynamic aspects of speech production* (pp. 251–275). Tokyo, Japan: University of Tokyo Press.

Nakata, K. (1959). Synthesis and perception of nasal consonants. *Journal of the Acoustical Society of America, 31*, 661–666.

Nearey, T. M. (1980). On the physical interpretation of vowel quality: Cinefluorographic and acoustic evidence. *Journal of Phonetics, 8*, 213–241.

Nearey, T. M. (1989). Static, dynamic, and relational properties in vowel perception. *Journal of the Acoustical Society of America, 85*, 2088–2113.

Neiman, G. S., Klich, R. J., & Shuey, E. M. (1983). Voice onset time in young and 70–year-old women. *Journal of Speech and Hearing Research, 26*, 118–123.

Nessel, E. (1962). Über das Tonfrequenz Spektrum der Pathologisch veränderten Stimme. *Acta Otolaryngologica, Suppl. 157*, 1–45.

Newman, R. A., & Emanuel, F. W. (1991). Pitch effects on vowel roughness and spectral noise for subjects in four musical voice classifications. *Journal of Speech and Hearing Research, 34*, 753–760.

Nittrouer, S., Studdert-Kennedy, M., & McGowan, R. S. (1989). The emergence of phonetic segments: Evidence from the spectral structure of fricative-vowel syllables spoken by children and adults. *Journal of Speech and Hearing Research, 32*, 120–132.

Novak, A., Dlouha, O., Capkova, B., & Vohradnik, M. (1991). Voice fatigue after theater performance in actors. *Folia Phoniatrica, 43*, 74–78.

O'Connor, J. D., Gerstman, L. J., Liberman, A. M., Delattre, P. G., & Cooper, F. S. (1957). Acoustic cues for the perception of initial /w, j, r, l/ in English. *Word, 13*, 24–43.

Ohde, R. N. (1984). Fundamental frequency as an acoustic correlate of stop consonant voicing. *Journal of the Acoustical Society of America, 75*, 224–230.

Ohde, R. N., & Sharf, D. J. (1992). *Phonetic analysis of normal and abnormal speech.* New York: Merrill.

Öhman, S. E. G. (1966). Coarticulation in VCV utterances: Spectrographic measurements. *Journal of the Acoustical Society of America, 39*, 151–168.

Öhman, S. E. G. (1967). Numerical model of coarticulation. *Journal of the Acoustical Society of America, 41*, 310–320.

Orlikoff, R. F., & Baken, R. J. (1993). *Clinical speech and voice measurement: Laboratory exercises.* San Diego, CA: Singular Publishing Group.

Orlikoff, R. F., & Kahane, J. C. (1996). Structure and function of the larynx. In N. J. Lass (Ed.), *Principles of experimental phonetics* (pp. 112–181). St. Louis, MO: Mosby-Year Book.

Orlikoff, R. F., & Kraus, D. H. (1996). Dysphonia following nonsurgical management of advanced laryngeal carcinoma. *American Journal of Speech-Language Pathology, 5*(3), 47–52.

Osberger, M. J. (1987). Training effects on vowel production by two profoundly hearing-impaired speakers. *Journal of Speech and Hearing Research, 30*, 241–251.

Ouellon, M., Ryalls, J., Lebeuf, J., & Joanette, Y. (1991). Le «voice onset time» chez des dysarthriques de Friedreich. *Folia Phoniatrica, 43*, 295–303.

Paige, A., & Zue, V. W. (1970a). Calculation of vocal tract length. *IEEE Transactions: Audio and Electroacoustics, AU18,* 268–270.

Paige, A., & Zue, V. W. (1970b). Computation of vocal tract area functions. *IEEE Transactions: Audio and Electroacoustics, AU18,* 7–18.

Parnell, M., Amerman, J. D., & Wells, G. B. (1977). Closure and constriction duration for alveolar consonants during voiced and whispered speaking conditions. *Journal of the Acoustical Society of America, 61,* 612–613.

Pentz, A., Gilbert, H. R., & Zawadzki, P. (1979). Spectral properties of fricative consonants in children. *Journal of the Acoustical Society of America, 66,* 1891–1893.

Peterson, G. E. (1959). Vowel formant measurements. *Journal of Speech and Hearing Research, 2,* 173–183.

Peterson, G. E. (1961). Parameters of vowel quality. *Journal of Speech and Hearing Research, 4,* 10–29.

Peterson, G. E., & Barney, H. L. (1952). Control methods used in a study of the vowels. *Journal of the Acoustical Society of America, 24,* 175–184.

Peterson, G. E., & Lehiste, I. (1960). Duration of syllable nuclei in English. *Journal of the Acoustical Society of America, 32,* 693–703.

Pickett, J. M. (1980). *The sounds of speech communication: A primer of acoustic phonetics and speech perception.* Baltimore, MD: University Park Press.

Pickett, J. M. (1999). *The acoustics of speech communication: Fundamentals, speech perception theory, and technology.* Needham Heights, MA: Allyn and Bacon.

Port, R. F., & Dalby, J. (1982). Consonant/vowel ratio as a cue for voicing in English. *Perception and Psychophysics, 32,* 141–152.

Port, R. F., & Rotunno, R. (1979). Relation between voice-onset time and vowel duration. *Journal of the Acoustical Society of America, 66,* 654–662.

Potter, R. K., Kopp, G. A., & Green, H. G. (1947). *Visible speech.* New York: Van Nostrand [reprinted by Dover Books, New York, 1966.] .

Potter, R. K., & Peterson, G. E. (1948). The representation of vowels and their movements. *Journal of the Acoustical Society of America, 20,* 528–535.

Potter, R. K., & Steinberg, J. C. (1950). Toward the specification of speech. *Journal of the Acoustical Society of America, 22,* 807–820.

Prestigiacomo, A. J. (1957). Plastic-tape sound spectrograph. *Journal of Speech and Hearing Disorders, 22,* 321–327.

Preston, M. S., & Port, D. K. (1969). Further results of voicing in stop consonants in young children. *Haskins Laboratories Status Report on Speech Research, SR13/14,* 181–184.

Preston, M. S., & Yeni-Komshian, G. (1967). Studies on the development of stop consonants in children. *Haskins Laboratories Status Report on Speech Research, SR-11,* 49–53.

Prosek, R. A., & Runyan, C. M. (1982). Temporal characteristics related to the discrimination of stutterers' and nonstutterers' speech samples. *Journal of Speech and Hearing Research, 25,* 29–33.

Pruszewicz, A., Obrebowski, A., Swindzinski, P., Demenko, G., Wika, T., & Wojciechowska, A. (1991). Usefulness of acoustic studies on the differential diagnostics of organic and functional dysphonia. *Acta Otolaryngologica, 111,* 414–419.

Ramig, L. A. (1986). Acoustic analyses of phonation in patients with Huntington's disease: Preliminary report. *Annals of Otology, Rhinology, and Laryngology, 95,* 288–293.

Ramig, L. O., Scherer, R. C., Klasner, E. R., Titze, I. R., & Horii, Y. (1990). Acoustic analysis of voice in amyotrophic lateral sclerosis: A longitudinal case study. *Journal of Speech and Hearing Disorders, 55,* 2–14.

Ramirez, R. W. (1985). *The FFT, fundamentals and concepts.* Englewood Cliffs, NJ: Prentice-Hall.

Raphael, L. J. (1972). Preceding vowel duration as a cue to the perception of the voicing characteristics of word-final consonants in American English. *Journal of the Acoustical Society of America, 51,* 1296–1303.

Raphael, L. J., & Dorman, M. F. (1980). Acoustic cues for a fricative-affricate contrast in word-final position. *Journal of Phonetics, 8,* 397–405.

Rastatter, M. P., & Jacques, R. D. (1990). Formant frequency structure of the aging male and female vocal tract. *Folia Phoniatrica, 42,* 312–319.

Recasens, D. (1983). Place cues for nasal consonants with special reference to Catalan. *Journal of the Acoustical Society of America, 73,* 1346–1353.

Remacle, M., & Trigaux, I. (1991). Characteristics of nodules through the high-resolution frequency analyzer. *Folia Phoniatrica, 43,* 53–59.

Repp, B. H. (1986). Perception of the [m]–[n] distinction in CV syllables. *Journal of the Acoustical Society of America, 79,* 1987–1999.

Revoile, S., Pickett, J. M., Holden-Pitt, L. D., Talkin, D., & Brandt, F. D. (1987). Burst and transition cues to voicing perception for spoken initial stops by impaired- and normal-hearing listeners. *Journal of Speech and Hearing Research, 30,* 3–12.

Riesz, R. R., & Schott, L. (1946). Visible speech cathode-ray translator. *Journal of the Acoustical Society of America, 18,* 50–61.

Rihkanen, H., Leinonen, L., Hitunen, T., & Kangas, J. (1994). Spectral pattern recognition of improved voice quality. *Journal of Voice, 8,* 320–326.

Robb, L., & Saxman, J. (1988). Acoustic observations in young children's noncry vocalizations. *Journal of the Acoustical Society of America, 83,* 1876–1882.

Rontal, E., Rontal, M., & Rolnick, M. I. (1975a). Objective evaluation of vocal pathology using spectrography. *Annals of Otology, Rhinology, and Laryngology, 84,* 662–671.

Rontal, E., Rontal, M., & Rolnick, M. I. (1975b). The use of spectrograms in the evaluation of vocal cord injection. *Laryngoscope, 85,* 47–56.

Rontal, E., Rontal, M., Leuchter, W., & Rolnick, M. I. (1978). Voice spectrography in the evaluation of myasthenia gravis of the larynx. *Annals of Otology, Rhinology, and Laryngology, 87,* 722–728.

Rothenberg, M. (1968). The breath-stream dynamics of simple released plosive production. *Bibliotheca Phonetica, 6,* 1–117.

Ryalls, J., & Larouche, A. (1992). Acoustic integrity of speech production in children with moderate and severe hearing impairment. *Journal of Speech and Hearing Research, 35,* 88–95.

Sáfrán, A. (1971). Vergleichende Untersuchungen der Leistung der normal-, Flüster- und Ösophagussprache sowie der Stimmprothese mit dem Sona-Graph. *Folia Phoniatrica, 23,* 323–332.

Sansone, F. E., Jr., & Emanuel, F. W. (1970). Spectral noise levels and roughness severity ratings for normal and simulated rough vowels produced by adult males. *Journal of Speech and Hearing Research, 13,* 489–502.

Sapir, S. (1989). The intrinsic pitch of vowels: Theoretical, physiological, and clinical considerations. *Journal of Voice, 3,* 44–51.

Sasaki, Y., Okamura, H., & Yumoto, E. (1991). Quantitative analysis of hoarseness using a digital sound spectrograph. *Journal of Voice, 5,* 36–40.

Sawashima, M. (1970). Glottal adjustments for English obstruents. *Haskins Laboratories Status Report on Speech Research, SR21/22*, 180–200.

Schäferskipper, P., Amorosa, H., von Benda, U., & Dames, M. (1986). Spektral-Energieverteilungen des /s/-Lautes bei sprachentwicklungsgestörten Kindern. *Folia Phoniatrica, 38*, 36–41.

Schlorhaufer, W., Müller, W. G., Hussl, B., & Scharfetter, L. (1972). Energieverteilung und Dynamik bei der Mutationsfistelstimme im Vergleich zur Normalstimme. *Folia Phoniatrica, 24*, 7–18.

Schönhärl, E. (1963). Beitrag zur Qualitativen Stimmanalyse. *Zeitschrift für Laryngologie, Rhinologie, und Otologie, 42*, 130–139.

Schroeder, M. R. (1967). Determination of the geometry of the human vocal tract by acoustic measurements. *Journal of the Acoustical Society of America, 41*, 1002–1010.

Scukanec, G., Petrosino, L., & Squibb, K. (1991). Formant frequency characteristics of children, young adult, and aged female speakers. *Perceptual and Motor Skills, 73*, 203–208.

Scully, C., Castelli, E., Brearley, E., & Shirt, M. (1992). Analysis and simulation of a speaker's aerodynamic and acoustic patterns for fricatives. *Journal of Phonetics, 20*, 39–51.

Seikel, J. A., Wilcox, K. A., & Davis, J. (1990). Dysarthria of motor neuron disease: Clinical judgments of severity. *Journal of Communication Disorders, 23*, 417–431.

Seikel, J. A., Wilcox, K. A., & Davis, J. (1991). Dysarthria of motor neuron disease: Longitudinal measures of segmental durations. *Journal of Communication Disorders, 24*, 393–409.

Sharf, D. J., & Benson, P. J. (1982). Identification of synthesized /r-w/ continua for adult and child speakers. *Journal of the Acoustical Society of America, 71*, 1008–1015.

Shewan, C. M., Leeper, H. A., Jr., & Booth, J. C. (1984). An analysis of voice onset time (VOT) in aphasic and normal subjects. In J. C. Rosenbek, M. R. McNeil, & A. E. Aronson (Eds.), *Apraxia of speech: Physiology, acoustics, linguistics, management* (pp. 197–220). San Diego, CA: Singular Publishing Group.

Shoup, J. E., Lass, N. J., & Kuehn, D. P. (1982). Acoustics of speech. In Lass, N. J., Northern, J. L., & Yoder, D. E. (Eds.), *Speech, language, and hearing*, vol. 1 (pp. 193–218). Philadelphia, PA: Saunders.

Shuster, L. I., Ruscello, D. M., & Smith, K. D. (1992). Evoking [r] using visual feedback. *American Journal of Speech-Language Pathology, 1*(3), 29–34.

Simmons, N. N. (1983). Acoustic analysis of ataxic dysarthria: An approach to monitoring treatment. In Berry, W. R. (Ed.), *Clinical dysarthria* (pp. 283–294). San Diego, CA: College-Hill Press.

Sirviö, P., & Michelsson, K. (1976). Sound spectrographic cry analysis of normal and abnormal newborn infants. *Folia Phoniatrica, 28*, 161–173.

Slawinski, E. B. (1994). Acoustic correlates of [b] and [w] produced by normal young to elderly adults. *Journal of the Acoustical Society of America, 95*, 2221–2230.

Slis, I. H., & Cohen, A. (1969a). On the complex regulating the voiced-voiceless distinction I. *Language and Speech, 12*, 80–102.

Slis, I. H., & Cohen, A. (1969b). On the complex regulating the voiced-voiceless distinction II. *Language and Speech, 12*, 137–155.

Smith, B. E., & Kenney, M. K. (1998). An assessment of several acoustic parameters in children's speech production development: Longitudinal data. *Journal of Phonetics, 26*, 95–108.

Smith, B., Marquardt, T. P., Cannito, M. P., & Davis, B. L. (1994). Vowel variability in developmental apraxia of speech. In J. A.

Till, K. M. Yorkston, & D. R. Beukelman (Eds.), *Motor speech disorders: Advances in assessment and treatment* (pp. 81–88). Baltimore, MD: Paul H. Brookes.

Soli, S. D. (1981). Second formants in fricatives: Acoustic consequences of fricative-vowel coarticulation. *Journal of the Acoustical Society of America, 70*, 976–984.

Sondhi, M. M., & Gopinath, B. (1971). Determination of the geometry of the human vocal tract by acoustic measurements. *Journal of the Acoustical Society of America, 49*, 1867–1873.

Sonninen, A. (1968). The external frame function in the control of pitch in the human voice. *Annals of the New York Academy of Sciences, 155*, 68–90.

Speaks, C. E. (1999). *Introduction to sound: Acoustics for the hearing and speech sciences* (3rd ed.). San Diego, CA: Singular Publishing Group.

Steinberg, J. C. (1934). Application of sound measuring instruments to the study of phonetic problems. *Journal of the Acoustical Society of America, 6*, 16–24.

Stetson, R. H. (1928). Motor phonetics. *Archives Néerlandaises de Phonétique Expérimentale, 3*, 1–216. [Reprinted as: J. A. S. Kelso & K. G. Munhall (Eds.), *R. H. Stetson's motor phonetics.* Boston, MA: Little, Brown, 1988.]

Stevens, K. N. (1971). Airflow and turbulence noise for fricative and stop consonants: Static considerations. *Journal of the Acoustical Society of America, 50*, 1182–1192.

Stevens, K. N., & Blumstein, S. E. (1978). Invariant cues for place of articulation in stop consonants. *Journal of the Acoustical Society of America, 64*, 1358–1368.

Stevens, K. N., & House, A. S. (1955). Development of a quantitative description of vowel articulation. *Journal of the Acoustical Society of America, 27*, 484–493.

Stevens, K. N., & House, A. S. (1961). An acoustical theory of vowel production and some of its implications. *Journal of Speech and Hearing Research, 4*, 303–320.

Stevens, K. N., Kasowski, S., & Fant, G. M. (1953). An electrical analog of the vocal tract. *Journal of the Acoustical Society of America, 25*, 734–742.

Stevens, K. N., & Klatt, D. H. (1972). Current models of sound sources for speech. In B. D. Wyke (Ed.), *Ventilatory and phonatory control systems.* New York: Oxford University Press.

Stevens, K. N., & Klatt, D. H. (1974). The role of formant transitions in the voiced-voiceless distinction for stops. *Journal of the Acoustical Society of America, 55*, 653–659.

Strange, W. (1989). Dynamic specification of coarticulated vowels spoken in sentence context. *Journal of the Acoustical Society of America, 85*, 2135–2153.

Strange, W., Verbrugge, R. R., Shankweiler, D. P., & Edman, T. R. (1976). Consonant environment specifies vowel identity. *Journal of the Acoustical Society of America, 60*, 213–224.

Strange, W., Jenkins, J. J., & Johnson, T. L. (1983). Dynamic specification of coarticulated vowels. *Journal of the Acoustical Society of America, 74*, 695–705.

Strevens, P. (1960). Spectra of fricative noise in human speech. *Language and Speech, 3*, 32–49.

Strube, H. W. (1977). Can the area function of the human vocal tract be determined from the speech wave? In M. Sawashima & F. S. Cooper (Eds.), *Dynamic aspects of speech production* (pp. 233–248). Tokyo, Japan: University of Tokyo Press.

Stuart, R. D. (1966). *An introduction to Fourier analysis.* London, UK: Chapman and Hall.

Summerfield, Q., & Haggard, M. (1977). On the dissociation of spectral and temporal cues to the voicing distinction in initial stop consonants. *Journal of the Acoustical Society of America, 62*, 435–448.

ŠSvec, J., & Pšák, J. (1994). Vocal breaks from the modal to falsetto register. *Folia Phoniatrica et Logopaedica, 46*, 97–103.

ŠSvec, J. G., Schutte, H. K. & Miller, D. G. (1996). A subharmonic vibratory pattern in normal vocal folds. *Journal of Speech and Hearing Research, 39*, 135–143.

Sweeting, P. M., & Baken, R. J. (1982). Voice onset time in a normal-aged population. *Journal of Speech and Hearing Research, 25*, 129–134.

Syrdal, A. K. (1984). Aspects of a model of the auditory representation of American English vowels. *Speech Communication, 4*, 121–135.

Syrdal, A. K., & Gopal, H. S. (1986). A perceptual model of vowel recognition based on the auditory representation of American English vowels. *Journal of the Acoustical Society of America, 79*, 1086–1100.

Tarnóczy, T. (1948). Resonance data concerning nasals, laterals, and trills. *Word, 4*, 71–77.

Tarnóczy, T., & Fant, G. (1964). Some remarks on the average speech spectrum. *Speech Transmission Laboratory Quarterly Progress and Status Report* (Royal Institute of Technology, Stockholm, Sweden), *4*, 13–14.

Tato, J. M., Mariani, N., DePiccoli, E. M. W., & Mirasov, P. (1954). Study of the sonospectrographic characteristics of the voice in laryngectomized patients. *Acta Otolaryngologica, 44*, 431–438.

Thomas-Kersting, C., & Casteel, R. L. (1989). Harsh voice: Vocal effort perceptual ratings and spectral noise levels of hearing-impaired children. *Journal of Communication Disorders, 22*, 125–135.

Tiffany, W. R. (1959). Nonrandom sources of variation in vowel quality. *Journal of Speech and Hearing Research, 2*, 305–317.

Till, J. A., & Stivers, D. K. (1981). Instrumentation and validity for direct-readout voice onset time measurement. *Journal of Communication Disorders, 14*, 507–512.

Titze, I. R. (1994). *Principles of voice production* (pp. 136–168). Englewood Cliffs, NJ: Prentice-Hall.

Titze, I. R. (1995). *Workshop on acoustic voice analysis: Summary statement* (36 pp.). Iowa City, IA: National Center for Voice and Speech, University of Iowa.

Titze, I. R., Baken, R. J., & Herzel, H. (1993). Evidence of chaos in vocal folds vibration. In I. R. Titze (Ed.), *Vocal fold physiology: Frontiers in basic science* (pp. 143–188). San Diego, CA: Singular Publishing Group.

Tjaden, K., & Turner, G. S. (1997). Spectral properties of fricatives in amyotrophic lateral sclerosis. *Journal of Speech, Language, and Hearing Research, 40*, 1358–1372.

Toner, M. A., Emanuel, F. W., & Parker, D. (1990). Relationship of spectral noise levels to psychophysical scaling of vowel roughness. *Journal of Speech and Hearing Research, 33*, 238–244.

Trullinger, R. W., Emanuel, F. W., Skenes, L. L., & Malpass, J. C. (1988). Spectral noise level measurements used to track voice improvement in one patient. *Journal of Communication Disorders, 21*, 447–457.

Turner, G. S., Tjaden, K., & Weismer, G. (1995). The influence of speaking rate on vowel space and speech intelligibility for individuals with amyotrophic lateral sclerosis. *Journal of Speech and Hearing Research, 38*, 1001–1013.

Tyler, A., & Saxman, J. H. (1991). Initial voicing contrast acquisition in normal and phonologically disordered children. *Applied Psycholinguistics, 12*, 453–479.

Tyler, A. A., & Watterson, T. L. (1991). VOT as an indirect measure of laryngeal function. *Seminars in Speech and Language, 12*, 131–141.

Uldall, E. (1964). Transitions in fricative noise. *Language and Speech, 7*, 13–14.

Umeda, N. (1975). Vowel duration in American English. *Journal of the Acoustical Society of America, 58*, 434–445.

Umeda, N. (1977). Consonant duration in American English. *Journal of the Acoustical Society of America, 61*, 846–858.

van Son, R. J. J. H., & Pols, L. C. W. (1990). Formant frequencies of Dutch vowels in a text, read at normal and fast rate. *Journal of the Acoustical Society of America, 88*, 1683–1693.

Verbrugge, R. R., Strange, W., Shankweiler, D. P., & Edman, T. R. (1976). What information enables a listener to map a talker's vowel space? *Journal of the Acoustical Society of America, 60*, 198–212.

Vilkman, E., Aaltonen, O., Raimo, I., Arajärvi, P., & Oksanen, H. (1989). Articulatory hyoid-laryngeal changes vs. cricothyroid muscle activity in the control of intrinsic F_0 of vowels. *Journal of Phonetics, 17*, 193–203.

Vilkman, E., Aaltonen, O., Laine, U., & Raimo, I. (1991). Intrinsic pitch of vowels—A complicated problem with an obvious solution? In J. Gauffin & B. Hammarberg (Eds.), *Vocal fold physiology: Acoustic, perceptual, and physiological aspects of voice mechanisms* (pp. 159–166). San Diego, CA: Singular Publishing Group.

Vilkman, E., Laine, U. K., & Klojonen, J. (1991). Supraglottal acoustics and vowel intrinsic fundamental frequency; An experimental study. *Speech Communication, 10*, 325–334.

Walton, J. H., & Pollack, K. E. (1993). Acoustic validation of vowel error patterns in developmental apraxia of speech. *Clinical Linguistics and Phonetics, 7*, 95–111.

Wang, W. S.-Y. (1959). Transition and release as perceptual cues for final plosives. *Journal of Speech and Hearing Research, 2*, 66–73.

Warren, D. W., & Hall, D. J. (1973). Glottal activity and intraoral pressure during stop consonant productions. *Folia Phoniatrica, 25*, 121–129.

Watterson, T., & Emanuel, F. (1981). Effects of oral-nasal coupling on whispered vowel spectral. *Cleft Palate Journal, 18*, 24–38.

Wedin, S., Leanderson, R., & Wedin, L. (1978). Evaluation of voice training. *Folia Phoniatrica, 30*, 103–112.

Wedin, S., & Ögren, J.-E. (1982). Analysis of the fundamental frequency of the human voice and its frequency distribution before and after a voice training program. *Folia Phoniatrica, 34*, 143–149.

Weinberg, B., Horii, Y., & Smith, B. E. (1980). Long-time spectral and intensity characteristics of esophageal speech. *Journal of the Acoustical Society of America, 67*, 1781–1784.

Weismer, G. (1979). Sensitivity of VOT measures to certain segmental features in speech production. *Journal of Phonetics, 7*, 197–204.

Weismer, G. (1984a). Acoustic descriptions of dysarthric speech: Perceptual correlates and physiological inferences. *Seminars in Speech and Language, 5*, 293–313.

Weismer, G. (1984b). Articulatory characteristics of Parkinsonian dysarthria: Segmental and phrase-level timing, spirantization, and glottal-supraglottal coordination. In J. C. Rosenbek, M. R. McNeil, & A. E. Aronson (Eds.), *Apraxia of speech: Physiology, acoustics, linguistics, management* (pp. 101–130). San Diego, CA: Singular Publishing Group.

Weismer, G., & Liss, J. M. (1991). Acoustic/perceptual taxonomies of speech production deficits in motor speech disorders. In C. A. Moore, K. M. Yorkston, & D. R. Beukelman (Eds.), *Dysarthria and apraxia of speech: Perspectives on management* (pp. 245–270). Baltimore, MD: Paul H. Brookes.

Weismer, G., Martin, R., Kent, R. D., & Kent, J. F. (1992). Formant trajectory characteristics of males with amyotrophic lateral sclerosis. *Journal of the Acoustical Society of America, 91*, 1085–1098.

Weiss, M. S., Yeni-Komshian, G. H., & Heinz, J. M. (1979). Acoustical and perceptual characteristics of speech produced with an electronic artificial larynx. *Journal of the Acoustical Society of America, 65,* 1298–1308.

Wendahl, R. W., Moore, P., & Hollien, H. (1963). Comments on vocal fry. *Folia Phoniatrica, 15,* 251–255.

Wendler, J., Doherty, E. T., & Hollien, H. (1980). Voice classification by means of long-term speech spectra. *Folia Phoniatrica, 32,* 51–60.

Waldstein, R. S. (1990). Effects of postlingual deafness on speech production: Implications for the role of auditory feedback. *Journal of the Acoustical Society of America, 88,* 2099–2114.

Whalen, D. H., Abramson, A. S., Lisker, L., & Mody, M. (1993). F_0 gives voicing information even with unambiguous voice onset times. *Journal of the Acoustical Society of America, 93,* 2152–2159.

Whitehead, R. L., & Emanuel, F. W. (1974). Some spectrographic and perceptual features of vocal fry, abnormally rough, and modal register phonations. *Journal of Communication Disorders, 7,* 305–319.

Whitehead, R. L., & Lieberth, A. K. (1979). Spectrographic and perceptual features of vocal tension/harshness in hearing-impaired adults. *Journal of Communication Disorders, 12,* 83–92.

Winitz, H. E., Scheib, M. E., & Reeds, J. A. (1972). Identification of stops and vowels from the burst portion of /p, t, k/ isolated from conversational speech. *Journal of the Acoustical Society of America, 51,* 1309–1317.

Wirz, S. L., Subtelny, J., & Whitehead, R. L. (1981). Perceptual and spectrographic study of tense voice in normal hearing and deaf subjects. *Folia Phoniatrica, 33,* 23–36.

Wolfe, V. I., & Bacon, M. (1976). Spectrographic comparison of two types of spastic dysphonia. *Journal of Speech and Hearing Disorders, 41,* 325–332.

Wolfe, V., Fitch, J., & Cornell, R. (1995). Acoustic prediction of severity in commonly occurring voice problems. *Journal of Speech and Hearing Research, 38,* 273–279.

Wolfe, V., Cornell, R., & Palmer, C. (1991). Acoustic correlates of pathologic voice types. *Journal of Speech and Hearing Research, 34,* 509–516.

Wolfe, V. I., & Ratusnik, D. L. (1981). Vocal symptomatology of postoperative dysphonia. *Laryngoscope, 91,* 635–643.

Wong, D., Ito, M. R., Cox, N. B., & Titze, I. R. (1991). Observation of perturbations in a lumped-element model of the vocal folds with application to some pathological cases. *Journal of the Acoustical Society of America, 89,* 383–394.

Wood, D. E., & Hewitt, T. L. (1963). New instrumentation for making spectrographic pictures of speech. *Journal of the Acoustical Society of America, 35,* 1274–1278.

Yanagihara, N. (1967a). Hoarseness: Investigation of the physiological mechanisms. *Annals of Otology, Rhinology, and Laryngology, 76,* 472–488.

Yanagihara, N. (1967b). Significance of harmonic changes and noise components in hoarseness. *Journal of Speech and Hearing Research, 10,* 531–541.

Yoon, K. M., Kakita, Y., & Hirano, M. (1984). Sound spectrographic analysis of the voice of patients with glottic carcinomas. *Folia Phoniatrica, 36,* 24–30.

Young, E. C., & Gilbert, H. R. (1988). An analysis of stops produced by normal children and children who exhibit velar fronting. *Journal of Phonetics, 16,* 243–246.

Yumoto, E. (1983). The quantitative evaluation of hoarseness. *Archives of Otolaryngology, 109,* 48–52.

Yumoto, E. (1988). Quantitative assessment of the degree of hoarseness. *Journal of Voice, 1,* 310–313.

Yumoto, E., Baer, T., & Gould, W. J. (1982). Harmonics-to-noise ratio as an index of the degree of hoarseness. *Journal of the Acoustical Society of America, 71,* 1544–1550.

Yumoto, E., Sasaki, Y., & Okamura, H. (1984). Harmonics-to-noise ratio and psychophysical measurement of the degree of hoarseness. *Journal of Speech and Hearing Research, 27,* 2–6.

Ziegler, W., & von Cramon, D. (1986). Disturbed coarticulation in apraxia of speech: Acoustic evidence. *Brain and Language, 29,* 34–37.

Zlatin, M. A. (1974). Voicing contrast: Perceptual and productive voice onset time characteristics of adults. *Journal of the Acoustical Society of America, 56,* 981–994.

Zlatin, M. A., & Koenigsknecht, R. A. (1975). Development of the voicing contrast: Perception of stop consonants. *Journal of Speech and Hearing Research, 18,* 541–553.

Zlatin, M. A., & Koenigsknecht, R. A. (1976). Development of the voicing contrast: A comparison of voice onset time in stop perception and production. *Journal of Speech and Hearing Research, 19,* 93–111.

Zwicker, E., Flottrop, G., & Stevens, S. S. (1957). Critical bandwidth in loudness summation. *Journal of the Acoustical Society of America, 29,* 548–557.

Air Pressure

The sounds of speech are the product of careful and precise use of the air pressure generated by the respiratory system. It is often useful to know what the air pressure is in a given region of the vocal tract (especially as compared with the pressure at some other location) and, often more important, to observe changes in air pressure values that result from speech activity. These observations, coupled with an understanding of vocal tract structure and function, permit the clinician to infer a great deal about the nature and degree of speech abnormality. The importance of air pressure measures has motivated the development of numerous measurement instruments and techniques. The most useful of these will be discussed in this section.

GENERAL PHYSICAL PRINCIPLES

Definition and Units of Measurement

Pressure is defined as the force per unit area acting perpendicular to a surface. Both the unit of force and the area may be selected to suit the application. One would not, for example, find it convenient to measure the pressure in a child's balloon in tons per square yard nor the pressure at the depths of the ocean in grams per square millimeter. Until fairly recently, in the field of speech and hearing the most common force unit has been the *dyne* (d) and the unit of area most frequently used has been the *square centimeter* (cm²). Revisions of the international system of weights and measures in 1982 have given more currency to a pressure unit called the *pascal* (Pa). One Pa (the equivalent of 10 d/cm²) is defined as the force of one newton (N) acting on a surface of one square meter. Older literature may refer to pressure using the unit *torr*, which is the exact equivalent of the pascal.

Important as it is to know and understand these units of measurement, they are not often encountered in descriptions of speech behavior. Rather, a simpler and more direct yardstick is usually applied. Its basis is exemplified by the U-tube manometer (shown in Figure 8–1), a simple tube partially filled with a liquid. When both ends of the tube are open, the level of the liquid will be the same in both sides because both sides are acted on equally by the pressure of the atmosphere. As a higher pressure is applied to the column of liquid on one side, it forces fluid out, causing the column of liquid on the other side to rise. The applied pressure can be described in terms of the height of the column of liquid it is supporting, which is the vertical distance between the two liquid levels. To say, for example, that a person's subglottal pressure for speech is 7 cmH₂O is to indicate that the air below the larynx exerts enough

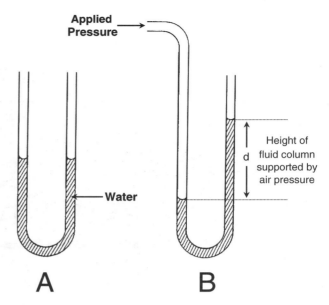

Figure 8–1. The U-tube manometer is simply a glass tube filled with water **(A)**. Pressure applied to one arm of the tube, as in **(B)**, causes the water to rise in the other arm. The difference in the level of the water in the two arms is a measure of the applied pressure.

force to elevate a column of water to a height of 7 cm. Thus, despite the fact that the current "standard" SI Unit is the pascal, most speech pressures continue to be expressed in centimeters of water (cmH₂O). Some literature, especially that published before the 1970s, may refer to pounds per square inch (psi) or ounces per square inch (oz/in²) and an occasional instrument (such as the Hunter oral manometer, still lurking in many clinics) may be calibrated this way. However, conversion from one pressure unit to another is relatively straightforward.

The height of the column of liquid in the U-tube manometer is really a function of two opposing forces: The air pressure applied to one side of the U-tube and whatever pressure might be acting on the other side. In Figure 8–1, while the pressure to be measured is applied to one side, the other is left open to the atmosphere. But the atmosphere itself exerts pressure (that is what a barometer measures), and this acts on the open side of the U-tube. The resultant height of the fluid column, therefore, represents not simply the applied air pressure, but rather the difference between it and the pressure of the atmosphere. The height of the fluid column in Figure 8–1 really should be said to be "d" units greater than atmospheric pressure. Engineers refer to this kind of measure as *gauge* (or *gage*) *pressure*. But it is also possible to measure pressure as compared with a vacuum (***absolute pressure***) or as compared with some other pressure (***differential pressure***). Absolute pressure is clearly of little everyday value to the speech clinician, and it will not generally be encountered. All three types of pressure measures are schematized in Figure 8–2.

The Influence of Flow on Pressure Measurement

If the air whose pressure is to be determined is not moving (as when maximum sustainable oral air pressure is to be assessed), its pressure is the same in all directions and the spatial orientation of the tube through which the pressure is sampled is irrelevant. The situation is very different if pressure must be measured during an air flow (as during speech). The force exerted against a surface by a stream of air is the result of two factors: The ***static air pressure*** (which is the component of interest) and the ***kinetic energy pressure*** (commonly called the ***stagnation pressure***) which is a result of the momentum of the air molecules. The latter is due to the speed of air movement rather than to the driving pressure itself. It must not be allowed to exert an influence on the pressure measurement. Figure 8–3 shows how the kinetic energy pressure alters the air pressure measurement. When the

pressure-sampling tube faces into the airflow (pointing upstream, as shown in Figure 8–3A), both the static and kinetic energy pressures impinge on the measurement system, giving a spuriously high reading. When the tube faces away from the airflow (pointing downstream, as shown in Figure 8–3B), the observed pressure is the static pressure *minus* the kinetic energy pressure, a value significantly below the static pressure alone. The solution to the measurement problem lies in orienting the probe tube so that its opening is perpendicular to the flow of air, as shown in Figure 8–3C. This orientation is more easily described than achieved with precision, but incorrect placement of the probe tube is a major threat to validity, so at least an approximation of perpendicularity must be obtained if useful pressure measures are to be taken. An interesting example of grossly inflated pressure values, no doubt due to stagnation pressure effects, may be seen in the intraoral pressure values obtained by Black (1950) and analyzed by Hardy (1965).

Static and Dynamic Pressure Measures

The choice of a measurement technique is very strongly influenced by whether the pressure to be observed is static (relatively stable) or dynamic (char-

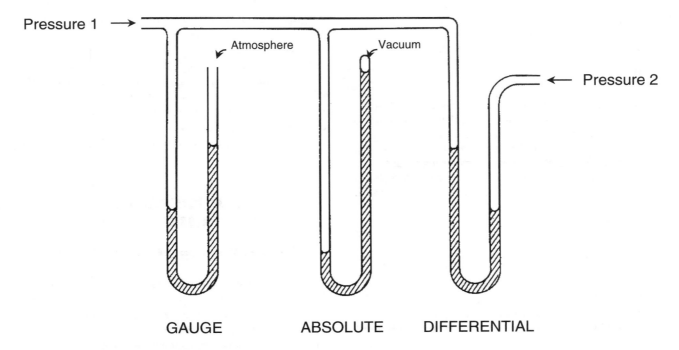

Figure 8–2. Different pressure measures.

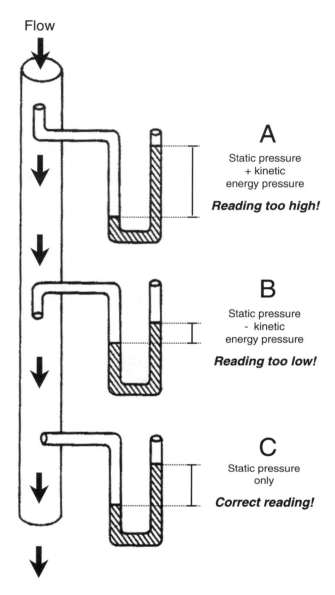

Flow

A

Static pressure
+ kinetic
energy pressure

Reading too high!

B

Static pressure
- kinetic
energy pressure

Reading too low!

C

Static pressure
only

Correct reading!

Figure 8–3. Effect on the pressure reading of different orientations of the sensing tube in a flow. If the sensing tube faces into the flow **(A)**, the reading represents static *plus* kinetic pressures. If it faces away from the flow **(B)**, the reading is of the static pressure *minus* the kinetic pressure. Only when the sensing tube faces perpendicular to the flow **(C)** does the reading reflect the static pressure alone.

acterized by fairly rapid change). For example, the determination of maximum oral breath pressure involves observation of a static pressure: The patient maintains an intraoral pressure for a relatively long time. On the other hand, determination of intraoral

air pressure during /p/ in running speech involves a dynamic pressure: The air pressure rises rapidly, is sustained for only a fraction of a second, if at all, and then is released. Static pressures are equivalent to DC electrical signals, whereas dynamic pressures represent AC events (see Chapter 2, "Analog Electronics"). Accurate recording of dynamic pressures will require instrumentation capable of faithfully reproducing even the fastest fluctuations. More precisely stated, the measurement system must have an adequate frequency response. The emphasis here is on the response of the *system*, the combination of transducer, amplifier, and readout device. (The influence of various system characteristics on measurement accuracy is analyzed by Fry, 1960.) Since most transducers are too big to be placed directly into the vocal tract where pressure is to be measured, a sensing probe tube of some sort will almost always be needed. This tube can and does limit the frequency response of the system, and its effects should be considered when interpreting results. Sensing tubes are described in greater detail in the discussion of instrumentation that follows.

For precise measurement of dynamic pressures it is important that the transducer neither expand nor contract as the pressure inside it changes. It should not, in other words, behave like an elastic balloon. When it does, air from the region in which the sensing tube lies will flow into the tube and transducer as pressure rises, and it will flow back out as pressure falls. These volumetric reactions reduce the amount of pressure change by the pneumatic equivalent of electronic integration. A system that smooths out the very pressure changes it should be detecting is said to be excessively compliant. Most electronic pressure transducers will not present the clinician with this problem since their volumetric displacement is on the order of 0.01 mL. But simpler devices, such as a U-tube manometer, may have a displacement in the milliliter range at typical vocal tract pressures, making them useless for dynamic measurements even if their other limitations could be remedied.

AIR PRESSURE INSTRUMENTATION

The Pressure Sensing Tube

As a rule, pressure transducers are located externally and are coupled to the vocal tract region in which pressure is to be observed by a probe or sensing tube. When measuring quasi-static pressures, or when the probe's interference with speech behavior is not a concern, the tube can be of any convenient type. Standard laboratory rubber tubing, for example, is commonly used with oral manometers and is suitable for use with other devices of this category.

Dynamic pressure measurements confront the clinician with more complex problems. The sensing tube will frequently have to be placed where the lip or tongue may jostle it as they move, so the sensing tube and the means of fastening it in place should ideally be as small and unobtrusive as possible. Any reduction of the tube's diameter, or increase in its length, increases its impedance, which limits frequency response and may interfere with measurement validity. Hardy (1965) felt that curvature of the sensing tube also affects system response, although this has not been borne out in tests conducted by Edmonds, Lilly, and Hardy (1971). All of these problems become more acute as the pressure fluctuations become more rapid (that is, there is progressive high-frequency loss). The choice of a sensing tube must inevitably reflect a compromise between minimization of deleterious factors and the important requirement that the measurement process not disrupt speech activity.

For most applications, a polyethylene tube having an internal diameter of 1.4 to 1.6 mm is used. This size will fit on a 17-gauge hypodermic needle, which is used to couple it to the fitting used on many pressure transducers. The sensing tube is shaped to minimize interference with articulatory contact and movement and to assure that the probe tube opening maintains a perpendicular orientation to the direction of speech airflow. Shaping the tube for specific applications is accomplished by inserting a length of relatively thick copper wire or solder into it and bending the tube-cum-wire to the desired shape. With the wire serving as the form, the tube is immersed in boiling water until softened, then it is removed and allowed to cool. The wire is then pulled out, leaving the sensing tube shaped as needed. To keep the length of the sensing tube to a minimum (no more than 15 cm, if at all possible), the pressure transducer should be located very close to the patient's face. Further details regarding this type of probe tube formation and fitting are provided by Orlikoff and Baken (1993).

Another sensing-tube option involves modifying bendable tubes used commonly in dentistry to remove oral secretions. Hygroformic saliva ejectors, available from dental supply dealers, are hollow small-diameter tubes that are very easily molded by hand at room temperature to almost any shape desired. They can also be cut to size and individually formed to accommodate the oral cavity of the person to be tested. They will maintain this shape, but can be modified as desired. Because saliva ejectors are disposable, they are very modestly priced.

Air Pressure Transducers

U-TUBE MANOMETER

Construction and Physical Principles

An extremely simple device, the U-tube manometer is available to any clinical facility. Although a U-tube can be bought, one is easily made in just a few minutes by mounting a bent section of laboratory glass tubing on a vertical surface. (If glass-bending skills or facilities are not available, two straight tubes can be connected at the bottom with rubber or plastic tubing.) The mounted tube is filled to half its height with water to which a *very* small amount of detergent is added to reduce surface-tension effects. Care must be taken to avoid trapping air bubbles in the tube during the filling operation. The sensing tube is attached to one arm and the device is ready for use.

The functioning of the U-tube manometer rests on fundamental physical principles; it is therefore inherently calibrated. Readings are taken of the difference between the heights of the liquid in the two arms of the tube. This distance is itself the pressure measurement. Due to surface tension the fluid level surfaces are not flat, but instead concave. The fluid level is measured at the bottom of the concavity, called the meniscus, in each arm of the U-tube. (A metric ruler is usually attached to the surface on which the U-tube is mounted to facilitate the measurement of the level difference.) Those unaccustomed to reading U-tube measurements often make the mistake of measuring the fluid's displacement within the right arm of the U-tube, between its rest position (especially when labeled "0") and the level assumed with an applied pressure. This reading, of course, will represent half of the applied pressure.

The choice of fluid for filling the U-tube is governed by the expected magnitude of the pressure to be measured. The denser the liquid the less displacement of the column per unit of force. That is, sensitivity diminishes with increased fluid density. The most commonly used liquid is water. Other fluids with densities lower than that of water could serve in cases where still greater sensitivity is needed. Measurement validity is dependent, at least in part, on the purity of the liquid used, but for clinical purposes ordinary tap water will suffice.

Implementation

Because it requires the movement of a large mass over a significant distance, the response of the U-tube manometer is inherently slow. Accordingly, it is useful only for static pressures. It is also difficult to read accurately with any speed. While schemes for electronically transducing the height of the column have been worked out, they are hardly worth the significant investment required. (Obviously, it would be better to purchase an electronic transduction system in the first place.) For all practical purposes, the U-tube cannot generate a permanent record.

Determination of Static Pressure

The U-tube manometer is most commonly used to measure static oral or nasal pressure. All that is required is that the sensing tube be fitted with a suitable mouthpiece—a short length of fire-polished glass tubing will do in many instances—or with a nasal olive. (If the latter is not available a substitute may be made by fashioning ear-mold plastic around the end of a glass tube.) The sensing tube is then simply held in the mouth or fitted to a naris.

Calibration of Other Pressure Transducers

Because it is inherently calibrated, the U-tube manometer is often used to calibrate other pressure transducers. It is this purpose, in fact, that the U-tube most commonly serves. Figure 8–4 shows how the U-tube and the device to be calibrated are connected in parallel to a source of air pressure (in this case, a hypodermic syringe). The air pressure acts equally on both devices, and thus the output of the device being calibrated represents the pressure shown by the U-tube.

BOURDON TUBE PRESSURE TRANSDUCER

Construction and Physical Principles

The device used in most dial-type pressure gauges is the Bourdon tube, which is one type of "elastic" pressure transducer. The Bourdon tube itself is a thin-walled metal tube whose cross section is a flattened circle (Figure 8–5A). Increased pressure within the tube causes it to bend outward as its cross section becomes more nearly circular. The resulting stress forces the free end of the tube to be displaced. The direction of this movement depends on the shape of the tube, and the "C" form, shown in Figure 8–5B is common. The movement of the free end of the Bourdon tube is used to drive a dial pointer via a mechanical linkage to permit pressure to be read directly. In cases where an electronic output is desirable the movement of the tube can be transduced in a number of ways, for example by linkage to a special transformer called a *linear variable differential transformer* (LVDT) or by having it move a shutter to vary the amount of light that shines on a photocell. These schemes, however, require considerable mechanical structure, which is likely to

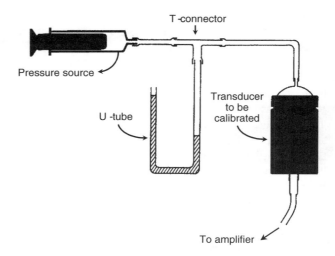

Figure 8–4. Connection of a U-tube manometer for calibrating a pressure transducer.

impair reliability, degrade frequency response, and reduce overall ruggedness. Despite its very real limitations in terms of resolution and frequency response, the Bourdon-type oral manometer (such as the one once produced by Hunter) can be "a useful clinical tool when it is used properly and when the obtained results are interpreted in ways which are consistent with our current knowledge of it" (Morris, 1966, p. 362).

STRAIN GAUGE PRESSURE TRANSDUCERS

Construction and Physical Principles

Strain gauges are devices that exhibit a change of some electrical property (most commonly resistance) when they are deformed (strained) by some external force (stress). Strain gauge pressure transducers take advantage of this property. The pressure sensing tube is connected to a chamber or cavity whose floor is a relatively flexible diaphragm. The diaphragm is deformed by the air pressure inside the chamber. It is this deformation (strain) that the system actually measures. Strain gauge pressure transducers thus contain a primary transducer (the diaphragm) and a secondary transducer (the strain gauges mounted on the diaphragm). In general, these transducers will contain four strain gauges wired in a Wheatstone bridge configuration (see Chapter 2, "Analog Electronics").

Unbonded Strain Gauge Transducers

Unbonded strain gauge transducers are generally of the form shown schematically in Figure 8–6A. During

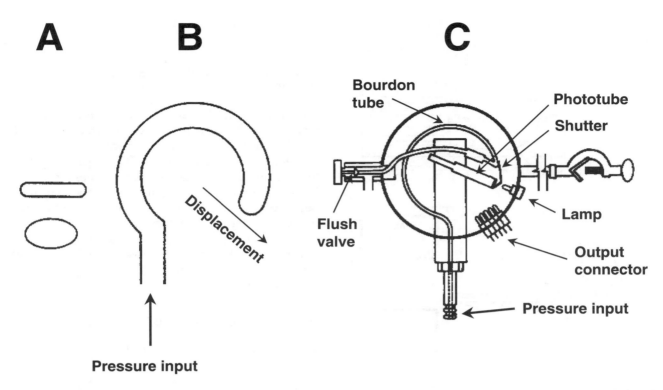

A   B   C

Bourdon tube

Phototube

Shutter

Displacement

Flush valve

Lamp

Output connector

Pressure input

Pressure input

Figure 8–5. A. Cross-section of a Bourdon tube when its internal (relative) pressure is zero (top), and when its internal pressure is high (bottom). **B.** Lateral view of a C-form Bourdon tube. When the cross-section shape changes, the resulting strain displaces the free end of the tube. **C.** The movement of the free end can be used to move a dial pointer.

use, the pressure gauge is clamped to a solid support, and the open end of the sensing tube is positioned in the region of the vocal tract where pressure is to be evaluated. That pressure will subsequently displace the diaphragm within the transducer. Movement of the diaphragm changes the amount of stretch of the gauge wires that are attached to it. This produces a change in the wires' resistances that is sensed by appropriate external circuitry. This type of transducer is very popular and widely available. It has good sensitivity and excellent reliability. It is, however, somewhat less rugged than some of the other transducer types and it may be damaged by severe physical shock—such as when dropped—or by even moderately forceful contact with the diaphragm.

Since strain gauge transducers use electrical bridge circuits, they require an excitation voltage. An amplifier is also needed to track the bridge output, which is usually very small (Figure 8–6B). Since the gauge system is resistive, either a DC or AC excitation can be used. (Note, however, that transducers with built-in amplifiers, such as the MicroSwitch pressure gauges discussed later, must be connected to a DC

source only.) It is critically important that the bridge supply be very stable: any change in bridge excitation will result in a proportional change in the bridge output, an artifact that will confound the pressure measurement. Although carrier amplifiers are widely available, highly miniaturized hybrid circuits (such as those available from Analog Devices Inc., Norwood, MA) make it fairly easy and very cheap to assemble one's own precision system for clinical use. Transducers that include a built-in amplifier do not need external bridge excitation (it is included as part of the built-in circuitry). Also, an external amplifier for these devices is not obligatory, but is useful for adjusting the system gain and center voltage.

Bonded Strain Gauge Transducers

In the bonded strain gauge transducer the elements that sense diaphragm movement are either bonded directly to the diaphragm or are special semiconductor elements that are actually part of it. An example of the latter, the MicroSwitch (Honeywell Inc., Freeport, IL), is shown in Figure 8–7A and its construction is shown

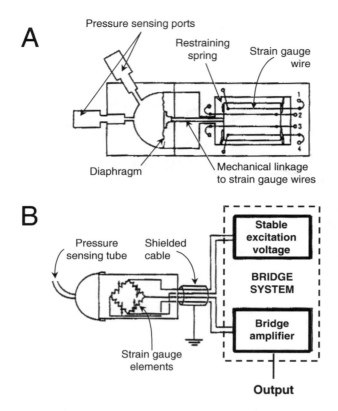

Figure 8–6. A. A cutaway schematic of a typical unbonded strain-gauge pressure transducer. Note that whenever wires 2 and 3 are stretched, wires 1 and 4 are shortened. The restraining springs protect the wires from overload. **B.** Block diagram of a strain-gauge transducer system.

in Figure 8–7B. This type of transducer was developed originally for use in automobile "cruise control" systems and features a compact size, exceptional ruggedness, and relative insensitivity to vibration in use. The sensing element of a MicroSwitch transducer consists of four piezoresistors in a Wheatstone bridge configuration integrated into the surface of a thin crystalline (silicon) diaphragm. The excellent response of this transducer is due to the inherent properties of the semiconductor elements which makes them much more sensitive than unbonded or other wire bonded strain gauges. The very small and exceptionally stiff diaphragm assures a good frequency response. Their cost is remarkably low, often one-fifth to one-tenth the cost other pressure transducer types. Indeed, the MicroSwitch device can powered by a single 9-V battery and simple circuitry will allow the user to zero the output (Figure 8–7C). Given their low cost and excellent performance, it is not surprising that semiconductor bonded strain gauges are quickly becoming the

transducer of choice for dynamic speech pressure measurement.

REACTANCE-BASED PRESSURE TRANSDUCERS

Pressure may also be sensed by causing it to alter the reactance of a capacitor or inductor (see Chapter 2, "Analog Electronics"). Variable capacitance transducers used for work in speech and hearing are generally confined to the role of condenser microphones for recording of airborne speech signals, although there have been descriptions of the use of capacitative pressure transducers for the measurement of dynamic vocal tract pressures (Fischer-Jørgensen & Hansen, 1959). On the other hand, inductive transducers have achieved moderate popularity and, therefore, warrant separate consideration.

Variable Inductance Transducers

Construction and Physical Principles

The inductance of a coil can be made to vary under the influence of changing air pressure in a number of ways. One of these (Figure 8–8A) is exemplified by a variable-reluctance pressure gauge made by VacuMed (Ventura, CA). (Reluctance is the magnetic equivalent of impedance.) Transducers of this type use two inductors in series. In this system, a diaphragm of a magnetically permeable material (such as stainless steel) is positioned so as to divide a small cavity into two equal and separate spaces, each of which can serve as a pressure chamber. In the wall of each of the cavities is a toroidal inductive coil (shown in section in Figure 8–8B). As the pressure in one chamber rises, the diaphragm is deflected (Figure 8–8C), moving away from the coil on the high-pressure side and toward the coil in the low-pressure chamber. Because the diaphragm has high magnetic permeability, the inductance of one coil increases as the diaphragm moves closer to it, while the inductance of the other decreases as the diaphragm moves away.

The advantages of the two-coil arrangement are significant. From an electrical point of view, half of a bridge circuit has been formed, with benefits similar to those of resistive bridges; that is, greatly improved sensitivity and inherent temperature compensation. Other benefits are gained as well. The transducer is quite rugged and will withstand considerable mechanical shock. In addition, it is fairly tolerant of serious overpressure, greatly reducing the possibility that it will be damaged by application of pressures beyond its operating range. Frequency response is also very good. Variable reluctance transducers, however, require AC

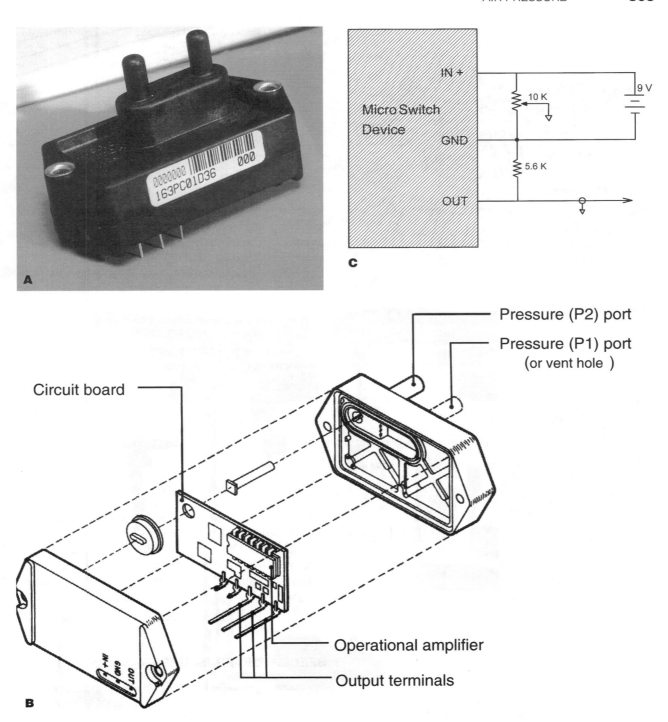

Figure 8-7. The MicroSwitch model 160PC strain-gauge pressure transducer **(A)** and a cutaway illustration showing its construction **(B)** (Courtesy of Honeywell, Inc., MicroSwitch Division, Freeport, IL). Circuitry that can be used to power the transducer and to zero its output is shown in **C**.

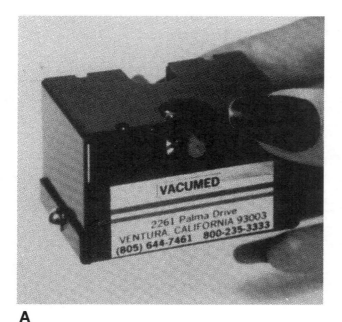

A

B

Figure 8–8. A VacuMed pressure transducer **(A)** and a diagramatic section through such a variable-reluctance transducer **(B)**. When pressure on one side of the diaphragm is higher than the pressure on the other side, the diaphragm is pushed to the low-pressure side **(C)**. This changes the inductive balance of the coils.

excitation (since the reactance at DC for any inductor is zero), and thus a carrier amplifier system (see Chapter 4, "General-Purpose Tools") will be needed. These transducers may also be susceptible to the presence of stray magnetic fields, which could be a problem (although not very serious) if they are used in conjunction with devices such as magnetometers (Chapter 12, "Speech Movements"). Their price is comparable to resistive strain gauge units.

Implementation

Variable reluctance transducers are used in exactly the same way as the resistive strain gauge devices already discussed. The inductive transducers, however, require somewhat different support electronics, schematized in Figure 8–9. Because transduction depends on variations of inductive reactance, the excitation must be a sine wave. This is provided by the carrier oscillator, shown on the left in the block diagram. It is critical that the amplitude of the excitation waveform be stable, and so a feedback loop is incorporated into the oscillator to control its output. The gauge itself contains only half of a bridge circuit, and thus the excitation is provided through a transformer in the carrier amplifier whose secondary winding provides the two fixed inductors needed to complete the bridge. The output of the bridge is amplified and demodulated to provide a voltage analog of the air pressure acting on the transducer's diaphragm. Excitation and demodulation systems (that is, carrier amplifiers) are generally available from the transducer manufacturer. A system such as the one shown requires only minor modification to permit it to be used with resistive strain gauge transducers as well.

Variable reluctance transducers have very good sensitivity. The Validyne MP45–871, for example, has a nominal output of 25 mV/V full scale. With the recommended 5-V excitation voltage at a frequency of 5000 Hz, its output would be 0.125 V at maximal transducible pressure.

SPECIALIZED PRESSURE TRANSDUCERS

Specialized pressure transducers are sensing devices of the types discussed above that have been adapted for a specific use. In particular, ultra-miniaturized pressure transducers have some history in the measurement of speech-related pressures. Hixon (1972), for instance, described transducers small enough to be placed in the esophagus and stomach for determination of trans-diaphragmatic pressure. Pressure gauges small enough to fit within the oral cavity have been designed. Subtelny, Worth, and Sakuda (1966), for instance, used a semiconductor strain gauge device that was about 10 mm in diameter and about 3 mm thick. This was pasted to the palate to sense intraoral pressure during running speech. Koike and Perkins (1968) also discuss an even smaller transducer—cylindrical in form, 3 mm in diameter and 4 mm long—that could be introduced into almost any space in the vocal tract. Koike and his coworkers measured precise pressure variations in the vicinity of the glottis, placing such a transducer in the laryngopharynx approximately 4 cm above the vocal folds (Koike, Imaizumi, Kitano, Kawasaki, & Hirano, 1983) as well as in the trachea about 4 cm below the glottis (Perkins & Koike, 1969; Koike & Hirano, 1973; Koike, 1981). Aside from the convenience afforded by these instruments, they have the advantages of relatively high sensitivity and excellent frequency response. Unfortunately, calibration of these types of transducers is more difficult than it is with more conventional devices, and they are prone to drift significantly in a way that is highly suggestive of sensitivity to the temperature difference of the egressive and ingressive tidal air flow. This, of course, casts doubt on the validity of the measurement (see the critique of the method by Hardy, 1967). Intraoral devices are probably no less encumbering of articulation than a sensing tube, and the electrical connections to intraoral gauges must pass the lips just as a sensing tube would. It is clear, then, that they offer little advantage over a standard pressure gauge, which is also usable for other kinds of measures.

CALIBRATION OF PRESSURE TRANSDUCERS

Manufacturers typically provide calibration data for their pressure transducers. There are two common formats in which this information may appear.

1. *Volts output per volt excitation per unit pressure.* A Statham model P23BB unbonded pressure gauge, for example, has a stated calibration factor of 268.7 μV/V/cmHg. This indicates that for each volt of bridge excitation the gauge produces 0.0002687 volt for each centimeter of mercury of applied pressure. We can easily convert this factor to use cmH_2O as the reference unit of measurement; Since 1 cmHg is the pressure equivalent of approximately 13.6 cmH_2O, each volt of bridge excitation produces 0.002687 × 13.6, or 0.00365 volt for each centimeter of water pressure. If an excitation voltage of 12 V is used and the gauge is sensing an air pressure to 2 cmH_2O, the amplifier at the bridge output will receive an input of 0.0876 V (which is, 0.00365 V × 12 V × 2 cmH_2O).

2. *Volts output per volt excitation, full scale.* This description indicates the voltage output for each volt of excitation at the maximum pressure for which the gauge is rated. Thus, a pressure gauge that can transduce pressures up to 25 cmH_2O with a stated sensitivity of 5 mV/V full scale would be expected to output 0.2 mV per volt of excitation per centimeter of water pressure (5 mV/V ÷ 25 cmH_2O = 0.2 mV/V/cmH_2O). With an excitation of 20 V the output would be 4 mV per cmH_2O (0.2 mV × 20 V = 4 mV).

Aside from providing a description of the overall sensitivity of the transducer, the manufacturer's calibration data are not really very useful. In the first place, the calibration of any device may change with time and use.

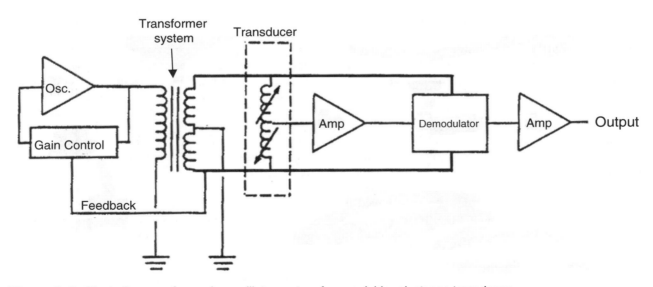

Figure 8–9. Block diagram of a carrier oscillator system for a variable-reluctance transducer.

Table 8–1. An Example of a Calibration Table Showing Sample Input Pressures and Corresponding System Output Values in Volts

System Input (Pressure, cmH$_2$O)	System Output (Volts)
0.0	−4.7
1.0	−4.0
4.0	−1.5
8.0	2.1
12.0	4.4

Second, the final output of the transduction system also depends on the gain of the amplifiers to which the transducer is connected, and the gauge's manufacturer cannot know what the user's amplifier is like. Fortunately, using a U-tube to calibrate a pressure transducer is so simple that it is easy to calibrate a pressure measurement system right in the setting in which it will be used.

Calibration requires that the pressure source, gauge, and U-tube be set up as in Figure 8–4. Pressures are generated over the entire range to which the gauge is sensitive, and, using a voltmeter, readings of the amplifer's output are taken at several pressure levels. A table is then constructed that shows the relationship of voltage output per pressure input, such as shown in the hypothetical example in Table 8–1.

From these data a regression equation can be generated (most hand calculators can handle this chore). Enough different pressures within the gauge's range should be tested to provide a good basis for estimating the system's linearity. In the above example, the correlation coefficient (r) is +.997. Given that the system is obviously very linear (despite some expected imprecision in the pressure and voltage readings), we can use linear regression to translate any amplifier output voltage within the range to the equivalent air pressure measure. For the example we are considering, the regression equation is cmH$_2$O = (1.27 × Volts) + 5.94. Therefore, an output of 3.5 volts represents a pressure of about 10.4 cmH$_2$O. (Determining the linear regression equation and the Pearson product-moment correlation coefficient for sample data is reviewed in Orlikoff and Baken (1993) and in many reviews of basic statistical methods.) Obviously, neither the excitation voltage nor the gain setting of the amplifier can be changed between calibration and use. Calibration should be repeated every time the system is set up or after it is altered in any way.

SUMMARY OF PRESSURE TRANSDUCERS

Important characteristics of the various types of pressure transducers are summarized in Table 8–2 as an aid to selecting the device most suitable in a given setting.

AIR PRESSURE MEASUREMENTS

Maximum Intraoral Air Pressure

The purpose of this nonspeech measurement is to assess a patient's ability to generate air pressure on demand. Also called the *maximum expiratory pressure* (PE$_{max}$), the test rests on the assumption that the pressure in the mouth is generated by the respiratory system (and special precaution must be taken to assure that this is the case). Since there is very little or no air flow and the glottis is open during the test, intraoral pressure is equal to lung pressure.

TECHNIQUE

Maximum intraoral air pressure is traditionally evaluated with a U-tube or Bourdon-type oral manometer. Any other pressure transducer with an adequate maximum-pressure rating can be used, however. The test requires the patient to blow into the sensing tube with as much force as possible. It is important that there be a tight lip seal around the sensing tube and a noseclip should be used to prevent nasal air escape. Hardy (1961) suggests that if there is lip paresis (for example, in cases of cerebral palsy) a face mask might be required. In fact, a mask should be considered in any case of facial muscle weakness. Cook, Mead, and Orzalesi (1964) argue that, even with normal lip control, when generating such high intraoral pressures a specialized mouthpiece is necessary to prevent air leakage. Several reports advocate having the clinician actively support the cheeks or compressing the lips and corners of the mouth during the task (Rubinstein et al., 1988; Fiz et al., 1992). When the clinician is satisfied that the patient is producing maximal expiratory effort, the highest pressure reading shown on the gauge, even momentarily, is recorded as the test result. Several studies have shown that the highest intraoral pressures are obtained when the patient is using a lung volume that is greater than 80% of the total lung capacity (Rahn, Otis, Chadwick, & Fenn, 1946; Cook, Mead, & Orzalesi, 1964; Derenne, Macklem, & Roussos, 1978; Gaultier & Zinman, 1983; Baydur, 1991), so the patient should be instructed to inhale to maximal, or near maximal, levels before blowing into the mouthpiece.

This test is intended to evaluate a capability of the respiratory system. But intraoral air pressure can also

Table 8–2. Summary of Pressure Transducer Characteristics

Transducer	Sensitivity	Frequency Response	Excitation	Support Electronics	Ruggedness
U-tube[1]	Varies	*Very* poor	None	None	Good
Bourdon tube[2]	Moderate	Poor	None	None (mechanical)	Moderate
Strain gauges:					
Unbonded[3]	Low	Good	AC or DC	Bridge excitation and instrumentation amplifier	Poor-to-Moderate
Bonded—Wire[4]	Low	Good	AC or DC	Same as unbonded	Moderate
Bonded—Semiconductor	Excellent	Excellent	DC usually	Same as unbonded[5]	Excellent
Inductive	Very good	Very good	AC only	Carrier amplifier	Excellent

[1]Cannot be read with precision; limited to static measures; no permanent record.

[2]Limited to static measures; no permanent record.

[3]Sensitive to vibration.

[4]May be temperature sensitive.

[5]May have support electronics incorporated into the transducer package.

be produced by sealing the oral cavity off from the pharynx with a linguavelar contact and using oral movement (buccal contraction) to compress the intra-oral air. The resulting pressure is not the measure of interest in this test. To prevent this action, a "bleed valve"is placed in the measurement system. This represents a shunt by which air is allowed to escape from the oral cavity. If pressure is being produced by oral valving, the loss of air will quickly cause the pressure to fall dramatically. Only if the air is constantly replenished from the lungs will it be possible for the patient to maintain a high intraoral pressure for a significant period of time. A bleed valve is built into commercially available Bourdon-type manometers. In other systems a T-tube with a very narrow opening in its side arm may be connected to the sensing tube to achieve the same effect. This arrangement is diagrammed in Figure 8–13A in the section "Subglottal Pressure." For the purposes of the present test, however, the opening of the bleed tube should be smaller than the one shown there.

ADVANTAGES AND LIMITATIONS

This test is extremely simple and requires minimal instrumentation. It does not, however, evaluate speech performance. Therefore, it is difficult to draw inferences from the results beyond the conclusion that adequate pressure for speech is at least possible. Usually several attempts are necessary to obtain the patient's greatest PE_{max}. There are admittedly rare, but nonetheless possible, attendant risks associated with multiple efforts to generate maximal alveolar pressure. The

PE_{max} maneuver raises the patient's blood pressure dramatically and there have been reports ranging from nose bleeds and hemorrhages of the conjunctiva of the eye (Rindqvist, 1966) to pneumothorax and subcutaneous emphysema (Rahn et al., 1946; Manco, Terra-Filho, & Silva, 1990), even in otherwise healthy individuals. Thus risk and benefit to the patient are important considerations before attempting to obtain measures of maximal pressure.

EXPECTED RESULTS

There have been numerous investigations of maximal pressure generation in the literature of respiratory physiology, although it has been difficult to compare results due to key differences in methodology. The summary data in Table 8–3 are derived from several studies following procedures similar to that described earlier. These and other data (Cook, Mead, & Orzalesi, 1964; Inkley, Oldenburg, & Vignos, 1974; Leech, Ghezzo, Stevens, & Becklake, 1983; Wilson, Cooke, Edwards, & Spiro, 1984; Chen & Kuo, 1989; Ordiales Fernández et al., 1995) suggest that PE_{max} increases during childhood and throughout young adulthood, begins to decline after the fifth decade, and the maximal pressures of females remains about 60 to 75% that of age-matched males. In a classic study, Black and Hyatt (1969) provided normal PE_{max} values and linear regression equations based on the maximal pressures generated by 120 normal men and women between the ages of 20 and 86 years. These are shown in Table 8–4.

Table 8–3. Mean Maximum Intraoral Air Pressure (PE$_{max}$)

| Age[†] | Number of Subjects | PE$_{max}$ (cmH$_2$O)* | | | Source[‡] |
		Mean	SD	Range	
Males					
7.4–8.6	26	99	23	—	1
9.0–10.8	26	123	27	—	1
11.0–13.0	23	161	37	—	1
14–17	29	166	44	—	2
18–39	31	167	37	96–244	3
21–40	14	242	41	–1	
55–73	40	173	41	105–280	4
69 ± 8	44	190	55	—	5
68–89	27	124	43	36–198	3
Females					
7.1–8.9	15	74	25	—	1
9.0–10.8	17	108	39	—	1
11.7–13.3	27	126	32	—	1
14–17	38	135	29	—	2
18–38	31	121	24	81–178	3
21–31	10	—	—	67–140	6
21–40	16	143	36	—	1
55–80	64	115	34	45–190	4
67 ± 8	57	125	36	—	5
66–93	35	88	37	25–188	3

*1 cmH$_2$O = 10.2 kPa

†Range of ages included or mean age ± SD (in years).

‡*Sources*:

1. Gaultier and Zinman, 1983. Strain gauge transducer used in measurement.

2. Szeinberg et al., 1987. Aneroid pressure gauge used for measurement.

3. Ptacek, Sander, Maloney, and Jackson, 1966. Data converted from inches of water and rounded to the nearest cmH$_2$O; Measurement done with a U-tube manometer.

4. McElvaney et al., 1989. Aneroid pressure gauge used for measurement; Range approximated from authors' scatterplot.

5. Berry, Vitalo, Larson, Patel, and Kim, 1996. Used both aneroid gauge and strain gauge transducers for pressure measurement.

6. Gibson, Edmonds, and Hughes, 1977. Esophageal balloon technique used for pressure measurement.

In general, maximal pressure data should be interpreted with extreme caution. Morris (1966) quite correctly points out that manometric results are not measures of intraoral breath pressure for speech. Although PE$_{max}$ measures have been used for some time as an indirect index of respiratory muscle force and strength, they have never been shown to be related to speech or voice competence in any appreciable way. The absolute values themselves have no utility since there is no criterion for "adequate," and normal speakers differ radically in their performance on this task—a fact demonstrated by the wide ranges cited in Table 8–3. The usefulness of breath pressure measures lies almost exclusively in the breath pressure ratios derived from them. These are discussed with respect to the assessment of velopharyngeal function in Chapter 11.

Dynamic Intraoral Pressure

The intraoral air pressures (P$_{io}$) that accompany speech provide insight into the function of the entire speech system. Abnormal pressure values might reflect inadequate or unstable ventilatory support. But they may also indicate inappropriate velopharyngeal status or abnormality in the degree, location, or timing of

Table 8–4. Normal PE_{max} Values (in cmH_2O) and Regression Equations Relating PE_{max} and Age*

	Age Range (years)	Normal Value		Regression Equation
		Mean	(SD)	
Men	20–54	233	(42)	$PE_{max} = 229 + 0.08 \times$ Age
	55–59	218	(35)	
	60–64	209	(35)	
	65–69	197	(35)	
	70–74	185	(35)	
	55–80			$PE_{max} = 353 - 2.33 \times$ Age
Women	20–54	152	(27)	$PE_{max} = 158 - 0.18 \times$ Age
	55–59	145	(20)	
	60–64	140	(20)	
	65–69	135	(20)	
	70–74	128	(20)	
	55–86			$PE_{max} = 210 - 1.14 \times$ Age

Source:

*Data and regression equations from "Maximal Respiratory Pressure: Normal Values and Relationship to Age and Sex," by L. F. Black and R. E. Hyatt, 1969, *American Review of Respiratory Disease, 99*, 696–702. Tables 1 and 2, p. 700.

vocal tract constrictions. There is some evidence that P_{io} is a key articulatory variable. That is, it is possible that speakers adjust other physiologic parameters (such as air flow) to maintain specific air pressures for high-pressure consonants (Warren, Hall, & Davis, 1981; Putnam, Shelton, & Kastner, 1986; Warren, 1986, 1996; Laine, Warren, Dalston, Hairfield, & Morr, 1988; Warren, Dalston, Morr, Hairfield, & Smith, 1989).

TECHNIQUE

Instrumentation

Generally, dynamic P_{io} is measured with a sensing tube placed in the posterior oral cavity or in the oropharynx. There are two common means of achieving this, each having its own disadvantages. The tube may be passed through the nasal cavity until its tip hangs somewhat below the velum, in much the same manner as a flexible fiberscope is placed for laryngoscopy. Since the end of the nasal tube points into the airstream, it is important that the tip be closed and that the tube walls be perforated near the tip region to provide sensing port openings that are perpendicular to the direction of airflow (see previous section, "Influence of Flow on Pressure Measurement").

The advantage of the nasal tube placement is that there is no interference with movement of the articulators, nor will vigorous tongue or lip activity displace the sensing tube. Velar movement does not seem to compromise the measurement significantly, nor is velopharyngeal closure measurably affected, provided the tube is thin enough. Polyethylene tubing with an outer diameter of about 2 mm works quite well.

Some patients may have trouble tolerating a nasal approach. In these cases a sensing tube may be molded to lie in the buccogingival sulcus and curve around the last molar so that the opening of the tube is approximately at the midline and oriented perpendicular to the airflow. (Recall the earlier discussion of the importance of tube orientation.) This orientation can be assured by tying the tube to a molar with dental floss. The tube exits the oral cavity at the corner of the lips. (This tube placement is illustrated in Figure 8–10.) While easy to implement and less invasive than nasal placement, this method leaves the tube more prone to displacement by tongue, cheek, and labial movements.

With either sensing-tube placement, the near end of the tube is connected to an external pressure transducer located close to the patient. The oral end of the tube is likely to fill with saliva, which interferes with accurate measurement. Therefore, it is advisable to connect the sensing tube to the pressure gauge via a three-way stopcock, as in Figure 8–11. A large hypodermic syringe connected to the stopcock assembly can be used to force a blast of air through the tube to clear it when necessary.

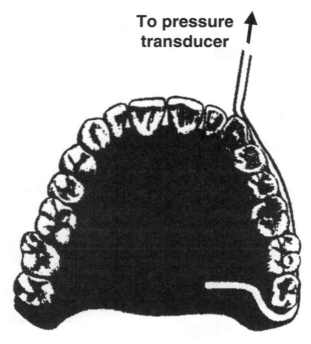

To pressure transducer

Figure 8–10. Placement of the intraoral pressure sensing tube around the last molar. The tube lies in the buccogingival sulcus and exits at the corner of the mouth. Note that the open end of the tube is perpendicular to the direction of airflow.

Method

P_{io} may be examined during running speech, but this procedure leaves too many potentially confounding variables uncontrolled. Variability of peak pressure for the same phoneme spoken by a given speaker is much greater during ordinary speech than during repetition of carefully specified test utterances (Miller & Daniloff, 1977). For this reason, testing usually involves having the patient repeat selected utterances—generally of the CVC or VCV type—a number of times. Usually it is the peak air pressure attained during the consonant that is of interest. To control testing further, the test utterances are commonly embedded in a carrier phrase, such as "It's a _____ again," and subjects are instructed to speak at a standard effort level. Often the patient is asked to talk so that the pointer of a sound level or VU-meter is deflected to within a few units of some preselected reading (perhaps representing 70 dB SPL). Several repetitions of each phoneme being tested are needed because the mean pressure and its variability (in the form of the standard deviation or coefficient of variation) are both important.

Pressure signals are commonly digitized and data are subsequently derived by computer software. Data may also be derived from an oscilloscope display or pen writer with an adequate frequency response. The transducer output can also be stored on an FM tape system or digital instrumentation recorder for later analysis if desired. When possible, the simultaneous sound pressure waveform should be stored and displayed with the pressure record in order to align the acoustic and pressure events in time. (Such a readout is shown in Figure 8–12.) Aligning a spectrogram to the pressure signal, in particular, can yield insight into articulatory dynamics (Agnello & McGlone, 1972; Karnell & Willis, 1982a), while simultaneous recording of other physiologic signals can prove useful as well. Interpretation of the pressure record is discussed in more detail in the next section.

EXPECTED RESULTS

The Output Record

Figure 8–12 shows P_{io} as measured via an intraoral catheter and bonded strain-gauge transducer for the utterance "time to buy a pot" spoken at a moderate rate and loudness. This output is typical of a normal speaker. Peaks indicate the consonants; during full vowels the P_{io} is essentially zero (atmospheric). The sound pressure (microphone) signal is used to identify the location of each phone, whose pressure is determined from the height of the pressure peak. Thus the P_{io} during the first /t/ was just under 7 cmH$_2$O, whereas the /t/ in "to" was produced with almost 8 cmH$_2$O pressure. In contrast, the final postvocalic /t/ in "pot" was associated with a minimal build-up of P_{io}—well below 1 cmH$_2$O—which is not uncommon in such contexts when plosive release may be reduced or omitted. Note that the peak pressure for /p/ was around 8 cmH$_2$O, whereas /b/ was generated with only 5 cmH$_2$O. The lower peak pressure of voiced cognates is to be expected. The relative uniformity of the durations of the pressure peaks is consistent with the nature of the utterance and may be considered an indicator of speech-timing stability.

The shape and duration of the pressure peaks can provide important information about articulatory function (Hutchinson & Smith, 1976; Gracco, Gracco, Löfqvist, & Marek, 1994; for an extensive review, see Müller and Brown, 1980). In this case, the sharp fall in P_{io} coincident with the plosive burst seen in the sound pressure record indicates normal function. That is, if the plosive release had been sluggish the pressure record would show it. Equally important is the fact that the sharp fall of the pressure trace demonstrates the adequacy of the measuring system's frequency response. To avoid erroneous interpretations of articulatory behavior, it is important to verify the response adequacy of the measurement system and to take note of any filtering used. (In Figure 8–12, for instance, the

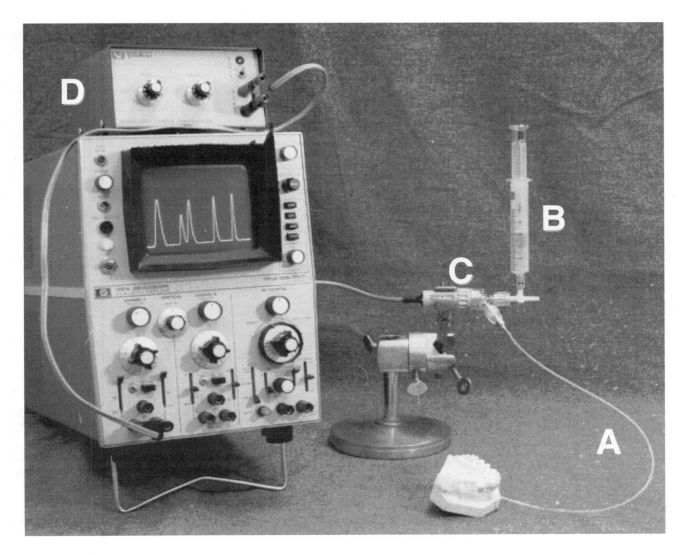

Figure 8–11. Setup for intraoral pressure measurement: **(A)** sensing tube; **(B)** hypodermic syringe mounted on a three-way stopcock; **(C)** pressure transducer; and **(D)** carrier amplifier.

intraoral pressure signal has been low-pass filtered with a 50-Hz cutoff frequency to minimize the voicing component.) The relative stability of the pressure baseline (the absence of drift) and the resolution of small pressure changes (for example the residual voice-related oscillation during /m/ and /b/ production) are also meaningful indicators of measurement accuracy and should be checked in any system before use.

Pressure Values

Data on a wide range of phones measured under the same conditions in children and adults continue to be scarce. Tables 8–5 and 8–6, however, can serve as a general guide for comparison of test results. The data in Table 8–6 were obtained with a special intraoral transducer and may be less than optimally valid (see

"Specialized Pressure Transducers," this chapter). Consequently these data should be compared to those of other research, such as the data in Tables 8–7 and 8–8.

Malécot (1966, 1968) also presents peak P_{io} values for many of the phonemes listed in the two preceding tables. His values, however, are consistently—and often significantly—higher than those presented above. This may be due, at least in part, to the loudness level ("one which is appropriate for talking to a person 4 feet away under ideal acoustic conditions") used by his subjects.

The question of why P_{io} changes with age is currently unresolved. Although studies have shown children to use higher pressures than older speakers (Subtelny, Worth, & Sakuda, 1966; Bernthal & Beukelman, 1978; Stathopoulos & Weismer, 1985; Netsell et al., 1994), Stathopoulos (1986) provided evidence that

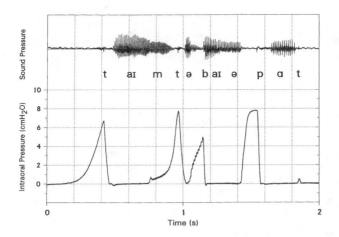

Figure 8–12. Intraoral pressure events during the utterance "Time to buy a pot." A simultaneous microphone (sound pressure) record is shown above.

the difference may simply reflect the fact that children tend to speak more loudly (see Table 8–7). Equivocal findings with respect to a P_{io} difference between adult male and female speakers may likewise be tied to known sex-related differences in speech intensity, which may be strongly subject to cultural differences.

Hixon, Minifie, and Tait (1967) have determined that vocal intensity level is approximately proportional to the 1.3 power of intraoral air pressure. That is,

$$SPL \propto P_{io}{}^{\sim 1.3}.$$

This relationship has been essentially confirmed by Ringel, House, and Montgomery (1967) and by Leeper and Noll (1972).

CONSISTENCY OF INTRAORAL PRESSURE MEASURES

Although peak pressure values have not been shown to be substantially influenced by syllable context (Karnell & Willis, 1982b) and stress (Netsell, 1970; Brown & McGlone, 1974; Flege, 1983), Miller and Daniloff (1977) found that, at least for the plosive consonants tested, mean peak P_{io} differed greatly depending upon whether the measurement came from a continuous speech sample or from repetitions of simple /CʌC/ syllables. In particular, the variability observed during extended monologue was much greater than that of the monosyllabic test words (see Table 8–8). Brown and McGlone (1969) determined that, under controlled conditions of vocal fundamental frequency and inten-

sity, adult speakers varied their peak P_{io} for /tʌ/ very little, even when repetitions over a period of 5 days were compared. Brown and Shearer (1970) found similar constancy for /s, z, p, and w/. Even varying the rate of syllable repetition seems to produce no consistent peak P_{io} effect (Hixon, 1966; Brown & McGlone, 1969). Hence, *when controlled testing conditions are used*, high intrasubject variability over time should be viewed as clinically suspect. Note, however, that esophageal speakers routinely have high intraoral pressure variability (Murry & Brown, 1975). Morris and Brown (1994) also reported significantly higher P_{io} variablity among a group of normal 75 to 90 year old women compared with a group of young female adults.

It is clear that P_{io} observed during speech varies as a function of a large number of variables. Most of these have not been fully explored. Table 8–9 summarizes these influences in cases where there are enough data to warrant at least a tentative judgment.

Subglottal Pressure

The subglottal pressure (P_s) represents the energy immediately available for creation of the acoustic signals of speech. It should be of appropriate magnitude and, perhaps even more important, it should be well regulated, that is, it should be *stable*. Inappropriate levels of P_s or inadequate pressure regulation can cause abnormal speech intensity levels or (to a lesser extent) sudden shifts in vocal fundamental frequency (for example, see Izdebski, 1984, or Shipp, Izdebski, Schutte, & Morrissey, 1988). Subglottal pressure may be adversely affected by problems of neuromuscular control of the chest wall (for example, athetosis or lower motoneuron paresis), by disorders that result in unacceptable vocal tract impedances (such as vocal fold paralysis) or by pulmonary pathology (such as advanced emphysema). Measurement of P_s is, therefore, potentially of great diagnostic and therapeutic value in a wide range of speech and related disorders (D'Antonio, Lotz, Chait, & Netsell, 1987; D'Antonio, Muntz, Province, & Marsh, 1988; Tanaka & Gould, 1985; Schutte, 1986; Iwata, 1988; Eibling & Gross, 1996). Clinical interpretation of findings requires a firm knowledge of the respiratory mechanics of speech.[1]

While it is an easy matter to obtain a nonspeech estimate of the subglottal pressure that might be used by a patient for speech, there is unfortunately no simple, direct, and convenient technique for actually measuring P_s during speech. Essentially three useful

---

[1]Good reviews of the rather complex interactions involved are provided by Mead, Bouhuys, and Proctor (1968), Hixon, Mead, and Goldman (1976), and Hixon (1973, 1987). More recent investigations in this area are reviewed by Orlikoff (1994).

Table 8–5. Mean Peak Intraoral Pressure (in cmH$_2$O)*

Phoneme	Men		Women		Children	
	Mean	SD	Mean	SD	Mean	SD
p	6.43	1.07	7.52	2.17	9.66	3.34
b	4.37	1.42	6.05	1.82	6.57	1.97
t	6.18	1.29	7.44	1.92	9.35	2.76
d	4.52	1.60	6.67	1.91	6.78	1.73
s	5.69	1.14	6.41	2.64	7.95	2.13
z	4.30	1.18	5.23	1.77	5.91	1.52
f	5.80	0.65	6.34	2.95	7.95	2.93
v	3.82	0.53	4.37	0.86	5.13	2.44
t	6.77	1.01	7.32	2.28	10.48	3.64
d	5.92	1.28	6.72	1.77	9.83	2.65
l	1.09	0.62	1.39	0.25	0.68	0.53
r	0.99	0.57	2.01	0.96	1.93	1.48
w	0.78	0.66	1.54	0.96	2.01	0.98
m	0.22	0.47	0.60	1.05	0.00	0.00
n	0.43	0.70	0.45	0.68	0.00	0.00

*Based on 10 men, 10 women, and 10 children (ages 6 to 10 years); VCV syllables, with V constant; Specialized intraoral transducer used for measurement. (1 cmH$_2$O = 10.2 kPa.)

Source: From "Intraoral Pressure and Rate of Flow During Speech," by J. D. Subtelny, J. H. Worth, and M. Sakuda, 1966, *Journal of Speech and Hearing Research, 9*, 498–519. Table 1, p. 505. © American Speech-Language-Hearing Association, Rockville, MD. Reprinted by permission.

Table 8–6. Mean Peak Intraoral Pressure in Children (in cmH$_2$O)*

Phoneme	Prevocalic	Intervocalic	Postvocalic
p	6.69	8.23	6.24
b	3.14	4.05	2.57
t	6.64	8.34	6.26
d	2.91	3.76	2.69
	6.25	7.18	5.22
	3.87	4.38	3.10
	5.77	6.62	5.15
	3.79	4.09	2.92
s	5.74	6.91	5.32
z	3.57	3.99	3.21
f	5.56	6.45	5.13
v	3.15	3.60	2.58

*Based on 6 boys and 4 girls, ages 8 years 2 months to 12 years 2 months (mean 10 years 0 months); /CʌC/ or /ʌCʌ/, three repetitions per phoneme; Normal pitch and loudness; Post-molar sensing tube and strain gauge transducer used for measurement. 1 cmH$_2$O = 10.2 kPa.

Source: From "Peak Intraoral Air Pressures During Speech," by H. J. Arkebauer, T. J. Hixon, and J. C. Hardy, 1967, *Journal of Speech and Hearing Research, 10*, 196–208. Table 1, p. 200. © American Speech-Language-Hearing Association, Rockville, MD. Reprinted by permission.

Table 8–7. Mean Peak Intraoral Pressure (in cmH₂O)* as a Function of Speech Intensity, Voicing, and Phonemic Position‡

Phoneme	Soft		Medium		Loud	
	Initial	Final	Initial	Final	Initial	Final
p						
Mean	8.02	8.00	11.60	11.20	15.68	15.28
(SD)	(4.04)	(3.98)	(5.18)	(4.92)	(6.18)	(5.54)
b						
Mean	5.82	4.46	8.92	6.72	12.86	8.06
(SD)	(4.06)	(2.78)	(4.58)	(3.44)	(6.26)	(3.48)

*1 cmH₂O = 10.2 kPa

‡Data derived from 10 boys and 10 girls, ages 8 to 10 years, and 10 men and 10 women, ages 22 to 34 years; /CᴧC/ embedded in carrier phrase "say _____ again" with three repetitions; Modified pitot tube and strain gauge transducer used for measurement; No significant age or sex effect, data are averaged across these variables.

Source: From "Relationship Between Intraoral Air Pressure and Vocal Intensity in Children and Adults," by E. T. Stathopoulos, 1986, *Journal of Speech and Hearing Research, 29,* 71–74. Table 1, p. 73. © American Speech-Language-Hearing Association, Rockville, MD. Reprinted by permission.

Table 8–8. Mean Peak Intraoral Pressure (in cmH₂O)* of CVC Syllables versus Spontaneous Speech‡

Phoneme	/CᴧC/ Syllable		Monologue	
	Mean	Range of Means	Mean	Range of Means
p	5.5	4.2–6.7	4.6	3.4–6.0
b	3.0	2.7–3.4	2.9	2.5–3.5
t	5.1	4.7–5.8	4.9	3.5–5.9
d	3.5	2.5–4.4	2.5	1.6–3.0
k	5.2	5.0–5.5	5.1	3.5–6.2
g	3.6	2.8–4.4	3.1	2.2–4.0

*1 cmH₂O = 10.2 kPa

‡Data derived from 3 "phonetically trained" men; Five repetitions each of /CᴧC/ words; 5-minute spontaneous monologue; Nasal catheter and strain gauge transducer used for measurement; Means averaged across prevocalic and postvocalic contexts.

Source: From "Aerodynamics of Stops in Continuous Speech," by C. J. Miller and R. Daniloff, 1977, *Journal of Phonetics, 5,* 351–360. Table 1, p. 356. Reprinted by permission.

methods have been developed, but each has very significant disadvantages or limitations. These three different methods are discussed separately below.

NONSPEECH ESTIMATES OF SUBGLOTTAL PRESSURE

Hixon and his coworkers, using the simplest possible instrumentation, have developed two methods of obtaining estimates of a patient's ability to generate and sustain subglottal pressure.

The first method, described by Netsell and Hixon (1978), is diagrammed in Figure 8–13A. Essentially it places the equivalent of a normal glottal resistance outside of the vocal tract. If the patient blows air through this artificial resistance with about the same effort as would be used for speech, the intraoral pressure will approximate speech subglottal pressure quite

Table 8–9. Summary of Mean Peak Intraoral Pressure Influences*

Higher Pressure Associated With:	Lower Pressure Associated With:	According to:
Voiceless plosives	Voiced plosives	Arkebauer et al. (1967) Netsell (1969) Lisker (1970)[†] Lubker & Parris (1970) Slis (1970) Warren & Hall (1973) Hutchinson & Smith (1976)[‡] Miller & Daniloff (1977) Karnell & Willis (1982b) Stathopoulos (1984) Stathopoulos & Weismer (1985) Stathopoulos (1986)
Voiceless plosives	Voiceless fricatives	Subtelny et al. (1966) Arkebauer et al. (1967) Andreassen, Smith, & Guyette (1991)
Voiceless fricatives	Voiced fricatives	Subtelny et al. (1966) Arkebauer et al. (1967) Slis (1970) Scully (1971) Hutchinson & Smith (1976)[‡] Warren, Hall, & Davis (1981)
Voiced fricatives	Voiceless fricatives	Stathopoulos (1984)
Intervocalic plosive	Prevocalic plosive	Arkebauer et al. (1967) Brown & Ruder (1972)
Prevocalic plosive	Postvocalic plosive	Malécot (1968) Brown, McGlone, Tarlow, & Shipp (1970) Bernthal & Beukelman (1978) Stathopoulos & Weismer (1985) Stathopoulos (1986)
High effort or SPL	Low effort or SPL	Hixon (1966) Hixon, Minifie, & Tait (1967) Ringel, House, & Montgomery (1967) Brown & McGlone (1969, 1974) Slis (1970) Brown & Brandt (1971) Leeper & Noll (1972) Klich (1982) Stathopoulos (1986)

*This summary table presents general trends; see specific data tables.
†With qualifications.
‡Subjects with severe-to-profound bilateral sensorineural hearing loss.

closely. One has only to measure the static intraoral pressure to obtain a good estimate of the patient's ability to generate Ps.

The artificial glottal resistance is formed by a **leak-** or **bleed-tube** in the measurement system. Originally, Netsell and Hixon suggested that the bleed tube have a resistance of 75 cmH$_2$O/L/s, which would be approximated by a glass tube 5 cm long having an internal diameter of 2 mm. Later research (Smitheran & Hixon, 1981) indicated that the resistance might more appropriately be in the range of 35 cmH$_2$O/L/s. Therefore, a tube of the same length with an internal diameter of about 2.75 cm would perhaps be more suitable as a substitute for the glottal resistance. A U-tube manometer is adequate for the measurement of the intraoral air pressure.

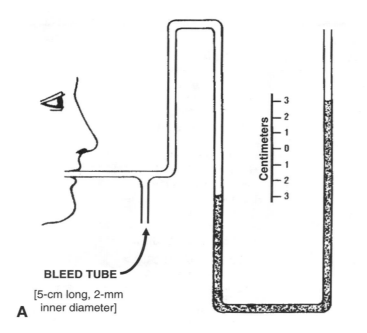

BLEED TUBE

[5-cm long, 2-mm inner diameter]

A

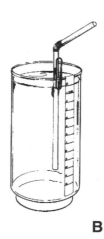

B

Figure 8–13. A. A method of estimating ability to generate subglottal pressure. The bleed tube has a resistance of about 75 cmH$_2$O/LPS. **B.** Apparatus for Ps estimation constructed of household objects (From "An Around-the-house Device for the Clinical Determination of Respiratory Driving Pressure: A Note on Making Simple Even Simpler," by T. J. Hixon, L. L. Hawley, and K. J. Wilson, 1982, *Journal of Speech and Hearing Disorders*, *47*, 413–415. Figure 1, p. 414. © 1982 American Speech-Language-Hearing Association, Rockville, MD. Reprinted by permission.)

To obtain the P$_s$ estimate, the patient is instructed to blow into the tube and to maintain a fixed level of pressure for a specified amount of time. Failure to achieve and hold adequate velopharyngeal closure, or a good lip seal to the inlet, violates the assumptions on which the test is based and, hence, will compromise validity of the results. It is also important that there be an air flow out of the leak-tube at the instant of measurement.

The other method, described by Hixon et al. (1982), involves extremely simple materials that are likely to be available around the house. The "instrument" (shown in Figure 8–13B) is made from a tall (at least 12 cm) jar or water glass. A centimeter ruler is attached vertically to the jar's outer surface, with the zero-centimeter mark at the top. (Alternatively, a strip of adhesive tape can be marked at half-centimeter increments and fixed to the jar.) A paper clip holds an ordinary drinking straw (the kind with an accordion pleat, which allows bending, is best) upright just inside the jar near the ruler. The jar is filled with water exactly to the level of the ruler's zero marking. The pressure at any given point in the water is determined by the point's depth below the surface. (In essence, the sys-

tem is a functionally inverted version of a U-tube.) If a patient can blow air out of the straw, his breath pressure must be greater than the pressure pushing water into the straw. That pressure is directly measured by the depth of the straw's open end.

The patient is asked to blow into the straw using an amount of effort that is comparable to speech. The straw is moved up or down until its open end is just at the depth at which bubbles are created and rise to the surface of the water. The oral breath pressure in cmH$_2$O is then just a bit greater than the depth of the open end of the straw (which can be read from the ruler). The patient must produce bubbles continuously for 5 seconds before the pressure reading is considered an indication of sustainable P$_s$. The same precautions that were associated with the leak-tube estimate apply in this case: There must be a good lip seal to the straw and velopharyngeal closure must be maintained. Because the patient is producing bubbles, air is being lost from the system, so a separate bleed valve to guard against oral valving is not really needed. However, it is probably wise to include a separate bleed resistance (in the form of a glass tube discussed above) if possible.

Advantages and Limitations

These techniques are extremely simple, inexpensive, and nonthreatening to the patient. They are valuable both for screening patients' performances and for providing feedback during the course of therapeutic management. Their chief limitation, of course, is that the measurements are not obtained during speech and, especially in the case of the straw and bubble technique, are, at best, approximate. Nonetheless, these methods are likely to be very useful in case management (for an example, see Netsell and Daniel, 1979).

Expected Results

Netsell and Hixon (1978) have found, after evaluating more than 120 dysarthric patients, that the ability to sustain a subglottal pressure of 5 cmH$_2$O for 5 seconds is a rule-of-thumb minimum for adequately meeting speech requirements. However, Netsell (1998) warns that significant laryngeal pathology or any speech disorder that reduces the "speed and range of articulatory movements (including those of the larynx and velopharynx) will rapidly 'drain' a 5 cmH$_2$O pressure head" (p. 107). Accordingly, Netsell suggests that the ability to develop a subglottal pressure of 10 cmH$_2$O and to sustain it for at least 10 seconds may be the more appropriate therapeutic target.

SUBGLOTTAL PRESSURE MEASUREMENT DURING SPEECH

Direct Methods

The most straightforward way of observing any pressure is to place the sensing tube right into the region where the pressure is. For the subglottic region this may be accomplished via the pharynx either with a specially configured sensing tube (van den Berg, 1956; Iwata, 1988) or with a special ultraminiature pressure transducer placed transglottally (Perkins & Koike, 1969; Koike & Hirano, 1973; Kitzing & Löfqvist, 1975; Koike, 1981; Kitzing, Carlborg, & Löfqvist, 1982; Schutte & Miller, 1986). Unfortunately these methods require that a tube remain between the vocal folds and, despite reports that this does not interfere with phonation, intubation techniques for direct evaluation of P$_s$ have not been widely accepted by speech professionals.

At present, the most common method of direct P$_s$ measurement involves piercing the trachea with a large-bore hypodermic needle. This can be left in place and the sensing tube attached to it, or it can be used as a sleeve through which a sensing tube is introduced into the trachea (the needle itself is then withdrawn). Netsell (1969), for example, reports using a needle about 4 cm long with an inner diameter of 0.055 cm

inserted between the first and second tracheal rings, while others have inserted the needle through the cricothyroid membrane to reach the subglottis (for example, Schutte & van den Berg, 1976; Bard, Slavit, McCaffrey, & Lipton, 1992; Plant & Hillel, 1998). The needle is attached to a pressure transducer by a polyethylene tube. The same instrumentation considerations previously discussed under dynamic intraoral pressure measurement apply in the case of direct measurement of P$_s$.

Advantages and Limitations

The prime advantage of the tracheal-puncture technique is its directness. In contrast to other methods that rely on observation of a correlate of P$_s$, this procedure requires no special calibration aside from that of the pressure transducer itself. All other factors being equal, it yields an inherently accurate measure. The drawbacks of the method, however, are obvious and significant. While not particularly painful, the procedure is very likely to provoke considerable patient anxiety. Technically a surgical procedure, placement of the sensing tube must be done by a physician and is attended by some risk of damage or bleeding. In extreme instances a painful subdermal air bubble can accidentally be produced. These problems have motivated the development of more innocuous indirect approaches.

Indirect Methods

Indirect measurement of P$_s$ entails the determination of a pressure that is analogous, or closely related, to the subglottal pressure. Subglottal pressure may be estimated from intraesophageal pressure or from the pressure in a sealed body plethysmograph. While neither method yields results as accurate as those obtained from an intratracheal probe, the fact that neither requires surgical placement of the sensing tube makes them more acceptable for clinical use. Finally, it is also possible to obtain a somewhat more approximate and discontinuous estimate of P$_s$ from the oral pressure during specially designed speech tasks.

Esophageal Pressure

The esophagus passes through the thorax and hence is influenced by the intrathoracic pressure. It also lies against the membranous, relatively compliant, posterior portion of the trachea. Thus, it is reasonable to assume that the pressure of a bolus of air in the esophagus might accurately reflect the tracheal (that is, subglottal) pressure.

While this reasoning is intuitively appealing, it overlooks a number of important factors that are considered in some detail by Bouhuys, Proctor, and Mead (1966), Lieberman (1968), and van den Berg (1956). The most significant problems arise from the fact that, while the esophagus runs through the thorax, it lies in the pleural space outside the lungs. The pressure in this region is *always* lower than the pressure in the lungs. It is not surprising, therefore, that esophageal pressure (P_{es}) does not equal P_s. Another consequence of the pleural location of the esophagus is that the lung recoil forces act in opposite directions on the alveolar air and on the esophagus. For example, at the lung volumes typical of speech, lung stretch causes an inward recoil of the lung membranes. That is, the lungs act like inflated balloons and tend to shrink back toward their uninflated size. This diminishes their volume, and compresses the air in them, raising its pressure. At the same time, however, shrinkage of the lungs increases the volume of the pleural space, lowering the pleural pressure. The degree to which the subglottal pressure is affected by lung recoil forces (and the extent to which esophageal pressure is changed in the opposite direction) varies with the lung volume. Therefore, a lung-volume-correction factor must be applied to P_{es} before it can serve as an estimate of P_s.

Instrumentation. Aside from the standard pressure transducer, the main item of instrumentation required for the measurement of intraesophageal pressure is a long sensing tube ending in a thin-walled rubber balloon. Several different designs have been tested; they vary primarily in the length of the balloon itself (Fry, Stead, Ebert, Lubin, & Wells, 1952; van den Berg, 1956; Milic-Emili, Mead, Turner, & Glauser, 1964; Lieberman, 1968). A common design includes a long (> 50 cm) polyethylene tube with a 2-mm diameter and a 1.5-mm bore. At one end is mounted a 11.5-cm long, 1-cm diameter balloon made of very thin rubber. The catheter tube is perforated with two 1.4-mm diameter holes for every centimeter of length enclosed by the balloon. The transducer end of the catheter is fitted with the appropriate connector for the pressure transducer that is used.

Procedure. Measuring esophageal pressure is a difficult procedure that will require the skills of a physician or similarly trained individual. The two critical aspects are placing the balloon and calibrating the output. The empty balloon is inserted via the nasal cavity into the esophagus. Patients quickly learn to swallow the balloon with ease, especially if aided by sips of water. Various placements for balloons of differing length have been proposed (Fry et al., 1952; Draper, Ladefoged & Whitteridge, 1960; Ladefoged, 1963; Siegert, 1969;

Schutte, 1986; Sundberg, Elliot, Gramming, & Nord, 1993). However, since the optimal balloon location is the one that results in the smallest artifacts (for instance, cardiac pulses) with the best pressure sample, it seems best to adjust the position of the balloon for each patient, rather than to depend on a fixed (and perhaps arbitrary) distance. The placement technique described by Lieberman (1968) seems particularly well suited to clinical work.

Calibration. While the pressure transducer itself may be calibrated against a U-tube manometer, the strong influence of lung volume on esophageal pressure makes it imperative that an additional calibration be done. There are two problems inherent in achieving the necessary correction. First, the actual recoil-induced pressure at any given lung volume is different in different people, and there is no way of predicting it a priori. Second, while the recoil pressure varies with lung volume in a fairly linear way in the mid-region of the vital capacity range, as one approaches the extremes of lung volume the relationship becomes markedly nonlinear, again in essentially unpredictable ways. This might not be a catastrophic problem in normal speakers, but patients in rehabilitation programs cannot be so categorized, and they are more likely to use lung volumes near the extremes of their vital capacities. For these reasons, different calibration techniques have been devised to delineate and compensate for the change in P_{es} due solely to change in lung volume in the specific patient being evaluated.

Ladefoged (1964) and Ladefoged and McKinney (1963) proposed a calibration method that rests on the following principle. If the glottis remains open and the velopharyngeal port closed, the intraoral air pressure must be essentially the same as the tracheal pressure when one exhales against a high resistance. Calibration for changes of esophageal pressure thus requires that intraoral air pressure be monitored along with esophageal pressure as the patient blows against an oral obstruction with different amounts of effort. Each esophageal pressure reading obtained can be paired with a measured intraoral air pressure to generate a table of equivalents. This procedure is repeated at several lung volumes. A sample oscillographic record of the results of this maneuver at a single lung volume is shown in Figure 8–14. Note that the procedure requires a second pressure-measuring system (for intraoral pressure) and a means of monitoring lung volume.

Lieberman (1968) used a calibration technique that is simpler to implement. While not as accurate as Ladefoged's method, it gives results which are sufficiently valid for everyday clinical use. It assumes, for the duration of an utterance lasting for 2 to 3 seconds,

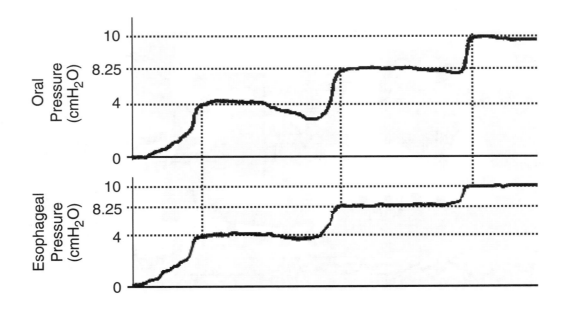

Figure 8–14. Calibration of the esophageal pressure according to the method recommended by Ladefoged and McKinney (1963). Known intraoral pressures are used to determine esophageal pressure equivalents. The P_{es} scale (bottom) is assigned values of the P_{io} pressures. Note that the P_{es} scale is nonlinear.

that the recoil pressure generated in the lungs is essentially a linear function of the lung volume and that the decrease in lung volume proceeds at a steady rate during speech. If the airway is unobstructed by glottal closure or oral constriction, the tracheal pressure must be zero when there is no airflow. During speech this condition is met at every transition from inspiration to expiration or vice versa. During the speech task, therefore, airflow is simultaneously recorded along with the esophageal pressure. A sample record, showing how the calibration is handled, is presented in Figure 8–15. Every point in the esophageal pressure trace that corresponds to a point of ventilatory phase transition (as shown by the flow record) is considered to represent $P_s = 0$. The subglottal pressure at any point in the record is read as the distance of the esophageal pressure trace (according to the transducer system calibration originally performed with a U-tube) above the zero-pressure baseline that is constructed by connecting the zero-pressure points with straight lines. In essence, the deduced baselines subtract out the lung-volume error. Since each breath group begins and ends with a ventilatory phase transition, each has its own (approximate) correction factor. Lieberman (1968) determined that this calibration method results in P_s estimates that are accurate within about 1 cmH$_2$O,

provided that the speaker does not use lung volumes near the extremes of his or her vital capacity.

Advantages and limitations. Using an esophageal balloon to sense a correlate of subglottal pressure has the obvious advantage of avoiding tracheal puncture, with its attendant risks, pain, and patient anxiety. But this method is not altogether anxiety-free either, and since it is itself somewhat invasive, its use is accompanied by reduced, but nonetheless real, risk. Clearly, the esophageal balloon should be placed by a physician.

The question of the validity of the resultant data has been debated at some length in the literature (van den Berg, 1956; Kunze, 1964; Ladefoged, 1964; McGlone, 1967; Rubin, LeCover, & Vennard, 1967; Baydur, Behrakis, Zin, Jaeger, & Milic-Emili, 1982; Baydur, Cha, & Sassoon, 1987). While the theoretical issues and practical problems discussed in these assessments certainly merit consideration, the clinician should bear in mind that the researchers participating in the published debate had measurement objectives very different from those that guide clinical rehabilitation. That is, the purpose behind their development of various subglottal pressure measurement procedures was the generation of highly accurate data that will permit testing

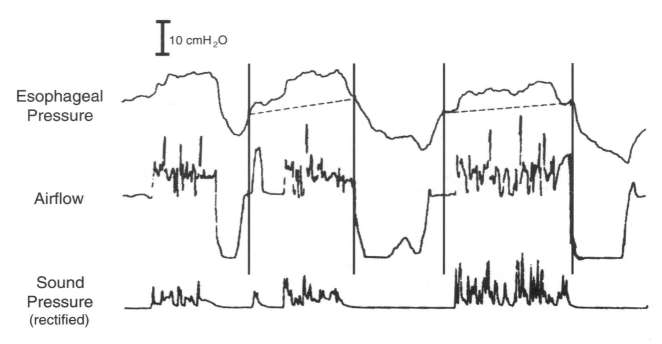

Figure 8–15. Calibration of an esophageal pressure record according to Lieberman's (1968) method. Respiratory phase transitions (shown in the flow record) are delineated by vertical lines. They are used to define points in the record when the tracheal pressure must be zero. For each breath-group the beginning and ending zero-pressure points are connected to form a pressure baseline (dashed lines). Pressure measures are then made in terms of the height of the trace above the pressure baseline.

hypotheses resulting from various physiological theories. In the research laboratory uncertainty of measurement often proves fatal to hypothesis confirmation. The clinician's objectives are very different, in that it is rare for small differences in P_s to be of clinical importance. In general the speech pathologist will be more interested in the patient's ability to generate subglottal pressures that at least fall into the usable range, to vary the pressure voluntarily, and, perhaps of supreme importance, to maintain the stability of whatever pressure is being used. With reasonable care, the accuracy of P_{es} measurements will be adequate for the purposes of the clinical rehabilitation specialist even if they are not sufficiently precise to satisfy the speech scientist. Thus it is the difficulty in balloon placement and calibration, rather than the issue of measurement precision, that continues to restrict the clinical popularity of this P_s estimation technique.

Plethysmography

Hixon (1972) and Warren (1976) have described a method for evaluating Ps using a body plethysmograph (described in Chapter 9, "Airflow and Volume"). For this measurement, a dome is hermetically clamped to the top of the body box, enclosing the patient's head (see Figure 8–16). In this arrangement, the plethysmo-graph forms a quasi-closed system with the patient inside, breathing to and from the space within the box. As the patient inhales (increasing his lung volume) the increase in the size of his body causes the amount of free space inside the box to diminish; the reverse is true on expiration. In short, since the closed system has a constant volume, an increase in the volume of one part (for instance, the lungs) will be exactly matched by a decrease in the volume of the other part (the free space within the box) if all other factors are constant.

Any change in lung volume occurs together with (and, indeed, is produced by) a change in alveolar pressure. Boyle's law states that the volume of a gas is inversely proportional to its pressure:

$$V = \frac{1}{P}.$$

If alveolar pressure increases somewhat, the volume of the lungs will diminish a little, and vice versa. This change of volume does *not* result in movement of air from one part of the closed system to the other and, therefore, the pressure in the space surrounding the patient will change by a proportional amount in the opposite direction. Because there is only a negligible difference between lung and subglottal pressures, the air pressure of the plethysmograph may serve as an index of P_s.

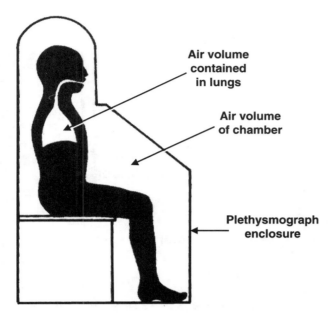

Figure 8–16. The body plethysmograph. When completely sealed within the box the subject's lungs and the surrounding space constitute two parts of a single volume of air. Assuming that the pressure inside the box does not change, expansion of one part of the air volume must be at the expense of the other part of the volume, since the total air volume in the box must remain constant.

Labels in figure:
- Air volume contained in lungs
- Air volume of chamber
- Plethysmograph enclosure

Unfortunately, the lung volume is very different from the volume of the air surrounding the patient and therefore, the magnitude of the box pressure change is proportional to, *but not equal to*, the change in lung pressure. This means that the method requires special calibration procedures, similar to those used for esophageal pressure estimates of P_s.

Instrumentation. The actual setup required is diagrammed in Figure 8–17. The patient normally breathes into the space within the chamber. There is, however, a special tube, closed at one end, mounted just in front of the patient's mouth. A transducer is connected to measure the pressure in this tube during calibration. Measurement of the box pressure, the correlate of P_s, is accomplished with another transducer that senses the pressure just inside of a screened opening in the box wall. The screen provides a moderate resistance to the flow of air, across which the pressure appears. The opening allows slow changes in pressure (equivalent to DC voltage) to be equalized, while allowing comparatively rapid (AC-type) changes to be measured. Functionally, then, the box can be considered to be sealed for high-frequency AC signals, but fully vented for DC.

Calibration. The system is calibrated by having the patient seal his lips around the mouth tube and, keep-

ing his glottis open, compress and expand the gas in his lungs by attempting to "pant" into it (DuBois, Botelho, Bedell, Marshall, & Comroe, 1956). The pressure transducer attached to the mouth tube records the intraoral pressure during this maneuver. Since the glottis is open and, because the mouth tube is sealed at the far end so that there is only negligible airflow, this matches the lung pressure quite closely. The intraoral pressures are then used to calibrate the box pressures that were simultaneously recorded.

Since the calibration thus obtained is valid only for the lung volume at which the calibrating maneuver was performed, the patient is usually asked to do the calibrating task, come off the mouth tube, and immediately speak the test utterances with no intervening inspiration or expiration. If the lung volume changes significantly during the utterance (because of its length or because of excessive air usage), a second calibration will be required at its end. In this case the patient is asked to hold his breath at the postsample lung volume and perform the "panting" maneuver into the mouth tube again. The change in calibration factor due to lung volume change can thereby be accounted for. A single calibration suffices for short utterances if air usage is essentially normal. Recent insights regarding the physics of body plethysmography have resulted in newer calibration techniques that do not require the patient to pant into a mouth tube (for example, see Agrawal & Agrawal, 1996), but these methods have yet to show their clinical validity and reliability or to gain currency in practice.

Boyle's law is valid for gases maintained at a constant temperature (see "The Gas Laws," Chapter 9). But in plethysmography, the box pressure is substantially influenced by heat radiated from the patient's body and by air temperature fluctuations associated with the patient's respiration (Bates, 1992). Tanaka and Gould (1983) suggested a correction for this (Figure 8–18). Assuming continuous heat radiation and a fairly stable expiratory flow rate, they draw a straight upward-sloping "baseline" on the pressure record beginning just prior to phonation and ending when the patient's lung pressure again approximates that of the box following phonation. This correction is performed for each calibration (that is, for each phonation or utterance breath group).

Advantages and limitations. The prime advantage of the plethysmographic method of estimating P_s is the fact that it is completely noninvasive. Not only does this eliminate risk, but it makes the measurement procedure far more acceptable to the patient. In fact, this method may be the only way to obtain P_s measures during speech in young children, for whom the plethysmograph may be decorated as a "space ship," and the measurement procedure made part of an appropriate game. While frequent calibrations are

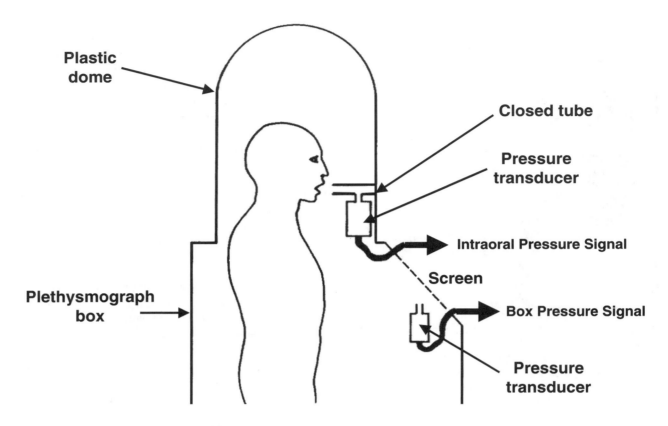

Figure 8–17. Use of the body plethysmograph to measure subglottal pressure.

required, the technique is based on fairly straightforward and well understood physical principles. With a modicum of care, measures of exceptional precision and excellent validity are possible. The cost of a body plethysmograph is relatively high, but since it may also be used for airflow and lung volume measurements, its versatility permits the higher capital investment to be amortized over greater use.

Estimation Using P_{io} During Plosive Production

When the vocal folds are abducted and the oral airway closed for a sufficiently long period during the production of a voiceless plosive, the intraoral air pressure rises to the value of the tracheal pressure. The two are, in fact, essentially equal when the intraoral pressure reaches its maximum (Netsell, 1969; Shipp, 1973; Kitajima & Fujita, 1990; Hertegård, Gauffin, & Lindestad, 1995). The magnitude of the oral pressure peak during plosive production can be considered, therefore, to be a good estimate of P_s if the speech task is carefully constructed and appropriately performed.

Method. While subject to certain limitations and problems (Smitheran & Hixon, 1981; Hixon & Smith-

eran, 1982; Rothenberg, 1982; Fisher & Swank, 1997), using intraoral pressure to estimate P_s has recently become especially popular with both researchers and clinicians. The typical protocol requires the patient to produce about 7 repetitions of the syllable /pi/—although /pɑ/ and /pæ/ have also been used—at a rate of 1.5 syllables per second. (A metronome set to 92 beats per minute can be used to help the patient maintain the desired rate.) Intraoral pressure is sensed by a polyethylene tube and pressure transducer. The patient is required to produce the syllable train, after an inhalation to twice normal depth, on a single continuous expiration. Normal pitch and loudness are used, and the syllables should all receive equal stress. Under these conditions, the peak intraoral pressures are considered to equal the subglottal pressure (Rothenberg 1973). Since P_s varies little during speech (Draper et al., 1960; Mead et al., 1968; Netsell, 1973; Gelfer, Harris, & Baer, 1987), the subglottal pressure used for the utterance can be estimated by drawing a line through the peak P_{io} of adjacent syllables (Figure 8–19). Specific examples and exercises are provided in Orlikoff and Baken (1993). For patients with velopharyngeal dysfunction, it is important to use a nose clip to eliminate nasal airflow when obtaining P_{io} measures.

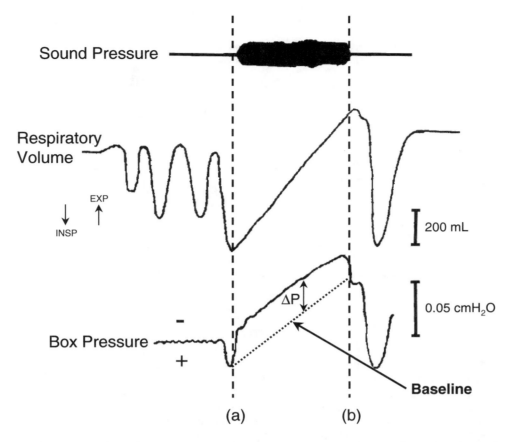

Figure 8–18. Calibration of a plethysmographic pressure record according to Tanaka and Gould's (1983) method. At the end of inspiration just prior to phonation, the subglottal pressure is equal to the pressure within the plethysmograph. A pressure baseline is determined by drawing a line from the prephonatory box pressure **(a)** to the box pressure just after phonation **(b)** when the subglottal pressure again approximates the pressure within the plethysmograph chamber. Subglottal pressure measures are then estimated by ΔP, the difference between the baseline and box pressures. (Adapted with permission from "Relationships Beween Vocal Intensity and Noninvasively Obtained Aerodynamic Parameters in Normal Subjects," by S. Tanaka and W. J. Gould, 1983, *Journal of the Acoustical Society of America, 73*, 1316–1321. Figure 2, p. 1317. © Acoustical Society of America, Woodbury, NY.

Advantages and limitations. This method does have the advantage of being very simple to use. It entails no significant invasiveness, requires only simple instrumentation, and involves a speech task that is within the competence of most patients. Although certain procedural points continue to be debated, Löfqvist, Carlborg, and Kitzing (1982) have shown that an acceptable estimate of P_s during vowel production results if the oral pressure reading is taken at the midpoint of a line connecting two successive pressure peaks. Kitajima and Fujita (1990) also found peak intraoral pressure to be nearly equivalent to P_s, but only when the subglottal pressure was smaller than 25 cmH$_2$O. P_s will rarely approach 25 cmH$_2$O during speech production but, since a number of factors can

influence oral pressure, caution should be exercised in interpreting the data in special cases. In addition to the making the necessary assumption that the P_s a given patient uses during the interconsonantal vowel reflects the bordering P_{io} pressure peaks (see, for instance, Plant and Hillel, 1998), there remains some question as to whether the P_s a patient uses during production of a syllable train at an even rate, pitch, and loudness provides an adequate reflection of the P_s that is used during spontaneous speech (McHenry, Kuna, Minton, & Vanoye, 1996).

Estimation Using P_{io} During Airway Interruption

Another way to force the oral air pressure to approxi-

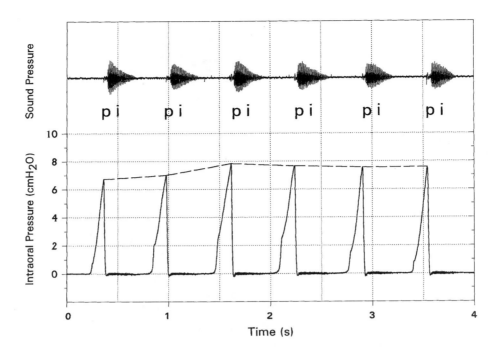

Figure 8–19. A microphone signal and intraoral pressure trace obtained during repetition of the syllable /pi/. A metronome set to 92 beats/min was used to assist the speaker to maintain a rate of approximately 1.5 syllables/s. The dotted line connecting sequential peak pressures approximates the subglottal pressure used over the course of the utterance. The stability of rate, waveshape, and peak pressures is typical of speakers with normal ventilatory and articulatory control.

mate P_s is to suddenly block the airway during phonation (van den Berg, 1956). This can be accomplished by closing a valve at the outlet of a mouthpiece or a face mask that the speaker wears. In essence, the valve closure constitutes an artificial plosive articulation.

Method. Sawashima and his coworkers (Sawashima et al., 1983, 1984; Sawashima, Niimi, Horiguchi, & Yamaguchi, 1988; Sawashima & Honda, 1987) implement this technique with a specially made, electrically operated shutter valve that achieves rapid and complete closure when the tester pushes a button. It takes up to 200 ms for the oral pressure to rise to the magnitude of the subglottal pressure. Since ventilatory and vocal tract adjustments can change the pressure if the closure persists (Baken & Orlikoff, 1987), the valve must not be kept closed too long. Sawashima and his colleagues recommend that closure be limited by an electronic timer to a maximum of 400 ms. The estimate of subglottal pressure is represented by the P_{io} at the point where it just levels off after valve closure. The reason is that, while air may be prevented from flowing through the mouth, glottal flow continues for a short time after valve closure due to the compliance of the upper respiratory system. A valid estimate of subglottal pressure can only be obtained once all airflow has ceased and P_s and P_{io} have equalized. To hasten the

stoppage of flow, some clinicians and investigators have advocated placing the palms of the hands against the cheeks of the patient (for example, Bates, Sly, Kochi, & Martin, 1987; Blosser et al., 1992). When the measurements are derived correctly, Bard and his colleagues (1992) found a high correlation ($r = .92$) between P_s estimated by airway interruption using an air-driven balloon valve and the pressure measured directly via tracheal puncture.

Advantages and limitations. The advantages that accrue from the noninvasiveness of this method are offset by the relative complexity and expense of the valve assembly and its electronic control system. Care must be taken to ensure that the valve closure does not cause a patient reaction that, by changing the subglottal pressure, would result in an invalid measure. Since the valve closure is quite disruptive of phonation, it is likely to cause the speaker to use abnormal or compensatory behaviors after the first trial. The patient must also be able to maintain a tight lip seal around the mouthpiece or to tolerate a firm fitting of the cushion of the face mask.

Although the application of airway interruption techniques for estimating P_s during speech has been fairly recent, it has had a long history in the measurement of nonspeech respiratory pressures and pulmonary airway resistance (von Neergaard & Wirz, 1927; Otis & Proctor, 1948; Mead & Wittenberger, 1954). Despite several superseding techniques, the advent of digital processing has again made the airway interruption method popular in respiratory physiology (Bates, Baconnier, & Milic-Emili, 1988; D'Angelo, Prandi, Tavola, Calderini, & Milic-Emili, 1994), except in cases where respiratory disease results in topographic pressure differences within the lower respiratory system (Valta, Corbeil, Chassé, Braidy, & Milic-Emili, 1996).

Expected Results

Murry (1971) reported that P_s was higher during pulse- than during modal-register phonation, although McGlone and Shipp (1971) found no significant difference between phonations sustained in these voice registers. However, pulse register phonation that normally occurs during terminal syllables in running speech seems to be characterized by a P_s that is considerably *lower* than that of the modal phonation that preceded it (Murry & Brown, 1971). Blomgren, Chen, Ng, and Gilbert (1998) recently compared the peak intraoral pressure during /pi/ repetition for syllables produced by 20 normal men and women using both the modal and pulse registers. They found that the peak pressure values for the modal productions (averaging roughly 7.5 cmH$_2$O) was significantly higher than those for the pulse register productions (with a mean of approximately 5.5 cmH$_2$O). Other studies have shown that P_s is consistently higher in loft-register phonation than in either the pulse or modal registers (Shipp & McGlone, 1971).

Within the modal voice register, P_s is more closely tied to vocal intensity than to frequency regulation (Monsen, Engebretson, & Vemula, 1978; Holmberg et al., 1988, 1989; Sawashima et al., 1988). The typical larynx produces about a 3- to 5-Hz change in vocal F_0 for each cmH$_2$O of P_s change (van den Berg, 1958; Ladefoged & McKinney, 1963; Lieberman, Knudson, & Mead, 1969; Hixon, Klatt, & Mead, 1971; Baer, 1979; Rothenberg & Mahshie, 1986; Baken & Orlikoff, 1987, 1988; Kitajima & Tanaka, 1995). Subglottal pressure, however, is held relatively stable during spoken utterances despite F_0 variations that are on the order of 75 to 100 Hz. Furthermore, data from Tanaka, Kitajima, and Kataoka (1997) suggest that, at typical speaking fundamental frequencies, F_0 regulation is less sensitive to changes in transglottal pressure. Nevertheless, changes in driving pressure may be important for the control of particularly low voice frequencies when vocal fold tension is greatly reduced (Atkinson, 1978; Holmberg et al., 1989; Titze, 1989). Conversely, in singing there appears to be a much closer association between vocal F_0 and the driving pressure (Schutte & Miller, 1986; Leanderson, Sundberg, & von Euler, 1987; Titze & Sundberg, 1992; Åkerlund & Gramming, 1994).

The Relationship of Subglottal Pressure to Vocal Intensity

Subglottal pressure varies directly with vocal intensity. The exact relationship is not linear, and it appears to differ quantitatively among individuals. Isshiki (1964) found (in a single male subject) that P_s, measured by tracheal puncture, varied from 3 to 25 cmH$_2$O as intensity increased from 65 to 95 dB SPL. The approximate relationship was

$$SPL \propto P_s^{3.3 \pm 0.7}.$$

Using a body plethysmograph, Tanaka and Gould (1983) report that, for 4 male and 6 female healthy subjects,

$$SPL = 31.8 \log(P_s) + 56.4.$$

Estimating P_s from intraoral pressure, Titze and Sundberg (1992) observed that once the normal speaker attains his or her phonation threshold pressure, SPL increases by 8 to 9 dB each time P_s is doubled. Considering only subglottal pressures between 10 and 30 cmH$_2$O, Ladefoged and McKinney (1963, p. 456) found that "peak subglottal pressure was proportional to the 0.6 power of the peak [rms] sound pressure." That is,

$$P_s \propto dB\ SPL^{0.6}.$$

The relationship of P_s and intensity is well illustrated in data presented in Table 8–10 and plotted in Figure 8–20. Although data are shown separately for men and women, several studies have failed to show a significant sex difference with respect to the subglottal pressures used (Schutte, 1986; Holmberg et al., 1988; Higgins & Saxman, 1991; Netsell et al., 1991; Stathopoulos & Sapienza, 1993; Holmes, Leeper, & Nicholson, 1994). Vocal frequency and intensity tend to covary during speech, but under controlled situations there seems to be no clear effect of vocal F_0 on subglottal pressure (Holmberg, Hillman, & Perkell, 1989; Sawashima et al., 1988).

The Relationship of Subglottal Pressure to Word Stress

Stress, or "prominencing" of syllables, is of two types: sentence-level and lexical. Lexical stress clarifies gram-

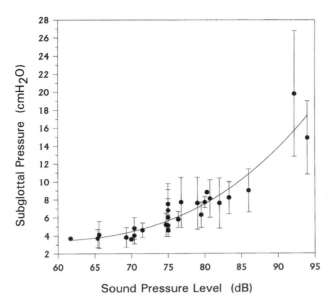

Figure 8–20. A plot of the data from Table 8–10 when both the mean SPL and Ps are reported. The range of P_s values is also shown, when provided by the authors. The curve represents a third-order regression fit to the mean P_s values.

matical function, as in the English words *con*duct (noun) versus con*duct* (verb). In sentence-level stress one word is chosen, for semantic or pragmatic reasons, as the focus of the sentence (as in "*She* did it," in which "she" is the stressed element). Sentence-level stress is almost always heavily marked for prominence, while, in conversation, lexical stress may be essentially unmarked. Only in careful, "citational" pronunciation is it the case that, as Ladefoged (1968, p. 143) notes, "accompanying every stressed syllable there is always an increase in the subglottal pressure." This observation receives support in the data of McGlone and Shipp (1972) who contrasted P_s during production of /p/ and /b/ in stressed (/əpa/, /əba/) and unstressed (/apə/, /abə/) positions. For the stressed productions of their 10 subjects, P_s was somewhat higher than average. The relationship between stress and P_s, however, is extremely complex. Because of the multiple cuing for word stress (of which subglottal pressure change is only a part), it is only partially understood.

Minimal Driving Pressure for Vocal Fold Oscillation

Phonation Threshold Pressure. The initiation of vocal-fold vibration requires a transglottal pressure drop of at least 3 to 5 cmH_2O, but a pressure 1 or 2 cmH_2O lower is then sufficient to sustain phonation already under way (Draper et al., 1960; Lieberman et al., 1969). A conservative clinical rule of thumb, there-

fore, is that minimally adequate speech requires that the patient be able to sustain a subglottal pressure of no less than 5 cmH_2O for at least 5 seconds (Netsell & Hixon, 1978; see also, Netsell & Daniel, 1979). The minimal P_s necessary to initiate voice production is called the ***phonation threshold pressure*** (PTP) (Titze, 1988, 1992). It has recently attracted some clinical interest in the wake of a few studies that have suggested that the PTP may be tied both to the viscoelasticity of the vocal fold mucosa and to the configuration of the glottis (Verdolini, Titze, & Fennell, 1994; see also, Chan, Titze, & Titze, 1997). Woodson and her coworkers (1996) have suggested that an elevated PTP may be related to the vocal effort and fatigue perceived by dysphonic patients.

Using a direct or indirect method of P_s measurement, PTP is assessed by having the patient attempt to sustain either phonation or a train of /pi/ syllables, respectively, just above a whisper. This is done to assure that the vocal folds are loosely adducted—as high medial fold compression will substantially influence the oscillation threshold, perhaps reflecting laryngeal conditions other than vocal fold status, such as thickness and viscosity. Often patients are instructed to perform the task below and then slightly above threshold before data recording. Both Gramming (1989) and Verdolini-Marston, Titze, and Druker (1990) have found a strong relationship between threshold pressures and vocal F_0. The normal subjects they tested had PTPs of approximately 3 cmH_2O at near-minimal vocal frequencies increasing to about 8 cmH_2O for F_0s close to the upper extremes of their phonational frequency ranges. Similar results were reported by McAllister and Sundberg (1998) for a group of children between 8 and 11 years of age.

Transglottal pressure during /b/ occlusion. Kitajima and his colleagues (Kitajima & Fujita, 1992; Kitajima & Tanaka, 1993) have suggested that the transglottal pressure prior to the release of /b/ occlusion can be used to approximate the PTP. Because the voicing of /b/ is associated with rather loose vocal fold adduction and with a markedly reduced amplitude of vibration (Sawashima & Hirose, 1981; Bickley & Stevens, 1987), Kitajima and Fujita (1992) have hypothesized that the driving pressure used would be quite similar to the minimal pressure necessary to promote fold oscillation. To derive an estimate of transglottal pressure during /b/ production, the general method of Smitheran and Hixon (1981) is used. The speaker first repeats /i:pi:/, followed by /i:bi:/, making sure that the same vocal intensity is used for both utterances. Because both utterances will use approximately the same P_s under these conditions, the difference between the peak pressure for /p/ and /b/ ($P_{/p-b/}$)

Table 8–10. Mean Estimated Subglottal Pressure (P_s) for Whisper and Phonation at Different Vocal Intensities

Condition	Sex	No.	Age[†]	Mean	(SD)	Mean	(SD)	Range	Source[‡]
		Subjects		**dB SPL**		**Estimated P_s (cmH$_2$O)***			
Whisper									
	F	5	22–24	—	—	4.0	(1.1)	—	1
	M	5	20–22	—	—	4.5	(1.9)	—	1
"Soft"									
	F	20	18–36	71.5	(4.9)	4.6	(0.8)	3.2–6.0	2
	F	10	20–30	65.4	(1.8)	3.7	(1.0)	—	3
	F	10	20–31	—	—	4.8	(0.7)	—	4
	F	8	22–29	65.6	(3.2)	4.1	(1.5)	2.6–6.3	5
	F	1	26	~70	—	3.6	(0.1)	—	6a
	F	10	25–57	61.7	—	3.7	—	—	7
	F	11	75±4	—	—	4.6	(0.9)	—	4
	M	25	17–30	75.0	(2.5)	5.1	(1.2)	3.3–7.6	2
	M	10	20–30	70.4	(3.2)	4.0	(0.9)	—	3
	M	10	20–31	—	—	4.5	(1.2)	—	4
	M	7	23–30	69.3	(8.1)	3.8	(1.1)	2.3–5.7	5
	M	10	75±5	—	—	5.3	(2.1)	—	4
"Normal"									
	F	10	4±1	—	—	8.4	(1.3)	—	8
	F	10	7±1	—	—	7.4	(1.5)	—	8
	F	10	11±1	—	—	7.1	(1.2)	—	8
	F	20	18–36	76.4	(4.0)	5.8	(0.9)	4.4–7.6	2
	F	5	22–24	—	—	4.6	(1.0)	—	1
	F	10	20–30	70.4	(1.9)	4.8	(1.2)	—	3
	F	10	20–31	—	—	6.5	(0.8)	—	4
	F	8	22–29	79.0	(3.6)	7.6	(2.9)	3.8–12.6	5
	F	1	26	~75	—	4.6	(0.2)	—	6a
	F	10	27±2	—	—	5.3	(1.2)	—	8
	F	15	27±4	—	—	5.4	(1.1)	—	9
	F	15	—	—	—	6.4	(1.9)	3.5–11.6	6b
	F	11	75±4	—	—	6.4	(1.7)	—	4
	M	10	4±1	—	—	8.4	(1.4)	—	8
	M	9	7±1	—	—	8.3	(2.0)	—	8
	M	10	10±1	—	—	7.9	(1.3)	—	8
	M	25	17–30	79.5	(3.3)	6.3	(1.4)	4.2–9.6	2
	M	5	20–22	—	—	6.3	(2.1)	—	1
	M	10	20–30	74.7	(3.1)	5.2	(1.3)	—	3
	M	10	20–31	—	—	5.8	(1.4)	—	4
	M	7	23–30	82.0	(7.2)	7.6	(2.8)	4.5–12.8	5
	M	10	28±5	—	—	6.0	(1.4)	—	8
	M	15	32±8	—	—	6.1	(1.4)	—	9
	M	10	75±5	—	—	8.0	(2.7)	—	4
	MF	?	4–7	~75	—	7.5	(2.3)	2.8–11.8	10
	MF	?	8–12	~75	—	6.8	(2.3)	3.3–13.7	10
	MF	?	13–15	~75	—	6.0	(2.1)	2.1–9.1	10
	MF	6	33–58	—	—	7.2	(1.3)	—	11

(Continued)

"Loud"

Sex	N	Age†	SPL	(SD)	Ps*	(SD)	Range	Source‡
F	20	18–36	83.3	(3.2)	8.2	(1.8)	6.5–13.1	2
F	10	20–30	76.8	(3.4)	7.7	(2.8)	—	3
F	10	20–31	—	—	8.0	(1.0)	—	4
F	8	22–29	92.2	(4.3)	19.8	(7.0)	9.1–27.7	5
F	1	26	~80	—	7.7	(0.6)	—	6a
F	15	27±4	—	—	8.0	(1.0)	—	8
F	10	25–57	80.3	—	8.8	—	—	7
F	11	75±4	—	—	8.8	(1.7)	—	4
M	25	17–30	86.0	(4.3)	9.0	(2.4)	5.9–15.4	2
M	10	20–30	80.7	(3.5)	8.1	(2.1)	—	3
M	10	20–31	—	—	7.9	(2.3)	—	4
M	7	23–30	94.0	(6.9)	14.9	(4.1)	7.3–24.4	5
M	10	75±5	—	—	10.6	(5.1)	—	4

*1 cmH_2O = 10.2 kPa

†Age range or mean age ± SD (in years).

‡*Sources*:

1. Stathopoulos, Hoit, Hixon, Watson, and Solomon, 1991. Subglottal pressure estimated from peak P_{io} averaged over 7 repetitions of /pi/ at a rate of 1.5 syllables/s using a "comfortable whisper" and then speaking at a "comfortable loudness, pitch, and quality." Data rounded to the nearest 0.1.

2. Holmberg, Hillman, and Perkell, 1988; and erratum [*Journal of the Acoustical Society of America, 85*, 1787 (1989)]. Subglottal pressure estimated from peak P_{io} averaged over 15 repetitions of /pæ/ at three levels of "vocal effort." Subjects instructed to avoid whispering and shouting.

3. Stathopoulos and Sapienza, 1993. Subglottal pressure estimated from peak P_{io} averaged over 7 repetitions of /pɑ/ at a rate of 1.5 syllables/s using a comfortable pitch: 1) at a comfortable loudness, 2) at 5±1 dB below the subject's comfortable SPL ("soft"), and 3) at 5±1 dB above the subject's comfortable SPL ("loud"). Data rounded to the nearest 0.1.

4. Higgins and Saxman, 1991. Subglottal pressure estimate based on repetition of /bæp/ at a rate of 3 syllables/s using a comfortable pitch: (1) at a comfortable loudness ("normal"), (2) at approximately 6 dB below the subject's comfortable SPL ("soft"), and (3) at approximately 6 dB above the subject's comfortable SPL ("loud"). Data rounded to the nearest 0.1.

5. Wilson and Leeper, 1992. Subglottal pressure estimated from peak P_{io} averaged over 7 repetitions of /pi/ at a rate of 1.5 syllables/s using a "normal pitch and quality." Subjects monitored peak SPL level to produce syllable strings at the 25th, 50th, and 75th percentiles of each their maximum SPL range. Subjects instructed to "inhale maximally" before beginning.

6. Leeper and Graves, 1984. (a) Subglottal pressure estimated from peak P_{io} averaged over 7 repetitions of /pi/ at three "controlled intensity conditions," nominally 70, 75, and 80 dB SPL. Data averaged over three trials per SPL condition and rounded to the nearest 0.1; (b) "Young adult women"; Subglottal pressure estimated from peak P_{io} averaged over 12 trials of 7 /pi/-syllable trains produced over two days and two times of day (morning and afternoon); "Appropriateness" of loudness, pitch, rate, and syllable stress judged by the tester; Data rounded to the nearest 0.1.

7. Åkerlund and Gramming, 1994. Subjects instructed to repeat /pɑ/ "three or four times in rapid succession, first as softly and then as loudly as possible over their entire vocal ranges." Data converted from kPa and averaged over the 196-, 220-, and 262-Hz conditions.

8. Netsell, Lotz, Peters, and Schulte, 1994. Subglottal pressure estimate based on repetition of /pi/ at 1.5 syllables/s using a "conversational" pitch and loudness. Significant main pressure effects found for age, sex (males higher than females; overall 7.9 vs 7.3 cmH_2O), rate of syllable production (3.0 syllables/s higher than 1.5 syllables/s; overall 7.9 vs. 7.2 cmH_2O), and syllable type (/pi/ higher than /pɑ/; overall 7.7 vs. 7.4 cmH_2O).

9. Netsell, Lotz, DuChane, and Barlow, 1991. Subglottal pressure estimate based on repetition of /pi/ and /pɑ/ at 1.5 and 3.0 syllables/s using a "normal" pitch and loudness. Data averaged across syllable rate and type.

10. Keilmann and Bader, 1995. Subglottal pressure estimate based on repetition of /ipipi/ using Frokjær-Jensen Aerophone II system. Mean P_s rounded to the nearest 0.1; range estimated from authors' scatterplot. No significant correlation between subglottal pressure and age or height. (Total of 100 children tested, number and sex of subjects in each age group not provided.)

11. Blosser, Wigley, and Wise, 1992. Subglottal pressure estimated using airway interruption method. Subjects sustained /ɑ/ at a "conversational" pitch and loudness. Shutter valve closures were triggered at 1-s intervals and lasted for 400 to 500 ms each. Data rounded to the nearest 0.1.

will reflect the driving pressure used during the voicing of /b/. With this technique, Kitajima and Fujita (1992) measured a $P_{/p-b/}$ of 4.8 ± 2.2 cmH$_2$O for 14 normal adult speakers, substantially lower than the $P_{/p-b/}$ recorded for several patients with laryngeal cancer. Nonetheless, the sensitivity of this measure, its correspondance to the PTP, and its clinical interpretation await further investigation.

The Stability of Subglottal Pressure

When speaking with uniform loudness, the normal speaker maintains a remarkably constant mean tracheal pressure (Draper et al., 1960; Gelfer et al., 1987; Moon, Folkins, Smith, & Luschei, 1993). Small variations due to sudden vocal tract impedance changes will occur, however. For example, Netsell (1969) measured P_s during production of /t/ and /d/ in the syllables /ʌːtʌ/ and /ʌːdʌ/ and found that the only observable difference between the pattern of P_s during the two was a sudden, but small, decrease of pressure during the plosive phase of /t/. The drop in pressure terminated with a return to the preplosive value when voicing resumed. A similar tendency is apparent for both /p/ and /b/ in the data of McGlone and Shipp (1972) and Murry and Brown (1979) as well as Slis (1970), who found that P_s dropped during /h/, a phoneme produced with very low vocal tract impedance. This kind of pressure drop is due to the sudden loss of significant vocal tract obstruction and is not a reflection of change in the generation of P_s. Also, of course, the subglottal pressure rises and falls slightly across the glottal cycle (Perkins & Koike, 1969; Koike & Hirano, 1973; Koike, 1981; Dejonckere & Lebacq, 1986; Ursino, Pardini, Panattoni, Matteucci, & Grosjacques, 1991; Hertegård et al., 1995). Aside from this kind of transient phenomenon, instability of subglottal pressure in the absence of intentional loudness changes or word stress should be seen as abnormal and clinically suspect. As a quick clinical test, Schutte (1992) has suggested that observing a patient's ability to sustain a steady /s/ production might provide some insight regarding the speaker's "breath control." It is of utmost importance, however, to ensure that variations of /s/ production due to changes in articulator position and posture are not confounded with variations due to alterations of driving pressure.

REFERENCES

Agnello, J. G., & McGlone, R. E. (1972). Distinguishing features of /p/ and /b/ from spectrographic intraoral air pressure comparison. *Journal of the Acoustical Society of America, 51,* 121.

Agrawal, A., & Agrawal, K. P. (1996). Body plethysmographic measurement of thoracic gas volume without panting against a shutter. *Journal of Applied Physiology, 81,* 1007–1011.

Åkerlund, L., & Gramming, P. (1994). Average loudness level, mean fundamental frequency, and subglottal pressure: Comparison between female singers and nonsingers. *Journal of Voice, 8,* 263–270.

Andreassen, M. L., Smith, B. E., & Guyette, T. W. (1991). Pressure-flow measurements for selected oral and nasal sound segments produced by normal adults. *Cleft Palate-Craniofacial Journal, 28,* 398–407.

Arkebauer, H. J., Hixon, T. J., & Hardy, J. C. (1967). Peak intraoral air pressures during speech. *Journal of Speech and Hearing Research, 10,* 196–208.

Atkinson, J. E. (1978). Correlation analysis of the physiological factors controlling fundamental voice frequency. *Journal of the Acoustical Society of America, 63,* 211–222.

Baer, T. (1979). Reflex activation of laryngeal muscles by sudden induced subglottal pressure changes. *Journal of the Acoustical Society of America, 65,* 1271–1275.

Baken, R. J., & Orlikoff, R. F. (1987). Phonatory response to step-function changes in supraglottal pressure. In T. Baer, C. Sasaki, & K. S. Harris (Eds.), *Laryngeal function in phonation and respiration* (pp. 273–290). Boston, MA: College-Hill Press.

Baken, R. J., & Orlikoff, R. F. (1988). Changes in vocal fundamental frequency at the segmental level: Control during voiced fricatives. *Journal of Speech and Hearing Research, 31,* 207–211.

Bard, M. C., Slavit, D. H., McCaffrey, T. V., & Lipton, R. J. (1992). Noninvasive technique for estimating subglottic pressure and laryngeal efficiency. *Annals of Otology, Rhinology and Laryngology, 101,* 578–582.

Bates, J. H. T. (1992). Correcting for the thermodynamic characteristics of a body plethysmograph. *Annals of Biomedical Engineering, 17,* 647–655.

Bates, J. H. T., Baconnier, P., & Milic-Emili, J. (1988). A theoretical analysis of interrupter technique for measuring respiratory mechanics. *Journal of Applied Physiology, 64,* 2204–2214.

Bates, J. H. T., Sly, P. D., Kochi, T., & Martin, J. G. (1987). The effect of a proximal compliance on interrupter measurements of resistance. *Respiration Physiology, 70,* 301–312.

Bates, J. H. T., Sly, P. D., Sato, J., Davey, B. L., & Suki, B. (1992). Correcting for the Bernoulli effect in lateral pressure measurements. *Pediatric Pulmonology, 12,* 251–256.

Baydur, A. (1991). Respiratory muscle strength and control of ventilation in patients with neuromuscular disease. *Chest, 99,* 330–338.

Baydur, A., Behrakis, P. K., Zin, W. A., Jaeger, M., & Milic-Emili, J. (1982). A simple method for assessing the validity of the esophageal balloon technique. *American Review of Respiratory Disease, 126,* 788–791.

Baydur, A., Cha, E. J., & Sassoon, C. S. (1987). Validation of esophageal balloon technique at different lung volumes and postures. *Journal of Applied Physiology, 62,* 315–321.

Bernthal, J. E., & Beukelman, D. R. (1978). Intraoral air pressure during the production of /p/ and /b/ by children, youths, and adults. *Journal of Speech and Hearing Research, 21,* 361–371.

Berry, J. K., Vitalo, C. A., Larson, J. L., Patel, M., & Kim, M. J. (1996). Respiratory muscle strength in older adults. *Nursing Research, 45,* 154–159.

Bickley, C. A., & Stevens, K. N. (1987). Effects of a vocal tract constriction on the glottal source: Data from voiced consonants. In D. M. Bless & J. H. Abbs (Eds.), *Vocal fold physiology: Contemporary research and clinical issues* (pp. 239–253). San Diego, CA: College-Hill Press.

Black, J. W. (1950). The pressure component in the speech production of consonants. *Journal of Speech Disorders, 15,* 207–210.

Black, L. F., & Hyatt, R. E. (1969). Maximal respiratory pressure: Normal values and relationship to age and sex. *American Review of Respiratory Disease, 99,* 696–702.

Blomgren, M., Chen, Y., Ng, M. L., & Gilbert, H. R. (1998). Acoustic, aerodynamic, physiologic, and perceptual properties of modal and vocal fry registers. *Journal of the Acoustical Society of America, 103,* 2649–2658.

Blosser, S., Wigley, F. M., & Wise, R. A. (1992). Increase in translaryngeal resistance during phonation in rhumatoid arthritis. *Chest, 102,* 387–390.

Bouhuys, A., Proctor, D. F., and Mead, J. (1966). Kinetic aspects of singing. *Journal of Applied Physiology, 21,* 483–496.

Brown, W. S., Jr., & Brandt, J. F. (1971). Effects of auditory masking on vocal intensity and intraoral pressure during sentence production. *Journal of the Acoustical Society of America, 49,* 1903–1905.

Brown, W. S., Jr., & McGlone, R. E. (1969). Constancy of intraoral air pressure. *Folia Phoniatrica, 21,* 332–339.

Brown, W. S., Jr., & McGlone, R. E. (1974). Aerodynamic and acoustic study of stress in sentence productions. *Journal of the Acoustical Society of America, 56,* 971–974.

Brown, W. S., Jr., McGlone, R. E., Tarlow, A., & Shipp, T. (1970). Intraoral air pressures associated with specific phonetic positions. *Phonetica, 22,* 202–212.

Brown, W. S., Jr., & Ruder, K. F. (1972). Phonetic factors affecting intraoral air pressure associated with stop consonants. In A. Rigault & R. Charbonneau (Eds.), *Proceedings of the seventh International Congress of Phonetic Sciences* (pp. 294–299). The Hague: Mouton.

Brown, W. S., Jr., & Shearer, W. M. (1970). Constancy of intraoral air pressure related to integrated pressure-time measures. *Folia Phoniatrica, 22,* 49–57.

Chan, R. W., Titze, I. R., & Titze, M. R. (1997). Further studies of phonation threshold pressure in a physical model of the vocal fold mucosa. *Journal of the Acoustical Society of America, 101,* 3722–3727.

Chen, H.-I., & Kuo, C.-S. (1989). Relationship between respiratory muscle function and age, sex, and other factors. *Journal of Applied Physiology, 66,* 943–948.

Cook, C. D., Mead, J., & Orzalesi, M. M. (1964). Static volume-pressure characteristics of the respiratory system during maximal efforts. *Journal of Applied Physiology, 19,* 1016–1022.

D'Angelo, E., Prandi, E., Tavola, M., Calderini, E., & Milic-Emili, J. (1994). Chest wall interrupter resistance in anesthetized paralyzed humans. *Journal of Applied Physiology, 77,* 883–887.

D'Antonio, L., Lotz, W., Chait, D., & Netsell, R. (1987). Perceptual-physiologic approach to evaluation and treatment of dysphonia. *Annals of Otology, Rhinology and Laryngology, 96,* 187–190.

D'Antonio, L. L., Muntz, H. R., Province, M. A., & Marsh, J. L. (1988). Laryngeal/voice findings in patients with velopharyngeal dysfunction. *Laryngoscope, 98,* 432–438.

Dejonckere, P. H., & Lebacq, J. (1986). Dynamique de la pression aérienne au cours du cycle vibratoire des cordes vocales chez le suject normal. *Acta Phoniatrica Latina, 8,* 191–196.

Derenne, J. P., Macklem, P. T., & Roussos, C. H. (1978). The respiratory muscles: Mechanics, control and pathophysiology. *American Review of Respiratory Disease, 188,* 119–133.

Draper, M. H., Ladefoged, P., & Whitteridge, D. (1960). Expiratory pressures and air flow during speech. *British Medical Journal, 18,* 1837–1843.

DuBois, A. B., Botelho, S.Y., Bedell, G. N., Marshall, R., & Comroe, J. H., Jr. (1956). A rapid plethysmographic method for measuring thoracic gas volume. *Journal of Clinical Investigation, 35,* 322–326.

Edmonds, T. D., Lilly, D. J., & Hardy, J. C. (1971). Dynamic characteristics of air-pressure measuring systems used in speech research. *Journal of the Acoustical Society of America, 50,* 1051–1057.

Eibling, D. E., & Gross, R. D. (1996). Subglottic air pressure: A key component of swallowing efficiency. *Annals of Otology, Rhinology and Laryngology, 105,* 253–258.

Fischer-Jørgensen, E., & Hansen, A. T. (1959). An electrical manometer and its use in phonetic research. *Phonetica, 4,* 43–53.

Fisher, K.V., & Swank, P. R. (1997). Estimating phonation threshold pressure. *Journal of Speech and Hearing Research, 40,* 1122–1129.

Fiz, J. A., Carrerers, A., Rosell, A., Montserrat, J. M., Ruiz, J., & Morera, J. M. (1992). Measurement of maximal expiratory pressure: Effect of holding the lips. *Thorax, 47,* 961–963.

Flege, J. E. (1983). The influence of stress, position, and utterance length on the pressure characteristics of English /p/ and /b/. *Journal of Speech and Hearing Research, 26,* 111–118.

Fry, D. L. (1960). Physiologic recording by modern instruments with particular reference to pressure recording. *Physiological Reviews, 40,* 753–787.

Fry, D. L., Stead, W. W., Ebert, R. V., Lubin, R. I., & Wells, H. S. (1952). The measurement of intraesophageal pressure and its relationship to intrathoracic pressure. *Laboratory and Clinical Medicine, 40,* 664–673.

Gaultier, C., & Zinman, R. (1983). Maximal static pressures in healthy children. *Respiration Physiology, 51,* 45–61.

Gelfer, C. E., Harris, K. S., & Baer, T. (1987). Controlled variables in sentence intonation. In T. Baer, C. Sasaki, & K. S. Harris (Eds.), *Laryngeal function in phonation and respiration* (pp. 422–435). Boston, MA: College-Hill Press.

Gibson, C. J., Edmonds, J. P., & Hughes, G. R. (1977). Diaphragm function and lung involvement in systemic lupus erythematosus. *American Journal of Medicine, 63,* 926–932.

Gracco, L. C., Gracco, V. L., Löfqvist, A., & Marek, K. P. (1994). Aerodynamic evaluation of Parkinsonian dysarthria. In J. A. Till, K. M. Yorkston, & D. R. Beukelman (Eds.), *Motor speech disorders: Advances in assessment and treatment* (pp 65–79). Baltimore, MD: Paul H. Brookes.

Gramming, P. (1989). Non-organic dysphonia. A comparison of subglottal pressures in normal and pathological voices. *Acta Oto-Laryngologica, 107,* 156–160.

Hardy, J. C. (1961). Intraoral breath pressure in cerebral palsy. *Journal of Speech Disorders, 26,* 309–319.

Hardy, J. C. (1965). Air flow and pressure studies. *ASHA Reports, 1,* 141–152.

Hardy, J. C. (1967). Techniques of measuring intraoral air pressure and rate of air flow. *Journal of Speech and Hearing Research, 10,* 650–654.

Hertegård, S., Gauffin, J., & Lindestad, P.-Å. (1995). A comparison of subglottal and intraoral pressure measurements during phonation. *Journal of Voice, 9,* 149–155.

Higgins, M. B., & Saxman, J. H. (1991). A comparison of selected phonatory behaviors of healthy aged and young adults. *Journal of Speech and Hearing Research, 34,* 1000–1010.

Hixon, T. J. (1966). Turbulent noise sources for speech. *Folia Phoniatrica, 19,* 168–182.

Hixon, T. J. (1972). Some new techniques for measuring the biomechanical events of speech production: One laboratory's experiences. *ASHA Reports, 7,* 68–103.

Hixon, T. J. (1973). Respiratory function in speech. In F. D. Minifie, T. J. Hixon, & F. Williams (Eds.), *Normal aspects of speech, hearing, and language* (pp. 73–125). Englewood Cliffs, NJ: Prentice-Hall.

Hixon, T. J. (1987). *Respiratory function in speech and song.* Boston, MA: Little, Brown.

Hixon, T. J., Hawley, J. L., & Wilson, K. J. (1982). An around-the-house device for the clinical determination of respiratory driving pressure: A note on making simple even simpler. *Journal of Speech and Hearing Disorders, 47,* 413–415.

Hixon, T. J., Klatt, D. H., & Mead, J. (1971). Influence of forced transglottal pressure changes on vocal fundamental frequency. *Journal of the Acoustical Society of America, 49,* 105.

Hixon, T. J., Mead, J., & Goldman, M. (1976). Dynamics of the chest wall during speech production: Function of the rib cage, diaphragm, and abdomen. *Journal of Speech and Hearing Research, 19,* 297–356.

Hixon, T. J., Minifie, F. D., & Tait, C. A. (1967). Correlates of turbulent noise production for speech. *Journal of Speech and Hearing Research, 10,* 133–140.

Hixon, T. J., & Smitheran, J. R. (1982). A reply to Rothenberg. *Journal of Speech and Hearing Disorders, 47,* 220–223.

Holmberg, E. B., Hillman, R. E., & Perkell, J. S. (1988). Glottal airflow and transglottal air pressure measurements for male and female speakers in soft, normal, and loud voice. *Journal of the Acoustical Society of America, 84,* 511–529.

Holmberg, E. B., Hillman, R. E., & Perkell, J. S. (1989). Glottal airflow and transglottal air pressure measurements for male and female speakers in low, normal, and high pitch. *Journal of Voice, 3,* 294–305.

Holmes, L. C., Leeper, H. A., & Nicholson, I. R. (1994). Laryngeal airway resistance of older men and women as a function of vocal sound pressure level. *Journal of Speech and Hearing Research, 37,* 789–799.

Hutchinson, J. M., & Smith, L. L. (1976). Aerodynamic functioning in consonant production by hearing impaired adults. *Audiology and Hearing Education, 2* (December-January), 16–25, 32.

Inkley, S. R., Oldenburg, F. C., & Vignos, P. J., Jr. (1974). Pulmonary function in Duchenne muscular dystrophy related to stage of disease. *American Journal of Medicine, 56,* 297–306.

Isshiki, N. (1964). Regulatory mechanism of voice intensity variation. *Journal of Speech and Hearing Research, 7,* 17–29.

Iwata, S. (1988). Aerodynamic aspects for phonation in normal and pathologic larynges. In O. Fujimura (Ed.), *Vocal physiology: Voice production, mechanisms, and functions* (pp. 423–431). New York: Raven Press.

Izdebski, K. (1984). Overpressure and breathiness in spastic dysphonia. *Acta Otolaryngologica, 97,* 373–378.

Karnell, M. P., & Willis, C. R. (1982a). The reliability of the Kay Agnellograph pressure translator in the study of consonantal intraoral air pressure. *Folia Phoniatrica, 34,* 53–56.

Karnell, M. P., & Willis, C. R. (1982b). The effect of vowel context on consonantal intraoral air pressure. *Folia Phoniatrica, 34,* 1–8.

Keilmann, A., & Bader, C.-A. (1995). Development of aerodynamic aspects in children's voice. *International Journal of Pediatric Otorhinolaryngology, 31,* 183–190.

Kitajima, K., & Fujita, F. (1990). Estimation of subglottal pressure with intraoral pressure. *Acta Otolaryngologica, 109,* 473–478.

Kitajima, K., & Tanaka, K. (1993). Intraoral pressure in the evaluation of laryngeal function. *Acta Otolaryngologica, 113,* 553–559.

Kitajima, K., & Tanaka, K. (1995). The effects of intraoral pressure change on F_0 regulation—Preliminary study for the evaluation of vocal fold stiffness. *Journal of Voice, 9,* 424–428.

Kitzing, P., Carlborg, B., & Löfqvist, A. (1982). Aerodynamic and glottographic studies of the laryngeal vibratory cycle. *Folia Phoniatrica, 34,* 216–224.

Kitzing, P., & Löfqvist, A. (1975). Subglottal and oral air pressures during phonation—Preliminary investigation using a miniature transducer system. *Medical and Biological Engineering,* 13, 644–648.

Klich, R. J. (1982). Effects of speech level and vowel context on intraoral air pressure in vocal and whispered speech. *Folia Phoniatrica, 34,* 33–40.

Koike, Y. (1981). Sub- and supraglottal pressure viariation during phonation. In K. N. Stevens & M. Hirano (Eds.), *Vocal fold physiology* (pp. 181–191). Tokyo, Japan: University of Tokyo Press.

Koike, Y., & Hirano, M. (1973). Glottal area time function and subglottal pressure variation. *Journal of the Acoustical Society of America, 54,* 1618–1627.

Koike, Y., Imaizumi, S., Kitano, Y., Kawasaki, H., & Hirano, M. (1983). Glottal area time function and supraglottal pressure variation. In D. M. Bless & J. H. Abbs (Eds.), *Vocal fold physiology: Contemporary research and clinical issues* (pp. 300–306). San Diego, CA: College-Hill Press.

Koike, Y., & Perkins, W. H. (1968). Application of a miniaturized pressure transducer for experimental speech research. *Folia Phoniatrica, 20,* 360–368.

Kunze, L. H. (1964). Evaluation of methods of estimating subglottal air pressure. *Journal of Speech and Hearing Research, 7,* 151–164.

Ladefoged, P. (1963). Some physiological parameters in speech. *Language and Speech, 6,* 109–119.

Ladefoged, P. (1964). Comment on "Evaluation of methods of estimating sub-glottal air pressure." *Journal of Speech and Hearing Research, 7,* 291–292.

Ladefoged, P. (1968). Linguistic aspects of respiratory phenomena. *Annals of the New York Academy of Sciences, 155,* 141–151.

Ladefoged, P., & McKinney, N. P. (1963). Loudness, sound pressure, and subglottal pressure in speech. *Journal of the Acoustical Society of America, 35,* 454–460.

Laine, T., Warren, D. W., Dalston, R. M., Hairfield, W. M., & Morr, K. E. (1988). Intraoral pressure, nasal pressure and airflow rate in cleft palate speech. *Journal of Speech and Hearing Research, 31,* 432–437.

Leanderson, R., Sundberg, J., & von Euler, C. (1987). Breathing muscle activity and subglottal pressure dynamics in singing and speech. *Journal of Voice, 1,* 258–261.

Leech, J. A., Ghezzo, H., Stevens, D., & Becklake, M. R. (1983). Respiratory pressure and function in young adults. *American Review of Respiratory Disease, 128,* 17–23.

Leeper, H. A., Jr., & Graves, K. K. (1984). Consistency of laryngeal airway resistance in adult women. *Journal of Communication Disorders, 17,* 153–163.

Leeper, H. A., Jr., & Noll, J. D. (1972). Pressure measurements of articulatory behavior during alterations of vocal effort. *Journal of the Acoustical Society of America, 51,* 1291–1295.

Lieberman, P. (1968). Direct comparison of subglottal and esophageal pressure during speech. *Journal of the Acoustical Society of America, 43,* 1157–1164.

Lieberman, P., Knudson, R., & Mead, J. (1969). Determination of the rate of change of fundamental frequency with respect to subglottal air pressure during sustained phonation. *Journal of the Acoustical Society of America, 45,* 1537–1543.

Lisker, L. (1970). Supraglottal air pressure in the production of English stops. *Language and Speech, 13,* 215–230.

Löfqvist, A., Carlborg, B., & Kitzing, P. (1982). Initial validation of an indirect measure of subglottal pressure during vowels. *Journal of the Acoustical Society of America, 72,* 633–635.

Lubker, J. F., & Parris, P. J. (1970). Simultaneous measurements of intraoral pressure, force of labial contact, and labial electromyography during production of the stop consonant cognates /p/ and /b/. *Journal of the Acoustical Society of America, 47,* 625–633.

Malécot, A. (1966). The effectiveness of intra-oral air pressure-pulse parameters in distinguishing between stop cognates. *Phonetica, 14,* 65–81.

Malécot, A. (1968). The force of articulation of American stops and fricatives as a function of position. *Phonetica, 18,* 95–102.

Manco, J. C., Terra-Filho, J., & Silva, G. A. (1990). Pneumomediastinum, pneumothorax and subcutaneous emphysema following the measurement of maximal expiratory pressure in a normal subject. *Chest, 98,* 1530–1532.

McAllister, A., & Sundberg, J. (1998). Data on subglottal pressure and SPL at varied vocal loudness and pitch in 8– to 11–year-old children. *Journal of Voice, 12,* 166–174.

McElvaney, G., Blackie, S., Morrison, N. S., Wilcox, P. G., Fairbarn, M. S., & Pardy, R. L. (1989). Maximal static respiratory pressures in the normal elderly. *American Review of Respiratory Disease, 139,* 277–281.

McGlone, R. E. (1967). Intraesophageal pressure during syllable repetition. *Journal of the Acoustical Society of America, 42,* 1208.

McGlone, R. E., & Shipp, T. (1971). Some physiological correlates of vocal fry phonation. *Journal of Speech and Hearing Research, 14,* 769–775.

McGlone, R. E., & Shipp, T. (1972). Comparison of subglottal air pressures associated with /p/ and /b/. *Journal of the Acoustical Society of America, 51,* 664–665.

McHenry, M. A., Kuna, S. T., Minton, J. T., & Vanoye, C. R. (1996). Comparison of direct and indirect calculations of laryngeal airway resistance in connected speech. *Journal of Voice, 10,* 236–244.

Mead, J., Bouhuys, A., & Proctor, D. F. (1968). Mechanisms generating subglottic pressure. *Annals of the New York Academy of Sciences, 155,* 177–181.

Mead, J., & Wittenberger, J. L. (1954). Evaluation of airway interruption technique as a method for measuring pulmonary airflow resistance. *Journal of Applied Physiology, 6,* 408–416.

Milic-Emili, J., Mead, J., Turner, J. M., & Glauser, E. M. (1964). Improved technique for estimating pleural pressure from esophageal balloons. *Journal of Applied Physiology, 18,* 208–211.

Miller, C. J., & Daniloff, R. (1977). Aerodynamics of stops in continuous speech. *Journal of Phonetics, 5,* 351–360.

Monsen, R. B., Engebretson, A. M., & Vemula, N. R. (1978). Indirect assessment of the contribution of subglottal air pressure and vocal-fold tension to changes of fundamental frequency in English. *Journal of the Acoustical Society of America, 64,* 65–80.

Moon, J. B., Folkins, J. W., Smith, A. E., & Luschei, E. S. (1993). Air pressure regulation during speech production. *Journal of the Acoustical Society of America, 94,* 54–63.

Morris, H. L. (1966). The oral manometer as a diagnostic tool in clinical speech pathology. *Journal of Speech and Hearing Disorders, 31,* 362–369.

Morris, R. J., & Brown, W. S., Jr. (1994). Age-related differences in speech variability among women. *Journal of Communication Disorders, 27,* 49–64.

Müller, E. M., & Brown, W. S., Jr. (1980). Variations in the supraglottal air pressure waveform and their articulatory interpretation. In N. J. Lass (Ed.), *Speech and language: Advances in basic research and practice* (pp. 317–389). New York: Academic Press.

Murry, T. (1971). Subglottal pressure and airflow measures during vocal fry phonation. *Journal of Speech and Hearing Research, 14,* 544–551.

Murry, T., & Brown, W. S., Jr. (1971). Subglottal air pressure during two types of vocal activity: Vocal fry and modal phonation. *Folia Phoniatrica, 23,* 440–449.

Murry, T., & Brown, W. S., Jr. (1975). Intraoral air pressure variability in esophageal speakers. *Folia Phoniatrica, 27,* 237–249.

Murry, T., & Brown, W. S., Jr. (1979). Aerodynamic interactions associated with voiced-voiceless stop consonants. *Folia Phoniatrica, 31,* 82–88.

Netsell, R. (1969). Subglottal and intraoral air pressures during the intervocalic contrast of /t/ and /d/. *Phonetica, 20,* 68–73.

Netsell, R. (1970). Underlying physiological mechanisms of syllable stress. *Journal of the Acoustical Society of America, 47,* 103.

Netsell, R. (1973). Speech physiology. In F. D. Minifie, T. J. Hixon, & F. Williams (Eds.), *Normal aspects of speech, hearing, and language* (pp. 211–234). Englewood Cliffs, NJ: Prentice-Hall.

Netsell, R. W. (1998). Speech rehabilitation for individuals with unintelligible speech and dysarthria: The respiratory and velopharyngeal systems. *Journal of Medical Speech-Language Pathology, 6,* 107–110.

Netsell, R., & Daniel, B. (1979). Dysarthria in adults: Physiologic approach to rehabilitation. *Archives of Physical Medicine and Rehabilitation, 60,* 502–508.

Netsell, R., & Hixon, T. J. (1978). A noninvasive method for clinically estimating subglottal air pressure. *Journal of Speech and Hearing Disorders, 43,* 326–330.

Netsell, R., Lotz, W. K., DuChane, A. S., & Barlow, S. M. (1991). Vocal tract aerodynamics during syllable productions: Normative data and theoretical implications. *Journal of Voice, 5,* 1–9.

Netsell, R., Lotz, W. K., Peters, J. E., & Schulte, L. (1994). Developmental patterns of laryngeal and respiratory function for speech production. *Journal of Voice, 8,* 123–131.

Ordiales Fernández, Fernández Moya, A., Colubi Colubi, L., Nisal de Paz, F., Allende González, J., Alvarez Asensio E., & Rodrigo Sáez, L. (1995). Presiones respiratorias estáticas máximas. Importancia del estudio de los valores de referencia normales. *Archivos de Bronconeumología, 31,* 507–511.

Orlikoff, R. F. (1994). Anatomy and physiology of respiration. *Current Opinion in Otolaryngology & Head and Neck Surgery, 2,* 220–225.

Orlikoff, R. F., & Baken, R. J. (1993). *Clinical speech and voice measurement: Laboratory exercises.* San Diego, CA: Singular Publishing Group.

Otis, A. B., & Proctor, D. F. (1948). Measurement of alveolar pressure in human subjects. *American Journal of Physiology, 152,* 106–112.

Perkins, W. H., & Koike, Y. (1969). Patterns of subglottal pressure variations during phonation: A preliminary report. *Folia Phoniatrica, 21,* 1–8.

Plant, R. L., & Hillel, A. D. (1998). Direct measurement of subglottic pressure and laryngeal resistance in normal subjects and in spasmodic dysphonia. *Journal of Voice, 12,* 300–314.

Ptacek, P. H., Sander, E. K., Maloney, W. H., & Jackson, C. C. (1966). Phonatory and related changes with advanced age. *Journal of Speech and Hearing Research, 9,* 353–360.

Putnam, A. H. B., Shelton, R. L., & Kastner, C. U. (1986). Intraoral air pressure and oral air flow under different bleed and bite-block conditions *Journal of Speech and Hearing Research, 29,* 37–49.

Rahn, H., Otis, A. B., Chadwick, L. E., & Fenn, W. O. (1946). The pressure-volume diagram of the thorax and lung. *American Journal of Physiology, 146,* 161–179.

Rindqvist, T. (1966). The ventilatory capacity in healthy subjects: An analysis of causal factors with special reference to the respiratory forces. *Scandinavian Journal of Clinical and Laboratory Investigation, 18* (Suppl. 88), 8–170.

Ringel, R. L., House, A. S., & Montgomery, A. H. (1967). Scaling articulatory behavior: Intraoral air pressure. *Journal of the Acoustical Society of America, 42,* 1209.

Rothenberg, M. (1973). A new inverse filtering technique for deriving the glottal airflow waveform during voicing. *Journal of the Acoustical Society of America, 53,* 1632–1645.

Rothenberg, M. (1982). Interpolating subglottal pressure from oral pressure. *Journal of Speech and Hearing Disorders, 47,* 219–220.

Rothenberg, M., & Mahshie, J. (1986). Induced transglottal pressure variations during voicing. *Journal of Phonetics, 14,* 365–371.

Rubin, H. J., LeCover, M., & Vennard, W. (1967). Vocal intensity, subglottic pressure, and air flow relationships in singers. *Folia Phoniatrica, 19,* 393–413.

Rubinstein, I., Slutsky, A. S., Rebuck, A. S., McClean, P. A., Boucher, R., Szeinberg, A., & Zamel, N. (1988). Assessment of maximal expiratory pressure in healthy adults. *Journal of Applied Physiology, 64,* 2215–2219.

Sawashima, M., & Hirose, H. (1981). Abduction-adduction of the glottis in speech and voice production. In K. N. Stevens & M. Hirano (Eds.), *Vocal fold physiology* (pp. 329–346). Tokyo, Japan: University of Tokyo Press.

Sawashima, M., & Honda, K. (1987). An airway interruption method for estimating expiratory air pressure during phonation. In T. Baer, C. Sasaki, & K. S. Harris (Eds.), *Laryngeal function in phonation and respiration* (pp. 439–447). Boston, MA: College-Hill Press.

Sawashima, M., Honda, K., Kiritani, S., Sekimoto, S., Ogawa, S., & Shirai, K. (1984). Further works on the airway interruption method of measuring expiratory air pressure during phonation. *Annual Bulletin of the Research Institute for Logopedics and Phoniatrics, 18,* 19–26.

Sawashima, M., Kiritani, S., Sekimoto, S., Horiguchi, S., Okafuji, K., & Shirai, K. (1983). The airway interruption technique for measuring expiratory air pressure during phonation. *Annual Bulletin of the Research Institute for Logopedics and Phoniatrics, 17,* 23–32.

Sawashima, M., Niimi, S., Horiguchi, S., & Yamaguchi, H. (1988). Expiratory lung pressure, airflow rate, and vocal intensity: Data on normal subjects. In O. Fujimura (Ed.), *Vocal physiology: Voice production, mechanisms, and functions* (pp. 415–422). New York: Raven Press.

Schutte, H. K. (1986). Aerodynamics of phonation. *Acta Oto-Rhino-Laryngologica Belgica, 40,* 344–357.

Schutte, H. K. (1992). Integrated aerodynamic measurements. *Journal of Voice, 6,* 127–134.

Schutte, H. K., & Miller, D. G. (1986). Transglottal pressure in professional singing. *Acta Otolaryngologica Belgica, 40,* 395–404.

Schutte, H. K., & van den Berg, Jw. (1976). Determination of the subglottic pressure and the efficiency of sound production in patients with disturbed voice production. In E. Loebell (Ed.), *Proceedings of the XVIth International Congress of Logopedics and Phoniatrics* (pp. 415–420). Basel: S. Karger.

Scully, C. (1971). A comparison of /s/ and /z/ for an English speaker. *Language and Speech, 14,* 187–200.

Shipp, T. (1973). Intraoral air pressure and lip occlusion in mid-vocalic stop consonant production. *Journal of Phonetics, 1,* 167–170.

Shipp, T., Izdebski, K., Schutte, H. K., & Morrissey, P. (1988). Subglottal air pressure in spastic dysphonia speech. *Folia Phoniatrica, 40,* 105–110.

Shipp, T., & McGlone, R. E. (1971). Laryngeal dynamics associated with vocal frequency change. *Journal of Speech and Hearing Research, 14,* 761–768.

Siegert, C. (1969). Der intrathorakale Druck und seine Beziehungen zur Stimmfunktion. *Folia Phoniatrica, 21,* 98–104.

Slis, I. H. (1970). Articulatory measurements on voiced, voiceless,

and nasal consonants. *Phonetica, 21,* 193–210.

Smitheran, J. R., & Hixon, T. J. (1981). A clinical method for estimating laryngeal airway resistance during vowel production. *Journal of Speech and Hearing Research, 46,* 138–146.

Stathopoulos, E. T. (1984). Oral air flow during vowel production of children and adults. *Cleft Palate Journal, 21,* 71–74.

Stathopoulos, E. T. (1986). Relationship between intraoral air pressure and vocal intensity in children and adults. *Journal of Speech and Hearing Research, 29,* 71–74.

Stathopoulos, E. T., Hoit, J. D., Hixon, T. J., Watson, P. J., & Solomon, N. P. (1991). Respiratory and laryngeal function during whispering. *Journal of Speech and Hearing Research, 34,* 761–767.

Stathopoulos, E. T., & Sapienza, C. (1993). Respiratory and laryngeal function of women and men during vocal intensity variation. *Journal of Speech and Hearing Research, 36,* 64–75.

Stathopoulos, E. T., & Weismer, G. (1985). Oral airflow and air pressure during speech production: A comparative study of children, youths and adults. *Folia Phoniatrica, 37,* 152–159.

Subtelny, J. D., Worth, J. H., & Sakuda, M. (1966). Intraoral pressure and rate of flow during speech. *Journal of Speech and Hearing Research, 9,* 498–519.

Sundberg, J., Elliot, N., Gramming, P., & Nord, L. (1993). Short-term variation of subglottal pressure for expressive purposes in singing and stage speech: A preliminary investigation. *Journal of Voice, 7,* 227–234.

Szeinberg, A., Marcotte, J. E., Roizin, H., Mindorff, C., England, S., Tabachnik, E., & Levison, H. (1987). Normal values of maximal inspiratory and expiratory pressures with a portable apparatus in children, adolescents, and young adults. *Pediatric Pulmonology, 3,* 255–258.

Tanaka, S., & Gould, W. J. (1983). Relationships between vocal intensity and noninvasively obtained aerodynamic parameters in normal subjects. *Journal of the Acoustical Society of America, 73,* 1316–1321.

Tanaka, S., & Gould, W. J. (1985). Vocal efficiency and aerodynamic aspects in voice disorders. *Annals of Otology, Rhinology and Laryngology, 94,* 29–33.

Tanaka, S., Kitajima, K., & Kataoka, H. (1997). Effects of transglottal pressure change on fundamental frequency of phonation: Preliminary evaluation of the effect of intraoral pressure change. *Folia Phoniatrica et Logopaedica, 49,* 300–307.

Titze, I. R. (1988). The physics of small-amplitude oscillation of the vocal folds. *Journal of the Acoustical Society of America, 83,* 1536–1552.

Titze, I. R. (1989). On the relationship between subglottal pressure and fundamental frequency in phonation. *Journal of the Acoustical Society of America, 85,* 901–906.

Titze, I. R. (1992). Phonation threshold pressure: A missing link in glottal aerodynamics. *Journal of the Acoustical Society of America, 91,* 2926–2935.

Titze, I. R., & Sundberg, J. (1992). Vocal intensity in speakers and singers. *Journal of the Acoustical Society of America, 91,* 2936–2946.

Ursino, F., Pardini, L., Panattoni, G., Matteucci, F., & Grosjacques, M. (1991). A study of Egg and simultaneous subglottal pressure signals. *Folia Phoniatrica, 43,* 220–225.

Valta, P., Corbeil, C., Chassé, M., Braidy, J., & Milic-Emili, J. (1996). Mean airway pressure as an index of mean alveolar pressure: Effect of expiratory flow limitation. *American Journal of Respiratory and Critical Care Medicine, 153,* 1825–1830.

van den Berg, Jw. (1956). Direct and indirect determination of the mean subglottic pressure. *Folia Phoniatrica, 8,* 1–24.

van den Berg, Jw. (1958). Myoelastic-aerodynamic theory of voice production. *Journal of Speech and Hearing Research, 1,* 227–244.

Verdolini, K., Titze, I. R., & Fennell, A. (1994). Dependence of phonatory effort on hydration level. *Journal of Speech and Hearing Research, 37,* 1001–1007.

Verdolini-Marston, K., Titze, I. R., & Druker, D. G. (1990). Changes in phonation threshold pressure with induced conditions of hydration. *Journal of Voice, 4,* 142–151.

von Neergaard, K., & Wirz, K. (1927). Die Messung der Strömungwiederstände in der Atemwege des Menschen, inbesondere beim Asthma und Emphysema. *Zeitschrift für Klinische Medicine, 195,* 51–82.

Warren, D. W. (1976). Aerodynamics of speech production. In N. J. Lass (Ed.), *Contemporary issues in experimental phonetics* (pp. 105–137). New York: Academic Press.

Warren, D. W. (1986). Compensatory speech behaviors in individuals with cleft palate: A regulation/control phenomenon? *Cleft Palate Journal, 23,* 251–260.

Warren, D. W. (1996). Regulation of speech aerodynamics. In N. J. Lass (Ed.), *Principles of experimental phonetics* (pp. 46–92). St. Louis, MO: Mosby.

Warren, D. W., Dalston, R. M., Morr, K. E., Hairfield, W. M., & Smith, L. R. (1989). The speech regulating system: Temporal and aerodynamic responses to velopharyngeal inadequacy. *Journal of Speech and Hearing Research, 32,* 566–575.

Warren, D. W., & Hall, D. J. (1973). Glottal activity and intraoral pressure during stop consonant productions. *Folia Phoniatrica, 25,* 121–129.

Warren, D. W., Hall, D. J., & Davis, J. (1981). Oral port constriction and pressure-airflow relationships during sibilant productions. *Folia Phoniatrica, 33,* 380–394.

Wilson, S. H., Cooke, N. T., Edwards, R. H. T., & Spiro, S. G. (1984). Predicted normal values for maximal respiratory pressures in caucasian adults and children. *Thorax, 39,* 535–538.

Wilson, J. V., & Leeper, H. A. (1992). Changes in laryngeal airway resistance in young adult men and women as a function of vocal sound pressure level and syllable context. *Journal of Voice, 6,* 235–245.

Woodson, G. E., Rosen, C. A., Murry, T., Madasu, R., Wong, F., Hengesteg, A., & Robbins, K. T. (1996). Assessing vocal function after chemoradiation for advanced laryngeal carcinoma. *Archives of Otolaryngology—Head and Neck Surgery, 122,* 858–864.

9

Airflow and Volume

The vocal tract is an **aerodynamic** sound generator and resonator system. Variations in the flow of air through it reflect changes in the "manner" of consonant and vowel articulations. Evaluation of air flow, then, can provide considerable insight into speech system dysfunction and efficiency. The data can be of great assistance in improving the precision of initial diagnosis, documenting change during therapy, and providing biofeedback to patients with pathologies of voice or articulation (Gordon, Morton, & Simpson, 1978; Amerman & Williams, 1979; Bastian, Unger, & Sasama, 1981; Fritzell, Hammarberg, Gauffin, Karlsson, & Sundberg, 1986; Woo, Colton, & Shangold, 1987; Dalston, Warren, & Dalston, 1991; Ruscello, Shuster, & Sandwisch, 1991; Tanaka, Hirano, & Terasawa, 1991; Watson & Alfonso, 1991; Rammage, Peppard, & Bless, 1992; Kotby, Shiromoto, & Hirano, 1993; Leeper, Gagne, Parnes, & Vidas, 1993; Miller & Daniloff, 1993; Warren, 1996).

GENERAL PHYSICAL PRINCIPLES

Good discussions of airflow phenomena and air volume characteristics of speech can be found in almost any elementary textbook of speech physiology or phonetics. This section will present a summary of pertinent information that will be important in applying or interpreting airflow or air volume measurements.

Airflow

Flow is a term used to describe the movement of a quantity (volume) of gas through a given area in a unit of time. As such, the rate of flow is also referred to as the *volume velocity*. As in the case of air pressure, several different units may serve to quantify a given flow. Liters or milliliters per second or per minute are the most common, the choice being made to suit the specific situation. Table 9–1 provides the required conversion factors for changing from one set of units to another.

FLOW-PRESSURE RELATIONSHIP

When a gas flows, its molecules are being driven from a region of relatively high pressure to one where the pressure lower. The pressure difference between the two areas is called the **driving pressure**. The rate of flow of a gas is directly proportional to the driving pressure and inversely proportional to the resistance of the conduit through which the gas is moving. That is,

$$U = \frac{P}{Z}, \tag{1}$$

where U = flow (volume velocity);
P = driving pressure; and
Z = impedance (resistance) of the pathway.

This is simply a pneumatic version of Ohm's law (see Chapter 2, "Analog Electronics"), and it may be rearranged in the same ways. Therefore,

$$Z = \frac{P}{U} \tag{2}$$

and

$$P = U \times Z. \tag{3}$$

These restatements of the flow-pressure-impedance relationship are particularly important. Equation 2 implies that the impedance of a system (for instance, the vocal tract) can be expressed in terms of flow through it and the driving pressure. In fact, impedance is often quantified in just such terms. One might, for example, describe a vocal tract as having an impedance of 30 cm of water pressure per liter per second (30 cmH$_2$O/LPS), meaning that impedance is high enough to produce a pressure drop of 30 cmH$_2$O for each liter per second of flow through it. (This does *not* mean that the flow ever actually has to be 1 L/s; A driving pressure of 3 cmH$_2$O at a flow of 0.1 L/s, for instance, represents an impedance of 30 cmH$_2$O/LPS.) An impedance of this magnitude is not uncommon for voicing. A much smaller figure might be indicative of, for example, laryngeal adductor paralysis, while a larger value might characterize hyperaddoction (see "Laryngeal Airway Resistance," Chapter 10).

Table 9–1. Conversion Factors for Flow Units*

	Milliliters per second (mL/s)	Liters per second (L/s)
Liters per minute (L/min)	0.06	60
Milliliters per minute (mL/min)	60	60,000

*To convert a value at the top to one at the side, *multiply* by the number in the appropriate box. To convert a value at the side to one at the top, *divide* by the number in the appropriate box. For example: 100 mL/s = ? L/min; 100 × 0.06 = 6 L/min.

The other alternative form of the relationship, $P = U \times Z$, states the principle upon which the most common method of measuring airflow is based. In simple terms, it says that the pressure difference (P) between two points along an air stream is a function of the flow (U) and of the system's impedance (Z). It also implies that a pressure difference will be created across any impedance placed in an airflow. This statement is important and must be kept in mind whenever one deals with airflow measurement. It will explain many of the phenomena to be discussed later.

Laminar and Turbulent Flow

When a sizable pressure forces a gas through a tube of relatively large diameter, the molecules all tend to move at the same speed along straight parallel paths. Pressure characteristics everywhere in the tube are stable and orderly. This kind of flow is described as *laminar*. It is the quiet flow of a large deep river between wide banks. If the tube becomes narrower (that is, if its impedance rises) or if the rate of flow becomes significantly greater, the flow pattern tends to change. The paths of the gas molecules become less universally parallel, and local velocity variations are produced. Irregularities of flow (eddy currents) appear, and there are small and random pressure fluctuations from point to point. The flow is said to be *turbulent*. It resembles the flow in a river as it becomes overswollen with too much rain. Turbulent airflow is characteristic of speech sounds (such as fricatives) that are produced by the high impedance of a tight vocal-tract constriction (Stevens, 1971; Catford, 1977; Miller & Daniloff, 1993). The degree of turbulence of an airflow is often significant. Some flow transducers—particularly the warm wire types—may yield inaccurate measures in the presence of a lot of turbulence, while certain measurement rationales are based on the assumption of laminar flow. In effect, turbulence represents pressure-flow noise, and, depending upon the impedance of interest, its increase or reduction may be critically important to speech production.

Air Volume

All of the air used for speech by a normal speaker is drawn from the same reservoir: the lungs. Therefore, air volumes used in speaking represent a change in lung volume, and some techniques for determining air usage actually monitor lung inflation status, instead of metering air passing out of the vocal tract. In general, the speech pathologist will be more interested in volume change than in lung volume itself. For instance,

we are only rarely concerned with the actual volume of the lungs (including, for example, the dead space) but rather with the level to which the lungs are inflated before, or deflated during, speech. To say that a patient used 1 L of air for a phonatory task is to indicate that the lung volume diminished by that amount. The variable of primary interest in this chapter is not how much air is in storage, but how much is moved in accomplishing a speech task. Colloquially speaking, the bank balance is usually of less interest than the size of the withdrawals.

FLOW-VOLUME RELATIONSHIP

Flow is the rate of change of volume. To return to the phonating patient just mentioned, if the one liter volume change occurred in 10 s of voice production, then it is apparent that the *mean* flow (volume velocity, U) was 100 mL/s. That is,

$$U = \frac{\mathrm{D}V}{\mathrm{D}t}, \tag{4}$$

flow is equal to the volume change (ΔV) divided by the time over which the change occurred (Δt). In our example, therefore, $U = 1$ L/10 s, which is 0.1 L (or 100 mL) per second. Thus, if one is interested in the average flow during some period of time, one need only divide the volume of air used by the amount of time in question.

All of this really means that the volume change per unit of time is the *slope* of the volume line on a graph, such as that shown in Figure 9–1A. Mathematically, the slope of the volume line is $\Delta V/\Delta t$. But the figure also illustrates a major problem with using a simple averaging technique. Both of the graphs shown represent 1 L (1000 mL) of air being used in 8 s. Therefore, the average flow for both recordings is 1000 mL/8 s or 125 mL/s. In 1A, air usage is relatively steady and the average flow for the 8 s is a good indicator of the actual flow *at any point in time* during the task. In 9–1B, however, the situation is very different. The rate at which the volume increases (that is, the slope of the line) fluctuates significantly. A liter of air has indeed been used in 8 s, but this average does not provide a good estimate of what the flow is likely to be at any given instant.

Clearly, what is needed is a way of expressing the average change of volume during successive, but exceptionally short, intervals of time. The shorter the time interval, the more accurate the representation of the real flow. In fact, it would be ideal if the change of volume could be computed for time intervals so short that they are zero seconds long. Then one could be sure that the actual flow at every instant was observed.

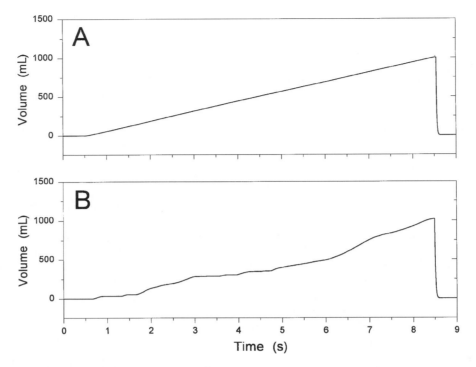

Figure 9–1. Each of the traces above represents 1 liter of air expired over a period of roughly 8 seconds. Trace A, however, shows a fairly uniform flow rate, while the varying slope of trace B indicates variations in flow rate.

While it might seem a bit strange, there is a way to find the slope of a line at a single point (that is, when $\Delta t = 0$). Such a measure is, in fact, one of the bases of the calculus. It is called the ***derivative***, and the process of determining the derivative is known as ***differentiation***. Flow, then, is the rate of change of the volume at every point in time. It is, in the language of the calculus, the derivative of the volume. The mathematical notation for this is

$$\text{Flow} = dV/dt,\text{[1]} \tag{5}$$

It is common to denote this function as $\dot{V}$, where the dot indicates ***derivative***. (Indeed $\dot{V}$, is a standard symbol for flow in the physiological literature.) Figure 9–2 shows the same volume traces from Figure 9–1, but with the inclusion of lines that represent the corresponding dV/dt—the derivative of the volume (that is, the flow) at every point in time. Note that, for 9–2B, the changes in flow from instant to instant are dramatic.

Fortunately, one need not master the calculus to generate a flow line from volume data. For years this was achieved by using a simple electronic circuit called a ***differentiator***, although this is now accomplished almost exclusively by computer software. Nonetheless, what is important to bear in mind is that flow data can be derived from volume data. The average flow can be calculated if one knows only how much air was used in a certain amount of time, or the instantaneous flow can be derived if the volume at every point in time is available. Both measures have their uses.

If the flow rate can be computed from the volume change, it is reasonable to assume that the process might be reversible. Given a flow, one should be able to find the volume change. It is indeed possible although, in cases where the flow changes very rapidly, it may be difficult. Volume is the product of flow and time:

$$V = U \times t. \tag{6}$$

If a steady flow persists for a know interval of time, determination of the volume of air moved is simple and direct. For example, if a patient phonated for 10 s using a (remarkably steady) flow of 150 mL/s, she must have used 150 mL $\times$ 10 s, or 1500 mL (1.5 L) of air. A

[1]The notation dV/dt is to be read as a symbol. It does not represent a fraction.

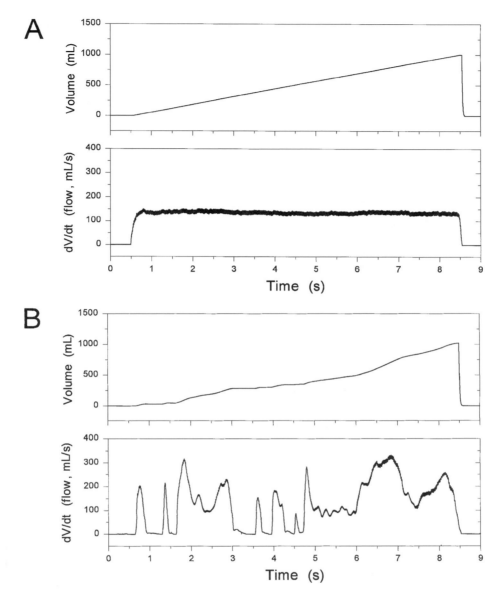

Figure 9–2. The same volume records as in Figure 9–1, but with the addition of a trace indicating the derivative of volume (that is, the *flow*) associated with each.

flow-versus-time graph of such rock-steady hypothetical phonation is shown in Figure 9–3. This graphic representation illustrates an important fact. Multiplying flow by time gives the area enclosed by the flow curve. Volume, then, could be defined as the area under the flow trace. Figure 9–4 demonstrates the obvious problem in applying this concept: How does one compute the actual area under a highly irregular trace? Again, the calculus provides a way in the form of the **integral**. In the present discussion the integral can be described as the cumulative area under the flow curve. (The notation for the integral of the flow is $\int \dot{V}$.) The process is called **integration**. Calculation of the inte-

gral can be very difficult. However, as was the case with the derivative, one need not bother. Computer programs, if not analog electronic *integrators* (Hardy & Edmonds, 1968), are readily available. If supplied with digitized flow data, an output representing the cumulative volume can be obtained quite simply. Figure 9–4 shows the integral of flow (B, below) resulting from the flow trace (A, above).

Thus, in summary, flow is the rate of change of volume. It is expressed as the *derivative* of volume. Volume is the product of flow and time. It is the *integral* of flow. The foregoing discussion leads to the conclusion that flow and volume change are essentially two sides

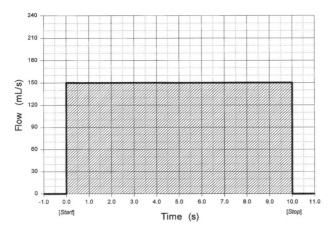

Figure 9–3. A graph of 10 s of phonation at an exceptionally constant flow of 150 mL/s. The air volume used is equal to flow × time, and is represented by the *area* under the flow line (shaded).

of the same coin and that instrumentation to measure one can often be used to determine the other. This is shown schematically in Figure 9–5, in which both flow and volume are derived from a single measurement device. The flow signal can be integrated to produce a volume output, or a volume signal can be differentiated to produce a flow signal.

In this chapter, instruments are categorized as either volume- or flow-measuring systems according to their primary output. It is important to keep in mind that integration or differentiation can be applied to that output to produce the complementary measure.

The Gas Laws

To a much greater extent than solids or liquids, the volume of a gas is affected by its pressure and tempera-

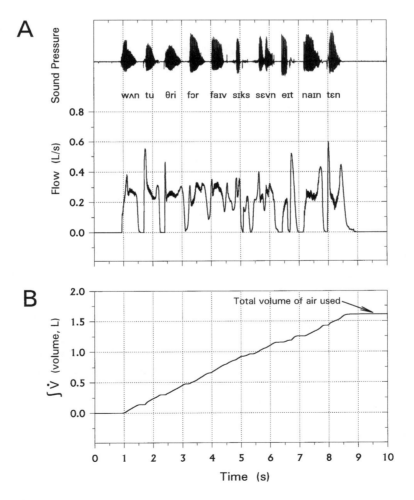

Figure 9–4. A. Airflow during counting from one to ten. **B.** A trace showing the integral of the flow (that is, the expired *volume*).

A

Pneumotachograph

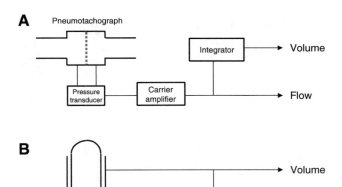

B

Spirometer

Figure 9–5. Alternative methods of deriving flow and volume from a single transducer: **A.** By integration of the output of a flow transducer (such as a pneumotachograph); **B.** By differentiation of the output of a volumetric devices (such as a spirometer).

ture.[2] Increasing the pressure diminishes gas volume very significantly. (A small SCUBA tank of highly compressed air can, therefore, contain enough gas to sustain a diver for a long time.) Conversely, increasing temperature causes a gas to expand. These effects may be of more than academic interest when it comes to measuring speech or lung volumes, especially for research purposes. The air in the lungs during speech is pressurized and is at body temperature (about 37°C). However, in a collecting device, such as a spirometer, that same air is at close to atmospheric pressure (0 cmH$_2$O) and at room temperature (about 20°C). Therefore, the volume of the air in the spirometer may not be the same as the volume that the same air occupied when it was still in the respiratory system.

Fortunately, under ordinary circumstances pressure and temperature differences are not so large as to create a clinically meaningful difference in air volume. For everyday clinical purposes, then, they can probably be safely ignored, especially if the values result from the same testing procedure, applied under essentially the same conditions. It is nonetheless wise to be aware of the principles that govern gas volumes, especially when comparing the results of different studies in the literature (in which correction factors may be used) or when designing clinical research studies. The most important "gas laws" that quantify volume changes are summarized next.

PRESSURE: BOYLE'S LAW

The effect of pressure on a gas is expressed by Boyle's law, which states that (if temperature does not change) the product of volume and pressure is constant. That is,

$$P_1V_1 = P_2V_2,$$

where the subscript 1 denotes the *original* value, and 2 indicates the *new* quantity. By dividing both sides of the equation by P_2, we can determine the new volume of a gas after a change in pressure:

$$V_2 = V_1 \left(\frac{P_1}{P_2}\right).$$

Put into words, Boyle's law says that the volume of a gas after a pressure change is equal to its former volume times the ratio of the original and new pressures.

TEMPERATURE: CHARLES' LAW

Charles' law states that the volume of a gas varies directly with temperature (assuming that pressure remains constant). Therefore, volume change with temperature can be calculated as

$$V_2 = V_1 \left(\frac{T_2}{T_1}\right).$$

where, as before, the subscripts denote original (1) and new (2) conditions. T, the temperature, must be expressed in absolute terms, as degrees **Kelvin** (°K). Zero degrees Kelvin equals −273°C.

COMBINED PRESSURE AND TEMPERATURE

Obviously, Boyle's and Charles' laws can be combined to a single volume-correction equation. Simple algebraic manipulation gives

$$V_2 = V_1 \left(\frac{T_2}{T_1}\right)\left(\frac{P_1}{P_2}\right).$$

WATER VAPOR

Each gas that makes up the mixture called **air** accounts for part of the air's total pressure. Dalton's law states that each gas makes an *independent* contribution to the total. Therefore, if one of the gases in the air mixture should be lost, the total pressure would diminish. The

---

[2]More complete discussions of the gas laws can be found in Comroe, Forster, Dubois, Brisco, and Carlson (1962); Abramson (1981); Vick (1984); Levitzky (1995); or in any elementary physics or physiology text.

other gases would not "compensate" for the loss. As air cools after exhalation, part of the water vapor in the air condenses. This represents a loss of some of the pressure contribution made by the water vapor and, therefore, a change in the volume of the gas. Hence, another correction factor is needed. Unfortunately, the "partial pressure" of water at different temperatures is not easily calculated: It must be found in a table of partial pressures.

BTPS

From all of the above, it becomes clear that different volume data can be compared with precision only if the temperature, pressure, and water-saturation conditions under which they are obtained are known. Rather than make the user of data perform the necessary calculations, it is common in the research literature to report volume data already converted to a set of standard conditions. These are body temperature, atmospheric pressure, and saturated with water vapor. The label **BTPS** (*body temperature and pressure, saturated*) is used to denote the fact that the volume being reported has been corrected to the standard conditions. BTPS values can be compared across test conditions, across subjects, or across research studies without further manipulation.

AIRFLOW INSTRUMENTATION

Face Masks

Evaluation of airflow requires that all of the air to be measured, and only the air to be measured, pass through the flow transducers. For evaluation of speech behavior it is important that the channeling of air be done in a way that does not alter the speaker's ventilatory or articulatory performance. In general these requirements are largely met by attaching the flow transducer to the outlet of an anesthesia-type face mask. This solution is not ideal, however, and a number of precautions must be taken and some compromises accepted.

It is vitally important that the face mask not leak around the edges, allowing air to escape without passing through the transducer. Although cushioning around the mask's periphery helps minimize this problem, it is still often necessary to use a substantial harness around the head to keep the edges of the mask tightly pressed against the face (as shown in Figure 9–6), especially for extended airflow recording.

Although Till, Jaffari, Crumley, and Law-Till (1992) provide evidence that the use of a face mask does not

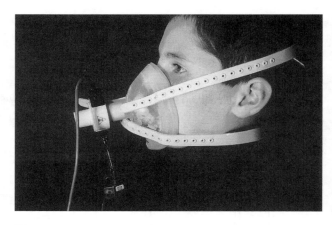

Figure 9–6. An anesthesia-type face mask held in place by an elastic head harness. A heated pneumotachograph is attached to the port opening of the mask.

significantly affect measured vocal perturbation or harmonics-to-noise ratio, Bond, Moore, and Gable (1989) found substantial change in the vowel formant center frequencies of mask-wearing subjects. The latter investigators report a general compression of the vowel space that, they speculate, is tied to both a restriction of jaw movement and the effective lengthening of the vocal tract by the mask enclosure. Lubker and Moll (1965) have also shown definite effects of a face mask on both mandibular and labial motion. In general they found that it lowered the maximal rate of syllable production, but not to such an extent that the speakers' conversational speech rate was affected. Although their subjects did not perceive a need to use greater effort for speech, the possibility that other speakers might perceive this need cannot be completely ignored.

The problem of contact with the articulators can be alleviated by using a very large mask that encloses the entire face (like a fencer's or baseball catcher's mask) as described, for instance, by Klatt, Stevens, and Mead (1968). Alternatively, a "space helmet" type of arrangement could be used, thereby completely eliminating contact with the face. This type of solution, however, exacerbates another difficulty of mask-type arrangements. Any air collector represents a volume added to the vocal tract that increases the ventilatory dead space through which the patient must breathe. Tidal breathing patterns will change to accommodate to this ventilatory situation. The volume of an adult-size anesthesia-type face mask is only about 150 mL when in place, but even that may be enough to cause noticeable ventilatory adaptation in some patients. While a small change in tidal breathing does not in itself have a meaningful impact on speech behavior, it is sometimes enough to frighten a patient sufficiently to cause his speech to be abnormal in some way. With very large face masks and helmet arrangements the degradation of ventilatory conditions may have a more deleterious effect on speech than the restriction of articulatory movements that they are designed to avoid (Hardy, 1965).

The dead space problem can be solved by providing a **bias airflow** (Klatt et al., 1968; Hixon, 1972). That is, a pump can be used to force a constant and steady flow of fresh air into the mask at a known rate. The fresh air leaves the mask via the flow transducer together with the ventilatory airflow. The magnitude of the bias flow is then subtracted from the flow measurement, leaving a remainder that represents vocal tract flow alone. In most cases the use of an ordinary small face mask will be acceptable for clinical evaluation. But, despite its added complexity, the bias flow system is advantageous in those cases (for example, very young children, highly anxious, or cerebral palsied patients) where a small, confining mask is poorly tolerated.

SEPARATING ORAL AND NASAL AIRFLOW

The interior of the mask can be divided in order to channel oral and nasal flows through different outlets, to either or both of which a flow transducer can be connected. Lubker and Moll (1965) used a plexiglass diaphragm, edged with a bumper of ¼-inch rubber tubing, to divide the interior of a face mask into two chambers, each provided with an outlet port. Similar arrangements have been described by others (Quigley, Webster, Coffee, Kelleher, & Grant, 1963; Quigley, Shiere, Webster, & Cobb, 1964; Hixon, 1966; Hixon, Saxman, & McQueen, 1967; Leiter & Baker, 1989). A set of commercially available split masks are shown in Figure 9–7. Also available are masks designed to channel nasal flow exclusively (see Chapter 11, "Velopharyngeal Function").

Airflow Transducers

Many different means can be used to transduce an airflow into an appropriate electrical signal, ranging from pin-wheel rotors to ultrasonic detectors (Ower & Pankhurst, 1977; Collatina, Barone, Monini, & Bolasco, 1980). The various methods have been applied in a very wide variety of devices. Only a few, however, are suitable to the needs of speech clinicians. The discussion to follow, therefore, will be limited to the pneumotachograph, warm-wire anemometer, plethysmograph, and electro-aerometer.

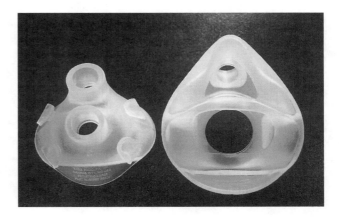

Figure 9–7. Split masks designed to channel oral and nasal airflows separately: Pediatric (left) and adult (right) models viewed from the front and back, respectively. [Large pediatric and medium adult dual port masks manufactured by Hans Rudolph, Inc., Kansas City, MO.]

PNEUMOTACHOGRAPHS

Construction and Physical Principles

Broadly speaking, a *pneumotachograph* (Figure 9–8), sometimes also called a *pneumotachometer*, is any primary transducer that takes advantage of one of the airflow principles discussed earlier: A pressure drop occurs across any resistance introduced into an airstream. The pneumotachograph generates a pressure proportional to flow, and this pressure must then be transduced (by a secondary transducer) to provide a proportional electrical signal. The pneumotachograph's resistance to airflow is created in one of two ways. Either a fine wire-mesh screen (or set of screens as shown in Figure 9–8B) is used, or else the air is channeled through a series of narrow tubes. In the former case, the resistance is a function of the wire mesh —the more wires per square centimeter of screening, the higher the resistance. The tube-type system, called a Fleisch pneumotachograph, has an impedance (Z) whose magnitude is governed by Poiseuille's law,

$$Z = \frac{8\mu l}{\pi r^4}$$

where μ = gas viscosity,

l = tube length, and

r = tube radius.

Therefore, the longer the tubes and the smaller their radius, the greater the resistance to airflow (Fleisch, 1925). Irrespective of specific construction, however, all pneumotachographs have pressure-sensing ports on either side of the resistive element. Through these, the

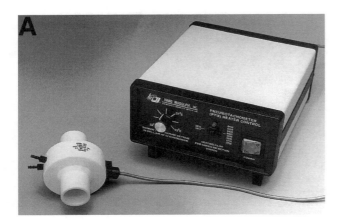

Figure 9–8. A. A screen pneumotachograph and a heater control unit, **B.** A exploded diagram showing the construction the screen pneumotachograph. (Courtesy of Hans Rudolph, Inc., Kansas City, MO.)

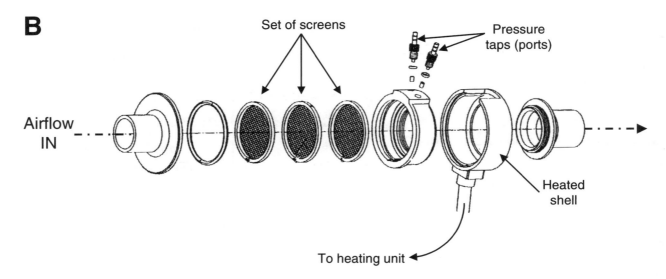

pressure drop created by the resistance is sampled. This pressure difference is the output of the pneumotachograph.[3]

The magnitude of the pressure drop within the pneumotachograph is governed by the aerodynamic principles discussed earlier: $P = U \times Z$. For a given airflow, U, the pressure drop, P, can be increased (making the pneumotachograph more sensitive) by increasing the impedance, Z. But a higher impedance will disrupt breathing more. (Try breathing through a soda straw, which represents a very high impedance.) For minimal interference with normal ventilatory (including speech) behavior, the transducer should have negligible impedance. But this, in a pneumotachograph, means low sensitivity. One is trapped between two conflicting requirements. The nature of the dilemma indicates that a single transducer will not be suitable for a wide range of flow rates and, therefore, pneumo-

tachographs are offered in different "sizes." Those intended for measuring low rates of flow have higher impedances than those designed for larger flows. When doing flow measurement it is important to select a device with enough impedance to get adequate measures, but not enough to interfere with the airflows being observed. Table 9–2 shows the characteristics of several sizes of pneumotachographs offered by OEM Medical (Richmond, VA), a major distributor of Fleisch transducers.

Under ordinary conditions of use, the pneumotachograph will be much cooler than the expiratory flow through it, and, because air coming from the lungs is saturated with water vapor, condensation will occur within it. As water droplets form on the resistive element they begin to block the small openings, raising the impedance, playing havoc with the device's calibration. To prevent this, a small current is passed

---

[3]The physics of pneumotachographs has been experimentally investigated by Fry, Hyatt, McCall, and Mallos (1957).

Table 9–2. Characteristics of Typical Fleisch Pneumotachographs[†]

Transducer Size	Useful Maximum Airflow (L/s)	Resistance (cmH$_2$O/L/s)	Dead Space (mL)
0000	0.02	75.00	1.7
000	0.05	30.00	1.7
00*	0.10	15.00	1.7
0*	0.30	5.00	4.7
1	1.00	1.50	15.0
2	3.00	0.50	40.0
3	6.00	0.25	92.0
4	14.00	0.11	200.0

*Units most useful for speech work.

[†]Data are for transducers manufactured by OEM, Inc., Corvallis, OR.

through the resistive element; the resultant heating eliminates the condensation problem. (A heater-current supply can be purchased from the transducer manufacturer as shown in Figure 9–8A, but simple transformers providing 6.3 V AC and having a current capability of about 2 A serve quite nicely and are available at electronics supply stores.) Calibration is best performed while the pneumotachograph is heated to the same temperature that it will be used during airflow measurement (Frye & Doty, 1990).

Despite the fact that it requires a face mask and imposes extra equipment requirements (that is, a secondary pressure transducer, appropriate amplifier, and current for the heater), the pneumotachograph has several features that make it the instrument of choice for airflow evaluation (van den Berg, 1962; Hardy, 1967; Lubker, 1970; Sullivan, Peters, & Enright, 1984). It is highly reliable and, because of its comparatively uncomplicated structure, relatively inexpensive. It is also rugged—virtually immune to mishandling—and easy to maintain. Its output is linear over the range for which it is designed, making it easy to calibrate, and it holds its calibration very well over time (Finucane, Egan, & Dawson, 1972; Miller & Pincock, 1986). It also differentiates between egressive and ingressive airflows (Orlikoff, Baken, & Kraus, 1997), a feature not characteristic of all flow systems.

Implementation

A block diagram of a typical pneumotachograph system is shown in Figure 9–9. A mask is fitted snugly to the patient's face with the pneumotachograph

attached to its outlet. It is important that the mask not leak; this should be checked carefully. It the mask outlet is closed off, the patient should be able to blow quite forcefully, generating a large positive pressure inside the mask, before air leakage occurs. The pneumotachograph's output is the pressure drop across its resistive element. This is sensed by attaching a *differential* pressure transducer (see Chapter 8, "Air Pressure") to its pressure ports by means of rubber or plastic tubing. The pressure transducer's output is the electrical analog of airflow. Because the impedance of the pneumotachograph must be kept low, the pressure difference to be measured will be quite small, probably far less than 1 cmH$_2$O. The pressure transducer must, therefore, be as sensitive as possible. The pneumotachograph's heater current must also be turned on, and the device allowed to warm up before use.

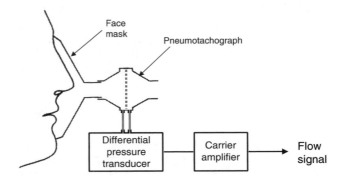

Figure 9–9. Block diagram of a typical pneumotachograph system.

Variations on the Pneumotachograph Principle

The basic principle of the pneumotachograph (the imposition of an impedance to produce a measurable pressure drop proportional to flow) has been incorporated into a number of special face-mask designs that provide special advantages. Klatt and his colleagues (1968), for instance, have used a very large mask that encloses the entire face, so as to minimize articulatory loading (Figure 9–10). Wire screens in front of the mask serve as the resistive element. The difference between the pressure inside the mask and atmospheric pressure is, therefore, proportional to flow. The problem of the approximate addition of 2 L to the ventilatory dead space is resolved by supplying a steady bias flow of 400 mL/s. Nonetheless, mandibular movement remains somewhat restricted by the mask. The investigators also report that articulatory movements tend to distort the mask, thus changing the volume of air within it.

Circumferentially Vented Pneumotachograph Mask

Rothenberg (1973) has constructed a primary flow transducer that consists of an anesthesia-type face mask circumferentially vented by several relatively large (roughly 1-cm diameter) holes covered by one or two layers of fine-mesh wire screening (Figure 9–11). The screens serve as resistive elements across which a pressure proportional to the flow is developed, and can be heated to prevent the condensation of water vapor. Although the frequency response of the typical pneumotachograph is quite good, the mask system provides an excellent time resolution of up to 0.25 ms. Therefore, very rapid changes in airflow can be transduced; the response is fast enough, in fact, to allow the detection of flow changes over the course of individual glottal pulses (see "Flow Inverse Filtering," Chapter 10). The total resistance of the screen elements is quite small, keeping pressure inside the "Rothenberg mask" generally under 1 cmH$_2$O/L/s. Originally, Rothenberg (1973, 1977) measured the transmask pressure with a pair of specially modified microphones connected to a differential amplifier that developed a voltage proportional to the instantaneous airflow. As currently marketed by Glottal Enterprises, Inc. (Syracuse, NY), these microphones have been replaced by highly sensitive bonded strain gauge differential pressure transducers. In addition to Rothenberg's design, other types of pneumotachograph masks have been described for flow measurement when reduction of the ventilatory dead space is of particular importance (Murty, Lancaster, & Kelly, 1991; Huber, Stathopoulos, Bormann, & Johnson, 1998). However, for most clinical purposes, such as mean airflow measurement, patients rarely wear flow masks for an extended length of time and they are often instructed to inhale before placing the mask over their face. Thus changes in ventilatory behavior due to the added dead space are not a common concern. Furthermore, flow signals are often lowpass filtered for later analysis, so that it may make little sense to employ a transducer with an extended fre-

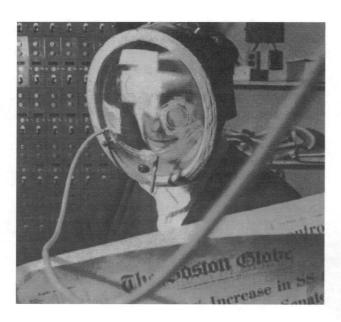

Figure 9–10. A special pneumotachograph helmet design used by Klatt (pictured), Stevens, and Mead (1968) to measure speech airflow. A set of fine wire screens in the mask allows the helmet itself to serve as a pneumotachograph. The tube leading to the mask supplies a steady bias airflow to minimize the effect of the added ventilatory dead space. (Photograph by John F. Cook, courtesy of the Massachusetts Institute of Technology Research Laboratory of Electronics, Cambridge, MA.)

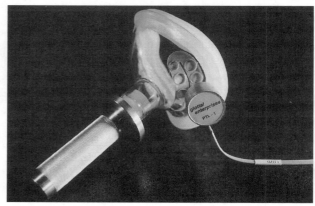

Figure 9–11. A circumferentially vented pneumotachograph (Rothenberg) mask.

quency response when it will not be used and is, in fact, unwanted.

WARM-WIRE ANEMOMETER

Construction and Physical Principles

The electrical resistance of any material changes in known ways with temperature. This fact is the basis for measurement of airflow by the warm-wire anemometer. When a ventilatory or speech airflow passes over it, an electrically heated wire will be cooled significantly.

The consequent change of the wire's resistance can be measured; it serves as an index of the magnitude of the flow.

There are a number of different ways in which this principle is actually exploited. In the simplest case (diagrammed in Figure 9–12A) a constant current is passed through a wire having a relatively high resistance. Doing this causes the wire to dissipate power as heat. (Power in watts is equal to the resistance times the square of the current.) The temperature of the wire therefore rises. Ohm's law states that $E = IR$. That is, if current, I, passes through a resistance, R, a voltage

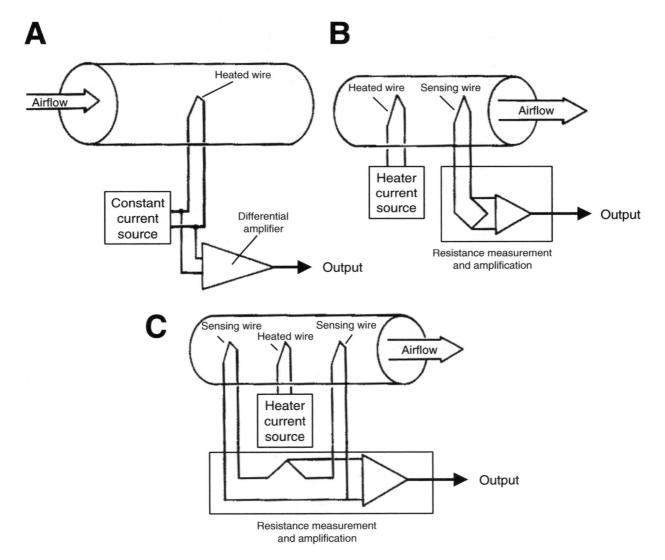

Figure 9–12. **A.** A simple warm-wire anemometer. The sensing wire is heated by a constant current. The voltage drop across it is proportional to its resistance, which is in turn related to its temperature. The differential amplifier senses the voltage drop and its output, therefore, indicates the flow rate. **B.** Two-wire anemometer system. **C.** Directionally sensitive warm-wire anemometer. Heat is transferred from the central heated element to one or the other of the sensing wires depending on the direction of airflow. The resulting changes in resistance are sensed and are converted to an analog voltage representing the magnitude and direction of flow.

difference, E, is produced across the resistance. If the current is constant, then any change in the resistance will show up as an equivalent change in the voltage difference. The resistance of the wire changes with temperature, and the temperature of a heated wire will change with alterations in the amount of air flowing past it. The reason for the latter effect is simple enough. Any flow of air past the wire carries heat away with it, thereby lowering the wire's temperature. The greater the airflow, the faster heat is lost, and the cooler the wire becomes. So the resistance of the wire should mirror the airflow. The resistance, in turn, can be tracked by monitoring the voltage drop across the wire.

There are a number of important problems with this simple system. Most significant is its nonlinearity. For a number of reasons the voltage drop changes in an irregular way as the flow changes. Either complex calibrating scales or, when possible, special electronic linearizing circuits are required. Beyond this is the fact that egressive air (essentially at body temperature) is considerably warmer than ingressive air (at room temperature) and, therefore, cools the wire less for the same rate of flow. Transducer sensitivity, in other words, differs with flow direction.

The latter problem has been addressed by Quigley et al. (1964) in a way diagrammed in Figure 9–12B. In this system, two wire filaments are used. One is unheated and senses any change in temperature of the passing air. A special electronic circuit provides just enough current to heat the other filament to an absolute temperature of about 120% of the unheated reference wire. The greater the airflow the faster the heated wire cools, and thus more current is required to keep it heated to the proper level. The magnitude of the heater current is an analog of airflow, irrespective of the temperature of the flowing air. This transduction scheme represents an improvement over the single heated wire, but it does not provide for discrimination of the direction of airflow. This is not a trivial problem, since small ingressive flows occur during speech articulation (Isshiki & Ringel, 1964; Lubker & Moll, 1965) and their detection is all but impossible in the absence of flow direction sensitivity.

It is possible, with relatively simple electronic circuitry, to use two heated wires to detect only the direction of airflow, without determining its magnitude (Micco, 1973). But, on the whole, it would obviously be better to determine magnitude and direction from a single instrument. A warm-wire flow meter that can achieve this has been created by Yoshiya, Nakajima, Nagai, and Jitsukawa (1975). It is schematized in Figure 9–12C. A platinum wire within the transducer is maintained at a temperature of about 375°C. A short distance away, upstream and downstream of this

heated element, are two other unheated sensing wires. Air flowing through the transducer passes over all three wire elements in series. In the absence of any airflow, the heated wire warms its vicinity and the two sensing wires are at the same temperature. As air flows, however, the upstream wire is cooled somewhat, and the air is then heated by the warm wire before passing to the second sensing element, whose temperature it raises. An airflow thus produces a significant temperature (and hence resistance) difference between the two sensing elements. The resistance change is monitored by appropriate circuitry that produces the final analog output voltage. If the direction of the airstream changes, the resistance difference between the two sensing wires reverses, and the polarity of the voltage output switches.

Despite some ingenious steps taken to minimize their deficiencies, warm-wire anemometers have typically exhibited a number of significant limitations (van den Berg, 1962; Hardy, 1967; Lubker, 1970). In particular, because they depend on relatively slow temperature change, their frequency response was limited so that rapid changes of flow were likely to be distorted or absent in the output. More recent engineering improvements have now overcome many of these limitations, to the point where the examination of very brief airstream events is often possible. It has been found (Isshiki, 1981) that the frequency response of the anemometer can be improved substantially by using a very fine wire that is kept at a near-constant temperature by a feedback circuit. This circuit allows compensation for the cooling effect of the airflow with a regulated increase of the electric current that maintains the wire at its original temperature. Both the Phonatory Function Analyzer® (Model PS − 77, Nagashima) and Phonation Analyzer® (Model PA 500, Minato Medical Science) use such modified anemometer systems to measure airflow (Isshiki, 1981; Wilson & Starr, 1985; Paynter, 1991; Kitajima & Fujita, 1992). Nonetheless, a careful check of transducer specifications is desirable before any purchase. As mentioned above, the relationship between airflow and wire resistance is by no means linear. While special electronics can handle this difficulty to some extent, it is generally necessary to generate special calibration tables for each transducer. This is a tedious and inconvenient process at best, and it may seriously inhibit collection of adequate data (van Hattum & Worth, 1967).

Finally, there remains a problem that is somewhat more subtle than those just reviewed, but potentially of great impact. The warm-wire system is really only sensitive to flow in the immediate vicinity of the sensing element. Since the wire itself occupies only a small fraction of the cross-sectional area of the tube, the transducer actually determines the flow of that small sample of the total stream that happens to pass near its sensing element. This sample is representative only to the extent that the flow is laminar. As turbulence increases, random eddy currents and local flow variations increase, making it more likely that the wire will be influenced by them. The result may be a measurement that represents the significant perturbations of a limited region with the airstream, rather than the more stable average magnitude of the entire flow. Laminar flow cannot be guaranteed under all circumstances and, unfortunately, there is no easy way to determine the extent to which turbulence may have confounded the system output.

Implementation

The warm-wire anemometer, with its associated electronics, represents a complete transducer. No secondary transducer is required, as with the pneumotachograph. Attempts have been made (Subtelny, Worth, & Sakuda, 1966; Subtelny, Kho, McCormack, & Subtelny, 1969) to place an array of anemometer wires in front of the mouth in order to eliminate the need for a face mask. The resulting measures, however, have very dubious validity, and so it is best to use one of the air-collecting systems described earlier.

While the warm-wire anemometer offers the advantage of a relatively simple setup compared with other flow-measuring systems, its problems and limitations outweigh this one benefit. Consequently, most clinicians, given a choice, will prefer an alternative method for evaluating airflow.

BODY PLETHYSMOGRAPH

The body plethysmograph, described by Mead (1960), can be modified to measure airflow (Hixon, 1972; Warren, 1976). This may be accomplished in two ways, illustrated in Figure 9–13. In the first method (Figure 9–13A), the patient's body is enclosed within the plethysmograph. A special collar forms an airtight seal around the neck. During inspiration and expiration the volume of the body increases and decreases, compressing and rarefying the air within the box. The pressure change causes air to flow through a screen in the wall of the box that serves as a resistance. The screen, therefore, functions like the resistive element of a pneumotachograph, so the pressure difference across it is proportional to the flow of air in or out of the lungs. In this case, of course, a differential pressure transducer is not

needed since it is ***gauge pressure*** that is being measured (see Chapter 8, "Air Pressure"). It should be clear that inspiration causes air to flow out of the plethysmograph (as the lungs enlarge, taking up more space in the box), while expiration results in an airflow into the box. In this sense the transducer flow is an *inverse* of the lung volume change.

What the plethysmograph actually measures is change in lung volume. Strictly speaking, this is not the same as flow. The reason is that the lung volume is altered by two effects. First, air is moved in or out of the ventilatory system: *This* is the phenomenon of interest. But, secondly, lung volume also changes as a function of changes in alveolar pressure, and this also contributes to the flow across the plethysmograph's resistive element. (This is discussed more fully in the discussion of subglottal pressure in Chapter 8.) The two components of the transducer output signal—lung volume change due to airflow into or out of the lungs and lung volume change due to alveolar pressure change—cannot be separated with the arrangement shown in Figure 9–13A. Hixon (1972) does describe a more elaborate plethysmographic arrangement that provides for separate measures of transglottal flow and alveolar pressure. However, the magnitude of the error is likely to be small and can be ignored for most clinical purposes.

Figure 9–13B shows how a plethysmograph can be used to measure flow alone. The box itself remains open, but the patient's head is enclosed in the plethysmograph dome. The collar is again used to form an airtight seal around the neck. As is the case when the body box is used, a screen (this time in the dome) serves as the resistance across which a pressure proportional to the flow is measured. This method actually uses the plethysmograph as a rather special modification of a face-mask and pneumotachograph system. In essence, the patient is placed inside the flow transducer. While one would not want to purchase a plethysmograph in order to be able to implement this technique, it is a good method to use if a plethysmograph is already available.

ELECTRO-AEROMETER

The electro-aerometer (Smith, 1960; van den Berg, 1962) represents a very different approach to the transduction of airflow. The primary transducer is a rubber flap valve through which the airstream must pass. The valve has a resistance of between 1.25 and 3.0 cmH_2O/LPS[4] that produces a pressure drop in the air

---

[4]LPS = liters per second (L/s).

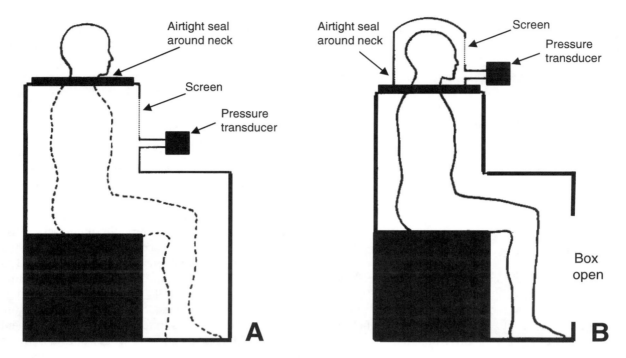

Figure 9–13. Using the body plethysmograph for airflow measurement. **A.** The flow signal from the body portion of the box represents airflow *and* intrathoracic pressure changes. **B.** Measuring pressure from the dome eliminates the influence of lung pressure.

flowing through it. This pressure causes the valve's two rubber flaps to separate. A light beam is directed through the valve to be sensed by a photodiode (the secondary transducer). The amount of light transmitted is proportional to the area of the valve opening, which is in turn proportional to the pressure drop and, therefore, to the airflow. The output of the photodiode is an analog of the flow rate. Each flap valve is a one-way device: One is required for ingressive air, and another for egressive air.

In the commercial version of this instrument the valves are mounted as part of the face-mask assembly. Manufacturer's specifications indicate a range of 0–1600 mL/s (with linearity best in the 0–1000 mL/s range) and a frequency response of DC to 200 Hz. Systems can be configured to measure oral and nasal airflow simultaneously. There are not yet enough reports on this instrument to evaluate its performance in routine use.

SUMMARY OF AIRFLOW TRANSDUCERS

Important characteristics of the various types of airflow transducers discussed in this section are summarized in Table 9–3. As can be seen, they vary widely in their frequency response, linearity, and in the additional equipment needed to complete the airflow system.

Calibration of Airflow Systems

Flow measuring systems are calibrated by observing the system output when airflows of precisely known magnitude are passed through the transducer. Calibration requires a source of compressed air and a precision metering device to monitor the flow rate.

ROTAMETER (FLOWMETER)

Metering of airflow is most easily done with a *rotameter*, also known as a *flowmeter*. This simple, reliable, and relatively inexpensive device works on a variable-area principle. As indicated in Figure 9–14, the rotameter consists of a glass tube, a small and precisely machined ball, and a measurement scale. The tube widens uniformly from bottom to top, while the ball within it has a diameter very nearly identical to the inner diameter of the tube's lower end. When a stream of air is introduced into the inlet, the ball (resting at the bottom) presents a very high resistance to the flow (since it effectively blocks the passage completely). A relatively high pressure develops beneath it, forcing the ball upward. Since the tube grows wider from bottom to top, there is an ever-growing gap between the ball (known as the *float*) and the tube walls as the ball rises. Air can, therefore, escape more easily around the

Table 9–3. Summary of Airflow Transducer Characteristics.

Transducer	Frequency Response	Linearity	Additional Equipment Needed
Pneumotachograph[a]	Good	Excellent	Differential pressure transducer system
Pneumotachograph (Rothenberg) mask	Excellent	Unknown[b]	Differential pressure transducer system
Warm-wire anemometer[c]	Poor	Very poor	None; Complete system
Body plethysmograph[d]	Good	Good-to-Excellent	Pressure transducer system
Electro-aerometer	Moderate	Fair	None; Complete system

[a]Preferred method; Stable, reliable, and rugged.

[b]Data from Hertegård and Gauffin (1992) suggest that the response of the model MA – 2N pneumotachograph mask (Glottal Enterprises, Syracuse, NY) is essentially linear from zero airflow to approximately 1600 Hz.

[c]Usually insensitive to direction of airflow; Frequency response and linearity may be improved by special construction and circuitry (see text).

[d]Large and expensive, but useful for other measures.

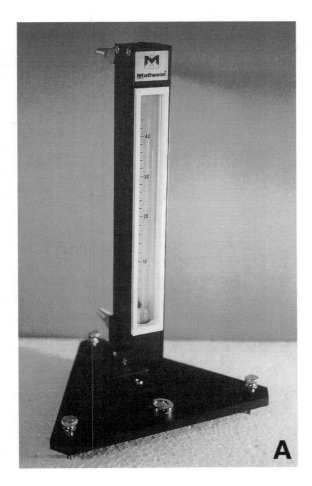

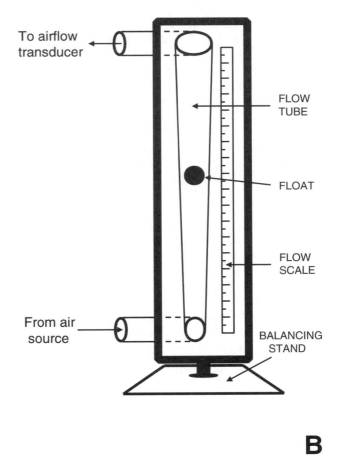

Figure 9–14. **A.** A typical rotameter and **B.** a schematic illustration of its construction. The rotameter consists of a tapered glass tube with a spherical float. Airflow from the bottom to the top of the tube causes the float to rise to a level proportional to the flow rate. A balancing stand is used to assure that the rotameter maintains a vertical orientation.

ball as it rises. In other words, as the ball moves upward it represents a constantly smaller resistance, so the pressure under it will remain at a level that is just sufficient to keep it suspended in the airstream. Clearly, the height of the ball can be read from the rotameter flow-rate scale. The scale marking that corresponds to the center of the elevated float is taken as the airflow value.

The sensitivity and range of the rotameter depend on the material of which the float is made (less dense materials yield greater sensitivity) and the taper of the tube (greater tapers provide extended ranges). Manufacturers offer rotameters of many sensitivities, and the clinician should select one appropriate to the sensitivity of the transducers to be calibrated. It should have a range that is not too wide (smaller ranges generally provide more accurate readings) and that is centered on a value within the range of actual airflows that will be measured in practice.

COMPRESSED AIR SOURCE

Accurate calibration demands that the calibrating airstream be free of observable fluctuations and that it not change slowly during the calibration period. The best source of an airstream is a large tank of compressed air (a SCUBA tank is sufficient). Gases other than air can be used, but inaccuracy will be introduced into the calibration to the extent that the density of the gas differs from that of air (Turney & Blumenfeld, 1973). Obviously, flammable gases should never be used, nor should oxygen, which also presents a fire hazard. The tank of compressed air should be fitted with a regulator so that the flow can be controlled. A good quality air compressor can be used to provide compressed air to a storage tank, but it must be fitted with a filter if there is any danger of it spraying oil, which will gum up the rotameter and the transducer.

A vacuum cleaner can serve as the compressor if it has an air-outlet connection, as many tank-types do. A filter of lightly-packed glass wool should be placed in the hose line between the vacuum cleaner and the transducer, and a valve should be added to the line to control airflow. The vacuum side of the vacuum cleaner can also be used as a "negative" airflow for calibration if the connections to the rotameter are reversed. That is, the vacuum line should be connected to what is normally the rotameter's output connection, while the transducer (through which the air will pass before going to the rotameter) is connected to the inlet connection.

FLOW CALIBRATION METHOD

Figure 9–15 shows how a calibrating setup is arranged. The rotameter and flow transducer are connected in

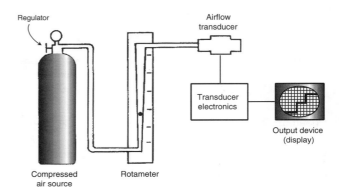

Figure 9–15. Setup for calibration of an airflow measurement system.

series, the airstream passing first through one and then the other. The airflow is adjusted at the tank to some convenient value, and the voltage output of the transducer system is noted. Airflow is then changed to a new value, and a new reading of the output is taken. This process is repeated at several different flow rates over the range of the system, generating a table of correspondence between flow and transducer output. If the transduction system is a highly stable one (such as a pneumotachograph) this calibration need be done only occasionally. It must, of course, be repeated whenever any system characteristic (such as amplifier gain) or component is changed.

It is exceptionally difficult to measure the frequency response of an airflow system, and for this reason the adequacy of the response is best estimated by evaluating the quality of the system output when measures are done on a normal speaker. (Examples of such records are provided for several of the measurements discussed below.) Alternatively, good approximations of a "step function" (or very sudden change) in airflow through the system can be achieved by attaching a balloon to the outlet of the flow transducer and blowing it up by coupling a relatively high-pressure air supply to the inlet. After the balloon has achieved maximal size, it is punctured, causing a sudden onset of airflow through the transducer. The readout of the flow reveals how quickly the system responds to a dramatic and almost instantaneous change. Other, more expensive and elaborate methods are also available (Jackson & Vinegar, 1979).

Flow Calibration Using a Syringe

Another method of calibrating an airflow system requires the use of a large 1- to 3-L syringe with a large bore opening (Hobbes, 1967; Yeh, Gardner, Adams, &

Yanowitz, 1982). The air-filled syringe is connected to the transducer inlet and emptied by hand at a fairly constant rate. For a 1-L syringe, for example, emptying speeds of 2 and 8 s represent mean flows of 500 and 125 mL/s, respectively. The transducer signal is sent to an electronic or digital integrator to derive the volume. The time-averaged a/d value obtained by the computer is the equivalent of the injected air volume divided by the injection time. When the temperature of the room air is measured, a BTPS correction can be approximated. Unlike the rotameter method, however, the syringe technique can only be applied to flow transducers that are known to be highly linear and have a fairly good frequency response, such as the pneumotachograph. Also, a flow system calibrated by the syringe method must have no DC offset; that is, the zero-flow condition must be represented by an a/d value of zero as well.

AIRFLOW MEASUREMENTS

If driving pressure is adequate and constant, then airflow measurements reflect on the integrity of the vocal tract. Increased flow must indicate a more dilated constriction and reduced airway resistance since, as pointed out earlier, air-path diameter and air-path impedance are inversely proportional to each other. The record of a dynamic airflow also indicates the time relationship of impedance changes, an important consideration in many speech disorders.

Airflow measurement requires a face mask or other air-collecting arrangement and a flow transducer with appropriate support electronics. If significant nasal escape of air is likely, it is best to use a modified face mask to collect only oral airflow, unless the total vocal tract flow is of interest. Nasal consonants, of course, will show predominantly nasal air emission. According to Lotz, D'Antonio, Chait, and Netsell (1993), with a bit of care, skill, and experience, valid and reliable aerodynamic measurements can be routinely obtained from children as young as 2 years of age.

Broadly speaking, there are three categories of airflow that are of maximal interest to the speech pathologist: (1) flow associated with consonants; (2) flow during sustained phonation; and (3) nasal airflow. The first evaluates oral articulatory events, while the second is an indicator of the functional efficiency of the laryngeal system. Nasal flow is primarily of use in assessing velopharyngeal function and is, therefore, discussed in Chapter 11, which deals with those issues.

Mean Peak Airflow

TECHNIQUE

Most frequently, measurement of the mean peak consonant airflow is obtained using test syllables of the CV or VC type, perhaps in a carrier phrase. The variable of interest is the *maximum flow* observed during the consonant being examined. Multiple repetitions are gathered, and the mean and standard deviation of the flow maxima are computed. High variability (large standard deviation) is as significant a finding as an abnormal mean.

Unlike relatively low-flow continuent speech sounds, such as vowels, sonorants, and nasals, the ability to release a quick and substantial airflow is critical to the manner of plosive and affricate production and, to a lesser extent, to fricative production as well. As such, peak airflow data are most commonly associated with these latter speech sounds.

Peak airflow varies as a function of speech intensity (Hixon, 1966). It is, therefore, of some importance that speech intensity be controlled during testing. Although Brown, Murry, and Hughes (1976) suggested that visual feedback to the patient (by means of a VU meter, for example) should be used to minimize intensity variations, Stathopoulos (1985) has shown that simply instructing the subject to maintain a comfortable speech loudness is just as effective in controlling SPL variability.

EXPECTED RESULTS

Output Record

Flow traces obtained with a heated screen pneumotachograph during production of the words "pay" and "ape" are shown in Figure 9–16. During the vocalic portion of each syllable the expiratory airflow is "chopped" by the action of the vocal folds; this is reflected in the flow trace whenever there is voicing.[5] There is a clear flow peak during /p/ associated with the plosive release. It is the height of this peak that is measured. Figure 9–17 shows similarly obtained flow traces during production of the words "say" and "ace."

---

[5]Evaluation of peak airflow requires that the sampling rate and frequency response of the instrumentation system be adequate: an inadequate frequency response will be signaled by a flattening of the peaks and a loss of the pulsatile character of the voiced segments in the flow trace. (Nonetheless, because consonant rather than phonatory airflow is of concern here, the flow signals have been low-pass filtered to minimize energy above 100 Hz in both Figures 9–16 and 9–17.)

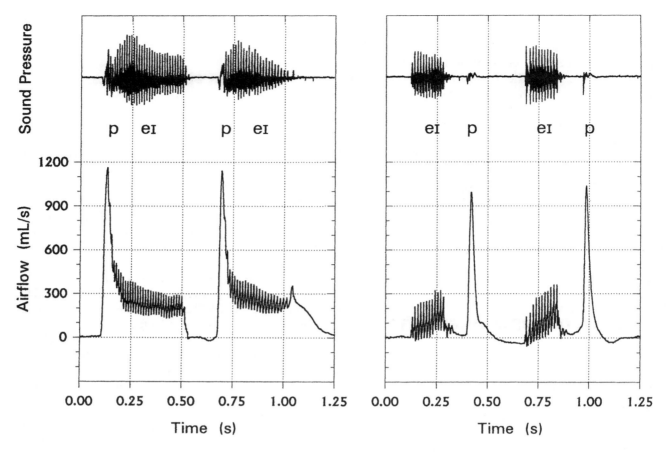

Figure 9-16. Speech airflow during repetition of the words "pay" (left) and "ape" (right).

Note that double peaks typify /s/ (and all fricative consonants). The first peak occurs before maximal tract constriction, while the second follows release of the articulatory occlusion (Scully, Castelli, Brearley, & Shirt, 1992). In reporting the peak airflow of fricative consonants, some investigators have used the highest peak (see, for instance, Klatt et al., 1968, and Horii and Cooke, 1978), while others have taken the average of the pre- and post-constriction peaks regardless of individual height (as did Stathopoulos and Weismer, 1985, for example).

Clearly, the evaluation of peak airflow requires that the frequency response of the instrumentation be adequate to the task. An inadequate response will cause a flattening of the airflow peaks and thus will result in erroneous peak flow data. Since the response characteristics are of such concern, most studies of peak consonant airflow have employed a pneumotachograph system to acquire the flow signal.

Typical Values

Tables 9–4 and 9–5 provide typical values for peak plosive airflow for normal men and children. These findings suggest that the peak airflows of the children's plosive productions follow essentially the same rank order as those reported for adult speakers. As with adults, higher airflows are associated with the children's voiceless plosives. Table 9–6 presents data from Stathopoulos (1980), who measured the peak airflow of both plosive and fricative consonants produced by both male and female children and adults. In this study, the adult speakers produced the plosives and fricatives with significantly greater peak airflow than the children. Like Trullinger and Emanuel (1983), Stathopoulos found no significant difference between the peak airflows of the boys and girls she tested. For adults, however, men typically show greater peak airflow than women (Stathopoulos, 1980; Stathopoulos

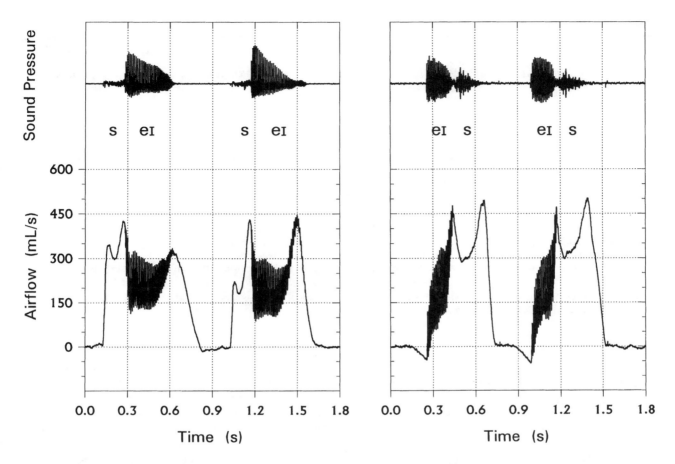

Figure 9–17. Speech airflow during repetition of the words "say" (left) and "ace" (right).

Table 9–4. Peak Airflow (in mL/s) for Plosive Consonants*

Plosive		Prevocalic		Intervocalic		Postvocalic	
Voiceless	**Voiced**	**Mean**	**SD**	**Mean**	**SD**	**Mean**	**SD**
p	—	1529	401	1266	464	1293	498
—	b	682	248	574	203	535	232
t	—	1789	391	1429	469	1259	484
—	d	973	248	738	224	602	226
k	—	1534	396	1240	488	1018	395
—	g	650	240	523	209	528	192

*Based on 9 adult males; three repetitions each of /CΛC/ or /ΛC/ syllables; pneumotachograph system used for flow measurement. Data converted from L/min. Significant differences were voiced vs. voiceless; prevocalic vs. postvocalic (except for /g/); prevocalic vs. intervocalic (except for /g/ and /b/); and intervocalic vs. postvocalic (only for /t/ and /d/).

Source: From "Oral Airflow During Stop Consonant Production," by H.R. Gilbert, 1973, *Folia Phoniatrica, 25,* 288–301, Table 1, p. 295. ©1973 S. Karger, Basel, Switzerland. Reprinted by permission.

Table 9–5. Mean Peak Airflow (in mL/s) for Plosive Consonants Produced by Children*

Plosive					Across Contexts	
Voiceless	Voiced	Prevocalic	Intervocalic	Postvocalic	Boys	Girls
p	—	1010	745	711	797	846
—	b	529	382	508	468	488
t	—	952	716	477	730	769
—	d	513	318	435	416	440
k	—	729	518	519	617	644
—	g	287	235	416	310	333

*Based on 15 boys and 15 girls, ages 8 through 10 years; four repetitions each of /Cɑ/ & /Ci/, /ɑC/ & /iC/, and /ɑCɑ/ & /iCi/ syllables; unheated pneumotachograph system used for flow measurement. Syllable context means derived from authors' line graph, averaged across vowel type and sex. Boy and girl means from Table 1, p. 205, averaged across syllable context and vowel type. Significant differences included voiced vs. voiceless; prevocalic vs. postvocalic; and prevocalic vs. intervocalic. The main effect for sex was not statistically significant.

Source: From "Airflow Characteristics of Stop-plosive Consonant Productions of Normal-speaking Children," by R.W. Trullinger and F.W. Emanuel, 1983, *Journal of Speech and Hearing Research, 26,* 202–208.

& Weismer, 1985). To produce plosive consonants, men appear to use roughly 30 to 40% greater peak airflow than women (Emanuel & Counihan, 1970; Stathopoulos, 1980; Stathopoulos & Weismer, 1985).

Mean Airflow Rate

The mean flow rate over the course of a speech sound, phonation, or utterance may be of value when assessing the general characteristics of speech and vocal function. Unlike the measurement of peak airflow, a transduction system with a good frequency response is not critical for the acquisition of valid mean airflow data; usually a simple spirometer or flow transduction system serves quite nicely. The improved frequency response offered by a Rothenberg mask, for instance, is of no particular benefit. Indeed for the typical mean flow measure, it is common to low-pass filter the flow signal to average across the more rapid flow changes that the pneumotachograph mask is specifically designed to transduce.

CONSONANT PRODUCTION

Consonants are distinguished by the degree, locus, and time course of the vocal tract constrictions that produce them, as well as by whether these articulatory gestures are accompanied by vocal fold vibration. Speech airflow is directly proportional to the driving pressure and inversely proportional to the resistance of the airway. To produce turbulent (fricative) and transient (plosive) articulatory sound sources, a stable regulation of the forces responsible for the generation and release of a sufficient back pressure is necessary (Stevens, 1971; Gilbert, 1973). For voiced fricatives, aerodynamic conditions that allow the maintenance of both periodic and turbulent sound sources must be supported. In particular, as Miller and Daniloff (1993) pointed out, "across the time course of sustained production for continuant speech sounds, a smooth, steady air flow pattern implies a constancy of the valving mechanism(s) involved and thus, appropriately coordinated control of the mechanisms for speech production. In contrast, major fluctuations in the air flow pattern, untoward or unusual ripples, etc., imply an unsteadiness of control" (p. 40). Thus the mean airflow used during the production of prolonged continuant consonants—particularly fricatives—may contribute profitable information regarding ventilatory, glottal, and supraglottal articulatory performance. This may be particularly useful for patients with neurologic impairments that disrupt ventilatory, laryngeal, and/or tongue coordination and stability.

Expected Results

Patient performance may be compared with the summary data shown in Table 9–7 from Isshiki and Ringel (1964). These values are likely to be substantially higher than those obtained from consonants produced in isolation. The flow rate has been shown to be sensi-

Table 9–6. Peak Airflow (mL/s) Associated with Plosive and Fricative Consonant Production in Children, Youths, and Adults*

Consonant	Position†	Adults	Youths	Children
p	I	1352.9	696.4	673.7
	F	462.1	343.7	333.8
b	I	316.1	295.8	290.2
	F	269.0	279.6	253.4
t	I	1891.5	1030.3	808.5
	F	310.8	308.7	209.7
d	I	569.8	443.0	318.2
	F	345.5	279.6	227.1
k	I	1537.7	855.6	670.7
	F	537.4	298.8	266.8
g	I	436.1	348.8	242.2
	F	311.0	225.5	188.1
f	I	570.7	351.7	332.8
	F	714.9	401.1	359.2
v	I	317.6	264.8	230.1
	F	375.0	281.4	216.0
	I	606.6	351.9	335.8
	F	751.9	332.9	377.7
	I	416.9	299.8	250.1
	F	373.3	299.8	239.6
s	I	545.5	380.2	402.1
	F	700.9	384.0	400.2
z	I	435.3	284.9	237.7
	F	380.2	275.2	216.0
	I	694.7	487.0	442.4
	F	848.6	507.9	438.1
	I	457.9	332.6	291.4
	F	444.4	296.7	271.3

*From *A Normative Air Flow Study of Children and Adults Using a Circumferentially-vented Pneumotachograph Mask,* by E. T. Stathopoulous, 1980, Unpublished doctoral dissertation, Indiana University, Bloomington, IN. Table 5, p. 46. Reprinted by permission.

*Based on 5 male and 5 female children, age 4–8 years, 5 male and 5 female youths, age 10–12 years, and 5 men and 5 women, age 18–30 years; Data represent mean of 3 productions of the target syllable /CᴧC/ embedded in the carrier phrase "Say _____ again". "In the case of a double-peaked air flow event, as sometimes occurs during adult fricative production, two peak air flow measurements were completed . . . and then an average was computed from the two values" (p. 34). Circumferentially vented pneumotachograph mask system used for flow measurement.

†I = initial consonant position; F = final consonant position.

Table 9–7. Average Airflow during Consonant Production (mL/s)*

Consonant		CV Syllables		VC Syllables	
Voiceless	Voiced	Mean	SD	Mean	SD
p	—	933	65	1019	57
—	b	472	159	675	229
t	—	968	136	821	157
—	d	410	147	481	259
k	—	940	159	882	226
—	g	372	103	455	263
f	—	352	73	525	113
—	v	95	59	338	108
	—	652	194	869	230
—		126	77	365	124
s	—	466	53	455	254
—	z	159	50	231	73
	—	583	128	479	108
—		249	39	303	119
t	—	881	106	583	183
—	d	525	119	424	101
—	m	168	80	287	145
—	n	155	64	244	113
—	l	133	72	213	108
—	r	143	47	132	84

*Based on 4 male and 4 female normal adults; "Normal vocal effort"; pitch and loudness uncontrolled; Single production of each syllable; Heated pneumotachograph system used for flow measurement.

Source: From "Air Flow During the Production of Selected Consonants," by N. Isshiki and R. Ringel, 1964, *Journal of Speech and Hearing Research, 7*, 233–244. Table 1, p. 235. © American Speech-Language-Hearing Association, Rockville, MD. Reprinted by permission.

tive to the class of speech sound, lexical context, and syllabic stress (Hutchinson & Smith, 1976; Löfqvist & Yoshioka, 1984; Löfqvist & McGarr, 1987; Löfqvist & McGowan, 1991, 1992; Stevens, 1991) and is likely to be greatly influenced by the speaker's native language (for example, see Nihalani, 1975; Dart, 1987; Ladefoged and Maddieson, 1996).

CONTINUOUS SPEECH

While observation of airflow for isolated phonemes provides valuable information about specific articulatory acts, it is very often desirable to obtain airflow records for running speech. During ongoing utterances, cognition, coarticulation, syntactic and semantic planning, and suprasegmental organization all conspire to make speech more difficult to control and more prone to breakdown. It is possible to construct stimuli that will facilitate evaluation of specific aspects of speech performance. For example, sentences can be loaded with voiced phonemes, with high-impedance sounds,

and the like. It may also be useful to compare the aerodynamic characteristics of a phoneme when spoken in an isolated syllable to those of the same phoneme produced in the context of a longer utterance.

The average airflow over the duration of a relatively long spoken passage might also be of use to the clinician—particularly for establishing a baseline against which the effect of therapy can be judged. From the data presented in the preceding tables it is clear that the mean flow will be strongly influenced by the content of the spoken material. To assure comparability of trials, most clinicians will wish to select some piece of prose to use as a standard. Over the years the Rainbow Passage (Fairbanks, 1960) has generally come to fill this need for English speakers. Patient performance may be compared with the summary data shown in Table 9–8 derived from values provided by Horii and Cooke (1975, 1978) for eight normal young adult speakers reciting the Rainbow Passage. Similar standard passages are available in many other languages as well, although the expected

Table 9–8. Average Airflow (mL/s) during Reading of the Rainbow Passage*

Sex	Expiratory			Inspiratory		
	Mean	**SD**	**Range of Means**	**Mean**	**SD**	**Range of Means**
Men	177	53	142–218	1109	257	1046–1234
Women	159	20	152–170	1105	175	963–1194
Combined	168	23	142–218	1107	86	963–1234

*Four male and four female "young adults." Single reading of the Rainbow Passage; Comfortable intensity. Face mask coupled to pneumotachograph; Flow signal low-pass filtered at 30 Hz before computer sampling and averaging.

Sources: From "Analysis of Airflow and Volume During Continuous Speech," by Y. Horii and P.A. Cooke, 1975, *Behavior Research Methods and Instrumentation, 7,* 477. Composite data were derived from Horii, Y., and Cooke, P. A. (1978). Some airflow, volume, and duration characteristics of oral reading. *Journal of Speech and Hearing Research, 21,* 470–481. Table 3, p. 475.

mean flow rates may be quite different from these few American speakers.

If the flow associated with any particular phoneme in the passage is not of interest, the average flow during reading can be easily determined with a spirometer. A face mask is used to collect the expired air, but the connection to the spirometer is through a special valve (available from suppliers of pulmonary testing equipment). This device, called a nonrebreathing valve, will pass expired air to the spirometer but will permit the patient to inhale room air, insuring that the spirometer volume is not reduced by inspiration (see Orlikoff & Baken, 1993). It is also possible to integrate the expiratory signals from a flow transduction system over the entire duration of the reading. In either case, the total expiratory volume divided by the expiratory time is the mean flow rate. Gross irregularities of flow will show as changes in the spirometer or integrator output record.

Although not thoroughly investigated, it is clear that many different speech phenomena may influence the ways in which airflow varies. Table 9–9 summarizes these influences in cases where there are enough data to warrant at least a tentative judgment.

SUSTAINED PHONATION

During production of a vowel, the upper airway resistance is very small compared to the resistance of the glottis. Since (other things being equal) airflow is a reciprocal function of resistance, measuring it during sustained phonation of a vowel should provide insight into glottal function. In fact, a number of investigations have confirmed that this is the case. There are even some data (Kelman, Gordon, Simpson, & Morton, 1975) indicating that certain dysphonic patients will demonstrate abnormal airflow even during quiet non-speech breathing.

The relationship among vocal fundamental frequency, intensity, and airflow is extremely complex. It would appear that, at low vocal F_0s, changes in the resistance of the glottis are used to regulate vocal intensity (Isshiki, 1964). Increases in subglottal pressure result in greater sound pressure but not necessarily in greater flow. At high vocal frequencies, however, flow does increase with increasing subglottal pressure and vocal intensity. But it is also important to note that different speakers use different regulatory techniques (Isshiki, 1965, 1969). These findings are confirmed by the work of Yanagihara and Koike (1967), Cavagna and Margaria (1965, 1968), and Schutte (1996) whose reports also provide a lucid discussion of the complexities of the relationships involved.

Given the variability that characterizes the data, caution should be exercised in drawing conclusions about normality of airflow across widely different vocal fundamental frequencies or intensities. A standard set of conditions for routine clinical assessment that meets the clinician's particular needs and clinical style should be consistently followed. (Dejonckere, Greindl, and Sneppe, 1985, provide an example.) The data summarized below, however, can serve as basic guidelines for clinical interpretation of the results of controlled testing under comparable conditions.

Expected Results

Modal Register

Based on a review of aerodynamic data available in the Japanese literature, Hirano (1981) concluded that the normal mean phonatory flow rates between 90 and 140 mL/s can be expected, although a given speaker's airflow may range anywhere between approximately 70 and 200 mL/s when voice is maintained at a comfortable pitch and loudness. Others (Wilson & Starr,

Table 9–9. Summary of Factors Affecting Consonant Airflow*

Greater Airflow Associated With:	Lesser Airflow Associated With:	According to:
Plosives	Fricatives	Isshiki & Ringel (1964) Hutchinson & Smith (1976)† Horii & Cooke (1978) Stathopoulos (1985) Stathopoulos & Weismer (1985)
Fricatives	"Vowel-like sounds"	Isshiki & Ringel (1964)
Voiceless phones	Voiced cognates	Isshiki & Ringel (1964) Emanuel & Counihan (1970) Scully (1971) Gilbert (1973) Hutchinson & Smith (1976)† Horii & Cooke (1978) Trullinger & Emanuel (1983) Whitehead & Barefoot (1983) Stathopoulos & Weismer (1985)
Prevocalic context	Postvocalic context	Gilbert (1973) Trullinger & Emanuel (1983)
Prevocalic context	Intervocalic context	Gilbert (1973) Trullinger & Emanuel (1983) Whitehead & Barefoot (1983)
Lingua-alveolars	Labiodentals	Emanuel & Counihan (1970) Gilbert (1973) Whitehead & Barefoot (1983)
High effort or SPL	Low effort or SPL	Hixon (1966) Brown & McGlone (1974) Stathopoulos (1985)
Adults	Children	Stathopoulos (1985) Stathopoulos & Weismer (1985)
Men	Women	Klatt et al. (1968) Emanuel & Counihan (1970) Horii & Cooke (1978) Whitehead & Barefoot (1983) Stathopoulos & Weismer (1985)

*This summary table presents general trends; see specific data tables.

†Subjects with severe-to-profound bilateral sensorineural hearing loss.

1985; Iwata, 1988; Dobinson & Kendrick, 1993; Schutte, 1996) have argued that "normal" airflows are highly variable and may well exceed Hirano's suggested upper limit. In addition, Iwata, von Leden, and Williams (1972) have stressed that the inability to maintain a steady flow rate, even in the face of an unremarkable mean flow rate, may provide the best aerodynamic indication of laryngeal dysfunction.

As discussed above, airflow does not change in a consistent way as vocal fundamental frequency and intensity are altered within the modal voice register.

The summary data presented in Tables 9–10, 9–11, and 9–12 should serve as general guidelines, not as norms. Some of the variability within and between studies may relate to the complex interaction between the flow rate and specific phonatory conditions (Hirano, Koike, & Joyner, 1969; Brown & McGlone, 1974; Kelman et al., 1975; Woo et al., 1987; Sawashima, Niimi, Horiguchi, & Yamaguchi, 1988; Löfqvist, 1992; Pedersen, 1995; Stemple, Stanley, & Lee, 1995), although other factors may substantially influence performance as well (Schutte, 1992). These include the instructions

Table 9–10. Mean Airflow (mL/s) during Sustained Phonation

| Age* | Number of Subjects | Airflow | | | Source† |
		Mean	(SD)	Range	
Females					
7.6	10	72	(21)	46–115	1
8	5	162	(38)	—	2
9	5	150	(24)	—	2
10	5	180	(39)	—	2
16–30	10	116	(26)	73–160	3
19–26	25	154	(71)	67–399	4
21–29	9	112	(16)	78–134	5
19–31	30	153	—	—	6a
19–31	30	123	—	—	6b
23	36	91	—	—	7
22–28	20	156	(23)	111–204	8
20–37	5	136	(36)	69–171	9
21–41	11	100	(23)	61–130	10
22–45	10	124	(46)	—	11
22–65	10	155	(39)	—	12
Adult	21	94	(32)	—	13
Adult	25	92	—	43–197	14
Adult	?	119	(25)	76–172	15
60–77	20	151	(63)	40–266	8
Males					
7.6	10	96	(24)	51–128	1
8	5	133	(54)	—	2
9	5	223	(36)	—	2
10	5	218	(82)	—	2
19–26	25	183	(54)	63–332	4
19–28	10	121	(16)	81–139	5
23	67	112	—	—	7
20–37	5	126	(21)	105–164	9
22–39	30	155	—	—	6a
22–39	30	133	—	—	6b
30–43	11	112	(30)	70–164	10
22–65	10	214	(77)	—	12
Adult	21	112	(36)	—	13
Adult	25	101	—	46–222	14
Adult	?	141	(22)	109–182	15
Adult	9	142	—	75–268	16

*Mean age or, if specified, range in years.

†*Sources*:

1. Beckett, Thoelke, and Cowan, 1971. Maximally sustained /ɑ/; Spirometer measurement; Flow data from child's "best effort" from a minimum of 3 trials. Data and rounded to the nearest integer. Airflow data were not statistically different between the boys and girls.

2. Trullinger and Emanuel, 1989. Four maximally sustained productions of the vowels /ɑ, æ, ʌ, u, and i/; Comfortable pitch, 75 ± 2 dB SPL; Airflow measured with pneumotachograph system, pediatric mask hand-held "tightly" against face by subject; Data averaged across trials and vowel-type; Vowel effect not statistically significant.

3. Peppard, Bless, and Milenkovic, 1988. Face mask connected to a Nagashima PS–77 Phonatory Function Analyzer (anemometer) used for flow measurement; Subjects sustained the vowels /ɑ, i, and u/ at a "normal pitch and loudness" for 3 s; Mean $F_0 = 212 \pm 27$ Hz. Data are averaged across vowels and rounded to the nearest integer.

4. Wilson and Starr, 1985. Flow measured using a Minato PA 500 Phonation Analyzer (anemometer); Three "detached" phonations of the vowel /a/ made into a tube mouthpiece at a comfortable pitch and loudness; Investigator "activated the equipment at a point where he judged the vowel production to be stable." Data are averaged across each subject's trials. For women, mean $F_0 = 219 \pm 37$ Hz, mean SPL = 74 ± 3 dB; for men, mean $F_0 = 115 \pm 17$ Hz, mean SPL = 75 ± 3 dB.

(Continued)

Table 9–10. Mean Airflow (mL/s) During Sustained Phonation (*continued*)

5. Rau and Beckett, 1984. Same method as Source 1.

6. Terasawa, Hibi, and Hirano, 1987. Nagashima PS – 77H Phonatory Function Analyzer (anemometer) used for flow measurement; Phonation made into mouthpiece at a comfortable pitch and loudness; (a) Three phonations maintained over a "comfortable duration" of 3–5 s, and (b) Three maximally sustained phonations following the subjects' "deepest inspiration"; Data averaged over each subject's trials; Significant average airflow difference between comfortable and maximal phonation duration for both sexes.

7. Prathanee, Watthanathon, and Ruangjirachuporn, 1994. Data for subjects sustaining the vowel /ɑ/ at a "habitual pitch" after taking a "deep inspiration." Spirometer measurement via mouthpiece with nasal occlusion; Intensity kept "stable" by VU-meter feedback. Mean age for male and female subjects combined; Across subjects, mean airflow was 105 mL/s (SD = 36). Data rounded to nearest integer.

8. Biever and Bless, 1989. Subjects sustained the vowel /i/ at a "normal pitch and loudness" for 3 s. For younger women, mean F_0 = 194 ± 11 Hz, mean SPL = 72 ± 2 dB; for older women, mean F_0 = 192 ± 14 Hz, mean SPL = 72 ± 2 dB. Nagashima model PS – 77 Phonatory Function Analyzer (anemometer) used for flow measurement. Data were not statistically different between the younger and older subjects.

9. Isshiki, Okamura, and Morimoto, 1967. Subjects instructed to "take a deep breath" and to sustain the vowel /ɑ/ for a long as possible at a comfortable pitch and loudness. Flow measured using a pneumotachograph; Data averaged across 3 trials per subject and rounded to the nearest integer.

10. Yanagihara, Koike, and von Leden, 1966. Subjects instructed to inhale "deeply" and to sustain the vowel /ɑ/ for a long as possible using a constant, but comfortable vocal pitch and loudness. For women, mean F_0 = 230 ± 33 Hz, mean SPL = 64 ± 3 dB; for men, mean F_0 = 118 ± 20 Hz, mean SPL = 67 ± 4 dB. Flow transduced using a screen pneumotachograph; mean flow determined by dividing the integrated flow signal (volume) by the duration of phonation.

11. Stemple, Stanley, and Lee, 1995. Mouthpiece attached to a Nagashima PS – 77H Phonatory Function Analyzer (anemometer) used for flow measurement; Maximum sustained phonation of the vowels /a, i, and u/ at a comfortable pitch (mean F_0 = 214 ± 19 Hz) and controlled sound pressure level (75–80 dB). Baseline data averaged across vowel-type, before induced vocal fatigue.

12. Blomgren, Chen, Ng, and Gilbert, 1998. Airflow measured using a circumferentially vented pneumotachograph mask system; flow rates were averaged across four sustained productions of the vowels /i, æ, u, and ɑ/ (no significant difference in mean flow for vowel type); Mean F_0 was 117.5 Hz for the men and 211.0 Hz for the women; Average airflow significantly higher for the men studied. Flow rates rounded to the nearest integer value.

13. Koike and Hirano, 1968. Same instructions and procedure as described in Source 10. Subjects described as "healthy adults," mostly "graduate students and laboratory personnel without professional training in singing;" No significant difference in average age between sexes; Data rounded to nearest integer; Average airflow statistically significant between male and female subjects.

14. Hirano, Koike, and von Leden, 1968. "Normal adults"; Same instructions and procedure as described in Source 10. Range represents 95% critical region.

15. Isshiki and von Leden, 1964. A total of 36 normal men and women served as subjects; Same instructions and procedures as described in Source 9.

16. McGlone and Shipp, 1971. Normal "young adult males"; Airflow measured with pneumotachograph system with subject in supine position; Phonation sustained at 10% of subject's modal-falsetto range at both 25% and 75% of his vocal intensity range; Flow data are averaged across intensity levels and rounded to the nearest integer; 2 s of "steady-state phonation" chosen for measurement.

and feedback provided to the speaker before and during the task (McCurrach, Evans, Smith, Gordon, & Cooke, 1991; Soman, 1997), voice onset characteristics (Koike, Hirano, & von Leden, 1967; Beckett, 1971; Murry & Schmitke, 1975), and whether the data are derived from phonation sustained over a comfortable or maximal duration (Terasawa, Hibi, & Hirano, 1987).

The vocal velocity index. Although not a consistent finding, Table 9–10 indicates that the mean flow rates of men tend to be slightly higher than those of women. This was hypothesized by Koike and Hirano (1968) to be related to the well-documented sex difference in vital capacity and they devised a measure to correct for this possible source of bias. Their *vocal velocity index* (VVI) is defined as the "ratio of the mean air flow rate [during sustained phonation of /ɑ/] to vital capacity . . . in pro mille" (p. 287). That is, the measure is derived by dividing the mean flow in milliliters per second by the vital capacity, expressed in liters. Values of the VVI from normal adults are provided in Table 9–13. Koike and Hirano (1968) established a 95% confidence interval for their data; VVI values greater than 44 or less than 14.3 should be considered abnormal. Iwata and von Leden (1970a) provided summary data regarding VVI in patients with various vocal pathologies (Table 9–14). The VVI, however, has not been widely used in research or clinical practice and it

Table 9–11. Relationship of Mean Airflow (mL/s) to Vocal Fundamental Frequency and Intensity*

	Fundamental Frequency Level		
Vocal Intensity Level†	*98 Hz ("low")*	*196 Hz ("medium")*	*392 Hz ("high")*
"Soft" (mean 70 dB)	113	66	88
"Loud" (mean 82 dB)	135	151	299

*Eleven male and 11 female adults, *most with at least some singing training*. Phonation at 98, 196, and 392 Hz (musical G3, G4, and G5); Pneumotachograph used for airflow measurement; Mean data for two trials in each condition used for grand means.

†Re: 0.002 Pa

Source: "Vocal Intensity and Air Flow Rate," by N. Isshiki, 1965, *Folia Phoniatrica*, *17*, 92–104. Table I, p. 95. Reprinted by permission.

Table 9–12. Mean Rate of Increase in Airflow (mL/s) for a 10-dB Increase in Vocal Intensity*

	Mean Rate of Increase in Airflow					
Vocal Frequency Level	Men			Women		
	Mean	*SD*	*Range*	*Mean*	*SD*	*Range*
"Low" (98 Hz)	1.05	0.26	0.65–1.70	1.04	0.33	0.56–1.60
"Medium" (196 Hz)	1.30	0.32	0.91–2.10	1.88	0.46	1.05–2.70
"High" (392 Hz)	1.80	0.60	1.05–3.50	1.94	0.55	0.56–2.70

*Conditions as for Table 9–11. *Reading the table*: The data entry represents the mean proportion of airflow at a given level to airflow during phonation at 10 dB lower intensity. Thus, at low frequency, if flow = 113 mL/s, an increase of 10 dB would cause flow to increase to 113 × 1.05 = 118.7 mL/s.

Source: "Vocal Intensity and Air Flow Rate," by N. Isshiki, 1965, *Folia Phoniatrica*, *17*, 92–104. Table II, p. 98. Reprinted by permission.

Table 9–13. Vocal Velocity Index in Normal Adults*

Group	*Mean*	*SD*
Men	23.5	7.45
Women	26.7	8.18
Combined	25.1	7.95

*Twenty-one male and 21 female adults; sustained phonation of /a/ at comfortable pitch and loudness.

Source: "Significance of Vocal Velocity Index," by Y. Koike and M. Hirano, 1968, *Folia Phoniatrica*, *20*, 285–296. Table III, p. 292. Reprinted by permission.

remains largely unknown how it varies with age and various phonatory characteristics (Dobinson & Kendrick, 1993).

Pulse Register

Table 9–15 demonstrates the significantly lower flow rates to be expected during pulse register phonation. In general, no consistent relationship between airflow and fundamental frequency has been observed. At comfortable intensity, airflow for men producing pulse-register vowels will range between 10 and approximately 72 mL/s, while women will use from 2 to about 63 mL/s (McGlone, 1967). Similar findings have been reported by Murry (1971) and, more recently, by Blomgren, Chen, Ng, and Gilbert (1998).

Falsetto (Loft) Register

McGlone (1970) has done a careful study of airflow during phonation in the "upper register," which he has defined as "that group of frequencies that occur above the modal register. This register may be falsetto"—or loft (p. 231). Eight college-age women sustained a

Table 9–14. Vocal Velocity Index in Vocal Pathology*

Condition	N	Mean	(SD)	Range
Chronic laryngitis	42	41.6	(14.9)	19.5–86.9
Vocal nodules	13	49.5	(6.2)	33.6–63.2
Contact ulcer granuloma	5	17.5	(5.2)	7.6–21.7
Laryngeal carcinoma				
pretreatment	9	47.7	(15.2)	31.8–73.5
postradiation	3	34.9	—	26.3–48.3
postoperative	2	40.6	—	20.2–46.7
Vocal-fold paralysis				
unilateral	25	91.6	(54.7)	25.5–243.3
bilateral	5	63.7	(40.0)	42.8–119.2
Spasmodic dysphonia	3	11.7	—	10.1–13.8
"Psychosomatic diseases"	17	47.2	(23.0)	20.9–108.4

*Same instrumentation and procedure used by Koike and Hirano (1968); Patients "sustained phonation of the vowel /ɑ/ at comfortable pitch and loudness as long as possible."

Source: Selected data from "Clinical Evaluation of Vocal Velocity Index in Laryngeal Disease," by S. Iwata and H. von Leden, 1970a, *Annals of Otology, Rhinology and Laryngology, 79*, 259–268. Table I, p. 260.

Table 9–15. Mean Airflow in Pulse and Modal Registers in Normal Men*

Voice Register	Fundamental Frequency (Hz)		Airflow (mL/s)	
	Mean	Range	Mean	Range
Pulse	34.4	18–65	40.4	‡–145.3
Modal	107.9	87–117	142.2	74.9–267.8

*Nine young adult men; phonations sustained for 2 s at 10% frequency and 25% and 75% intensity levels in each subject's range; Flow data averaged across intensity level; Pneumotachograph measurement.

‡Too small to be measured.

Source: "Some Physiologic Correlates of Vocal Fry Phonation," by R.E. McGlone and T. Shipp, 1971, *Journal of Speech and Hearing Research, 14*, 769–775. Table 1, p. 772. (c) American Speech-Language-Hearing Association, Rockville, MD. Reprinted by permission.

vowel for 4 s at 10% intervals of their intensity range and at 10% intervals of their frequency range, within this register. Flow rate was derived by dividing the volume of air used by the duration of phonation. The resultant data are summarized in Table 9–16.

Vocal Pathology

The expectation that the mean airflow rate should reflect the degree of laryngeal dysfunction is generally borne out by research reported in the literature. This is particularly true in those instances when adequate glottal closure is not achieved (Hirano, Koike, & von Leden, 1968; Yanagihara, 1970; Hippel &

Mrowinski, 1978; Coelho, Gracco, Fourakis, Rossetti, & Oshima, 1994; Omori, Slavit, Kacker, & Blaugrund, 1996). Airflow data, then, are useful in initial diagnosis or evaluation of the degree of dysfunction (Murry & Bone, 1978; Hirano, Hibi, Terasawa, & Fujiu, 1986; Hirano, Kurita, & Matsuoka, 1987; Rammage et al., 1992; Woodson et al., 1996) and may also serve as an indicator of therapeutic progress (Werner-Kukuk, von Leden, & Yanagihara, 1968; Fritzell, Hallén, & Sundberg, 1974; Murry, Bone, & Von Essen, 1974; Woo, Colton, Casper, & Brewer, 1992; Woo, Casper, Colton, & Brewer, 1994; Cragle & Brandenburg, 1993; Vavares, Montgomery, & Hillman, 1995; Lockhart, Paton, & Pearson, 1997; McFarlane, Watterson, Lewis, & Boone, 1998).

Table 9–16. Mean Airflow in Loft (Falsetto) Register in Normal Women*

Intensity Level (percentage intervals)	Frequency Level (percentage intervals)									Mean for Intensity Level
	10	20	30	40	50	60	70	80	90	
10	92.4	96.9	91.7	87.8	100.8	132.8	130.7	121.9	131.8	109.6
20	121.1	120.6	114.4	123.4	133.9	149.2	154.4	151.8	158.6	136.4
30	162.0	158.6	138.0	154.2	144.3	165.6	167.2	159.1	180.2	158.8
40	185.7	187.8	177.3	164.6	148.7	183.3	169.5	173.9	186.1	175.2
50	208.9	200.5	174.2	203.1	179.4	184.1	198.4	182.0	188.5	191.0
60	207.5	217.4	183.9	216.4	188.8	200.5	227.8	190.1	188.8	202.4
70	242.4	232.0	194.3	224.5	205.5	220.6	229.7	215.2	206.2	218.9
80	239.8	240.4	211.5	246.4	202.6	237.8	242.2	223.1	216.4	228.9
90	266.4	249.7	223.9	249.0	198.4	232.9	268.7	213.3	224.0	236.3
Mean for Frequency Level	191.8	189.8	167.7	185.5	166.9	189.6	198.7	181.2	186.7	

Source: "Air Flow in the Upper Register," by R.E. McGlone, 1970, *Folia Phoniatrica*, *22*, 231–238. Table II, p. 234. Reprinted by permission.

The data presented in Table 9–17 are drawn from comparable studies of patients with various laryngeal pathologies. Measurements were made during sustained /ɑ/ at a pitch and loudness deemed "comfortable" for the patient. In some cases, post-treatment measurements were also made and these, too, are included in the table.

Note that the airflow values for any given group show very wide dispersion, and the standard deviations demonstrate that airflow measurements in these cases of pathology frequency overlap the normal range. Thus, an airflow value far beyond the normal is clearly indicative of disorder, but a value within the expected range is not presumptive evidence of normal laryngeal function. The results of measurement are always useful, however, in targeting therapeutic goals and in choosing clinical courses of action.

Correlates of Mean Phonatory Airflow

For a given driving pressure, the flow rate measured during vocalization provides a reflection of the speaker's ability to regulate the mean resistance of the glottal airway. As is clear from Table 9–17, laryngeal dysfunction is often associated with excessive airflow, and thus air loss, during phonation. It follows that, for a given volume of air available for phonation, an increase in air usage should reduce the *maximal* length of time that a speaker could sustain vocalization on a single expiration. This has led a number of researchers and clinicians to propose a variety of maximum duration measures as

approximate indices of phonatory airflow and thus, hopefully, of vocal dysfunction (Johnson, 1985).

Unfortunately, as attractive as such measures may at first seem, they are fraught with several shortcomings—and, in some instances, a few untenable assumptions—that pose a serious threat to their reliability if not to their validity as gauges of phonatory competence. Nonetheless, the popularity and ubiquity of these duration-based correlates of the mean volume velocity warrant a careful discussion of their relative strengths and weaknesses.

Maximum Phonation Time

To estimate a speaker's *maximum phonation time* (MPT) measure, he is asked to inhale as deeply as he can and then to sustain a steady vowel production for as long as possible. The MPT (sometimes also called the *maximum phonation duration*) is thus the greatest length of time over which voice can be prolonged. Like Ptacek and Sander (1963a) before them, Yanagihara, Koike, and von Leden (1966) found that men produce significantly longer MPTs than women. They attributed this sex difference to well documented differences in the amount of air available for phonation (see "Phonation Volume," this chapter). Yanagihara and his colleagues (1966) also noted very large variations between speakers of the same sex, which they ascribed largely to differences in mean phonatory airflow. Thus, like flow measures themselves, MPT has been applied as a gauge of air *consumption* and, by extension, of the

Table 9–17. Mean Airflow (mL/s) During Sustained Phonation in Vocal Pathology

Condition	Untreated			Treatment	Posttreatment			Source[†]
	N	Mean	(SD)		N	Mean	(SD)	
Vocal fold paralysis								
unilateral	10	442	(204)	Teflon injection	4	200	(35)	1
	11	313	(155)	Teflon injection	3	148	(46)	2
	19	353	(155)					3a
	16	249	(156)					3b
	16	475	(213)					4
	49	470	(390)	Thyroplasty	49	260	(200)	5
	10	490	(230)	Arytenoid adduction	10	300	(310)	5
bilateral	7	234	(194)					3c
mixed	17	469	(271)					6
Glottic insufficiency	15	343	—	Thyroplasty	15	304	—	7
Vocal nodules	8	154	(36)					1
	8	161	(66)					2
	23	177	(53)					
	3							
	10	226	(97)					
	8							
	6	275	—	Surgery	6	140	—	9
Polyps	4	478	(182)					1
	10	218	(92)					2
	18	162	(123)					3
	7	224	(37)	Surgery	4	162	(27)	10
Contact ulcer granuloma	5	98	(37)					2
	5	69	(24)					3
	?	144	(42)					13
Laryngeal carcinoma	4	236	(27)					1
	5	224	(172)	Radiation	4	90	(32)	2
	13	170	(70)	Radiation	6	99	(24)	3
				Surgery	2	136	—	3
	26	269	(120)					6
	19	198	—					11
				Radiation	20	143	(52)	12
				Surgery	14	204	—	14
Inflammation								
minor	11	134	(29)					1
edema	3	198	(32)					10
	?	173	(94)					13
Chronic laryngitis	5	212	(80)					2
	68	146	(44)					3
Spasmodic dysphonia								
adductor	8	110	(50)					2
	17	89	(23)					15
	13	72	—	Nerve block	6	232	—	16
				Botox injection	12	138	—	16
Laryngeal fatigue	25	203	(89)					17a
	40	143	(54)					17b

(*Continued*)

Sources:

1. Yanagihara and von Leden, 1967. Means and SDs compiled from individual case data.

2. Hirano, Koike, and von Leden, 1968. Means and SDs compiled from individual case data.

3. Iwata and von Leden, 1970b. Of 42 patients with laryngeal paralysis (23 men and 19 women): a. Nineteen had complete unilateral paralysis with the vocal fold in intermediate position; b. Sixteen had an incomplete unilateral paralysis with the vocal fold in the median or paramedian position; and c. Seven had bilateral abductor paralysis.

4. McFarlane, Watterson, Lewis, and Boone, 1998. Baseline condition for 8 men and 8 women (age 37–77 years) with unilateral vocal fold paralysis who "could initiate a productive cough" and who had "demonstrated a reduction in airflow rate in response to at least 1 facilitation technique, and reported little or no aspiration during swallowing" (p. 188). Mean airflow for the last of four prolonged phonations of the vowel /i/.

5. Bielamowicz, Berke, and Gerratt, 1995.

6. Woo, Colton, and Shangold, 1987. Some patients had unilateral and other bilateral vocal fold paralyses; Glottic cancer staging T1 to T4, two had prior biopsy and radiation therapy.

7. Ford, Bless, and Prehn, 1992. Patients with "glottic insufficiency" included those with vocal fold paresis or paralysis, sulcus vocalis, and bowing.

8. Peppard, Bless, and Milenkovic, 1988.

9. Benninger and Jacobson, 1995.

10. Tanaka and Gould, 1985.

11. Iwata, 1988. Laryngeal cancer staging: Five T1, six T2, six, T3, and two T4. Flow ranged from 65 to 280 mL/s; Mean vocal intensity = 75.3 dB, ranging from 57.1 to 91.0 dB.

12. Lehman, Bless, and Brandenburg, 1988.

13. Isshiki and von Leden, 1964.

14. Cragle and Brandenburg, 1993. Comparable patients with T1 glottic cancer treated with laser cordectomy compared with post-radiotherapy patients studied in Source 11.

15. Murry and Woodson, 1995.

16. Woo, Colton, Casper, and Brewer, 1992.

17. Eustace, Stemple, and Lee, 1996. "Patients with a primary complaint of chronic laryngeal fatigue in the absence of other pathologies." a. men, age 19—80 years; and b. women, age 15–74 years.

degree of laryngeal dysfunction, especially when inadequate glottal airway resistance is suspected (Arnold, 1955, 1958; Hirano, Kurita, & Matsuoka, 1987; Hirano, 1989). It is also common for MPT to be used as an indicator of the "physiologic support" for speech (Canter, 1965; Mueller, 1971; Ramig, 1986; Hillel, Yorkston, & Miller, 1989; Ramig, Scherer, Klasner, Titze, & Horii, 1990), of the severity of dysphonia (Ptacek & Sander, 1963b; Lehman, Bless, & Brandenburg, 1988; Von Doersten, Izdebski, Ross, & Cruz, 1992; LaPointe, Case, & Duane, 1994; Leeper, Millard, Bandur, & Hudson, 1996; Raes & Clement, 1996; Dagli, Mahieu, & Festen, 1997), or of therapeutic change in vocal function (Arnold, 1963; von Leden, Yanagihara, & Werner-Kukuk, 1967; Hirano, 1989; Ford, Bless, & Prehn, 1992; LaBlance & Maves, 1992; Adams, Hunt, Charles, & Lang, 1993; Dromey, Ramig, & Johnson, 1995; Countryman, Hicks, Ramig, & Smith, 1997).

However, the MPT alone cannot serve to distinguish inefficient glottal valving from reduced volume availability or from difficulty in sustaining adequate driving pressure—problems that may well have entirely different pathological bases (Boshes, 1966; Hillel et al., 1989; Ramig et al., 1990). This may partially account for why MPT has been reported to be less sensitive than the mean flow rate in reflecting laryngeal dysfunction (Woo et al., 1994). Indeed, although Hirano, Koike, and von Leden (1968) reported a significant negative correlation between MPT and the flow rate, the relationship could be considered moderate at best. For the normal men that they tested, $r = -.76$ ($R^2 = .58$), whereas for their group of normal women, $r = -.67$ ($R^2 = .49$), leaving much of the variance unaccounted for. Yanagihara and Koike (1967) reported similar results which, in addition to their own analyses, led Isshiki, Okamura, and Morimoto (1967) to conclude that, because of the many uncontrolled or unknown factors involved, MPT measurement "permits only an incomplete evaluation of the glottal condition" and is thus "of limited clinical use as a vocal function test."

As with the mean flow rate, the relationship between the maximum vowel duration and vocal fundamental frequency and intensity appears to be very complex (Ptacek & Sander, 1963a; Stone, 1983). Despite exceptionally high variability both between and within individuals (even when vocally trained), Schmidt, Klingholz, and Martin (1988) have shown that the MPT tends to be substantially shorter when phonation is sustained at an elevated vocal intensity. They found little influence of an increased vocal F_0 on the speaker's MPT, although several other investigators report substantially shorter maximal phonations under such conditions (Yanagihara, Koike, & von Leden, 1966; Yanagihara & Koike, 1967; Dobinson & Kendrick, 1993; Stemple, Stanley, & Lee, 1995; Eustace, Stemple, & Lee, 1996). Likewise, Schmidt and her colleagues (1988) reported no significant effect for the type of vowel used for MPT measurement, but this, too, has not been a universal finding (Kreul, 1972; Harden & Looney, 1984; Prathanee, Watthanathon, & Ruangjirachuporn, 1994).

Although advocating the use of MPT as a "criterion for the general quality of the voice," Arnold (1955) noted that maximum vowel duration can be expected to vary depending on a number of respiratory, neuromuscular, laryngeal, and articulatory factors as well as on physiologic and pathologic variations tied to health, training, and physical condition. However, despite the number of influences that may or may not be accounted for, the biggest threat to the validity of MPT and its interpretation would appear to be the number of trials necessary to obtain a speaker's "true" maximal performance. For instance, Ptacek and Sander (1963a) reported that, for the normal men that they tested, the average absolute difference between first two MPT attempts was 3.3 s (ranging from 0.1 to 17.6 s). For the women who participated in their study, the average absolute difference was 2.9 s (ranging from 0.2 to 9.4 s). In a study of MPT in children, Finnegan (1985) found that, on average, only 16% of the boys and 23% of the girls achieved their longest vowel prolongation by their third trial, the majority requiring at least nine attempts. Among 21 normal adults, Stone (1983) found only one subject to be able to produce the longest phonation by the third attempt. Just over half of Stone's subjects acheived their maximum phonation length by the ninth trial, with improvement noted in some through at least 15 trials. For 40 normal children, Lewis, Casteel, and McMahon (1982) reported substantial lengthening of maximum vowel durations through at least 20 trials. Many explanations for such a "practice effect" have been proposed, including subject differences in motivation, task understanding, and need for performance feedback. In general, subjects achieve longer phonation lengths and require fewer attempts if they are provided with explicit instructions, are given a complete model of the task by the examiner, and are supportively and enthusiastically coached during maximal inhalation and vowel prolongation (Reich, Mason, & Polen, 1986; Soman, 1997). Even under these conditions, Neiman and Edeson (1981) found that, on average, the 40 normal adults they tested required between four to six trials to produce

their longest phonation. Nonetheless, as with Stone's (1983) subjects, improvement in performance was noted through the 15 trials conducted. Soliciting the number of performances that appears to be necessary, however, can be clinically problematic. Regardless of the time needed to obtain a given patient's best effort, most will find the repeated effort fatiguing, if not uncomfortable or perhaps even vocally deleterious.

Nonetheless, there remains no standard procedure for eliciting MPT (Neiman & Edeson, 1981; Kent, Kent, & Rosenbek, 1987; Kent, Sufit, et al., 1991; Soman, 1997). The data shown in Table 9–18 come from studies where, in general, vocally normal subjects sustained the vowel /ɑ/ for as long as possible at a self-selected comfortable pitch and loudness following a maximal inhalation. Usually, the MPT reported is for the *longest* of three phonation, although some researchers and clinicians have reported the speaker's *average maximal duration* or the length of phonation for a particular preselected trial. Since vital capacity (VC) is related to body size and is known to be reduced in advanced age, it is perhaps not surprising that the mean MPT shows a marked tendency to be shorter in the youngest and oldest subjects. Yet, given a "normal" range of 6.6 to to as much as 69.5 s among *healthy* young adults, it is probably prudent to use these data only as a rough indication of how the typical speaker might perform on a maximum vowel duration task under similar circumstances. As Finnegan (1985) concluded, such "large intra- and intersubject variability prevent[s] valid individual to group mean comparison of MPT." At best, the interpretation of MPT data remains tenuous and their clinical utility questionable (Schutte, 1992; Treole & Trudeau, 1997).

The Phonation Quotient

Hirano, Koike and von Leden (1968) described a measure that would account for the effect of the size of a speaker's moveable air supply on the maximal vowel duration. Called the *phonation quotient* (PQ), it is obtained by dividing the vital capacity by the MPT. Since the value is derived by dividing a volume by time, the PQ (like the phonatory flow rate) is reported in mL/s. Among other things, Hirano et al. (1968) found a higher correlation between the PQ and the mean flow than that found between the flow and the MPT alone. For the normal subjects they tested, $r = .86$ ($R^2 = .74$) and $r = .75$ ($R^2 = .56$), for men and women, respectively. Based on these results and on those obtained from 73 patients with various vocal pathologies, they concluded that "clinically, we may use the phonation quotient as an indicator of air consumption if direct measurements of air flow during phonation are not feasible" (p. 188). Iwata and von

Table 9–18. Maximum Phonation Time (MPT, in seconds) for Normal Speakers

Subjects		Maximum Phonation Time			
Age*	N	Mean	(SD)	Range	Source†
Females					
3	5	6.3	(1.8)	2.8–9.7	1
4	10	8.7	(1.8)	5.3–12.5	1
5	10	10.5	(2.6)	5.4–15.5	1
6	9	13.8	(3.6)	6.7–21.0	1
6	58	10.6	(6.3)	6.2–30.6	2
7	10	13.7	(2.4)	8.9–18.5	1
7	10	15.4	(2.7)	12.0–22.0	3
8	10	17.1	(4.6)	8.1–26.2	1
8	10	19.1	—	11.9–23.0	4
8–10	7	16.7	(3.0)	—	21
10	9	14.5	(3.8)	7.1–21.9	1
10	10	15.9	(6.0)	4.1–27.6	1
10	10	16.5	—	12.9–21.8	4
11	10	14.8	(2.1)	10.7–18.8	1
12	10	15.2	(3.9)	7.6–22.7	1
13	10	19.2	(4.6)	10.3–28.2	1
14	10	18.8	(5.2)	8.8–28.9	1
15	10	19.5	(4.7)	10.4–29.9	1
16	10	21.8	(4.5)	13.1–30.6	1
17	10	22.0	(6.3)	9.6–34.3	1
16–30	10	22.0	(4.2)	17.0–30.0	5
20–25	30	21.5	(6.4)	10.7–39.2	6
21–29	9	24.6	(5.4)	19.0–37.5	7
18–38	31	20.9	(5.7)	11.8–32.0	8
20–37	5	18	(7.7)	11–36	9
18–40	40	17.9	(6.4)	8.4–39.7	10
21–40	11	22.5	(6.1)	16.4–32.7	11
22–45	10	26	(8)	—	12
20–58	41	18.4	(7.3)	6.6–40.4	13
Adults	25	25.7	—	14.3–40.4	14
49–72	5	13.0	—	—	15
65–76	12	14.6	(5.8)	—	16
68	7	17.9	(5.0)	8.5–26.2	17
55–84	4	16.8	(2.8)	13–25	18
66–93	36	14.2	(5.6)	7.0–24.8	8
70–89	30	12	(5)	4–20	19
85–96	18	10	—	6–18	20
Males					
3	5	7.9	(1.8)	4.4–11.5	1
4	10	10.0	(2.5)	5.1–14.9	1
5	10	10.1	(3.0)	4.2–16.1	1
6	9	13.9	(3.0)	8.1–19.7	1
6	44	10.4	(5.1)	3.8–16.8	2
7	9	14.6	(2.8)	9.1–20.2	1
7	10	14.2	(3.3)	9.0–19.0	3
8	10	16.8	(4.5)	8.0–25.6	1
8	10	20.0	—	11.5–24.5	4
9	10	16.8	(6.1)	4.9–28.7	1
10	10	22.2	(4.7)	12.9–31.5	1
10	10	24.9	—	15.9–39.0	4
11	10	19.8	(3.8)	12.4–27.3	1
12	9	20.2	(5.7)	9.0–31.4	1

(Continued)

Table 9–18. Maximum Phonation Time (MPT, in seconds) for Normal Speakers (*continued*)

Subjects		Maximum Phonation Time			
Age*	N	Mean	(SD)	Range	Source†
13	10	22.3	(8.2)	6.3–38.3	1
14	10	22.3	(6.9)	8.8–35.8	1
15	10	20.7	(5.3)	10.3–31.2	1
16	10	21.0	(4.4)	12.4–29.7	1
17	10	28.7	(7.1)	14.8–42.6	1
20–25	30	28.4	(11.1)	13.7–69.5	6
19–28	10	31.6	(7.9	20.0–47.0	7
18–39	31	24.6	(6.7)	12.5–36.0	8
20–37	5	32	(7.5)	24–46	9
17–41	40	24.9	(9.5)	12.3–59.0	10
20–55	35	22.2	(9.2)	7.7–49.2	13
30–43	11	30.2	(9.7)	20.4–50.7	11
Adults	25	34.6	—	15.0–62.3	14
35–75	17	20.6	—	14.8–42.4	22
51–65	5	15.4	—	—	15
65–75	10	14.6	(5.9)	—	16
49–87	16	18.6	(0.1)	12–25	18
68–89	27	18.1	(6.6)	10.0–37.2	8
72	7	17.4	(5.6)	8.5–26.2	17
73–89	10	20	(9)	11–39	19

*Mean age or, if specified, range in years.

†*Sources*:

1. Finnegan, 1985. MPT measured as the mean of the "three longest sustained phonations" (of a total of 14) produced by each child. Vowel /ɑ/ maintained at a "habitual pitch level" while child self-monitored a VU meter to maintain a level and stabile intensity. Range data represent 95% confidence interval. All data rounded to the nearest 0.1 s. "On average, males sustained phonation 2 sec longer than females . . . In addition, males tended to be more motivated to increase the length of phonation over repeated trials than females" (p. 315).

2. Harden and Looney, 1984. Kindergarten children with a mean age of 6.2 years; Vowels /ɑ, i, and u/ maintained at a "habitual pitch level" while child self-monitored a VU meter to maintain a level and stabile intensity. Authors report a significant vowel effect; mean, SD and range reported in table are for the vowel /ɑ/. MPT was not significantly different between the boys and girls tested.

3. Beckett, Thoelke, and Cowan, 1971. "Best effort" from a minimum of 3 maximally sustained phonations of the vowel /ɑ/.

4. Lewis, Casteel, and McMahon, 1982. Longest of 20 sustained prolongations of the vowel /ɑ/ "while controlling for pitch and intensity."

5. Peppard, Bless, and Milenkovic, 1988. Subjects sustained the vowels /ɑ, i, and u/; data averaged across vowel-type.

6. Shanks and Mast, 1977. Longest of 10 prolongations of the vowel /ɑ/ sustained at a "comfortable pitch and loudness." Mean, SD and range calculated from authors' raw data. MPT significantly longer for men tested.

7. Rau and Beckett, 1984. "Best effort" of minimum of 3 maximally sustained phonations of the vowel /ɑ/, using a "comfortable" pitch and loudness.

8. Ptacek, Sander, Maloney, and Jackson, 1966. MPT data derived from 3 maximal phonations of the vowel /ɑ/ sustained while self-monitoring vocal frequency and sound pressure level. Mean F_0 = 210 ± 30 Hz and 130 ± 20 Hz for the women and men, respectively; Mean SPL = 82 ± 4 dB. Older adults had significantly shorter MPTs than younger adult subjects.

9. Isshiki, Okamura, and Morimoto, 1967. Subjects "sustained the vowel /ɑ/ as long as possible at a comfortable pitch and intensity while they were expiring into a spirometer." Data represent the longest of three MPT attempts.

10. Ptacek and Sander, 1963a. Subjects instructed to "take a deep breath" and to "phonate the vowel [ɑ] as long as possible at a comfortable pitch and level of intensity." Mean, SD and range data in table from third maximal prolongation with vocal frequency and intensity uncontrolled (and thus assumed to be "comfortable"). Median F_0s were between 225 and 228 Hz for the women and between 124 and 130 Hz for the men.

11. Yanagihara and Koike, 1967. Subjects produced 3 maximally sustained phonations of the vowel /ɑ/, "at the most comfortable and easiest pitch" and using "the most appropriate loudness of voice for maximum continuation of phonation." For the women, mean F_0 = 230 Hz with an average vocal intensity of 64 ± 3.0 dB; For the men, mean F_0 = 118 Hz with an average vocal intensity of 67 ± 3.9 dB. MPT data represent the mean of subject's first and second MPT attempts.

(Continued)

12. Stemple, Stanley, and Lee, 1995. Maximum sustained phonation of the vowels /ɑ, i, and u/ at a "comfortable pitch" (mean F_0 = 214 ± 19 Hz) and "controlled sound pressure level" (75–80 dB). Baseline data averaged across vowel-type, before induced vocal fatigue.

13. Dobinson and Kendrick, 1993. "British Caucasian subjects"; mean, SD and range data for the vowel /ɑ/ sustained at a "comfortable pitch."

14. Hirano, Koike, and von Leden, 1968. "Normal adult" subjects instructed to "sustain the vowel [ɑ] at the easiest pitch and intensity as long as possible after maximum inspiration." Phonations were repeated "several times and the longest sustained phonation and the greatest vital capacity measurements were adopted for further evaluation." Range represents 95% critical region.

15. Mueller, 1971. Control subjects produced single maximum sustained phonation of the vowel /ɑ/ while wearing a divided oral/nasal face mask.

16. Kreul, 1972. Subjects sustained the vowels /ɑ, o, and i/; Data reported in the table are for the vowel /ɑ/.

17. Fox and Ramig, 1997. Subjects sustained the vowel /ɑ/ six times in each of three sessions. "A clock with a second hand was provided for the subjects to watch, and each subject was encouraged to monitor his or her performance. No instructions for loudness level were given for this task." Data in table represent longest mean MPT for subject group from the 3 sessions (women, session 3; men, session 2). MPT rounded to the nearest 0.1 s; range data are for the women and men combined. For the women and men, mean SPL was 71.7 ± 6.0 dB and 74.6 ± 5.4 dB, respectively.

18. Dagli, Mahieu, and Festen, 1997. Normal control subjects maximally sustained the vowel /ɑ/; best of three efforts.

19. Morsomme, Jamart, Boucquey, and Remacle, 1997. Subjects sustained "a long a 5 times on the usual speaking tone . . . The intensity (60 dB) was controlled by a decibelmeter placed near the microphone . . . placed 30 cm from the subject's mouth." MPT significantly longer for the men than for the women studied.

20. Mueller, 1982. Subjects sustained /ɑ/ at a "constant pitch and loudness . . . for as long as possible."

21. Reich, Mason, and Polen, 1986. "Normal third-grade girls" produced "three maximal-effort /ɑ/ prolongations" in each of two sessions. "Subjects were encouraged to employ their typical pitch level," although phonations were maintained between 65 and 75 dB by means of an SPL meter. Data represent average maximum duration for subjects during the second experimental session who received "verbal encouragement (coaching)."

22. Canter, 1965. Normal control subjects produced three maximal prolongations of the vowel /ɑ/; MPT determined as the *mean* length of the three phonations. Average MPT in the table represents the *median* MPT for the group of men.

Leden (1970b) later evaluated PQ with 192 patients with various laryngeal pathologies and found the measure a useful clinical index, but one that proved, much like MPT, to be "a less sensitive indicator [of laryngeal dysfunction] than the mean air flow rate." Using a large database of patients with many different voice disorders, Hirano (1989) obtained similar results and reached the same conclusions regarding PQ, MPT, and the mean phonatory airflow rate.

PQ data from several selected studies are provided in Table 9–19. Although both the PQ and mean airflow are reported in mL/s, they should not be expected to be identical. PQs are typically higher than the measured flow rate, largely because speakers are unable to use all of their VC in a maximum sustained phonation task (see "Phonation Volume," this chapter). It is also important to keep in mind that the MPT and VC used to derive PQ come from two separate series of expiratory tasks. And, because PQ depends on obtaining a measure of maximal vowel duration, the procedural pitfalls of valid and reliable MPT apply to PQ as well. Like MPT, accurate VC measurement requires several attempts with clear instructions, task modelling, and constant coaching to solicit a maximal performance. Often the time commitment and exertion required to obtain a patient's PQ precludes its routine use, especially as pneumotachograph and anemometer

systems have become more widely available in the clinical setting. Furthermore, if one has access to a recording spirometer, then it can be used to obtain accurate and reliable mean airflow measures (Isshiki, Okamura, & Morimoto, 1967), thus obviating the need for PQ.

The S/Z Ratio

Schutte (1992) has suggested that requiring a speaker to sustain /s/ for as long as possible might provide useful "information on breath control and the amount of available air." Earlier, with much the same idea, Boone (1977) proposed comparing a speaker's maximum duration of /s/ production with that of its cognate /z/, which differs solely with respect to voicing. By dividing the maximum duration of /s/ by the maximum duration of /z/, the resulting *s/z ratio* presumably allows one to distinguish the ventilatory from laryngeal factors associated with a voice disorder (Eckel & Boone, 1981). The s/z ratio has thus been proposed as a tool to screen speakers for vocal fold pathology (Boone, 1977; Shearer, 1983; Perkins, 1985; Gamboa, Nieto, del Palacio, Rivera, & Cobeta, 1995) or to document improvement in laryngeal function (LaBlance & Maves, 1992).

According to Eckel and Boone (1981), the rationale behind the use of this ratio is as follows: Normal

Table 9–19. Phonation Quotient (PQ, in mL/s) for Normal Speakers

Subjects		Phonation Quotient			
Age*	N	Mean	(SD)	Range	Source†
Females					
7	10	90	(16)	66–123	1
8	10	82	—	—	2
8	5	82	—	—	2
10	10	106	—	—	2
Adults	25	137	—	78–241	3
21–29	9	126	(16)	87–148	4
18–38	31	168	—	—	5
68–89	27	134	—	—	5
70–89	30	154	(87)	17–450	6
Males					
7	10	112	(21)	81–147	1
8	10	78	—	—	2
10	10	84	—	—	2
Adults	25	145	—	69–307	3
19–28	10	135	(19)	93–156	4
18–39	31	195	—	—	5
68–89	27	171	—	—	5
73–89	10	153	(48)	74–250	6

*Mean age or, if specified, range in years.

†*Sources*:

1. Beckett, Thoelke, and Cowan, 1971. Mean PQ, SD, and range derived from authors' VC and MPT data. For girls and boys respectively, mean airflow was 71.6 ± 19.6 mL/s and 95.9 ± 22.6 mL/s and mean VC was 1.346 ± 0.146 L and 1.548 ± 0.190 L.

2. Lewis, Casteel, and McMahon, 1982. Mean PQ derived from authors' mean VC and MPT data after conversion of VC from cubic inches to L. For the 8-year-old children, mean VC was 1.573 L and 1.557 L for the girls and boys, respectively; for the 10-year-old children, mean VC was 1.754 L and 2.098 L for the girls and boys, respectively.

3. Hirano, Koike, and von Leden, 1968. "Normal adults"; Range represents 95% critical region. Mean airflow was 92 mL/s and 101 mL/s for women and men, respectively.

4. Rau and Beckett, 1984. PQ data rounded to nearest integer. For women: mean VC = 3.019 ± 0.319 L; mean flow = 112.4 ± 15.7 mL/s. For men: mean VC = 4.185 ± 0.875 L; mean flow = 120.6 ± 16.1 mL/s. Mean PQ significantly greater for male subjects.

5. Ptacek, Sander, Maloney, and Jackson, 1966. Mean PQ derived from authors' mean VC and MPT data. For younger and older groups of female subjects, mean VC was 3.5 ± 0.6 L and 1.9 ± 0.4 L, respectively; for younger and older groups of male subjects, mean VC was 4.8 ± 0.6 L and 3.1 ± 0.7 L, respectively.

6. Morsomme, Jamart, Boucquey, and Remacle, 1997. Mean VC was 1.6 ± 0.6 L and 2.7 ± 0.7 L for women and men, respectively. Mean PQ not significantly different between male and female subjects.

speakers can be expected to be able to sustain voicing for a period of time equal to that of sustained voiceless airflow; that is, the s/z ratio should approximate 1.0. However, for any pathology which sacrifices glottal efficiency, the speaker should have a reduced ability to sustain the voiced /z/ without a concomitant loss of ability to sustain the voiceless /s/. Indeed, in a comparison of normal speakers with two groups of dysphonic patients, both with and without laryngeal pathology, Eckel and Boone (1981) found no significant difference between them in their ability to prolong /s/, while only the voice patients with laryngeal pathology showed a significant reduction in maximum /z/ duration. The

resulting s/z ratios, then, were substantially higher for the speakers with laryngeal pathology than for the other two groups. In fact, the s/z ratios exceeded 1.4 for 95% of these patients. Boone and McFarlane (1988) later suggested that a value of 1.2 could serve as the upper limit to which the s/z ratio should be considered normal. Such results have since inspired a great deal of clinical interest in the measure, especially for instances when airflow and volume measurement were not feasible or equipment was unavailable.

In some respects, the s/z ratio can be considered a wholly time-based equivalent of the phonation quotient. That is, assuming a relatively steady expiratory flow, the maximum duration of /s/ should vary directly with the size of the speaker's vital capacity. By using the maximum duration of /z/ to represent the maximum duration of the speaker's "vocalization," the s/z ratio thus represents a dimensionless counterpart of the PQ, and one that does not require a spirometric measure to normalize for the speaker's overall ventilatory capacity. This has made the s/z ratio particularly appealing, especially as a means of detecting laryngeal disorder in and outside the clinic. Unfortunately subsequent investigations have largely failed to replicate Eckel and Boone's (1981) results and the use of s/z as a screening tool has not been particularly promising (Rastatter & Hyman, 1982; Hufnagle & Hufnagle, 1988; Sorensen & Parker, 1992; Trudeau & Forrest, 1997). This may be due to differences in measurement procedure, the pathologies tested, or to certain assumptions underlying the ratio that may not be tenable.

For one thing, there may be no reason to expect the s/z ratio of the normal speaker to approximate unity. As indicated previously in Table 9–7, a greater mean airflow is to be expected for voiceless cognates. The consonant /z/, for instance, is produced with two impedances in series, one glottal and the other lingua-alveolar. Its cognate /s/ is, of course, produced without a substantial glottal constriction. Because, at similar intensities, both sounds can be expected to be produced with roughly the same subglottal pressure, the flow rate will be lower (and therefore the phoneme duration longer) for /z/. It is not surprising, then, that some investigations of normal speakers have observed s/z ratios lower than 1 (Tait, Michel, & Carpenter, 1980; Young & Bless, 1983; Sorensen & Parker, 1992; Gamboa, Jiménez-Jiménez, Nieto et al., 1997, 1998) and that ratios from dysphonic patients, although apparently reliable for a given speaker, are nonetheless quite variable between individuals (Fendler & Shearer, 1988; Larson, Mueller, & Summers, 1991; see also Madison & Seikel, 1990, and Shearer, 1990). Shearer (1983), for instance, using the s/z ratio to screen school children for laryngeal pathology found that "values near 1.0 would suggest a nearly equal probability for the presence or absence of nodules." Such results call the sensitivity of this index into serious question. Furthermore, if normal and many abnormal speakers may be expected to prolong /z/ longer than /s/, then the use of a maximal /s/ production to reflect ventilatory capacity may not be appropriate. Like the MPT and PQ, the s/z ratio suffers from the difficulties inherent in eliciting a speaker's maximal performance (Kent, Kent, & Rosenbek, 1987; Soman, 1997). In addition, the need to sustain a a high-flow consonant introduces several possible (supraglottal) articulatory influences on a measure that ostensibly assesses laryngeal function. Christensen, Fletcher, and McCutcheon (1992),

for instance, provide evidence that speakers may alter linguapalatal contact patterns for /s/ and /z/ to maintain the integrity of the sibilant in response to decreased ventilatory capability. Thus, unlike a VC measure, the maximal duration of /s/ depends on the extent to which a speaker can sufficiently pressurize (or depressurize) the available lung volume and can maintain sufficient oral impedance to produce steady frication.

Table 9–20 provides some summary data on the s/z ratios of normal speakers and of patients with vocal pathology. The values provide some indication of the the variability that can be expected and of the potential difficulty differentiating normal and abnormal speakers on the basis of the ratio alone. Table 9–21, from a study by Trudeau and Forrest (1997), provides airflow, air volume, and duration data for 32 adults with vocal-fold lesions who maximally sustained /s/ and /z/. These data do not support the hypothesis that patients with vocal fold pathology will tend toward elevated s/z ratio values.

AIR VOLUME INSTRUMENTATION

Spirometers (Respirometers)

WET SPIROMETERS

The classic instrument for evaluation of air volumes is the *wet spirometer*, an extremely simple device that has not changed much since its invention well over 100 years ago. It consists of an air-collecting "bell" inverted in a vessel of water. At the start of a test, water fills the bell, but air from the patient is channelled into it, and the water is displaced. This causes the bell to float, so that its height is directly proportional to the amount of air in it. A pointer linked to the bell indicates the volume of air. Most spirometers also have a pen, moved by the bell via a pulley arrangement, that marks moving chart paper to produce a permanent record of the volume events. Many spirometers are also equipped with a system to provide an electrical output proportional to the volume of air contained.

Although spirometers are widely available and are virtually unsurpassed for measurement of ventilatory volumes, their inherent characteristics limit their usefulness for observing small, rapid volume changes, such as those that may occur during speech (Hardy & Edmonds, 1968). Because they are mechanical devices, there is significant resistance to be overcome before bell displacement is achieved. Even when this is minimized, as it can be with careful design, the device still suffers from the effects of its inherently large inertia. That is, the spirometer is sluggish in its response. Therefore, rapid speech events are likely to be

Table 9–20. Duration (in seconds) of Maximally Sustained /s/ and /z/ for Normal and Abnormal Speakers

| Subjects | | /s/ | | | /z/ | | | s/z ratio | | | |
Age*	N	Mean	(SD)	Range	Mean	(SD)	Range	Mean	(SD)	Range	Source†
					Normal Speakers						
5	6	7.9	(1.4)	5–10	8.6	(2.1)	7–13	0.92	—	0.82–1.08	1a
5	9	8.3	(4.0)	5–18	10.0	(3.3)	5–16	0.83	—	0.50–1.14	1b
6	?	—	—	—	—	—	—	1.42	(0.52)	0.51–2.66	2a
6	?	—	—	—	—	—	—	1.31	(0.38)	0.48—2.02	2b
7	6	9.3	(1.7)	7—12	13.2	(3.6)	9—20	0.70	—	0.52–0.97	1c
7	8	10.2	(2.6)	7–16	13.1	(4.0)	9—20	0.78	—	0.51–1.10	1d
7	?	—	—	—	—	—	—	1.13	(0.33)	0.53–2.13	2c
7	?	—	—	—	—	—	—	1.19	(0.31)	0.52–2.34	2d
9	15	16.7	(8.5)	7–44	18.1	(6.8)	10—33	0.92	—	0.66–1.50	1e
9	8	14.4	(3.1)	9–21	15.8	(5.2)	8–24	0.91	—	0.75–1.26	1f
24–27	11	28.0	(14.5)	18–69	26.6	(9.6)	10—55	1.05	—	—	3a
8–88	86	17.7	(7.6)	5–38	18.6	(7.0)	5–37	0.99	(0.36)	0.41–2.67	4
19–41	22	20.8	(9.2)	—	18.9	(5.8)	—	1.11	(0.31)	—	5
73±4	11	20.2	(13.4)	6–51	24.5	(8.0)	15–37	0.82	—	—	3b
77±6	11	14.7	(4.4)	8–22	19.3	(8.4)	10–36	0.76	—	—	3c
					Vocal Pathology						
"Functional dysphonia"											
4–15	32	5.4	(3.0)	—	6.5	(3.2)	—	0.87	—	—	6a
4–15	22	5.6	(2.8)	—	6.0	(3.0)	—	0.97	—	—	6b
9–79	36	16.8	(5.5)	4–30	16.8	(5.4)	5–26	1.03	(0.23)	0.69–2.00	4
Nodules or Polyps											
5–8	8	5.3	(1.2)	—	6.5	(1.6)	—	0.81	—	—	7a
5–8	8	4.5	(1.4)	—	4.8	(1.5)	—	0.93	—	—	7b
3–12	50	4.7	(2.3)	—	5.9	(3.1)	—	0.84	—	—	6c
3–12	19	5.7	(3.1)	—	5.8	(2.4)	—	1.03	—	—	6d
8–60	28	19.9	(4.6)	10–31	13.7	(5.5)	4–22	1.65	(0.63)	0.91–3.60	4
20–50	13	—	—	—	—	—	—	1.44	(0.66)	0.90–3.30	8a
20–50	13	—	—	—	—	—	—	1.13	(0.20)	0.78–1.60	8b
Unilateral paralysis											
21–75	8	—	—	—	—	—	—	1.86	(0.69)	—	9a
21–75	8	—	—	—	—	—	—	1.19	(0.31)	—	9b

*Mean age ± SD or, if specified, range in years.

†Sources:

1. Tait, Michel and Carpenter, 1980. Subjects were 53 physically normal school children. Data derived from longest /s/ and /z/ from three maximal prolongations of each. a. 5-year-old boys; b. 5-year-old girls; c. 7-year-old boys; d. 7-year-old girls; e. 9-year-old boys; and f. 9-year-old girls. No difference between the boys and girls with respect /s/ or /z/ duration or the s/z ratio; Significant age effect for maximal fricative duration, but not for the s/z ratio.

2. Fendler and Shearer, 1988. Subjects were 78 vocally normal first and second grade elementary school children; ages, sex distribution, and number of children in each grade not provided. Data derived from longest /s/ and /z/ from three maximal prolongations of each. a. First grade boys; b. First grade girls; c. Second grade boys; and d. Second grade girls. Overall mean s/z ratio for first and second graders was 1.36 and 1.16, respectively.

3. Young, 1982; Young and Bless, 1983. Data derived from longest /s/ and /z/ from three maximal prolongations of each. a. Normal "active" young women; b. "Active geriatric" women; and c. "Sedate geriatric" women. Subjects used a "a comfortable pitch and loudness level." Duration data for /s/ and /z/ are rounded to the neareast 0.1 s; range rounded to nearest integer. Unlike the "sedate geriatric" subjects, the "performance of the active geriatric subjects [were] comparable to that of the young subjects" in their ability to sustain /s/ and /z/ (Young, 1982, p. 167).

(Continued)

4. Eckel and Boone, 1981. Data derived from longest /s/ and /z/ from two maximal prolongations of each. Subjects instructed to use a "comfortable pitch and loudness level." Patients with "functional dysphonia" were reportedly "without laryngeal pathology"; Other group of patients studied had either vocal fold "nodules or polyps." Duration data for /s/ and /z/ are rounded to the nearest 0.1 s.

5. Larson, Mueller and Summers, 1991. Data in table from subjects who prolonged /s/ three times followed by three trials of /z/. Subjects used a "a comfortable pitch and loudness level." Duration data for /s/ and /z/ are rounded to the nearest 0.1 s.

6. Hufnagle and Hufnagle, 1988. Subjects produced three maximal prolongations of /s/ and /z/ and were provided "encouragement during the task." a. Boys and b. girls diagnosed with "functional dysphonia . . . with no vocal cord lesions"; c. Boys and d. girls diagnosed with vocal nodules. Duration data for /s/ and /z/ are rounded to the nearest 0.1 s.

7. Rastatter and Hyman, 1982. Children with "bilateral vocal nodules (located at the juncture of the anterior or middle third of the vocal cord)" were instructed to maximally prolong /s/ and /z/ while "disregarding loudness." Five prolongations of each sound obtained. Duration data for /s/ and /z/ are rounded to the nearest 0.1 s.

8. Treole and Trudeau, 1997. Data for women diagnosed with bilateral vocal fold nodules: a. Prior to treatment and b. Following successful voice therapy that resulted in the "elimination" of the lesion. Ratios derived from maximally sustained /s/ and /z/ "after several practice trials and clinician models." No statistically significant difference in s/z ratio as a function of treatment.

9. LaBlance and Maves, 1992. Data derived from longest sustained /s/ and /z/ from three trials of each, prior to and following surgery. Patients with unilateral vocal fold paralysis due to "thyroidectomy, idiopathic causes, meningioma, and vagal neuroma." a. Untreated (preop) and b. Following type I thyroplasty to medialize the paralyzed fold.

Table 9–21. Mean Airflow (mL/s), Volume (mL), and Duration (s) of Maximally Sustained /s/ and /z/ for Patients with Mass Vocal Fold Lesions*

	/s/		/z/		
	Mean	**(SD)**	**Mean**	**(SD)**	**Ratio (s/z)**
Men					
Airflow	218	(118)	179	(74)	1.24
Volume	3437	(716)	3380	(645)	1.03
Duration	19.7	(9.4)	21.3	(8.2)	**0.99**
Women					
Airflow	132	(50)	147	(50)	0.89
Volume	2192	(793)	2195	(791)	1.00
Duration	17.8	(5.9)	15.6	(5.9)	**1.15**
Combined					
Airflow	150	(77)	154	(56)	0.98
Volume	2464	(927)	2255	(901)	1.00
Duration	18.2	(7.8)	16.8	(6.8)	**1.09**

*Based on 7 men, 34–56 years of age (4 with bilateral vocal nodules, 1 with leukoplakia, & 2 with vocal polyps) and 25 women, 19–75 years of age (23 with bilateral vocal nodules, 1 with a unilateral nodule, & 1 with a unilateral polyp). Patients trained to produce maximum sustained vowel phonation before obtaining 3 trials each of /s/ and /z/ prolonged maximally at a "comfortable" loudness. Data were obtained using a face mask coupled to a Nagashima Phonatory Function Analyzer; Airflow values derived by dividing volume used by the duration of each prolongation; Flow and volume data are averaged across trials and rounded to the nearest integer; Maximum durations are averaged across trials and rounded to the nearest 0.1 s. Average s/z ratios appear in boldface.

Source: "The Contributions of Phonatory Volume and Transglottal Airflow to the S/Z Ratio," by M.D. Trudeau and L.A. Forrest, 1997, *American Journal of Speech-Language Pathology, 6*(1), 65–69. Table 1, p. 67. © American Speech-Language-Hearing Association, Rockville, MD. Reprinted by permission.

completely obscured by mechanical integration. The spirometer is not the instrument of choice for most evaluative tasks. Providing, however, that the duration of phonatory or speech acts can be accurately marked on the spirometric record, it is quite acceptable in the determination of phonation volume or of total speech volume (Beckett, 1971). And, of course, the spirometer is the classic instrument for assessment of gross respiratory volumes.

DRY SPIROMETERS

Hand-held, or *dry*, spirometers are compact and portable devices that do not depend on the displacement of water from a bell. Two types are in current use. One kind—exemplified by the Propper spirometer—is purely mechanical. A small turbine within its case is driven by the air blown into the mouthpiece. Its rotation moves a pointer around a dial on the outside of the case. Air volume is read from the position of the pointer at the end of the task. The instrument is rugged and reliable, but it may not be equally valid at all flow rates.

The other kind of portable spirometer is actually a flow transducer-and-integrator-circuit system. A digital readout shows volume. These electronic instruments are less rugged and more expensive than their purely mechanical counterparts, and they tend to be relatively insensitive to low flows, such as frequently occur during speech.

Compact spirometers are useful only for gross assessments of air volume, such as the vital capacity. Rau and Beckett (1984) have determined that VC measures done with several hand-held units (including the Propper spirometer) compare quite well with VCs obtained with a standard water-displacement spirometer. For clinical purposes, then, compact spirometers may be confidently used in situations where only a gross measure is needed and a paper record is not required.

Chest Wall Measurement

Lung volume changes can be determined from the changes in rib cage and abdominal size. Devices for transducing size changes include magnetometers (Mead, Peterson, Grimby, & Mead, 1967; Stagg, Goldman, & Newsom-Davis, 1978; Reich & McHenry, 1990), mercury strain gauges (Baken & Matz, 1973; van Lieshout, Hulstijn, & Peters, 1996), and inductive plethysmographs (Sackner, 1980; Chadha et al., 1982; Russell & Stathopoulos, 1988; Boliek, Hixon, Watson, & Morgan, 1996, 1997). The technology of these systems is discussed in Chapter 12 ("Speech Movements").

The chest wall's two parts contribute independently to the total lung volume changes, and the contributions need not be in the same direction. It is entirely possible, for example, for the rib cage to be enlarging (moving in an inspiratory direction) while the abdominal wall is forcing the diaphragm upward (in an expiratory direction). Therefore, derivation of a lung volume estimate requires that the separate motions of the rib cage and abdomen be added. Unfortunately, the different geometric properties of the two chest-wall components cause them to make unequal contributions to the net lung volume change. That is, a 1-cm change in the diameter of the abdomen does not alter the lung volume as much as a similar change in rib cage diameter. Taking these factors into account (but ignoring changes due to air compression), estimating lung volume change from movements of the chest wall entails solving an equation of the form

$$\Delta LV = k(\Delta RC + m\Delta Ab),$$

where ΔRC and ΔAb are the observed size changes of the rib cage and abdomen, respectively. The coefficient m expresses the relative effectiveness of abdominal to rib cage motion, while k is a scaling constant to convert the sum of the terms to liters. Motion can be defined as the change in anteroposterior diameter (Mead et al., 1967; Konno & Mead, 1967), anterior hemicircumference (Baken, 1977), or torso circumference (Sackner, Nixon, Davis, Atkins, & Sackner, 1980).

CALIBRATION

Because individuals differ in their anatomy, the rib-cage and abdominal equivalence ratio, m, varies greatly from one body to another (Fugl-Meyer, 1974; Sharp, Goldberg, Druz, & Danon, 1976). There is no practical way to predict it for a given person. Also, the scaling factor, k, changes as a function of system characteristics. This might seem to imply that application of this measurement method would require an inordinate amount of calibration for each subject. This is not the case, however. In practice, the equation can be solved electronically using very simple circuitry. It is not even necessary to determine the actual value of any of the unknowns. The method is as follows.

The transduction system is attached to the subject, and its electrical outputs are connected to the inputs of a variable summing amplifier, as shown in Figure 9–18. This simple operational amplifier circuit (specific details are available in any elementary electronics text) produces an output representing the difference of the separate inputs. By using a variable resistance for the rib cage input, it is easy to adjust its

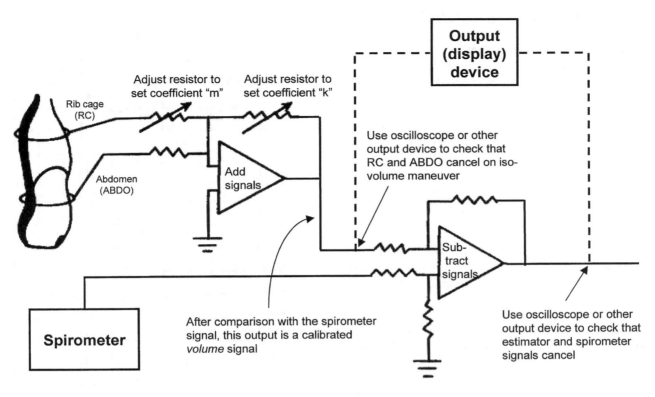

Figure 9–18. Diagram of the method of obtaining a lung-volume estimate from chest-wall signals (see text; also "Chest-wall Movement," Chapter 12).

contribution to the final output. The setting of the variable resistor, in short, represents m in the equation. Adjusting the feedback resistor changes the scaling factor, k. Thus, the simple circuit is an analog computer that, in voltage terms, solves for $k(\Delta RC + m\Delta Ab)$ when the m and k resistors are properly set.

To set the m resistor, the subject performs a series of *isovolume maneuvers*: after inhaling a moderate quantity of air, he closes his glottis ("holds his breath") and alternately contracts and relaxes his abdominal wall. Since, when the glottis is closed, no air can enter or leave the lungs, the net volume change during the isovolume maneuver must be zero. Any contraction of the abdomen will cause an equivalent expansion of the rib cage. While the subject performs the isovolume maneuver, the tester adjusts the m resistor until the summing amplifier's output shows minimal change. This indicates that the abdomen's voltage signal is cancelling that of the rib cage, thus the summing amplifier reflects no net lung volume change.

When the m resistor has been set, the output of the summing amplifier will be *proportional* to lung volume change, but it needs to be calibrated to actual volume values. This can be done in two ways. One is to match the output with that of an already calibrated volume transducer (spirometer, pneumotachograph and integrator, etc.). The two can be compared visually on an oscilloscope while the k (scaling) resistor is adjusted to make them match. More precise calibration can be obtained by subtracting one system output from the other (using a subtracting amplifier, also shown in Figure 9–18) while adjusting k until the two signals cancel each other completely. When k is properly adjusted, the volume calibration of the chest-wall system is the same as that of the volume instrumentation to which it has been compared, and the second system can be removed.

The other method of calibration is easier, but less exact. The subject can simply be asked to inhale and exhale a known volume of air (to and from a spirometer, or into and out of a nonstretchable plastic bag of known capacity) while noting the change in the output voltage, from which the volts per liter calibration of the system is easily determined. (A detailed description and comparison of several calibration methods is provided by Chadha et al., 1982).

AIR VOLUME MEASUREMENTS

In theory, all of the instrumentation used for measurement of ventilatory volumes can be made to serve for observation of the volumes associated with specific articulatory events or phonatory tasks. But the volumes at issue in speech tasks may be very small and may be expended in very brief time intervals. This situation imposes special requirements with respect to resolution and frequency response that might not be met by traditional instruments used in respiratory assessment. Any limitations along these lines must be considered in the light of the speech task to be evaluated so as to be certain that necessary compromises do not invalidate the data.

The shortcomings of the spirometer have been discussed above, but other volumetric instrumentation may have similar limitations. Several types are also sensitive to compressional lung volume changes which is undesirable if articulatory or phonatory volumes are to be examined. The method of choice for observing articulatory and phonatory volumes is integration of the output of a pneumotachograph. This instrumentation can show very small volume changes in time periods of only a fraction of a second. The improvement in resolution is clearly illustrated in Figure 9–19, in which the outputs of a spirometer and a pneumotachograph-integrator system are compared during production of the same utterance. Currently integration is most likely to be done by computer software after digitizing the flow signal.

Given the relationship between flow and volume (see "General Physical Principles," this chapter), it is clear that volume may always be calculated by multiplying the mean flow during an event by the event's duration. This indirect approach might not always be convenient, however, and it may not always be possible to determine the mean flow, particularly in the case of the flow pulses that characterize many articulatory gestures. Nevertheless, specific *volume* measures are often useful.

Articulatory Volumes

The volume of air used during a particular articulatory event depends on the subglottal pressure, the vocal tract impedance, and the duration of the event. While generally a less useful measure than the flow rate for understanding articulatory coordination, volumetric evaluation may provide special insights in particular cases.

Volume usage can be determined for whole syllables or for individual phonemes. In the former case, a

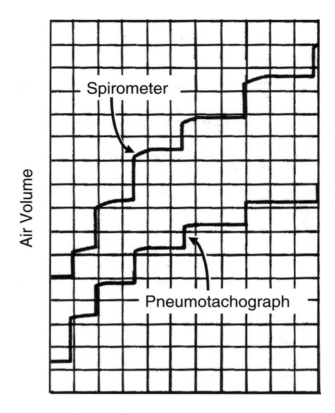

Figure 9–19. Comparison of the outputs of a spirometer (upper trace) and a pneumotachograph-integrator system (lower trace) for rapid incremental increases of air. The greater "squareness" of the corners in the pneumotachograph record indicates its superior frequency response.

spirometer can be used to determine the *mean* volume per syllable by having the patient repeat the test utterance fairly rapidly on a single breath while the spirometer records the volume of air expired. The mean volume per syllable is the total volume expended divided by the number of syllables produced—assuming that there is no airflow between syllable repetitions. This technique produces only approximate results. It obscures any significant variability among the syllables and may be very misleading if rapid, nonspeech inspirations are interspersed within the spoken text. (Itoh and Horii, 1985, have shown this to be characteristic of some deaf speakers, for instance.) Nonetheless, the method is often sufficiently discriminating for clinical purposes. Hardy (1961), for example, found that it demonstrated differences in production of /ba/ by dysarthric and nondysarthric spastic children. More refined measures, however, will require better temporal and volumetric resolution than can be provided by a spirometer.

CONTINUOUS SPEECH

As mentioned in the discussion of airflow during running speech, measures of average expiratory and inspiratory volumes are best assessed by having the speaker read a standard passage. For English speakers, the "Rainbow Passage" continues to be the almost-universal choice for this purpose. Horii and Cooke (1978), using an analog pneumotachograph-integrator system and a special computer program (Horii & Cooke, 1975), have carefully generated relevant data (summarized in Table 9–22) that may be useful as broad guidelines in the evaluation of disorder.

SPECIFIC SPEECH EVENTS

Volume per Speech Sound

Determining the air volume used during production of a phoneme will, ideally, involve three data signals: flow, volume, and sound pressure. The flow and sound pressure channels are used to delineate the phoneme being tested. A carrier phrase should be constructed to provide a clear contrast between the event of interest and the surrounding phones. The flow data are most commonly generated with a face mask-pneumotachograph system, while the sound pressure signal is derived from a microphone mounted on or within the face mask. Volume is usually subsequently derived by integrating the flow signal using computer software.

The phoneme of interest is placed in a syllable which is in turn embedded in a carrier phrase. For example, /t/ might be tested in the syllable /tɪp/ in the phrase "Say tip again." It is the usual practice to have the patient speak with comfortable loudness and pitch, although other conditions may be useful in special circumstances (see, for instance, Reich & McHenry, 1987). Several repetitions are spoken, and the mean and standard deviation of the trials are the data of interest.

Figure 9–20 shows a typical output record. In this case, the air volume used for /t/ before a stressed and an unstressed vowel was of concern, so the test phrase was "It's a tat again." The initial (pre-stressed vowel) and final (pre-unstressed vowel) /t/s of "tat" are measured. The flow and sound pressure traces are used to mark the start of flow for /t/ and the beginning of post-plosive voicing. The change in the integrator (volume) signal between these two points is the volume expended during /t/. Measurement of several repetitions of the phrase would be done in order to derive a mean and standard deviation for these phones.

Typical Values

The data presented in Table 9–23 were derived by Warren and Wood (1969) according to the method described above. Thirteen men and seven women, all speakers of "Southern [U.S.A.] dialect," spoke the carrier phrase "Say /Cæt/ again," where C was each of the consonants shown.

Volume per Syllable

Hardy and Arkebauer (1966) employed a spirometer to measure the mean air volume per syllable used by 32 normal children, aged 6 to 13 years. A face mask collected oral and nasal air. The mean volume per syllable was determined by division of the spirometer volume change during the task by the number of syllables produced. The resulting data are summarized in Table 9–24.

Boliek and her colleagues (1997) recently used a respiratory inductive plethysmograph to assess the speech breathing of 40 normal children between the ages of 18 months and 3 years. During spontaneous utterances, the children used substantially higher per-syllable volumes than the older children studied by Hardy and Arkebauer (1966); The preschool children used 46 to 207 mL of air per syllable, averaging roughly 100 mL/syllable. It was determined that these children were expending between 4 and 20% of their predicted vital capacities per syllable produced (mean = 8.8% PVC).

Table 9–22. Average Air Volume (in mL) Used per Breath During Reading of the Rainbow Passage*

	Expiratory			Inspiratory		
Sex	**Mean**	**SD**	**Range of Means**	**Mean**	**SD**	**Range of Means**
Men	650.5	99.4	541.8–782.5	640.3	101.4	422.8–770.1
Women	636.4	31.4	599.0–670.4	623.9	35.9	596.5–676.6
Combined	643.5	68.7	541.8–782.5	632.1	71.0	422.8–770.1

Source: Data compiled from Horii and Cooke (1978). Four male and four female "young adults"; single reading of the Rainbow Passage at comfortable intensity.

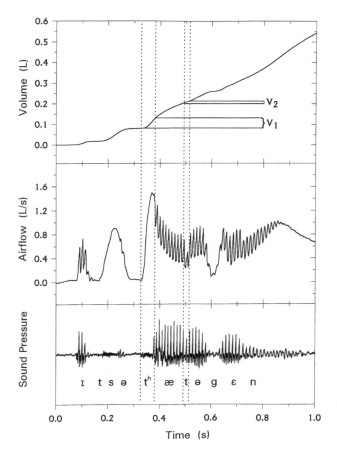

Figure 9–20. Volume usage during pre- and postvocalic /t/ in the phrase "It's a tat again." The flow and microphone trace are used to delimit the onset (sudden increase in flow) and termination (initiation of voicing) of each /t/. The change in the volume trace between onset and termination is the volume used. Note that the (aspirated) prevocalic /t/ was produced using approximately 50 mL of air (V₁), while the (unaspirated) postvocalic /t/ used a volume of about 10 mL (V₂).

Hoit, Hixon, Watson, and Morgan (1990) used a magnetometer system to assess speech breathing in 40 children between 7 and 16 years of age. Comparable to the data of Hardy and Arkebauer (1966), Hoit and her colleagues found that, in general, the average volume per syllable tended to increase with age (from roughly 35 to 60 mL/syllable), but that the per-syllable volume represented an increasingly smaller percentage of the children's vital capacities. Using the same methodology, Hoit, Hixon, Altman, and Morgan (1989) assessed 30 normal women grouped by age (25, 50, and 75 years). The average volume per syllable used by these women did not differ substantially and was similar to that observed for the female adolescents in the Hoit et al. (1990) study. As to be expected, however, with increasing age the per-syllable volume represented an increasingly larger percentage of the women's vital capacities.

Phonation Volume

Determining the volume of air used during a prolonged phonation is relatively easy since the absence of sudden flow changes means that the dynamic response of the measurement system is not of great concern. Therefore, the volume can be accurately measured with a spirometer which is, in fact, the preferred instrument in this case. Unfortunately, phonatory volume is not, of itself, a very useful measure. It represents only the long-term integral of the flow (the mean flow times the phonatory duration), and thus it merges two variables of clinical interest. From a clinical point of view, the flow rate and its stability during the task are much more important. (The former can be derived from the volume measure, while the latter is not easily observed in the spirometric record.)

Table 9–23. Mean Air Volume (in mL) for Selected Consonants

Sex	/b, d/ Mean	(SD)	/p, t/ Mean	(SD)	/z, v/ Mean	(SD)	/s, f/ Mean	(SD)
Men	53	(17)	93	(22)	76	(29)	106	(28)
Women	40	(13)	84	(21)	50	(17)	75	(14)

Significant differences: men vs. women and voiced vs. voiceless.

Source: "Respiratory Volumes in Normal Speech: A Possible Reason for Intraoral Pressure Differences Among Voiced and Voiceless Consonants," by D.W. Warren and M.T. Wood, 1969, *Journal of the Acoustical Society of America, 45,* 466–469. Table 1, p. 468. Reprinted by permission © Acoustical Society of America.

Table 9–24. Mean Volume (in mL, BTPS) per Syllable in Children's Speech

Speech Activity	Utterance	Mean	(SD)
Counting	1–10	32	(10)
Syllable Repetition	/pʌ/	39	(17)
	/tʌ/	35	(17)
	/kʌ/	37	(16)
	/sʌ/	56	(18)
	/tʃʌ/	42	(16)
	/fʌ/	52	(18)

Instructions: "Say _____ as fast as you can." Authors report a modest correlation ($r = -.40$) between rate of repetition and air volume. Data converted to mL/syllable.

Source: "Development of a Test for Velopharyngeal Competence During Speech," by J.C. Hardy and H.J. Arkebauer, 1966, *Cleft Palate Journal, 3,* 6–21.

A measure that is likely to be of great value to the speech pathologist is called the **phonation volume** (PV). It has been defined by Yanagihara and Koike (1967, p. 5) as "the maximum amount of air which is available for maximally sustained phonation." It is evaluated by requiring the patient to inhale maximally and then phonate for as long as possible, keeping vocal pitch and loudness constant. Volume is measured by spirometer or by integrating a digitized flow signal. Clearly the PV is related to measures of the MPT and mean phonatory airflow (von Leden, 1968). In theory, a speaker's PV should be equal to the product of his or her maximum phonation duration and mean flow rate (that is, PV = MPT × Flow). Thus the PV is generally affected by the same factors that influence maximum phonation and fricative duration measures (especially vital capacity, which in turn varies with age, sex, and stature).

EXPECTED RESULTS

Phonation volume has been evaluated in 22 men and women by Yanagihara, Koike, and von Leden (1966) and by Yanagihara and Koike (1967). They had each of their subjects phonate at three pitch levels: (1) "most comfortable and easiest"; (2) "highest pitch in chest register sustainable without special effort"; and (3) "lowest [modal] pitch sustainable without special effort." Comfortable loudness was used at all pitches, and three trials were performed at each level. Yanagihara and his coworkers (Yanagihara et al., 1966; Yanagihara & Koike, 1967) established that there is, under all pitch conditions, a significant correlation (ranging from $r = .59$ to $r = .90$) between a speaker's one-stage VC and PV. The following regressions were computed to quantify this relationship:

1. At high pitch, PV = 0.85VC − 1133;

2. At comfortable pitch, PV = 0.86VC − 891; and

3. At low pitch, PV = 0.94VC − 1186.

These equations may be used to generate a predicted PV (for either men or women) that can be compared with the individual's measured PV. Nonetheless, in light of the modest correlations behind the equations, the predicted PV value should be liberally interpreted and not be construed as a rigid standard.

By dividing the PV by the patient's VC (the *PV/VC ratio*), Yanagihara et al. (1966) and Yanagihara and Koike (1967) determined that a given adult speaker can expect to be able to sufficiently pressurize (or, perhaps at high lung volumes, to sufficiently depressurize) about 45 to 80% of the VC to produce voice under most phonatory conditions. Their volume and ratio data are shown in Table 9–25. Isshiki, Okamura, and Morimoto (1967) and Rau and Beckett (1984) report similar PV data and likewise observed that men used higher volumes than the women they tested. For both, however, somewhat higher mean PV/VC ratios of 86 and 90% (ranging from 69% to as much as 97%) are reported or can be derived from their data, respectively. These ratios do not appear to be appreciably different between men and women. Nonetheless, it should be noted that normal speech production characteristically employs a fairly small percentage of the speaker's movable lung volume. Hoshiko (1965), for instance, noted that normal speakers tend to initiate speech at approximately 50% of their VCs and use only about 20% of the VC for the typical utterance.

Beckett, Thoelke and Cowan (1971) provide PV data for 7-year-old children who maximally sustained phonation at a comfortable loudness. These data are shown in Table 9–26. Given their smaller stature, it is not surprising that the PVs used by children are substantially less than those reported for adults. No normative PV equations are as yet available for children, although both VC and PV can be expected to increase as the child ages, according to their sex and commensurate with their height and weight (Weng & Levison, 1969; Trullinger & Emanuel, 1989). Note, however, that the PV/VC ratios derived from Beckett et al.'s (1971) volume data are not unlike those of adults.

Vocal Onset

Different types of **vocal initiation** (or **attack**) result in different flow rates during the vocal rise time (see Chapter 5, "Speech Intensity"). The nature of these differences has been explored in men by Koike, Hirano,

Table 9–25. Mean Phonation Volume (in Liters) and PV/VC Ratio (in Percent) for Normal Adult Men and Women*

Pitch Level Condition	Mean F_0 (Hz)	Phonation Volume			PV/VC Ratio		
		Mean	(SD)	Range	Mean	(SD)	Range
Men							
High	208	3.359	(0.498)	2.690–4.400	68	(5.2)	59–77
Comfortable	118	3.256	(0.602)	2.200–4.255	67	(6.5)	57–78
Low	95	2.946	(0.408)	2.540–3.550	63	(8.0)	50–76
Women							
High	390	2.161	(0.451)	1.480–2.980	60	(9.6)	47–77
Comfortable	230	2.146	(0.345)	1.520–2.723	59	(7.3)	50–70
Low	209	1.879	(0.782)	1.020–2.880	53	(18.1)	33–69

*Eleven men, age 30–43 years, and 11 women, age 21–40 years; See text for method; PVs of men and women are significantly different.

Sources: Compiled from "Phonation and Respiration: Function Study in Normal Subjects," by N. Yanagihara, Y. Koike, and H. von Leden, 1966, *Folia Phoniatrica*, *18*, 323–340 (Table II, p. 330); and from "The Regulation of Sustained Phonation, by N. Yanagihara and Y. Koike, 1967, *Folia Phoniatrica*, *19*, 1–18 (Tables I and II, p. 6).

Table 9–26. Phonation Volume (PV), Vital Capacity (VC), and PV/VC Ratio for Normal 7-year-old Boys and Girls*

	Subject Height (cm)	Subject Weight (kg)	Phonation Volume (Liters)	Vital Capacity (Liters)	PV/VC Ratio (percent)
Boys					
Mean	126.2	25.7	1.310	1.548	84
(SD)	(4.2)	(4.3)	(0.280)	(0.190)	(8.7)
Range	119.0–134.0	20.9–34.1	0.900–1.650	1.150–1.825	63–92
Girls					
Mean	124.0	22.8	1.069	1.346	79
(SD)	(4.2)	(1.9)	(0.227)	(0.126)	(11.8)
Range	118.5–130.5	19.5–25.0	0.700–1.500	1.175–1.600	57–94

*Ten boys and 10 girls, average age 7.6 years; "selected on the basis of normal height for their age level." Maximally sustained /ɑ/; Spirometer measurement; data from "best effort" of a minimum of 3 trials. Weight converted to kg, PV and VC to liters. PV/VC data calculated from authors' original data. PV not significantly different between the boys and girls studied.

Source: Data derived from "A Normative Study of Airflow in Children," by R.L. Beckett, W. Thoelke, and L. Cowan, 1971, *British Journal of Disorders of Communication*, *6*, 13–16. Tables I and II, p. 14.

and von Leden (1967) and Koike (1967) who compared the amount of air consumed in the first 200 ms of phonations initiated with different attacks. The data (Table 9–27) may be useful in evaluation of voice onset characteristics and assessment of therapeutic progress. Note, however, that intrasubject variability tends to be high. Koike, Hirano, and von Leden (1967) noted small or negligible "air leakage" prior to phonations initiated with either a "soft" or "hard" attack, but did measure losses of 45 to 600 mL (mean = 207 mL) prior to vocalization with a "breathy" onset. Table 9–28 demonstrates how air consumption during the first 200 ms of phonation is elevated in at least some types of vocal pathologies.

Table 9–27. Air Consumption (in mL) During the First 200 ms of Phonation in Normal Men*

Vocal Onset (Attack)	Mean	SD	Range
"Breathy"	97	52.1	23–215
"Soft" (normal)	23	5.0	15–33
"Hard"	46	16.4	29–77

*Fourteen men, phonation of /ɑ/ for "several seconds" for "over 200 samples." Pneumotachograph-integrator system. Air consumption significantly different for type of vocal attack.

Source: "Vocal Initiation: Acoustic and Aerodynamic Investigations of Normal Subjects," by Y. Koike, M. Hirano, and H. von Leden, 1967, *Folia Phoniatrica*, *19*, 173–182. Table II, p. 177. Reprinted by permission.

Table 9–28. Air Consumption (in mL) During the First 200 ms of Phonation in Laryngeal Pathology*

Vocal Disorder	(Number, Sex)	Mean	Range
Laryngeal carcinoma	(3 M)	55.5	37–90
Unilateral paralysis	(2 M; 1 F)	135.3	77–184
Papilloma	(1 M; 1 F)	34.0	29–39

*Phonation of /ɑ/ with patients using their best vocal attack. Pneumotachograph-integrator system. Patients with carcinoma had vocal-fold disease.

Source: "Experimental Studies on Vocal Attack," by Y. Koike, 1967, *Practica Otologica Kyoto, 60*, 663–688. Table 5, p. 675. Reprinted by permission.

REFERENCES

Abramson, J. (1981). *Practical application of the gas laws to pulmonary physiology*. Scottsdale, AZ: Holcomb Hathaway.

Adams, S. G., Hunt, E. J., Charles, D. A., & Lang, A. E. (1993). Unilateral versus bilateral botulinum toxin injections in spasmodic dysphonia: Acoustic and perceptual results. *Journal of Otolaryngology, 23,* 171–175.

Amerman, J. D., & Williams, D. K. (1979). Implications of respirometric evaluation for diagnosis and management of vocal fold pathologies. *British Journal of Disorders of Communication, 14,* 153–160.

Arnold, G. E. (1955). Vocal rehabilitation of paralytic dysphonia. II. Acoustic analysis of vocal function. *Archives of Otolaryngology, 62,* 593–601.

Arnold, G. E. (1958). Vocal rehabilitation of paralytic dysphonia. IV. Paralytic dysphonia due to unilateral recurrent nerve paralysis. *Archives of Otolaryngology, 68,* 284–300.

Arnold, G. E. (1963). Alleviation of aphonia or dysphonia through intracordal injection of Teflon paste. *Annals of Otology, Rhinology and Laryngology, 72,* 385–395.

Baken, R. J. (1977). Estimation of lung volume change from torso hemicircumferences. *Journal of Speech and Hearing Research, 20,* 808–812.

Baken, R. J., & Matz, B. J. (1973). A portable impedance pneumograph. *Human Communication, 2,* 28–35.

Bastian, H.-J., Unger, E., & Sasama, R. (1981). Pneumotachologische Objektivierung von Behandlungsverläufen und Ergibnissen. *Folia Phoniatrica, 33,* 216–226.

Beckett, R. L. (1971). The respirometer as a diagnostic and clinical tool in the speech clinic. *Journal of Speech and Hearing Disorders, 36,* 235–241.

Beckett, R. L., Thoelke, W., & Cowan, L. (1971). A normative study of airflow in children. *British Journal of Disorders of Communication, 6,* 13–16.

Benninger, M. S., & Jacobson, B. (1995). Vocal nodules, microwebs, and surgery. *Journal of Voice, 9,* 326–331.

Bielamowicz, S., Berke, G. S., & Gerratt, B. R. (1995). A comparison of type I thyroplasty and arytenoid adduction. *Journal of Voice, 9,* 466–472.

Biever, D. M., & Bless, D. M. (1989). Vibratory characteristics of the vocal folds in young adult and geriatric women. *Journal of Voice, 3,* 120–131.

Blomgren, M., Chen, Y., Ng, M. L., & Gilbert, H. R. (1998). Acoustic, aerodynamic, physiologic, and perceptual properties of modal and vocal fry registers. *Journal of the Acoustical Society of America, 103,* 2649–2658.

Boliek, C. A., Hixon, T. J., Watson, P. J., & Morgan, W. J. (1996). Vocalization and breathing during the first year of life. *Journal of Voice, 10,* 1–22.

Boliek, C. A., Hixon, T. J., Watson, P. J., & Morgan, W. J. (1997). Vocalization and breathing during the second and third years of life. *Journal of Voice, 11,* 373–390.

Bond, Z. S., Moore, T. J., & Gable, B. (1989). Acoustic-phonetic characteristics of speech produced in noise and while wearing an oxygen mask. *Journal of the Acoustical Society of America, 85,* 907–912.

Boone, D. R. (1977). *The voice and voice therapy* (pp. 86–87). Englewood Cliffs, NJ: Prentice-Hall.

Boone, D. R., & McFarlane, S. C. (1988). *The voice and voice therapy* (4th ed.). Englewood Cliffs, NJ: Prentice-Hall.

Boshes, B. (1966). Voice changes in parkinsonism. *Journal of Neurosurgery, 24,* 286–288.

Brown, W. S., Jr., & McGlone, R. E. (1974). Aerodynamic and acoustic study of stress in sentence productions. *Journal of the Acoustical Society of America, 56,* 971–974.

Brown, W. S., Jr., Murry, T., & Hughes, D. (1976). Comfortable effort level: An experimental variable. *Journal of the Acoustical Society of America, 60,* 696–699.

Canter, G. J. (1965). Speech characteristics of patients with Parkinson's disease: II. Physiological support for speech. *Journal of Speech and Hearing Disorders, 30,* 44–49.

Catford, J. C. (1977). *Fundamental problems in phonetics.* Bloomington: Indiana University.

Cavagna, G. A., & Margaria, R. (1965). An analysis of the mechanics of phonation. *Journal of Applied Physiology, 20,* 301.

Cavagna, G. A., & Margaria, R. (1968). Airflow rates and efficiency changes during phonation. *Annals of the New York Academy of Sciences, 155,* 152–163.

Chadha, T. S., Watson, H., Birch, S., Jenouri, G. A., Schneider, A. W., Cohn, M. A., & Sackner, M. A. (1982). Validation of respiratory inductive plethysmography using different calibration procedures. *American Review of Respiratory Disease, 125,* 644–649.

Christensen, J. M., Fletcher, S. G., & McCutcheon, M. J. (1992). Esophageal speaker articulation of /s,z/: A dynamic palatometric assessment. *Journal of Comunication Disorders, 25,* 65–76.

Coelho, C. A., Gracco, V. L., Fourakis, M., Rossetti, M., & Oshima, K. (1994). Application of instrumental techniques in the assessment of dysarthria: A case study. In J. A. Till, K. M. Yorkston, & D. R. Beukelman (Eds.), *Motor speech disorders: Advances in assessment and treatment* (pp. 103–117). Baltimore, MD: Paul H. Brookes.

Collatina, S., Barone, E., Monini, S., & Bolasco, P. (1980). Realizzazione di un flussometro ad ultrasuoni e sua applicazione nella misura del flusso fonatorio: Primi risultati. *Acta Phonatrica Latina, 2,* 61–68.

Comroe, J. H., Jr., Forster, R. E. II, DuBois, A. B., Briscoe, W. A., & Carlsen, E. (1962). *The lung: Clinical physiology and pulmonary function tests* (2nd ed.). Chicago: Year Book Medical Publishers.

Countryman, S., Hicks, J., Ramig, L. O., & Smith, M. E. (1997). Supraglottal hyperadduction in an individual with Parkinson disease: A clinical treatment note. *American Journal of Speech-Language Pathology, 6*(4), 74–84.

Cragle, S. P., & Brandenburg, J. H. (1993). Laser cordectomy or radiotherapy: Cure rates, communication, and cost. *Otolaryngology—Head and Neck Surgery, 108,* 648–654.

Dagli, A. S., Mahieu, H. F., & Festen, J. M. (1997). Quantitative analysis of voice quality in early glottic laryngeal carcinomas treated with radiotherapy. *European Archives of Otorhinolaryngology, 254,* 78–80.

Dalston, R. M., Warren, D. W., & Dalston, E. T. (1991). The temporal characteristics of aerodynamic phenomena associated with patients manifesting varying degrees of velopharyngeal adequacy. *Folia Phoniatrica, 43,* 226–233.

Dart, S. N. (1987). An aerodynamic study of Korean stop consonants: Measurements and modeling. *Journal of the Acoustical Society of America, 81,* 138–147.

Dejonckere, Ph., Greindle, M., & Sneppe, R. (1985). Debitmetrie aerienne a parametres phonatoires standardises. *Folia Phoniatrica, 37,* 58–65.

Dobinson, C. H., & Kendrick, A. H. (1993). Normal values and predictive equations for aerodynamic function in British Caucasian subjects. *Folia Phoniatrica, 45,* 14–24.

Dromey, C., Ramig, L. O., & Johnson, A. B. (1995). Phonatory and articulatory changes associated with increased vocal intensity in Parkinson disease: A case study. *Journal of Speech and Hearing Research, 38,* 751–764.

Eckel, F. C., & Boone, D. R. (1981). The s/z ratio as an indicator of laryngeal pathology. *Journal of Speech and Hearing Disorders, 46,* 147–149.

Emanuel, F. W., & Counihan, D. T. (1970). Some characteristics of oral and nasal air flow during plosive consonant production. *Cleft Palate Journal, 7,* 249–260.

Eustace, C. S., Stemple, J. C., & Lee, L. (1996). Objective measures of voice production in patients complaining of laryngeal fatigue. *Journal of Voice, 10,* 146–154.

Fairbanks, G. (1960). *Voice and articulation drill book* (2nd ed.). New York: Harper.

Fendler, M., & Shearer, W. M. (1988). Reliability of the s/z ratio in normal children's voices. *Language, Speech, and Hearing Services in Schools, 19,* 2–4.

Finnegan, D. E. (1985). Maximum phonation time for children with normal voices. *Folia Phoniatrica, 37,* 209–215. (Reprinted as: Finnegan, D. E. [1985]. Maximum phonation time for children with normal voices. *Journal of Communication Disorders, 17,* 309–317)

Finucane, K. E., Egan, B. E., & Dawson, S. V. (1972). Linearity and frequency response of pneumotachographs. *Journal of Applied Physiology, 32,* 121–126.

Fleisch, A. (1925). Der Pneumotachograph—ein Apparat zur Beischwindigkeitregistrierung der Atemluft. *Pflügers Archiv, 209,* 713–722.

Ford, C. N., Bless, D. M., & Prehn, R. B. (1992). Thyroplasty as primary and adjunctive treatment of glottic insufficiency. *Journal of Voice, 6,* 277–285.

Fox, C. M., & Ramig, L. O. (1997). Vocal sound pressure level and self-perception of speech and voice in men and women with idiopathic Parkinson disease. *American Journal of Speech-Language Pathology, 6*(2), 85–94.

Fritzell, B., Hallén, O., & Sundberg, J. (1974). Evaluation of Teflon injection procedures for paralytic dysphonia. *Folia Phoniatrica, 26,* 414–421.

Fritzell, B., Hammarberg, B., Gauffin, J., Karlsson, I., & Sundberg, J. (1986). Breathiness and insufficient vocal fold closure. *Journal of Phonetics, 14,* 549–553.

Fry, D. L., Hyatt, R. E., McCall, C. B., & Mallos, A. J. (1957). Evaluation of three types of respiratory flowmeters. *Journal of Applied Physiology, 10,* 210–214.

Frye, R. E., & Doty, R. L. (1990). A comparison of response characteristics of airflow and pressure transducers commonly used in rhinomanometry. *IEEE Transactions on Biomedical Engineering, 37,* 937–944.

Fugl-Meyer, A. R. (1974). Relative respiratory contributions of the rib cage and the abdomen in males and females with special regard to posture. *Respiration, 31,* 240–251.

Gamboa, F. J., Nieto, A., del Palacio, A. J., Rivera, T., & Cobeta, I. (1995). El indice s/z en los defectos de cierre glotico. *Acta Otorrinolaringologica Española, 46,* 45–48.

Gamboa, J., Jiménez-Jiménez, F. J., Nieto, A., Montojo, J., Ortí-Pareja, M., Molina, J. A., García-Albea, E., & Cobeta, I. (1997). Acoustic voice analysis in patients with Parkinson's disease treated with dopaminergic drugs. *Journal of Voice, 11,* 314–320.

Gamboa, J., Jiménez-Jiménez, F. J., Nieto, A., Cobeta, I., Vegas, A., Ortí-Pareja, M., Gasalla, T., Molina, J. A., & García-Albea, E. (1998). Acoustic voice analysis in patients with essential tremor. *Journal of Voice, 12,* 444–452.

Gilbert, H. R. (1973). Oral airflow during stop consonant production. *Folia Phoniatrica, 25,* 288–301.

Gordon, M. T., Morton, M., & Simpson, I. C. (1978). Air flow measurements in diagnosis, assessment and treatment of mechanical dysphonia. *Folia Phoniatrica, 30,* 161–174.

Harden, J. R., & Looney, N. A. (1984). Duration of sustained phonation in kindergarten children. *International Journal of Pediatric Otorhinolaryngology, 7,* 11–19.

Hardy, J. C. (1961). Intraoral breath pressure in cerebral palsy. *Journal of Speech and Hearing Disorders, 26,* 309–319.

Hardy, J. C. (1965). Air flow and pressure studies. *ASHA Reports, 1,* 141–152.

Hardy, J. C. (1967). Techniques of measuring intraoral air pressure and rate of air flow. *Journal of Speech and Hearing Research, 10,* 650–654.

Hardy, J. C., & Arkebauer, H. J. (1966). Development of a test for velopharyngeal competence during speech. *Cleft Palate Journal, 3,* 6–21.

Hardy, J. C., & Edmonds, T. D. (1968). Electronic integrator for measurement of partitions of the lung volume. *Journal of Speech and Hearing Research, 11,* 777–786.

Hertegård, S., & Gauffin, J. (1992). Acoustic properties of the Rothenberg mask. *Speech Transmission Laboratory—Quarterly Progress and Status Report* (Royal Institute of Technology, Stockholm, Sweden), 2/3, 9–18.

Hillel, A. D., Yorkston, K., & Miller, R. M. (1989). Using phonation time to estimate vital capacity in amyotrophic lateral sclerosis. *Archives of Physical Medicine and Rehabilitation, 70,* 618–620.

Hippel, K., & Mrowinski, D. (1978). Untersuchung stimmgesunder und stimmkranker Personen nach der Methode der Pneumotachographie. *Hals-, Nasen-, und Ohrenheilkunde, 26,* 421–423.

Hirano, M. (1981). *Clinical examination of voice* (pp. 25–42). New York: Springer-Verlag.

Hirano, M. (1989). Objective evaluation of the human voice: Clinical aspects. *Folia Phoniatrica, 41,* 89–144.

Hirano, M., Hibi, S., Terasawa, R., & Fujiu, M. (1986). Relationship between aerodynamic, vibratory, acoustic and psychoacoustic correlates in dysphonia. *Journal of Phonetics, 14,* 445–456.

Hirano, M., Koike, Y., & Joyner, J. (1969). Style of phonation: An electromyographic investigation of some laryngeal muscles. *Archives of Otolaryngology, 89,* 902–907.

Hirano, M., Koike, Y., & von Leden, H. (1968). Maximum phonation time and air usage during phonation. *Folia Phoniatrica, 20,* 185–201.

Hirano, M., Kurita, S., & Matsuoka, H. (1987). Vocal function following hemilaryngectomy. *Annals of Otology, Rhinology and Laryngology, 96,* 586–589.

Hixon, T. J. (1966). Turbulent noise sources for speech. *Folia Phoniatrica, 19,* 168–182.

Hixon, T. J. (1972). Some new techniques for measuring the biomechanical events of speech production: One laboratory's experiences. *ASHA Reports, 7,* 68–103.

Hixon, T. J., Saxman, J. H., & McQueen, H. D. (1967). A respirometric technique for evaluating velopharyngeal competence during speech. *Folia Phoniatrica, 19,* 203–219.

Hobbes, A. F. T. (1967). A comparison of methods of calibrating the pneumotachograph. *British Journal of Anaesthesia, 39,* 899–907.

Hoit, J. D., Hixon, T. J., Altman, M. E., & Morgan, W. J. (1989). Speech breathing in women. *Journal of Speech and Hearing Research, 32,* 353–365.

Hoit, J. D., Hixon, T. J., Watson, P. J., & Morgan, W. J. (1990). Speech breathing in children and adolescents. *Journal of Speech and Hearing Research, 33,* 51–69.

Horii, Y., & Cooke, P. A. (1975). Analysis of airflow and volume during continuous speech. *Behavior Research Methods and Instrumentation, 7,* 477.

Horii, Y., & Cooke, P. A. (1978). Some airflow, volume, and duration characteristics of oral reading. *Journal of Speech and Hearing Research, 21,* 470–481.

Hoshiko, M. S. (1965). Lung volume for initiation of phonation. *Journal of Applied Physiology, 20,* 480–482.

Huber, J. E., Stathopoulos, E. T., Bormann, L. A., & Johnson, K. (1998). Effects of a circumferentially vented mask on breathing patterns of women as measured by respiratory kinematic techniques. *Journal of Speech, Language, and Hearing Research, 41,* 472–478.

Hufnagle, J., & Hufnagle, K. K. (1988). S/Z ratio in dysphonic children with and without vocal cord nodules. *Language, Speech, and Hearing Services in Schools, 19,* 418–422.

Hutchinson, J. M., & Smith, L. L. (1976). Aerodynamic functioning in consonant production by hearing impaired adults. *Audiology and Hearing Education, 2*(Dec-Jan), 16–25, 32.

Isshiki, N. (1964). Regulatory mechanism of voice intensity variation. *Journal of Speech and Hearing Research, 7,* 17–29.

Isshiki, N. (1965). Vocal intensity and air flow rate. *Folia Phoniatrica, 17,* 92–104.

Isshiki, N. (1969). Remarks on mechanism for vocal intensity variation. *Journal of Speech and Hearing Research, 12,* 665–672.

Isshiki, N. (1981). Vocal efficiency index. In K. N. Stevens & M. Hirano (Eds.), *Vocal fold physiology* (pp. 193–203). Tokyo, Japan: Tokyo University Press.

Isshiki, N., Okamura, H., & Morimoto, M. (1967). Maximum phonation time and air flow rate during phonation: Simple clinical tests for vocal function. *Annals of Otology, Rhinology and Laryngology, 76,* 998–1007.

Isshiki, N., & Ringel, R. (1964). Air flow during the production of selected consonants. *Journal of Speech and Hearing Research, 7,* 233–244.

Isshiki, N., & von Leden, H. (1964). Hoarseness: Aerodynamic studies. *Archives of Otolaryngology, 80,* 206–213.

Itoh, M., & Horii, Y. (1985). Airflow, volume, and durational characteristics of oral reading by the hearing-impaired. *Journal of Communication Disorders, 18,* 393–407.

Iwata, S. (1988). Aerodynamic aspects for phonation in normal and pathologic larynges. In O. Fujimura (Ed.), *Vocal physiology: Voice production, mechanisms, and functions* (pp. 423–431). New York: Raven Press.

Iwata, S., & von Leden, H. (1970a). Clinical evaluation of vocal velocity index in laryngeal disease. *Annals of Otology, Rhinology and Laryngology, 79,* 259–268.

Iwata, S., & von Leden, H. (1970b). Phonation quotient in patients with laryngeal diseases. *Folia Phoniatrica, 22,* 117–128.

Iwata, S., von Leden, H., & Williams, D. (1972). Air flow measurement during phonation. *Journal of Communication Disorders, 5,* 67–79.

Jackson, A. C., & Vinegar, A. (1979). A technique for measuring frequency response of pressure, volume, and flow transducers. *Journal of Applied Physiology, 47,* 462–467.

Johnson, T. S. (1985). Voice disorders: The measurement of clinical progress. In J. M. Costello (Ed.), *Speech disorders in adults: Recent advances* (pp. 127–152). San Diego, CA: College-Hill Press.

Kelman, A. W., Gordon, M. T., Simpson, I. C., & Morton, F. M. (1975). Assessment of vocal function by air-flow measurements. *Folia Phoniatrica, 27,* 250–262.

Kent, R. D., Kent, J. F., & Rosenbek, J. C. (1987). Maximum performance tests of speech production. *Journal of Speech and Hearing Disorders, 52,* 367–387.

Kent, R. D., Sufit, R. L., Rosenbek, J. C., Kent, J. F., Weismer, G., Martin, R. E., & Brooks, B. R. (1991). Speech deterioration in amyotrophic lateral sclerosis: A case study. *Journal of Speech and Hearing Research, 34,* 1269–1275.

Kitajima, K., & Fujita, F. (1992). An airflow study of pathologic larynges using a constant temperature anemometer: Further experience. *Annals of Otology, Rhinology and Laryngology, 101,* 675–678.

Klatt, D. H., Stevens, K. N., & Mead, J. (1968). Studies of articulatory activity and airflow during speech. *Annals of the New York Academy of Sciences, 155,* 42–55.

Koike, Y. (1967). Experimental studies on vocal attack. *Practica Otologica Kyoto, 60,* 663–688.

Koike, Y., & Hirano, M. (1968). Significance of vocal velocity index. *Folia Phoniatrica, 20,* 285–296.

Koike, Y., Hirano, M., & von Leden, H. (1967). Vocal initiation: Acoustic and aerodynamic investigations of normal subjects. *Folia Phoniatrica, 19,* 173–182.

Konno, K., & Mead, J. (1967). Measurements of the separate volume changes of rib cage and abdomen during breathing. *Journal of Applied Physiology, 22,* 407–422.

Kotby, M. N., Shiromoto, O., & Hirano, M. (1993). The accent method of voice therapy: Effect of accentuations on F0, SPL, and airflow. *Journal of Voice, 7,* 319–325.

Kreul, E. J. (1972). Neuromuscular control examination (NMC) for Parkinsonism: Vowel prolongations and diadochokinetic and reading rates. *Journal of Speech and Hearing Research, 15,* 72–83.

LaBlance, G. R., & Maves, M. D. (1992). Acoustic characteristics of post-thyroplasty patients. *Otolaryngology—Head and Neck Surgery, 107,* 558–563.

Ladefoged, P., & Maddieson, I. (1996). *The sounds of the world's languages.* Cambridge, MA: Blackwell.

LaPointe, L. L., Case, J. L., & Duane, D. D. (1994). Perceptual-acoustic speech and voice characteristics of subjects with spasmodic torticollis. In J. A. Till, K. M. Yorkston, & D. R. Beukelman (Eds.), *Motor speech disorders: Advances in assess-*

ment and treatment (pp. 57–64). Baltimore, MD: Paul H. Brookes.

Larson, G. W., Mueller, P. B., & Summers, P. A. (1991). The effect of procedural variations on the s/z ratio. *Journal of Communication Disorders, 24,* 135–140.

Leeper, H. A., Gagne, J.-P., Parnes, L. S., & Vidas, S. (1993). Aerodynamic assessment of the speech of adults undergoing multichannel cochlear implantation. *Annals of Otology, Rhinology, and Laryngology, 102,* 294–302.

Leeper, H. A., Millard, K. M., Bandur, D. L., & Hudson, A. J. (1996). An investigation of deterioration of vocal function in subgroups of individuals with ALS. *Journal of Medical Speech-Language Pathology, 4,* 163–181.

Lehman, J. J., Bless, D. M., & Brandenburg, J. H. (1988). An objective assessment of voice production after radiation therapy for Stage I squamous cell carcinoma of the glottis. *Otolaryngology—Head and Neck Surgery, 98,* 121–129.

Leiter, J. C., & Baker, G. L. (1989). Partitioning of ventilation between nose and mouth: The role of nasal resistance. *American Journal of Orthodontics and Dentofacial Orthopedics, 95,* 432–438.

Levitzky, M. G. (1995). *Pulmonary physiology* (4th ed.). New York: McGraw-Hill.

Lewis, K., Casteel, R., & McMahon, J. (1982). Duration of sustained /ɑ/ related to the number of trials. *Folia Phoniatrica, 34,* 41–48.

Lockhart, M. S., Paton, F., & Pearson, L. (1997). Targets and timescales: A study of dysphonia using objective assessment. *Logopedics Phonology Vocology, 22,* 15–24.

Löfqvist, A. (1992). Aerodynamic measurements of vocal function. In A. Blitzer, M. F. Brin, C. T. Sasaki, S. Fahn, S., & K. S. Harris (Eds.), *Neurologic disorders of the larynx* (pp. 98–107). New York: Thieme Medical Publishers.

Löfqvist, A., & McGarr, N. S. (1987). Laryngeal dynamics in voiceless consonant production. In T. Baer, C. Sasaki, & K. S. Harris (Eds.), *Laryngeal function in phonation and respiration* (pp. 391–402). Boston, MA: Little, Brown.

Löfqvist, A., & McGowan, R. S. (1991). Voice source variations in running speech. In J. Gauffin & B. Hammarberg (Eds.), *Vocal fold physiology: Acoustic, perceptual, and physiological aspects of voice mechanisms* (pp. 113–120). San Diego, CA: Singular Publishing Group.

Löfqvist, A., & McGowan, R. S. (1992). Influence of consonantal environment on voice source aerodynamics. *Journal of Phonetics, 20,* 93–110.

Löfqvist, A., & Yoshioka, H. (1984). Intrasegmental timing: Laryngeal-oral coordination in voiceless consonant production. *Speech Communication, 3,* 279–289.

Lotz, W. K., D'Antonio, L. L., Chait, D. H., & Netsell, R. W. (1993). Successful nasoendoscopic and aerodynamic examinations of children with speech/voice disorders. *International Journal of Pediatric Otorhinolaryngology, 26,* 165–172.

Lubker, J. F. (1970). Aerodynamic and ultrasonic assessment techniques in speech-dentofacial research. *ASHA Reports, 5,* 207–223.

Lubker, J. F., & Moll, K. L. (1965). Simultaneous oral-nasal air flow measurements and cinefluorographic observations during speech production. *Cleft Palate Journal, 2,* 257–272.

Madison, C. L., & Seikel, J. A. (1990). Reliability or difference? A comment on the reliability of the s/z ratio. *Language, Speech, and Hearing Services in Schools, 21,* 60.

McCurrach, G., Evans, A. L., Smith, D. C., Gordon, M. T., & Cooke, M. B. D. (1991). Real-time air flow measurement system for use by speech therapists. *Medical and Biological Engineering and Computing, 29,* 98–101.

McFarlane, S. C., Watterson, T. L., Lewis, K., & Boone, D. R. (1998). Effect of voice therapy facilitation techniques on airflow in unilateral paralysis patients. *Phonoscope, 1,* 187–191.

McGlone, R. E. (1967). Air flow during vocal fry phonation. *Journal of Speech and Hearing Research, 10,* 299–304.

McGlone, R. E. (1970). Air flow in the upper register. *Folia Phoniatrica, 22,* 231–238.

McGlone, R. E., & Shipp, T. (1971). Some physiological correlates of vocal fry phonation. *Journal of Speech and Hearing Research, 14,* 769–775.

Mead, J. (1960). Volume displacement body plethysmograph for respiratory measurements in human speech. *Journal of Applied Physiology, 15,* 736–740.

Mead, J., Peterson, N., Grimby, G., & Mead, J. (1967). Pulmonary ventilation measured from body surface movements. *Science, 156,* 1383–1384.

Micco, A. J. (1973). A sensitive flow direction sensor. *Journal of Applied Physiology, 35,* 420–422.

Miller, C. J., & Daniloff, R. (1993). Airflow measurements: Theory and utility of findings. *Journal of Voice, 7,* 38–46.

Miller, M. R., & Pincock, A. C. (1986). Linearity and temperature control of the Fleisch pneumotachograph. *Journal of Applied Physiology, 60,* 710–715.

Morsomme, D., Jamart, J., Boucquey, D., & Remacle, M. (1997). Presbyphonia: Voice differences between the sexes in the elderly. Comparison by maximum phonation time, phonation quotient and spectral analysis. *Logopedics Phonology Vocology, 22,* 9–14.

Mueller, P. B. (1971). Parkinson's disease: Motor-speech behavior in a selected group of patients. *Folia Phoniatrica, 23,* 333–346.

Mueller, P. B. (1982). Voice characteristics of octogenerian and nonagenerian persons. *Ear, Nose, and Throat Journal, 61,* 204–207.

Murry, T. (1971). Subglottal pressure and airflow measures during vocal fry phonation. *Journal of Speech and Hearing Research, 14,* 544–551.

Murry, T., & Bone, R. C. (1978). Aerodynamic relationships associated with normal phonation and paralytic dysphonia. *Laryngoscope, 88,* 100–109.

Murry, T., Bone, R. C., & Von Essen, C. (1974). Changes in voice production during radiotherapy for laryngeal cancer. *Journal of Speech and Hearing Disorders, 39,* 194–201.

Murry, T., & Schmitke, L. K. (1975). Air flow onset and variability. *Folia Phoniatrica, 27,* 401–409.

Murry, T., & Woodson, G. E. (1995). Combined-modality treatment of adductor spasmodic dysphonia with botulinum toxin and voice therapy. *Journal of Voice, 9,* 460–465.

Murty, G. E., Lancaster, P., & Kelly, P. J. (1991). Cough intensity in patients with a vocal cord palsy. *Clinical Otolaryngology, 16,* 248–251.

Neiman, G. S., & Edeson B. (1981). Procedural aspects of eliciting maximum phonation time. *Folia Phoniatrica, 33,* 285–293.

Nihalani, P. (1975). Air flow rate in the production of stops in Sindhi. *Phonetica, 31,* 198–205.

Omori, K., Slavit, D. H., Kacker, A., & Blaugrund, S. M. (1996). Quantitative criteria for predicting thyroplasty type I outcome. *Laryngoscope, 106,* 689–693.

Orlikoff, R. F., & Baken, R. J. (1993). *Clinical speech and voice measurement: Laboratory exercises.* San Diego, CA: Singular Publishing Group.

Orlikoff, R. F., Baken, R. J., & Kraus, D. H. (1997). Acoustic and physiologic characteristics of inspiratory phonation. *Journal of the Acoustical Society of America, 102,* 1838–1845.

Ower, R., & Pankhurst, R. C. (1977). *The measurement of air flow.* Oxford: Pergamon Press.

Paynter, E. T. (1991). Phonatory function analyzer. *Seminars in Speech and Language, 12,* 98–107.

Pedersen, M. F. (1995). Stimmfunktion vor und nach Behandlung von Hirngeschädigten. Mit Stroboskopie, Phonetographie und Luftstromanalyse durchgeführt. *Sprache Stimme Gehör, 19,* 84–89.

Peppard, R. C., Bless, D. M., & Milenkovic, P. (1988). Comparison of young adult singers and nonsingers with vocal nodules. *Journal of Voice, 2,* 250–260.

Perkins, W. H. (1985). Assessment and treatment of voice disorders: State of the art. In J. M. Costello (Ed.), *Speech disorders in adults: Recent advances* (pp. 79–111). San Diego, CA: College-Hill Press.

Prathanee, B., Watthanathon, J., & Ruangjirachuporn, P. (1994). Phonation time, phonation volume and air flow rate in normal adults. *Journal of the Medical Association of Thailand, 77,* 639–645.

Ptacek, P. H., & Sander, E. K. (1963a). Maximum duration of phonation. *Journal of Speech and Hearing Disorders, 28,* 171–182.

Ptacek, P. H., & Sander, E. K. (1963b). Breathiness and phonation length. *Journal of Speech and Hearing Disorders, 28,* 267–272.

Ptacek, P. H., Sander, E. K., Maloney, W. H., & Jackson, C. C. (1966). Phonatory and related changes with advanced age. *Journal of Speech and Hearing Research, 9,* 353–360.

Quigley, L. F., Jr., Shiere, F. R., Webster, R. C., & Cobb, C. M. (1964). Measuring palatopharyngeal competence with the nasal anemometer. *Cleft Palate Journal, 1,* 303–314.

Quigley, L. F., Jr., Webster, R. C., Coffey, R. J., Kelleher, R. E., & Grant, H. P. (1963). Velocity and volume measurements of nasal and oral airflow in normal and cleft palate speech utilizing a warm-wire flowmeter and two-channel recorder. 2. *Journal of Dental Research, 42,* 1520–1527.

Raes, J. P. F., & Clement, P. A. R. (1996). Aerodynamic measurements of voice production. *Acta Oto-Rhino-Laryngologica Belgica, 50,* 293–298.

Ramig, L. A. (1986). Acoustic analyses of phonation in patients with Huntington's disease. *Annals of Otology, Rhinology and Laryngology, 95,* 288–293.

Ramig, L. A., Scherer, R. C., Klasner, E. R., Titze, I. R., & Horii, Y. (1990). Acoustic analysis of voice in amyotrophic lateral sclerosis. *Journal of Speech and Hearing Disorders, 55,* 2–14.

Rammage, L. A., Peppard, R. C., & Bless, D. M. (1992). Aerodynamic, laryngoscopic, and perceptual-acoustic characteristics in dysphonic females with posterior glottal chinks: A retrospective study. *Journal of Voice, 6,* 64–78.

Rastatter, M. P., & Hyman, M. (1982). Maximum phoneme duration of /s/ and /z/ by children with vocal nodules. *Language, Speech, and Hearing Services in Schools, 13,* 197–199.

Rau, D., & Beckett, R. L. (1984). Aerodynamic assessment of vocal function using hand-held spirometers. *Journal of Speech and Hearing Disorders, 49,* 183–188.

Reich, A. R., Mason, J. A., & Polen, S. B. (1986). Task administration variables affecting phonation-time measures in third-grade girls with normal voice quality. *Language, Speech, and Hearing Services in Schools, 17,* 262–269.

Reich, A. R., & McHenry, M. A. (1987). Respiratory volumes in cheerleaders with a history of dysphonic episodes. *Folia Phoniatrica, 39,* 71–77.

Reich, A. R., & McHenry, M. A. (1990). Estimating respiratory volumes from rib cage and abdominal displacements during ventilatory and speech activities. *Journal of Speech and Hearing Research, 33,* 467–475.

Rothenberg, M. (1973). A new inverse-filtering technique for deriving the glottal waveform during voicing. *Journal of the Acoustical Society of America, 53,* 1632–1645.

Rothenberg, M. (1977). Measurement of airflow in speech. *Journal of Speech and Hearing Research, 20,* 155–176.

Ruscello, D. M., Shuster, L. I., & Sandwisch, A. (1991). Modification of context-specific nasal emission. *Journal of Speech and Hearing Research, 34,* 27–32.

Russell, N. K., & Stathopoulos, E. (1988). Lung volume changes in children and adults during speech production. *Journal of Speech and Hearing Research, 31,* 146–155.

Sackner, J. D., Nixon, A. J., Davis, B., Atkins, N., & Sackner, M. A. (1980). Noninvasive measurement of ventilation during exercise using a respiratory inductive plethysmograph. *American Review of Respiratory Disease, 122,* 867–871.

Sackner, M. A. (1980). Monitoring of ventilation without a physical connection to the airway. In M. A. Sackner (Ed.), *Diagnostic techniques in pulmonary disease* (Part 1, pp. 503–537). New York: Dekker.

Sawashima, M., Niimi, S., Horiguchi, S., & Yamaguchi, H. (1988). Expiratory lung pressure, airflow rate, and vocal intensity: Data on normal subjects. In O. Fujimura (Ed.), *Vocal physiology: Voice production, mechanisms, and functions* (pp. 415–422). New York: Raven Press.

Schmidt, P., Klingholz, F., & Martin, F. (1988). Influence of pitch, voice sound pressure, and vowel quality on the maximum phonation time. *Journal of Voice, 2,* 245–249.

Schutte, H. K. (1992). Integrated aerodynamic measurements. *Journal of Voice, 6,* 127–134.

Schutte, H. K. (1996). *The efficiency of voice production: An aerodynamic study of normals, patients and singers* (2nd ed.). San Diego, CA: Singular Publishing Group.

Scully, C. (1971). A comparison of /s/ and /z/ for an English speaker. *Language and Speech, 14,* 187–200.

Scully, C., Castelli, E., Brearley, E., & Shirt, M. (1992). Analysis and simulation of a speaker's aerodynamic and acoustic patterns for fricatives. *Journal of Phonetics, 20,* 39–51.

Shanks, S. J., & Mast, D. (1977). Maximum duration of phonation: Objective tool for assessment of voice. *Perceptual and Motor Skills, 45,* 1315–1322.

Sharp, J. T., Goldberg, N., Druz, W. S., & Danon, J. (1976). Relative contributions of rib cage and abdomen to breathing in normal subjects. *Journal of Applied Physiology, 39,* 608–618.

Shearer, W. M. (1983). S/Z ratio for detection of vocal nodules. In *Proceedings of the XIXth Congress of the International Association of Logopedics and Phoniatrics* (4 pp.). Edinburgh, UK: IALP.

Shearer, W. M. (1990). Reply to comment on the reliability of the s/z ratio in normal children's voices. *Language, Speech, and Hearing Services in Schools, 21,* 61.

Smith, S. (1960). The electro aerometer. *Speech Pathology and Therapy, 3,* 27–33.

Soman, B. (1997). The effect of variations in method of elicitation on maximum sustained phoneme duration. *Journal of Voice, 11,* 285–294.

Sorensen, D. N., & Parker, P. A. (1992). The voiced/voiceless phonation time in children with and without laryngeal pathology. *Language, Speech, and Hearing Services in Schools, 23,* 163–168.

Stagg, D., Goldman, M., & Newsom-Davis, J. (1978). Computer-aided measurement of breath volume and time components using magnetometers. *Journal of Applied Physiology, 44,* 623–633.

Stathopoulos, E. T. (1980). *A normative air flow study of children and adults using a circumferentially-vented pneumotachograph mask.* Unpublished doctoral dissertation, Indiana University, Bloomington, IN.

Stathopoulos, E. T. (1985). Effects of monitoring vocal intensity on oral air flow in children and adults. *Journal of Speech and Hearing Research, 28,* 589–593.

Stathopoulos, E. T., & Weismer, G. (1985). Oral airflow and air pressure during speech production: A comparative study of children, youths and adults. *Folia Phoniatrica, 37,* 152–159.

Stemple, J. C., Stanley, J., & Lee, L. (1995). Objective measures of voice production in normal subjects following prolonged voice use. *Journal of Voice, 9,* 127–133.

Stevens, K. N. (1971). Airflow and turbulence noise for fricative and stop consonants: Static considerations. *Journal of the Acoustical Society of America, 50,* 1180–1192.

Stevens, K. N. (1991). Vocal-fold vibration for obstruent consonants. In J. Gauffin & B. Hammarberg (Eds.), *Vocal fold physiology: Acoustic, perceptual, and physiological aspects of voice mechanisms* (pp. 29–36). San Diego, CA: Singular Publishing Group.

Stone, R. E., Jr. (1983). Issues in clinical assessment of laryngeal function: Contraindications for subscribing to maximum phonation time and optimum fundamental frequency. In D. M. Bless & J. H. Abbs (Eds.), *Vocal fold physiology: Contemporary research and clinical issues* (pp. 410–424). San Diego, CA: College-Hill Press.

Subtelny, J., Kho, G., McCormack, R. M., & Subtelny, J. D. (1969). Multidimensional analysis of bilabial stop and nasal consonants—cineradiographic and pressure-flow analysis. *Cleft Palate Journal, 6,* 263–289.

Subtelny, J. D., Worth, J. H., & Sakuda, M. (1966). Intraoral pressure and rate of flow during speech. *Journal of Speech and Hearing Research, 9,* 498–519.

Sullivan, W. J., Peters, G. M., & Enright, P. L. (1984). Pneumotachographs: Theory and clinical application. *Respiratory Care, 29,* 736–749.

Tait, N. A., Michel, J. F., & Carpenter, M. A. (1980). Maximum duration of sustained /s/ and /z/ in children. *Journal of Speech and Hearing Disorders, 45,* 239–246.

Tanaka, S., & Gould, W. J. (1985). Vocal efficiency and aerodynamic aspects in voice disorders. *Annals of Otology, Rhinology and Laryngology, 94,* 29–33.

Tanaka, S., Hirano, M., & Terasawa, R. (1991). Examination of air usage during phonation: Correlations among test parameters. *Journal of Voice, 5,* 106–112.

Terasawa, R., Hibi, S. R., & Hirano, M. (1987). Mean airflow rates during phonation over a comfortable duration and maximum sustained phonation. Results from 60 normal adult subjects. *Folia Phoniatrica, 39,* 87–89.

Till, J. A., Jafari, M., Crumley, R. L., & Law-Till, C. B. (1992). Effects of initial consonant, pneumotachographic mask, and oral pressure tube on vocal perturbation, harmonics-to-noise, and intensity measurements. *Journal of Voice, 6,* 217–223.

Treole, K., & Trudeau, M. D. (1997). Changes in sustained production tasks among women with bilateral vocal nodules before and after voice therapy. *Journal of Voice, 11,* 462–469.

Trudeau, M. D., & Forrest, L. A. (1997). The contributions of phonatory volume and transglottal airflow to the s/z ratio. *American Journal of Speech-Language Pathology, 6*(1), 65–69.

Trullinger, R. W., & Emanuel, F. W. (1983). Airflow characteristics of stop-plosive consonant productions of normal-speaking children. *Journal of Speech and Hearing Research, 26,* 202–208.

Trullinger, R. W., & Emanuel, F. W. (1989). Airflow, volume, and duration characteristics of sustained vowel production of normal-speaking children. *Folia Phoniatrica, 41,* 297–307.

Turney, S. Z., & Blumenfeld, W. (1973). Heated Fleisch pneumotachometer: A calibration procedure. *Journal of Applied Physiology, 34,* 117–121.

van den Berg, Jw. (1962). Modern research in experimental phoniatrics. *Folia Phoniatrica, 14,* 81–149.

van Hattum, R., & Worth, J. H. (1967). Air flow rates in normal speakers. *Cleft Palate Journal, 4,* 137–147.

van Lieshout, P. H. H. M., Hulstijn, W., & Peters, H. F. M. (1996). Speech production in people who stutter: Testing the motor plan assembly hypothesis. *Journal of Speech and Hearing Research, 39,* 76–92.

Vavares, M. A., Montgomery, W. W., & Hillman, R. E. (1995). Teflon granuloma of the larynx: Etiology, pathophysiology, and management. *Annals of Otology, Rhinology and Laryngology, 104,* 511–515.

Vick, R. L. (1984). *Contemporary medical physiology.* Menlo Park, CA: Addison-Wesley.

Von Doersten, P. G., Izdebski, K., Ross, J. C., & Cruz, R. M. (1992). Ventricular dysphonia: A profile of 40 cases. *Laryngoscope, 102,* 1296–1301.

von Leden, H. (1968). Objective measures of laryngeal function and phonation. *Annals of the New York Academy of Sciences, 155,* 56–67.

von Leden, H., Yanagihara, N., & Werner-Kukuk, E. (1967). Teflon in unilateral vocal cord paralysis. *Archives of Otolaryngology, 85,* 110–118.

Warren, D. W. (1976). Aerodynamics of speech production. In N. J. Lass (Ed.), *Contemporary issues in experimental phonetics* (pp. 105–137). New York: Academic Press.

Warren, D. W. (1996). Regulation of speech aerodynamics. In Lass, N. J. (Ed.), *Principles of experimental phonetics* (pp. 46–92). St. Louis: Mosby.

Warren, D. W., & Wood, M. T. (1969). Respiratory volumes in normal speech: A possible reason for intraoral pressure differences among voiced and voiceless consonants. *Journal of the Acoustical Society of America, 45,* 466–469.

Watson, B. C., & Alfonso, P. J. (1991). Noninvasive instrumentation in the treatment of stuttering. In D. Vogel & M. P. Cannito (Eds.), *Treating disordered speech motor control: For clinicians by clinicians* (pp. 319–340). Austin, TX: Pro-Ed.

Weng, T., & Levison, H. (1969). Standards of pulmonary function in children. *American Review of Respiratory Disease, 99,* 879–894.

Werner-Kukuk, E., von Leden, H., & Yanagihara, N. (1968). The effects of radiation therapy on laryngeal function. *Journal of Laryngology and Otology, 82,* 1–15.

Whitehead, R. L., & Barefoot, S. M. (1983). Airflow characteristics of fricative consonants produced by normally hearing and hearing-impaired speakers. *Journal of Speech and Hearing Research, 26,* 185–194.

Wilson, F. B., & Starr, C. D. (1985). Use of the phonation analyzer as a clinical tool. *Journal of Speech and Hearing Disorders, 50,* 351–356.

Woo, P., Casper, J., Colton, R., & Brewer, D. (1994). Aerodynamic and stroboscopic findings before and after microlaryngeal phonosurgery. *Journal of Voice, 8,* 186–194.

Woo, P., Colton, R., Casper, J., & Brewer, D. (1992). Analysis of spasmodic dysphonia by aerodynamic and laryngostroboscopic measurements. *Journal of Voice, 6,* 344–351.

Woo, P., Colton, R. H., & Shangold, L. (1987). Phonatory airflow analysis in patients with laryngeal disease. *Annals of Otology, Rhinology and Laryngology, 96,* 549–555.

Woodson, G. E., Rosen, C. A., Murry, T., Madasu, R., Wong, F., Hengesteg, A., & Robbins, K. T. (1996). Assessing vocal function after chemoradiation for advanced laryngeal carcinoma. *Archives of Otolaryngology—Head and Neck Surgery, 122,* 858–864.

Yanagihara, N. (1970). Aerodynamic examination of the laryngeal function. *Studia Phonologica, 5,* 45–51.

Yanagihara, N., & Koike, Y. (1967). The regulation of sustained phonation. *Folia Phoniatrica, 19,* 1–18.

Yanagihara, N., Koike, Y., & von Leden, H. (1966). Phonation and respiration: Function study in normal subjects. *Folia Phoniatrica, 18,* 323–340.

Yanagihara, N., & von Leden (1967). Respiration and phonation: The functional examination of laryngeal disease. *Folia Phoniatrica, 19,* 153–166.

Yeh, M. P., Gardner, R. M., Adams, T. D., & Yanowitz, F. G. (1982). Computerized determination of pneumotachometer characteristics using a calibrated syringe. *Journal of Applied Physiology, 53,* 280–285.

Yoshiya, I., Nakajima, T., Nagai, I., & Jitsukawa, S. (1975). A bidirectional respiratory flowmeter using the hot-wire principle. *Journal of Applied Physiology, 38,* 360–365.

Young, M. (1982). *Acoustic and aerodynamic correlates of age-related voice changes.* Unpublished master's thesis, University of Wisconsin, Madison, WI.

Young, M., & Bless, D. M. (1983). Relation of physical condition to age-related voice changes. *Proceedings of the XIXth Congress of the International Association of Logopedics and Phoniatrics.* Edinburgh, UK: IALP.

10

Laryngeal Function

Evaluation of dysphonia and of problems of vocal control is a complex undertaking (Hirano, 1981; Feudo, 1984; Kelly, 1984; Sundberg, 1987; Isshiki, 1989; Baken, 1991; Titze, 1994; Colton & Casper, 1996; Orlikoff & Kahane, 1996; Baken & Orlikoff, 1997; Harris, Harris, Rubin, & Howard, 1998; Andrews, 1999). It must include careful observation of the phonatory performance of the larynx and, in particular, of the vocal folds. Other, more indirect, means of assessment, including aerodynamic, spectrographic, intensity, and fundamental frequency evaluation also provide a great deal of useful information upon which inferences can be based and they are critically important.

This chapter explores several techniques currently available for obtaining information about the exact function of the larynx, including photographic, photoelectric, impedance, and acoustic methods. The value of these techniques to the therapist lies in their ability to provide a close-up view of the relatively fine details of the movement and contact patterns of the vocal folds themselves. In other words, these methods offer the means for watching the abnormal activity which is the real target of therapy and which may change before the perceptual aspects of voice do. In cases of unilateral paralysis, for example, the degree to which the normal vocal fold is managing to effectuate a compensatory displacement can easily be estimated long before final success results in a clear vocal signal. Thus, progress can be evaluated throughout the course of therapy. Several of the techniques to be discussed below also lend themselves to biofeedback approaches to vocal rehabilitation, and so they can be used as both diagnostic and therapeutic tools.

VISUALIZATION OF VOCAL FOLD MOVEMENT

In the final analysis, the only way to know what the larynx is actually doing is to look at it more or less directly. Laryngeal observation is also the only way to rule out specific structural or functional pathologies. Not very long ago laryngoscopy was a task left solely to the physician, whose role it is to detect tissue abnormality and evaluate functional deficits that are amenable to medicosurgical intervention. But the procedure is now routinely done by speech pathologists (at least in the United States), to whom commonly falls the task of remediating abnormal laryngeal functions (perhaps including those that led to tissue pathology in the first place). The need for careful observation and documentation by the voice rehabilitation specialist has been strengthened as our understanding of the relationship between vocal fold action and the final acoustic product has improved (Broad, 1973, 1979;

Titze, 1973, 1974, 1976, 1984, 1985; Hirano, 1974, 1975, 1977; Titze & Talkin, 1979; Baer, 1981; Baer, Titze, & Yoshioka, 1983; Isshiki, 1989).

What is wanted, in most cases, is an accurate assessment of the phonatory behavior at the glottal level. There are, in addition to laryngoscopy, many ways of obtaining this information. These can, and should, be part of the vocal therapist's diagnostic armamentarium. In general, the needed information can be obtained from what might be termed "glottographic waveforms": changes in any one of a number of variables that can be related to activity at the level of the vocal folds. Examples of such data include the glottal area function, glottal pressure waveform, glottal volume velocity, and electroglottogram. (Titze and Talkin, 1981, provide a brief, but excellent, overview of the relationship among these.)

While perhaps useful for detecting gross abnormalities of structure and position, simple indirect laryngoscopy cannot provide much information about vocal fold vibration. At the speeds characteristic of phonation, the moving edge of the vocal fold appears as a blur to the unaided eye. There are two fundamentally different ways in which the problem may be solved: high-speed cinematography—digital or analog —and stroboscopy. Both approaches, however, require that the larynx be illuminated by a bright light source and that there be a line-of-sight from the larynx to the outside. That is, before anything else, one must be able to see the larynx and it must reflect enough light to permit photography or video recording.

The basic elements of the simplest system for visualizing and photographing the functioning of the larynx are shown in Figure 10–1. An intense beam of light is reflected through a mirror onto a second, laryngeal, mirror. The observer (or a motion picture or TV camera) sees the larynx through an aperture in the first mirror. Incandescent light sources tend to produce a great deal of radiation in the infrared region of the spectrum. Some form of filtering must be used to eliminate this light, or excessive heating of the larynx may result (possibly entailing serious damage). This kind of observation system is relatively inexpensive and, from a technological point of view, quite easy to set up. It is even possible to attach the perforated mirror to the end of the camera lens (Ferguson & Crowder, 1970) to create a very simple photographic system.

Sophisticated work, however, requires better illumination methods that may entail considerable technological complexity. One relatively simple enhancement, however, requires only that the larynx be illuminated from below by a white light source applied to the pretracheal region while, from above, the larynx is illuminated by a blue light (Hess, Ludwigs, Gross, & Orglmeister; 1997; Ludwigs, Hess, Gross, & Orglmeis-

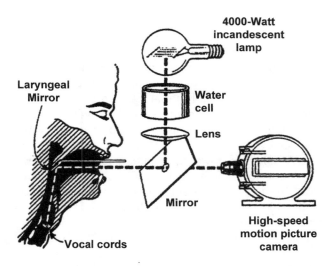

Figure 10–1. Simple arrangement for laryngeal photography. From *Speech and Hearing in Communication* (Figure 14, p. 18), by H. Fletcher, 1953, Princeton, NJ: van Nostrand. Reprinted by permission.

ter, 1997). Because the vibrating medial edges of the vocal folds are generally quite thin in the vertical dimension, they transmit the light shining up from the trachea. They therefore appear red, in contrast to the surrounding blue structures. This allows an evaluation of their shape and the extent of thinning, providing clinically-important information about oscillatory control.

Cinematography

Motion pictures of the functioning vocal folds provide an excellent means of evaluating the details of glottal function. Relatively fast filming (at about 50 frames per second) provides sufficient "slow motion" to determine many of the details of laryngeal articulatory behavior. Using ultrahigh speeds (that is, greater than 4,000 frames per second) allows the finer aspects of vocal fold motion during each vibratory cycle to be explored at a speed reduction of 1:250 or more when the film is viewed with a standard projector. The production and analysis of ultrahigh-speed films is not easy, and it requires much more complex instrumentation than the simple system of Figure 10–1 might suggest. But the extra effort (and expense) was occasionally deemed justified in settings that dealt with a large volume of difficult vocal rehabilitation cases.

Newer methods of observing the phonating larynx have made laryngeal cinematography unnecessary in clinical practice. But the cinematographic methods are worth examining because they produced an important corpus of research literature (upon which much of

our understanding of phonation rests) and because the problems that they addressed are the same problems that have motivated the compromises upon which current observational techniques are based. Paul Moore, a pioneer in ultrahigh-speed laryngeal filming, is shown in Figure 10–2 as he obtains images of his own vocal fold activity for later analysis.

ULTRAHIGH-SPEED PHOTOGRAPHY

Ultrahigh-speed laryngeal photography, done at an exposure rate of more than 4,000 frames per second (fps), was developed at Bell Telephone Laboratories (Bell Telephone Laboratories, 1937; Farnsworth, 1940). It was being used to quantify vocal fold movement just a few years later (Brackett, 1948). The technique is expensive, in terms of the requisite equipment and operating costs. Film analysis—even if partly assisted by computer technology—is tedious and time-consuming. It could not, therefore, ever have been a preferred approach to the evaluation of most cases. On the other hand, early workers found that

> there is often a puzzling disproportion between subjective symptoms and objective findings during a routine laryngoscopic examination. Many patients with moderate or severe voice changes present little visible evidence in the larynx to explain their vocal abnormalities. In these cases, ultra high speed photography of the larynx often discloses physiologic

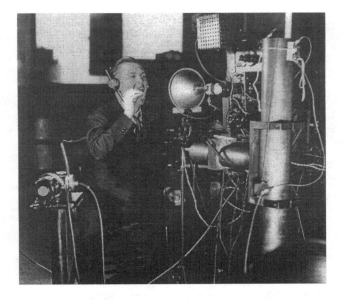

Figure 10–2. Instrumentation used in early attempts to use ultrahigh-speed filming to visualize vocal fold behavior during phonation. From *Flash! Seeing the Unseen by Ultra High-speed Photography*, H. E. Edgerton and J. R. Killian, Jr., 1939, Boston, MA: Hale, Cushman, & Flint.

variations in the vibratory patterns which account for the acoustic manifestations. This diagnostic information has also proved of value in the determination of treatment and in supervision of the indicated therapeutic measures. (Moore, White, & von Leden, 1962, p. 167)

Ordinary camera shutter and film-transport mechanisms are simply incapable of the speeds required for ultrahigh-speed work. The shutter is therefore replaced by a rotating prism that, as it turns, projects successive images onto the continuously-moving film. The very short exposure time requires an extremely bright light source if there is to be adequate exposure of the film. Meeting this need entailed significant improvements in photographic light sources.

Figure 10–3 schematizes a modern, more sophisticated illumination system developed by Metz, Whitehead, and Peterson (1980). In this arrangement, the light source is a 300 W xenon arc lamp, equipped with ultraviolet filters, that produces bursts of very intense light, adequate for film speeds up to 6,000 fps. On its way to the laryngeal mirror the light beam encounters three special "cold" mirrors that remove more than 90% of the infrared radiation. The noise of the camera is controlled by locating it in a separate soundproof room and filming through a window.

The advantages gained by the very high frame rate are significant. Consider, for example a larynx phonating at 100 Hz. Each glottal cycle lasts 10 ms. Standard film speed is 16 fps, meaning that 62.5 ms elapses from the start of one frame to the start of the next. In this period, more than 6 glottal cycles will have occurred. Furthermore, the camera shutter is open for a significant portion of the frame-to-frame period—certainly long enough for a full glottal cycle to be completed. The record on the standard-speed film will therefore be just as much a smear as the blur seen by the unaided eye.

At 4,000 fps, however, the situation is very different. The frame-to-frame interval is only 1/4 ms, which provides 40 successive exposures during each 10 ms period of the 100 Hz phonation. The high-speed "shutter" is open about 40% of the time, or about 0.1 ms, so there is relatively little blurring of the picture. When the film is viewed at the standard projector speed of 16 fps vocal fold motion is slowed by a factor of 250. The 10 ms glottal cycle takes 2,500 ms when projected, and fine details of vocal fold displacements are observable. If the vocal F_0 is, let us say, 250 Hz (approximately that of the average woman), only 16 exposures will be made during each glottal cycle. This is not as good, although there will still be quite a bit of movement detail. As the F_0 rises it may be necessary to increase filming speed. Cameras are available that can expose more than 8,000 fps.

Ultrahigh-speed photography using a laryngeal mirror has proven to be an extraordinary means of getting information about vocal function. Many improvements and modifications of the original technique have been made to overcome limitations or to meet special requirements (Rubin & LeCover, 1960; von Leden, LeCover, Ringel, & Isshiki, 1966; Soron, 1967; Hirano, Yoshida, Matsushita, & Nakajima, 1974; Metz & Whitehead, 1982). While perhaps superseded in its utility in most circumstances, there remain both research and special clinical situations in which ultrahigh-speed cinematography still has much to offer.

DIGITAL HIGH-SPEED IMAGING

Advances in solid-state electronics, in digital processing, and in integrated circuit fabrication have made it possible to build very much faster video cameras. Although none can yet match the speeds attainable by film-based cinematography, in some cases true high-speed frame rates have been achieved. Beginning in the mid–1980s, Kiritani, Hirose, and their associates (Imagawa, Kiritani, & Hirose, 1984; Honda, Kiritani, Imagawa, & Hirose, 1987; Hirose, 1988; Hirose, Kiritani, & Imagawa, 1988; Kiritani, Imagawa, & Hirose, 1988; Hirose, Kiritani, & Imagawa, 1991) examined vocal-fold oscillation at a frame rate of 2,000 frames per second (which could be pushed to as much as 4,000 frames per second by narrowing the size of the observational field), but with quite limited resolution.

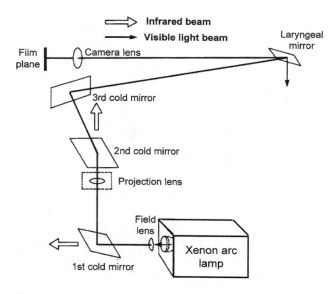

Figure 10–3. Improved illumination system for ultrahigh-speed filming of the larynx. From "An Optical-illumination System for High-speed Laryngeal Cinematography," by D. E. Metz, R. L. Whitehead, and D. H. Peterson, 1980, *Journal of the Acoustical Society of America, 67*, 719–720, Figure 2, p. 719. Reprinted by permission.

By 1993 the frame rate had improved somewhat and resolution had quadrupled (Hirose, 1993; Kiritani, Hirose, & Imagawa, 1993a, 1993b). At about the same time Hess, Gross, and their colleagues were using a new digital camera that achieved frame rates of up to 6,000 frames per second with moderately good resolution to explore subtle changes in vocal fold function (Hess & Gross, 1993; Maurer, Hess, & Gross, 1996; Hess, Herzel, Köster, Scheurich, & Gross, 1996).

High-speed videoendoscopy shows significant promise, and the improvement that it will need is certain to be made. At the present time, though commercially available, these systems remain relatively inconvenient and far too expensive for widespread clinical adoption.

ENDOSCOPY

The presence of a laryngeal mirror effectively precludes studying laryngeal actions during anything but a sustained vowel. Further, it is poorly tolerated by many patients, is difficult to position, and often does not provide an adequate view of the entire length of the vocal folds. These problems have provided the impetus for the development of a number of endoscopic devices—telescopic systems that are inserted into the pharynx via the oral cavity or nasal airway.

Early endoscopes had a light source at the distal end that illuminated the field of view. The optical system, composed of a prism and lenses, provided some magnification. The instrument also generally had some provision for coupling to a camera lens (Taub, 1966a, 1966b; Hahn & Kitzing, 1978). The major problem was the light source. A bulb that was sufficiently bright to produce enough light for even moderately fast photography would get very hot and therefore could not be placed in the oropharynx. One could replace the incandescent bulb with a very intense, but relatively cool electrical discharge flash tube (Bjuggren, 1960), but it requires very high voltages and so exposes the patient to serious electrical risk.

One way out of the dilemma is to use optical fibers to deliver the light (Gould, 1973). The light source itself can then be located outside of the instrument (where its heat is dissipated) and can be very bright and properly filtered. The optical fibers form a cable that is channelled through the shaft of the endoscope, generally ending in two bundles that project light onto the larynx from either side of the objective lens. The instrument is otherwise conventional (Figure 10–4). Because of the

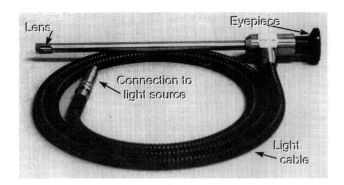

Figure 10–4. A simple rigid laryngeal endoscope.

brilliant illumination, high-speed filming is possible (Gould, Jako, & Tanabe, 1974; Gould, 1977).

Endoscopes with fiberoptic illumination systems solve the problem of safe and adequate lighting, but they are just as encumbering of the oral cavity as more conventional instruments. A means of circumventing this problem was reported by Sawashima, Hirose, and Fujimura (1967) and by Sawashima and Hirose (1968), who designed an endoscope that had two fiberoptic bundles formed into a single cable. One bundle provides illumination, while the other conveys the image of the larynx back to the eyepiece.[1] The entire fiber cable is only about 5 mm in diameter and is quite flexible. A set of controls in the instrument's handle allows the distal portion of the cable system to be bent and thereby guided into position (Figure 10–5).

The fiberoptic endoscope, commonly called a **fiberscope**, is inserted through the nasal cavity and, using the positioning controls, is visually guided through the velopharyngeal port, across the oropharynx, and into the hypopharynx. There, the tip is brought to the level of the epiglottis and angled to provide an unobstructed view of the vocal folds (Sawashima, Abramson, Cooper, & Lisker, 1970; Sawashima & Ushijima, 1972; Davidson, Bone, & Nahum, 1974; Saito, Fukuda, Kitahara, & Kokawa, 1978; Hirano & Bless, 1993; Karnell, 1994), as shown in Figure 10–6. The patient does not have to be specially positioned, and so the view is of the functioning larynx in its normal postural relationship to other structures. The fiberscope may also be used to observe velopharyngeal activity (see Chapter 11, "Velopharyngeal Function"). The ease with which patients tolerate the fiberscope and the excellent view of the larynx that it affords (for example, see Yanagisawa, Strothers, Owens, & Honda, 1983)

---

[1]In passing, it should be noted that the fiber bundles must be organized quite differently. The image-carrying fibers must be parallel to each other. If they were randomly organized the picture at the eyepiece would be a scrambled version of the image entering at the pick-up end. For the illuminating fibers, such "coherence" is immaterial.

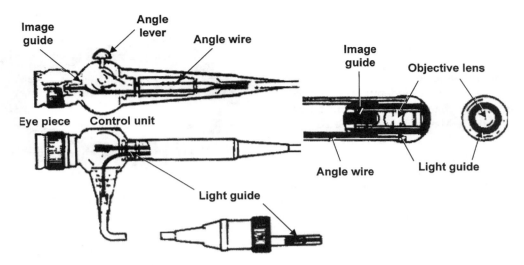

Figure 10–5. Organization of the fiberoptic bundles and positioning control of a fiberoptic endoscope. From "Fiberoptic Observation of the Larynx and Other Speech Organs." In M. Sawashima and F. S. Cooper (Eds.), *Dynamic Aspects of Speech Production* (pp. 31–46). Figure 1, p. 33. Tokyo, Japan: University of Tokyo Press. Reprinted by permission.

makes it an instrument of choice in routine clinical assessment of disorders (Brewer & McCall, 1974; Casper, Brewer, & Conture, 1982; Gould 1983; Blaugrund, Gould, Tanaka, & Kitajima, 1983; Rosevear & Hamlet, 1991; Havas & Priestley, 1993).

The fiberscope does not interfere with oral articulation and does not significantly hinder velar closure. It is therefore of enormous value in assessing the articulatory performance of the larynx. It has proven its worth in research that has provided new insights into how the larynx works in concert with the rest of the vocal tract system (Sawashima, 1970; Kagaya, 1974; Sawashima, Hirose, & Niimi, 1974; Benguerel & Bhatia, 1980; Löfqvist & Yoshioka, 1980; Yoshioka, Löfqvist, & Hirose, 1980).

Some progress has also been made in the development of stereoscopic endoscopes. A double fiberscope that yields a stereo image has been constructed (Niimi & Fujimura, 1976; Fujimura, 1977; Fujimura, Baer, & Niimi, 1979; Sawashima et al., 1983). It allows vertical movement of laryngeal structures to be quantified, a feat hitherto all but impossible. Other stereoscopic endoscopes, such as those described by Sawashima et al. (1983) and by Kakita, Hirano, Kawasaki, & Matsuo (1983) are of the standard telescope type. Since they are not introduced via the nasal passage and do not penetrate deep into the pharynx they entail significantly less invasion. Stereoscopic techniques may ultimately play a role in the clinical assessment of laryngeal function.

The significant advantages of the fiberscope come at a real price: the transmissive capabilities of the instrument will not permit enough light for high-speed filming. Frame rates are limited to about 50 fps with sensitive film (Sawashima, 1977; Fujimura, 1981). Articulatory movements may also change the position of the viewing tip, creating ultimate measurement artifacts, and backward motion of the tongue may interfere with visualization of the glottis. Lastly, the standard method for determining the absolute dimensions of the laryngeal structures cannot be used with the fiberscope.

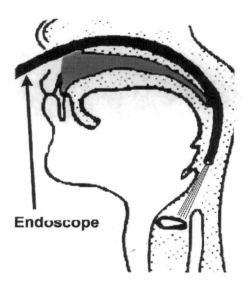

Figure 10–6. Position of the fiberscope in the hypopharynx for viewing the larynx.

Stroboscopy

Under favorable circumstances, one can avoid ultra-high-speed filming, with all of its special illumination and photographic requirements, when the oscillatory motions of the vocal folds must be visualized. Vocal fold motion can be apparently slowed, or even stopped, through the optical illusion of stroboscopy. (It is the same illusion that makes the blades of a moving electric fan seem to slowly revolve in reverse under certain lighting conditions.) The technique depends on rapidly sampling vocal fold position at selected time intervals. When conditions are right, extraordinarily useful insight into vocal fold motion can be obtained,

as in Figure 10–7. But the moving image or sequence of still photographs that is obtained is synthetic in that it is a composite of samples of different cycles. Because of the way in which the illusion is created it is important that the user understand the stroboscopic method well in order to avoid invalid, misleading, and sometimes foolish conclusions.

BASIC PRINCIPLES

Imagine some very rapid event, such as the phonatory opening and closing of the glottis, occurring too fast for the eye to follow. Imagine also that the event occurs in a poorly lit area. Assume further that the repetition

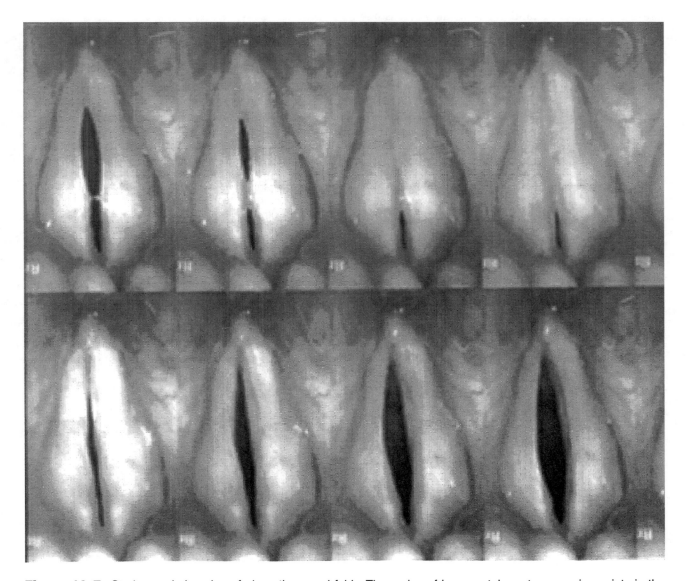

Figure 10–7. Stroboscopic imaging of phonating vocal folds. The series of images, taken at successive points in the glottal cycle, are read from the upper left to the lower right.

rate is about 100 per second, and that each vocal fold cycle is exactly like every other one in every detail.

Now imagine that the moving vocal folds are suddenly lit with an exceptionally brief burst of bright light, lasting perhaps 0.1 ms. The observing eye (or a camera) will see a clear image of the structures at a single point in time. Because the light flash was so brief, the vocal folds will not have moved an appreciable amount during the time that they were lit up, and so the image of them will be relatively sharp. Thanks to persistence of vision, the image will last about a fifth of a second in the observer's eye.

Finally, suppose that the short flashes are repeated at a rate that precisely matches the repetition rate of the vocal fold cycle—that is, 100 flashes per second are produced. Since the flash and repetition rates are exactly matched (and we have already assumed that every vocal fold cycle is precisely like every other one) each flash illuminates the vocal folds at exactly the same point in their cycle. They are always in the same position when a flash of light happens. The human eye cannot discriminate separate flashes 1/100 of a second apart, so the observer sees what appears to be constantly lit and *stationary* vocal folds. It seems that the vocal folds have been stopped dead and locked into position at a single point in their vibratory cycle. This is of course not the case, but the illusion offers a fairly good way of getting a clear view of what the folds look like while they are in motion.

The trick can be refined a bit. Again, suppose that the vocal fold cycle repeats at a rate of exactly 100 per second, but this time let the flash rate be only 99 flashes per second. The vocal fold cycle requires 1/100 = 0.01 s, but the flash rate of 99 per second means that the bursts of illumination are 1/99 = 0.0101 s apart. Because of this discrepancy each flash is delivered slightly later in the vocal fold cycle than the one before. (In other words, the phase difference between the vocal cycle and the flash cycle steadily increases.) The position of the vocal folds shown by the first flash will not be shown again until the 101st flash. Until then, 100 successive positions of the vocal folds will have been illuminated.

This process is demonstrated in Figure 10–8. At the top (A) a schematic diagram illustrates when samples ("light flashes," shown as black circles) are taken of a periodic waveform. When the sample points are joined together a slow-motion (drawn-out, or time-expanded) version of the sampled waveshape is obtained. In the lower illustration (B) blank spots represent sampled points against the background of a relatively high frequency wavetrain. Notice how the flashes recreate (apparent) cycles at a rate that is very much lower than the actual F_0 of the sampled wavetrain. The apparent frequency of the wave reconstructed from the sampled points, delta f (Δf or Df), is

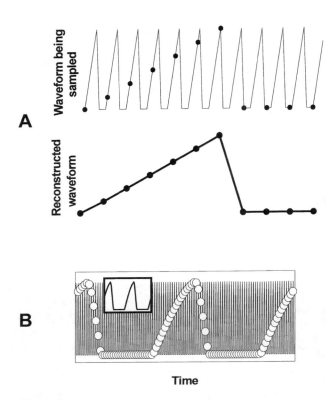

Figure 10–8. A. Sample points taken at regular intervals of a periodic wave (top) can be used to reconstruct the periodic waveform (bottom). **B.** Blank circles represent sampled points of a relatively high-frequency waveform (shown expanded in the inset), which fills the background. The reconstructed wave has a very much lower frequency than the original.

equal to the difference between the wavetrain frequency (f_o) and the sampling ("flash") frequency (f_f):

$$\Delta f = f_o - f_f.$$

At this much lower repetition rate it would be very much easier for the eye to follow the action of, let us say, the vocal folds (and it would be possible to film and maybe even to videotape the action). But the resulting image would not really show vocal fold oscillations. It would, rather, be a depiction of tiny bits of many such cycles, joined together by persistence of vision. Therein lies a host of potential, and too-often-overlooked, problems.

Figure 10–9 demonstrates some of the pitfalls of stroboscopy that can confound the unwary. Figure 10–9A illustrates what happens if the flash rate is too long. The longer the period of illumination, the more the waveform changes while it is illuminated. The result is exactly analogous to a long-exposure photograph of a moving object: the image is blurred. The flash duration, therefore, must be short relative to the speed of the structures being observed. In practice, this should not be a problem with commercially-available equipment: stroboscope flash lamps produce *very* brief bursts of light.

A more subtle problem is shown in Figure 10–9B in which the flash rate is just a bit *higher* than the waveform repetition rate. The result is that the stroboscopic illumination creates an apparent reversal of the wave. The equation for apparent frequency indicates that this should occur. Suppose that the flash rate is 101 per second, while the frequency of, let us say, vocal fold oscillation is 100 per second. Then

$$\Delta f = f_o - f_f$$
$$= 100 - 101$$
$$\Delta f = -1 \text{ cycles per second}$$

The negativity of Δf indicates that the apparent movement will be a reversal of the true movement. The experience is common in everyday life. If an electric fan is turned off there will be a time, as it slows down, when the revolution-per-second rate of the blades is just slightly less than the flicker rate of, say, a fluorescent lamp that illuminates it. At that time the blades will seem to reverse direction and to rotate slowly backwards. (A similar relationship between the frames-per-second rate of an adventure movie and the rotational rate of the rescuing helicopter's rotors results in the same rather odd effect.) Under appropriate conditions the vocal folds might seem to move backwards—surface waves, for example, will seem to propagate *toward* the glottis. The naïve examiner might be led to some very strange conclusions indeed.

Figure 10–9C demonstrates an effect that is insidious. In this case the flash rate remains constant, but the waveform repetition rate varies. There is, in other words, some frequency jitter. The reconstructed stroboscopic waveform varies in waveshape and amplitude, rather than simply in frequency as is actually the case. This effect might, in the clinical context, cause the observer to conclude that the movement pattern of the vocal folds was highly abnormal, when actually only the fundamental frequency was changing.

A moment's reflection shows why this last problem is so serious. In reality, the fundamental frequency of phonation is far from perfectly stable. It is, in fact, highly perturbed in patients with many voice disorders (see Chapter 6, "Vocal Fundamental Frequency") and these are the very people to whom stroboscopy is most likely to be applied. *The magnitude of fundamental frequency perturbation and the associated likelihood that the observed movement pattern is an artifact need to be assessed before relying on the stroboscopic observation for clinical purposes.* And, it should go without saying, if the phonation being observed is not of Type 1

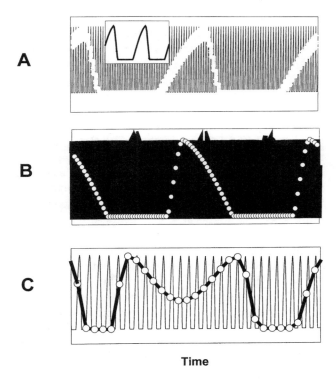

Figure 10–9. Possible pitfalls of stroboscopy: **A.** When the flash rate is too long, the reconstruction of the original waveform (shown in the inset) is blurred, **B.** If the interflash interval is too short—so that the flash rate is higher than the waveform's F_0—the reconstruction will be a reversal of the original wave. **C.** Instability of the flash frequency or of the waveform frequency will result in distortion in the reconstruction.

(described in Chapter 6) the stroboscopic movement pattern is likely to have no validity at all.

The problem of changing vocal F_0 motivated the development of the synchronstroboscope, whose flash rate varies with the patient's fundamental frequency in an attempt to make the flashes occur with a phase lag that steadily increases at a constant increment. (Or at least the equipment *tries* to track the vocal F_0. The key portion of the synchronstroboscope is a circuit that generates a Df that is added to the patient's F_0 as transduced by a contact microphone or by an electroglottograph (van den Berg, 1959; von Leden, 1961; Winckel, 1965; Pedersen, 1977; Anastaplo & Karnell, 1988; Karnell, 1989; Roch, Comte, Eyraud, & Dubreuil, 1990; Sercarz et al., 1992).

Laryngeal stroboscopy was originally performed by flashing a beam of light focused on a laryngeal mirror, and observation was by indirect laryngoscopy. Today, of course, a fiberscopic endoscope is used, and its high-power lamp is controlled by the stroboscope—a scheme first developed by Saito and his colleagues

(1978). And the image is not merely observed, it is almost always videotaped. Furthermore, in a modern system (such as that shown in Figure 10–10) the light control, camera control, recording, and display systems are all under the control of a central computer, which also allows for on-screen annotation and extraction of images for printing.

Video recording, however, creates a very special problem. Much in the way that a motion picture is made up of a series of still frames shown in rapid succession, so the video image is also really a series of still images. The video "frame rate"—depending on the particular national standard—is either 25 or 30 complete frames per second. Because of this, the timing of light flashes for videostroboendoscopy is governed not only by the need to have a constantly increasing phase delay, but by the fact that two flashes must not occur during the same video frame. (Because of the way in which video images are built up, having two "exposures" in the same frame might produce some very novel distortions indeed.) Thus, videostroboscopic systems need not only to advance the time of each flash, but need also to hold off the next flash until a new video frame has started. Given that the video frame rate is 25 or 30 Hz, and that phonatory F_0s vary from about 100 to a few hundred hertz, the requirement of a fresh screen for each exposure dictates that videostroboscopy cannot sample successive vocal cycles. Since the required inter-exposure interval is not likely to be an integer submultiple of the video frame rate, the videostroboscopic light flashes cannot even occur at regular—if relatively long—intervals. A well-designed videostroboscopic system can manage all the competing requirements, but the user should be aware of how distant the reconstructed image is from the real-time laryngeal reality.

Videokymography

A television image is different from a photograph. In photography the film is exposed to all points of a scene at the same time, but television is based on a "raster scan." The process is illustrated in Figure 10–11. The television picture is actually composed of a set of lines that are written on the screen by a "dot" that moves from left to right. After writing a line, the dot's writing capability is turned off while it returns to the left and writes a new line just a bit lower on the screen. This repeats until a complete picture has been produced on the screen. If each line is sufficiently thin, and if the image is represented by a large number of lines, a relatively crisp and detailed picture results. If new images are created in rapid-enough succession, motion can be smoothly shown. North American broadcast standards, for example, call for 525 lines per screen, and a total of 30 complete images per second.[2] There are thus

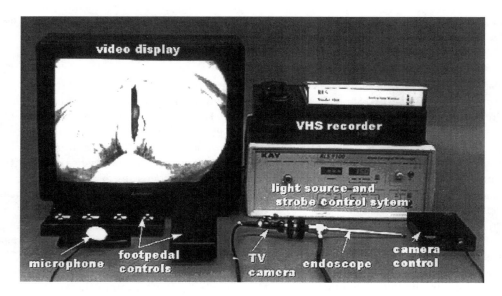

Figure 10–10. A modern computer-controlled videostroboscopic system, the Kay Elemetrics RhinoLaryngoStroboscope. (Courtesy of Kay Elemetrics Corp., Lincoln Park, NJ.)

[2]For various reasons the scanning is actually done in two passes. First, all of the odd-numbered lines are scanned, and then, 1/60th of a second later, the even-numbered lines are drawn on the screen between the odd-numbered lines. There are thus 30 images per second, but each screen is a mélange of two "exposures" taken 1/60ths apart. European broadcast standards call for similarly-interlaced imaging with a total of 625 lines, completely redrawn 25 times per second.

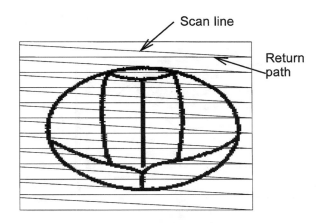

Figure 10–11. A television image is formed by a "raster scan," here diagrammed superimposed on an image of the larynx. A modulated spot of light moves from left to right across the screen, and then is turned off as it follows a return path back to the left. Lines are written in this way, from the top to the bottom of the screen, to make a complete image. There are different standards that govern how many lines an image will contain.

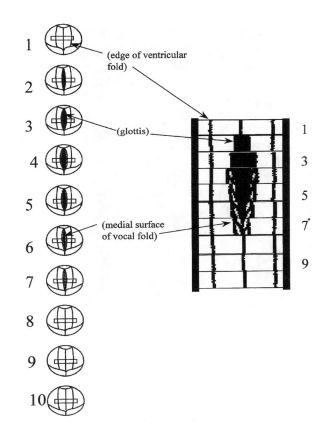

Figure 10–12. In videokymography a single line of the field of view is scanned repeatedly and the resulting one-dimensional images are displayed, each below the previous one, on the TV screen. The result is an image of the changes over time at the level of the scanned line. See text for details.

15,750 lines generated every second.[3] Because a large number of lines must be devoted to depicting a full two-dimensional plane, and because there are real limits to the speed with which a screen can be filled with lines, the number of complete images that can be shown every second is seriously limited, and so an ordinary television system cannot provide clear images of the moving vocal folds.

Videokymography was developed as a means of using television technology to accomplish some of what ultrahigh-speed filming can achieve (Gall, Gall, & Hanson, 1971; Gall & Hanson, 1973; Gall, 1978, 1984; Gross, 1985, 1988; Švec & Schutte, 1996; Schutte, Svec, & Šram, 1997; Šram, Schutte, & Svec, 1997; Švec, Schutte, & Šram, 1997). Videokymography sacrifices two-dimensionality in order to gain speed. It does that by ignoring all of the field of view and limiting scanning of the endoscopic image to rapid repetition of a single line. Each new scan of the same line in the field of view is displayed on the screen just under the previous scan, so that a screen image is built up, with time (advancing downward) as the vertical dimension. Figure 10–12 schematizes the process, using simplified views of the vocal folds at ten successive points in time during a single oscillatory

cycle. The rectangle in each image outlines the contents of the "line" being scanned. If the rectangles are lined up, one below the other, the equivalent of a videokymographic image results. Note how the margins of the ventricular folds remain fixed as time progresses (from top to bottom in the videokymographic reconstruction), while the dark "glottis" and the stippled regions representing the visible portion of the medial surface of the vocal folds expand and contract.[4]

The video camera that is used for kymography is a modified commercial solid-state unit. In its videokymographic mode, it is capable of scanning at a rate of almost 8,000 lines/s. At an F_0 of 200 Hz this means that

---

[3]For the sake of technical accuracy it should be noted that not all of the lines generated are actually projected on the screen. In North America even-numbered lines 242 through 262, and odd-numbered lines 505 through 525 (which should form the bottom of the image) are turned off during a "blanking interval" in which the trace is returned to the top of the screen. A similar blank period is built into other national standards.

[4]While a rectangular area is used in the figure for illustrative purposes, in actual practice a very thin line is scanned, resulting in a very much more detailed image.

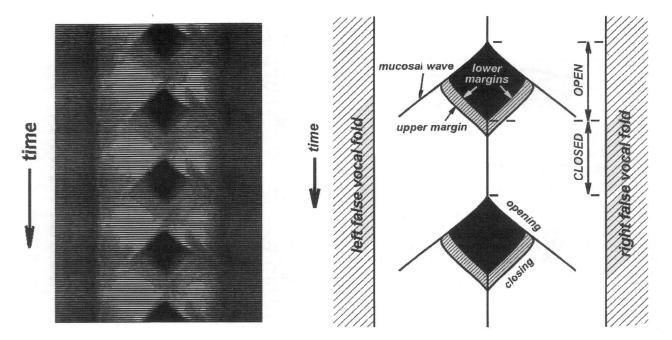

Figure 10–13. Top: Videokymogram of normal vocal fold oscillation. (The resolution of the original image is better than what can be produced in this reproduction.) Bottom: Schematic illustration of the features depicted in the videokymogram. (Courtesy of Drs. JŠvec and FŠram, Prague, Czech Republic, and Dr. H. Schutte, Groningen, The Netherlands.)

a single glottal cycle will occupy 40 lines—more than enough to show significant details of motion. The camera can also be set to function normally, producing a two-dimensional image of the field of view in which the line that is to be visualized during high-speed scanning is highlighted in the image. In this way the position of the scan along the length of the vocal folds can be selected. A major shortcoming, however, is that there is no way to assure that movement of either the endoscope or the larynx does not change the locus being observed.

The videokymogram is a new kind of image, and it requires some practice and acclimation before one can read it easily. But it contains a wealth of information not easily obtained in any other way. Because it displays the actual motion of the structures, rather than a reconstruction (as stroboscopy does), there is no requirement that the vocal fold motions be periodic or regular in any way. With the exception of ultrahigh-speed filming, it is the only means of visualization that can do this, and thus it is the sole practical means of assessing vocal fold movements associated with dysphonia.

Figure 10–13 shows how the movements of normal vocal folds are depicted by videokymography. The image on the left is composed of sequential scans (lines) done at a single transverse position on the vocal folds. A bit more than four glottal cycles are shown, with time progressing from top to bottom. The illustration on the right schematizes the features that are shown in the videokymogram. The dark central regions

are the glottal space, which widens and narrows with each glottal cycle. During the opening portion of each cycle the glottis is (vertically) convergent, so their medial surfaces are hidden. As a consequence the opening phases have a sharp edge delineating the glottal space. During the time that the vocal folds are returning to the midline, however, the glottis is (vertically) divergent, and the medial surfaces of the vocal folds can be seen from above. The grayish margin of the glottis during the closing intervals represents the temporarily-visible medial surfaces. The glottis remains closed for a period of time before another opening phase begins. During this closed interval a lighter-colored band can be seen radiating away laterally. This is the mucosal surface wave. It is clear that the videokymogram allows easy measurement of opening time, closing time, and the duration of the closed interval—characteristics which, as will be discussed shortly, are important in characterizing vocal fold function and which previously could only be obtained reliably from high-speed films.

The depiction of the irregular oscillations of the vocal folds in a case of unilateral vocal fold paralysis demonstrates the very significant value of videokymography (Figure 10–14). The two vocal folds oscillate at different frequencies. Although it is clear that there is a mutual coupling between them, the separate oscillatory frequencies are not fully independent. Furthermore, the motions of the two vocal folds are obviously different. The healthy fold has rapid, sharply delineated

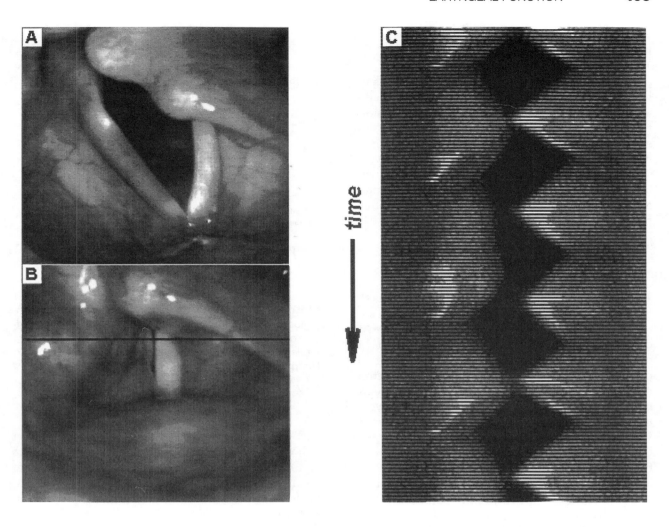

Figure 10–14. Videokymogram of vocal fold oscillation in a case of unilateral paralysis: **A.** Overall view of the larynx, **B.** The black bar indicates the region of the vocal folds that has been scanned, **C.** The videokymogram shows the vocal folds to be oscillating at different frequencies, but there is mutual coupling. The displacements of the paralyzed side are not are "sharp" or as regular as those of the normal vocal fold. [Note: The resolution of this reproduction is not as good as the that of the original image.] (Courtesy of Drs. JŠvec and FŠram, Prague, Czech Republic.)

opening and closing gestures, whereas the paralyzed fold appears "sluggish" in its movements. Close inspection—especially of the original image, which has significantly greater resolution than this copy—reveals other features of interest, including in particular the fact that the medial surface of the healthy vocal fold is visible during the closing gestures, but that of the paralyzed vocal fold is not. This, of course, suggests that the impaired vocal fold does not show the normal alternation between a convergent and divergent glottal margin. Stroboscopy could not be relied on to reveal these motions because the irregularity of glottal closures would fail to provide a timing reference point for controlling the light flashes. Thus, in the practical world of clinical practice, it is very likely that only

videokymography would be capable of capturing the important details of vocal fold motion in this case.

CORRELATES OF VOCAL FOLD MOTION

While visualization of the larynx is a sine qua non of assessing tissue disorders, much crucial information is provided by measures that do not reveal what the vocal folds actually look like. An example is the glottal area function (discussed more fully later on) which is the area of the glottal opening as a function of time. In general, these measures can be derived from ultrahigh-speed films, and that is the means by which many were, in fact, originally obtained. But doing so is tedious, terribly time-consuming, and relatively costly. These considerations, and a desire to probe more deeply into the physiology of vocal fold oscillation, have motivated a search for simpler methods that rely as much as possible on correlates of vocal fold motion that can be easily transduced with a minimum of invasion. None of the techniques discussed under this heading replaces good visual assessment of laryngeal status. Instead, they provide a more complete quantitative and qualitative understanding that is vital to assessment and to the design of an appropriate therapeutic regimen.

Photoglottography (PGG)

The principle on which photoglottography rests is simple enough. The glottis can be considered to be a shutter through which light passes in proportion to the degree of opening. In theory, if a light is made to shine on the glottis, the amount of light passing through it is directly proportional to the glottal area. Optoelectronic devices are more than adequate to transduce changes in luminous intensity at the rates typical of laryngeal function. It is possible, therefore, to obtain an electrical voltage proportional to the glottal area—at least in theory. A moment's reflection indicates where the difficulties lie in the translation of principle to practice: arranging for adequate illumination of the larynx and devising a system to pick up and transduce the transmitted light. Fortunately, today's instrumentation makes meeting these needs quite simple.

Modern photoglottography began with Sonesson (1959, 1960) and has been modified or combined with other techniques in a number of ways by others (Lisker, Abramson, Cooper, & Schvey, 1966, 1969; Kitzing, 1977; Kitzing & Löfqvist, 1978; Löfqvist, 1980; McGarr & Löfqvist, 1982, 1988; Hanson, Gerratt, & Ward, 1983; Gerratt, Hanson, & Berke, 1987; Doyle & Wallace, 1990; Alfonso, Kalinowski, & Story, 1991; Murty & Carding, 1991; Slavit & Maragos, 1994; Lin, Jiang, Hone, & Hanson, 1999). A basic photoglottographic setup, as originally used by Sonesson, is shown in Figure 10–15. A bright light source is placed against the neck just below the cricoid cartilage. The lamp causes the subglottal space to be suffused with the light that filters through the tissues of the neck. A pickup probe, either a curved plastic rod or a fiberoptic bundle, transmits any of this light that passes to the pharynx to a photosensor. The result, after amplification, is a voltage that should be proportional to the area of the glottic opening.

It makes no difference what the direction of the light path is, so the light source can be placed on the

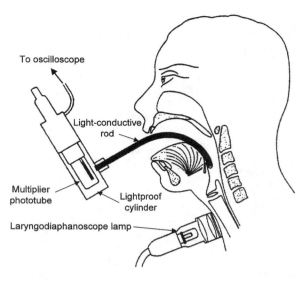

Figure 10–15. Sonesson's original technique for photoglottography. From "On the anatomy and vibratory pattern of the human vocal folds," by B. Sonesson, 1960, *Acta Otolaryngologica*, *Suppl. 156*, 1–80. Figure 22, p. 47. Reprinted by permission.

neck and the detector in the oropharynx (as Sonesson did) or the light can shine onto the larynx from above and the photosensor can be placed on the surface of the neck (Gerratt, Hanson, & Berke, 1986; Gerratt, Hanson, Berke, & Precoda, 1991; Doyle & Fraser, 1993). Better yet, illumination can be provided by a fiberscope, inserted via the nasal cavity into the lower pharynx. This has the advantage of permitting normal articulatory movements (Lisker et al., 1966, 1969; Löfqvist, 1980). In today's clinical environment, fiberscopic endoscopy of the larynx is routine, and thus the light source for photoglottography is in place during part of the exam. Only the addition of a photosensor over the trachea is needed for PGG to be routinely included in the laryngeal examination.

There are problems with photoglottography, and its validity has been questioned. Specifically, Wendahl and Coleman (1967) and Coleman and Wendahl (1968) reported on simultaneous determinations of changes in glottal area using ultrahigh-speed filming and photoglottography. In some cases, the curves produced by the two methods were highly congruent, but in many instances they were markedly dissimilar. The discrepancies were particularly serious if the waveforms were used to derive glottal source spectra, as they sometimes have been (Ohala, 1967). The conclusion was that "relating photoglottographic waveforms . . . to glottal area is not only hazardous but invalid in many cases" (Coleman & Wendahl, 1968, p. 1734).

A later study by Harden (1975) using very similar methods obtained completely different results. She found that, for 5 subjects sustaining vowels in each of the three vocal registers, the photoglottograph provided "essentially the same information on glottal area function as that provided by ultrahigh-speed photography" (Harden, 1975, p. 734). Although the curves generated by the two methods were not identical, photoglottography was judged to provide "reasonably approximate information." In still another study comparing high-speed filming and photglottography, Baer, Löfqvist, and McGarr (1983) concluded that the two methods provide comparable data about peak glottal opening and glottal closure.

There is no clear explanation for the different results of these studies. It is possible, for instance, that some light is transmitted through the greatly thinned edge of the vocal folds under some adjustment conditions. It is clear that a number of extrinsic factors do influence the photoglottogram, and the user must keep them in mind in order to control them rigorously. Vallancien and his colleagues (Vallancien, Gautheron, Pasternak, Guisez, & Paley, 1971) summarized them as follows:

1. The amount of light projected on the larynx. This varies with lateral and angular displacement of both the illumination source and the photoelectric transducer. Displacements can be produced by activity of the articulators.

2. Changes in light-transmissive characteristics of the neck tissues due to vertical movement of the larynx.

3. Changes in the shape and volume of the hypopharynx caused by tongue retraction during certain productions.

In short, the normal structural displacements of speech may threaten the validity of the photoglottographic measurements. Accordingly, the part of the photoglottograph that is placed inside the vocal tract should be located in such a way as to assure stability. This argues strongly for a fiberscopic light source that can be inserted via the nasal cavity, because it is least likely to be moved by the tongue and its tip placement in the laryngeal vestibule promises a relatively good line of sight to the vocal folds. The fiberscope also has the advantage of allowing the examiner to monitor the adequacy of placement visually and to signal the intrusion of any obstruction, such as the epiglottis, that temporarily invalidates the data.

Analysis of Glottal Status

Beyond purely qualitative description, high-speed cinematography, photoglottography, videokymography, and (using very great caution) videostroboscopy can provide quantitative data upon which graphic or numeric analysis of vocal fold function can be performed.

VOCAL FOLD EXCURSION AND GLOTTAL WIDTH

A frame-by-frame analysis of the width of the glottis as seen in ultrahigh-speed films or in videostroboscopic recordings[5] is a useful means of quantifying peculiarities of vocal fold movement. The distance of a point along the length of the vocal fold (usually the midpoint) is plotted over time or, equivalently, over frame number. Using ultrahigh-speed film, Hirano, Kakita, Kawasaki, Gould, and Lambiase (1981) tracked the horizontal excursion of three blood vessels on the superior surface and the edge of a subject's right vocal fold during phonation. However, note that, as Smith (1954) originally pointed out, complex movements of the *medial* surface of the vocal folds are only intermittently visible in high-speed films. The most medial point of the vocal fold, as seen in a given frame, may not be on the edge of the superior surface. If a relative scale is used the distance of maximum opening is usually designated 100% and all other values are scaled accordingly.

This technique was extensively explored by Timcke, von Leden, and Moore (1958, 1959), von Leden, Moore, and Timcke (1960), and von Leden and Moore (1961). Examples of their analyses (Figure 10–16) show how strikingly it can demonstrate movement abnormality. Trace A shows a normal glottal width function. Opening takes less time than closing, and there is a period of obviously complete closure. The vocal folds move symmetrically. Trace B, on the other hand, is the glottal width function of a patient with left recurrent nerve paralysis. The paralyzed vocal fold never reaches midline, but its movements seem otherwise fairly normal. The healthy vocal fold passes the midline during what should be the closed phase, but no direct contract of the two vocal folds is achieved. A wider range of abnormal width functions will be considered later on.

Only videokymography or frame-by-frame analysis of ultrahigh-speed films can provide graphic records like the ones of Figure 10–16 because, at the moment, those are the only techniques that can track

---

[5]Using the videostroboscopic image requires significant caution and *very* serious consideration of the possibility of imaging artifacts. See the previous discussion of the limitations of stroboscopy.

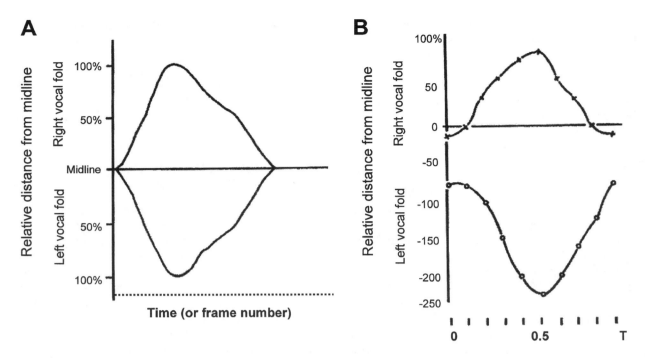

Figure 10–16. A. Normal glottal width function. The distance of the midpoint of each vocal fold from the midline is plotted from successive frames of an ultrahigh-speed film. **B.** Glottal width function in a case of left recurrent nerve paralysis. The left vocal fold never reaches the midline. Its vibratory excursion is greater than that of the right vocal fold, which crosses the midline slightly, since the paralyzed fold is not there to arrest its medial motion. From "Laryngeal vibrations: Measurements of the glottic wave. Part III: The pathologic larynx," by H. von Leden, H. Moore, and R. Timcke, 1960, *Archives of Otolaryngology, 71,* 16–35. Figure 3, p. 19. Reprinted by permission.

each vocal fold separately. Plotting the width function one frame at a time is enormously tedious and time-consuming, so videokymography is clearly the method of choice for evaluating and providing documentation of abnormalities of glottal behavior.

THE GLOTTAL AREA FUNCTION

The glottal area function is the area of the glottal opening plotted over time. It is strongly correlated to the glottal width function (defined for the present purposes as the distance from the middle of one vocal fold to the middle of the other). Koike and Hirano (1973) computed an average discrepancy between the two of less than 2%. Given this close correspondence the width is often used as an estimate of the relative glottal area, since it is much easier to derive. In fact, it is the glottal width that is represented by the dark space in a videokymogram. If, however, the absolute area is needed, the actual area must be computed. This cannot be done from a videokymogram, because the geometry of the glottal opening is important, and is not represented in the kymographic image. Deriving the area using a planimeter is possible, but even short sequences

of film can take hours of measurement time. Efforts to automate the process using special computer programs and video processors have met with some success (Hayden & Koike, 1972; Childers, Paige, & Moore, 1976; Gould, 1977; Hirano, Kawasaki, Gould, & Lambiase, 1981). But, in general, automated methods remain either slow or of dubious reliability. Fortunately, the absolute area is rarely needed: it is usually the *pattern* of glottal area change that is of interest. For this, a relative measure is perfectly adequate.

Parameters of the Glottal Area Function

A number of parameters have been devised to quantify important aspects of the glottal area (or glottal width) waveshape. They are based on the durations of various phases of the wave, and are schematized in Figure 10–17.

The open phase, during which the glottal area is greater than zero, is divided into an opening (closed-to-open; C→O) part and a closing (open-to-closed, O→C) part. The duration of the cycle (its period) is designated T. The durations of these phases are used to compute the following indices:

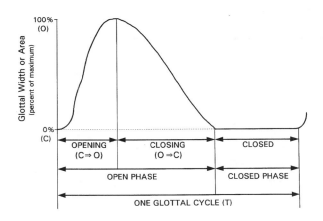

Figure 10–17. Divisions of the glottal area or glottal width functions.

1. The *open quotient* (O_q) is the proportion of the period during which the glottis is open. That is,

$$O_q = \frac{\text{open phase}}{T}.$$

When there is no glottal closure the duration of the open phase equals the period, and therefore $O_q = 1$.

2. The *speed quotient* (S_q) measures the symmetry of the opening (C → O) and closing (O → C) parts of the open phase:

$$S_q = \frac{C \to O}{O \to C}.$$

An S_q of 1 indicates that the opening and closing parts take the same amount of time. An $S_q < 1$ results when closing takes longer than opening, whereas an $S_q > 1$ signals the reverse.

3. The *speed index* (SI) is another way of describing the symmetry of the opening and closing phases (Hirano, 1981). It is the ratio of the durational differences of the two to the total duration of the open phase. That is,

$$SI = \frac{[(C \to O) - (O \to C)]}{\text{open phase}}$$

$$= \frac{[(C \to O) - (O \to C)]}{[(C \to O) + (O \to C)]}.$$

The value of SI is related to the speed quotient, just discussed:

$$SI = \frac{(S_q - 1)}{(S_q + 1)}.$$

The speed index has certain advantages over the somewhat more popular speed quotient. Figure 10–18 and Table 10–1 show these by comparing the behavior of SI *and* S_q. Symmetry of the open phase is indicated by an S_q of 1.00. As the wave is increasingly skewed to the right the S_q decreases to a limit of zero, but the limit of S_q for extreme left-skewing is infinite. The S_q grows exponentially as skewness increases to the right. The SI, on the other hand, extends from -1 to $+1$ as skewing goes from extreme right to extreme left. Thus, a negative value shows a shorter opening than closing part, and a positive value shows a relatively short closing period. Equality of these two parts of the glottal width function is indicated by SI = 0. Although the two parameters are mathematically equivalent and interconvertible, the behavior of SI seems more in keeping with intuitive notions of scaling, and may well come to replace S_q.

4. The *rate quotient* (R_q) is yet another glottal index that has been proposed. It is defined as

$$R_q = \frac{[\text{closed phase} + (C \to O)]}{(O \to C)}.$$

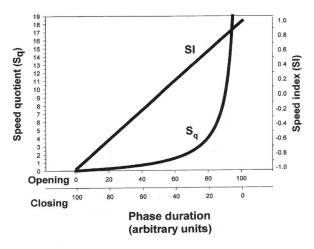

Figure 10–18. Comparison of the growth of S_q and SI.

Table 10–1. The Relationship of the Opening and Closing Parts of the Open Phase to the Speed Quotient (S_q) and Speed Index (SI)*

Duration (Arbitrary Units)		Glottal Area Index		
Glottal Opening (C → O)	Glottal Closing (O → C)	S_q	SI	
0	100	0.000	−1.0	
5	95	0.053	−0.9	
10	90	0.111	−0.8	
15	85	0.176	−0.7	
20	80	0.250	−0.6	
25	75	0.333	−0.5	
30	70	0.429	−0.4	
35	65	0.538	−0.3	
40	60	0.667	−0.2	
45	55	0.818	−0.1	
50	50	1.000	0.0	
55	45	1.222	0.1	
60	40	1.500	0.2	
65	35	1.857	0.3	
70	30	2.333	0.4	
75	25	3.000	0.5	
80	20	4.000	0.6	
85	15	5.667	0.7	
90	10	9.000	0.8	
95	5	19.000	0.9	
100	0	∞	1.0	

*Based on Hirano (1981).

It describes the relative duration of the closed and opening phases to the closing interval. Introduced by Kitzing and Sonesson (1974), it has not gained widespread use.

Expected Values

Normal Function. The variations of several glottographic parameters with changes in F_0 and vocal intensity have been systematically studied by ultrahighspeed filming and by photoglottography. The general accuracy of these data has been confirmed by other photoglottographic studies (Kitzing & Sonesson, 1974; Hanson, Gerratt, & Berke, 1990) and by ultrahighspeed filming (Moore & von Leden, 1958; von Leden, 1961; Timcke, von Leden, & Moore, 1958). Some of the data of Sonesson, provided in Table 10–2 are representative. Taken together, these investigations support the following generalizations:

1. The open quotient increases with vocal F_0 in modal register. At higher (loft or falsetto register) F_0s, glottal closure may not occur, so that $O_q = 1$. Pulse register has very long closed periods (Hollien, Girard, & Coleman, 1977; Whitehead, Metz, & Whitehead, 1984), so O_q will be very small. O_q tends to vary inversely with vocal intensity.

2. The speed quotient varies directly with vocal intensity. It is essentially unaffected by F_0.

3. The overall pattern of the glottal width function changes dramatically with register (Figure 10–19). In fact, the change is part of the definition of register itself (Hollien, 1974).

Vocal Disorder. Most of the value of the glottal area function in assessment of voice disorders lies in its depiction of possible anomalies of vocal-fold movement. Obviously, videokymography is the method of

Table 10–2. Mean Open Quotient (O_q), Speed Quotient (S_q), and Speed Index (SI) for Normal Speakers*

Approximate Vocal F_0 (Hz)	O_q		S_q		SI†	
	Mean	Range	Mean	Range	Mean	Range
Low Vocal Intensity†						
120	0.57	0.38–0.80	0.92	0.80–1.06	−0.04	−0.11–+0.03
175	0.68	0.49–0.77	0.89	0.72–1.13	−0.06	−0.16–+0.06
225	0.71	0.51–1.00	0.91	0.69–1.18	−0.05	−0.18–+0.08
275	0.80	0.47–1.00	0.85	0.61–1.16	−0.08	−0.24–+0.07
325	0.82	1.54–1.00	0.92	0.59–1.19	−0.04	−0.25–+0.09
High Vocal Intensity‡						
120	0.47	0.37–0.58	0.99	0.77–1.44	0.00	−0.97–+0.19
175	0.58	0.38–0.72	0.99	0.86–1.46	0.00	−0.07–+0.19
225	0.64	0.49–1.00	0.95	0.59–1.29	−0.03	−0.26–+0.13
275	0.70	0.46–1.00	0.95	0.71–1.18	−0.03	−0.17–+0.08
325	0.77	0.44–1.00	0.97	0.81–1.62	−0.01	−0.10–+0.24

*From "On the anatomy and vibratory pattern of the human vocal folds," by B. Sonesson, 1960, *Acta Otolaryngologica, Suppl. 156,* 1–80. Table 2, p. 62. Reprinted by permission. Data derived from photoglottographic signals; 25 normal speakers, age 18 to 21 years. Subjects sustained /ɛ/, matching provided tones.
†Computed from author's data.
‡Intensity difference approximately 6 dB.

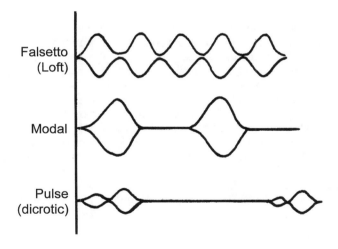

Figure 10–19. Vocal fold excursion patterns in the three voice registers.

choice for getting this information. The next best option, from the point of view of validity, is ultrahigh-speed filming, but its labor-intensiveness makes it impractical. Videostroboscopy is thus the next practical alternative but, as has already been repeated many times, it must be used with a very healthy awareness of the possibility of artifact.

Figure 10–20 illustrates the kinds of glottal width functions that may be encountered in some common pathologies. Failure to achieve glottal closure (A), abnormal excursion of a vocal fold across the midline (B), and phase differences between the displacements of the two vocal folds (C and D) are typical findings. On the basis of analysis of a great many cases, von Leden, Moore, and Timcke (1960) and Yanagihara (1967) have drawn the following conclusions:

1. Benign lesions do not prevent vibration of the vocal fold on which they are located. Both folds vibrate at the same frequency.

2. In general, abnormal vibration patterns are typical of disease, with the possible exception of very small lesions.

3. The most common (almost ubiquitous) symptom of disease is frequent and rapid changes in vibratory rate. These may be detectable by perturbation analysis (see Chapter 6, "Vocal Fundamental Frequency").

4. Damping of vocal fold vibration is caused by all but the very smallest lesions (see, for instance, Figure 10–20B).

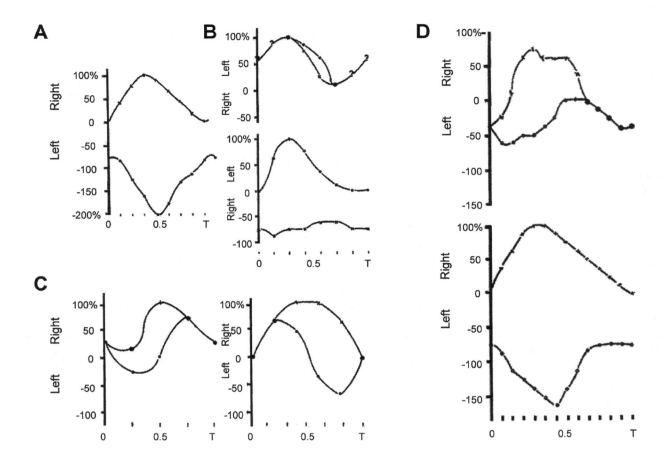

Figure 10–20. Vocal fold excursion patterns (glottal width functions) in some common pathologies: **A.** Left vocal fold paralysis. The paralyzed fold does not come to the midline to effect glottal closure. Its excursion is greater than that of the healthy fold. **B.** Sessile polyp and diffuse edema of the right vocal fold. Measurement at the center of the lesion (upper traces) shows how, at this location, the diseased fold follows the movements of the healthy one. The glottal width function measured at the posterior end of the membranous folds (lower traces) demonstrates the failure to achieve glottal closure in this area. **C.** Fixation of the left cricoarytenoid joint at the midline (traces at left) results in a constant phase shift of about 90° throughout the cycle. For a patient with anterior webbing (traces at right) there is a constant phase shift of about 115° (left side lagging). **(D)** A patient with bilateral polyps, larger on the left vocal fold. When measured in the vicinity of the lesions (upper traces) the glottal width function show a phase shift of about 90° (left side leading) and a highly abnormal open phase. Closure is to the left of the midline. Measurement posterior to the lesions (lower traces) shows an abnormal excursion pattern of the left vocal fold and a failure to achieve glottal closure in this area. From "Laryngeal vibrations: measurements of the glottic wave. Part III: The pathologic larynx," by H. von Leden, P. Moore, and R. Timcke, 1960, *Archives of Otolaryngology, 71*, 16–35. Figure 5, p. 21; Figure 7, p. 24; Figure 9, p. 27; and Figure 12, p. 32. Reprinted by permission.

5. Great increases in excursion are often associated with lower motoneuron paralysis (see Figure 10–20A).

6. There is almost always asynchronism of vibration of the two vocal folds. That is, they will move out of phase.

    a. The phase shift may be constant during the cycle, or it may change. If constant, the open period will show the pattern of Figure 10–20C.

    b. If the phase shift affects the closed phase, the approximated edges of the vocal folds will deviate from the midline, as in Figure 10–20C.

7. It is common for either the normal or the diseased vocal fold to cross the midline during part of the glottal cycle (see Figure 10–20C).

8. Projecting soft tumors tend to follow the motions of the opposing healthy vocal fold (as in Figure 10–20B). Firm tumors do not.

9. The period of closure is prolonged at the site of a projecting tumor. The projection, however, prevents any approximation in adjoining areas (see Figure 10–20B and D).

10. The open quotient is often increased.

Hirano, Gould, Lambiase, and Kakita (1981) have confirmed many of these findings in cases of unilateral vocal fold polyps. They also have stressed concurrent changes of the traveling wave of the mucosa. Cycle-to-cycle waveform variability is considerable in many cases of laryngeal pathology, and rapid alterations of the glottal waveform contribute significantly to the perception of vocal roughness (Coleman, 1971).

Many of the defects listed above can be seen in, or inferred from photoglottograms. Unfortunately, the photoglottograph cannot differentiate the contribution of each vocal fold to the observed signal, so much information is lost. Attempts to correlate photoglottogram patterns with specific disorders are still far from complete (Kitzing & Löfqvist, 1979).

Electroglottography (Electrolaryngography, EGG)

Because it is entirely noninvasive, electroglottography (EGG) has attracted a great deal of interest. It was very early applied by researchers to probe the function of the normal larynx (Chevrie-Muller, 1967; Holm, 1971; Ondráckova, 1972; Reinsch & Gobsch, 1972; Kelman, 1981; Rothenberg, 1981), including attempts to confirm the neurochronaxic theory of voice production (Chevrie-Muller & Grémy, 1962; van Michel, 1964, 1966; Grémy & Guérin, 1963) or to refute it (Decroix & Dujardin, 1958; Lebrun & Hasquin-Deleval, 1971). It was also quite soon developed as a means of diagnosing vocal pathology (Chevrie-Muller, 1964; van Michel, 1967; Jentzsch, Sasama, & Unger, 1978; Croatto & Ferrero, 1979; Lecluse, Tiwari, & Snow, 1981; Berry, Epstein, Fourcin et al., 1982; Berry, Epstein, Freeman, MacCurtain, & Noscoe, 1982; Gleeson & Fourcin, 1983; Smith & Childers, 1983; Childers, Smith, & Moore, 1984) and as a tool in voice therapy (Fourcin & Abberton, 1971, 1976; Abberton, 1972; Abberton & Fourcin, 1972, 1975; Fourcin, 1974, 1981; Abberton, Parker, & Fourcin, 1977; Jentzsch, Unger, & Sasama, 1981; Reed, 1982). EGG has become a preferred tool of voice specialists. Given that it is likely to be increas-

ingly important in vocal rehabilitation, it is considered here in some detail.[6]

The electroglottograph has been improved very significantly since it was developed by Fabre (1957) as an extension of early investigations into peripheral blood flow (Mann, 1937; Fabre, 1940). What seemed at first so simple and straightforward a procedure needed considerable modification before it was to become a useful clinical tool. Early electroglottographs were fairly simple devices using vacuum tubes or just passive elements. They often required a separate highly stable oscillator and an outboard amplifier and demodulator (van Michel, 1967; Vallancien & Faulhaber, 1966). A transistorized device appeared in 1960 (Gougerot, Grémy, & Marstal, 1960; Decroix & Dujardin, 1958). A major advance was the mark IV Electroglottometer (van Michel & Raskin, 1969) which was quite sensitive and contained all the circuitry (some of it integrated) required to function as a free-standing unit.

Today's electroglottographs are sensitive, safe, and convenient to use. But there is as yet no "standard" electroglottograph. The various modifications have led to a number of different varieties of electroglottograph that may, under certain circumstances, produce different outputs for the same event. It is wise to understand the differences among the various devices being offered in the marketplace in order to better judge the validity of findings in the literature and to select for purchase the one most suited to the intended use.

ELECTRICAL FLOW IN BIOLOGICAL MATERIALS

Human tissue is a moderately good conductor of electricity (Dalziel, 1956; Geddes & Baker, 1967, 1989). The degree to which a tissue or organ impedes the flow of electrical current (that is, the magnitude of its resistance) depends mostly on its chemical composition. But resistance also varies as the shape of a structure changes, and the total resistance of a group of structures varies as their relationship to each other is altered. By using an appropriate electrical circuit it is possible to transduce the resistance changes that occur as a result of a wide range of biological processes, from the dilatation of blood vessels (Fabre, 1940) to movements of the velum (Chouard, Meyer, & Chabolle, 1987).

Ohm's law implies that a current must flow through a system if its resistance is to be measured (see Chapter 2, "Analog Electronics"). Special cautions and limitations apply if the resistance of living material is at

---

[6]General reviews of the clinical application of electroglottography are available in Childers and Krishnamurthy (1985), Colton and Conture (1990), Kitzing (1990), Baken (1992a), and Orlikoff (1998).

issue (Dalziel, 1956; Geddes, Baker, Moore, & Coulter, 1969). Aside from the obvious—that the current must be small enough to avoid damage—there are two other limiting considerations. First is the fact that many tissues are irritable, which means that passing an electrical flow through them can elicit a physiological response. Nerve fibers, for instance, will discharge and muscles will contract when electrically stimulated. To avoid these undesirable reactions the current must be kept very small. Furthermore, it is a matter of everyday experience that a current flow may be easily perceptible—and often unpleasantly so. The strength of the sensation is fortunately a function of stimulus frequency: very high frequencies are generally imperceptible unless the current is quite large. For these reasons, a small high-frequency alternating current is used for electroglottography, and, technically, the variable assessed is the tissue's *impedance*.[7]

Electrical Resistance of the Laryngeal Region

In the course of phonation the vocal folds are periodically separated by an air-filled space, the **glottis**. Although tissue is a relatively good conductor of electricity, air is an extremely poor conductor. Therefore the electrical impedance across the phonating larynx rises when the glottis opens and falls as the vocal folds come into increasingly broad contact. Transducing the impedance across the larynx would therefore seem to be ideally suited to showing the details of laryngeal function. But there are special challenges that must be surmounted to make that transduction practical, and the ways in which they are met conditions and restricts interpretation of the resulting electroglottograms.

In Figure 10–21 the vocal folds are shown in their anatomical context, surrounded by the muscles and cartilages of the larynx, the esophagus, the extralaryngeal musculature of the neck, superficial fascia, and the skin (which, quite commonly, has a fat layer of appreciable thickness below it). The larynx in the figure, as in many people, is not very prominent. Electrodes are shown by heavy rectangular bars on the neck surface; they have been located on the skin in approximately the position they would occupy for electroglottography.

For electroglottography a current is passed from one electrode to the other. An important problem is that the current will not take a simple straight-line path between the electrodes. The neck is a "volume

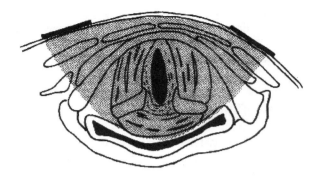

Figure 10–21. Transverse section of the neck showing the larynx in its anatomical context. Black bars on the neck surface represent electroglottograph electrodes; the shaded region shows the zone through which most of the inter-electrode current might be expected to flow.

conductor" and the electrical current spreads out in all directions (including vertically, which is not shown in this section). If the neck were a homogeneous mass the geometry of the current pathway might perhaps be knowable.[8] However, it is anything but homogeneous, and different kinds of tissues have different resistive properties. So the pattern of electrical flow is largely unpredictable, although it is certain to be irregular, and current flow will be more densely concentrated in some areas than in others. The result is that the electrical current does not simply traverse the region of the vocal folds; it also passes through many structures in the neck that are of no particular relevance to evaluating vocal function.

Any impedance measurement must therefore include all the neck structures in the vicinity of the electrodes. A change in any of these—such as an alteration of the shape of an extralaryngeal muscle caused by its contraction—will result in some change of the electrical path and will therefore be reflected in the resulting electroglottogram. More importantly, the spread of current in the neck allows it to flow around the vocal folds. Therefore, changes in the region of the glottis affect only a part of the total current. So the large impedance changes that might be expected to result from the periodic development of an insulating glottal air space prove to be a disappointingly minor part of the overal electroglottographic signal. In fact, they may account for as little as 1% or 2% of the gross transneck impedance.

---

[7]For more detailed discussion of the broader aspects of bioimpedance measurements, see Bagno and Liebman (1959), Allison (1970), or Geddes and Baker (1989).

[8]Titze (1990) has performed some experimental studies to provide preliminary insight into the shape of the electrical field in the neck during electroglottography.

Then, too, the larynx is not fixed in its relationship to other neck structures. The laryngeal cartilages can change their orientation with respect to each other, and the entire larynx can be raised, lowered, and tilted. These actions not only alter the characteristics of the transneck electrical pathway, they also modify the relationship between the larynx and the measuring electrodes. The effect of all of this, given the irregular shape of the current field and the variability of current densities within it, is to add uninterpretable features to the output of any impedance-measuring system.

Electroglottographs are designed to cope with these problems. In particular, they include circuit elements that are intended to minimize the impact on the electroglottogram of changes in perilaryngeal structures; to ignore or compensate for motion of the larynx with respect to the electrodes; to maximize the contribution of the periglottal region to the output; to compensate for slow changes in overall impedance (resulting, for example, from changes in head posture); and to adjust to impedance differences associated with normal anatomical variation across subjects.

THE ELECTROGLOTTOGRAPH

The anatomy of the neck and the characteristics of phonatory motions make it possible to use relatively simple methods to transduce transneck impedance. Figure 10–22 is a block diagram of a "generic" electroglottograph. A stable oscillator produces a high-frequency current that is fed to the electrodes on the neck.[9] In general, the current frequency will be anywhere between about 300 kHz and several megaherz.

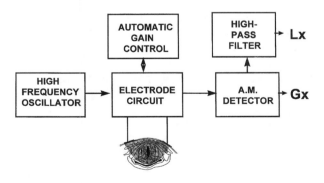

Figure 10–22. A block diagram of a typical electroglottograph.

It will be limited to 10 mA or less, which typically results in a transneck voltage of about 0.5 V. If the impedance of the current path changes, the magnitude of the alternating current will change. Equivalently, there will be a change in the voltage drop between the electrodes (see Chapter 2, "Analog Electronics"). In either case, what results is technically known as an "amplitude modulation of a carrier frequency." It is a simple matter to decode this signal by "demodulation": rectification and low-pass filtering. The resulting signal reflects all of the changes in the region of the neck between the electrodes, including those that are unrelated to glottal behavior.

Electroglottographs may include an "automatic gain control" that adjusts the system's sensitivity to compensate for baseline impedance differences among subjects and for inevitable differences in electrode placement. It also aids in the elimination of the gradual baseline drift that might, for instance, be caused by slow changes in the characteristics of the electrode-skin interface.

Figure 10–23 shows the signal that results from the processing described to this point. At the top, the traces labeled *Gx* show the sound pressure of a sustained /ɑ/ (lower trace) and phonatory events at the glottal level (upper trace). The latter are represented by the very small sawtooth-like variations in the upper trace. A much larger slow impedance change occurs across the duration of phonatory event: the baseline impedance drifts significantly. This record highlights the fact that the impedance changes associated with vocal fold contact patterns are quite small compared to the total impedance variation in the neck region under observation.

In general, however, it is only the function of the vocal folds that is of interest, and, in any case, it is essentially impossible to interpret unambiguously the slower perilaryngeal changes.[10] All electroglottographs therefore provide at least one more stage of signal processing. In general this takes the form of a high-pass filter, which serves to eliminate the slow changes and to pass the more rapid impedance variations for final amplification. The result is shown in the lower part of Figure 10–24, labeled *Lx*. The large slow impedance change is essentially eliminated, and the small phonatory signal has been amplified considerably, allowing its details to be evaluated. Fourcin (1974) has proposed the symbol "Gx" to designate the raw EGG signal, while "Lx" denotes the high-pass-filtered version. That terminology has been widely accepted, and will be used in discussion that follows.

---

[9]Strictly speaking, only two electrodes are required. Some instruments have a third electrode. In Fourcin's Laryngograph, for example, it takes the form of a grounded "guard ring" around each of the active electrodes, shielding it somewhat from noise and restricting the influence of surface current.

[10]Note, however, that electroglottography has been applied to evaluation of some non-speech functions of the upper airway, such as swallowing. See, for instance, Pouderoux, Logemann, and Kahrilas (1996).

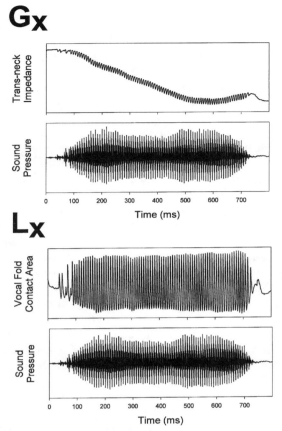

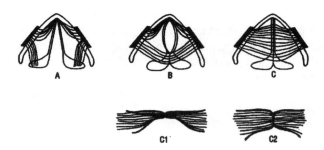

Figure 10–24. Current flow (represented by the solid lines) between electrodes applied to the thyroid alae: **A.** Ventilatory position of the vocal folds, **B.** During the open phase of the phonatory cycle, **C.** During the closed phase of the phonatory cycle; (**C1** and **C2**) At different degrees of vocal fold contact during the closed phase, as seen in coronal section.

Figure 10–23. The unfiltered EGG output (upper trace) shows large, slow impedance changes on which the high-frequency changes associated with vocal fold contacts are imposed. The unfiltered mode is designated *Gx*. High-pass filtering removes the slow changes, which are usually not of interest, and allows the signal representing vocal fold oscillation to be amplified. This mode is called *Lx*.

The Electroglottogram

While there were some questions about a few of the earlier instruments (Smith, 1977, 1981) there is no doubt that modern electroglottographs transduce impedance changes in the area between the electrodes. The major question, however, has centered on what those changes represent.

Physiological Origin of the EGG Signal

The electroglottogram is only minimally influenced, if at all, by the vowel being produced (Fabre, 1958; Vallancien & Faulhaber, 1967; Orlikoff, 1995), which implies that it is insensitive to vocal tract shape. But the hypothesis was advanced by Smith (1977, 1981) that

the impedance changes being observed are produced mostly by compression of the perilaryngeal tissue by the acoustic waves in the vocal tract. That is, the EGG, in Smith's view, functions as a complex microphone. Yet a simple demonstration by Baken (1992a) shows that this is not likely to be the case. When an electrolarynx applied to the neck surface is used to provide acoustic excitation of the vocal tract during breath-holding (when the vocal folds are in contact) the EGG record fails to show oscillations, although an accelerometer on the neck clearly shows that the perilaryngeal tissues are being affected. It seems clear that the EGG is not a microphonic record.

Despite Fabre's (1958) original assertion that "the [electro]glottogram primarily shows the progression of vocal fold contact during each glottal closure,"[11] and confirmatory opinions by several early investigators (Köster & Smith, 1970; Vallancien, 1972; Lecluse, Brocaar, & Verschuure, 1975; Kelman, 1981) there has been a strong and lamentable tendency to treat the electroglottogram as a correlate of glottal width or area (Chevrie-Muller & Grémy, 1962; Grémy & Guérin, 1963). Yet a number of studies involving vocal fold tissue modeling (Rothenberg, 1981; Titze & Talkin, 1981; Titze, 1984; Childers, Hicks, Moore, & Alsaka, 1986; Childers, Alsaka, Hicks, & Moore, 1987; Cranen, 1991), comparison of Lx to glottal volume velocity (Scherer, Druker, & Titze, 1988), and in vitro comparisons of measured contact area to Lx magnitude (van Michel, Pfister, & Luchsinger, 1970) strongly support Fabre's original assumption. So have studies that used high-speed filming or photoglottography to compare Lx to direct measures of glottal width (Croatto, Ferrero, &

---

[11]"La glottogramme révèle d'abord la progressivité de l'accolement des cordes vocales lors de chaque fermeture glottique."

Arrigoni, 1980; Dejonckere, 1981; Childers, Naik, Larar, Krishnamurthy, & Moore, 1983). Perhaps the most telling demonstration was performed by Gilbert, Potter, and Hoodin (1984) who inserted a plastic insulating strip between the vocal folds during phonation. This reduced the length of electrical contact of the vocal folds by 5 mm, although it did not impede physical contact. Their records clearly show the very significant extent to which this electrical isolation of a region of the vocal folds reduced the magnitude of the resulting EGG signal.

It seems abundantly clear that electroglottography transduces the *vocal fold contact area*. Because of this the electroglottogram contains information only about those parts of the vocal fold oscillatory cycle during which there is some contact. It reveals nothing, in short, about the open phase. There is unfortunately, a great deal of casual terminological sloppiness which has encouraged widespread confusion, such that electroglottograms are commonly described in terms of "open" and "closed" phases, implying a transduction of the glottal status. No such representation can be derived from the electroglottogram. Accordingly, in the discussion that follows, reference will be made not to "closing" and "opening", but rather to "contacting" and "decontacting" phases of the vibratory cycle.

Figure 10–24 shows, in a highly schematic way, the form of the laryngeal "resistor" as seen by an electroglottograph. The lines represent the paths taken by current flowing between the two electrodes applied over the alae of the thyroid cartilage. In Figure 10–24A, the vocal folds are abducted to a nonphonatory position. Air is an excellent electrical insulator and the electrical current cannot traverse the glottal space. The current pathways are therefore greatly lengthened, and the impedance of the pathway thereby greatly increased, as electrons flow (in three dimensions) around the glottis. When the arytenoids adduct and contact each other (Figure 10–24B) the current pathway is simplified and shortened, causing the impedance to drop. Even when the glottis opens during part of the phonatory cycle there is a moderately good conducting path through the arytenoids (and also a longer path through the perilaryngeal tissues). During the closed phase of vocal fold oscillation (Figure 10–24C) the electrical pathway is optimized by the contact of the vocal folds. There are, however, degrees of contact. Over the course of the "closed" phase of each glottal cycle (at least in modal register) the contact of the vocal folds varies from minimal (Figure 10–24C1) to maximal (Figure 10–24C2) as contact involves more of the vertical dimension of the vocal folds. Electrical resistance increases with the total length of the current path and decreases as the area of contact grows. Thus, one would expect the translaryngeal resistance to con-

stantly (but not linearly) drop as the laryngeal status changed from status A through C2 in the figure. This expectation is, in fact, borne out in practice, including the change of resistance during the closed phase.

Because the output is not an analog of the glottal area, but represents instead the status of the larynx as a unit, Fourcin has proposed that the instrument be called an *electrolaryngograph*, rather than an electroglottograph (Fourcin & Abberton, 1971, 1976; Fourcin, 1981; Abberton, Howard, & Fourcin, 1989; Fourcin, 1993; Fourcin, Abberton, Miller, & Howells, 1995; Abberton & Fourcin, 1997). While Fourcin's point is well taken, laryngography has long been used by radiologists to refer to contrast-medium visualization of the larynx (Landman, 1970). To prevent any confusion it seems wiser to retain the term, which, despite its literal inaccuracy, has long been prevalent in the literature.

Electroglottographic Procedure

Although specific details differ according to the particular model of electroglottograph being used, the technique of electroglottography is straightforward. The measuring electrodes are attached according to the manufacturer's recommendations. (Some units, for instance, require that electrode paste be used.) There is no firm rule for the exact location of the electrodes, but in general they should be superficial to the thyroid cartilage at a level that approximates the position of the vocal folds. Positioning is optimized by watching the waveforms generated during trial phonations and moving the electrodes until the best signal is obtained. It should have maximal amplitude, be free of extraneous noise, and have a moderately stable baseline. Although all EGGs have circuitry that is designed to reject nonphonatory signals and to compensate for baseline drift, to some extent they are all still sensitive to movement artifacts. The patient should therefore be positioned (perhaps with a head support) so as to minimize movement during testing.

Interpretation of Electroglottographic Waveforms

The Lx waveform (that is, the electroglottogram after high-pass filtering to remove the slower articulatory and other influences) is shown together with the sound pressure record for sustained /ɑ/ by a normal male speaker in Figure 10–25. Increasing impedance (that is, a smaller vocal fold contact area) is downward. This is the orientation that has been recommended internationally (Baken, 1992a) because it satisfies our intuitive sense that higher values should be closer to the top of the graph; it emphasizes the fact that the variable being plotted is not, in fact, glottal width; and

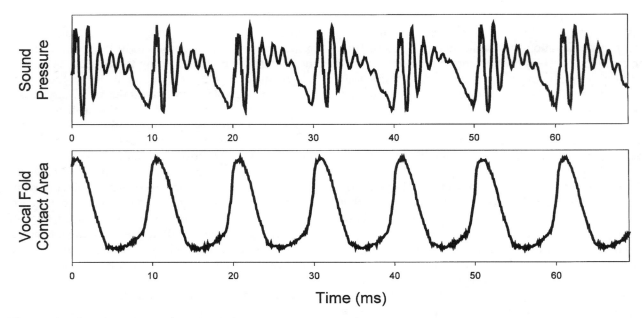

Figure 10–25. Bottom: Lx of modal register phonation at comfortable pitch as produced by a normal adult speaker. Increasing resistance (decreasing vocal fold contact area) is downward. Top: The sound pressure signal.

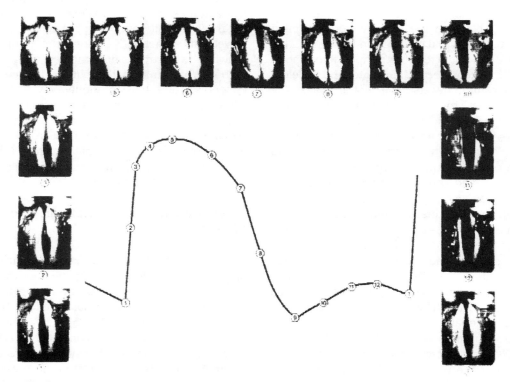

Figure 10–26. Lx with simultaneous stroboscopic views of the vocal folds. The photographs correspond to the number points in the Lx wave. (Courtesy of Dr. F. L. E. Lecluse, Amsterdam, The Netherlands.)

it makes for a more easily-interpreted data representation when Lx is plotted along with other traces, especially the photoglottogram. The literature contains numerous examples oriented the other way (that is, with larger vocal fold contact area toward the bottom). It is therefore important to check the captions in research reports and—because there remain some clinical centers that prefer the alternative presentation style—to indicate the direction of increasing vocal fold contact on clinical EGG records.

The Lx waveform is not of interest in itself: Its importance lies in the vocal fold behavior that it represents. Considerable research effort has been devoted to establishing what the important features of the waveform are and what they correspond to. As mentioned earlier, it is very clear that the curve does not reflect glottal width, but rather vocal fold contact area. Because of the complex motion of the vocal fold margin during the phonatory cycle, the contact area function is a very complicated one and is itself far from perfectly understood. It is therefore not surprising that the interpretation of Lx is still subject to significant debate. Both elucidation and revision of currently held views are likely in the future.

Lecluse and his coworkers (Lecluse, Brocaar, & Verschuure, 1975; Lecluse, 1974, 1977) did simultaneous electroglottography and synchronstroboscopy on normal subjects, with results illustrated in Figure 10–26. That there is an overall relationship between the size of the glottic opening and the translaryngeal impedance is apparent, but the correspondence is clearly very imperfect. Significant details of vocal fold movement appear to have been missed.

This is hardly surprising, and is easily explained by the fact that the vocal folds do not meet in the midline as two monolithic masses. Rather, the medial surface of each vocal fold is constantly deforming and, during the closed phase each vocal fold "rolls" against its opposite. In the normal larynx, closure thus begins at the bottom of the vocal fold and spreads upward. In other words, after the glottis has been closed (by meeting of the lower margins of the vocal folds), contact area—and hence the magnitude of the electroglottographic signal—continues to increase. But soon the lower margins begin to separate, and the contact area —and the electroglottogram's amplitude—decreases, although the glottis remains closed above the area of growing separation. Thus, although looking down from above reveals an apparently-stable glottal closure, there is a great deal taking place.

Further complicating the picture is the fact that vocal fold contact is a gradual process in the transverse plane as well. That is, the vocal folds do not suddenly meet all at once along their full length. There is, instead, a "zippering," such that contact is initiated at one point and then spreads horizontally to close (in the normal larynx) the full length of the glottis.

In summary, the electroglottogram is sensitive to the covert changes of contact area occurring during glottal closure, and it also reflects the growth and loss of contact area along the length of the vocal folds as glottal closure and opening succeed each other. It is easy to see why the electroglottogram corresponds only poorly to the glottal width function.

Figure 10–27, based on the work of Rothenberg (1981) and of MacCurtain and Fourcin (1982) depicts

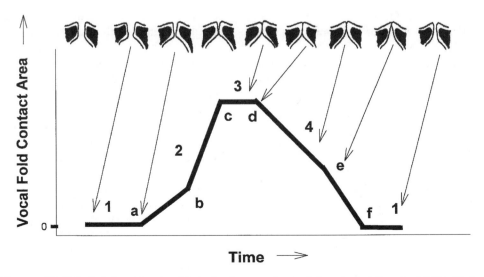

Figure 10–27. Relationship of points in the Lx wave to medial contact of the vocal folds. (Illustration based on the work of Rothenberg, 1981, and MacCurtain and Fourcin, 1982.)

the changes in the coronal plane that help clarify the Lx wave a bit. In this figure, an idealized Lx wave is shown (with decreasing resistance, or greater vocal fold contact area, upward) but various points have been labeled to correspond with positions of the vocal folds as seen in *coronal* section, primarily during the closed phase. With this understanding one can construct an "ideal" Lx wave and consider the significance of its features. The various inflection points are labelled with letters, while the intervals between them are numbered.

The relationship between gross features of Lx and the major phases of the glottal cycle is reasonably well established and generally agreed upon:

- A flat **segment 1** represents minimal contact of the vocal folds. It is considered to show the period during which the vocal folds are separated, and it is during this phase that peak glottal flow occurs.
- During **segment 2** interelectrode impedance falls rapidly, marking the growing contact of the vocal folds.
- **Segment 3** is the period of maximal vocal fold contact. An important caution must be kept in mind: "maximal contact" means just that—it does not imply total overall contact and hence does not signal glottal closure. In many situations—pathological and occasionally normal—the glottis remains somewhat patent throughout this period.
- Vocal fold contact is lost during **segment 4** until a minimum is again reached, ending the glottal cycle.

Research by several investigators (Rothenberg, 1981; Titze & Talkin, 1981; Baer, Löfqvist, & McGarr, 1983; Childers et al., 1986, 1987; Titze, 1989; Cranen, 1991) allows a more complete interpretation of the idealized waveform:

Point a: The lower margins of the vocal folds make initial contact, signaling the start of the glottal closing phase. Fourcin (1981) believes that vocal fold contact is often initiated by the sudden establishment of a mucus bridge between the two vocal folds, which results in a very abrupt onset of the contacting phase.

Interval a–b: Lower margin approximation proceeds. In some instances of closure the folds remain virtually parallel and closure occurs very rapidly along their entire length. Under these circumstances the slope of the a–b interval is great. Often, however, the folds form an acute angle, giving the glottis a V shape, and causing a "zippering" closure. When this happens, the slope of the a–b interval is less.

Point b: The upper margins of the vocal folds make initial contact.

Interval b–c: Upper margin approximation spreads anteroposteriorly; glottal closure is achieved during this interval.

Point c: Maximal contact is achieved. The closing phase ends. Note that this does NOT mean that no glottal gap remains.

Interval c–d: The surface area of contact remains maximal. Minimal glottal size persists. "Minimal glottal size" might be zero (no glottal opening), but it might not.

Point d: Separation of the lower margins of the vocal folds begins, initiating the opening phase.

Interval d–e: Lower margin separations proceeds gradually.

Point e: Separation of the lower margin completed. The upper margins begin to separate, with opening often proceding in a posterior-to-anterior direction. The exact significance of this inflection point, commonly referred to as a *knee*, in the opening phase, has been a matter of considerable interest and dispute. There is evidence to show that the abrupt change in slope occurs at the time when a bridge of mucus linking the vocal folds suddenly ruptures. But the data of some investigators (Baer, Titze, & Yoshioka, 1983; Fourcin, 1986; Childers et al., 1987; Berke, Moore, Gerratt, Aly, & Tantisira, 1988) suggest an explanation more dependent on the upward excursion of the vocal lip just before opening, at least under certain circumstances.

Interval e–f: The upper margins of the vocal folds continue to separate. Glottal opening occurs somewhere in this interval, following which glottal length and (perhaps) glottal width increase. Note that the exact time within this interval at which a glottal space first appears is unknowable from the EGG record.

Point f: Contact between the vocal folds reaches its minimum. Glottal length is presumed to be maximal.

Interval f–a: No change in vocal fold contact occurs, although glottal width is likely to increase to a maximum and then reduce again during this time period. Because the vocal folds are not in contact the electroglottogram provides no information about glottal events during this interval.

The following general conclusions seem justified by our current understanding of laryngeal function and electroglottographic transduction:

1. The electroglottogram depicts *relative* vocal fold contact area. This implies that maximal contact does not necessarily indicate glottal closure. It is entirely possible and, especially in loft (falsetto) phonation, it is not uncommon, for there to be no glottal closure at all.

2. Obliteration of the glottis probably occurs before maximal vocal fold contact is attained. Therefore, even when there is complete glottal closure, it is not possible, on the basis of the EGG signal, to specify the precise time at which it is first achieved.

3. Because phonation requires a transglottal airflow it is safe to conclude that there is a glottal opening during the f–a interval. But the exact instant at which that opening first appears (and at which airflow first begins) cannot be determined by inspection of the Lx record.

4. Although there is an interval of minimal vocal fold contact area, and although it represents glottal opening, that minimum is influenced in no predictable way by the extent of vocal fold separation. Therefore, the f–a interval does not reflect glottal width, nor can it show movements of the vocal folds.

5. Events that occur during the period of vocal fold contact should be evident in the Lx record. In particular, aberrations during the period of maximal contact should be clearly indicated.

6. A knee during the decontacting phase is common, but it is by no means universal. Its significance, particularly for clinical evaluation, is not definitively known.

7. Lx amplitude is not a valid correlate of vocal intensity.

8. The F_0 of Lx matches the vocal F_0 exactly.

Effect of Vocal Register on Lx. On the whole, each of the three normal vocal registers has a recognizable electroglottographic signature, illustrated in Figure 10–28. The waveform of normal modal register is of large amplitude and shows a distinct asymmetry: contacting progresses more rapidly than decontacting. There is also a period of sustained minimal contact. (It is this pattern that has previously been used to illustrate the Lx waveform in this chapter.)

Pulse register (glottal fry) is produced with very lax vocal folds that contact each other over a large medial surface area. The result is a large-amplitude Lx wave. Unique to pulse register in normal voices is a "dicrotic" waveform. Small-amplitude contact peaks alternate with large-amplitude contact peaks.[12] Loft register (falsetto), on the other hand, is generated by very tense vocal folds whose medial surfaces are extremely narrowed. The area of contact is therefore very reduced, producing small-amplitude Lx waves. (In fact, it is not uncommon for loft register phonation to be produced without the vocal folds meeting at the midline.) The Lx waveform during loft register is more symmetrical than modal register phonation, commonly achieving a very sinusoidal waveshape.

The Interpretation of Lx Geometry. The EGG signal provides only an overall *summary* of what is happening at the level of the glottis. That is because the activities of all of the separate structures and areas involved in vocal fold oscillation are inextricably blended together to create the Lx signal. It is therefore not possible to infer the movement of any particular point along the length of the vocal fold. Nonetheless, modeling and observation suggest that changes of certain basic geometric properties of the Lx wave are indicative of specifiable alterations of vocal fold adjustment and behavior (Gleeson, Pearson, Armistead, & Yates, 1984; Titze, 1984, 1989; Childers et al., 1986; Lesser, Williams, & Hoddinott, 1986; Gómez Gonzáles, & del Cañizo Alvarez, 1988; Lesser & William, 1988; Painter, 1988, 1990; Larson, Ramig, & Scherer, 1994). Titze (1990) has described four geometric characteristics

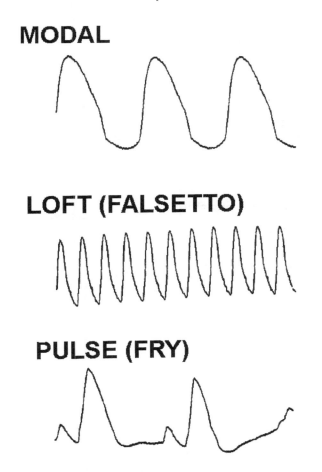

MODAL

LOFT (FALSETTO)

PULSE (FRY)

Figure 10–28. Typical appearance of the Lx electroglottogram for the three voice registers.

---

[12]There is disagreement about whether phonation can be labelled pulse register only when this "dicrotic" pattern is observed. The term "creak" is often reserved to distinguish pulse–register-like phonation without dicrotic wavetrains.

that are likely to result from clinically meaningful alterations of vocal fold status or behavior. They are summarized in Figure 10–29A, which depicts various idealized Lx waveshapes on the left, and associates them with glottal characteristics, schematized on the right in the coronal plane. The topmost curve and vocal fold diagrams (1) represent the normal adjustment of the vocal folds for modal register phonation and the Lx wave (with increasing vocal fold contact area shown as an upward excursion) associated with it. It is assumed that, for normal phonation, the vocal folds barely contact each other at their most medial edges (the upper lips of the vocal folds) when at rest. During the vibrational cycle various forces cause them to move laterally, and they are separated for a significant period of time.

After achieving a maximal lateral displacement each vocal fold accelerates toward the midline, and momentum forces ultimately cause them to collide and to deform against each other. Their contact during this phase is indicated by the non-zero portion of the idealized EGG, whose amplitude increases as the size of the deformed "front" of each vocal fold grows. Ultimately, however, the medializing momentum is spent and lateralizing forces again become dominant. The vocal folds begin to separate as the medial edges bounce away from each other, decreasing the size of the contacting face. The Lx wave loses amplitude during this time. Ultimately the folds lose contact, and the Lx wave resumes a zero amplitude.

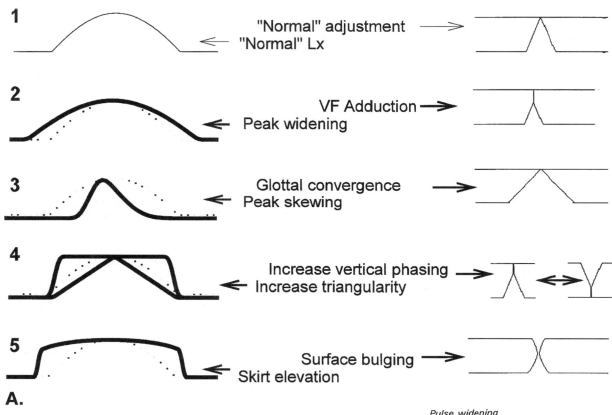

Figure 10–29. **A.** Variations in the geometry of the Lx wave and their relationship to glottal adjustment. The curves on the left are idealizations of different Lx geometries. The top curve—of normal phonation—is superimposed on each of the lower four curves to highlight the geometric change that is involved. The outlines on the right schematize (in coronal section) the related glottal configuration characteristics. **B.** Various Lx waveforms showing differences in pulse widening, peak skewing, skirt bulging, and overall triangularity. See text for details.

Peak widening. Now assume that the vocal folds are more adducted than "normal" (schematized by (2) in Figure 10–29A). That is, the vocal folds retain their geometry, but each one's entire mass is moved toward the midline. Instead of merely touching at their upper margins they are significantly compressed against each other. The lateralizing forces will succeed in separating the folds, but there is more "opening work" to be done. Furthermore, the glottal opening that is achieved will not be as wide, and thus will be more quickly closed once the restoring medializing forces again come to predominate. The result is that the vocal folds spend a greater proportion of each cycle in contact with each other (or alternatively, they spend relatively less time apart). The Lx wave therefore shows a contacting (non-zero amplitude) segment that occupies a greater proportion of the cycle (Figure 10–29B). The Lx peak, in other words, has been widened in proportion to the cycle's duration.

Peak skewing. The glottis at rest is convergent. That is, it is wider in cross section at the bottom than it is at the top. The angle of convergence can be varied as a function, for instance, of the tensional forces operating at the edge of the vocal fold. During vibration, however, there is also a phase lag between the position of the upper and lower margins. That is, they do not medialize and lateralize at the same time, and thus there are times during the glottal cycle when the glottis is divergent (wider at the top than at the bottom). The combination of convergence and phase lag produce asymmetry (skewing) of the Lx waveform (schematized by (3) in Figure 10–29A). This is because, as the vocal folds meet and deform each other the leading edges, which are convergently wedge-shaped in cross section, square up against each other, thus rapidly increasing the contact area, which is reflected in a rapid rise of the Lx wave (Figure 10–29B). During the separation phase, however, the convergent shape is resumed as the vocal folds separate. The decontacting is therefore a somewhat slower process, and the Lx wave loses amplitude more gradually.

Ramping. The "ramping" of the Lx wave is due to the time delay (phase lag) between approximation of the lower and upper lips of the vocal folds. (It therefore implies the convergent glottal shape just discussed.) If the phase lag (time difference between the start of contact of the lower lip and the start of contact of the upper lip) is small, the contact must grow very rapidly and, in the decontacting phase, will diminish just as quickly. The Lx wave will therefore tend to be more

rectangular. Conversely, a larger phase difference will cause the Lx wave to be more triangular, since contact changes will occur more gradually.

Skirt elevation. Skirt elevation refers to the presence of a "knee" in the rising and falling phases of the Lx wave. The knee is produced by the presence of a bulge in the vocal fold's medial surface. The bulging area is similar to a vertical segment in the wall of the otherwise sloped medial surface. As the vocal folds begin their contact, the contact surface area increases very rapidly in the region of the bulge, causing the Lx wave to grow quickly. As contact increases, however, the contribution of the bulging areas is exhausted and further contact increase is produced by the sloping surfaces. This contact develops more slowly. Hence, the Lx amplitude increases more gradually. The reverse, of course, occurs during the decontacting behavior of vocal fold separation. The result is an Lx wave whose knees are produced by the switch between rapid contact change (at onset and offset) and more gradual contact variation.

Deviations from the Ideal Lx Waveshape. Electroglottography is undertaken to assess abnormal

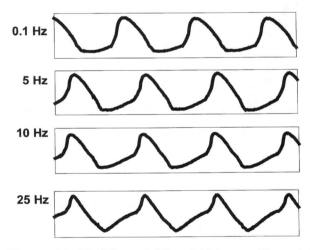

Figure 10–30. Effect of different high-pass filter cutoff frequencies (F_c) on the appearance of the Lx waveform. Most prominent is the change in the "open" (minimal contact) portion of the wave, which, in principle, should be flat but which becomes increasingly sloped as the cutoff frequency rises. Note also that the Lx peak grows sharper with increasing F_c and, in this example, the decontacting phase becomes noticeably more linear, giving the Lx waveshape greater triangularity.

---

[13]Unfortunately, several manufacturers do not specify the cutoff frequency used by their instrument, making signal evaluation somewhat uncertain in some circumstances.

[14]On some instruments the cutoff frequency can be selected by the user, while in others it is fixed and, in general, unspecified.

voice production, which is commonly characterized by Lx waves that differ not only from the normal form but, indeed, often present abnormalities not accounted for by the principles discussed above. Some of these are unavoidable artifact, but others can serve as the basis of reasonable inference founded on a solid appreciation of the principles of electroglottography, awareness of the characteristics of the measuring instrument, and a firm understanding of vocal physiology.

The effect of filtering. All of the electroglottographs currently on the market include high-pass filtering and display the Lx waveform. (Some also provide access to the unfiltered Gx signal.) The high-pass cutoff frequency varies from one manufacturer to another.[13]

The benefits of high-pass filtering to obtain the Lx wave are not obtained without a cost. The filtering produces a certain amount of waveform distortion, a fact noted quite early in the history of electroglottography by van Michel, Pfister, and Luchsinger (1970). Figure 10–30 illustrates how the Lx wave obtained from a single male subject changes as the cutoff frequency is varied within the range available in modern electroglottographs.[14] The most obvious effect is on the open-glottis (maximal

impedance, minimal contact) portion of the wave, which, in principle, should be flat. As the high-pass cutoff frequency rises this portion of the wave develops an increasing slope. Aside from changing one's visual impression of the character of the Lx wave, this distortion can have serious consequences for the validity of measurement of EGG parameters, such as the "contact quotient" (discussed later), that are derived by voice analysis software. Close examination also shows that raising the cutoff frequency also causes the Lx wave to have a sharper peak and the decontacting phase to become less "rounded" and more linear. These effects can be particularly serious if they are not taken into account when assessing the implications of the waveform geometry according to the principles just discussed.

Irregularity of EGG amplitude. Like all physiologic signals, Lx has a certain amount of normal cycle-to-cycle variability of frequency and amplitude. Frequency instability is the same as that measured by jitter (see Chapter 6, "Vocal Fundamental Frequency"), but Lx amplitude perturbation, which reflects period-to-period changes in maximal vocal fold contact area, is not at all related to the variations of the sound pressure

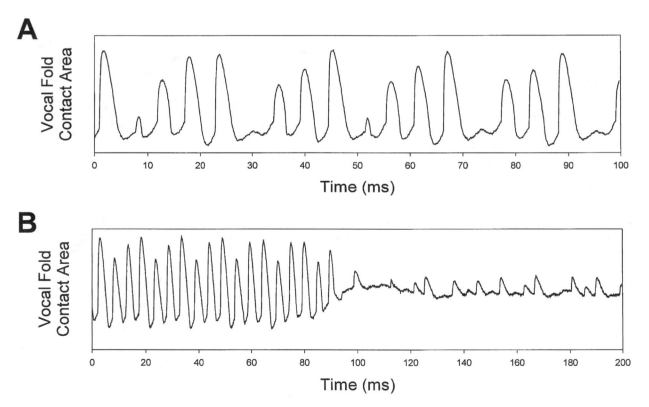

Figure 10–31. The sudden change in maximal vocal fold contact area, implied by the change in Lx amplitude, betrays a bifurcation in the function of the oscillatory system. **A.** This repeated tetrad of 4 Lx cycles, each with a greater maximal vocal fold contact area, shows the sort of complex behavior that is typical of chaotic systems. **B.** Complex patterns—in this case Lx triplets—are usually unstable and abruptly give way to regular phonatory oscillation, other complex patterns, or to random oscillation (aphonia).

of the radiated speech signal that are assessed by shimmer (see Chapter 5, "Speech Intensity"). The exact relationship of Lx amplitude variations to other characteristics of the vocal signal is, in fact, unknown. Lx amplitude may be influenced by changes of larynx height and posture. (Automatic gain control circuits in some EGG instruments, however, may minimize or completely hide these effects if the change is accomplished slowly.)

Changes in Lx amplitude that are effected over the space of only a cycle or two may indicate a clinically significant shift in vibratory behavior (Sopko, 1986; Orlikoff & Kraus, 1996) especially if the change is suggestive of what nonlinear dynamics theory refers to as a "bifurcation" of oscillatory function. Patterned changes of Lx amplitude (Figure 10–31A) indicate the dominance of a chaotic (in the technical sense) mode of function (Awrejcewicz, 1990; Baken, 1990, 1992b, 1993, 1994,1995a, 1995b; Herzel, Steinecke, Mende, & Wermke, 1991; Mende, Herzel, & Wermke, 1990; Titze, Baken, & Herzel, 1993). Quite commonly, the complexly patterned mode of oscillation is unstable, and the oscillation soon shows another bifurcation. In the case of Figure 10–31B, a pattern of Lx triplets changes abruptly to an erratic, apparently-random "flopping" of the vocal folds.

Some preliminary evidence (Haji, Horiguchi, Baer, & Gould, 1986; Horiguchi, Haji, Baer, & Gould, 1987) suggests that the perturbation of Lx amplitude may be a more sensitive gauge of perceived vocal disorder than acoustic perturbation measures. It presumably reflects the cycle-to-cycle variability of the extent of vocal fold contact, which may be a more powerful correlate of phonatory stability (Orlikoff, 1991, 1995; Linders, Massa, Boersma, & Dejonckere, 1995; Orlikoff, Baken, & Kraus, 1997). For the normal voice Lx amplitude perturbation is typically about 0.2 dB, considerably less than the shimmer measured from a microphone signal. It is, however, crucial to keep in mind that the Lx and sound pressure perturbation measures are not at all comparable. The former assesses vocal physiology, whereas the latter is a metric of the acoustic yield. Beyond the fact that high variability in physiological systems is always suspect, not enough is yet known about Lx amplitude variability to make it useful in clinical evaluation.

Irregularities of Lx geometry. Aside from the changes in the geometric conformation of the Lx wave discussed earlier, the intrusion of irregular features into the wave is not uncommon in cases of vocal pathology. That is, there are often assorted "bumps" and "dips" in the waveshape. Given the complexity of the motion of the glottal margin and the myriad possibilities for abnormality of tissue structure or biomechanics, it is not surprising that efforts to formulate simple rules

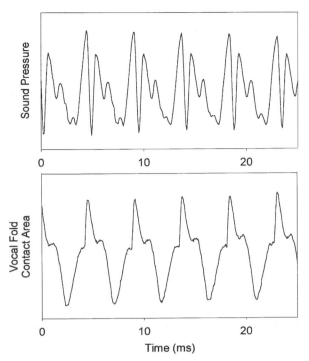

Figure 10–32. Sound pressure (above) and Lx electroglottogram (below) for a speaker with vocal fold nodules.

relating abnormal details to specific pathologies have not met with notable success (van Michel, 1967; Neil, Wechsler, & Robinson, 1977; Hanson, Gerratt, & Ward, 1983; Smith & Childers, 1983; Childers et al., 1984; Rambaud-Pistone, 1984; Dejonckere & Lebacq, 1985; Motta, Cesari, Lengo, & Motta, 1990). In many cases, however, reasoning based on a solid understanding of glottal mechanics will lead to a useful interpretation of the source of waveshape irregularities.

The Lx signal shown in Figure 10–32, from a patient with vocal-fold nodules, may provide an example of how such contact-pattern irregularities my be interpreted. Note how vocal fold contact area increases rather linearly before a distinct "shoulder" appears in the contacting phase. The shoulder probably results from a momentary decrease in the growth of contact as the "open" spaces on each side of the well-developed nodule are compressed. Once these paranodular regions are approximated, the contact area continues to increase, now with a rate that is even greater. During the decontacting phase the situation is reversed, except that the nodule seems to "bounce" back into contact, causing the contact area to increase a bit at the shoulder of the decontacting phase. This may be due to the release of the paranodular zones, allowing the nodule to elastically recoil toward the midline. Decontacting then proceeds unremarkably. There is no evidence of a true "open" phase although it is clear that the glottis must be open at some time. This is therefore also a good example of why "open" and "closed" must not be inferred from Lx waves.

Contact-Based Measures of Vocal Fold Behavior

The configuration of the glottis is tied to the position and configuration of the vocal-fold edges. But electroglottography provides no useful information about any portion of the vocal fold that is not in contact with its opposite member, since electrical impedance is in no way related to the size of the glottis. It is not surprising, then, that measures of glottal dynamics (such as O_q and S_q) measured from the Lx wave do not correspond well to those obtained from the glottal area function (Reinsch & Gobsch, 1972; Kelman, 1981; Unger, Unger, & Tietze, 1981; Hacki, 1989; Dromey, Stathopoulos, & Sapienza, 1992; Nieto, Cobeta, & Kitzing, 1993). Baer, Titze, and Yoshioka (1983) showed quite clearly that *glottal* and *contact* landmarks identified through simultaneously obtained glottal-area and EGG waveforms do not coincide. That is, there are substantial changes in glottal dimensions during the relatively flat minimal (or lost) contact portion of the EGG, while there is significant contact area change during the flat (closed glottis) phase of the glottal area function. In particular, the beginning of glottal closure precedes the increasing-contact Lx interval and glottal opening continues long after the folds apparently lose contact.

Such data raise the question of what, exactly, is meant by "glottal opening" and "glottal closure." Measures of glottal behavior depend critically on identifying when and whether the glottis is closed or open. Before researchers and clinicians had identified the importance of the vocal fold mucosal wave and vertical contact dynamics in the maintenance of phonation, these terms were quite clear—defined by the 2-dimensional glottal width/area function or visually by a endoscopic view of the superior surface. But it is now well recognized that the vocal folds typically assume a divergent configuration during approximation and become convergent during separation. For this reason, contemporary descriptions of glottal dynamics necessarily refer to the separate behavior of the upper and lower "portions" of the glottis (Gauffin, Binh, Ananthapadmanabha, & Fant, 1983; Scherer & Guo, 1991), recognizing that at a particular instant one portion might be growing wider while the other is growing narrower.

To derive measures of vocal fold contact behavior, it is best to destinguish the *vibratory cycle*, defined by contact phenomena and schematized in Figure 10–33, from the more commonly depicted *glottal cycle* as shown earlier in Figure 10–18. Discussing the contact area waveform in terms of the vibratory cycle elimi-

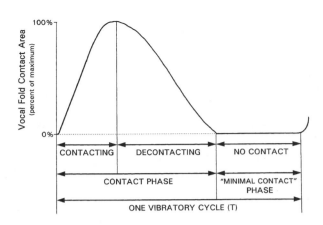

Figure 10–33. Divisions of the vibratory or vocal-fold contact cycle.

nates the need to refer to opening and closing behavior that cannot be verified using EGG alone (Baer, Löfqvist, & McGarr, 1983; Orlikoff, 1998). Unfortunately, most quantitative EGG measures assume a waveshape that, more or less, approximates the one shown in Figure 10–33. Although such an assumption may be safe to make in the absence of pathology, it may be untenable for many dysphonic patients. For instance, consider once again the rapid and often unpredictable Lx changes shown in Figure 10–31 or the "peculiar" Lx waveshape in Figure 10–32. At present, there is no way to characterize the salient features of the signal beyond the sort of informed interpretation discussed earlier. Thus, for any vocal pathology, it is critically important to evaluate any quantitative electroglottographic measure in light of a qualitative assessment of the vibratory pattern.

Relative Contact Duration. For purposes of computer synthesis and analysis, Titze (1984, 1989) defined the ***abduction quotient*** as the ratio of the half distance between the vocal processes to the amplitude of vocal fold vibration. This parameter is thought to reflect the degree of medial fold compression along a hypoadducted "breathy" to a hyperadducted "pressed" (or "tight") voice continuum (Scherer & Titze, 1987). In actual practice, however, it is not possible to obtain quick and precise information in vivo about the width of the cartilaginous glottis and the vibratory amplitude. Thus, some investigators have turned to the EGG for an indirect assessment of adductory adjustment. The derived measure, usually referred to as the ***contact quotient*** (or ***CQ***), is defined as the percent of the entire vibratory cycle wherein vocal fold contact area is greater than some "minimal level" (Rothenberg & Mahshie, 1988; Scherer, Druker, & Titze, 1988; Scherer, Gould, Titze, Meyers, & Sataloff, 1988; Orlikoff, 1991;

Houben, Buekers, & Kingma, 1992). (In Figure 10–33, $CQ\%$ = Contact Phase/Vibratory Cycle, multiplied by 100.) This measure has also been called the EGG *closed quotient*, although it is probably best to suppress this usage for the reasons outlined above regarding the inappropriate application of glottal terminology. Preliminary evidence indicates that the CQ provides a fairly good metric of vocal fold adduction (Scherer et al., 1995).

Under normal vocal circumstances, CQ typically varies between 40 and 60% and there does not appear to be a significant sex effect (Robb & Simmons, 1990; Orlikoff, 1991; Scherer et al., 1995; Orlikoff et al., 1997). Given the propensity for a posterior glottal chink and a "breathier" voice quality in women, several investigators have sought to document a substantially lower CQ in female subjects (Lindsey, Breen, & Fourcin, 1988; Higgins & Saxman, 1991). But, as with any measure derived from the Lx signal, the CQ reflects the relative degree of vocal fold contact and is unlikely to be sensitive to unvarying glottal gaps or chinks that may substantially influence mean phonatory airflow but not the contact pattern.

It has been observed that the CQ tends to increase with F_0 in women, although the contact duty cycle is apparently unrelated to vocal frequency in men (Lindsey et al., 1988; Howard, Lindsey, & Allen, 1990; Howard, 1995). Nonetheless, an increase in the CQ with vocal intensity has been documented for both men and women (Kempster, Preston, Mack, & Larson, 1987; Hacki, 1989; Orlikoff, 1991; Dromey et al., 1992), consistent with data that show a strong relationship between vocal intensity and the adductory presetting of the vocal folds (Titze, 1988; Hacki, 1996).

Relative Contact Rise Time. It has been hypothesized that the relative duration or slope of the increasing-contact portion of the vibratory cycle might provide greater information about vocal fold dynamics directly associated with the acoustic excitation of the vocal tract (Kelman, 1981). Vocal intensity is strongly related to the maximal rate of transglottal airflow declination (see "Maximum Flow Declination Rate," this chapter), which appears to be closely related to the rate at which vocal fold contact is made (Titze, 1988; Orlikoff, 1991). Thus not only the CQ, but the rate of gained contact can be useful in documenting vocal effort (Kakita, 1988). It has been suggested also that analysis of the ascending leg of the contact interval can be useful for describing the specific effects of a mass lesion on vocal physiology (Colton & Conture, 1990; Orlikoff, 1991).

Investigators have defined the contact rise time (or slope) in a number of ways. Some of the proposed measures attempt to assess the relative steepness of the most linear portion of the increasing-contact interval. For example, Orlikoff (1991) derived a slope measure for the rise between 25% and 75% (the middle 50%) of the maximum contact area, while Fisher and her colleagues (Fisher, Scherer, Swank, Giddens, & Patten, 1995) focused their measure on the increase from 10% to 90% (the middle 80%) of the peak contact. Other studies, however, have examined the duration of the entire increasing-contact interval, relative to that of the full vibratory cycle (Wechsler, 1977; Houben, et al., 1992; Orlikoff et al., 1997). The use of the time-differentiated electroglottogram (dEGG) to examine the rapidity of contact change (or to define the beginning and end of the contact interval) has also enjoyed some popularity among researchers (Childers & Krishnamurthy, 1985; Dromey et al., 1992; Houben et al., 1992). Unfortunately, as the EGG signal is prone to high-frequency noise, experience has shown that it is not practicable for routine clinical use, especially for computer-automated data extraction of contact parameters. Determining the most clinically relevant measure of contact rise and the most reliable method of measurement will require further investigation.

Contact Symmetry. For the typical modal-register electroglottogram, the contact phase is asymmetrical: that is, the contacting phase is shorter than the decontacting phase. The degree of contact asymmetry is thought to reflect vocal fold tonus and to be particularly sensitive to vertical mucosal dynamics (Hirano, 1981; Titze & Talkin, 1981; Childers et al., 1986). Orlikoff (1991) defined a dimensionless ratio to describe EGG symmetry called the ***contact index (CI)***. The CI is the time difference between the contacting and decontacting phases divided by the duration of the full contact phase. The CI will vary between –1 (for a negligibly short contacting phase) and +1 (for a negligibly short decontacting phase), such that CI = 0 represents a perfectly symmetrical contact phase. Under normal vocal circumstances, CI seems to vary between –0.6 to –0.4 for men and women (Orlikoff, 1991; Orlikoff et al., 1997). It is inversely related to vocal intensity (Orlikoff, 1991) and can be expected to vary with voice register (Gougerot et al., 1960; Fourcin, 1981; Kitzing, 1982; Roubeau, Chevrie-Muller, & Arabia-Guidet, 1987; Schutte & Seidner, 1988; Fisher et al., 1995; Orlikoff et al., 1997) or with the specific mode of vocal fold vibration (Welch, Sergeant, & MacCurtain, 1989; Kitzing, 1990).

Ultrasonography

Although ultrasound techniques (discussed in Chapters 11, "Velopharyngeal Function", and 12, "Speech

Movements") can be adapted for laryngeal examination, the size of the vocal folds, their location, the complexity of their movements, and the small distances they traverse during phonation create very special difficulties in doing so. Since the edges of the vocal folds constitute a very small target, the ultrasonic beam must be very narrow and well defined. The laws of physics conspire to make such a beam very difficult to obtain. A small ultrasound transmitter crystal produces a small beam, but the angle of divergence increases with decreasing crystal size. At the depth of the vocal folds, the beam will likely have enlarged too much. A large crystal produces a less diverging beam, but one that is too large to be optimal in the first place. Higher frequency is associated with less beam spread, but absorption by intervening tissue is increased. Thus, the final design of the transducer system has to represent a compromise that balances all of these factors. Optimization must be undertaken with an eye to the specific measures to be obtained, which explains the very different designs that have been proposed.

Typically, ultrasound transducers range from 5 to 18 mm (circular or rectangular) in size, and the frequencies used are commonly in the range of 1 to 7.5 MHz (Hertz, Linström, & Sonesson, 1970; Hamlet & Reid, 1972; Holmer, Kitzing, & Linström, 1973; Holmer & Kitzing, 1975; Hamlet, 1980, 1981; Raghavendra et al., 1987; Böhme, 1989; Miles, 1989; Garel, Contencin, Polonovski, Hassan, & Narcy, 1992; Ueda, Yano, & Okuno, 1993; Friedman, 1997; Harries, Hawkins, Hacking, & Hughes, 1998). Two resolution factors are of vital importance in examining the larynx via ultrasonic means:

1. When transducers are placed on the side of the neck, the opening and closing of the glottis represents a change of the axial distance of the edge of the vocal fold. Resolution in this dimension is theoretically limited to $1/2$ the ultrasound wavelength. If, for instance, the speed of ultrasound in muscle is about 1500 m/s, a 2.5 MHz wave has a wavelength of 0.6 mm. The best resolution attainable would be close to 0.3 mm—and no system comes close to the theoretical limit of resolution. Therefore, fine detail of glottal opening and closing cannot be discriminated with certainty.

2. Lateral resolution depends on the size of the ultrasound beam at the target. It is clear from the earlier discussion of beam size that fine lateral resolution is exceptionally difficult to achieve. Details of vertical motions at the edge of the vocal folds still lie beyond the resolving power of ultrasound instrumentation.

ECHOGLOTTOGRAPHY

Vocal fold position can be tracked using the same principles as sonar (*so*und *na*vigation and *r*anging) in a process called *echoglottography*. During phonation, the velocity of the edges of the vocal folds is moderately great. Tracking them adequately requires that the ultrasound pulses be very short and their repetition rate high. Generally, medical ultrasound reflectoscopes are inadequate with respect to these requirements, and special instruments have been designed (Hertz et al., 1970; Holmer et al., 1973; Homer & Kitzing, 1975) that provide up to 10,000 pulses per second and offer better characteristics for time-motion displays.

Echoglottography has successfully shown glottal motion in the form of an undulating echo curve in the T-M mode (Figure 10–34A). While the opening and closing phases are discernible, the closed and open intervals are not well demonstrated. Hertz, Linström, and Sonesson (1970) have measured vocal fold excursions on the order of 1 mm with their system and have been able to calculate approximate open and speed quotients. Kaneko and coworkers (1981) have used two probes to view both vocal folds simultaneously, permitting evaluation of the symmetry of their motion. They have also been able to use their dual-probe system to resolve both lateral and vertical displacements of a single vocal-fold edge.

Unfortunately, the edge of the vocal fold does not move as a single flat reflecting plane (Saito, Fukuda, Isogai, & Ono, 1981; Fukuda et al., 1983). The complexity of the changes in its shape creates very confusing echoes, as shown in Figure 10–34B–E. When the vocal folds are in position A, the ultrasound beam encounters only one reflecting surface. The A-mode representation is as in Figure 10–34C. But when the vocal folds are configured like position B, the beam is reflected from two tissue-air interfaces, one at the upper surface of the fold and the other, a bit further away, at the edge. The resulting A-mode display (Figure 10–34D) therefore has two peaks. In the T-M mode the multiple-echo pattern fades in and out (Figure 10–34E) as the folds change shape. Clearly, interpretation of the echoglottogram is not likely to be a simple matter.

On the other hand, the echoglottograph can provide relatively clear-cut data (within the limits of its resolution) if the actual movement pattern of the vocal folds is not at issue. Hamlet (1972b), for instance, used simple A-mode displays to show that the glottis is narrower during whispered /ɑ/ than during whispered /s/, while Munhall and Ostry (1983) have successfully timed laryngeal articulatory behaviors.

Improvements in transducers, such as scanned arrays (Kaneko et al., 1983; Zagzebski & Bless, 1983; Zagzebski, Bless, & Ewanowski, 1983), in support electronics, and in data enhancement through computer-

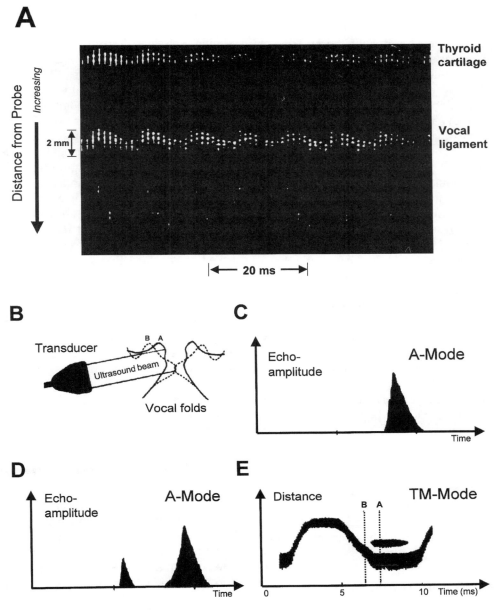

Figure 10–34. Ultrasonic scans of the vocal folds. **A.** T-M display during phonation. From "Ultrasonic recording of the vibrating vocal folds," by C. H. Hertz, K. Linström, and B. Sonesson, 1970, *Acta Otolaryngologica, 69,* 223–230. Figure 4, p. 228. Reprinted by permission. **B–E.** The relationship of the ultrasonic beam to the vocal folds. the complex movements of the free edge of the vocal fold (points A and B) produce A-mode displays of C and D, while the T-M mode pattern may resemble that of E. From "Echo glottography," by N.G. Holmer, P. Kitzing, and K. Linström, 1973, *Acta Otolaryngologica, 75,* 454–463. Figure 8, p. 461. Reprinted by permission.

interfacing bode well for further development and useful clinical implementation of ultrasonic scanning techniques.

CONTINUOUS WAVE GLOTTOGRAPHY

Ultrasonic waves can be constantly applied to the neck, and the magnitude of transmission from one side to the other determined. Such a *continuous wave*

(*CW*) technique is analogous to electroglottography. Air is an extremely poor ultrasound transmission medium. Therefore, if an ultrasound beam is projected across the larynx from one side of the neck, it will be interrupted by the air in the open glottis, and a receiver on the other side will pick up no signal. When the vocal folds are in contact, however, a transmission path exists. Continuous wave glottography should show an "on-off" pattern that corresponds to the closed and open phases, respectively. The technique was first used by Bordone-Sacerdote and Sacerdote (1965) and has been more fully developed and exploited by Hamlet (1971, 1973). She has shown, for instance, that the open quotient varies with vowel nasalization (Hamlet, 1973), and she has also explored laryngeal excitation of the vocal tract (Hamlet, 1971). Holmer and Rundqvist (1975) have used CW ultrasound to obtain a simple waveform for the extraction of vocal fundamental frequency.

One would expect that the amplitude of the transmitted CW signal would increase in rough proportion to the degree of vocal fold contact. That is (again analogous to electroglottography), change in vocal fold contact area should result in amplitude modulation of the ultrasonic carrier. Hamlet and Palmer (1974) have shown this to be the case. It has also been found that a demodulated waveform can even show features suggestive of the vertical phase difference in the movements of the edge of the vocal fold (Hamlet, 1980).

This degree of resolution requires a very narrow ultrasound beam (Hamlet, 1972a). Such a beam is very sensitive to changes in the position of the larynx in the neck. If the larynx moves either up or down, the transmission bridge across the airway—the vocal folds—moves out of the path and transmission is lost. Therefore, narrowbeam CW ultrasound can be used to determine the exact level of the vocal folds. Their position when adducted is betrayed by a maximum-amplitude ultrasound signal when the transducers are moved along the neck. Hamlet (1980) has used this fact to confirm the findings of Shipp (1975) on vertical larynx height. The use of ultrasound arrays, with a row of transducers excited in very rapid sequence, may provide an effective means of continuously tracking larynx height (Hamlet & Reid, 1972; Hamlet, 1981).

COMBINED ECHO AND TRANSMISSION

In an attempt to extract maximum information from ultrasonic probing of the larynx, Kaneko and his coworkers (1976) created a new, combined ultrasound technique. Adopting the premise that laryngeal behavior can best be evaluated only when the glottal area and the movement pattern of the vocal folds are both known, they combined CW and pulse-echo along with simultaneous measures of the subglottal pressure. While a great deal of information is obtained this way, the method is complex and does not seem to offer greater insight than can be attained by other means.

DOPPLER ULTRASOUND MONITORING

Attempts have been made to use the Doppler frequency shift of the ultrasound echoes to determine the actual velocity of the edge of the vocal folds during phonation. This method was first tried in a series of pilot studies by Minifie, Kelsey, and Hixon (1968) that were soon followed by comparisons of the ultrasound data to simultaneous ultrahigh-speed films (Beach & Kelsey, 1969). While the procedure has intuitive appeal, the experimental results were disappointing. Ultrasound-based velocities and displacements (found by integrating the velocity data) differed from those derived by measurement of the films in timing, magnitude, and overall patterns. There was also significant ambiguity and inconsistency in the ultrasound data. This is not surprising: the movement of the edge of the vocal folds is nonuniform and complex, and the returned echoes probably represent different motions occurring at the same time in different places. The researchers were forced to conclude that the quality of the data made "positive identification of a particular type of vocal fold motion by inspection of the associated Doppler signal impossible" (Beach & Kelsey, 1969, p. 1047).

Ultrasound nonetheless holds promise as a noninvasive means of laryngeal monitoring, all of its current problems notwithstanding. Studies of the last several years have confirmed its potential and pointed the way to needed improvements (Kitzing, 1986; Böhme, 1988a, 1988b, 1989; Miles, 1989; Schindler, Gonella, & Pisani, 1990; Ooi, Chan, & Soo, 1995; Friedman, 1997).

GLOTTAL AERODYNAMICS

To produce phonation, the vocal folds must be suitably adducted toward the midline in the presence of a sufficient transglottal airflow. This flow of air induces pressure variations within the laryngeal airway that interact with the movements of the vocal folds to produce sustained periodic vibration. Although vocal-fold oscillation is of obvious significance to voice production, it is nonetheless important to remember that the vocal signal itself is produced as a consequence of that oscillation as it modulates the relatively steady flow of air from the lungs. Thus a more detailed assessment of glottal aerodynamics is likely to provide valuable information regarding a speaker's vocal function.

Acoustic Extraction of the Glottal Wave

This *glottal wave* may be defined as the pattern of the glottal volume velocity—the changes in glottal airflow with time. The major reason why this waveform is of interest is that it constitutes the vocal tract excitation. It is, in the purest sense of the word, the voice. Anything heard by a listener is the product of this voice excitation and the vocal tract's acoustic characteristics. It is possible to derive the glottal wave from the sound pressure signal. In doing so, two different approaches are readily applicable: neutralization of vocal tract characteristics by a reflectionless tube and by inverse filtering. Once extracted, the glottal wave can be acoustically analyzed to provide significant information about the vocal component of speech.

THE REFLECTIONLESS (SONDHI) TUBE

Vocal tract modification of the glottal waveform into the final voice signal is achieved through the effect of nonuniformities of the vocal tract diameter and, more importantly, through the sudden change at the lips from a small diameter system to the infinite diameter of the free space around the mouth. Any sudden change in the size of a tube implies a discontinuity in its acoustic impedance, and at any such impedance shift some of the signal is transmitted, but the rest is reflected back toward the source. The discontinuity of the vocal tract at the lips creates a very sudden and exceptionally large change in acoustic impedance, called the *lip-radiation impedance*. A significant portion of the egressive speech signal is, therefore, reflected from the lips back toward the larynx. The glottal waveform interacts with its own reflections in the vocal tract to produce the signal heard by the listener as a distinctive speech sound. If the vocal tract could be made fairly uniform in its cross-sectional shape, and if the lip-radiation impedance could be eliminated, the emergent signal would be the unaltered glottal wave itself.

Sondhi (1975) proposed a conceptually simple way of achieving the necessary modifications of a speaker's vocal tract. Uniformity of the tube is approximated during production of a neutral, schwa-like vowel. The elimination of the radiation impedance is trickier. For this a special metal tube is needed (Figure 10–35), about 2 m in length with a diameter that approximates that of the speaker's vocal tract, that is, roughly between 2 and $2^3/_4$ cm. The speaker seals his lips around the open end of the tube and phonates a neutral vowel[15] with good velopharyngeal closure. The signal is picked up by a precision miniature microphone inserted through the tube wall.

What makes the system work is a long (1-m) wedge of sound-absorbent material that closes the distal end of the tube. If properly shaped, this will soak up essentially all of the impinging sound energy and, therefore, none will be reflected back into the vocal tract. Such a (quasi-) reflectionless tube essentially extends the acoustic length of the vocal tract to the functional equivalent of infinity and eliminates the radiation impedance.

If the system were sealed, with no way for the expired air to escape, the pressure inside the tube would quickly rise to the level of the subglottal pressure, and in the resultant absence of a transglottal pressure drop, airflow would cease and phonation would stop. Therefore, provision must be made for venting the tube to the outside. The way in which this is done is important. If the vent is not large enough, air pressure in the Sondhi tube will rise, and laryngeal behavior may be changed in compensation. On the other hand, the vent must be small enough, and so placed, as to avoid creating reflections that defeat the purpose of the system. Hillman and Weinberg (1981a) have evaluated different venting methods (Figure 10–35 incorporates their recommendations). While Sondhi's original device used fiberglass as the absorbent material, polyurethane

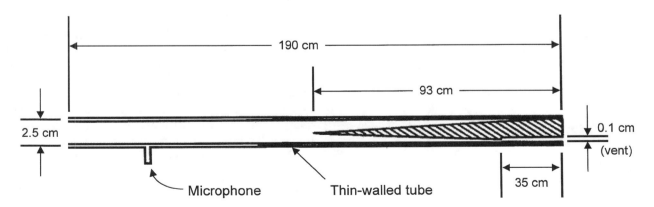

Figure 10–35. Design of a reflectionless (Sondhi) tube.

---

[15]Hillman, Oesterle, and Feth (1983) have also used the reflectionless tube to assess glottal turbulence produced during the production of whispered vowels.

foam is now the material of choice. Details for constructing a reflectionless tube system have been published by Monsen and Engebretson (1977), Monsen (1981), and Hillman and Weinberg (1981a). The construction itself is not difficult, but the system must then be tested to verify its lack of resonances across a sufficiently broad bandwidth. This requires coupling sinusoidal signals across the frequency spectrum to the mouth-end of the tube and measuring the amplitude and phase-shift of the tube's response to the injected signals (Schneider & Baken, 1984; Howell & Williams, 1988). Details of the calibration procedure are provided by Hillman, Weinberg, and Tree (1978).

The Sondhi Tube Glottal Waveform

Examples of waveforms sensed in a Sondhi tube at different loudness levels are shown in Figure 10–36. The pressure wave has a simple shape that, to a certain degree, resembles the glottal area function measured from ultrahigh-speed films or the photoglottogram. There is, however, a disturbing difference. In most cases, there is a distinct closed phase during the glottal cycle. During this period the vocal folds are in medial contact and, since there is no glottal opening, the air-

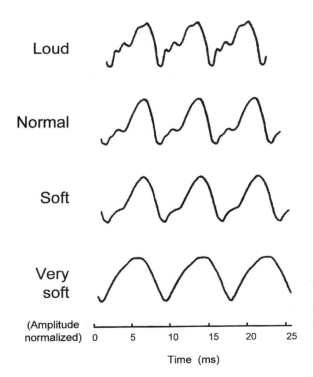

Figure 10–36. Glottal pressure waves sensed by a reflectionless tube. Increasing pressure is upward. From "The use of a reflectionless tube to assess vocal function," by R. B. Monsen, 1981, *ASHA Reports*, *11*, 141–150. Figure 8, p. 145. Reprinted by permission.

flow must be zero. The closed phase takes a significant amount of time—typically at least one-third of the glottal cycle. Furthermore, as will be discussed later, the relative duration of the closed phase increases with vocal intensity.

Except for a momentary minimum, the glottal waves of Figure 10–36 fail to show such a closed phase. The problem is not unique to Monsen's data. Other researchers (Sondhi, 1975; Tanabe, Isshiki, & Kitajima, 1978; Howell & Williams, 1988) have published similar traces. Hillman and Weinberg (1981b) have explored the causes of imperfections in the Sondhi-tube representation of the glottal volume velocity and have concluded that the closed-phase problem is caused by the influence of the first formant. The Sondhi tube's validity rests on the assumption that the vocal tract being tested has a uniform diameter. This is obviously not the case with a real human structure, so the uniform-diameter assumption is never met in practice. Apparently, the deviation of the real from the ideal is sufficiently great to produce the closed-phase distortion that is so commonly seen.

The Sondhi tube is imperfect in other ways, too. Clearly, no real tube is absolutely without reflections, and it is unlikely that the tube diameter actually matches (and is therefore a good extension of) the cross-sectional diameter of the speaker's vocal tract. Despite the designer's best efforts, there is likely to remain a sudden change in the system diameter where the Sondhi tube meets the lips. The net result of any of these deviations from the assumptions of the rationale is the occurrence of resonances that distort the glottal waveform.

If it is the examiner's intention to quantify important aspects of the glottal waveform for comparison to normative data generated by other means, the reflectionless tube is probably not the best method to use. Under laboratory conditions, the tube's output can approximate synthetic waves generated by a mathematical vocal-fold model (Monsen, Engebretson, & Vemula, 1978). It is also recognized that the waveform does show abnormalities in cases of confirmed vocal disorder (Tanabe et al., 1978). But, given the poorly understood and poorly predicted distortions produced by the measurement system, it is not really possible to relate waveform irregularities back to distinct aberrations of laryngeal function, and not enough research on the waveform differences—whatever they may represent—has been done to allow their use for the unequivocal assessment of glottal dynamics.

ACOUSTIC INVERSE FILTERING

The idea of inverse filtering is to derive the vocal tract transfer function and construct a filter that is its inverse. If the (voiced) speech signal is subjected to such a filter, the acoustic effects of the vocal tract are negated, and the original glottal waveform is restored. The method was first proposed by Miller (1959) who initially implemented it with analog filter circuits, although computer techniques were soon applied to assist in the generation of inverse-filter equations (Miller & Mathews, 1963). Since that time, more advanced computational techniques have been developed (Wong, Markel, & Gray, 1979; Matausek & Batalov, 1980; Veeneman & DeMent, 1985; Krishna-murthy & Childers, 1986; Javkin, Antoñanzas-Barroso, & Maddieson, 1987; Price, 1989; Alku & Vilkman, 1992; Howell & Williams, 1992; Alku, Vilkman, & Pekkarinen, 1993; Vilkman, Alku, & Laukkanen, 1995; Alku, Strik, & Vilkman, 1997; Vilkman, Lauri, Alku, Sala, & Sihvo, 1997; Alku, Vilkman, & Laukkanen, 1998).

To derive an adequate estimate of the glottal pressure wave, the lip-radiated signal must be transduced using a microphone with a superior low-frequency response (Javkin et al., 1987; Löfqvist, 1991; Alku & Vilkman, 1992, 1995). If inverse filtering is to be done on stored signals, they must first be recorded using an FM or digital tape recorder or digitized using an adequate sampling rate (see Chapter 3, "Digital Systems"). Although automated methods can simplify the application of inverse filtering, the technique can still be quite complex to implement and prone to unintended distortion of the true glottal wave, especially when the voiced samples are highly nasalized. As such, the clinical application of acoustic inverse filtering has been rather meager.

Flow Glottography

Rothenberg (1972, 1973, 1977) described an inverse-filtering method to extract the glottal wave that returns to the use of analog filter techniques. The difference is that the input used is the volume-velocity (flow) waveform radiated from the mouth, rather than the radiated pressure wave sensed by a microphone. The volume-velocity wave is transduced using the principle of the pneumotachograph (see Chapter 9, "Airflow and Volume") in a special modification. The primary transducer in Rothenberg's system is a face mask circumferentially vented by relatively large holes that are covered by fine-mesh wire screening. These serve as resistive elements across which a pressure proportional to the flow is generated (Figure 10–37). Whereas the frequency response of a pneumotachograph is quite poor, the mask system has a time resolution of less than 0.5 ms. Therefore, very rapid changes in airflow—over the course of a single

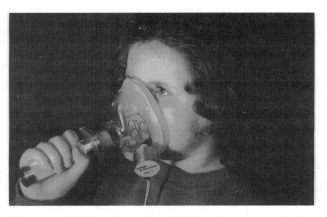

Figure 10–37. A circumferentially vented pneumotacho-graph (Rothenberg) mask held firmly against the face by the speaker. Attached is a strain-gauge transducer that compares pressures within and outside the mask.

glottal cycle—can be transduced.[16] The total resistance of the screen elements is very small, keeping pressure inside the mask under 0.3 cmH$_2$O/L/s. The pressure difference across the screen elements created by the airflow was originally sensed by a pair of specially modified microphones, but in its more recent incarnation of the mask system that is marketed by Glottal Enterprises, Inc. (Syracuse, NY), these have been replaced by a differential strain gauge pressure transducer (see Chapter 8, "Air Pressure").

The inverse filter network is a special circuit with essentially no phase shift to distort the signal. The filter characteristics are initially set on the basis of spectrographic analysis (see Chapter 7, "Sound Spectrography") of the oral flow waveform. They are then adjusted to produce a final glottal flow waveform, sometimes called the *flow glottogram*, that appears to show minimal evidence of the effect of vocal-tract formants. Precise knowledge of vocal tract formants is not often possible in practice, however. To a significant degree, fine adjustment of the filter characteristics is based on the clinician's notion of how the flow waveform, once free of supraglottal influences, should appear. As Titze (1994) noted, "one major criterion for success is to eliminate formant ripple in the closed phase of the glottal cycle, assuming no flow exists there" (p. 224). In vocal pathology, however, such an assumption may be one that wise clinicians are loath to make. Nonetheless, more automatic means of deriving inverse-filter characteristics using linear predictive coding among other techniques are currently being developed and refined with

---

[16]Hertegård and Gauffin (1992) and Alku and Vilkman (1995), however, question whether the circumferentially vented mask system has an adequate bandwidth to derive a reasonable glottal wave for certain types of voices or for phonation produced at especially high fundamental frequencies.

an eye toward facilitating more widespread clinical implementation (Perkell, Holmberg, & Hillman, 1991; Rothenberg & Nezelek, 1991; Södersten, Hammarberg, & Håkansson, 1996). The accuracy and reliability of such systems remain to be tested, however.

THE FLOW GLOTTOGRAM

It might be anticipated that the inverse-filtered glottal waveform and glottal area function (derived, for instance, from the photoglottogram or from high-speed filming) would be quite similar to each other. After all, if we assume that the driving pressure is relatively constant, as the glottal area increases the resistance to the flow of air should decrease. Nevertheless, the two glottograms are not identical. That is because when the glottis first opens, the inertia of the subglottal air column retards the onset of transglottal flow. Furthermore, as the glottis closes, the momentum of the moving air column retards the subsequent return of the flow to zero (Rothenberg, 1973, 1981, 1983). The delays caused by air acceleration and deceleration result in a phase lag and a skewing of the waveform relative to the measured glottal area function.[17] Although it has become common to derive certain

glottal measurements such as the open, closing, and speed quotients from the flow glottogram (Holmberg, Hillman, & Perkell, 1988, 1989; Hilman, Holmberg, Perkell, Walsh, & Vaughan, 1989; Dromey et al., 1992; Stathopoulos & Sapienza, 1993a, 1993b; Alku & Vilkman, 1995; Hertegård & Gauffin, 1995; Sapienza & Stathopoulos, 1995; Sulter & Wit, 1996; Alku et al., 1997; Ng, Gilbert, & Lerman, 1997), the lack of conformity to the glottal area function will likely render measures that are palpably different from those derived from the photoglottogram or from high-speed film data.

Figure 10–38 shows a fairly typical flow glottogram derived by inverse-filtering the output from a circumferentally vented pneumotachograph mask system. The acoustic signal, obtained from a condenser microphone placed within the mask, is shown at the top. The line drawn on the flow trace represents the maximal (negative) slope during the glottal-flow cycle. Since it is the sudden stoppage of flow (causing a rapid fall in supraglottal pressure) that corresponds to the source of vocal-tract excitation, several investigators have suggested that the rate at which the descending portion of the flow glottogram falls is of critical importance to the nature and quality of the sound produced

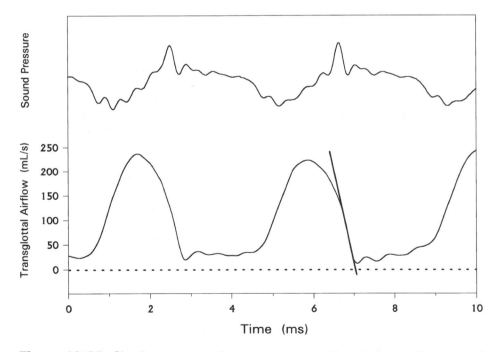

Figure 10–38. Simultaneous sound pressure wave and flow glottogram for a normal woman comfortably sustaining production of the vowel /ɑ/. The line in the transglottal flow trace represents the sharpest negative slope for that glottal cycle. Note that this corresponds to the major aerodynamic disruption seen in the microphone signal above.

---

[17]Other influences on the shape of the glottal flow waveform include that of the vertical and horizontal phase differences in vocal-fold movement (see, for instance, Hertegård, Gauffin, and Karlsson, 1992).

by the larynx (Rosenberg, 1971; Fant, 1979; Sundberg & Gauffin, 1979; Gauffin & Sundberg, 1980, 1989; Rothenberg, 1981; Fritzell, Gauffin, Hammarberg, Karlsson, & Sundberg, 1984; Fritzell, Hammarberg, Gauffin, Karlsson, & Sundberg, 1986; Colton, 1985; Fant, Liljencrants & Lin, 1985; Javkin et al., 1987; Price, 1989; Hertegård & Gauffin, 1995). The flow "ripple" that can be seen during the presumed closed phase is due to the failure of the inverse filter to cancel the influence of energy at and above the third formant. Unlike the glottal wave derived using acoustic inverse filtering, the flow signal used for filtering may be calibrated to provide an absolute scale (see Chapter 9, "Airflow and Volume"); Note that, for this speaker, glottal leakage is suggested by the fact that the transglottal flow remains above zero during the "closed" phase. Such leakage is actually quite common among speakers and, unless excessive, should not be construed as an indication of vocal pathology (Karlsson, 1986, 1991; Hillman et al., 1989; Hertegård et al., 1992; Hertegård & Gauffin, 1995; Ng et al., 1997).

The Maximum Flow Declination Rate

By differentiating the flow glottogram (see Chapter 2, "Analog Electronics"), the rate of change in glottal airflow at each point in the glottal cycle can be deter-mined. Accordingly, Holmberg, Hillman, and Perkell (1988) defined the *maximum flow declination rate* (*MFDR*) as the maximum negative peak measured from the first derivative of the glottal flow wave. The earliest measures of the MDFR (Holmberg et al., 1988, 1989; Hillman et al., 1989, 1990) indicated that it was strongly related to vocal effort, particularly when associated with an increase in vocal SPL. Perkell, Hillman, and Holmberg (1994) were able to replicate their earlier results, but found that the 900-Hz low-pass filtering they had originally used to minimize the effects of formants above F1 prior to inverse filtering had the consequence of lowering MFDR values. The robust relationship between vocal SPL and MFDR has been documented in several studies of normal and some dysphonic speakers (Stathopoulos & Sapienza, 1993a, 1993b; Holmberg, Hillman, Perkell, & Gress, 1994a, 1994b; Holmberg, Hillman, Perkell, Guiod, & Goldman, 1995; Sapienza & Stathopoulos, 1995; Södersten, Hertegård, & Hammarberg, 1995; Sulter & Wit, 1996). Data from such studies of normal adults is shown plotted in Figure 10–39.

Owing largely to differences in laryngeal anatomy, investigations have consistently shown men to have a significantly higher MFDR than women, with differences typically over 100 LPS/s at a given sound pressure level. In a series of studies conducted by

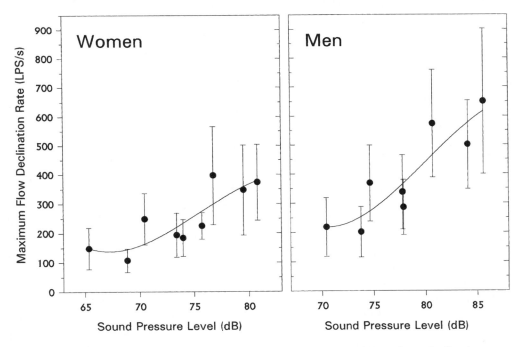

Figure 10–39. The relationship between SPL and the maximum flow declination rate (MFDR) for normal women and men. The data plotted are those reported by Stathopoulos and Sapienza (1993a), Perkell, Hillman, and Holmberg (1994), and Sapienza and Stathopoulos (1994, 1995) in studies that used comparable methodology. The error bars represent the standard deviation associated with each mean datum, whereas the curves represent a third-order regression fit to the mean values.

Stathopoulos and Sapienza, MFDR data from groups of 4- and 8-year-old boys and girls were compared with those from young adults. They reported significantly lower MFDRs for the children, who nonetheless showed the expected increase in flow deceleration with increased vocal SPL (Stathopoulos & Sapienza, 1993a; Sapienza & Stathopoulos, 1994).

Peak Glottal Flow

Vocal intensity may be increased by more sharply truncating the expiratory airflow (as assessed by the MFDR) or by boosting the subglottal pressure (see Chapter 8, "Air Pressure") which, all things being equal, increases the overall rate of glottal airflow. It has thus become common when assessing the flow glottogram to measure both the MFDR and the peak glottal flow. Numerous studies have shown that normal speakers typically increase both the MFDR and the peak glottal flow with increasing vocal effort and intensity. Unfortunately, the peak flow rate is related both to the subglottal pressure and the degree of medial compression of the speaker's vocal folds. Thus peak glottal flow reflects both the SPL and type of phonation—from whisper to what has been referred to as a "pressed" voice (Sundberg & Gauffin, 1979; Sundberg, 1987; Södersten, Hertegård, & Hammarberg, 1995). Alone, the measure tells the clinician little about glottal dynamics, but may be useful when combined with other aerodynamic indices.

Vocal Efficiency

The efficiency of any mechanical system is defined simply by the ratio of output power to input power. As far as the laryngeal generator is concerned, we can translate this as the amount of physical or bodily effort required to produce a given amount of acoustic energy at the glottal outlet. Since physiologic power cannot be measured practicably, pulmonic or subglottal power is typically substituted (van den Berg, 1956; Isshiki, 1964). *Subglottal power* is the product of the subglottal pressure and tracheal airflow. Because it is difficult to measure acoustic energy at the level of the glottis (Koyama, Harvey, & Ogura, 1972), the lip-radiated acoustic energy (that is, the vowel intensity measured at a fixed distance from the mouth) is adopted as the measure of power output. Such measurements, therefore, more correctly relate to *vocal* efficiency, rather than to *glottal* efficiency. Both van den Berg (1956) and Cavagna and Margaria (1968) found that vocal efficiency increases with subglottal power. However, the vocal tract is known to absorb a variable amount of acoustic energy, and the degree of mouth-opening surely affects the intensity detected at the microphone (Fairbanks, 1950; House, 1959; Ladefoged & McKinney, 1963; Isshiki,

1964). Isshiki (1964) has accordingly recommended that a mouthpiece be used to stabilize the configuration of the vocal tract during phonation.

The AC/DC Ratio. While the utility of vocal efficiency measures in the description of normal phonatory function has yet to be demonstrated, their application to dysphonic populations would seem self-evident. To dispense with the need to obtain a measure of subglottal pressure, Isshiki (1981, 1985) has proposed a pseudo-efficiency measure, the *vocal efficiency index* (otherwise known as the *AC/DC ratio*) based on aerodynamic measurement alone. In short, the measure compares the *effective* glottal flow (that is, the root mean square of the alternating "AC" portion of the flow signal) to the mean flow rate (see Chapter 2, "Analog Electronics"). This ratio reflects the ability of the glottis to convert an unmodulated or "DC" pulmonary airflow into a modulated or AC supraglottal airstream. If the vocal folds do not make complete contact over their entire length, there may be an increase in the level of unmodulated airflow emerging from the glottis, which would result in an abnormally low AC/DC ratio. Unmodulated airflow does not contribute to the glottal waveform and thus, in terms of voice production, represents wasted air and energy. Excessive DC flow may in fact result in unwanted turbulence noise (Isshiki, Yanagihara, & Morimoto, 1966; Yanagihara, 1967, 1970), a decrease in relative acoustic energy (Fant, 1979; Holmberg et al., 1988; Gauffin & Sundberg, 1989), and the perception of a "breathy" voice (Fritzell et al., 1984, 1986; Södersten & Lindestad, 1990). It should be noted once again, however, that even speakers with a perceptually normal voice may have incomplete vocal-fold contact, especially at the posterior glottis (Schönhärl, 1960; Koike & Hirano, 1973; Cavagna & Camporesi, 1974; Biever & Bless, 1989; Holmberg et al., 1989; Södersten & Lindestad, 1990; Linville, 1992; Södersten et al., 1995). For normal phonation, the amount of DC glottal flow does not appear to dramatically affect acoustic voice measures (Holmberg et al., 1995).

Unfortunately, normal to high AC/DC ratios can be obtained from inefficient voices of a so-called hyperfunctional nature (Isshiki, 1981; Hillman et al., 1989). These factors, coupled with the high intrasubject variability typically observed in efficiency measures, have severely limited their ability to discriminate pathology when used alone (Wilson & Starr, 1985; Schutte, 1986; Hillman et al., 1989). However, when used in conjunction with other measures, they may serve quite effectively to provide a more descriptive assessment of phonatory function (Schutte & van den Berg, 1976; Hiki, 1983; Tanaka & Gould, 1985; Schutte, 1986; Woo, Colton, & Shangold, 1987; Hillman et al., 1989; Woo, Casper, Colton, & Brewer, 1994).

Laryngeal Airway Resistance

Phonatory airflow is induced by the driving pressure and moderated by the resistance to the flow at the glottal constriction. An abnormally high flow rate, then, may be tied to an increase in subglottal pressure, to a decrease in glottal resistance, or, quite often, to a combination of the two (Isshiki, 1969). For this reason, flow measures alone confound aspects of ventilatory and glottal behavior that, according to D'Antonio, Netsell, and Lotz (1988), may "offer a partial and often erroneous impression of laryngeal function." A more descriptive analysis is provided when both the flow rate and driving pressure are known. In accordance with Ohm's law, these values can be used to measure the mean *laryngeal airway resistance* (R_{law}), also known as the *glottal resistance* (R_g), defined as the ratio of translaryngeal pressure to the translaryngeal airflow (van den Berg, Zantema, & Doornenbal, 1957).

Although R_{law} can be measured for a prolonged phonation, it is typically assessed using a /pʊ/ syllable-repetition task to facilitate P_s estimation and to approximate values that may be more representative of the voiced segments within connected speech (Netsell, Lotz, & Shaughnessy, 1984; D'Antonio et al., 1988; Netsell, Lotz, DuChane, & Barlow, 1991; but see also McHenry, Kuna, Minton, & Vanoye, 1996). Figure 10–40 shows a short portion of a typical pressure-flow data trace from which an estimate of the mean R_{law} may be derived. Note that the peak intraoral pressure for /p/ varies slightly from syllable to syllable. This suggests that the P_s is changing relatively slowly. A line that connects the peak pressure (the dashed line in the figure) can therefore serve as an estimate of P_s over the course of the syllable repetitions (see Chapter 8, "Air Pressure"). The transglottal (driving) pressure at the midpoint of the vowel (the vertical dotted line in the figure) can estimated by subtracting the intraoral pressure at that point—which represents the supraglottal pressure during vowel production—from the estimated midvowel P_s. The midvowel transglottal airflow is measured from a flow trace obtained using a face mask coupled to pneumotachograph system.[18] Since all of the airflow through the glottis must exit through the nose and mouth, a face mask-based assessment of the mean flow rate will provide the required transglottal airflow measure. Because only mean vowel airflowdata are needed, the flow signal is typically low-pass filtered (as in Figure 10–40) to minimize the voicing"ripple"in the trace and thus to facilitate flow measurement. (For this reason, the improved frequency response provided by a pneumotachograph mask system is unnecessary and, perhaps,

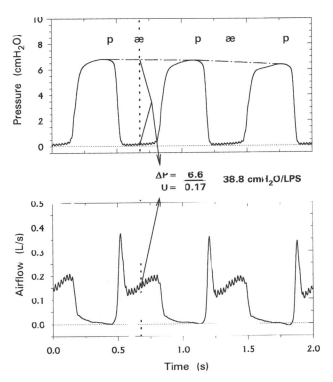

Figure 10–40. Intraoral pressure (top) and speech airflow (bottom) during repetition of the syllable /pæ/. The dashed line that connects the peak pressure for /p/ approximates the subglottal pressure over the course of the utterance. To estimate the pressure drop across the glottis, the intraoral pressure during the vowel production is subtracted from the estimated subglottal pressure. The laryngeal airway resistance may be determined by dividing the transglottal pressure by the simultaneous flow rate, as shown.

undesirable.) The mean R_{law} is determined by averaging the pressure/flow ratio from the middle of a train of several syllable repetitions. Smitheran and Hixon (1981), for instance, estimated the midvowel glottal resistance from the middle three /pi/ syllables of a 7-syllable utterance. Many researchers and most clinicians have adopted Smitheran and Hixon's method as the standard technique.

EXPECTED RESULTS

The flow resistance of the glottis has been shown to be substantially higher in both the loft (falsetto) and pulse voice registers (Isshiki, 1964; McGlone & Shipp, 1971) than is typical in the modal register, at least for speech produced at near-comfortable levels of pitch and loudness. For utterances produced under similar phonatory

---

[18]The measurement of subglottal pressure and mean phonatory airflow are discussed in Chapters 8 ("Air Pressure") and 9 ("Airflow and Volumes"), respectively. Greater detail regarding this method of R_{law} estimation is provided in Smitheran and Hixon (1981) and in Orlikoff and Baken (1993).

conditions, a number of studies have documented a larger R_{law} in women than in men, presumably due to the smaller dimensions of the female larynx. It is not surprising, then, that children have been shown to have a significantly higher glottal resistance than the average adult speaker (Keilmann & Bader, 1995). For instance, for trains of syllables produced at "conversational levels of pitch and loudness," Netsell, Lotz, Peters, and Schulte (1994) reported average R_{law} values of 116, 94, and 69 cmH₂O/LPS for groups of normal preschoolers, school-age children, and preadolescents, respectively.

The summary data in Table 10–3 are derived from several studies following similar R_{law} estimation procedures. While it has been shown that airflow does not change in a consistent way with vocal intensity within the modal voice register, a fairly clear relationship between vocal SPL and R_{law} has been documented in numerous reports owing, largely, to the affinity of P_s and intensity. Thus, as Leeper and Graves (1984) suggested, "it would appear that control of intensity, either intuitively or via direct monitoring, may be a key factor to consider in attempts to establish norms for a variety of age and sex groups from which to compare patients with laryngeal dysfunction" (p. 159). At present, such normative data do not exist, but Table 10–3 may serve to provide a rough guideline. Note in particular the generally higher glottal resistance values for women as well as the tendency toward a greater increase in R_{law} with increasing vocal SPL.

Vocal Pathology

Normal phonation requires appropriate vocal-fold adduction and adequate glottal opening and sealing. The laryngeal airway resistance must, therefore, be neither so low as to cause excessive air loss, nor so high as to hinder glottal function. For instance, a mass lesion that develops on the margin of the vocal fold might interfere with glottal closure, thus decreasing flow resistance (Isshiki & von Leden, 1964; Isshiki et al., 1966). Because lesions of this sort often hinder the speaker's ability to sufficiently increase R_{law}, it is not surprising that such patients typically show high phonatory flow rates and an inability to increase vocal intensity above a relatively low level. Alternatively, large mass lesions (Iwata, 1988), laryngospasm (Gracco, Gracco, Löfqvist, & Marek, 1994; Plant & Hillel, 1998), or laryngeal trauma (D'Antonio, Lotz, Chait, & Netsell, 1987) may greatly increase glottal resistance. In these patients the flow rate may be normal or slightly reduced in the face of an excessively large subglottal pressure that the speaker supplies in an attempt to compensate for an overly constricted airway. Vocal intensity may be inappropriately high or low, but the most salient characteristic (beyond a degraded voice quality) is often a marked restriction in both speaking pitch and loudness.

Blosser, Wigley, and Wise (1992) reported a significantly higher R_{law} for a group of patients with rheumatoid arthritis (mean = 65 ± 8 cmH₂O/LPS) compared with a group of healthy speakers (mean = 38 ± 7 cmH₂O/LPS). Since arthritic ankylosis of the cricoarytenoid joints is known to cause adducted fixation of the vocal folds, it is not surprising that these patients had elevated airway resistance. However, it is interesting to note that few of the patients complained of voice symptoms. Such results highlight the ability of speakers to maintain functional voice characteristics despite what may be substantial airway disturbance. Nonetheless resistance measures may well document important aspects of vocal effort and efficiency (Netsell et al., 1984; Melcon, Hoit, & Hixon, 1989; Hoit & Hixon, 1992; Woodson et al., 1996; Kostyk & Rochet, 1998).

Table 10–3. Laryngeal Airway Resistance (R_{law}, in cmH₂O/LPS), Derived from the Estimated Transglottal Pressure (in cmH₂O) and Transglottal Airflow (U_g, in L/s), for Normal Adult Speakers

Speaking Condition	R_{law}		Estimated Transglottal Pressure		U_g		Source*
	Mean	(SD)	Mean	(SD)	Mean	(SD)	
Men							
Whisper	9.6	(5.7)	4.5	(1.9)	0.53	(0.22)	1
"Soft"	23.6	(10.4)	5.1	(1.2)	0.25	(0.11)	2
25% SPL	27.5	(21.6)	3.8	(1.1)	0.210	(0.096)	3
25% SPL	23.3	(8.5)	3.8	(1.7)	0.189	(0.076)	4a
25% SPL	29.8	(12.4)	4.5	(1.1)	0.191	(0.102)	4b
25% SPL	27.9	(16.3)	4.7	(1.4)	0.209	(0.103)	4c
"Normal"	44.6	(14.0)	6.3	(2.1)	0.15	(0.06)	1
"Normal"	37.7	(16.7)	6.3	(1.4)	0.19	(0.07)	2

(Continued)

Speaking Condition	R_{law}		Estimated Transglottal Pressure		U_g		Source[*]
	Mean	(SD)	Mean	(SD)	Mean	(SD)	
"Normal"	35.7	(3.3)	—	—	—	—	5
"Normal"	31.7	(7.8)	5.9	(1.4)	0.193	(0.047)	6
"Normal"	32.6	(13.7)	5.9	(1.1)	0.20	(0.06)	7
"Normal"	39.4	(6.4)	—	—	—	—	8a
"Normal"	35.7	(5.3)	—	—	—	—	8b
"Normal"	40.7	(4.6)	—	—	—	—	8c
"Normal"	24.4	(13.3)	4.0	(1.0)	0.249	(0.140)	4a
"Normal"	36.0	(7.1)	—	—	—	—	8d
"Normal"	27.7	(14.4)	4.3	(1.7)	0.200	(0.079)	4b
"Normal"	38.1	(7.5)	—	—	—	—	8e
"Normal"	26.0	(24.4)	4.1	(1.6)	0.186	(0.066)	4c
"Normal"	28.6	(4.4)	—	—	—	—	8f
50% SPL	33.8	(19.3)	7.6	(2.8)	0.275	(0.093)	3
50% SPL	29.2	(14.8)	6.2	(2.3)	0.306	(0.219)	4a
50% SPL	37.1	(28.4)	7.4	(2.0)	0.371	(0.408)	4b
50% SPL	33.2	(14.9)	6.6	(1.4)	0.259	(0.134)	4c
75% SPL	49.2	(26.8)	14.2	(5.4)	0.346	(0.130)	3
75% SPL	34.0	(18.1)	11.0	(2.9)	0.489	(0.375)	4a
75% SPL	35.4	(17.6)	12.2	(2.0)	0.485	(0.292)	4b
75% SPL	45.4	(22.5)	11.1	(2.6)	0.324	(0.143)	4c
"Loud"	48.6	(19.4)	9.0	(2.4)	0.20	(0.06)	2
"Loud"	41.4	(18.7)	8.7	(2.4)	0.24	(0.09)	7
Women							
Whisper	8.0	(1.9)	4.0	(1.1)	0.50	(0.08)	1
"Soft"	29.5	(10.3)	4.6	(0.8)	0.17	(0.04)	2
25% SPL	39.4	(18.3)	4.1	(1.5)	0.136	(0.060)	3
25% SPL	35.0	(14.9)	3.6	(0.4)	0.125	(0.041)	4a
25% SPL	44.0	(18.7)	3.9	(1.4)	0.140	(0.104)	4b
25% SPL	53.0	(33.4)	4.2	(1.7)	0.130	(0.115)	4c
"Normal"	34.5	(13.6)	4.6	(1.0)	0.14	(0.03)	1
"Normal"	42.2	(8.1)	5.8	(0.9)	0.14	(0.03)	2
"Normal"	42.7	(9.3)	5.3	(1.2)	0.127	(0.027)	6
"Normal"	30.8	(9.4)	5.5	(1.3)	0.20	(0.08)	7
"Normal"	38.3	(9.2)	6.4	(1.9)	0.200	(0.066)	9
"Normal"	48.8	(8.7)	9.1	(2.8)	0.190	(0.049)	10
"Normal"	27.2	(11.1)	3.6	(0.5)	0.158	(0.067)	4a
"Normal"	41.7	(24.4)	4.0	(1.2)	0.125	(0.056)	4b
"Normal"	51.0	(32.2)	3.8	(1.8)	0.111	(0.066)	4c
50% SPL	51.7	(31.1)	7.6	(2.9)	0.174	(0.047)	3
50% SPL	52.8	(24.6)	5.9	(1.4)	0.138	(0.064)	4a
50% SPL	55.2	(25.5)	5.8	(2.4)	0.172	(0.104)	4b
50% SPL	88.7	(52.0)	7.0	(4.2)	0.140	(0.119)	4c
75% SPL	97.3	(69.5)	16.9	(6.6)	0.222	(0.109)	3
75% SPL	70.3	(47.3)	8.0	(2.3)	0.150	(0.060)	4a
75% SPL	72.0	(26.7)	9.7	(4.8)	0.160	(0.073)	4b
75% SPL	112.9	(66.1)	10.2	(4.8)	0.160	(0.198)	4c
"Loud"	60.9	(20.6)	8.2	(1.8)	0.15	(0.04)	2
"Loud"	46.4	(21.3)	7.6	(1.8)	0.19	(0.07)	7

[*]Sources:

1. Stathopoulos, Hoit, Hixon, Watson, and Solomon, 1991. Five men (age 20–22 years) and 5 women (age 22–24 years) repeated the syllable /pi/ using a "comfortable whisper" and then using a "comfortable loudness, pitch, and quality." R_{law} and P_s data rounded to the nearest 0.1.

2. Holmberg, Hillman, and Perkell, 1988. Twenty-five men (age 17–30 years) and 20 women (age 18–36 years). Speakers repeated the syllable /pæ/ at a self-selected "comfortable" level for each loudness condition.

3. Wilson and Leeper, 1992. Seven men (age 23–30 years) and 8 women (age 22—29 years) repeated the syllable /pi/ with a "normal pitch and quality" at the 25th, 50th, and 75th percentile of their total SPL ranges. Airflow data converted to L/s.

4. Holmes, Leeper, and Nicholson, 1994. Thirty men and 30 women divided into three age groups: *a. 55–64; b. 65–74; and c. 75+* years. Speakers repeated the syllable /pi/ at four SPLs: "comfortable voice" and at the 25th, 50th, and 75th percentile of their total SPL range. There was a significantly lower mean R_{law} for the 75+ year-old women than for the two younger groups of women at each SPL; The 75+ year-old men had a significantly lower mean R_{law} than the younger groups of men at the 75th SPL percentile. Airflow data in table converted to L/s.

5. Smitheran and Hixon, 1981. Fifteen normal men, age 21 to 40 years, produced a train of 7 /pi/ syllables using a "continuous expiration at normal loudness, pitch, and quality, with equal stress on each syllable, with each of the seven vowels in the train prolonged slightly, and at an utterance rate of 1.5 syllables/sec. (as paced externally)" (p. 140). Range of R_{law} values = 30.0–43.1 cmH$_2$O/LPS.

6. Netsell, Lotz, DuChane, and Barlow, 1991. Fifteen men (mean age 32 ± 8 years) and 15 women (mean age 27 ± 4 years) repeated the syllables /pi/ and /pa/ at two different rates. Data in the table are for the syllable /pi/ repeated at 1.5 syllables/s. Airflow data converted to L/s; R_{law} values derived using estimated P$_s$ as measure of driving pressure; Data rounded to the nearest 0.1.

7. Perkell, Hillman, and Holmberg, 1994. Fifteen men (age 20–56 years) and 15 women (age 20–49 years). Speakers repeated the syllable /pæ/ at a self-selected "comfortable" level for each loudness condition.

8. Melcon, Hoit, and Hixon, 1989. Sixty men divided into six age groups: a. 25 ± 2; b. 35 ± 2; c. 45 ± 2; d. 55 ± 2; e. 65 ± 2; and f. 75 ± 2 years. There was a significantly lower mean R_{law} for the 75+ year-old men than for the younger groups. Same method as Source 5.

9. Leeper and Graves, 1984. Fifteen "normal, nonsmoking" women (age 23–32 years) repeated the syllable /pi/ using a "consistent 'conversational' level of effort." A "simultaneous flash and audible click from an electronic metronome" was used to help maintain a rate of 1.5 syllables/s. Data in table are values averaged across four experimental sessions conducted over two days, at two different times of day (no significant differences were noted across days or for time of testing). Airflow data converted to L/s; R_{law} and pressure data rounded to the nearest 0.1.

10. Kostyk and Rochet, 1998. Seven female schoolteachers (age 33 ± 7 years), "who reported experiencing no more than one symptom of vocal fatigue one time per week," repeated the syllable /pi/ with even stress. Data are for control group compared with female schoolteachers who reported "five or more symptoms of vocal fatigue at least once per week." No significant differences in pressure, flow or R_{law} were noted between the groups. Airflow data converted to L/s; R_{law} and pressure data rounded to the nearest 0.1.

REFERENCES

Abberton, E. (1972). Visual feedback and intonation learning. In A. Rigault & R. Charbonneau (Eds.), *Proceedings of the Seventh International Congress of Phonetic Sciences* (pp. 813–819). The Hague: Mouton.

Abberton, E., & Fourcin, A. J. (1972). Laryngographic analysis and intonation. *British Journal of Disorders of Communication, 7,* 24–29.

Abberton, E., & Fourcin, A. J. (1975). Visual feedback and the acquisition of intonation. In E. H. Lenneberg & E. Lenneberg (Eds.), *Foundations of language development: A multidisciplinary approach* (Vol. 2, pp. 157–165). New York: Academic Press.

Abberton, E., & Fourcin, A. (1997). Electrolaryngography. In M. J. Ball & C. Code (Eds.), *Instrumental clinical phonetics* (pp. 119–148). San Diego, CA: Singular Publishing Group.

Abberton, E. R. M., Howard, D. M., & Fourcin, A. J. (1989). Laryngographic assessment of normal voice: A tutorial. *Clinical Linguistics and Phonetics, 3,* 281–296.

Abberton, E., Parker, A., & Fourcin, A. J. (1977). Speech improvement in deaf adults using laryngograph displays. In J. M. Pickett (Ed.), *Papers from the research conference on speech analyzing aids for the deaf* (pp. 172–188). Washington, DC: Gallaudet.

Alfonso, P. J., Kalinowski, J. S., & Story, R. S. (1991). The effect of speech motor training on stutterers' speech physiology. *Haskins Laboratories Status Report on Speech Research (SR 107/108,* pp. 111–122).

Alku, P., Strik, H., & Vilkman, E. (1997). Parabolic spectral parameter—A new method for quantification of the glottal flow. *Speech Communication, 22,* 67–97.

Alku, P., & Vilkman, E. (1992). Preliminary experiences in using automatic inverse filtering of acoustical signals for the voice source analysis. *Scandinavian Journal of Logopedics and Phoniatrics, 17,* 128–135.

Alku, P., & Vilkman, E. (1995). Effect of bandwidth on glottal airflow waveforms estimated by inverse filtering. *Journal of the Acoustical Society of America, 98,* 763–767.

Alku, P., Vilkman, E., & Laukkanen, A.-M. (1998). Parameterization of the voice source by combining spectral decay and amplitude features of the glottal flow. *Journal of Speech, Language, and Hearing Research, 41,* 990–1002.

Alku, P., Vilkman, E., & Pekkarinen, E. (1993). PAAPPA: A flexible computer environment for the analysis of the voice source. *Scandinavian Journal of Logopedics and Phoniatrics, 18,* 51–56.

Allison, R. D. (1970). Bioelectric impedance measurements—Introduction to basic factors in impedance plethysmography. In R. D. Allison (Ed.), *Basic factors in bioelectric impedance measurements* (pp. 1–70). Pittsburgh, PA: Instrument Society of America.

Anastaplo, S., & Karnell, M. P. (1988). Synchronized videostroboscopic and electroglottographic examination of glottal opening. *Journal of the Acoustical Society of America, 83,* 1883–1890.

Andrews, M. L. (1999). *Manual of voice treatment: Pediatrics through geriatrics* (2nd ed.). San Diego, CA: Singular Publishing Group.

Awrejcewicz, J. (1990). Bifurcation portrait of the human vocal cord oscillations. *Journal of Sound and Vibration, 136,* 151–156.

Baer, T. (1981). Investigation of the phonatory mechanism. *ASHA Reports, 11,* 38–47.

Baer, T., Löfqvist, A., & McGarr, N. S. (1983). Laryngeal vibrations: A comparison between high-speed filming and glottographic techniques. *Journal of the Acoustical Society of America, 73,* 1304–1308.

Baer, T., Titze, I. R., & Yoshioka, H. (1983). Multiple simultaneous measures of vocal fold activity. In D. M. Bless & J. H. Abbs (Eds.), *Vocal fold physiology: Contemporary research and clinical issues* (pp. 229–237). San Diego, CA: College-Hill Press.

Bagno, S., & Liebman, F. M. (1959). Impedance measurements of living tissue. *Electronics, 32,* 62–63.

Baken, R. J. (1990). Irregularity of vocal period and amplitude: A first approach to the fractal analysis of voice. *Journal of Voice, 4,* 185–197.

Baken, R. J. (1991). An overview of laryngeal function for voice production. In R. T. Sataloff (Ed.), *Professional voice: The science and art of clinical care* (pp. 19–47). New York: Raven Press.

Baken, R. J. (1992a). Electroglottography. *Journal of Voice, 6,* 98–109.

Baken, R. J. (1992b). Géométrie «fractale» et évaluation de la voix: Application préliminaire à la dysphonie. *Bulletin d'Audiophonologie: Annales Scientifiques de l'Université de Franche-Comté (Médecine et Pharmacie), VII NS,* 731–749.

Baken, R. J. (1993). L'Analyse de la voix: Présent et avenir. *Bulletin d'Audiophonologie: Annales Scientifiques de l'Université de Franche-Comté (Médecine et Pharmacie), X* (1/2), 37–56.

Baken, R. J. (1994). The aged voice: A new hypothesis. *Voice, 3,* 57–73.

Baken, R. J. (1995a). Epilogue: Into a chaotic future. In W. J. Gould, J. S. Rubin, G. Korovin, & R. T. Sataloff (Eds.), *Diagnosis and treatment of voice disorders* (pp. 502–509). New York: Igaku-Shoin.

Baken, R. J. (1995b). Between organization and chaos: A different view of the human voice. In F. Bell-Berti & L. J. Raphael (Eds.), *Producing speech: Contemporary issues. For Katherine Safford Harris* (pp. 233–245). New York: American Institute of Physics.

Baken, R. J., & Orlikoff, R. F. (1997). Voice measurement: Is more better? *Logopedics Phoniatrics Vocology, 22,* 147–151.

Beach, J. L., & Kelsey, C. A. (1969). Ultrasonic doppler monitoring of vocal-fold velocity and displacement. *Journal of the Acoustical Society of America, 46,* 1045–1047.

Bell Telephone Laboratories. (1937). *High speed motion pictures of the vocal cords* [motion picture]. (Bell Telephone Laboratories Bureau of Publications, New York.)

Benguerel, A.-P., & Bhatia, T. K. (1980). Hindi stop consonants: An acoustic and fiberoptic study. *Phonetica, 37,* 134–148.

Berke, G. S., Moore, D. M., Gerratt, B., Aly, A., & Tantisira, J. (1988). Transtracheal stimulation of the recurrent laryngeal nerve. *American Journal of Otolaryngology, 8,* 12–17.

Berry, R. J., Epstein, R., Fourcin, A. J., Freeman, M., MacCurtain, F., & Noscoe, N. (1982). An objective analysis of voice disorders: Part one. *British Journal of Disorders of Communication, 17,* 67–76.

Berry, R. J., Epstein, R., Freeman, M., MacCurtain, F., & Noscoe, N. (1982). An objective analysis of voice disorders: Part two. *British Journal of Disorders of Communication, 17,* 77–85.

Biever, D. M., & Bless, D. M. (1989). Vibratory characteristics of the vocal folds in young adult and geriatric women. *Journal of Voice, 3,* 120–131.

Bjuggren, G. (1960). Device for laryngeal phase-determinable flash photography. *Folia Phoniatrica, 12,* 36–41.

Blaugrund, S. M., Gould, W. J., Tanaka, S., & Kitajima, K. (1983). The fiberscope: Analysis and function of laryngeal reconstruction. In I. R. Titze & R. C. Scherer (Eds.), *Vocal fold physiology: Biomechanics, acoustics, and phonatory control* (pp. 252–255). Denver, CO: Denver Center for the Performing Arts.

Blosser, S., Wigley, F. M., & Wise, R. A. (1992). Increase in translaryngeal resistance during phonation in rheumatoid arthritis. *Chest, 102,* 387–390.

Böhme, G. (1988a). Ein Beitrag zur Methode der Ultraschalldiagnostik des Kehlkopfes. *Laryngologie, Rhinologie, Otologie, 67,* 551–558.

Böhme, G. (1988b). Ultraschalldiagnostik der phonatorischen Leistungen des Laryngektomierten. *Laryngologie, Rhinologie, Otologie, 67,* 651–665.

Böhme, G. (1989). Ein klinischer Beitrag zur Ultraschalldiagnostik des Kehlkopfes (Echolaryngographie). *Laryngologie, Rhinologie, Otologie, 68,* 510–515.

Bordone-Sacerdote, C., & Sacerdote, G. (1965). Investigations on the movement of the glottis by ultrasound. *Proceedings of the Fifth International Congress on Acoustics,* Liege, Belgium.

Brackett, I. P. (1948). The vibration of vocal folds at selected frequencies. *Annals of Otology, Rhinology, and Laryngology, 57,* 556–558.

Brewer, D. W., & McCall, G. (1974). Visible laryngeal changes during voice therapy: Fiberoptic study. *Annals of Otology, Rhinology, and Laryngology, 83,* 423–427.

Broad, D. J. (1973). Phonation. In F. D. Minifie, T. J. Hixon, & F. Williams (Eds.), *Normal aspects of speech, hearing, and language* (pp. 127–167). Englewood Cliffs, NJ: Prentice-Hall.

Broad, D. J. (1979). The new theories of vocal fold vibration. In N. J. Lass (Ed.), *Speech and language: Advances in basic research and practice* (Vol. 2., pp. 203–256). New York: Academic Press.

Casper, J., Brewer, D. W., & Conture, E. G. (1982). Speech therapy patient evaluation techniques with the fiberscope. In V. Lawrence (Ed.), *Transcripts of the Tenth Symposium on Care of the Professional Voice* (Part II, pp. 136–140). New York: The Voice Foundation.

Cavagna, G. A., & Camporesi, E. (1974). Glottal aerodynamics and phonation. In B. Wyke (Ed.), *Ventilatory and phonatory control systems* (pp. 76–92). New York: Oxford University Press.

Cavagna, G. A., & Margaria, R. (1968). Airflow rates and efficiency changes during phonation. *Annals of the New York Academy of Sciences, 155,* 152–163.

Chevrie-Muller, C. (1964). Etude de fonctionnement laryngé chez les bègues par la méthode glottographique. *Revue de Laryngologie, 85,* 763–774.

Chevrie-Muller, C. (1967). Contribution à l'étude des traces glottographiques chez l'adulte normal. *Revue de Laryngologie, 88,* 227–244.

Chevrie-Muller, C., & Grémy, F. (1962). Etude de l'électro-glottogramme en période de "mue vocale." *Annales d'Oto-Laryngologie, 79,* 1035–1044.

Childers, D. G., Alsaka, Y. A., Hicks, D. M., & Moore, G. P. (1987). Vocal fold vibrations: An EGG model. In T. Baer, C. Sasaki, & K. S. Harris (Eds.), *Laryngeal Function in phonation and respiration* (pp. 181–202). Boston, MA: Little, Brown.

Childers, D. G., Hicks, D. M., Moore, G. P., & Alsaka, Y. A. (1986). A model for vocal fold vibratory motion, contact area, and the electroglottogram. *Journal of the Acoustical Society of America, 80,* 1309–1320.

Childers, D. G., & Krishnamurthy, A. K. (1985). A critical review of electroglottography. *CRC Critical Reviews in Biomedical Engineering, 12,* 131–161.

Childers, D. G., Naik, J. M., Larar, J. N., Krishnamurthy, A. K., & Moore, G. P. (1983). Electroglottography, speech, and ultrahigh speed cinematography. In I. R. Titze & R. C. Scherer (Eds.), *Vocal fold physiology: Biomechanics, acoustics, and phonatory control* (pp. 202–220). Denver, CO: Denver Center for the Performing Arts.

Childers, D. G., Paige, A., & Moore, G. P. (1976). Laryngeal vibration patterns: Machine-aided measurements from high-speed film. *Archives of Otolaryngology, 102,* 407–410.

Childers, D. G., Smith, A. M., & Moore, G. P. (1984). Relationships between electroglottograph, speech, and vocal cord contact. *Folia Phoniatrica, 36,* 105–118.

Chouard, C.-H., Meyer, B., & Chabolle, F. (1987). The veloimpedancemetry. *Acta Otolaryngologica, 103,* 537–545.

Coleman, R. F. (1971). Effect of waveform changes upon roughness perception. *Folia Phoniatrica, 23,* 314–322.

Coleman, R. F., & Wendahl, R. W. (1968). On the validity of laryngeal photosensor monitoring. *Journal of the Acoustical Society of America, 44,* 1733–1735.

Colton, R. H. (1985). Glottal waveform variations associated with different vocal intensity levels. In V. L. Lawrence (Ed.), *Transcripts of the Thirteenth Symposium on the Care of the Professional Voice* (pp. 39–47). New York: The Voice Foundation.

Colton, R. H., & Casper, J. K. (1996). *Understanding voice problems: A physiological persepctive for diagnosis and treatment* (2nd ed.). Baltimore, MD: Williams and Wilkins.

Colton, R. H., & Conture, E. G. (1990). Problems and pitfalls of electroglottography. *Journal of Voice, 4,* 10–24.

Cranen, B. (1991). Simultaneous modelling of EGG, PGG, and glottal flow. In J. Gauffin & B. Hammarberg (Eds.), *Vocal fold physiology: Acoustic, perceptual, and physiological aspects of voice mechanisms* (pp. 57–64). San Diego, CA: Singular Publishing Group.

Croatto, L., & Ferrero, F. E. (1979). L'esame elettroglottografico appliato ad alcuni casi di disodia. *Acta Phoniatrica Latina, 1,* 247–258.

Croatto, L., Ferrero, F. E., & Arrigoni, L. (1980). Comparazione fra segnale elettroglottografico e segnale fotoglottografica: Primi resultati. *Acta Phoniatrica Latina, 2,* 213–224.

Dalziel, C. F. (1956). Effects of electric shock in man. *IRE Transactions on Medical Electronics, PGME − 5,* 44–62.

D'Antonio, L., Lotz, W., Chait, D., & Netsell, R. (1987). Perceptual-physiologic approach to evaluation and treatment of dysphonia. *Annals of Otology, Rhinology and Laryngology, 96,* 187–190.

D'Antonio, L., Netsell, R., & Lotz, W. (1988). Clinical aerodynamics for the evaluation and management of voice disorders. *Ear, Nose and Throat Journal, 67,* 394–399.

Davidson, T. M., Bone, R. C., & Nahum, L. M. (1974). Flexible fiberoptic laryngobronchoscopy. *Laryngoscope, 84,* 1876–1882.

Decroix, G., & Dujardin, J. (1958). Etude des accolements glottiques au cours de la phonation par la glottographie e haute fréquence. *Journal Français d'Oto-Rhino-Laryngologie, 7,* 493–499.

Dejonckere, P. H. (1981). Comparison of two methods of photglottography in relation to electroglottography. *Folia Phoniatrica, 33,* 338–347.

Dejonckere, P. H., & Lebacq, J. (1985). Electroglottography and vocal nodules: An attempt to quantify the shape of the signal. *Folia Phoniatrica, 37,* 195–200.

Doyle, P. C., & Fraser, S. C. (1993). A simplified clinical procedure for the acquisition of photoglottographic waveforms from children and adults. *American Journal of Speech-Language Pathology, 2*(3), 36–40.

Doyle, P. C., & Wallace, W. J. B. (1990). Application and clinical use of the Kay Elemetrics Waveform Display System for photoglottographic (PGG) assessment of vocal function. *Computer Users in Speech and Hearing, 6,* 122–129.

Dromey, C., Stathopoulos, E. T., & Sapienza, C. M. (1992). Glottal airflow and electroglottographic measures of vocal function at multiple intensities. *Journal of Voice, 6,* 44–54.

Edgerton, H. E., & Killian, J. R., Jr. (1939). *Flash! Seeing the unseen by ultra high-speed photography.* Boston, MA: Hale, Cushman, & Flint.

Fabre, P. (1940). Sphygmographie par simple contact d'électrodes cutanées, introduisant dans l'artère de faibles courants de haute fréquence détecteurs de ses variations volumétriques. *Comptes Rendus de la Société de Biologie, 133,* 639–641.

Fabre, P. (1957). Un procédé électrique percutané d'inscription de l'accolement glottique au cours de la phonation: glottographie de haute fréquence. Premiers résultats. *Bulletin de l'Académie Nationale de Médecine, 141,* 66–69.

Fabre, P. (1958). Etude comparée des glottogrammes et de phonogrammes de la voix humaine. *Annales d'Oto-Laryngologie, 75,* 767–775.

Fairbanks, G. (1950). A physiological correlative of vowel intensity. *Speech Monographs, 17,* 390–395.

Fant, G. (1979). Glottal source and excitation analysis. *Speech Transmission Laboratory—Quarterly Progress and Status Report* (Royal Institute of Technology, Stockholm), *1,* 85–107.

Fant, G., Liljencrants, J., & Lin, Q. (1985). A four-parameter model of glottal flow. *Speech Transmission Laboratory—Quarterly Progress and Status Report* (Royal Institute of Technology, Stockholm), *4,* 1–13.

Farnsworth, D. W. (1940). High-speed motion pictures of the human vocal cords. *Bell Telephone Laboratories Record, 18,* 203–208.

Ferguson, G. B., & Crowder, W. J. (1970). A simple method of laryngeal and other cavity photography. *Archives of Otolaryngology, 92,* 201–203.

Feudo, P. (1984). Evaluation and rehabilitation voice disorders. *Otolaryngologic Clinics of North America, 17*(1), 81–89.

Fisher, K., Scherer, R., Swank, P., Giddens, C., & Patten, D. (1995). Electroglottographic tracking of phonatory response to Botox. *NCVS Status and Progress Report, 8,* 97–111.

Fletcher, H. (1953). *Speech and hearing in communication.* Princeton, NJ: van Nostrand.

Fourcin, A. J. (1974). Laryngographic examination of vocal fold vibration. In B. Wyke (Ed.), *Ventilatory and phonatory control systems* (pp. 315–333). New York: Oxford University Press.

Fourcin, A. J. (1981). Laryngographic assessment of phonatory function. *ASHA Reports, 11,* 116–127.

Fourcin, A. (1986). Electrolaryngographic assessment of vocal fold function. *Journal of Phonetics, 14,* 435–442.

Fourcin, A. J. (1993). Normal and pathological speech: Phonetic, acoustic and laryngographic aspects. In W. Singh & D. S. Soutar (Eds.), *Functional surgery of the larynx and pharynx* (pp. 31–51). Oxford, UK: Butterworth-Heinemann.

Fourcin, A. J., & Abberton, E. (1971). First applications of a new laryngograph. *Medical and Biological Illustration, 21,* 172–182. (Reprinted in *Volta Review* [1972], *74,* 161–176; and in J. M. Levitt & R. A. Houde (Eds.), *Sensory aids for the hearing impaired* [pp. 376–386] [1980]. New York: John Wiley.)

Fourcin, A. J., & Abberton, E. (1976). The laryngograph and the Voiscope in speech therapy. In E. Loebell (Ed.), *Proceedings of the Sixteenth International Congress of Logopedics and Phoniatrics* (pp. 116–122). Basel, Switzerland: S. Karger.

Fourcin, A. J., Abberton, E., Miller, D., & Howells, D. (1995). Laryngograph: Speech pattern element tools for therapy, training and assessment. *European Journal of Disorders of Communication, 30,* 101–115.

Friedman, E. M. (1997). Role of ultrasound in the assessment of vocal cord function in infants and children. *Annals of Otology, Rhinology and Laryngology, 106,* 199–209.

Fritzell, B., Gauffin, J., Hammarberg, B., Karlsson, I., & Sundberg, J. (1984). Measuring insufficient vocal fold closure during phonation. *Speech Transmission Laboratory—Quarterly Progress and Status Report* (Royal Institute of Technology, Stockholm), *4,* 50–59.

Fritzell, B., Hammarberg, B., Gauffin, J., Karlsson, I., & Sundberg, J. (1986). Breathiness and insufficient vocal fold closure. *Journal of Phonetics, 14,* 549–553.

Fujimura, O. (1977). Stereo-fiberscope. In M. Sawashima & F. S. Cooper (Eds.), *Dynamic aspects of speech production* (pp. 133–137). Tokyo, Japan: University of Tokyo Press.

Fujimura, O. (1981). Fiberoptic observation and measurement of vocal fold movement. *ASHA Reports, 11,* 59–69.

Fujimura, O., Baer, T., & Niimi, S. (1979). A stereofiberscope with a magnetic interlens bridge for laryngeal observation. *Journal of the Acoustical Society of America, 65,* 478–480.

Fukuda, H., Saito, S., Kitahara, S., Isogai, Y., Makino, K., Tsuzuki, T., Kogawa, N., & Ono, H. (1983). Vocal fold vibration in excised larynges viewed with an x-ray stroboscope and an ultra-high-speed camera. In D. M. Bless & J. H. Abbs (Eds.), *Vocal fold physiology: Contemporary research and clinical issues* (pp. 238–252). San Diego, CA: College-Hill Press.

Gall, V. (1978). Fotokymografische Befunde bei funktionellen Dysphonien: Kehlkopflähmungen und Stimmlippentumoren. *Folia Phoniatrica, 30,* 28–35.

Gall, V. (1984). Strip kymography of the glottis. *Archives of Otorhinolaryngology, 240,* 287–293.

Gall, V., Gall, D., & Hanson, J. (1971). Larynx-Fotokymographie. *Archiv für klinische und experimentelle Ohren-, Nasen- und Kehlkopfheilkunde, 200,* 34–41.

Gall, V., & Hanson, J. (1973). Bestimmung physikalischer Parameter der Stimmlippenschwingungen mit Hilfe der Larynxphotokymographie. *Folia Phoniatrica, 25,* 450–459.

Gauffin, J., Binh, N., Ananthapadmanabha, T. V., & Fant, G. (1983). Glottal geometry and volume velocity waveform. In D. M. Bless & J. H. Abbs (Eds.), *Vocal fold physiology: Contemporary research and clinical issues* (pp. 194–201). San Diego, CA: College-Hill Press.

Gauffin, J., & Sundberg, J. (1980). Data on the glottal voice source behavior in vowel production. *Speech Transmission Laboratory—Quarterly Progress and Status Report* (Royal Institute of Technology, Stockholm), *2–3,* 61–70.

Gauffin, J., & Sundberg, J. (1989). Spectral correlates of glottal voice source waveform characteristics. *Journal of Speech and Hearing Research, 32,* 556–565.

Garel, C., Contencin, P., Polonovski, J. M., Hassan, M., & Narcy, P. (1992). Laryngeal ultrasonography in infants and children: A new way of investigating. Normal and pathological findings. *International Journal of Pediatric Otorhinolaryngology, 23,* 107–115.

Geddes, L. A., & Baker, L. E. (1967). The specific resistance of biological material—A compendium of data for the biomedical engineer and physiologist. *Medical and Biological Engineering, 5,* 271–293.

Geddes, L. A., & Baker, L. E. (1989). *Principles of applied biomedical instrumentation* (3rd ed.). New York: John Wiley.

Geddes, L. A., Baker, L. E., Moore, A. G., & Coulter, T. W. (1969). Hazards in the use of low frequencies for the measurement of physiological events by impedance. *Medical and Biological Engineering, 7,* 289–296.

Gerratt, B. R., Hanson, D. G., & Berke, G. S. (1986). A non-invasive transoral technique for glottography. In M. Hirano & S. R. Hibi (Eds.), *Proceedings of the International Conference on Voice* (pp. 85–87). Kurume, Japan: Kurume University Press.

Gerratt, B. R., Hanson, D. G., & Berke, G. S. (1987). Glottographic measures of laryngeal function in individuals with abnormal motor control. In T. Baer, C. Sasaki, & K. S. Harris (Eds.), *Laryngeal function in phonation and respiration* (pp. 521–532). Boston, MA: Little, Brown.

Gerratt, B. R., Hanson, D. G., Berke, G. S., & Precoda, K. (1991). Photoglottography: A clinical synopsis. *Journal of Voice, 5,* 98–105.

Gilbert, H. R., Potter, C. R., & Hoodin, R. (1984). Laryngograph as a measure of vocal fold contact area. *Journal of Speech and Hearing Research, 27,* 178–182.

Gleeson, M. J., & Fourcin, A. J. (1983). Clinical analysis of laryngeal trauma secondary to intubation. *Journal of the Royal Society of Medicine, 76,* 928–932.

Gleeson, M. J., Pearson, R. C., Armistead, S., & Yates, A. K. (1984). Voice changes following cricothyroidotomy. *Journal of Laryngology and Otology, 98,* 1015–1019.

Gómez Gonzáles, J. L., & del Cañizo Alvarez, C. (1988). Nuevas tecnicas de exploración funcional laríngea: la electroglotografia. *Anales Oto-Rino-Laryngologica Ibero-Americana, 15,* 239–262.

Gougerot, L., Grémy, F., & Marstal, N. (1960). Glottographie à large bande passante. Application à l'étude de la voix de fausset. *Journal de Physiologie, 52,* 823–832.

Gould, W. J. (1973). The Gould laryngoscope. *Transactions of the American Academy of Ophthalmology and Otolaryngology, 77,* 139–141.

Gould, W. J. (1977). Newer aspects of high-speed photography of the vocal folds. In M. Sawashima & F. S. Cooper (Eds.), *Dynamic aspects of speech production* (pp. 139–144). Tokyo, Japan: Tokyo University Press.

Gould, W. J. (1983). The fiberscope: Flexible and rigid for laryngeal function evaluation. In I. R. Titze & R. C. Scherer (Eds.), *Vocal fold physiology: Biomechanics, acoustics, and phonatory control* (pp. 249–251). Denver, CO: Denver Center for the Performing Arts.

Gould, W. J., Jako, G. J., & Tanabe, M. (1974). Advances in high-speed motion picture photography of the larynx. *Transactions of the American Academy of Ophthalmology and Otolaryngology, 78,* 276–278.

Gracco, L. C., Gracco, V. L., Löfqvist, A., & Marek, K. P. (1994). Aerodynamic evaluation of Parkinsonian dysarthria: Laryngeal and supralaryngeal manifestations. In J. A. Till, K. M. Yorkston, & D. R. Beukelman (Eds.), *Motor speech disorders: Advances in assessment and treatment* (pp. 65–79). Baltimore, MD: Paul H. Brookes.

Grémy, F., & Guérin, C. (1963). Etude du glottogramme chez l'enfant sourd en cours de rééducation vocale. *Annales d'Oto-Laryngologie, 80,* 803–815.

Gross, M. (1985). Larynxfotokymographie. *Sprache-Stimme-Gehör, 9,* 112–113.

Gross, M. (1988). *Endoscopische Larynx-Fotokymografie.* Bingen, Germany: Renate Gross.

Hacki, T. (1989). Klassifizierung von Glottisdysfunktionen mit Hilfe der Elecktroglottographie. *Folia Phoniatrica, 41,* 43–48.

Hacki, T. (1996). Electroglottographic quasi-open quotient and amplitude in crescendo phonation. *Journal of Voice, 10,* 342–347.

Hahn, C., & Kitzing, P. (1978). Indirect endoscopic photography of the larynx. *Journal of Audiovisual Media in Medicine, 1,* 121–130.

Haji, T., Horiguchi, S., Baer, T., & Gould, W. J. (1986). Frequency and amplitude perturbation analysis of electroglottograph during sustained phonation. *Journal of the Acoustical Society of America, 80,* 58–62.

Hamlet, S. L. (1971). Location of slope discontinuities in glottal pulse shapes during vocal fry. *Journal of the Acoustical Society of America, 50,* 1561–1562.

Hamlet, S. L. (1972a). Interpretation of ultrasonic signals in terms of phase difference of vocal fold vibration. *Journal of the Acoustical Society of America, 51,* 90–91.

Hamlet, S. L. (1972b). Vocal fold articulatory activity during whispered sibilants. *Archives of Otolaryngology, 95,* 211–213.

Hamlet, S. L. (1973). Vocal compensation: An ultrasonic study of vocal fold vibration in normal and nasal vowels. *Cleft Palate Journal, 10,* 267–285.

Hamlet, S. L. (1980). Ultrasonic measurement of larynx height and vocal vibratory pattern. *Journal of the Acoustical Society of America, 68,* 121–126.

Hamlet, S. L. (1981). Ultrasound assessment of phonatory function. *ASHA Reports, 11,* 128–140.

Hamlet, S. L., & Palmer, J. M. (1974). Investigation of laryngeal trills using the transmission of ultrasound through the larynx. *Folia Phoniatrica, 26,* 362–377.

Hamlet, S. L., & Reid, J. M. (1972). Transmission of ultrasound through the larynx as a means of determining vocal-fold activity. *IEEE Transactions in Biomedical Engineering, 19,* 34–37.

Hanson, D. G., Gerratt, B. R., & Berke, G. S. (1990). Frequency, intensity, and target matching effects on photoglottographic measures of open quotient and speed quotient. *Journal of Speech and Hearing Research, 33,* 45–50.

Hanson, D. G., Gerratt, B. R., & Ward, P. H. (1983). Glottographic measurement of vocal dysfunction: A preliminary report. *Annals of Otology, Rhinology and Laryngology, 92,* 413–420.

Harden, R. J. (1975). Comparison of glottal area changes as measured from ultrahigh-speed photographs and photoelectric glottographs. *Journal of Speech and Hearing Research, 18,* 728–738.

Harries, M., Hawkins, S., Hacking, J., & Hughes, I. (1998). Changes in the male voice at puberty: Vocal fold length and its relationship to the fundamental frequency of the voice. *Journal of Laryngology and Otology, 112,* 451–454.

Harris, T., Harris, S., Rubin, J. S., & Howard, D. M. (1998). *The voice clinic handbook.* London: Whurr Publishers.

Havas, T., & Priestley, J. (1993). The revised Australian fiberscopic profile. *Journal of Voice, 7,* 377–381.

Hayden, E. H., & Koike, Y. (1972). A data processing scheme for frame by frame film analysis. *Folia Phoniatrica, 24,* 169–181.

Hertegård, S., & Gauffin, J. (1992). Acoustic properties of the Rothenberg mask. *Speech Transmission Laboratory—Quarterly Progress and Status Report* (Royal Institute of Technology, Stockholm), 2–3, 9–18.

Hertegård, S., & Gauffin, J. (1995). Glottal area and vibratory patterns studied with simultaneous stroboscopy, flow glottography, and electroglottography. *Journal of Speech and Hearing Research, 38,* 85–100.

Hertegård, S., Gauffin, J., & Karlsson, I. (1992). Physiological correlates of the inverse filtered flow glottogram. *Journal of Voice, 6,* 224–234.

Hertz, C. H., Linström, K., & Sonesson, B. (1970). Ultrasonic recording of the vibrating vocal folds. *Acta Otolaryngologica, 69,* 223–230.

Herzel, H., Steinecke, I., Mende, W., & Wermke, K. (1991). Chaos and bifurcations during voiced speech. In E. Mosekilde (Ed.), *Complexity, chaos and biological evolution* (pp. 41–50). New York: Plenum Press.

Hess, M. M., & Gross, M. (1993). High-speed, light-intensified digital imaging of vocal fold vibrations in high optical resolution via indirect microlaryngoscopy. *Annals of Otology, Rhinology and Laryngology, 102,* 502–507.

Hess, M. M., Herzel, H., Köster, O., Scheurich, F., & Gross, M. (1996). Endoskopische Darstellung von Stimmlippenschwingungen. *HNO, 44,* 685–693.

Hess, M., Ludwigs, M., Gross, M., & Orglmeister, R. (1997). Bidirectional stroboscopy—double information? Clinical aspects. In T. Wittenberg, P. Mergell, M. Tigges, & U. Eysholdt (Eds.), *Advances in quantitative laryngoscopy using motion-, image-, and signal-analysis* (pp. 83–90). Göttingen, Germany: University of Göttingen.

Higgins, M. B., & Saxman, J. H. (1991). A comparison of selected phonatory behaviors of healthy aged and young adults. *Journal of Speech and Hearing Research, 34,* 1000–1010.

Hiki, S. (1983). Relationship between efficiency of phonation and the tonal quality of speech. In D. M. Bless & J. H. Abbs (Eds.), *Vocal fold physiology: Contemporary research and clinical issues* (pp. 333–343). San Diego, CA: College-Hill Press.

Hillman, R. E., Holmberg, E. B., Perkell, J. S., Walsh, M., & Vaughan, C. (1989). Objective assessment of vocal hyperfunction: An experimental framework and initial results. *Journal of Speech and Hearing Research, 32,* 373–392.

Hillman, R. E., Holmberg, E. B., Perkell, J. S., Walsh, M., & Vaughan, C. (1990). Phonatory function associated with hyperfunctionally related vocal fold lesions. *Journal of Voice, 4,* 52–63.

Hillman, R. E., Oesterle, E., & Feth, L. L. (1983). Characteristics of the glottal turbulent noise source. *Journal of the Acoustical Society of America, 74,* 691–694.

Hillman, R. E., & Weinberg, B. (1981a). A new procedure for venting a reflectionless tube. *Journal of the Acoustical Society of America, 69,* 1449–1451.

Hillman, R. E., & Weinberg, B. (1981b). Estimation of glottal volume velocity waveform properties: A review and study of some methodological assumptions. In N. J. Lass (Ed.), *Speech and language: Advances in basic research and practice* (Vol. 6, pp. 411–473). New York: Academic Press.

Hillman, R. E., Weinberg, B., & Tree, D. (1978). *Glottal waveform measurement: Equipment, calibration, and application.* Paper presented at the annual convention of the American Speech-Language-Hearing Association. San Francisco, CA.

Hirano, M. (1974). Morphological structure of the vocal cord as a vibrator and its variations. *Folia Phoniatrica, 26,* 89–94.

Hirano, M. (1975). Phonosurgery: Basic and clinical investigations. *Otologia Fukuoka, 21,* 239–440.

Hirano, M. (1977). Structure and vibratory behavior of the vocal folds. In M. Sawashima & F. S. Cooper (Eds.), *Dynamic aspects of speech production* (pp. 13–30). Tokyo, Japan: University of Tokyo Press.

Hirano, M. (1981). *Clinical examination of voice.* New York: Springer-Verlag.

Hirano, M., & Bless, D. M. (1993). *Videoendoscopic examination of the larynx.* San Diego, CA: Singular Publishing Group.

Hirano, M., Gould, W. J., Lambiase, A., & Kakita, Y. (1981). Vibratory behavior of the vocal folds in a case of a unilateral polyp. *Folia Phoniatrica, 33,* 275–284.

Hirano, M., Kakita, Y., Kawasaki, H., Gould, W. J., & Lambiase, A. (1981). Data from high-speed motion picture studies. In K. N. Stevens & M. Hirano (Eds.), *Vocal fold physiology* (pp. 85–93). Tokyo, Japan: University of Tokyo Press.

Hirano, M., Yoshida, Y., Matsushita, H., & Nakajima, T. (1974). An apparatus for ultra highspeed cinematography of the vocal cords. *Annals of Otology, Rhinology and Laryngology, 83,* 12–18.

Hirose, H. (1988). High-speed digital imaging of vocal fold vibration. *Acta Otolaryngologica, Suppl. 458,* 151–153.

Hirose, H. (1993). Use of high-speed digital imaging system for the analysis of abnormal patterns of vocal fold vibration associated with diplophonia. In T. Hacki (Ed.), *Aktuelle phoniatrisch-pädaudiologische Aspekte 1993* (Vol. 1, pp. 118–125). Berlin, Germany: Renate Gross.

Hirose, H., Kiritani, S., & Imagawa, H. (1988). High-speed digital image analysis of laryngeal behavior in running speech. In O. Fujimura (Ed.), *Vocal physiology: Voice production, mechanisms, and functions* (pp. 335–345). New York: Raven Press.

Hirose, H., Kiritani, S., & Imagawa, H. (1991). Clinical application of high-speed digital imaging of vocal fold vibration. In J. Gauffin & B. Hammarberg (Eds.), *Vocal fold physiology: Acoustic, perceptual, and physiological aspects of voice mechanisms* (pp. 213–217). San Diego, CA: Singular Publishing Group.

Hoit, J. D., & Hixon, T. J. (1992). Age and laryngeal airway resistance during vowel production in women. *Journal of Speech and Hearing Research, 35*, 309–313.

Hollien, H. (1974). On vocal registers. *Journal of Phonetics, 2*, 125–143.

Hollien, H., Girard, G. T., & Coleman, R. F. (1977). Vocal fold vibratory patterns of pulse register. *Folia Phoniatrica, 29*, 200–205.

Holm, C. (1971). L'évolution de la phonation de la première enfance à la puberté: Une étude électroglottographique. *Journal Français d'Oto-Rhino-Laryngologie, 20*, 437–440.

Holmberg, E. B., Hillman, R. E., & Perkell, J. S. (1988). Glottal airflow and transglottal air pressure measurements for male and female speakers in soft, normal, and loud voice. *Journal of the Acoustical Society of America, 84*, 511–529.

Holmberg, E. B., Hillman, R. E., & Perkell, J. S. (1989). Glottal airflow and transglottal air pressure measurements for male and female speakers in low, normal, and high pitch. *Journal of Voice, 3*, 294–305.

Holmberg, E. B., Hillman, R. E., Perkell, J. S., & Gress, C. (1994a). Relationships between intra-speaker variation in aerodynamic measures of voice production and variation in SPL across repeated recordings. *Journal of Speech and Hearing Research, 37*, 484–495.

Holmberg, E. B., Hillman, R. E., Perkell, J. S., & Gress, C. (1994b). Individual variation in measures of voice. *Phonetica, 51*, 30–37.

Holmberg, E. B., Hillman, R. E., Perkell, J. S., Guiod, P. C., & Goldman, S. L. (1995). Comparisons among aerodynamic, electroglottographic, and acoustic spectral measures of female voice. *Journal of Speech and Hearing Research, 38*, 1212–1223.

Holmer, N.-G., & Kitzing, P. (1975). Localization of the vocal folds and registration of their movements by ultrasound. In E. Kazner (Ed.), *Ultrasonics in medicine* (pp. 349–354). Amsterdam: Excerpta Medica.

Holmer, N.-G., Kitzing, P., & Linström, K. (1973). Echo glottography. *Acta Otolaryngologica, 75*, 454–463.

Holmer, N.-G., & Rundqvist, H. E. (1975). Ultrasonic registration of the fundamental frequency of a voice during normal speech. *Journal of the Acoustical Society of America, 58*, 1073–1077.

Holmes, L. C., Leeper, H. A., & Nicholson, I. R. (1994). Laryngeal airway resistance of older men and women as a function of vocal sound pressure level. *Journal of Speech and Hearing Research, 37*, 789–799.

Honda, K., Kiritani, S., Imagawa, H., & Hirose, H. (1987). High-speed digital recording of vocal fold vibrations using a solid-state image sensor. In T. Baer, C. Sasaki & K. S. Harris (Eds.), *Laryngeal function in phonation and respiration* (pp. 485–491). Boston, MA: Little, Brown.

Horiguchi, S., Haji, J., Baer, T., & Gould, W. J. (1987). Comparison of electroglottographic and acoustic waveform perturbation measures. In T. Baer, C. Sasaki, & K. S. Harris (Eds.), *Laryngeal function in phonation and respiration* (pp. 509–518). San Diego, CA: College-Hill Press.

Houben, G. B., Buekers, R., & Kingma, H. (1992). Characterization of the electroglottographic waveform: A primary study to investigate vocal fold functioning. *Folia Phoniatrica, 44*, 269–281.

House, A. S. (1959). A note on optimal vocal frequency. *Journal of Speech and Hearing Research, 2*, 55–60.

Howard, D. M. (1995). Variation of electrolaryngographically derived closed quotient for trained and untrained adult female singers. *Journal of Voice, 9*, 163–172.

Howard, D. M., Lindsey, G. A., & Allen, B. (1990). Towards the quantification of vocal efficiency. *Journal of Voice, 4*, 205–212.

Howell, P., & Williams, M. (1988). The contribution of the excitatory source to the perception of neutral vowels in stuttered speech. *Journal of the Acoustical Society of America, 84*, 80–89.

Howell, P., & Williams, M. (1992). Acoustic analysis and perception of vowels in children's and teenagers' stuttered speech. *Journal of the Acoustical Society of America, 91*, 1697–1706.

Imagawa, H., Kiritani, S., & Hirose, H. (1984). High-speed digital image recording system for observing vocal fold vibration using an image sensor. *Japanese Journal of Medical Electronics and Biological Engineering, 25*, 284–290.

Isshiki, N. (1964). Regulatory mechanism of vocal intensity variation. *Journal of Speech and Hearing Research, 7*, 17–29.

Isshiki, N. (1969). Remarks on mechanism for vocal intensity variation. *Journal of Speech and Hearing Research, 12*, 665–672.

Isshiki, N. (1981). Vocal efficiency index. In K. N. Stevens & M. Hirano (Eds.), *Vocal fold physiology* (pp. 193–207). Tokyo, Japan: University of Tokyo Press.

Isshiki, N. (1985). Clinical significance of a vocal efficiency index. In I. R. Titze & R. C. Scherer (Eds.), *Vocal fold physiology: Biomechanics, acoustics, and phonatory control* (pp. 230–238). Denver, CO: The Denver Center for the Performing Arts.

Isshiki, N. (1989). *Phonosurgery*. New York: Springer-Verlag.

Isshiki, N., & von Leden, H. (1964). Hoarseness: Aerodynamic studies. *Archives of Otolaryngology, 80*, 206–213.

Isshiki, N., Yanagihara, N., & Morimoto, M. (1966). Approach to the objective diagnosis of hoarseness. *Folia Phoniatrica, 18*, 393–400.

Iwata, S. (1988). Aerodynamic aspects for phonation in normal and pathologic larynges. In O. Fujimura (Ed.), *Vocal physiology: Voice production, mechanisms, and functions* (pp. 423–431). New York: Raven Press.

Javkin, H. R., Antoñanzas-Barroso, N., & Maddieson, I. (1987). Digital inverse filtering for linguistic research. *Journal of Speech and Hearing Research, 30*, 122–129.

Jentzsch, H., Sasama, R., & Unger, E. (1978). Elektroglottographische Untersuchungen zur Problematik des Stimmeinsatzes bei zusammenhängenden Sprechen. *Folia Phoniatrica, 30*, 59–66.

Jentzsch, H., Unger, E., & Sasama, R. (1981). Elektroglottographische Verlaufskontrollen bei Patienten mit funktionellen Stimmstörungen. *Folia Phoniatrica, 33*, 234–241.

Kagaya, R. (1974). A fiberoptic and acoustic study of Korean stops, affricates, and fricatives. *Journal of Phonetics, 2*, 161–180.

Kakita, Y. (1988). Simultaneous observation of the vibratory pattern, sound pressure, and airflow signals using a physical model of the vocal folds. In O. Fujimura (Ed.), *Vocal physiology: Voice production, mechanisms, and functions* (pp. 207–218). New York: Raven Press.

Kakita, Y., Hirano, M., Kawasaki, H. & Matsuo, K. (1983). Stereolaryngoscopy: A new method to extract vertical movement of the vocal fold during vibration. In I. R. Titze & R. C. Scherer (Eds.), *Vocal fold physiology: Biomechanics, acoustics, and phonatory control* (pp. 191–201). Denver, CO: Denver Center for the Performing Arts.

Kaneko, T., Kobayashi, N., Tachibana, M., Naito, J., Hayawaki, K., Uchida, K., Yoshioka, T., & Suzuki, H. (1976). L'ultrasonoglottographie; L'aire neutre glottique et la vibration de la corde vocale. *Revue de Laryngologie, 97*, 363–369.

Kaneko, T., Suzuki, H., Uchida, K., Kanesaka, T., Komatsu, K., & Shimada, A. (1983). The movement of the inner layers of the vocal fold during phonation—Observation by ultrasonic method. In D. M. Bless & J. H. Abbs (Eds.), *Vocal fold physiology: Contemporary research and clinical issues* (pp. 223–237). San Diego, CA: College-Hill Press.

Kaneko, T., Uchida, K., Suzuki, H., Komatsu, K., Kanesaka, T., Kobayashi, N., & Naito, J. (1981). Ultrasonic observations of vocal fold vibration. In K. N. Stevens & M. Hirano (Eds.), *Vocal fold physiology* (pp. 107–117). Tokyo, Japan: University of Tokyo Press.

Karlsson, I. (1986). Glottal wave forms for normal female speakers. *Journal of Phonetics, 14,* 415–419.

Karlsson, I. (1991). Dynamic voice quality variations in natural female speech. *Speech Communication, 10,* 481–490.

Karnell, M. P. (1989). Synchronized videostroboscopy and electroglottography. *Journal of Voice, 3,* 68–75.

Karnell, M. P. (1994). *Videoendoscopy: From velopharynx to larynx.* San Diego, CA: Singular Publishing Group.

Keilmann, A., & Bader, C.-A. (1995). Development of aerodynamic aspects in children's voice. *International Journal of Pediatric Otorhinolaryngology, 31,* 183–190.

Kelly, J. H. (1984). Methods of diagnosis and documentation. *Otolaryngologic Clinics of North America, 17*(1), 29–34.

Kelman, A. W. (1981). Vibratory pattern of the vocal folds. *Folia Phoniatrica, 33,* 73–99.

Kempster, G., Preston, J., Mack, R., & Larson, C. (1987). A preliminary investigation relating laryngeal muscle activity to changes in EGG waveforms. In T. Baer, C. Sasaki, & K. S. Harris (Eds.), *Laryngeal function in phonation and respiration* (pp. 339–348). Boston, MA: Little, Brown.

Kiritani, S., Hirose, H., & Imagawa, H. (1993a). High-speed digital image analysis of vocal fold vibration in diplophonia. *Speech Communication, 13,* 23–32.

Kiritani, S., Hirose, H., & Imagawa, H. (1993b). Vocal fold vibration and the speech waveform in diplophonia. *Annual Bulletin of the Research Institute for Logopedics and Phoniatrics, 25,* 55–62.

Kiritani, S., Imagawa, H., & Hirose, H. (1988). High-speed digital image recording for the observation of vocal cord vibration. In O. Fujimura (Ed.), *Vocal physiology: Voice production, mechanisms, and functions* (pp. 261–269). New York: Raven Press.

Kitzing, P. (1977). Methode zur kombinierten photo- und elecktroglottographischen Registrierung von Stimmlippenschwingungen. *Folia Phoniatrica, 29,* 249–260.

Kitzing, P. (1982). Photo- and electroglottographical recording of the laryngeal vibratory pattern during different registers. *Folia Phoniatrica, 34,* 234–241.

Kitzing, P. (1986). Glottography, the electrophysiological investigation of phonatory biomechanics. *Acta Otorhinolaryngologica Belgica, 40,* 863–878.

Kitzing, P. (1990). Clinical applications of electroglottography. *Journal of Voice, 4,* 238–249.

Kitzing, P., & Löfqvist, A. (1978). Clinical application of combined electro- and photoglottography. *Proceedings of the Seventeenth Congress of Logopedics and Phoniatrics.* Copenhagen, Denmark.

Kitzing, P., & Löfqvist, A. (1979). Evaluation of voice therapy by means of photoglottography. *Folia Phoniatrica, 31,* 103–109.

Kitzing, P., & Sonesson, B. (1974). A photoglottographical study of the female vocal folds during phonation. *Folia Phoniatrica, 26,* 138–149.

Koike, Y., & Hirano, M. (1973). Glottal-area time function and subglottal pressure variation. *Journal of the Acoustical Society of America, 54,* 1618–1627.

Köster, J.-P., & Smith, S. (1970). Zur Interpretation elektrischer und photoelektrischer Glottogramme. *Folia Phoniatrica, 22,* 92–99.

Kostyk, B. E., & Rochet, A. P. (1998). Laryngeal airway resistance in teachers with vocal fatigue: A preliminary study. *Journal of Voice, 12,* 287–299.

Koyama, T., Harvey, J. E., & Ogura, J. H. (1972). Mechanics of voice production: III. Efficiency of voice production. *Laryngoscope, 82,* 210–217.

Krishnamurthy, A. K., & Childers, D. G. (1986). Two-channel speech analysis. *IEEE Transactions in Acoustics and Speech Signal Processing, 34,* 730–743.

Ladefoged, P., & McKinney, N. P. (1963). Loudness, sound pressure, and subglottal pressure in speech. *Journal of the Acoustical Society of America, 35,* 454–460.

Landman, G. H. M. (1970). *Laryngography and cinelaryngography.* Baltimore, MD: Williams and Wilkins.

Larson, K. K., Ramig, L. O., & Scherer, R. C. (1994). Acoustic and glottographic voice analysis during drug-related fluctuations in Parkinson disease. *Journal of Medical Speech-Language Pathology, 2,* 227–239.

Lebrun, Y., & Hasquin-Deleval, J. (1971). On the so-called 'dissociations' between electroglottogram and phonogram. *Folia Phoniatrica, 23,* 225–227.

Lecluse, F. L. E. (1974). Laboratory investigations in electroglottography. In E. Loebell (Ed.), *Proceedings of the Sixteenth International Congress of Logopedics and Phoniatrics* (pp. 294–296). Basel, Switzerland: S. Karger.

Lecluse, F. L. E. (1977). *Elektroglottographie.* Utrecht, The Netherlands: Drukkerijelinkwijk, B. V.

Lecluse, F. L. E., Brocaar, M. P., & Verschuure, J. (1975). The electroglottography and its relation to glottal activity. *Folia Phoniatrica, 27,* 215–224.

Lecluse, F. L. E., Tiwari, R. M., & Snow, G. B. (1981). Electroglottographic studies of Staffieri neoglottis. *Laryngoscope, 91,* 971–975.

Leeper, H. A., Jr., & Graves, D. K. (1984). Consistency of laryngeal airway resistance in adult women. *Journal of Communication Disorders, 17,* 153–163.

Lesser, T. H. J., & William, G. (1988). Laryngographic investigation of postoperative hoarseness. *Clinical Otolaryngology, 13,* 37–42.

Lesser, T. H. J., Williams, R. G., & Hoddinott, C. (1986). Laryngographic changes following endotracheal intubation in adults. *British Journal of Disorders of Communication, 21,* 239–244.

Lin, E., Jiang, J., Hone, S., & Hanson, D. G. (1999). Photoglottographic measures in Parkinson's disease. *Journal of Voice, 13,* 25–35.

Linders, B., Massa, G. G., Boersma, B., & Dejonckere, P. H. (1995). Fundamental voice frequency and jitter in girls and boys measured with electroglottography: Influence of age and height. *International Journal of Pediatric Otorhinolaryngology, 33,* 61–65.

Lindsey, G., Breen, A. P., & Fourcin, A. J. (1988). Glottal closed time as a function of prosody, style and sex in English. *Proceedings of the Seventh International FASE Symposium* (Vol. 3, pp. 1101–1103). Edinburgh, UK.

Linville, S. E. (1992). Glottal gap configurations in two age groups of women. *Journal of Speech and Hearing Research, 35,* 1209–1215.

Lisker, L., Abramson, A. S., Cooper, F. S., & Schvey, M. H. (1966). Transillumination of the larynx in running speech. *Journal of the Acoustical Society of America, 39,* 1218.

Lisker, L., Abramson, A. S., Cooper, F. S., & Schvey, M. H. (1969). Transillumination of the larynx in running speech. *Journal of the Acoustical Society of America, 45,* 1554–1546.

Löfqvist, A. (1980). Interarticulator programming in stop production. *Journal of Phonetics, 8,* 475–490.

Löfqvist, A. (1991). Inverse filtering as a tool in voice research and therapy. *Scandinavian Journal of Logopedics and Phoniatrics, 16,* 8–16.

Löfqvist, A., & Yoshioka, H. (1980). Laryngeal activity in Icelandic obstruent production. *Haskins Laboratories Status Report on Speech Research, SR 63/64,* 275–292.

Ludwigs, M., Hess, M., Gross, M., & Orglmeister, R. (1997). Bidirectional stroboscopy—double information? Technical considerations. In T. Wittenberg, P. Mergell, M. Tigges, & U. Eysholdt (Eds.), *Advances in quantitative laryngoscopy using motion-, image-, and signal-analysis* (pp. 75–82). Göttingen, Germany: University of Göttingen.

MacCurtain, F., & Fourcin, A. J. (1982). Applications of the electrolaryngograph wave form display. In V. L. Lawrence (Ed.), *Transcripts of the Tenth Symposium on the Care of the Professional Voice* (Part II, pp. 51–57). New York: The Voice Foundation.

Mann, H. (1937). Study of the peripheral circulation by means of an alternating current bridge. *Proceedings of the Society for Experimental Biology and Medicine, 36,* 670–673.

Matausek, M. R., & Batalov, V. S. (1980). A new approach to the determination of the glottal waveform. *IEEE Transactions in Acoustics and Speech Signal Processing, 28,* 616–622.

Maurer, D., Hess, M., & Gross, M. (1996). High-speed imaging of vocal fold vibrations and larynx movements within vocalizations of different vowels. *Annals of Otology, Rhinology, and Laryngology, 105,* 975–981.

McGarr, N. S., & Löfqvist, A. (1982). Obstruent production by hearing-impaired speakers: Interarticulator timing and acoustics. *Journal of the Acoustical Society of America, 72,* 34–42.

McGarr, N. S., & Löfqvist, A. (1988). Laryngeal kinematics in voiceless obstruents produced by hearing-impaired speakers. *Journal of Speech and Hearing Research, 31,* 234–239.

McGlone, R. E., & Shipp, T. (1971). Some physiologic correlates of vocal-fry phonation. *Journal of Speech and Hearing Research, 14,* 769–775.

McHenry, M. A., Kuna, S. T., Minton, J. T., & Vanoye, C. R. (1996). Comparison of direct and indirect calculations of laryngeal airway resistance in connected speech. *Journal of Voice, 10,* 236–244.

Melcon, M. C., Hoit, J. D., & Hixon, T. J. (1989). Age and laryngeal airway resistance during vowel production. *Journal of Speech and Hearing Disorders, 54,* 282–286.

Mende, W., Herzel, H., & Wermke, K. (1990). Bifurcations and chaos in newborn children. *Physics Letters A, 145,* 418–424.

Metz, D. E., & Whitehead, R. L. (1982). Simultaneous collection of multiple physiologic data with high-speed laryngeal film data. In V. L. Lawrence (Ed.), *Transcripts of the Tenth Symposium on the Care of the Professional Voice* (Part II, pp. 73–77). New York: The Voice Foundation.

Metz, D. E., Whitehead, R. L., & Peterson, D. H. (1980). An optical-illumination system for high-speed laryngeal cinematography. *Journal of the Acoustical Society of America, 67,* 719–720.

Miles, K. A. (1989). Ultrasound demonstration of vocal cord movements. *British Journal of Radiology, 62,* 871–872.

Miller, J. E., & Mathews, M. V. (1963). Investigation of the glottal waveshape by automatic inverse filtering. *Journal of the Acoustical Society of America, 67,* 1876.

Miller, R. L. (1959). Nature of the vocal cord wave. *Journal of the Acoustical Society of America, 31,* 667–677.

Minifie, F. D., Kelsey, C. A., & Hixon, T. J. (1968). Measurement of vocal fold motion using an ultrasonic Doppler velocity monitor. *Journal of the Acoustical Society of America, 43,* 1165–1169.

Monsen, R. B. (1981). The use of a reflectionless tube to assess vocal function. *ASHA Reports, 11,* 141–150.

Monsen, R. B., & Engebretson, A. M. (1977). Study of variations in male and female glottal wave. *Journal of the Acoustical Society of America, 62,* 981–993.

Monsen, R. B., Engebretson, A. M., & Vemula, N. R. (1978). Indirect assessment of the contribution of subglottal air pressure and vocal-fold tension to changes of fundamental frequency in English. *Journal of the Acoustical Society of America, 64,* 65–80.

Moore, P., & von Leden, H. (1958). Dynamic variation of the vibratory pattern in the normal larynx. *Folia Phoniatrica, 10,* 205–238.

Moore, G. P., White, F. D., & von Leden, H. (1962). Ultra high speed photography in laryngeal physiology. *Journal of Speech and Hearing Disorders, 27,* 165–171.

Motta, G., Cesari, U., Iengo, G., & Motta, G., Jr. (1990). Clinical application of electroglottography. *Folia Phoniatrica, 42,* 111–117.

Munhall, K. G., & Ostry, D. J. (1983). Ultrasonic measurement of laryngeal kinematics. In I. R. Titze & R. C. Scherer (Eds.), *Vocal fold physiology: Biomechanics, acoustics, and phonatory control* (pp. 145–162). Denver, CO: Denver Center for the Performing Arts.

Murty, G. E., & Carding, P. N. (1991). An outpatient clinic system for glottographic measurement of vocal fold vibration. *British Journal of Disorders of Communication, 26,* 115–123.

Neil, W. F., Wechsler, E., & Robinson, J. M. P. (1977). Electrolaryngography in laryngeal disorders. *Clinical Otolaryngology, 2,* 33–40.

Netsell, R., Lotz, W. K., DuChane, A. S., & Barlow, S. M. (1991). Vocal tract aerodynamics during syllable productions: Normative data and theoretical implications. *Journal of Voice, 5,* 1–9.

Netsell, R., Lotz, W. K., Peters, J. E., & Schulte, L. (1994). Developmental patterns of laryngeal and respiratory function for speech production. *Journal of Voice, 8,* 123–131.

Netsell, R., Lotz, W., & Shaughnessy, A. L. (1984). Laryngeal aerodynamics associated with selected voice disorders. *American Journal of Otolaryngology, 5,* 397–403.

Ng, M. L., Gilbert, H. R., & Lerman, J. W. (1997). Some aerodynamic and acoustic characteristics of acute laryngitis. *Journal of Voice, 11,* 356–363.

Nieto, A., Cobeta, I., & Kitzing, P. (1993). La electroglotografía en la investigación y la clínica laríngea. *Acta Otorrinolaringolocia Española, 44,* 257–263.

Niimi, S., & Fujimura, O. (1976). *Stereo-fiberscope investigation of the larynx.* Presentation at the Conference on the Care of the Professional Voice, New York, NY.

Ohala, J. (1967). Studies of variations in glottal aperture using photoelectric glottography. *Journal of the Acoustical Society of America, 41,* 1613.

Ondráckova, J. (1972). Vocal chord activity: Its dynamics and role in speech production. *Folia Phoniatrica, 24,* 405–419.

Ooi, L. L., Chan, H. S., & Soo, K. C. (1995). Color Doppler imaging for vocal cord palsy. *Head and Neck, 17,* 20–23.

Orlikoff, R. F. (1991). Assessment of the dynamics of vocal fold contact from the electroglottogram: Data from normal male subjects. *Journal of Speech and Hearing Research, 34,* 1066–1072.

Orlikoff, R. F. (1995). Vocal stability and vocal tract configuration: An acoustic and electroglottographic investigation. *Journal of Voice, 9,* 173–181.

Orlikoff, R. F. (1998). Scrambled EGG: The uses and abuses of electroglottography. *Phonoscope, 1,* 37–53.

Orlikoff, R. F., & Baken, R. J. (1993). *Clinical speech and voice measurement: Laboratory exercises.* San Diego, CA: Singular Publishing Group.

Orlikoff, R. F., Baken, R. J., & Kraus, D. H. (1997). Acoustic and physiologic characteristics of inspiratory phonation. *Journal of the Acoustical Society of America, 102,* 1838–1845.

Orlikoff, R. F., & Kahane, J. C. (1996). Structure and function of the larynx. In N. J. Lass (Ed.), *Principles of experimental phonetics* (pp. 112–181). St. Louis, MO: Mosby-Year Book.

Orlikoff, R. F., & Kraus, D. H. (1996). Dysphonia following non-surgical management of advanced laryngeal carcinoma. *American Journal of Speech-Language Pathology, 5*(3), 47–52.

Painter, C. (1988). Electroglottogram waveform types. *Archives of Otolaryngology, 245,* 116–121.

Painter, C. (1990). Electroglottogram waveform types of untrained speakers. *European Archives of Oto-Rhino-Laryngology, 247,* 168–173.

Pedersen, M. F. (1977). Electroglottography compared with synchronized stroboscopy in normal persons. *Folia Phoniatrica, 29,* 191–199.

Perkell, J. S., Hillman, R. E., & Holmberg, E. B. (1994). Group differences in measures of voice production and revised values of maximum airflow declination rate. *Journal of the Acoustical Society of America, 96,* 695–698.

Perkell, J. S., Holmberg, E. B., & Hillman, R. E. (1991). A system for signal processing and data extraction from aerodynamic, acoustic, and electroglottographic signals in the study of voice production. *Journal of the Acoustical Society of America, 89,* 1777–1781.

Plant, R. L., & Hillel, A. D. (1998). Direct measurement of subglottic pressure and laryngeal resistance in normal subjects and in spasmodic dysphonia. *Journal of Voice, 12,* 300–314.

Pouderoux, P., Logemann, J. A., & Kahrilas, P. J. (1996). Pharyngeal swallowing elicited by fluid infusions: Role of volition and vallecular containment. *American Journal of Physiology, 270,* G347–G354.

Price, P. J. (1989). Male and female voice source characteristics: Inverse filtering results. *Speech Communication, 8,* 261–277.

Raghavendra, B. N., Horii, S. C., Reede, D. L., Rumancik, W. M., Persky, M., & Bergeron, T. (1987). Sonographic anatomy of the larynx, with particular reference to the vocal cords. *Journal of Ultrasound in Medicine, 6,* 225–230.

Rambaud-Pistone, E. (1984). Place de l'étude instrumentale dans le bilan vocal. *Bulletin d'Audiophonologie, 17,* 43–58.

Reed, V. W. (1982). The electroglottograph in voice teaching. In V. L. Lawrence (Ed.), *Transcripts of the Tenth Symposium on the Care of the Professional Voice* (pp. 58–65). New York: The Voice Foundation.

Reinsch, M., & Gobsch, H. (1972). Zur quantitativen Auswertung-elektroglottographischer Kurven bei Normalpersonen. *Folia Phoniatrica, 24,* 1–6.

Robb, M. P., & Simmons, J. O. (1990). Gender comparisons of children's vocal fold behavior. *Journal of the Acoustical Society of America, 88,* 1318–1322.

Roch, J. B., Comte, F., Eyraud, A., & Dubreuil, C. (1990). Synchronization of glottography and laryngeal stroboscopy. *Folia Phoniatrica, 42,* 289–295.

Rosenberg, A. E. (1971). Effect of glottal pulse shape on the quality of natural vowels. *Journal of the Acoustical Society of America, 49,* 583–590.

Rosevear, W., & Hamlet, S. (1991). Flexible fiberoptic laryngoscopy used to assess swallowing function. *Ear, Nose and Throat Journal, 70,* 498–500.

Rothenberg, M. (1972). The glottal volume velocity waveform during loose and tight voiced glottal adjustments. In A. Rigault & R. Charbonneau (Eds.), *Proceedings of the Seventh International Congress of Phonetic Sciences* (pp. 380–388). The Hague: Mouton.

Rothenberg, M. (1973). A new inverse-filtering technique for deriving the glottal air flow waveform during voicing. *Journal of the Acoustical Society of America, 53,* 1632–1645.

Rothenberg, M. (1977). Measurement of airflow in speech. *Journal of Speech and Hearing Research, 20,* 155–176.

Rothenberg, M. (1981). Some relations between glottal air flow and vocal fold contact area. *ASHA Reports, 11,* 88–96.

Rothenberg, M. (1983). An interactive model for the voice source. In D. M. Bless & J. H. Abbs (Eds.), *Vocal fold physiology: Contemporary research and clinical issues* (pp. 155–165). San Diego, CA: College-Hill Press.

Rothenberg, M., & Mahshie, J. J. (1988). Monitoring vocal fold abduction through vocal fold contact area. *Journal of Speech and Hearing Research, 31,* 338–351.

Rothenberg, M., & Nezelek, K. (1991). Airflow-based analysis of vocal function. In J. Gauffin & B. Hammarberg (Eds.), *Vocal fold physiology: Acoustic, perceptual, and physiological aspects of voice mechanisms* (pp. 139–148). San Diego, CA: Singular Publishing Group.

Roubeau, C., Chevrie-Muller, C., & Arabia-Guidet, C. (1987). Electroglottographic study of the changes of voice registers. *Folia Phoniatrica, 39,* 280–289.

Rubin, H. J., & LeCover, M. (1960). Technique of high-speed photography of the larynx. *Annals of Otology, Rhinology, and Laryngology, 69,* 1072–1083.

Saito, S., Fukuda, H., Isogai, Y., & Ono, H. (1981). X-ray stroboscopy. In K. N. Stevens and M. Hirano (Eds.), *Vocal fold physiology* (pp. 95–106). Tokyo, Japan: University of Tokyo Press.

Saito, S., Fukuda, H., Kitahara, S., & Kokawa, N. (1978). Stroboscopic observation of vocal fold vibration with fiberoptics. *Folia Phoniatrica, 30,* 241–244.

Sapienza, C. M., & Stathopoulos, E. T. (1994). Comparison of maximum flow declination rate: Children versus adults. *Journal of Voice, 8,* 240–247.

Sapienza, C. M., & Stathopoulos, E. T. (1995). Speech task effects on acoustic and aerodynamic measures of women with vocal nodules. *Journal of Voice, 9,* 413–418.

Sawashima, M. (1970). Glottal adjustments for English obstruents. *Haskins Laboratories Status Report on Speech Research, SR 21/22,* 180–200.

Sawashima, M. (1977). Fiberoptic observation of the larynx and other speech organs. In M. Sawashima & F. S. Cooper (Eds.), *Dynamic aspects of speech production* (pp. 31–46). Tokyo, Japan: University of Tokyo Press.

Sawashima, M., Abramson, A. S., Cooper, F. S., & Lisker, L. (1970). Observing laryngeal adjustments during running speech by use of a fiberoptics system. *Phonetica, 22,* 193–201.

Sawashima, M., & Hirose, H. (1968). A new laryngoscopic technique by use of fiberoptics. *Journal of the Acoustical Society of America, 43,* 168–169.

Sawashima, M., Hirose, H., & Fujimura, O. (1967). Observation of the larynx by a fiberscope inserted through the nose. *Journal of the Acoustical Society of America, 42,* 1208.

Sawashima, M., Hirose, H., Honda, K., Yoshioka, H., Hibi, S. R., Kawase, N., & Yamada, M. (1983). Stereoscopic measurement of the laryngeal structure. In D. M. Bless & J. H. Abbs (Eds.), *Vocal fold physiology: Contemporary research and clinical issues* (pp. 265–276). San Diego, CA: College-Hill Press.

Sawashima, M., Hirose, H., & Niimi, S. (1974). Glottal conditions in articulation of Japanese voiceless consonants. In E. Loebell (Ed.), *Proceedings of the Sixteenth International Congress of Logopedics and Phoniatrics* (pp. 409–414). Basel, Switzerland: S. Karger.

Sawashima, M., & Ushijima, T. (1972). The use of fiberscope in speech research. In J. Hirschberg, Gy. Szèpe, & E. Vass-Kovács (Eds.), *Papers in interdisciplinary speech research* (pp. 229–231). Budapest, Hungary: Akadèmiai Kiadö.

Scherer, R. C., Druker, D. G., & Titze, I. R. (1988). Electroglottography and direct measurement of vocal fold contact area. In

O. Fujimura (Ed.), *Vocal physiology: Voice production, mechanisms, and functions* (pp. 279–291). New York: Raven Press.

Scherer, R. C., Gould, W. J., Titze, I. R., Meyers, A. D., & Sataloff, R. T. (1988). Preliminary evaluation of selected acoustic and glottographic measures for clinical phonatory function analysis. *Journal of Voice, 2*, 230–244.

Scherer, R. C., & Guo, C.-G. (1991). Generalized translaryngeal pressure coefficient for a wide range of laryngeal configurations. In J. Gauffin & B. Hammarberg (Eds.), *Vocal fold physiology: Acoustic, perceptual, and physiological aspects of voice mechanisms.*(pp. 83–90). San Diego, CA: Singular Publishing Group.

Scherer, R. C., & Titze, I. R. (1987). The abduction quotient related to vocal quality. *Journal of Voice, 1*, 246–251.

Scherer, R. C., Vail, V. J., & Rockwell, B. (1995). Examination of the laryngeal adduction measure EGGW. In F. Bell-Berti & L. J. Raphael (Eds.), *Producing speech: Contemporary issues for Katherine Stafford Harris* (pp. 269–289). New York: AIP Press.

Schindler, O., Gonella, M. L., & Pisani, R. (1990). Doppler ultrasound examination of the vibration speed of vocal folds. *Folia Phoniatrica, 42*, 265–272.

Schneider, P., & Baken, R. J. (1984). Influence of lung volume on the airflow-intensity relationship. *Journal of Speech and Hearing Research, 27*, 430–435.

Schönhärl, E. (1960). *Die Stroboskopie in der praktischen Laryngologie.* Stuttgart, Germany: Thieme Verlag.

Schutte, H. K. (1986). Aerodynamics of phonation. *Acta Oto-Rhino-Laryngologica Belgica, 40*, 344–357.

Schutte, H. K., & Seidner, W. W. (1988). Registerabhängige Differenzierung von Elektroglottogrammen. *Sprache Stimme Gehör, 12*, 59–62.

Schutte, H. K.,Śvec, J. G., &Śram, F. (1997). Videokymography: Research and clinical issues. *Logopedics Phoniatrics Vocology, 22*, 152–156.

Schutte, H. K., & van den Berg, Jw. (1976). Determination of the subglottic pressure and the efficiency of sound production in patients with disturbed voice production. In E. Loebell (Ed.), *Proceedings of the Sixteenth International Congress of Logopedics and Phoniatrics* (pp. 415–420). Basel, Switzerland: S. Karger.

Sercarz, J. A., Berke, G. S., Gerratt, B. R., Kreiman, J., Ming, Y., & Natividad, M. (1992). Synchronizing videostroboscopic images of human laryngeal vibration with physiological signals. *American Journal of Otolaryngology, 13*, 40–44.

Shipp, T. (1975). Vertical laryngeal position during continuous and discrete vocal frequency change. *Journal of Speech and Hearing Research, 18*, 707–718.

Slavit, D. H., & Maragos, N. E. (1994). Arytenoid adduction and type I thyroplasty in the treatment of aphonia. *Journal of Voice, 8*, 84–91.

Smith, A. M., & Childers, D. G. (1983). Laryngeal evaluation using features from speech and the electroglottograph. *IEEE Transactions on Biomedical Engineering, 30*, 755–759.

Smith, S. (1954). Remarks on the physiology of the vibrations of the vocal cords. *Folia Phoniatrica, 6*, 166–178.

Smith, S. (1977). Electroglottography. *Proceedings of the Seventeenth Congress of the International Association for Logopedics and Phoniatrics.* Copenhagen, Denmark.

Smith, S. (1981). Research on the principle of electroglottography. *Folia Phoniatrica, 33*, 1–10.

Smitheran, J. R., & Hixon, T. J. (1981). A clinical method for estimating laryngeal airway resistance during vowel production. *Journal of Speech and Hearing Disorders, 46*, 138–146.

Södersten, M., Hammarberg, B., & Håkansson, A. (1996). Comparison between automatic and manual inverse filtering procedures for healthy female voices. *Phoniatric and Logopedic Progress Report* (Karolinska Institute, Huddinge University Hospital), *10*, 19–36.

Södersten, M., Hertegård, S., & Hammarberg, B. (1995). Glottal closure, transglottal airflow, and voice quality in healthy middle-aged women. *Journal of Voice, 9*, 182–197.

Södersten, M., & Lindestad, P.-Å. (1990). Glottal closure and perceived breathiness during phonation in normally speaking subjects. *Journal of Speech and Hearing Research, 33*, 601–611.

Sondhi, M. M. (1975). Measurement of the glottal waveform. *Journal of the Acoustical Society of America, 57*, 228–232.

Sonesson, B. (1959). A method for studying the vibratory movements of the vocal folds. *Journal of Laryngology and Otology, 73*, 732–737.

Sonesson, B. (1960). On the anatomy and vibratory pattern of the human vocal folds. *Acta Otolaryngologica, Suppl. 156*, 1–80.

Sopko, J. (1986). Zur Objecktivierung der Stimmlippenschwingungen mittels synchroner elektroglottographischer und stroboskopischer Untersuchung. *Sprache-Stimme-Gehör, 10*, 83–87.

Soron, H. (1967). High-speed photography in speech research. *Journal of Speech and Hearing Research, 10*, 768–776.

Śram, F., Schutte, H. K., &Śvec, J. G. (1997). Clinical applications of videokymography. In G. McCafferty, W. Coman, & R. Carroll (Eds.), *XVI World Congress of Otorhinolaryngology Head and Neck Surgery* (pp. 1681–1684). Bologna, Italy: Monduzzi.

Stathopoulos, E. T., Hoit, J. D., Hixon, T. J., Watson, P. J., & Solomon, N. P. (1991). Respiratory and laryngeal function during whispering. *Journal of Speech and Hearing Research, 34*, 761–767.

Stathopoulos, E. T., & Sapienza, C. (1993a). Respiratory and laryngeal measures of children during vocal intensity variation. *Journal of the Acoustical Society of America, 94*, 2531–2543.

Stathopoulos, E. T., & Sapienza, C. (1993b). Respiratory and laryngeal function of women and men during vocal intensity variation. *Journal of Speech and Hearing Research, 36*, 64–75.

Sulter, A. M., & Wit, H. P. I. (1996). Glottal volume velocity waveform characteristics in subjects with and without vocal training, related to gender, sound intensity, fundamental frequency, and age. *Journal of the Acoustical Society of America, 100*, 3360–3373.

Sundberg, J. (1987). *The science of the singing voice.* DeKalb, IL: Northern Illinois University Press.

Sundberg, J., & Gauffin, J. (1979). Waveform and spectrum of the glottal voice source. In B. Lindblom & S. Öhman (Eds.), *Frontiers of speech communication research* (pp. 301–320). New York: Academic Press.

Śvec, J. G., & Schutte, H. K. (1996). Videokymography: High speed line scanning of vocal fold vibration. *Journal of Voice, 10*, 201–205.

Śvec, J. G., Schutte, H. K., &Śram, F. (1997). Videokymography: High-speed line scanning of vocal fold vibration. In G. McCafferty, W. Coman, & R. Carroll (Eds.), *XVI World Congress of Otorhinolaryngology Head and Neck Surgery* (pp. 1685–1688). Bologna, Italy: Monduzzi.

Tanabe, M., Isshiki, N., & Kitajima, K. (1978). Application of reflectionless acoustic tube for extraction of the glottal waveform. *Studia Phonologica, 12*, 31–38.

Tanaka, S., & Gould, W. J. (1985). Vocal efficiency and aerodynamic aspects in voice disorders. *Annals of Otology, Rhinology and Laryngology, 94*, 29–33.

Taub, S. (1966a). The Taub oral panendoscope: A new technique. *Cleft Palate Journal, 3*, 328–346.

Taub, S. (1966b). Oral panendoscope for direct observation and audiovisual recording of velopharyngeal areas during phonation. *Transactions of the American Academy of Ophthalmology and Otolaryngology, 70*, 855–857.

Timcke, R., von Leden, H., & Moore, P. (1958). Laryngeal vibrations: Measurements of the glottic wave. Part I: The normal vibratory cycle. *Archives of Otolaryngology, 68*, 1–19.

Timcke, R., von Leden, H., & Moore, P. (1959). Laryngeal vibrations: Measurements of the glottic wave. Part II: Physiologic variations. *Archives of Otolaryngology, 69*, 438–444.

Titze, I. R. (1973). The human vocal cords: A mathematic model: I. *Phonetica, 28*, 129–170.

Titze, I. R. (1974). The human vocal cords: A mathematic model: II. *Phonetica, 29*, 1–21.

Titze, I. R. (1976). On the mechanics of vocal-fold vibration. *Journal of the Acoustical Society of America, 60*, 1366–1380.

Titze, I. R. (1984). Parameterization of the glottal area, glottal flow, and vocal fold contact area. *Journal of the Acoustical Society of America, 75*, 570–580.

Titze, I. R. (1985). Mechanisms of sustained oscillation of the vocal folds. In I. R. Titze & R. C. Scherer (Eds.), *Vocal fold physiology: Biomechanics, acoustics, and phonatory control* (pp. 349–357). Denver, CO: Denver Center for the Performing Arts.

Titze, I. R. (1988). Regulation of vocal power and efficiency by subglottal pressure and glottal width. In O. Fujimura (Ed.), *Vocal physiology: Voice production, mechanisms and functions* (pp. 279–291). New York: Raven Press.

Titze, I. R. (1989). A four parameter model of the glottis and vocal fold contact area. *Speech Communication, 8*, 191–201.

Titze, I. R. (1990). Interpretation of the electroglottographic signal. *Journal of Voice, 4*, 1–9.

Titze, I. R. (1994). *Principles of voice production*. Englewood Cliffs, NJ: Prentice-Hall.

Titze, I. R., Baken, R. J., & Herzel, H. (1993). Evidence of chaos in vocal fold vibration. In I. R. Titze (Ed.), *Vocal fold physiology: New frontiers in basic science* (pp. 143–188). San Diego, CA: Singular Publishing Group.

Titze, I. R., & Talkin, D. (1979). A theoretical study of the effect of various laryngeal configurations on the acoustics of phonation. *Journal of the Acoustical Society of America, 66*, 60–86.

Titze, I. R., & Talkin, D. (1981). Simulation and interpretation of glottographic waveforms. *ASHA Reports, 11*, 48–55.

Ueda, D., Yano, K., & Okuno, A. (1993). Ultrasonic imaging of the tongue, mouth, and vocal cords in normal children: Establishment of basic scanning positions. *Journal of Clinical Ultrasound, 21*, 431–439.

Unger, E., Unger, H., & Tietze, G. (1981). Stimmuntersuchungen mittels der elektroglottographischen Einzelkurven. *Folia Phoniatrica, 33*, 168–180.

Vallancien, B. (1972). Nouvelles recherches sur le mécanism vibratoire du larynx. *Acta Oto-Rhino-Laryngologica, 26*, 725–740.

Vallancien, B., & Faulhaber, J. (1966). Causes d'erreurs en glottographie. *Journal Français d'Oto-Rhino-Laryngologie, 15*, 383–394.

Vallancien, B., & Faulhaber, J. (1967). What to think of glottography. *Folia Phoniatrica, 19*, 39–44.

Vallancien, B., Gautheron, B., Pasternak, L., Guisez, D., & Paley, B. (1971). Comparaison des signaux microphoniques, diaphanographiques et glottographiques avec application au laryngographe. *Folia Phoniatrica, 23*, 371–380.

van den Berg, Jw. (1956). Direct and indirect determination of the mean subglottic pressure. *Folia Phoniatrica, 8*, 1–24.

van den Berg, Jw. (1959). A Δf-generator and movie adapter unit for laryngo-stroboscopy. *Practica Oto-Rhino-Laryngologica, 21*, 355–363.

van den Berg, Jw., Zantema, J., & Doornenbal, P. (1957). On the air resistance and Bernoulli effect of the human larynx. *Journal of the Acoustical Society of America, 29*, 626–631.

van Michel, C. (1964). Etude, par la méthode électroglottographique, des comportements glottiques de type phonatoire en dehors de toute émission sonore. *Revue de Laryngologie, 7–8*, 469–475.

van Michel, C. (1966). Mouvements glottiques phonatoires sans Etude, par émission sonore: Etude électroglottographique. *Folia Phoniatrica, 18*, 1–18.

van Michel, C. (1967). Morphologie de la courbe glottographique dans certains troubles fonctionels du larynx. *Folia Phoniatrica, 19*, 192–202.

van Michel, C., Pfister, K. A., & Luchsinger, R. (1970). Electroglottographie et cinématographie laryngée ultra-rapide: Comparaison des résultats. *Folia Phoniatrica, 22*, 81–91.

van Michel, C., & Raskin, L. (1969). L'électroglottomètre Mark 4, son principe, ses possibilités. *Folia Phoniatrica, 21*, 145–157.

Veeneman, D. E., & DeMent, S. (1985). Automatic glottal inverse filtering from speech and electroglottographic signals. *IEEE Transactions in Acoustics and Speech Signal Processing, 33*, 369–377.

Vilkman, E., Alku, P., & Laukkanen, A.-M. (1995). Vocal-fold collision mass as a differentiator between registers in the low-pitch range. *Journal of Voice, 9*, 66–73.

Vilkman, E., Lauri, E.-R., Alku, P., Sala, E., & Sihvo, M. (1997). Loading changes in time-based parameters of glottal flow waveforms in different ergonomic conditions. *Folia Phoniatrica et Logopaedica, 49*, 247–263.

von Leden, H. (1961). The electronic synchron-stroboscope. *Annals of Otology, Rhinology, and Laryngology, 70*, 881–893.

von Leden, H., LeCover, M., Ringel, R. L., & Isshiki, N. (1966). Improvements in laryngeal cinematography. *Archives of Otolaryngology, 83*, 482–487.

von Leden, H., & Moore, P. (1961). Vibratory patterns of the vocal cords in unilateral laryngeal paralysis. *Acta Oto-Laryngologica, 53*, 493–506.

von Leden, H., Moore, P., & Timcke, R. (1960). Laryngeal vibrations: Measurements of the glottic wave. Part III: The pathologic larynx. *Archives of Otolaryngology, 71*, 16–35.

Wechsler, E. (1977). A laryngographic study of voice disorders. *British Journal of Disorders of Communication, 12*, 9–22.

Welch, G. F., Sergeant, D. C., & MacCurtain, F. (1989). Xeroradiographic-Electrolaryngographic analysis of male vocal registers. *Journal of Voice, 3*, 244–256.

Wendahl, R. W., & Coleman, R. F. (1967). Vocal cord spectra derived from glottal-area waveforms and subglottal photocell monitoring. *Journal of the Acoustical Society of America, 41*, 1613.

Whitehead, R. L., Metz, D. E., & Whitehead, B. H. (1984). Vibratory patterns of the vocal folds during pulse register phonation. *Journal of the Acoustical Society of America, 75*, 1233–1237.

Wilson, F. B., & Starr, C. D. (1985). Use of the phonation analyzer as a clinical tool. *Journal of Speech and Hearing Disorders, 50*, 351–356.

Wilson, J. V., & Leeper, H. A. (1992). Changes in laryngeal airway resistance in young adult men and women as a function of vocal sound pressure level and syllable context. *Journal of Voice, 6*, 235–245.

Winckel, F. (1965). Phoniatric acoustics. In R. L. Luchsinger & G. E. Arnold (Eds.), *Voice-speech-language* (pp. 24–55). Belmont CA: Wadsworth.

Wong, D. Y., Markel, J. D., & Gray, A. H., Jr. (1979). Least squares glottal inverse filtering from the acoustic speech waveform. *IEEE Transactions in Acoustics and Speech Signal Processing, 27*, 350–355.

Woo, P., Casper, J., Colton, R., & Brewer, D. (1994). Aerodynamic and stroboscopic findings before and after microlaryngeal phonosurgery. *Journal of Voice, 8*, 186–194.

Woo, P., Colton, R. H., & Shangold, L. (1987). Phonatory airflow analysis in patients with laryngeal disease. *Annals of Otology, Rhinology and Laryngology, 96*, 549–555.

Woodson, G. E., Rosen, C. A., Murry, T., Madasu, R., Wong, F., Hengesteg, A., & Robbins, K. T. (1996). Assessing vocal function after chemoradiation for advanced laryngeal carcinoma. *Archives of Otolaryngology—Head and Neck Surgery, 122*, 858–864.

Yanagihara, N. (1967). Hoarseness: Investigation of the physiological mechanisms. *Annals of Otology, Rhinology and Laryngology, 76*, 472–489.

Yanagihara, N. (1970). Aerodynamic examination of the laryngeal function. *Studia Phonologica, 5*, 45–51.

Yanagisawa, E., Strothers, G., Owens, T., & Honda, K. (1983). Videolaryngoscopy: A comparison of fiberscopic and telescopic documentation. *Annals of Otology, Rhinology, and Laryngology, 92*, 430–436.

Yoshioka, H., Löfqvist, A., & Hirose, H. (1980). Laryngeal adjustments in Japanese voiceless sound production. *Haskins Laboratories Status Report on Speech Research, SR 63/64*, 293–308.

Zagzebski, J. A., & Bless, D. M. (1983). Correspondence of ultrasonic and stroboscopic visualization of vocal folds. In I. R. Titze & R. C. Scherer (Eds.), *Vocal fold physiology: Biomechanics, acoustics, and phonatory control* (pp. 163–168). Denver, CO: Denver Center for the Performing Arts.

Zagzebski, J. A., Bless, D. M., & Ewanowski, S. J. (1983). Pulse echo imaging of the larynx using rapid ultrasonic scanners. In D. M. Bless & J. H. Abbs (Eds.), *Vocal fold physiology: Contemporary research and clinical issues* (pp. 210–222). San Diego, CA: College-Hill Press.

11

Velopharyngeal Function

Nasality and nasal emission of air are symptoms of many different kinds of speech disorders. Not only are they the central concern in cases of cleft palate and similar maxillofacial defects (Spriestersbach, 1965; Shprintzen et al., 1978; Shprintzen, Goldberg, Young, & Wolford, 1981; Peterson-Falzone, 1988; Haapanen & Somer, 1993), but they may be concomitants of dysarthria (Darley, Aronson, & Brown, 1969; Netsell, 1969; Cohn et al., 1982; Enderby, 1986; Kleppe, Katayama, Shipley, & Foushee, 1990; Theodoros, Murdoch, Stokes, & Chenery, 1993; Theodoros, Murdoch, & Thompson, 1995; Thompson & Murdoch, 1995; Åkefeldt, Åkefeldt, & Gillberg, 1997) and dyspraxia (Itoh, Sasanuma, & Ushijima, 1979; Ziegler & von Cramon, 1986) as well. Nasality also figures prominently in the speech of the hearing impaired (Colton & Cooker, 1968; Leder & Spitzer, 1990) and of those with various congenital syndromes (Sedláčková, 1967; Montague & Hollien, 1973; Sparks, 1984; Moran, 1986; Bradley, 1989). Nasality and nasal emission clearly are problems that clinicians encounter often. Because of the complexity of these symptoms and the many different approaches to their evaluation, they are considered separately here.

Nasalization may be defined as the existence of significant communication between the nasal cavity and the rest of the vocal tract. When inappropriate in degree or timing, such communication can result in two related, but clinically different, problems. **Nasal emission** refers to the abnormal escape of air via the nasal route. The abnormal "shunt" may reduce intraoral pressure, causing distortion of consonants. When the nasal air escape results in an audible "snort," the nasal emission becomes even more obtrusive and the speech is more seriously impaired. **Nasality** (more properly **hypernasality**) refers to the unacceptable vowel quality that results from inappropriate acoustic coupling of the nasal airway to the vocal tract. In contrast to nasal emission, nasality does not necessarily involve large nasal airflows, nor does it significantly change intraoral pressure. Obviously, nasality and nasal emission are often associated, and they may represent two facets of the same problem. It is possible for a patient to show one symptom and not the other. Both disorders of velopharyngeal function will be considered in this chapter.

Nasal emission is a fairly straightforward concept, not subject to much debate. On the other hand, while reliably perceived, nasality is an ill-defined phenomenon. Its basis lies in nasalization, and it is useful to consider nasality as nasalization that is inappropriate in degree or in timing. Such an operational definition places the full burden on the velopharyngeal port and would seem to point the way to fairly easy assessment methods. This, alas, is not the case.

Nasality is a *perceptual attribute* whose detection requires the judgment of a listener (Bell, 1890; Bradford, Brooks, & Shelton, 1964; Moll, 1964; Counihan & Culligan, 1970; Shelton & Trier, 1976; McWilliams et al., 1981; Bzoch, 1989; Haapanen, 1991a). The degree of nasality reflects the complex interaction of a number of factors. There is general agreement that, as expected, the most important of these is the size of the velopharyngeal opening. But the degree of nasality is not by any means a direct function of this alone (Subtelny, Koepp-Baker, & Subtelny, 1961). For example, Massengill and Bryson (1967) found that, in normal speakers, the amount of velopharyngeal opening was significantly correlated to the perceived nasality of /i/, /u/, and /æ/, but not of /ɑ/. Spriestersbach and Powers (1959a) have provided complementary findings in cleft palate children to the effect that isolated productions of high vowels are perceived as more nasal than similar productions of low vowels. The explanation for this seems to lie in the fact that, in normal speakers, the tongue posture of the high vowels facilitates velopharyngeal closure, while the low-vowel tongue positions reduce closure effectiveness (Harrington, 1944, 1946; Hess, 1959; Lintz & Sherman, 1961; Moll, 1962; Hardy & Arkebauer, 1966; Moll & Shriner, 1967; Bzoch, 1968; Lubker, 1968; Fritzell, 1969; Bell-Berti, 1976; Sawashima, 1977; Bell-Berti, Baer, Harris, & Niimi, 1979; Abramson, Nye, Henderson, & Marshall, 1981; Whalen, 1990; Kuehn & Moon, 1998). Schwartz (1968a) has presented sound pressure level data that support this contention. Listeners have learned to be expectant of, and tolerant toward, greater nasalization of low vowels, but are "surprised" by it in high vowels and are more attentive to it. Thus, if an isolated vowel is used to judge nasality, the choice of vowel may substantially influence the severity rating.

Defectiveness of a speaker's articulation also affects listeners' perceptions of nasality (Sherman, 1954; McWilliams, 1954; Spriestersbach, 1955; van Hattum, 1958; Spriestersbach & Powers, 1959b). So does his vocal pitch and intensity (Sherman & Goodwin, 1954; Hess, 1959; Lintz & Sherman, 1961; Fletcher & Bishop, 1970) and, possibly, his speech rate as well (Bzoch, 1968; Colton & Cooker, 1968; Brancewicz & Reich, 1989). In short, while nasality is fundamentally a matter of velopharyngeal function, the judgment of the severity of velopharyngeal malfunction is known to be confounded by many other aspects of speech that nonetheless remain poorly documented or understood.

Lest all of this leave the impression that nasality results from incomplete velopharyngeal closure alone, let it be added immediately that timing is also a critical variable (Netsell, 1969; Zimmerman, Karnell, & Rettaliata, 1984; Karnell, Folkins, & Morris, 1985). A perfectly competent velopharyngeal mechanism is of little value if it is closed at the wrong times during an utterance; perceived nasality can result from nasal coupling that is too early or too late. Since velar movement shows very extensive coarticulation (Ali, Gallagher, Goldstein, & Daniloff, 1971; Moll & Daniloff, 1971; McClean, 1973; Benguerel, Hirose, Sawashima, & Ushijima, 1977a, 1977b; Sawashima, 1977; Bell-Berti et al., 1979; Thompson & Hixon, 1979; Larson & Hamlet, 1987; Flege, 1988; Bell-Berti & Krakow, 1991; Bell-Berti, 1993; Kollia, Gracco, & Harris, 1995; Stone & Vatikiotis-Bateson, 1995; Engelke, Bruns, Striebeck, & Hoch, 1996; Zajac & Mayo, 1996; Zajac, Mayo, & Kataoka, 1998), the opening and closure timing patterns in running speech can be quite complex. It would be surprising if this complicated coordination were not disrupted in the dysarthric or dyspraxic speaker (Itoh et al., 1979; Itoh, Sasanuman, Hirose, Yoshiyoka, & Sawashima, 1983; Ziegler & von Cramon, 1986; Hoodin & Gilbert, 1989; Katz, Machetanz, Orth, & Schönle, 1990). Unfortunately, a clinician would require superhuman ability for her to reliably discriminate the nasality of mistiming from the nasality of velopharyngeal incompetence simply by listening to a patient's running speech. Furthermore, even among patients deemed "incompetent," there remains a great deal of variability of velopharyngeal function that may not be discernible perceptually. With regard to patients with marginal velopharyngeal abilities, Morris (1984), for instance, discriminates between those who "sometimes-but-not-always" (SBNA) and "almost-but-not-quite" (ABNQ) obtain adequate and appropriate closure during speech.

It is likely that "the perception of nasality, while dependent upon listener judgment, is a complex phenomenon, and that attempts to explain nasal speech through perceptual measures alone may be limited" (Counihan, 1972). Since the goal of speech therapy is to *modify* perceived nasality, the first task of the speech pathologist is to isolate its basic causes. To achieve this, the contributing factors need to be sorted out. Because they are more or less inextricably confounded in the perceptual judgment, objective tests will be needed. They are particularly important when data are required for informing decisions about surgical or prosthetic management. Instrumental measures of nasality can also be used to track the progress of therapy (Moser, 1942) and to provide feedback (Garber, Burzynski, Vale, & Nelson, 1979; Netsell & Daniel, 1979), especially to patients who, like the hearing-impaired, cannot make good use of auditory cues (Stevens, Nickerson, Boothroyd, & Rollins, 1976).

The field of speech pathology has been greatly concerned with the problem of nasality for a long time, and a great many observational methods have been devised. Some of these, for example, the Rheadeik of Vealey, Bailey, and Belknap (1965), the airflow paddle described by Bzoch (1989), or modified rotameters such as the Scapescope (Shprintzen, McCall, Skolnick, & Lencione, 1975) or See-Scape devices (Glaser & Shprintzen, 1979; Dworkin, 1991), are perhaps useful for patient motivation, but they do not greatly enhance the diagnostician's insight into the precise nature of the patient's speech impairment. These methods will not be discussed here. Rather, this chapter will focus on techniques that facilitate evaluation of the mechanisms of nasality or allow quantification of its severity. The prime emphasis will be on the measurement of the effectiveness and timing of velopharyngeal closure during speech production.

BACKGROUND CONSIDERATIONS

Decisions concerning the testing procedures to be used must be made carefully and with full consideration of the peculiar circumstances of any given case. The velopharyngeal port is a very complex system whose specific functional modalities are not well understood. It is known that activity patterns differ from task to task and from subject to subject. In the face of this variability are the common observations that most clinical measures of "velopharyngeal ability" show a great deal of inconsistency from trial to trial and that measures obtained by different instrumental means often do not agree. The "recurring problem in the evaluation of velopharyngeal function for speech," in the view of McWilliams, Morris, and Shelton (1990), is that "we have no single measure of velopharyngeal competence that can be used with confidence as a valid criterion for answering all clinical questions" (p. 190). Accordingly they would advise the clinician, for example, that "velopharyngeal function studied radiographically is a different thing than velopharyngeal function studied aerodynamically" (p. 193). Without a "gold standard," a multidimensional approach that employs several techniques may be requisite to evaluate velopharyngeal performance adequately (Schwartz, 1975; McWillams & Witzel, 1994).

In particular, the following points should be kept in mind when planning the evaluation procedure:

1. The principle of *motor equivalence* is fully applicable to velar and pharyngeal function. At our present level of understanding, ordinary testing procedures cannot clearly indicate the specific contributions of the several muscles of the system (Bell-Berti, 1976, 1980, 1993; Seaver & Kuehn, 1980).

2. The relationship between the size of the velopharyngeal port and perceived nasality is not, by any stretch of the imagination, a direct or linear one. Furthermore, openings of less than approximately 20 mm² generally do not seem to cause perceptible nasality (Warren, 1964a, 1967, 1979; McWilliams et al., 1981) or articulatory defectiveness (Shelton, Brooks, & Youngstrom, 1964; Isshiki, Honjow, & Morimoto, 1968; Shelton & Blank, 1984). Also, the effects of larger port openings can be masked by variations of oral port size, nasal airway resistance, and respiratory effort (Warren & Ryon, 1967).

3. Circumspection is required in generalizing from data gathered on normal speakers to those with maxillofacial defects. Closure mechanisms may be very different in the two groups (Buck, 1954; Hagerty, Hill, Pettit, & Kane, 1958a; Moll, 1965a). Nor can the nature of the maxillofacial deformity be considered a predictor of the closure pattern that will be used (Shelton, Brooks, & Youngstrom, 1964).

4. Nonspeech tasks are generally poor indicators of velopharyngeal behavior during speech. Impounding of intraoral air and sucking can be accomplished by linguapalatal valving. Cleft palate patients who cannot achieve velopharyngeal closure during speech routinely do so when swallowing (Moll, 1965a). Blowing, whistling, and sucking tasks (Chase, 1960; Fox & Johns, 1970; Wells, 1971) are particularly suspect. Several studies (Moll, 1965a; McWilliams & Bradley, 1965; Calnan & Renfrew, 1961; Kuehn & Moon, 1994) have indicated that velar elevation—and hence velopharyngeal closure—is significantly greater during blowing tasks than during speech, perhaps because the high intraoral pressure assists in forcing the velum more tightly against the pharyngeal wall.

5. Measurement of static productions (for example, of a sustained vowel) may yield results that differ from those obtained during speaking tasks (Powers, 1962) since crucial timing elements are not being tested.

Research Versus Clinical Measurement Tools

Not all of the techniques available for assessment of velopharyngeal function are suitable for routine clinical use. Electromyography, for example, has been of great value to the researcher (Li & Lundervold, 1958; Broadbent & Swinyard, 1959; Basmajian & Dutta, 1961; Harris, Schvey, & Lysaught, 1962; Fritzell, 1963, 1969, 1979; Cooper, 1965; Hering, Hoppe, & Kraft, 1965; Lubker, 1968; Shelton, Harris, Sholes, & Dooley, 1970; Bell-Berti, 1976; Fritzell & Kotby, 1976; Ushijima,

Sawashima, Hirose, Abe, & Harada, 1976; Kuehn, Folkins, & Cutting, 1982; Kuehn, Folkins, & Linville, 1988). But it is highly invasive, generally painful, and often disruptive of normal speech behaviors (see Chapter 12, "Speech Movements").

Likewise, a number of special X-ray techniques have been devised for visualizing palatal activity (Carrell, 1952; Hagerty, Hill, Pettit, & Kane, 1958b; Moll, 1960, 1965a, 1965b; Blackfield, Miller, Owsely, & Lawson, 1962; Powers, 1962; Massengill, 1966, 1972; Massengill, Quinn, Barry, & Pickrell, 1966; Bzoch, 1970; McKerns & Bzoch, 1970; Skolnick, 1970; Skolnick & McCall, 1972; Massengill & Brooks, 1973; Zwitman, Gyepes, & Sample, 1973; Kuehn & Dolan, 1975; Croatto, Cinotti, Moschi, & Toti-Zattoni, 1980; Iglesias, Kuehn, & Morris, 1980; Williams & Eisenbach, 1981; Stringer & Witzel, 1985, 1986, 1989; MacKenzie-Stepner, Witzel, Stringer, & Laskin, 1987; Moon & Smith, 1987). A substantial amount of research has also combined such X-ray observation with electromyography (Fritzell, 1963; Lubker, 1968; Subtelny et al., 1968), with sound spectrography (Björk & Nylén, 1961), with transvelar photodetection (Zimmerman et al., 1987), and with airflow measurement (Lubker & Moll, 1965). Indeed, assessment via cinefluoroscopy, videofluoroscopy, and computed tomography have proven quite valuable to researchers' ability to describe articulatory processes and to define patterns of normal and abnormal velopharyngeal function (Subtelny, Li, Whitehead, & Subtelny, 1989). But, while they have been employed in differential diagnosis of velopharyngeal insufficiency and in subsequent management decisions (Williams, 1989), there remains—in addition to the significant health risk associated with prolonged exposure to ionizing radiation—a lack of standardization of technique, of procedure, and of interpretation that limits clinical utility.

The latest development in radiographic examination of speech function has been the **X-ray microbeam** (Fujimura, Kiritani, & Ishida, 1973; Kiritani, Itoh, & Fujimura, 1975; Stone, 1990; Westbury, 1991; Ostry & Munhall, 1994; de Jong, 1997). It uses a very thin X-ray beam to track the movement of small radio-opaque pellets that are affixed in the midsagittal plane to one or to several articulators, which may include the velum (Vaissière, 1988; Fujimura, 1990). These pellets, that range from 2- to 3-mm in diameter, are made of a dense metal (such as gold) and are attached to several "fleshpoints" along the articulator(s) of interest using a dental adhesive. The greater the number of pellets used, the better the microbeam system may render the (midsagittal) shape and contour of the articulator. The system employs a rather low radiation level, maintained by using an extremely thin X-ray beam to scan the attached pellets. A sophisticated computer system is used to track the microbeam as the pellets are displaced during speech. Two-dimensional plots of pellet position over time are computer generated. The rapid tracking capability of the microbeam system allows for very accurate determination of fleshpoint position. Unfortunately, as promising as the X-ray microbeam may be for the assessment of speech movement, extensive studies of velar function have been precluded largely due to the difficulty of attaching pellets (or any other type of radio-opaque marker) to the velum (Kent, Carney, & Severeid, 1974; Kuehn, 1976) and the tendency of pellet placement to trigger a strong gag reflex (Stone, 1996). Furthermore, the tremendous expense of the microbeam system has not only limited its widespread application but has even prevented the few research sites that developed the technology from continuing to maintain their facilities.

Most practicing clinicians will require less invasive, time-consuming, and/or expensive means of clinical assessment. Horii (1980) has pointed out that an ideal technique for the evaluation of the physical correlates of nasality would meet the following criteria:

1. Psychological and physical noninvasiveness;

2. Capability of assessing velopharyngeal function during speech;

3. Nondisruptive of articulatory, phonatory, or ventilatory processes;

4. Noninterference with sensory feedback of speech activity;

5. Excellent correlation with perceived nasality;

6. Low cost, ease of operation, and portability; and

7. Ease of interpretation.

From the early flame, cold-mirror tests, and stretched-diaphragm systems (Moser, 1942) to the present sophisticated technology, no method meets all of these requirements. Compromise is always necessary: The criteria must be prioritized for each case and setting. The rest of this chapter will explore those techniques that are most likely to meet the priorities of speech clinicians.

DIRECT ASSESSMENT OF VELOPHARYNGEAL FUNCTION

Intuitively, it would seem that the easiest means of evaluating velopharyngeal function might be to watch the velum and the neighboring posterior and lateral pharyngeal walls during speech or to take motion pictures of them for fine analysis. Unfortunately, such simple methods are quite problematic. One study by Eisenbach and Williams (1984), for example, found that adequacy judgments made from simple visual observations showed relatively poor agreement with judgments based on cinefluorographic examination.

Aided Visualization of the Velopharynx

ENDOSCOPY

Part of the difficulty surrounding the observation of velopharyngeal activity is due to the fact that the working velopharynx is inaccessible to direct visual inspection.[1] It is therefore necessary to insert some sort of telescopic device into the pharyngeal area—a technique referred to as *endoscopy*. The endoscope may be either a rigid or flexible instrument that can be inserted into the patient's nose or mouth to view the movement of the velum and pharyngeal walls from either a superior (nasopharyngeal) or inferior (oropharyngeal) vantage point. While visual observations of velopharyngeal *structures* accord well with radiographic findings (Zwitman, Gyepes, & Ward, 1976), careful evaluation of velopharyngeal *activity* will likely require a relatively minute analysis of sound-synchronized images, a procedure that is, at best, laborious and time-consuming. But even careful endoscopic observation is incomplete since it provides a two-dimensional view of a three-dimensional mechanism which more or less resembles a vertical collapsible tube (Skolnick, McCall, & Barnes, 1973). That's to say that not all velopharyngeal movement occurs in a neat horizontal plane and any activity below the viewed surface—perhaps critical to closure—may go undocumented. Nonetheless, with continuing technological advances, endoscopy (often complemented by multiview video-

---

[1]Except in those rare cases in which a maxillofacial defect (usually created surgically) provides an opening through which the posterior oral cavity can be seen. Several of the early investigations of velopharyngeal valving indeed took advantage of such situations (see, for example, Harrington, 1944, Bloomer, 1953; also the classic text by West and Ansberry, 1968). While some insights into palatal function were gained, conclusions based on grossly abnormal oropharyngeal structures may have little applicability to more anatomically normal structures.

fluoroscopy and various aerodynamic measures) has increasingly found its way into the routine evaluation of velopharyngeal structure and function (Ibuki, Karnell, & Morris, 1983; Riski, Hoke, & Dolan, 1989; Shprintzen, 1989; D'Antonio, Achauer, & Vander Kam, 1993).

Rigid Endoscopy

The *oral panendoscope* is an early rigid endoscope that was designed specifically to observe the velopharyngeal port. The long shaft of the scope is inserted into the patient's mouth until its distal end lies in the oropharynx. The side-viewing telescope within its plastic shield is then rotated to view the velopharynx above, while a small light source next to the viewing lens provides illumination. The examiner can observe directly, or the panendoscope can be mounted on a camera. Since its introduction by Taub (1966a, 1966b), the panendoscope has been used with video recording or other monitoring systems to obtain simultaneous audio and visual records (Willis & Stutz, 1972) and to provide patients with immediate feedback of their own velar activity (Shelton, Paesani, McClelland, & Bradfield, 1975; Shelton, Baumont, Trier, & Furr, 1978).

Despite excellent optics and a relatively broad field of view, the disadvantages of an endoscope are readily apparent. Many subjects gag if the tongue base, faucial region, velum, or pharyngeal wall is touched by the instrument, as is almost inevitable. Less disturbing to the patient, but much more important to the clinician, is the fact that a fairly large instrument must traverse the length of the oral cavity pretty much in the midline. With the oral cavity thus encumbered, articulation is limited to labial phones and to low or neutral vowels. This is problematic since, at least for some patients, velopharyngeal competence may vary with vowel type (Finck, Gaspard, & Melon, 1987; Smith & Guyette, 1996). Unfortunately, the development of much thinner oral endoscopes that use fiberoptic bundles has diminished problems of speech interference only a little (Zwitman, Sonderman, & Ward, 1974; McWilliams et al., 1990), although moving the light source out of the working end of the instrument has placed the source of considerable heat far away from the oral tissues. The greatly reduced diameter of the fiberoptic shaft will often allow the nasal insertion of these rigid scopes, but such placement is usually performed with a flexible instrument, the *nasendoscope*, expressly designed for that purpose (Karnell, 1994).

Flexible Nasendoscopy

The advent of improved fiberoptic instruments, ranging in diameter from 1 to 3 mm, has allowed nasendoscopy (also called *flexible fiberoptic nasopharyngoscopy*) to become a standard procedure for many professionals who evaluate and manage velopharyngeal dysfunction (Shprintzen, 1989; D'Antonio, Achauer, & Vander Kam, 1993). The nasendoscope is passed via the naris into the nasopharynx to allow the velopharyngeal region to be viewed from above or within (Pigott, 1969; Pigott, Bensen, & White, 1969; Sawashima & Ushijima, 1971, 1972; Sawashima, 1977; Miyazaki, Matsuya, & Yamaoka, 1975; Itoh et al., 1979; Niimi, Bell-Berti, & Harris, 1982; Pigott & Makepeace, 1982; D'Antonio, Muntz, Marsh, Grames, & Backensto-Marsh, 1988; Karnell, 1998). Nasendoscopes may be of an *end-viewing* or *side-viewing* variety; the former may be directed into the velopharyngeal passage, whereas the latter type can only be positioned above it. Thus the end-viewing instrument may allow a better appreciation of vertical as well as horizontal velopharyngeal dynamics.

In either case, the *per nasum* approach has the advantage of leaving the articulators unencumbered. But this comes at the price of greater invasiveness that is apt to provoke considerable anxiety for some patients. Although the application of a topical anesthetic or vasoconstrictor to the nasal mucosa may not be a necessary precondition to successful viewing (Leder, Ross, Briskin, & Sasaki, 1997), good nasendoscopic technique requires both practice and the ability to ease the patient's anxiety. It has been reported that, with a bit of skill, direct visualization of velopharyngeal structure and function can be performed reliably even on young preschoolers (Lotz, D'Antonio, Chait, & Netsell, 1993; D'Antonio, Chait, Lotz, & Netsell, 1986; D'Antonio et al., 1988; Shprintzen, 1989; Karnell & Seaver, 1990; Karnell, 1994).

Like those used to observe the larynx (see Chapter 10, "Laryngeal Function"), flexible fiberscopes used in nasendoscopy consist of two bundles of thin glass fibers. One bundle of fibers conducts light from a bright source (usually from a xenon or mercury halide bulb) to illuminate the field of view, whereas the other bundle, made up of carefully aligned (or "coherent") fibers, transmits the image from the objective lens within the velopharynx back to the viewer's eyepiece (which can be connected, in turn, to a videocamera).

One notable shortcoming of nasendoscopy concerns the image distortion that results as a consequence of the wide-angle objective lens that must be used so that the field of view can encompass both the velum and the posterior and lateral pharyngeal walls. In particular, these lenses induce a "barrel-type" or "convergence" effect (Figure 11–1), whereby the center of the image appears larger, and thus closer, than the periphery (Pigott & Makepeace, 1982; Hibi, Bless, Hirano, & Yoshida, 1988; Muntz, 1992). In general, the

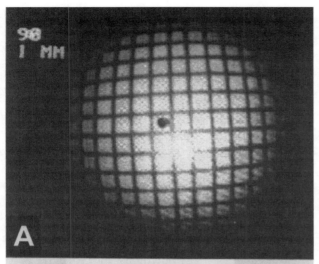

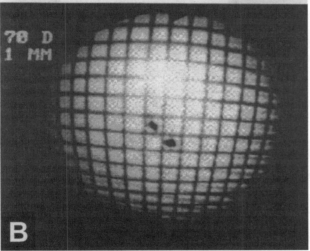

Figure 11–1. Oblique angle and barrel-shaped distortions of fiberscopic images. **(A)** Image of a 1–mm grid as seen through a fiberscope held perpendicular (90°) to the grid at a distance of 10 mm. **(B)** Same grid viewed from the same distance but with the scope oriented at a 60° angle. From "Distortions of Videofiberoscopy Imaging: Reconsideration and Correction," by S. R. Hibi, D. M. Bless, M. Hirano, & T. Yoshida, 1988, *Journal of Voice, 2,* 168–175. Figure 3, p. 171. Reprinted by permission.

distortion increases as the lens approaches the visualized object or deviates from a perpendicular orientation. This image distortion—coupled with the inherent difficulties in controlling for scope position and objective lens alignment—largely precludes accurate measurement of velopharyngeal area or of structural movement which must instead be expressed in arbitrary rather than absolute distance or area units (Sawashima, 1977; Pigott & Makepeace, 1982; Karnell,

Linville, & Edwards, 1988). Although some correction for this systematic image distortion is possible (Hibi et al., 1988; Engelke, Hoch, Bruns, & Striebeck, 1996), the computer-based techniques that are necessary are not easily adapted to the clinical setting. Nonetheless, while perhaps not well suited to deriving area or displacement measures, many clinicians have found the wide-angle image and flexible positioning of the nasendoscope extremely valuable in the documention of normal and abnormal velopharyngeal valving patterns (see, for example, Witzel & Posnick, 1989) and for providing therapeutic biofeedback to the patient (Siegel-Sadewitz & Shprintzen, 1982; Witzel, Tobe, & Salyer, 1988a, 1988b; Brunner et al., 1994).

ULTRASOUND IMAGING

Ultrasound techniques (discussed in Chapter 12, "Speech Movements" have been used to examine lateral pharyngeal wall movement during speech (Kelsey, Minifie, & Hixon, 1969; Minifie, Hixon, Kelsey, & Woodhouse, 1970; Skolnick, Zagzebski, & Watkin, 1975; Ryan & Hawkins, 1976). The ultrasound transducer is directed toward the pharyngeal wall at the level of the velopharynx usually by placing it against the neck just below the ear and behind the ramus of the mandible. Since the high-frequency ultrasound pulses are strongly reflected when they reach the interface between the pharyngeal mucosa and the air within the pharynx, the technique can be exploited to track pharyngeal wall position and movement. Visualization of both lateral pharyngeal walls requires a bilateral pair of transducers. However, lateral resolution remains plagued by the same problems encountered when attempting to examine the vocal folds via ultrasound imaging (see Chapter 10, "Laryngeal Function"). These include the limited width of the ultrasound beam which restricts the field of view and the difficulty of maintaining a stable and perpendicular transducer placement (Lubker, 1970; Miles, 1989). Furthermore, as most of the signal is reflected back toward the transducer when it encounters either an air-tissue boundary or a hard surface such as the bony palate, adequate visualization of the velum is problematic at best (Hawkins & Swisher, 1978).

MAGNETIC RESONANCE IMAGING

Magnetic resonance imaging (MRI) can be used to provide finely detailed three-dimensional images of the vocal tract and articulatory structures (Baer, Gore, Boyce, & Nye, 1987; Baer, Gore, Gracco, & Nye, 1991; Moore, 1992; Dang, Honda, & Suzuki, 1994). (MRI is discussed more fully in Chapter 12, "Speech Movements.") Although the technique has recently been used to assess nasal cavity volume (Corey, Gungor, Nelson, Fredberg, & Lai, 1997), morphology (Dang et al., 1994), and patency (Malm, 1997a), to date there has been little study of the velum or of the velopharyngeal orifice using MRI. This is due to the fact that the standard MR technique requires several seconds to several minutes to produce an image (thus obliging the speaker to maintain a static vocal tract posture). Also, the construction of current MRI units force the speaker to assume a supine position. Although there may be specific concerns about the effects of gravity on the velum, Whalen (1990) reports minimal gravity-dependent positional change, at least with regard to velar height. Ultrafast MRI techniques have been developed recently (Di Girolamo et al., 1996; Jäger et al., 1996; Yokoyama et al., 1996) so that dynamic assessments of velopharyngeal function are now possible (Wein, Drobnitzky, Klajman, & Angerstein, 1991; McGowan, Hatabu, Yousem, Randall, & Kressel, 1992; Yamawaki, Nishimura, & Suzuki, 1996; Yamawaki, Nishimura, Suzuki, Sawada, & Yamawaki, 1997). Especially if future units can allow the subject to maintain an upright posture, MRI holds great clinical promise in the assessment of velopharyngeal behavior.

INDIRECT ASSESSMENT OF VELOPHARYNGEAL FUNCTION

The limited utility of endoscopic/photographic techniques and the drawbacks associated with electromyography and with radiographic, MRI, and ultrasound imaging encourage the use of indirect assessment methods. These involve measuring correlates of velopharyngeal function so that inferences about malfunction may be drawn.

Articulation Tests

Obviously, one could use articulatory performance as an indirect index of velopharyngeal function. This has the appeal of a certain straightforwardness. Leakage of air through an incompetent port would be expected to interfere with high-pressure consonants and to produce perceptible nasality. Conversely, inadequate opening should severely distort /m/, /n/, and /ŋ/. Different phonemes might be expected to suffer in varying degrees according to the nature and magnitude of the malfunction. Differential diagnosis and severity scaling might, therefore, be possible.

Interest in the articulation profiles of cleft palate children is hardly recent (see, for example, Spriestersbach, Darley, & Rouse, 1956). Some attempts have been made to devise articulation tests that will, in fact,

provide a firm basis for drawing conclusions about actual or potential velopharyngeal valving function (Van Demark, 1970, 1979; McCabe & Bradley, 1973; Bzoch, 1989). Morris, Spriestersbach, and Darley (1961) created the Iowa Pressure Articulation Test (IPAT), a subset of items from the Templin-Darley test, in an attempt to do just this. While its correlation with other tests of velopharyngeal valving is only fair (Barnes & Morris, 1967), such articulation tests do seem to show promise as an indicator of the need for secondary management (Van Demark, 1974; Van Demark & Morris, 1977; Van Demark, Morris, & VandeHaar, 1979; Van Demark & Swickard, 1980; Hardin, Van Demark, & Morris, 1990) or of therapeutic progress (Van Demark & Hardin, 1985; Van Demark, 1997).

Appealing as such methods may be, they are fraught with problems. For one thing, velopharyngeal malfunction may induce speech changes other than the outright distortion of speech sounds, and, for another, misarticulations may be due, in whole or in part, to abnormalities other than those that involve the velopharyngeal port (Pitzner & Morris, 1966; Jones, 1991; Moller, 1991). In general, one cannot accurately measure and describe the specific movements of the velopharyngeal system that are defective on the basis of articulatory deficits. Instead, the clinician must have recourse to correlates of velopharyngeal action whose relationships to system functioning are stronger or better understood.

Acoustic Measures

Quantification of nasalization by means of acoustic measures would be very convenient. Because no invasive instrumentation would be required, speech performance would not be changed by the evaluation procedure and patient anxiety would be minimized. In principle, measurement could even be done from tape recordings. It is, therefore, not surprising that considerable effort has been devoted to the search for valid and reliable acoustic measures of velopharyngeal function. While a definitive method has yet to be established, considerable progress continues to be made and several options are now available for routine clinical use.

VOCAL TRACT DAMPING

If, during phonation, the supraglottal airway is suddenly blocked, the air pressure above the vocal folds will quickly rise to a level close to the subglottal pressure. Since this eliminates the transglottal pressure drop, transglottal flow ceases and vocal fold vibration must stop (van den Berg, 1956; Titze, 1980, 1985). The time required for the supraglottal pressure to reach a value sufficient to inhibit phonation depends on a number of inherent physical characteristics, including the volume of the vocal tract and its compliance. At least equally important, however, is the fact that air leakage around the blockage (that is, a shunt or "bleed" airflow) will significantly retard the rise in supraglottal pressure and, therefore, will delay the arrest of phonation. The greater the shunt airflow, the longer the delay should be.

Zemlin and Fant (1972) applied this reasoning to the development of a simple and completely non-invasive measure of velopharyngeal closure. Called the *Zemlin Index of Palatopharyngeal Opening* (**ZIPPO**), the measure can be done with a relatively simple apparatus. A mouthpiece, fitted with a special valve, is connected to a rotameter-type flowmeter (see Chapter 9, "Airflow and Volume"). The valve is kept open by an electromagnet that holds a stopper away from its seat. When current to the electromagnet is interrupted, the stopper drops and prevents egressive airflow. A microphone mounted on the outside of the valve system picks up the sound produced by the valve closure that signals airflow interruption. A contact microphone placed on the thyroid cartilage detects laryngeal vibrations, and both amplified microphone signals are displayed.

The test requires that the subject phonate /i/ into the mouthpiece while maintaining an airtight lip seal around it. Consistency of test conditions across trials is maintained by providing the patient with feedback of phonatory airflow and vocal intensity via a rotameter and a VU meter. When the tester presses a button, the valve closes. For the normal speaker, supraglottal pressure builds rapidly following valve closure and laryngeal vibration soon stops.

The relevant measure is the *damping time*, the interval between the acoustic event associated with the sudden valve closure and the disappearance of the laryngeal waves. Zemlin and Fant (1972) tested this system with normal speakers and found that the average damping time was about 100 ms. When shunts were added to the valve, the damping time increased as predicted.

Plattner, Weinberg, and Horii (1980) tested ZIPPO on a group of 15 normal young adult women. Using a computer, damping times were determined for 100 trials each, requiring about a half an hour of testing. The times ranged from 5 to 900 ms (mean = 108 ms; *SD* = 68 ms). Ninety-five percent of the measured times were less than 300 ms. These results are consistent with the damping times reported for other studies (Sawashima, Kiritani, et al., 1983; Sawashima, Honda, et al., 1984; Baken & Orlikoff, 1987; Sawashima & Honda, 1987) which used airway interruption during phonation to assess subglottal pressure (see Chapter 9, "Airflow and Volume"). Unfortunately, whereas the valve closure technique may provide a reasonable means of estimating lung pressure in the normal speaker, the time it takes to squelch phonation appears to be quite variable. Plattner et al. (1980), for instance, reported that while most of their subjects had a fairly narrow range of damping times, others showed wide variation. Both improvement and deterioration of performance over successive trials were noted.

Although valve closure instrumentation has enjoyed some recent clinical and research popularity in subglottal pressure estimation, the use of ZIPPO for the assessment of velopharyngeal function remains uncommon. Nonetheless, its "sound theoretical basis and ease of . . . administration provide sufficient grounds to prompt needed additional research into its clinical application" (Plattner et al., 1980, p. 215). Perhaps with such investigation, ZIPPO may become an important addition to the clinician's battery of diagnostic tests.

SPECTRAL FEATURES OF NASALIZATION

Abnormal nasalization can be reliably perceived. Therefore, the acoustic content of nasalized speech must be different from that of normal speech. When the velopharyngeal valve is opened, the nasal cavity is coupled to the rest of the vocal tract. One would, therefore, expect that nasalization might be the perception of the simple addition of a *nasal resonance* to the other resonance characteristics of the vocal tract.

This reasoning led to a search for relatively simple and invariant changes in the acoustic spectrum attributable to a nasal resonance that would signal nasalization. So, for example, Hattori, Yamamoto, and Fujimura (1958) found that the spectra of nasalized vowels showed distinct attenuation at 500 Hz owing to "the antiresonance of the nasal cavity acting as a side branch connected to the major vocal tract at its midpoint" (p. 269). Still other "nasalization phenomena" have been identified, but these tended to vary from one speaker to another (Bloomer & Peterson, 1955; Dickson, 1962; Weatherley-White, Dersch, & Anderson, 1964), were different for different vowels (Stevens et al., 1976), and generally failed to correlate well with the degree of perceived nasality. Using synthetic speech stimuli, investigators have confirmed that the perception of nasality depends on highly complex and very variable acoustic cues (House & Stevens, 1956; Farnetani, 1979) that may be language- and context-specific (Beddor & Strange, 1982; Beddor, 1993; Cohn, 1993; Maddieson & Ladefoged, 1993; Solé, 1995; Ladefoged & Maddieson, 1996). It is now clear that the discovery of "precise acoustic correlates of nasalization appears to be a far more formidable and perhaps questionable task than [had been] suspected (Schwartz, 1972, p. 198).

In fact, the search for invariant acoustic features of nasalization is almost certain to be fruitless. The reasoning behind this conclusion was excellently presented by Curtis (1968, 1970), and is summarized here. The basic flaw in earlier research is the assumption that the nasal space represents one more fixed resonator that appends it own distinct contribution to the combined acoustic properties of the other relatively autonomous resonators that make up the vocal tract. In other words, the difficulty lies in the assumption of a separate "nasal resonance" that is added to other independent resonances. Dunn (1950) has presented a model of the vocal tract that has been shown to be more explanatory of speech acoustics. According to his construct, the vocal tract can be said to consist of a set of cylinders arranged in series. Each of these, in some sense, has acoustic properties but, because the cylinders are connected in a string, they are enormously interdependent. None makes an identifiable isolated contribution to the final acoustic product. Quite the contrary: the contribution of any given region of the vocal tract is very much a function of all of the other regions. The final result is very different from the simple sum of a set of independent parts. Consequently, side-branch coupling of the nasal cavity to the rest of the system does not add an invariant resonator, but rather it just changes the overall nature of a complex acoustic system. Furthermore, as Maeda (1993) points out, a lowered velum associated with an open velopharyngeal orifice will also significantly modify the area function in the region of the velopharynx. The resonance characteristics of the nasal cavity thus *interact with* the variations in vocal tract shaping required for different vowels. Because of this, different vowels have different acoustic "nasalization" characteristics. Similarly, individual variations in vocal tract anatomy lead to differences in the acoustic correlates of nasality from one speaker to another. "The conclusion," according to Curtis (1970),

> seems self-evident. An adequate theoretical model for vocal resonance gives little reason to predict that nasalization will lead to invariant changes in the acoustic spectra of speech. On the contrary, the spectral changes which are to be expected will depend very considerably on what is happening in other portions of the vocal cavity system. If one accepts this conclusion the apparent inconsistency and lack of invariance in the data concerning the acoustic effects of nasalization are not mystifying. This lack of invariance is in fact consistent with theory and should have been expected." (p. 71)

Faced with a long history of acoustic research that largely offers equivocal findings, Feng and Castelli (1996, p. 3695) quite succinctly explain that "the difficulty in studying the acoustic behavior of nasal vowels arises from the fact that we do not know what exactly characterizes a nasal sound." However, despite inconsistency among speakers and among the phones produced by a single individual, certain spectral features are generally agreed to be associated with nasalization. While not useful for differential diagnosis (Dickson, 1962; Accordi, Croatto-Accordi, & Cassin, 1981; Plante, Berger-Vachon, & Kauffmann, 1993; Garnier, Gallego, Collet, & Berger-Vachon, 1996), change in any such feature in a standard speech context may serve as a useful, although perhaps tentative, means for observing the effect of therapy for a given patient. It is entirely conceivable that the speech spectrum will show changes that are real but too subtle for reliable perceptual detection. The more-or-less "established" features of nasalization are summarized in Table 11–1. Figure 11–2 shows how nasalization of a vowel might appear in a standard wide-band spectrogram (see Chapter 7, "Sound Spectrography"). More extensive discussion of the acoustics of nasalization is available in Schwartz (1968b, 1972), Curtis (1970), and in Pickett (1980).

ORAL AND NASAL SOUND PRESSURE

Lowering the velum increases the acoustic coupling of the nasal cavity to the rest of the vocal tract. More of the vocal signal is then propagated through the nose. In somewhat simpler terms, velopharyngeal opening increases the intensity of nasal sound emission. Increased nasal sound pressure at the nares provides a rather direct indication of a lowered velum, and the audio signal from a nasal microphone can be used to provide a patient with instantaneous feedback of nasalization (Hultzen, 1942).

Nasal sound pressure level can be measured fairly easily by inserting a probe microphone just inside the naris (Hirano, Takeuchi, & Hiroto, 1966) or by erecting a barrier that will separate oral and nasal signals (Hyde, 1968). The microphone output can be amplified, rectified, and filtered (Figure 11–3) to produce a signal representing the nasal sound amplitude. This can be displayed on an oscilloscope or computer screen (where the signal can be used for feedback to the patient) or recorded on paper. While simple, this method has a number of problems that limit its use as an evaluative tool. Even in normal speakers, supposedly non-nasal vowels are routinely produced with measurable nasal sound emission, the intensity of which varies, but not very predictably, with the vowel being produced (Schwartz, 1968a). Also, the sensitivity of the probe microphone to airflow through the nose can confound the measurement. Finally, the nasal sound pressure is not simply a function of the degree

Table 11–1. Spectral Features of Nasalization

Effect of Nasalization:	*According to:*
Increase in formant bandwidth	Bloomer & Peterson (1955) House (1957) Dickson (1962) Kent, Liss & Philips (1989)
[first formant]	Delattre (1954, 1955) House & Stevens (1956) Hawkins & Stevens (1985)
Formant frequency shift	Dickson (1962) Gonay (1972) Stevens et al. (1976) Watterson & Emanuel (1981)
[first formant higher]	House & Stevens (1956) Fujimura (1960, 1962) Kent, Liss, & Philips (1989)
[third formant higher]	Hanson (1964)
[second and third formants lower]	Bloomer & Peterson (1955) Kent, Liss & Philips (1989)
Extra resonances	Bloomer & Peterson (1955) House (1957) Dickson (1962) Watterson & Emanuel (1981) Hawkins & Stevens (1985)
[at approximately 250 Hz]	Tarnóczy (1948) Delattre (1954, 1955) House & Stevens (1956) Hattori et al. (1958)
[between about 250 and 500 Hz]	Kent, Liss, & Philips (1989)
Diminished resonances [first formant]	Dickson (1962) Delattre (1954, 1955) House & Stevens (1956)
Anti-resonances (acoustic zeros; antiformants)	Fujimura (1960, 1962) Dickson (1962) Dillenschneider, Zaleski, & Grenier (1973) Hawkins & Stevens (1985)
[at approximately 500 Hz]	Hattori et al. (1958)
[at about the first formant]	Stevens, Fant, & Hawkins (1987)
[at about the third formant]	Bloomer & Peterson (1955) House & Stevens (1956) Kent, Liss, & Philips (1989)
Noise between formants	Bloomer & Peterson (1955) Hattori et al. (1958)
Generally decreased vowel or speech intensity	House & Stevens (1956) Dickson (1962) Bernthal & Beukelman (1977) Kent, Liss, & Philips (1989)

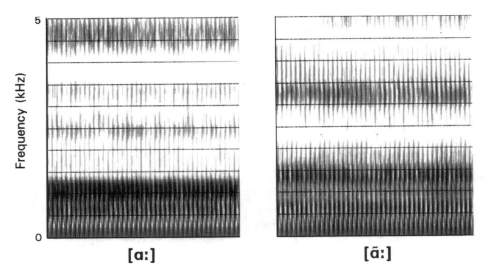

Figure 11–2. Wide-band spectrograms of [ɑ:] and ɑ̃:] spoken by the same normal speaker. Note the strong formant at about 3200 Hz (and the absence of energy around 2500 Hz and 4500 Hz) in the nasalized vowel.

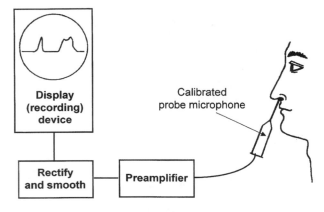

Figure 11–3. Set-up to measure nasal sound pressure.

of nasal coupling: it obviously also reflects the vocal intensity. Thus, an increase of intranasal sound intensity might represent nothing more than increased phonatory effort. Something of a solution to the last problem can be achieved by separately and simultaneously measuring intranasal and oral sound pressure levels and comparing them.[2] As vocal intensity changes, the oral and nasal signals would presumably change together, maintaining a constant relationship. The difference between the oral and nasal sound pressures (in dB) has been used, as has the ratio of one to the other (Shelton, Knox, Arndt, & Elbert, 1967;

Fletcher, 1970; Dejonckere, 1984). For patient feedback purposes, rectified oral and nasal signals can both be applied to a stereo balance meter (available at many audio equipment shops) to provide a real-time visual indication of oral-to-nasal balance (Yules, Josephson, & Chase, 1969).

Appealing though its theoretical basis may be, the results of nasal-to-oral sound pressure comparisons do not correspond very closely to listener judgments of nasality. Shelton and his colleagues (1967) found that the correlation between listener ratings of nasality and nasal sound pressure level was .47; between listener ratings and the difference of oral and nasal sound pressures, .41; and between listener ratings and the ratio of the two pressures, .37. These coefficients are significant ($p < .01$) from the standpoint of inferential statistics, but the relationship is clearly too weak to permit the use of such measures as indices of the severity of perceived nasality. (They may, however, reflect nasalization itself fairly well.) It should also be noted that the nasal-to-oral sound pressure ratio may show sex differences (Clarke, 1975, 1978).

Nasalance

When nasal sound pressure is obtained by positioning a microphone in or near the nares, the amplitude of the signal is influenced not only by the degree of nasal coupling, but by the overall speech intensity as well.

---

[2]A brief review of the rationale, advantages, and difficulties of this method has been prepared by Counihan (1972). Note also that the HONC index, described later, can be implemented with microphone pickups.

However, the simultaneous measurement of oral sound pressure can be used to account for variation in speech intensity by expressing the strength of the nasal signal as a proportion of the total acoustic energy radiated from the nose and mouth. Automatic derivation of such a ratio ($\frac{nasal}{nasal\ +\ oral}$) was accomplished by means of an electronic system named ***The Oral Nasal Acoustic Ratio*** (***TONAR***) by its developer (Fletcher, 1970). Performing a somewhat more complex function than its name might at first imply, the basic organization of the TONAR system is diagrammed in Figure 11–4B.

Inputs obtained from nasal and oral microphones —partitioned by a sound-separating baffle that is held in place by the specially-designed headgear shown in Figure 11–4A—are individually amplified and conditioned by identical bandpass (350–650 Hz) filters. Rectification and smoothing of the filtered signals results in DC voltages proportional to the amplitude of that part of each input within the filters' pass-band. A special circuit performs an analog summation and division function. Its output is the ratio of the (filtered) nasal amplitude to the sum of the filtered nasal and (identically filtered) oral amplitude. The ratio is then multiplied by 100 and expressed as a percentage score. However, the filtering done to the microphone input signals results in a complex output product: the relative nasal amplitude within a limited range of the speech frequency spectrum. The term ***nasalance*** has been coined to describe this measure and, depending upon the nature of the spoken utterance, it has been found to correlate moderately with perceived nasality (Fletcher & Bishop, 1970; Dalston & Warren, 1986; Dalston & Seaver, 1992; Hardin, Van Demark, Morris, & Payne, 1992; Nellis, Neiman, & Lehman, 1992; Watterson, McFarlane, & Wright, 1993; Vallino-Napoli & Montgomery, 1997; Watterson, Lewis, & Deutsch,

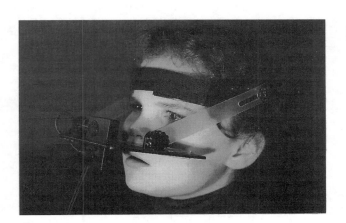

A

Figure 11–4. (A) Oral and nasal microphones separated by a baffle and held in place by a head harness for the measurement of nasalance. **(B)** A functional block diagram of the TONAR system.

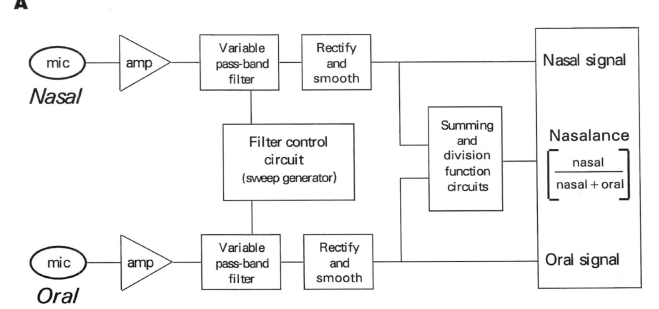

B

1998). Although the developer obviously attached importance to the frequency-limitation capability of the instrument and found it to be useful (Fletcher, 1970, 1973), the specific advantages conferred have not been clearly demonstrated. The first commercial incarnation of the system, TONAR II, was used for biofeedback and contingency-management therapies (Fletcher, 1972) and to conduct early nasalance studies of esophageal (Colyar & Christensen, 1980) and hearing-impaired (Fletcher & Daly, 1976) speakers, among others, with hypernasal speech (Fletcher, Sooudi, & Frost, 1974; Kahane, 1979). The TONAR II has since been supplanted by the **Nasometer** (marketed by Kay Elemetrics Corp., Lincoln Park, NJ), a computer-based TONAR system under software control that has become particularly popular among speech clinicians who have found the device to be useful for patient assessment and management.

The Nasometer has been used quite extensively to obtain and compare nasalance scores from a number of speakers for whom inappropriate nasalization is a primary concern (Parker, Maw, & Szallasi, 1989; González Landa, Santos Terrón, Miro-Viar, & Sánchez-Ruiz, 1990; Williams, Eccles, & Hutchings, 1990; Andreassen, Leeper, & MacRae, 1991; Andreassen, Leeper, MacRae, & Nicholson, 1994; Haapanen, 1991a; LaPine, Stewart, & Tatchell, 1991; LaPine, Stewart, Settle, & Brandow, 1992; Tatchell, Stewart, & LaPine, 1991; Dalston & Seaver, 1992; Nellis et al., 1992; Haapanen & Somer, 1993; Watterson et al., 1993; Stellzig, Heppt, & Komposch, 1994; Karnell, 1995; Hong, Kwon, & Jung, 1997; Kotby, Abdel Haleem, Hegazi, Safe, & Zaki, 1997; Vallino-Napoli & Montgomery, 1997; Pinborough-Zimmerman, Canady, Yamashiro, & Morales, 1998). But, despite its relative popularity, there have been surprisingly few studies of normal speakers. This exacerbates the difficulty of interpreting nasalance data (Seaver & Dalston, 1990; Hardin et al., 1992; Litzaw & Dalston, 1992; Nellis et al., 1992). As yet, studies are largely equivocal with respect to whether the sex of the speaker influences mean nasalance and it is unknown to what extent any intersex variability may be tied to the fixed bandpass filtering used in the analysis (Seaver, Dalston, Leeper, & Adams, 1991; Watterson et al., 1993; Zajac, Lutz, & Mayo, 1996). It also remains unclear how nasalance is affected by the physical characteristics of the oral and nasal cavities (Parker, Clarke, Dawes, & Maw, 1990; Williams et al., 1990; Dalston, Warren, & Dalston, 1991a, 1991b; Williams, Preece, Rhys, & Eccles, 1992; Mayo, Floyd, Warren, Dalston, & Mayo, 1996; Scarsellone, Rochet, & Wolfaardt, 1999), by the integrity of the velopharyngeal valve, and by the phonetic demands of the spoken utterance (Watterson, York, & McFarlane, 1994; Watterson, Lewis, & Foley-Homan, 1999). Per-

haps more importantly, it is not known to what degree turbulent nasal and/or oral airflow may affect nasalance—especially among speakers with velopharyngeal incompetence who are, after all, likely to be the subjects of nasometry. This uncertainty is particularly consequential since the Zoo Passage, while without nasal phones, is replete with high pressure and flow consonants. Karnell (1995) did, in fact, find significant differences in mean nasalance for some patients reading a set of high-pressure sentences from the Zoo Passage and another set of utterances devoid of both nasal and high-pressure consonants. Watterson et al. (1998), however, could not confirm this effect.

The limited data summarized in Table 11–2 provide some indication of nasalance values that can be expected from normal speakers of English, at least for selected speech stimuli. As a clinical rule of thumb, Dalston, Warren, and Dalston (1991c) have suggested that mean nasalance scores should be 32% or lower for speakers reciting the Zoo Passage, although other investigators have argued that the optimum cutoff would be closer to 26% (Fletcher, Adams, & McCutcheon, 1989; Hardin et al., 1992; Watterson et al., 1993). On the other hand, the Rainbow Passage and nasally-biased test stimuli appear to be most useful when assessing hyponasal speakers (Dalston et al., 1991b; Dalston & Seaver, 1992; Nellis et al., 1992; Watterson et al., 1993; Vallino-Napoli & Montgomery, 1997).

Not surprisingly, nasalance is known to be influenced by the speaker's native language (Haapanen, 1991b; Heppt, Westrich, Strate, & Mohring, 1991; Santos Terrón, González Landa, & Sánchez-Ruiz, 1991; Anderson, 1996; Kotby et al., 1997; Nichols, 1999) and may be affected by his regional dialect as well (Seaver et al., 1991; Dalston, Neiman, & González Landa, 1993; Kavanaugh, Fee, Kalinowski, Doyle, & Leeper, 1994). For this reason, clinicians are well advised to gather their own sets of normative data for those subgroups within the general population to which their patients belong.

Because many young children find it difficult to read or recite the Rainbow or Zoo Passages, there have been attempts to simplify test material. Watterson, Hinton, and McFarlane (1996), for instance, tested twenty 4- to 6-year-old children who read passages designed to be at an appropriate level for young, early readers. The nasalance scores they obtained indeed suggested that the simplified material could be substituted for the more difficult Rainbow and Zoo passages that are more typically used in nasometry.

MacKay and Kummer (1994) have designed a nasalance protocol to be used with young children and others for whom reading is difficult or impossible. Their ***Simplified Nasometric Assessment Procedures***

Table 11–2. Nasalance Scores (in %) Obtained for Normal English Speakers

Subjects		Sustained /ɑ/		Rainbow Passage[a]		Nonnasal Passage[b]		Highly "Nasal" Sentences[c]		
Age[d]	N	Mean	(SD)	Mean	(SD)	Mean	(SD)	Mean	(SD)	Source[e]
Children										
4–6	20	—	—	32.6	(6.7)	15.4	(3.3)	—	—	1
3–9	246	—	—	—	—	—	—	56.1	(7.4)	2a
3–9	76	—	—	—	—	15.4	(2.8)	—	—	2b
3–9	76	—	—	—	—	10.8	(3.1)	—	—	2c
4–9	238	—	—	—	—	13.1	(5.9)	—	—	3a
4–9	243	—	—	—	—	—	—	59.6	(8.1)	3b
5–12	117	—	—	35.7	(5.2)	15.5	(4.9)	61.1	(6.9)	4
Men										
18–38	11	8.0	(10.6)	16.8	(5.8)	8.7	(1.9)	32.9	(13.0)	5
23±5	40	—	—	—	—	17.2	(4.7)	58.8	(7.4)	6
24±2	15	—	—	36	(4)	19	(4)	63	(4)	7
38–63	56	—	—	35	(6)	15	(7)	61	(6)	8
50–80	50	16.2	(6.8)	23.5	(5.1)	16.7	(4.2)	38.2	(8.4)	9
Women										
18–38	11	6.5	(9.4)	18.8	(5.8)	8.3	(2.5)	38.9	(14.5)	5
23±6	40	—	—	—	—	18.1	(5.1)	59.8	(6.7)	6
28±8	15	—	—	37	(4)	19	(4)	64	(4)	7
16–50	92	—	—	36	(6)	16	(7)	63	(6)	8
50–80	50	23.6	(4.4)	32.0	(10.7)	27.3	(8.4)	47.5	(14.5)	9

[a]Fairbanks, 1960. The "Rainbow Passage" is phonemically balanced to represent the typical phonetic content of English; 11% of the passage consists of nasal phonemes.

[b]Except where noted in the source description, the nonnasal material used was the "Zoo Passage" (Fletcher, 1972).

[c]Nasally-biased sentences (Fletcher, 1978) included: "Mama made some lemon jam," Ten men came in when Jane rang," "Dan's gang changed my mind," "Ben can't plan on a lengthy rain," and "Amanda came from Bounding, Maine." Thirty-five percent of these sentences are represented by nasal phonemes.

[d]Age range (or mean ± SD) in years.

[e]Sources:

1. Watterson et al., 1996. Nasometer used for measurement of nasalance. Subjects were 7 normal girls and 13 normal boys from northern Nevada [USA]. Because the children showed difficulty reading the Rainbow Passage, a simpler paragraph (the Mouse Passage) that likewise contained 11% nasal phonemes was substituted. Boys produced slightly higher nasalance scores: For the Zoo Passage, nasalance was 17.0 ± 3.1% and 14.6 ± 3.2% for the boys and girls, respectively; For the Mouse Passage, nasalance was 36.4 ± 6.9% and 30.5± 5.8% for the boys and girls, respectively.

2. MacKay and Kummer, 1994. Nasometer measures. Subjects were normal children from the Cincinnati, Ohio [USA] area; Sex distribution not reported. Specially designed speech materials used: *a.* nasal sentences were "Mama made some mittens," "Mama made some muffins," and "Mama made some lemonade." For literate children, nonnasal reading passages were: *b.* Bobby and Billy Play Ball, and *c.* A School Day for Suzy.

3. van Doorn and Purcell, 1998. Nasometer measures. Subjects were normal children "from a variety of schools and preschools across the Sydney [Australia] metropolitan region . . . The children all spoke Australian English with no trace of foreign accent." *a.* For the 121 girls and 117 boys who read the Zoo Passage, the mean nasalance was 12.6 ± 5.6% and 13.6 ± 6.2%, respectively (range: 3.06–44.17%). *b.* For the 123 girls and 120 boys who read the nasal sentences, the mean nasalance was 58.6 ± 8.6% and 60.7 ± 7.5%, respectively (range: 31.40–77.74%). The authors report no significant age or sex effect on nasalance values.

4. Fletcher et al., 1989. Nasometer measures. Subjects were normal children "enrolled in kindergarten through the fifth grades in a suburban Birmingham, Alabama [USA] public school." Average age was 8.5 ± 1.8 years, sex distribution of children not provided. The authors report no significant age or sex effect on nasalance values.

5. Fletcher, 1976. TONAR II used for measurement. Unpublished study cited by Hutchinson, Robinson, and Nerbonne (1978). [See note for Source 9.]

6. Mayo et al., 1996. Nasometer used for measurement. Subject groups were divided equally by European ("white" American) and African ("African-American") ancestry. All speakers used a Mid-Atlantic American English dialect. No effects of speaker sex were noted. For the nasal sentences, the white subjects had significantly higher nasalance scores (60.9±6.6%) than the African-American subjects (57.7 ± 5.3%), whereas for the Zoo Passage, the effect was noted only for the male subjects: White men had significantly higher mean nasalance (18.9 ± 4.4%) than the African-American men (15.4 ± 4.4%).

(Continued)

Table 11–2. Nasalance Scores (in %) Obtained for Normal English Speakers (*continued*)

7. Litzaw and Dalston, 1992. Nasometer measures. Subjects were normal white adult American English speakers over the age of 18 years who used a "Mid-Atlantic dialect." No significant nasalance difference between men and women; Nasalance scores did not vary systematically as a function of the speakers' mean speaking fundamental frequency or measured nasal cross-sectional area.

8. Seaver et al., 1991. Nasometer measures. Subjects were normal white adult English speakers who had "speech patterns characteristic of one of four [North American] geographical regions (Mid-Atlantic, Southern, Mid-Western, Ontario Canada)." Some effects of speaker sex and regional dialect noted.

9. Hutchinson, Robinson, and Nerbonne, 1978. TONAR II used for nasalance measurement. Scores were significantly different between men and women; No significant age effect. [Fletcher et al. (1989) maintain that, because of differences between the TONAR II and Nasometer systems, nasalance measured with the two devices may not be comparable; Note, for instance, the lower TONAR II nasalance for the highly nasal utterances.]

(*SNAP*) test consists of three separate tasks. The first requires the patient to repeat 14 different CV syllables at a rate of about 3–5 per second. The second subtest is designed to elicit five speech samples each made up of three sentences spoken twice. The patient repeats a short carrier phrase and is cued to complete the sentence with one of three simple line drawings of common objects. Four of the cued passages are designed to elicit nasal-free, largely high-pressure sounds, while the last is heavily biased toward nasal consonants. Lastly, for appropriate patients, the third SNAP subtest requires the reading of a set of two paragraphs, each constructed to be "semantically, pragmatically, and lexically simple." Both passages contain a high proportion of high-pressure consonants and no nasal phonemes. MacKay and Kummer (1994) provide explicit instructions for scoring the SNAP test, based on a comparison to 246 children who speak a Midwestern dialect of American English. Selected summary data derived by MacKay and Kummer (1994) using their protocol are included in Tables 11–2 and 11–3.

Rather than serving to directly gauge velopharyngeal competence or nasal patency, the clinical value of nasalance would seem to lie largely in its ability to characterize the speech of patients with velopharyngeal inadequacy and/or upper airway impairment (Colyar & Christensen, 1980; Fletcher & Higgins, 1980; McWilliams et al., 1990; Dalston, Warren, & Dalston, 1991b; Hardin et al., 1992; Dalston et al., 1993; Stellzig et al., 1994; Pinborough-Zimmerman et al., 1998). Because different classes of speakers may show distinct patterns of nasalance change (Fletcher et al., 1989), an examination of both the intended and unintended variation in a patient's speech nasalance scores may be of clinical relevance. The **nasogram** (formerly **tonagram**), a time-history display of nasalance values, allows both long- and short-term assessment of nasalance. Especially when accompanied by additional physiologic data, it has been found to provide useful information about velopharyngeal timing and coarticulation (Flege, 1988; Dalston, 1989; Dalston & Seaver, 1990; Hong et al., 1997). Figure 11–5, for instance, shows the nasogram

obtained from a dysarthric patient during repetition of the syllable /mɑ/. The peaks correspond to the production of /m/, while the troughs are associated with the vowel. The acoustic consequence of muscle discoordination and progressive weakness is signalled by the substantial irregularity in degree and pattern of peak nasalance and by the progressive increase in vowel nasalance over the course of the CV-repetition task.

Recently the **NasalView** (Awan, 1996, 1998; Awan, Bressman, Sader, Busch, & Horch, 1998), another computer-based "nasalance acquisition system," has become commercially available (Tiger DRS, Inc., Seattle, WA). Unlike the Nasometer, however, the NasalView system does not bandpass filter the oral and nasal input signals and uses an RMS (see "Root-Mean-Square AC", Chapter 2) procedure in reporting nasalance values. Nasalance data derived with this system are, as yet, scarce, but are likely—given the difference in signal processing—to vary somewhat from those obtained with TONAR-based units (Awan, 1998).

NASAL ACCELEROMETRY

Nasal sounds induce vibration of the soft tissue of the nose that is easily detectable. Using accelerometers (see Chapter 4, "General Purpose Tools") to pick up the nasal vibration has two major advantages over the use of microphones to monitor the airborne nasal sound. First, the accelerometer is negligibly affected by normal nasal airflow that can confound microphone signals. Second, because the accelerometer is insensitive to airborne waves, it is minimally influenced by simultaneous oral sound emission. This means that better separation of the nasal signal from the total speech output can be achieved. Lippmann (1981) has shown that even relatively inexpensive ultraminiature accelerometers (such as those available from Knowles Electronics, Itasca, IL) can be used reliably for the detection of nasalization. To be sure, accelerometers are not without problems. Detection obviously varies with different tissue transmission characteristics, the angle of attachment to the nose, the nasal patency, and the

Table 11–3. Nasalance Scores (in %) for CV Syllable Repetition: Normal English-Speaking Children*

Syllable	Mean	(SD)		Syllable	Mean	(SD)
/pɑ/	7.2	(2.3)		/si/	17.1	(5.9)
/pi/	17.6	(6.2)		/ʃɑ/	7.5	(2.7)
/tɑ/	8.3	(2.8)		/i/	16.1	(5.9)
/ti/	19.0	(6.1)		/mɑ/	58.4	(7.8)
/kɑ/	8.6	(3.0)		/mi/	78.7	(7.4)
/ki/	19.4	(6.5)		/nɑ/	59.3	(8.6)
/sɑ/	7.1	(2.4)		/ni/	79.1	(6.9)

*MacKay and Kummer, 1994. Subjects were 246 normal children from the Cincinnati, Ohio [USA] area; Age ranged from 3 to 9 years; Sex distribution of children not reported. Authors report that "a small age effect and a small sex effect were found, but they were determined to be irrelevant for purposes of clinical evaluation" (p. 6). Syllables were repeated 6 to 10 times over a 2-s sample.

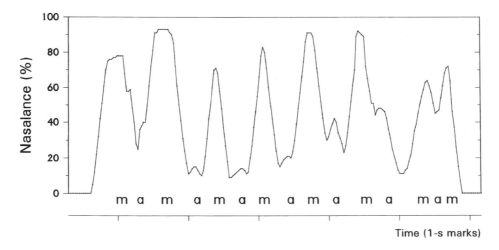

Figure 11–5. Nasalance record (nasogram) of a dysarthric patient during a /mɑ/-syllable repetition task.

degree of contact intimacy achieved (Horii, 1990; Moon, 1990). Therefore, it is not possible to compare absolute values of outputs between subjects nor, in fact, from one test session to another with the same subject. It has also been suggested that the strength of the nasal accelerometer signal tends to be greater for high vowels due to the relatively low-frequency energy of their first formant (Stevens et al., 1976; Larson & Hamlet, 1987). For this reason, nasal accelerometry is not well suited to the direct comparison of isolated sounds. The drawbacks, however, can be circumvented by careful design of the evaluation procedure.

Stevens, Kalikow, and Willemain (1975) have successfully used a very small accelerometer attached to the nose to provide feedback (via an oscilloscope) for management of nasality in deaf children. Also using this method, Stevens and his colleagues (1976) noted that, while the accelerometer signal reflected changes of vocal intensity as well as of varying nasalization, the problem was not serious. In particular, they found that changes in vocal intensity were not likely to amount to more than about ±2 dB, whereas nasalization increased accelerometer output by 10 to 20 dB. The problem of changing vocal intensity was investigated further by Garber and Moller (1979) and subsequently addressed by Horii and Monroe (1983), who described a very simple system that displays the ratio of the nasal accelerometer and oral microphone signals on an oscilloscope screen in a form that can easily be used to provide visual feedback during therapy.

The Horii Oral Nasal Coupling Index

Horii (1980) has devised an analog electronic system for producing the ratio of nasal-to-oral accelerometer output during running speech. The **Horii Oral Nasal Coupling (HONC)** index is a relative scale, with a value of 1 representing maximal nasalization.[3] HONC values have also been expressed in percent, simply by multiplying the ratio by 100 (Theodoros et al., 1993; Theodoros et al., 1995; Thompson & Murdoch, 1995), and in dB (Horii & Lang, 1981; Horii, 1983; Redenbaugh & Reich, 1985; Sussman, 1995; Mra, Sussman, & Fenwick, 1998). In any case, HONC data can be compared across speakers. The scaling procedure also compensates for changes in accelerometer mounting characteristics and tissue attenuation properties, thereby providing comparability of one test session with another for the same patient. There is also evidence of a high correlation between HONC and perceived nasality/denasality (Horii & Lang, 1981; Horii, 1983; Redenbaugh & Reich, 1985; Reich & Redenbaugh, 1985), especially when the ratios are averaged over relatively long speech samples (Jones, Folkins, & Morris, 1990).

The HONC index can be defined mathematically as follows

$$\text{HONC} = k \left(\frac{A_{\text{rms}(n)}}{A_{\text{rms}(v)}} \right),$$

where $A_{\text{rms}(n)}$ is the *root mean square amplitude* (see Chapter 2, "Analog Electronics") of the output of a *nasal* accelerometer and $A_{\text{rms}(v)}$ is a similar value for a *vocal* (neck-mounted) accelerometer. The constant, k, is a number (determined for each test condition) that causes the ratio to equal 1 when maximal nasalization occurs. The HONC index can be continuously derived either by a relatively uncomplicated analog system (Redenbaugh & Reich, 1985) or by a computer. Implementation is, therefore, quite simple and direct.

The block diagram of Horii's (1980) original instrumentation (Figure 11–6) illustrates its operating principles. A master amplifier is provided for separately boosting the output of both accelerometers, but the signal from the neck transducer is first amplified by a variable preamplifier. This additional gain represents k in the mathematical equation. After amplification, the signals from the two channels are independently rectified and smoothed to provide the DC amplitude of each. An analog divider circuit then generates the ratio, $k(A_{\text{rms}(n)}/A_{\text{rms}(v)})$, of the two voltages. A special circuit acts as a voice detector and produces an output only when the neck accelerometer is active. This output is used to control an electronic switch that cuts off the divider output if a voiceless sound is being produced. The display system therefore shows the ratio only during phonated speech segments. Of late, such analog circuitry has largely been replaced by interactive computer manipulation of the digitized accelerometric signals.

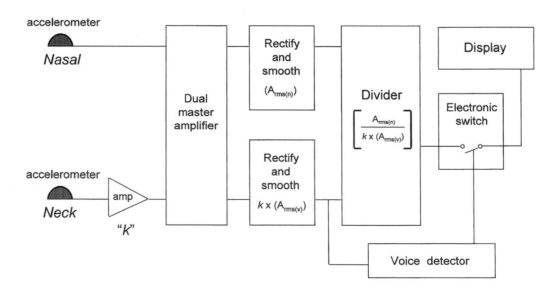

Figure 11–6. Functional block diagram of the HONC system.

---

[3]This ratio has also been called the *nasal accelerometric vibrational index* (*NAVI*).

Test Method

The nasal accelerometer is attached with adhesive tape to the external surface of the nose, somewhat above the ala. Redenbaugh and Reich (1985) pointed out that the accelerometer site should be chosen with some care. Septal deviation, for instance, is not uncommon in patients with velopharyngeal insufficiency. The nasal accelerometer should be located on the more patent side (Horii, 1990). The vocal accelerometer should be located between the thyroid cartilage and the sternal notch or at any location where tactile evaluation shows strong vibration during phonation. The patient then sustains /m/ or /n/ at a loud, but still comfortable vocal level as the variable (voice) amplifier (whose gain represents k) is adjusted until the display shows a maximal output. This represents a ratio of 1, indicating maximal nasalization. It is important that a moderately loud /m/ or /n/ be used for this adjustment to insure that the system will not later be overdriven by greater degrees of vocal effort. If necessary, the master amplifier may be adjusted to change the scale width on the display device without altering the relationship of nasal and vocal signals. Full-scale deflection on the display represents complete nasalization (HONC = 1 or 100%) and

no deflection indicates total denasalization (HONC = 0). Using /m/ or /n/ as the basis for calibration allows the system to be employed with normal subjects and with those who have velopharyngeal incompetence. The fully nasalized reference condition also provides a basis for comparison of results over time and across subjects. If there is a need to evaluate denasality, a fully oralized sound can be used as the baseline reference.

Output

A sample HONC output is shown in Figure 11–7. Horii (1980) also described the simultaneous display of the HONC trace with a corresponding speech spectrogram to facilitate phonetic segmentation. However, mean HONC data have only been reported rarely and are often difficult to compare to published reports that have expressed values in both dB and as a percentage score.

HONC Index in dB. Horii and Lang (1981) provide average HONC values of -22.8 ± 2.7 and -17.2 ± 2.6 dB for 10 young women reciting the Zoo and Rainbow passages, respectively. For similar spoken material, Sussman (1995) reported similar scores for both men and women, whereas, for nasal utterances,

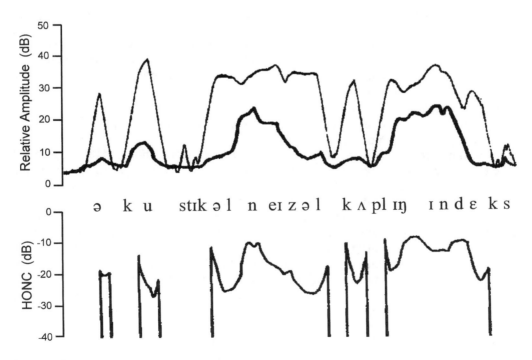

Figure 11–7. Examples of HONC output. The upper trace shows nasal (heavy line) and oral (thinner line) sound pressure levels. The lower trace is the corresponding HONC index in dB. Discontinuities are produced by the electronic switch that disables the instrument during voiceless sounds. Adapted from "An Accelerometric Approach to Nasality Measurement: A Preliminary Report," by Y. Horii, 1980, *Cleft Palate Journal, 17,* 254–261. Figure 6, p. 259. Used with permission.

HONC values of about −7 dB appear to be typical. For a normal group of ten boys and girls (4–6 years of age), Mra, Sussman, and Fenwick (1998) derived mean HONC values consistent with those of adults; roughly −6.3 and −19.3 dB for nasal and nonnasal sentences, respectively. As with the adults, there was no significant sex effect. For sustained /ɑ/ productions, Sussman (1995) reported mean HONC values of −21.7 ± 8.9 dB for 20 normal men and −22.0 ± 9.2 dB for 20 normal women, and significantly different scores for sustained /i/, that averaged −15.7 ± 4.9 and − ± 5.4 dB for the same men and women, respectively.

HONC Index in percent. In a study of 19 older adults (mean age 71 ± 9 years), Thompson and Murdoch (1995) derived mean percent HONC values of 26.6 ± 12.9% for nonnasal and 96.4 ± 31.5% for highly-nasal test utterances. Theodoros, Murdoch and Thompson (1995) found similar results for the 23 adults in their control group (mean 67 ± 8 years) and additionally report mean values of 32.1 ± 22.7, 43.8 ± 24.7, and 41.7 ± 25.5% for the vowels /ɑ/, /i/, and /u/, respectively, repeated at a rate of approximately 3 syllables per second.

Interpretation of the HONC index. The results of both Thompson and Murdoch (1995) and of Sussman (1995) are consistent with studies that have documented a relatively greater nasal accelerometric signal for high vowels (Stevens et al., 1976; Larson & Hamlet, 1987). As Larson and Hamlet (1987) point out, it is important to remember that, while the amplitude of the nasal accelerometer signal "reflects the degree of *acoustical* coupling," it cannot be used to directly assess "comparative velopharyngeal openness across vowels" (p. 289). Because some vocal energy is always transmitted to the nasal tissues (even during normally non-nasal speech) the HONC value only rarely reaches 0 in actual practice. In addition, since tissue transmission characteristics and the orientation of the transducer can change with patient movement and with muscle tension adjustments, it is possible for the HONC ratio to slightly exceed a value of 1. Furthermore, additional study is needed to document the extent to which the amplitude of the throat accelerometric signal may be influenced by factors other than vocal intensity, such as the quality and mode of phonation (Matthies, Perkell, & Williams, 1991; Krakow & Huffman, 1993) and artifacts attributable to laryngeal movement associated with changes in vocal frequency and supraglottal articulatory behavior (Horii, 1990).

The Accelerometric Difference Index

Citing the known and potential problems associated with dual throat and nasal accelerometer methods, Horii (1987, 1990) has suggested using only a nasal transducer while controlling for the effect of vocal intensity through careful selection of speech materials and tasks. Indeed, Till, Jafari, and Law-Till (1994) have recently proposed a measure that requires only a single nasal accelerometer. Noting no significant difference in the accelerometric output between a prolonged /m/ and the production of a sentence loaded with nasal consonants, they reasoned that a nasal sentence of this type could serve as a calibration reference for a given speaker. Thus, the accelerometric output for a highly-nasal utterance ("No more moms near") is compared with a signal obtained for a non-nasal sentence ("Show boats bob well") spoken with similar speech intensity. The measure, a decibel pressure ratio they call the ***Accelerometric Difference Index (ADI)***, is defined as

$$\text{ADI(dB)} = 20 \times \log\left(\frac{A_{\text{rms}(+n)}}{A_{\text{rms}(-n)}}\right),$$

where $A_{\text{rms}(+n)}$ is the root mean square amplitude of the nasal accelerometer output for the "nasal" utterance and $A_{\text{rms}(-n)}$ is the rms output for the "non-nasal" utterance. Like the HONC procedure, voiceless and silent intervals are excluded from the rms averaging. The limited data that Till and his colleagues (1994) obtained from 5 normal and 5 hypernasal subjects are promising with regard to the correspondence of ADI and listeners' direct magnitude estimation ratings of nasality, but further investigation and refinement of technique will clearly be necessary before it finds utility in the clinical setting.

Velopharyngeal Timing

Using instrumentation and procedure similar to that of Horii (1980), Zimmerman, Karnell and Rettaliata (1984) assessed the time between the onset of the neck accelerometric signal and the onset of the nasal accelerometric signal. Their results suggested that the perception of disordered nasalization may be related to the timing between voice onset and velopharyngeal closure. Specifically, they showed that nasal speakers with cleft palate may achieve velopharyngeal closure after the onset of voicing, whereas cleft palate speakers whose speech is normal attain closure before voice onset. Should further investigation show this measure to provide a reasonable estimate of whether velopharyngeal closure occurs before or after the onset of voicing and should it be shown that onset differences of short duration are indeed relevant to perceived hypernasality, accelerometric timing measures of this sort may gain greater currency in the clinical assessment of velopharyngeal function.

The Nasal Oral Ratio Meter

Karling and his colleagues (Karling, Lohmander, de Serpa-Leitão, Galyas, & Larson, 1985; Karling, Larson, Leanderson, Galyas, & de Serpa-Leitão, 1993) describe an instrument, the **Nasal Oral RAtio Meter (NORAM)**, that uses signals from a pair of nasal and throat accelerometers to assess nasality. Unlike the accelerometric measures described previously, NORAM determines the ratio of the duration of *nasalized* segments to the total duration of *vocalized* segments over the course of a spoken utterance. It is the belief of the developers that, by relying on the duration of the signals rather than on their respective amplitudes, the sensitivity of the resulting measure to the influences of speaker anatomy and accelerometer placement will be reduced. The veracity of this assumption, as well as the supposed superiority of NORAM over other accelerometric methods of evaluating nasality, remain largely untested, however.

With accelerometers positioned over the nasal and laryngeal alae, the NORAM device amplifies and conditions both the nasal and laryngeal signals equally. The signals are lowpass filtered at 500 Hz, rectified, and lowpass filtered once again at 15 Hz before being sent to a comparator (see Chapter 2, "Analog Electronics") that is used to detect the presence or absence of significant accelerometric energy (Figure 11–8.) The "significance" of the energy is determined both by the user and the instrument. In particular, the duration of the laryngeal signal is recorded when it exceeds a certain threshold level (set by the examiner to avoid residual instrumentation noise) and the duration of the

nasal signal is measured when its amplitude differs from the laryngeal signal by no more than 9 dB. The device then provides a **nasal percentage (n%)** measure, defined as

$$n\% = \frac{t_N}{t_L} \times 100,$$

where t_N is total time over which the nasal signal is detected and t_L is total time that the laryngeal signal is greater than the set threshold.

In a study of 18 normal Swedish speakers, Karling et al. (1985) reported a mean nasal percentage of 5.6% for passages of three 6-word sentences containing no nasal phonemes. The mean n% subsequently increased to 14.5 and 25.7% when the sentences included one and two nasal consonants, respectively. Karling et al. (1993) have since suggested that a nasal percentage greater than 10% appears to represent an unacceptable level of nasality for any spoken utterance devoid of nasal phones. Preliminary clinical tests suggest that NORAM may be best used to compare hypernasal patients before and after medical or behavioral management (Karling et al., 1993; Lohmander-Agerskov, Dotevall, Lith, & Söderpalm, 1996).

Aerodynamic Tests

Lowering the velum not only results in the propagation of the phonatory signal through the nasal cavity, it also diverts at least part of the airstream through the

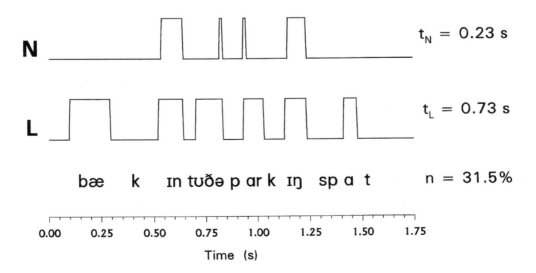

Figure 11–8. An example of a NORAM display for the utterance "back into the parking spot." The nasal (N, above) and laryngeal (L, below) signals represent comparator outputs (see text).

nose. Nasal escape of air, and the attendant rise of the intranasal air pressure can, therefore, serve as indicators of nasalization. The physics of air pressure and flow is reviewed in Chapters 8 and 9, as are the principles of their measurement. This section will deal primarily with the special application of specific airflow, air volume, and air pressure methods for the evaluation of velopharyngeal activity.

NASAL AIRFLOW

Nasal airflow measurement is done in order to detect and quantify **nasal emission** (alternatively called **nasal escape**) of air. McDonald and Koepp-Baker (1951, p. 12) have suggested that this term "be restrictively employed to describe the escape of air through the nasal passages when the speaker attempts to produce any sound requiring intra-oral breath pressure such as plosives or fricatives." Nasal emission may be monitored with a pneumotachograph (Warren, 1967; Lubker & Schweiger, 1969; Warren, Duany, & Fischer, 1969; Lubker, Schweiger, & Morris, 1970; Dickson, Barron, & McGlone, 1978; Thompson & Hixon, 1979; Gilbert & Hoodin, 1984; Laine, Warren, Dalston, & Morr, 1988a, 1988b; Hoodin & Gilbert, 1989; Ruscello, Shuster, & Sandwisch, 1991; Hoit, Watson, Hixon, McMahon, & Johnson, 1994; Woisard et al., 1998) or with a warm-wire anemometer (Kelleher, Webster, Coffey, & Quigley, 1960; Quigley, Webster, Coffey, Kelleher, & Grant, 1963; Quigley, Shiere, Webster, & Cobb, 1964; Ellis, Flack, Curle, & Selley, 1978; Hutters & Bróndsted, 1992) fitted to a nose mask or a divided oral/nasal face mask (also called a **split mask**).[4] Masks of these types can be purchased commercially or custom fabricated by the clinician. (Kastner, Putnam and Shelton (1985), for instance, provide detailed instructions for constructing different types of masks that may be necessary for certain patients with facial anomalies or for those who are otherwise difficult to fit adequately with a standard mask assembly.)

At first glance it might seem that the amount of nasal emission might be very directly related to the degree of velopharyngeal opening and would, therefore, serve by itself as an excellent index of the degree of nasalization. More careful consideration of the relationship of oral and nasal pathway aerodynamics, schematized in Figure 11–9, shows why such an expectation in unlikely to be realized. Assume that the vocal tract posture is fixed, as indicated in the figure. There is

a small velopharyngeal opening between essentially wide-open nasal and oral airways. Air under pressure streams up from the lower pharynx. Because the oral airway is unobstructed, it presents very little resistance to this flow. But some small fraction of the airstream will be pushed by the pressure through the slightly open velopharyngeal orifice. (The resistance through the opening is high, but it is not infinite; some small amount of air gets through.) The flow-pressure relationship (discussed in Chapter 9, "Airflow and Volume") indicates that the flow through the velopharyngeal port will be

$$U_n = \frac{P_{io}}{R_{vp}}.$$

That is, the airflow through the nose, U_n, is equal to the intraoral pressure, P_{io}, divided by the resistance of the velopharyngeal port, R_{vp}. (It is assumed for the moment that the nasal passage, being totally unobstructed, has no resistance of its own to complicate the situation.) The nasal airflow, then, will vary not only because of a change in the velopharyngeal resistance (which, in turn, reflects the amount of port opening), but with a change in oropharyngeal pressure as well (Warren, Hinton, Pillsbury, & Hairfield, 1987; Laine et al., 1988a, 1988b). Since a given speaker's oral pressure varies from phone to phone and also changes with the amount of vocal effort, it is clear that these variables

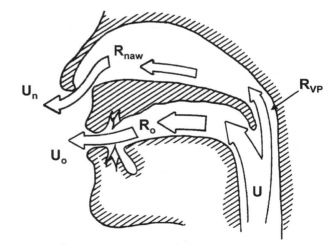

Figure 11–9. Airflows (U) and resistances (R) in the upper vocal tract.

---

[4]Although there are some reports of the use of warm-wire systems arranged in front of the nostrils without the use of a nose or split face mask (Subtelny et al., 1968; Subtelny, Kho, McCormack, & Subtelny, 1969; Worth, Runyon, & Subtelny, 1968; Ellis et al., 1978), the validity of such instrumentation is highly questionable (see Hardy, 1967).

likewise significantly affect the rate of nasal airflow. There is also reason to believe that velopharyngeal insufficiency may actually induce greater respiratory effort (Warren, Wood, & Bradley, 1969; Minsley, Warren, & Hinton, 1988) and vocal strain (Sapienza, Brown, Williams, Wharton, & Turner, 1996; McHenry, 1997).

The problems do not end here, however. Even if the intraoral air pressure were to remain constant, the amount of air being forced through the velopharyngeal port would vary according to the degree of oral constriction—including, for example, the amount of lip rounding or tongue elevation. This is because increasing oral constriction implies higher oral pathway resistance. As the oral resistance rises, more and more of the air finds it less "inconvenient" to squeeze through the velopharyngeal resistance. Hence, nasal airflow also reflects oral port constriction, which changes not only for different phones, but also from one production to another of the same phone (Selley, Zananiri, Ellis, & Flack, 1987). Furthermore, oral port constriction can be abnormal in cleft palate patients (Warren & Mackler, 1968; Honjo & Isshiki, 1971; Claypoole, Warren, & Bradley, 1974; Trost, 1981; Kawano et al., 1997). A way out of the tangle, namely the simultaneous measurement of *nasal and oral* airstream dynamics, will be discussed later.

There remains yet another difficulty. It was assumed earlier that the nasal passages were wide open and presented no resistance of their own to the flow of nasal air. In the anatomically normal individual this is a useful approximation of the truth. But patients with structural anomalies of the velopharynx (who are, after all, very likely to be the subjects of evaluation) are also likely to have nasal defects such as a deviated septum, bony spurs, mucous membrane thickening, and the like (Powers, 1962; Morris, 1968). They are, in short, the very individuals for whom the assumption of a wide open nasal cavity is least likely to be valid. Transnasal flow will decrease as nasal resistance increases, even if the velopharyngeal port is wide open. A speaker with a relatively high nasal resistance to airflow, therefore, will require less respiratory effort to produce nonnasal consonants—and will therefore generate less nasal air emission—than another speaker with the same degree of incompetency but with negligible nasal resistance. Thus, because nasal airway resistance is a function of the patency of both the velopharynx and the nasal passages, nasal airflow measures may reflect many aspects of vocal tract structure and function, all confounded in ways that can be very complex (Warren & Ryon, 1967).

Despite all the caveats and limitations, nasal airflow measures are likely to be useful if interpreted conservatively (Laine et al., 1988b). They seem particularly suited for assessing the effects of speech therapy or medicosurgical management in a given case (Smith, Skef, Cohen, & Dorf, 1985; Woisard et al., 1998). Emanuel and Counihan (1970) studied peak oral and nasal airflows using a split face mask and calibrated warm-wire anemometers. Normal adult subjects produced the six English plosives in combination with /i/ or /ɑ/; measurement was at the point of maximal oral flow. Their data are summarized in Table 11–4.

Thompson and Hixon (1979) also evaluated nasal airflow. Their subjects were 92 normal boys and girls aged 3 to 18 years and 20 men and women aged 18 to 37 years, who sustained /i, s, z, n/, repeated /ti, di, si, zi, ni/, and produced repetitions of /iti, idi, isi, izi, ini/ in a carrier phrase. Flow was measured with a nasal mask and pneumotachograph. Like Machida (1967), Emanuel and Counihan (1970), and Mueller (1971) before them, they detected no nasal flow at all except during utterances with a nasal phoneme. Therefore, they concluded, "the anticipated clinical observation in normal velopharyngeal closure on oral sounds would be no flow. However, a small amount of flow should not be interpreted to mean velopharyngeal incompetence" (p. 419). Lotz, Shaughnessy, and Netsell (1981) also warn that "most normal adults close completely for oral productions, but small and inconsistent leaks can be expected." In a study of 80 normal men and women 22 to 97 years of age, Hoit et al. (1994) reported similar findings in oral contexts with no significant age-related differences in nasal airflow.

Warren (1967) has explored the relationship of nasal emission to the area of the velopharyngeal port. He studied 28 subjects, aged 8 to 47 years, with surgically repaired or prosthetically closed palatal clefts, who produced the word /pɑpɑ/ while peak nasal airflow of the initial /p/ was measured with a pneumotachograph. Simultaneous estimates of the velopharyngeal orifice area (by a method discussed later) were derived. His results indicate that the degree of nasal emission is strongly correlated to velopharyngeal port size only when the area of the latter is less than 20 mm². When the area of the opening is greater, the nasal airflow is a poor indicator. The same situation seems to prevail in cases of oronasal fistulas (Shelton & Blank, 1984).

Even if nasal airflow is not highly valid as a discriminator of the degree of velopharyngeal opening, there is little reason to doubt that it can distinguish competent from incompetent velopharyngeal closure (Hoodin & Gilbert, 1989). Lubker and Schweiger (1969), whose data are summarized in Table 11–5, illustrated the magnitude of the differences that may be observed. The peak airflow during the several utterances was obtained by a nose mask and pneumotachograph. Normal subjects were free of speech defect

Table 11–4. Mean Peak Oral and Nasal Airflow in Normal English Speakers*

Target Syllable	Mean Peak Airflow (in mL/s)†			
	Men		**Women**	
	Oral	**Nasal**	**Oral**	**Nasal**
/pi/	936	17	690	26
/ti/	1045	5	798	16
/ki/	644	2	576	8
/bi/	437	6	324	10
/di/	370	14	215	15
/gi/	293	6	216	4
/pɑ/	1103	26	880	18
/tɑ/	1324	6	1162	16
/kɑ/	1144	7	904	5
/bɑ/	598	8	346	7
/dɑ/	425	23	232	17
/gɑ/	415	9	258	5
/ipi/	304	10	237	20
/iti/	324	4	276	7
/iki/	221	3	189	4
/ibi/	166	8	103	5
/idi/	112	12	66	10
/igi/	116	10	85	7
/ɑpɑ/	357	17	270	14
/ɑtɑ/	441	7	420	5
/ɑkɑ/	363	8	310	6
/ɑbɑ/	218	12	110	6
/ɑdɑ/	148	18	77	11
/ɑgɑ/	118	9	82	4

*Modified from Emanuel and Counihan, 1970. Twenty-five men and 25 women, ages 20 to 36 years. Split face mask, calibrated warm-wire anemometer used for flow measurement. Conversational loudness, comfortable pitch. Data derived at point of maximal oral airflow.

†Data converted from L/min.

or distortion; cleft palate subjects were all prosthetically managed by means of a fixed-type obturator and their speech quality was perceptually categorized as "good, fair, or poor." For all but one of the tasks the cleft palate subjects had significantly higher nasal flow rates ($p < .01$) than the normal speakers. The exception, surprisingly, occurred for /m/, during which the prosthetically managed cleft palate speakers had significantly lower ($p < .05$) nasal flow rates than normals. This probably reflects the restriction of velopharyngeal port size by the prosthesis.

In summary, nasal airflow rate, like any solitary measure, is only a fair predictor of how a listener will judge the severity of nasality. It is nonetheless an important contributor to that judgment. It can also serve grossly to differentiate good, fair, and poor velopharyngeal function in cleft palate speakers, and it can clearly distinguish such speakers from normals. However, as Warren (1989) points out, while peak nasal flow rates above 150 mL/s or so during nonnasal consonant production may indicate velopharyngeal incompetence, nasal airflows well under 150 mL/s do not necessarily portend adequate velopharyngeal function. That is, it is quite possible that a speaker with gross velopharyngeal incompetence can produce low nasal airflows when there is substantial nasal cavity obstruction and/or speech is produced using reduced respiratory effort.

Table 11–5. Mean Peak Nasal Airflow for Normal and Prosthetically Managed Cleft Palate Speakers*

| | Mean Peak Nasal Airflow (in mL/s)[†] | |
Utterance	Normal Adults	Prosthetically Managed Adults
/ɑ/	1.8	4.8 ±5
/i/	0.3	65.8 ±65
/u/	1.8	48.3 ±46
/æ/	1.3	8.3 ±24
/s/	0.3	164.0 ±188
/z/	6.3	137.5 ±143
/isi/	2.8	187.7 ±184
/izi/	6.5	162.8 ±157
/ipi/	2.8	206.7 ±176
/ibi/	4.8	121.8 ±104
/æsæ/	7.5	154.2 ±175
/æzæ/	5.3	123.5 ±155
/æpæ/	7.7	176.7 ±172
/æbæ/	6.7	117.8 ±106
/m/	211.5	168.0 ±75

*Modified from Lubker and Schweiger, 1969. Thirty-six subjects (18 men, 18 women) in each group; ages 8 to 44 years (mean 19 years). Nose mask and pneumotachograph used for flow measurement.

[†]Data converted from L/min. Airflow for prosthetically managed subjects reported as mean ± SD (rounded to the nearest integer).

NASAL PATENCY

Of the several threats to valid nasal airflow measures, the nasal resistance factor is the most difficult to control for in testing. It can, however, be measured. Clinicians might wish to do so in order to determine the extent to which the resistance of the nasal cavity facilitates nonnasal speech. Nasal patency is also of obvious importance in cases of clinical denasality, where the clinician must determine if the problem is tied to velopharyngeal malfunction or to nasal obstruction.

Nasal/Oral Air Volume Ratios

A fairly simple screening test for nasal patency can be performed with a spirometer (Davies, 1978). The maximal volume that can be inhaled in 0.5 s (the half-second *forced inspiratory volume*, $FIV_{0.5}$) is measured, first through the nose alone ($N-FIV_{0.5}$), and then through the mouth alone ($M-FIV_{0.5}$). The *Nasal*

Patency Index (*NPI*) is defined as the ratio of nasal to oral forced inspiratory volume:

$$\text{NPI} = \frac{N-FIV_{0.5}}{M-FIV_{0.5}}.$$

Because the resistance of the nasal passage is normally greater than that of the oral airway, the NPI is much less than unity in normal subjects. Davies (1978) found the NPI to range from 0.19 to 0.74 (mean = 0.47; SD = 0.15) in 11 healthy men. Values below this range may signal nasal obstruction.

More recently, Oluwole, Gardiner, and White (1997) assessed nasal patency using a ratio of nasal to oral *one-second* forced inspiratory volumes (that is, N-FIV_1/M-FIV_1) that they call the **naso-oral index**. For 10 patients who underwent rhinosurgery from nasal obstruction, the naso-oral index increased from a preoperative average of 0.52 to 0.55 following surgery. Based on their results, Oluwole and his colleages concluded that the naso-oral index "correlates acceptably well" with rhinomanometric measures of nasal airway resistance and may be *"potentially* useful in measuring patients' benefit from surgery."

Rhinomanometry

Rhinomanometry is the most commonly used procedure to measure the resistance of the nasal airway. The technique requires the measurement of airflow through the nose along with the simultaneous driving pressure (Tonndorf, 1958; Cass, 1967; Glass & Teller, 1969; Ingelstedt, Jonson, & Rundcrantz, 1969; Kortekangas, 1972; Kern, 1973; Cockcroft, MacCormack, Tarlo, Hargreave, & Pengelly, 1979; Hamilton, 1979; Kumlien & Schiratzki, 1979; Broms, Ivarsson, & Jonson, 1982; Connell, 1982; Warren, 1984; Pallanch, McCaffrey, & Kern, 1985; Berkinshaw, Spalding, & Vig, 1987; Smith, Fiala, & Guyette, 1989; Shelton & Eiser, 1992; Lai & Corey, 1993; Naito & Iwata, 1997).

Posterior Rhinomanometry

The resistance of the entire nasal airway can be measured using the instrumentation diagrammed in Figure 11–10 with a technique known as **posterior rhinomanometry**. One catheter is used to sense oropharyngeal pressure, while another is attached to a tightly fitting nose mask, as shown. The two catheters are connected to a differential pressure transducer that senses the pressure difference (ΔP) between the oropharynx and the nares. A pneumotachograph at the outlet of the nose mask measures the nasal airflow (U_n). The total nasal airway resistance (R_{naw}) can then be determined as

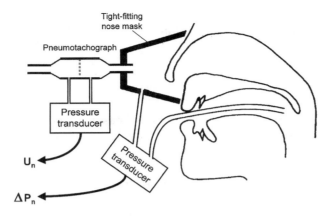

Figure 11–10. Determination of nasal airway resistance using posterior rhinomanometry.

Table 11–6. Nasal Airway Resistance (in cmH$_2$O/L/s)*

Age Range	Normal		Cleft Palate	
	Mean	SD	Mean	SD
9–11	3.0	0.4	4.9	2.1[†]
12–13	2.4	0.6	3.6	1.1
Over 15	2.0	1.1	3.5	1.8[†]

*Compiled from raw data in Warren, Duany, and Fischer, 1969. Male and female subjects combined; Resistance measured when nasal flow = 0.5 L/s.

[†]Difference between normal and cleft palate group statistically significant ($p<.05$). No significant sex differences. Note that there is a clear tendency for nasal resistance to diminish with age.

$$R_{naw} = \frac{\Delta P}{U_n}.$$

The resistance of the velopharyngeal orifice is coupled in series to the parallel resistances of the right and left nasal passages of the nasal cavity. The total nasal airway resistance is thus the sum of resistances of the velopharynx and the nasal cavity.

Among clinical and experimental rhinologists, it has become common practice to assess nasal airway during quiet breathing. Unfortunately, as the absolute flow rate increases, nonuniformities in the dimensions of the nasal airway cause the transnasal flow to become increasingly turbulent. This results in a curvilinear (sigmoid) pressure-flow relationship. Consequently, when derived using the equation above (that assumes a wholly laminar flow), R_{naw} increases nonlinearly with the flow rate. Because R_{naw} data have been reported using a variety of transnasal pressures and flows, resistance values have been difficult to interpret and to compare. While some clinicians and investigators have derived R_{naw} at the prevailing pressures and flows at peak expiration or inspiration (Hasegawa, Kern, & O'Brien, 1979; Vig & Zajac, 1993), others have reported various measures derived from the $\Delta P/U_n$ curve (Solomon & Stohrer, 1965; Broms, Jonson, & Lamm, 1982; Newcombe, O'Neill, Tolley, & Montgomery, 1997). Most others, however, have attempted to standardize the measure by using a reference differential pressure (usually 1.5 cmH$_2$O) or, more commonly, a fixed flow reference (usually 250 or 500 mL/s). If the patient is a child, her age is also important for purposes of data comparison, as nasal resistance values have been shown to decrease dramatically from infancy to young adulthood (Polgar & Kong, 1965; Principato & Wolf, 1985; Vig & Zajac, 1993). Warren and his coworkers (1969) measured the R_{naw} of 29 nor-

mal subjects and of 27 patients with different types of repaired and untreated palatal clefts when the transnasal flow was 500 mL/s. The resultant data, summarized in Table 11–6, may be useful when evaluating other clinical cases.

There have also been attempts to measure nasal airway resistance during specially selected speech tasks. Lotz and her colleagues (1981), for instance, used a nose mask, pneumotachograph, and oral pressure probe to assess nasal airway resistance in 15 men and 15 women, all normal speakers. Their measurement of a mean resistance of 3.1 cmH$_2$O/L/s ($SD = 0.3$) at the midpoint of sustained /m/ production and 3.9 cmH$_2$O/L/s ($SD = 0.4$) at peak pressure and flow during quiet breathing confirmed their assumption that velopharyngeal resistance can be considered negligible during production of a nasal phone. It is, as these researchers put it, a "happy finding" in that it demonstrates that an accurate measure of minimal nasal cavity resistance can be obtained during a few seconds of sustained /m/. This is much easier to achieve than trying to get subjects to breathe quietly while maintaining an open velopharynx without disturbing the oral pressure sensing tube with their tongue. Allison and Leeper (1990) found similar results for 20 normal young women in a study that placed tighter control over the flow rates used in R_{naw} measurement. Using reference flow rates of 150 and 250 mL/s, they, too, found no significant difference between the speech and breathing tasks, reporting a mean resistance of 2.4 cmH$_2$O/L/s ($SD = 1.4$) and 2.2 cmH$_2$O/L/s ($SD = 1.1$) for sustained /m/ and quiet breathing, respectively.

Anterior Rhinomanometry

If the patency of each of the nasal passages is of particular interest, another technique called *anterior rhi-*

nomanometry may be used. As illustrated in Figure 11–11, one nostril is occluded by a connector to a pressure transducer. Since that nasal passage is now blocked, the pressure recorded there (P_n) is the same as at the nasopharynx; that is, at the opposite choana—the entrance to the unoccluded nasal passage for which airway resistance is to be measured. Transnasal airflow (U_n) can be transduced using a pneumotachograph connected via a nasal mask (as shown) or a "flow nozzle" inserted into the unoccluded naris.

The combined (binasal) resistance of the nasal cavity (R_{nc}) may be calculated using the equation for the sum of parallel resistances (see Chapter 2, "Analog Electronics"). That is,

$$R_{nc} = \frac{R_{nr} \times R_{nl}}{R_{nr} + R_{nl}},$$

where R_{nr} and R_{nl} are the unilateral resistances of the right and left nasal passages, respectively. The caveats that apply to posterior rhinomanometry apply here as well. It is therefore very important that the pressure be measured at the same flow rate on both sides for the calculated R_{nc} value to be a valid indicator of nasal cavity resistance. Also, for obvious reasons, anterior rhinomanometry cannot be used with patients who have a perforated nasal septum or a complete obstruction of a nasal passage.

Based on an assessment of 974 patients using anterior rhinomanometry, McCaffrey and Kern (1979) reported that a unilateral nasal resistance greater than approximately 7 cmH$_2$O/L/s tends to be associated with "definite sympoms of nasal obstruction." However, in cases where the obstruction is binasal, symptoms tend to occur at lower levels of unilateral resistance.

Although the technique leaves the oral cavity unencumbered, it requires the insertion of at least one plug into the patient's nostril. Because the plug must be positioned well within the naris to ensure an airtight seal, significant distortion of the cartilaginous part of the nose, especially of the septum, can result (Craig, Dvorak, & McIlreath, 1965; Kern, 1973; Broms et al., 1982). This, of course, will affect the resistance of the opposite nasal passage which, of course, is what we are attempting to measure.

Acoustic Rhinometry

Hilberg and his colleagues (Hilberg, Jackson, Swift, & Pedersen, 1989) first reported the use of an acoustic reflection technique to assess nasal patency. Called ***acoustic rhinometry***, the procedure involves directing a short, wide-band acoustic impulse into a nostril by means of a nosepiece. The impulse is then reflected by changes in acoustic impedance that result from differences in nasal cross-sectional area. By comparing the time course of outgoing and incoming waves it becomes possible to determine the size of, and distance to, each change in cross-sectional area. In this way, acoustic rhinometry provides a 2-dimensional topographical portrait of nasal geometry—that is, the cross-sectional area as a function of distance from the tested naris. The area-by-distance portrait generated by the rhinometer has been referred to as a ***rhinogram*** (Figure 11–12). By integrating the rhinogram, the nasal volume can be determined (Corey, Gungor, Nelson, Fredberg, & Lai, 1997; Corey, Kemker, Nelson, & Gungor, 1997; Gilain et al., 1997; Shemen & Hamburg, 1997; Kim, Kang, & Yoon, 1998), whereas the symmetry of the nasal passages can be assessed by comparing right and left rhinograms (Kunkel & Hochban, 1994a, 1994b; Roithmann, Cole, Chapnik, Bareto, Szalai, &

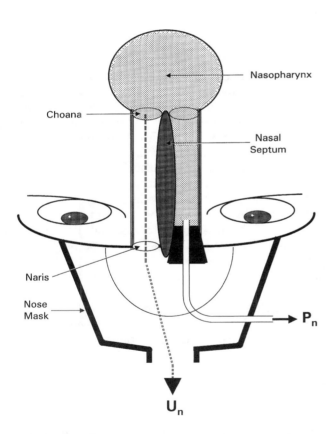

Figure 11–11. Measuring unilateral nasal passage resistance using anterior rhinomanometry. The drawing is a highly schematized view of the nasal passages and nasopharynx viewed from above. Because, in this case, the left naris is occluded, the pressure sensed there is equal to the pressure in the nasopharynx (shaded area). By measuring the nasopharyngeal pressure (P_n) and the flow through the unoccluded passage (U_n), the resistance of the right nasal passage (R_{nr}) can be determined.

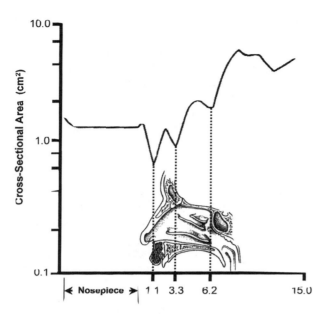

Figure 11-12. An example of a normal nasogram documenting the cross-sectional area across a single nasal passage and the nasopharynx. Structures are shown schematically below the area-distance function. From left to right, the first dashed line represents the point of minimal cross-sectional area, the second line represents the beginning of the inferior turbinate, and the last line indicates the posterior end of the assessed nasal passage. The substantial increase in cross-sectional area beyond approximately 7 cm reflects the dimensions of the nasopharynx. (Based on the work of Grymer et al., 1989, and Seaver et al., 1995.)

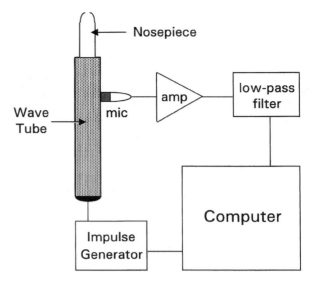

Figure 11-13. A functional block diagram of an acoustic rhinometry system.

Zamel, 1994; Kunkel, Wahlmann, & Wagner, 1997; Malm, 1997b). Furthermore, since the technique specifies cross-sectional area, nasal resistance can also be determined (Roithmann et al., 1994; Shemen & Hamburg, 1997).

Despite the novelty of acoustic rhinometry, it has spawned a fairly substantial international literature and has led to the development of several commercially available units, such as the ***Eccovision*** (Hood Laboratories, Pembroke, MA), ***Rhin2000*** (RhinoMetrics A/S, Lynge, Denmark), and ***Rhinoklack*** (Stimotron Medizinische Geräte, Wendelstein, Germany) acoustic rhinometers. Although the specific designs and specifications may vary, rhinometer systems, such as schematized in Figure 11-13, consist of an impulse (spark) generator, a long wave tube connected to a nosepiece, a microphone, an amplifier, and a computer.

There are several reasons why this new technique continues to gain popularity. Not only can the procedure can be performed quickly—a single measurement takes less than 10 ms—and simply, but it is also

relatively comfortable for the patient who, furthermore, does not need to learn or perform a specific task or maneuver (Grymer, Hilberg, Elbrønd, & Pedersen, 1989; Hilberg, Grymer, Pedersen, & Elbrønd, 1990; Elbrønd, Hilberg, & Felding, 1991). This makes acoustic rhinometry particularly well suited for the assessment of newborn and young children (Riechelmann, Rheinheimer, & Wolfensberger, 1993; Buenting, Dalston, & Drake, 1994; Pedersen, Berkowitz, Yamagiwa, & Hilberg, 1994; Djupesland & Lyholm, 1997; Kim et al., 1998). Because the assessment of nasal patency by acoustic rhinometry does not depend on transnasal airflow, the technique may be applied to patients with severe or even complete nasal obstruction. Also, unlike rhinomanometric methods that only provide information about the *smallest* cross-sectional area of the nasal airway, acoustic rhinometry specifies not only the size, but the location of local area fluctuations. This is particularly important to the speech pathologist, since resonance characteristics are likely to be quite different for constrictions in the anterior nasal cavity as opposed to those in the proximity of the velopharyneal orifice.

Although a nosepiece must be used to channel the acoustic energy into the nasal cavity, an *acoustic* rather than an *air-tight* seal is required. Thus significant anterior nasal distortion may be avoided since the wavetube connector does not need to be inserted into the nasal vestibule, especially if petroleum jelly or a silicone-based sealant is used (Fisher, Morris, Biemans, Palmer, & Lund, 1995; Hamilton, McRae, & Jones, 1997). Work nonetheless continues toward improving nosepiece design and minimizing artifacts attributable to breathing, head movement, and posture (Kase, Hilberg, & Pedersen, 1994; Fisher et al., 1995; Roithmann, Cole, Chapnik, Shpirer, Hoffstein, & Zamel, 1995; Roithmann, Shpirer, Cole, Chapnik, Szalai, & Zamel, 1997; Tomkinson & Eccles, 1995; Djupesland, Kaastad, & Franzen, 1997; Djupesland & Lyholm, 1997).

Experimental and clinical data suggest that even small variations in cross-sectional area can be reliably measured by acoustic rhinometry (Lenders & Pirsig, 1990; Yamagiwa, Hilberg, Pedersen, & Lundqvist, 1990; Kase et al., 1994; Kunkel & Hochban, 1994a; Roithmann et al., 1994; Grymer, 1995). In vivo data indicate that the technique provides a resolution of at least 7 mm (Fisher, Daly, Morris, & Lund, 1994), allowing for the determination of nasal obstruction, congestion, or septal abnormalities. Although methodological issues remain, initial studies have indicated that an equivalent or superior assessment of nasal airway geometry or patency can be obtained with acoustic rhinometry when compared with anterior rhinomanometry (Scadding, Darby, & Austin, 1994), posterior rhinomanometry (Austin & Foreman, 1994), plethysmography (Roithmann et al., 1997), and with CT (Lenders, Pentz, Brunner, & Pirsig, 1994; Min & Yang, 1995; Djupesland et al., 1997; Gilain et al., 1997) and MRI (Hilberg, Jensen, & Pedersen, 1993; Corey, Gungor, Nelson, Fredberg, & Lai, 1997) imaging.

AIR VOLUME MEASURES

Since air volume is the product of airflow and time, determination of the volume of nasal escape represents an alternative approach to velopharyngeal assessment that is sometimes simpler. Kantner (1947) seems to have been the first to suggest using a set of vital capacity tasks to assess nasal leakage. He recommended that the patient first do several vital capacity trials to stabilize the reading. The patient's nares are then occluded with a clip, and the vital capacity again determined. The nasal clip is removed, and the vital capacity is measured one last time. It is assumed that inadequacy of the velopharyngeal seal will result in nasal escape when the nares are open, and so the variable of interest is the ratio of the two vital capacity measures: with nares open and with nares occluded. A unity ratio would indicate no difference between the two conditions and hence (presumably) no nasal escape of air. As the ratio diminishes, air escape is assumed to be increasing. The test shares the advantages of the *oral pressure ratio* (discussed subsequently) to which it is logically related. It is quick and easy and poses no threat to a patient who may have experienced countless failures when confronted with speech tasks. At least in terms of group comparisons, the test seems to have validity. Spriestersbach and Powers (1959b)

tested 103 cleft palate children, aged 5 to 15 years, and found that those who could achieve velopharyngeal closure (as determined by X-ray studies) had a mean ratio of 0.99, while those who could not achieve such closure had ratios that were significantly smaller, averaging only 0.68 ($p < .01$).

Unfortunately, velar function is evaluated under conditions of higher-than-normal intraoral pressure which, as noted earlier, may promote a degree of closure not achieved in speech. It also evaluates a static velar posture, thereby ignoring the fact that it is the adequacy of rapid velar movements that is of prime concern in speech. Other methodological problems reside, for instance, in the assumption that equal effort underlies both nares-open and nares-occluded vital capacity trials and that there is no active middle-ear disorder (Morris, 1966).

Hardy and Arkebauer (1966) proposed a different method of respirometric testing that obviates some of these limitations. To the extent that the velopharyngeal port leaks air, they reasoned, the volume of oral emission should be less than the total (oral + nasal) air volume used during a speech task devoid of nasal phonemes. The test they proposed requires that the patient produce at least 25 repetitions of each of the following CV syllables: /pʌ, tʌ, kʌ, sʌ, tʌ, fʌ/. A mouth mask is used to collect the orally-emitted air in a recording spirometer. The spirometer chart is hand marked to indicate the beginning and the end of each task. The volume of air expired is divided by the number of syllables produced to derive the mean oral volume used per syllable. The entire process is then repeated, but this time a full-face mask is used, allowing the spirometer to record total air volume. The oral volume per syllable is divided by the total volume per syllable, generating a ratio that serves as an index of velopharyngeal closure.

Hardy and Arkebauer (1966) assessed their technique with 32 normal children, aged 6 to 13 years, using a 9-L spirometer and kymograph. In addition to performing the task described, the children counted from 1 to 11. The presence of 5 /n/s in the 11 syllables of the count allowed a test of the sensitivity of the method to the presence of nasalization. Indeed, the lower ratio they obtained for the counting task suggests that the method is a moderately good detector of relatively small amounts of nasalization. Furthermore, the comparatively low ratio standard deviations attest to acceptable intersubject reliability. It was also determined that simple hand marking of the spirometer record was adequate and that trial-to-trial reliability was acceptable. Although there was some relationship ($r = -.40$) between syllable rate and mean syllable volume, more troublesome was the fact that several of their mean ratios were greater than 1. This implies that the volume of orally expired air exceeded the total air usage—a logical impossibility. The fault, no doubt, lies in the fact that two separate trials are measured. Different respiratory effort on each trial could account for the error. But, despite the obvious (and relatively minor) flaw, Hardy and Arkebauer felt that the method held promise as an assessment technique. It requires only simple instrumentation, and is non-invasive. Children do not have to meet any difficult performance criteria as they need only be instructed to "say _____ as fast as you can." Each task is done three times and the results averaged.

The Respirometric Quotient

At the expense of considerably more elaborate instrumentation, Hixon, Saxman, and McQueen (1967) have modified the Hardy and Arkebauer test to eliminate the possibility of ratios greater than unity. At the same time they achieved lower ratio variability. The task to be performed by the patient remains essentially unchanged: three sets of 25 repetitions of /tʌ, kʌ, sʌ, ʃʌ, fʌ/. Air usage variation due to rate of utterance is controlled by pacing the repetitions with a metronome set for 4 beats per second. The patient is instructed to inspire maximally before each task and to produce all repetitions on a single breath. A split-face mask channels oral and nasal air to two separate spirometers. In their system, a dual electromechanical marker apparatus controlled by the tester puts reference marks on both spirometer charts to provide common time references. A ratio, sometimes referred to as the **respirometric quotient (RQ)**, is obtained by dividing the oral spirometer volume by the sum of the two volume records. In order to control for voice onset and offset phenomena, only repetitions 4 through 23 of each utterance (20 syllables) are used in the measurement. Shaw and Gilbert (1982) have tested this evaluation method on normal children, while Gilbert and Ferrand (1987) measured RQ in 10 normal adult speakers and in 10 cleft palate speakers who were assessed both with and without their oropharyngeal prostheses. Both these investigations used comparable methodology: 3 sets of 15 repetitions each of several CV syllables at a rate of 3 syllables per second and counting from 1 to 10.

The results of these validation studies is summarized in Table 11–7. When compared with the original data provided by Hardy and Arkebauer (1966), they clearly show the improvement achieved by the subsequent test modifications. None of the ratios exceeds 1, and the difference between the syllable repetition and counting ratios is more pronounced, indicating greater sensitivity to the presence of nasalization. Note that children do not appear to generate ratios that are much different from those of adults. The limited data on speakers with demonstrated velopharyngeal deficits provide some cause for cautious optimism that such spirometric tests may find wider use in clinical evaluation.

AIR PRESSURE MEASURES

It is common for speakers to use an intraoral pressure of 3 to 8 cmH$_2$O when producing fricative and plosive consonants (see Chapter 8, "Air Pressure"). Assuming a patent nasal airway, this buildup of pressure depends critically on adequate velopharyngeal sealing. Thus, one way of assessing velopharyngeal competence is to characterize the patient's ability to generate or to maintain intraoral pressure.

The Oral Breath Pressure Ratio

The **oral breath pressure ratio** has enjoyed considerable popularity among speech pathologists. It is defined as the ratio of intraoral pressure with the nares open to the pressure with the nares occluded (P_{open}/P_{sealed}). A ratio of 1 is assumed to demonstrate that occlusion of the nares has no effect, an indication that the velopharyngeal seal is effective. Ratios less then 1 (lower oral air pressure with the nares open) are considered demonstrative of nasal air leakage and hence are presumptive evidence of poor velopharyngeal closure.

Test Method

The U-tube manometer or Bourdon-type manometer is traditionally employed (however, any standard pressure transducer will serve adequately). The maximum intraoral pressure is measured by having the patient blow as forcefully as possible into the sensing tube. Two trials are typically run: one with a nose clip in place, and the other without it. It is important that a bleed valve be used during both trials to prevent the oral trapping of air via linguapalatal contacts (Morris, 1966; Barnes & Morris, 1967; Moore & Sommers, 1974). It is possible to obtain breath pressure ratios using negative pressure by having the patient generate a maximal inspiratory effort on both trials (Weinberg & Shanks, 1971; Noll, Hawkins, & Weinberg, 1977), but not only is the task difficult to describe, most patients will find it more difficult to perform than blowing. One is, therefore, best advised to restrict testing to positive (expiratory) pressure.

Table 11–7. Mean Respirometric Quotients (Oral ÷ Total Oral and Nasal Spirometric Volume) for Normal and Cleft-Palate Speakers During Syllable Repetition and Counting. (Standard Deviations Are in Parentheses, Below Each Mean Datum.)

Speech Task	Normal Speakers			Cleft-Palate Speakers[a]	
	Children[b]	Adults[c]	Mixed[d]	With Prosthesis	Without Prosthesis
Syllables					
/pʊ/	0.96 (0.01)		0.94 (0.08)	0.92 (0.08)	0.77 (0.16)
/tʊ/	0.96 (0.02)	0.99 (0.04)	0.95 (0.03)	0.91 (0.09)	0.74 (0.19)
/kʊ/	0.96 (0.02)	0.94 (0.05)	0.97 (0.02)	0.93 (0.08)	0.82 (0.19)
/fʊ/			0.94 (0.14)	0.86 (0.04)	0.72 (0.20)
/sʊ/	0.95 (0.01)	0.91 (0.05)	0.94 (0.05)	0.90 (0.08)	0.72 (0.22)
/ʃʊ/	0.96 (0.02)	0.92 (0.03)	0.96 (0.02)	0.88 (0.11)	0.76 (0.18)
/tʃʊ/	0.95 (0.01)		0.96 (0.03)	0.91 (0.08)	0.74 (0.21)
/mʊ/			0.49 (0.18)	0.77 (0.10)	0.74 (0.11)
Counting					
1–10	0.84 (0.06)	0.80 (0.06)	0.85 (0.05)	0.84 (0.11)	0.71 (0.17)

[a]From Gilbert and Ferrand, 1987. Three male and 7 female speakers, age 10–45 years (mean = 17.9). All subjects had repaired clefts of the hard and soft palate and were "fitted with a prosthetic appliance at an early age."

[b]From Shaw and Gilbert, 1982. Five normal boys and 5 girls, age 6–10 years; RQ data averaged to nearest 0.01.

[c]From Hixon, Saxman, and McQueen, 1967. Eight men and 1 woman, age 22–32 years, with "normal articulation, voice and hearing, and no known anatomical or physiological abnormalities"; RQ data averaged to nearest 0.01.

[d]From Gilbert and Ferrand, 1987. Six male and 4 female "normal speakers," age 7–40 years (mean = 22.8).

Advantages and Limitations

Morris and Smith (1962) point out that, by avoiding a speech activity, the breath pressure ratio procedure avoids arousing feelings of frustration and defeatism in severely disabled speakers. Furthermore, the task lends itself to easy quantification and comparison of evaluations done at different times in the therapeutic course. On the other hand, the nonspeech nature of the task severely constrains the interpretation of the results. The static measure is not necessarily reflective of a patient's ability to achieve the rapid velopharyngeal closure needed for speech, a fact demonstrated by McWilliams and Bradley (1965). Van Demark (1966), for

instance, found a correlation of only .3 between the breath pressure ratio and the degree of perceived hypernasality in the speech of 154 children with cleft palate. Furthermore, neither Shelton, Brooks, and Youngstrom (1965) nor Van Demark (1971) could document a post-therapeutic improvement in pressure ratios despite improved articulatory function and notably reduced hypernasality.

The air pressures involved in testing the breath pressure ratio are very different from those needed for speech production. This point is related to a more subtle problem discussed by Hardy (1965), who points out that the test rests on the assumption that the patient is producing a maximum (or at least equal) expiratory effort during the nares-open and nares-occluded conditions. The examiner cannot be certain that this is so when the ratio is significantly less than unity. Furthermore, maximal lung pressure is strongly influenced by lung volume, and a difference in maximal oral pressure may, therefore, reflect differences in lung inflation. It is probably wise, then, to measure maximal oral pressure under standardized ventilatory conditions—for instance, at the end of a maximal inspiration or at the resting end-expiratory level.

Lastly, the oral breath pressure ratio may be adversely affected by active disorders of the middle ear. When an individual with auditory tube malfunction blows into the manometer with the nares occluded, pain or discomfort may be felt in the ear, causing him to blow less forcefully. The result is that the nares-occluded pressure is spuriously lowered, raising the open-to-closed ratio. If velopharyngeal closure is indeed normal, the ratio may exceed 1. More serious, however, is the fact that the ratio may benefit from this artifact and approach unity in cases where there actually is a degree of velopharyngeal incompetence that would have been detected if the tympanic problem did not exist. Morris (1966) discusses this particular problem of "false negatives" more fully. The limitations of this test, then, are very real and have caused Shelton, Brooks, and Youngstrom (1965), among others, to exercise caution when attempting to base clinical decisions on simple, nonspeech manometric tests.

Expected Results

Spriestersbach and Powers (1959b) used a Bourdon-type manometer to determine oral breath pressure ratios in two groups of cleft palate boys and girls, ages 5 to 15 years. Those who could achieve adequate velopharyngeal closure (demonstrated by lateral X-rays) achieved a mean ratio of 0.98, while those with deficient velopharyngeal closure had a mean ratio of 0.70. Note, however, that test results are typically interpreted on the basis of an "adequate/inadequate dichotomy." At present, there is no justification for interpreting a ratio of, say, 0.80 as necessarily indicating better function than a ratio of 0.75.

Pitzner and Morris (1966) have found that cleft palate children who have breath pressure ratios less than 0.89 "display poorer articulation [as measured by the Templin-Darley Diagnostic Test] not only on plosives, fricatives, and affricates, but also on vocalic /r/ and /l/" (p. 39). Cleft palate children with higher ratios had articulation abilities similar to those of normal children. As a clinical rule of thumb, then, clinicians often take a ratio of 0.90 as the dividing point between "adequate" and "inadequate."

Noll et al. (1977) evaluated the breath-pressure ratios of 40 normal 6- and 7-year-old boys. They reported a mean ratio of 0.93 ± 0.11, although individual ratios ranged from 0.38 to 1.27. In fact, 11 of the children had mean ratios that exceeded 1.00. As with the air-volume ratios described earlier, values greater than unity violate the logical principles upon which the measure is based. Based on these results, Noll and his coworkers concluded that "the imprecise nature of the methodological procedures routinely used in manometric testing make it unreasonable to expect ratios of 1.00 from a large number of children . . . [such that] oral manometric ratios may be of questionable diagnostic value in predicting velopharyngeal adequacy for speech" (pp. 204–205).

Intranasal Pressure

Airflow through the nose necessarily implies elevated intranasal pressure. Logically, then, nasal air pressure reflects velopharyngeal opening. Simple nasal-pressure detection methods—a nasally-connected water manometer (Hess & McDonald, 1960) or strain-gauge transducer (Condax et al., 1974)—can be used to signal nasalization. While their simplicity suggests possible use in biofeedback-based therapies, these techniques provide no information about the size of the velopharyngeal port. Although provision of a variable "bleed" in the pressure measurement system might improve resolution, the results of such a method have been disappointing (Hess, 1976).

Oral-Nasal Differential Pressure

Intraoral pressure tends to decrease as the size of the velopharyngeal orifice increases. Nonetheless adequate oral pressures may be preserved even in the face of velopharyngeal insufficiency through increased respiratory effort or modification of upper airway valving (Warren & Mackler, 1968; Warren, Wood, & Bradley, 1969; Dalston, Warren, Morr, & Smith, 1988; Laine et al., 1988a; Minsley et al., 1988; Hinton & Warren, 1995; Zajac, Mayo, Kataoka, & Kuo, 1996; Sapineza et al., 1996; McHenry, 1997; Mayo, Warren, & Zajac, 1998). Warren (1979) hypothesized that, because nasal pressure increases as orifice size becomes larger, the resulting oral-nasal differential pressure would be more closely related to changes in velopharyngeal function than would measures of intraoral pressure alone. In essence, subtracting the intraoral pressure from the pressure generated in the nose serves to desensitize the assessment to differences in aerodynamic effort. Warren accordingly recommended using the difference between intraoral and intranasal pressures during production of /p/ as an index of ***palatal efficiency***.

In Warren's system, one pressure probe is placed in the posterior area of the mouth, while another is secured in the patient's nostril by means of a cork. After studying 75 cleft palate speakers, Warren (1979) concluded that an oral-nasal difference less than 3 cmH$_2$O or more during plosive production indicates adequate closure, whereas a difference less than 1 cmH$_2$O demonstrates inadequacy. Pressure differences between these cutoff points are presumed to signal "borderline" closure. Not only is the borderline region problematic, but it must also be understood that the method does not evaluate actual speech performance. Further, valid measures are not possible in the presence of incomplete lip closure, such as might be seen in cases of severe open bite or flaccid labial paralysis, or in severe cases of upper airway obstruction. The simplicity of the test, however, might recommend it to some practitioners for a well-selected subset of patients. A special computer-interfaced and software-controlled instrument, dubbed the ***Palatal Efficiency Rating Computed Instantaneously (PERCI)***, has been designed to facilitate differential pressure measurement (PERCI-PC, Microtronics, Inc., Carrboro, NC).

ORAL PRESSURE AND NASAL AIRFLOW

Observing nasal flow and oral pressure at the same time greatly enhances the potential for drawing inferences about the function of the velopharyngeal valve. The intraoral air pressure is the force tending to drive air through the port, while the nasal flow represents the failure of the velopharyngeal system to withstand that pressure. The simultaneous recording of P$_{io}$ and U$_n$ thus provides an excellent illustration of the effectiveness of velar closure during all the combinations of oral and velopharyngeal status needed for speaking. Furthermore, the timing characteristics of velar function are readily apparent.

Implementation of this observation method is straightforward and simple. Intraoral air pressure is sensed with an oral probe tube and pressure transducer while a nose mask (Figure 11–14) and pneumotachograph monitor nasal airflow. The speech signal, picked up by a microphone in front of the speaker's mouth, is also displayed in the output to facilitate the identification of speech events. A typical record for a normal speaker might look like that shown in Figure 11–15. Rapid and well-timed movements of the velum are apparent in the brief bursts of appropriate nasal expiration. Negligible nasal emission occurs, even during high-pressure speech sounds. However, note the nasal flow associated with the /v/ in "five" in anticipa-

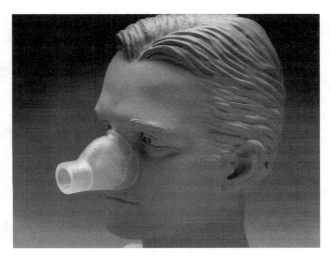

Figure 11–14. A nose mask for channeling nasal airflow. (Photo courtesy of Hans Rudolph, Inc., Kansas City, MO.)

tion of the /n/ that follows. This type of coarticulatory effect is to be expected in such nasal contexts. Although there are some carryover effects, rapid velopharyngeal closure is suggested by the relatively quick decrease in nasal flow prior to the peak pressure associated with the /θ/ phone in "three." Of course without a substantial reduction of nasal air escape, the speaker's ability to generate an adequate intraoral driving pressure for high-pressure speech sounds such as plosives and fricatives can be significantly compromised.

Warren (1964a, 1964b) compared nasal airflow with the oral-nasal differential pressure using a transoral pressure probe placed in the posterior oral cavity along with a second pressure probe and pneumotachograph, each secured firmly in the patient's nostrils (such as described for anterior rhinomanometry and illustrated in Figure 11–11).[5] Warren has used this system to evaluate the velopharyngeal adequacy of cleft palate individuals during running speech. He points out that incomplete velopharyngeal closure is frequently signaled by a reversal of the flow and pressure patterns. Normally, stop consonants are characterized by a relatively high transvelar pressure and very little, if any, nasal airflow. An incompetent velopharyngeal valve, however, often causes a severe reduction of the pressure and a great increase in the transnasal flow (Warren & Devereux, 1966; Laine et al., 1988a).

Consider, for instance, the pressure-flow records shown in Figure 11–16. They were obtained from a preteen girl with multiple articulatory deficits and serious

---

[5]Note that, as with anterior rhinometry, the assumption of equal patency of the two nasal passages must be valid.

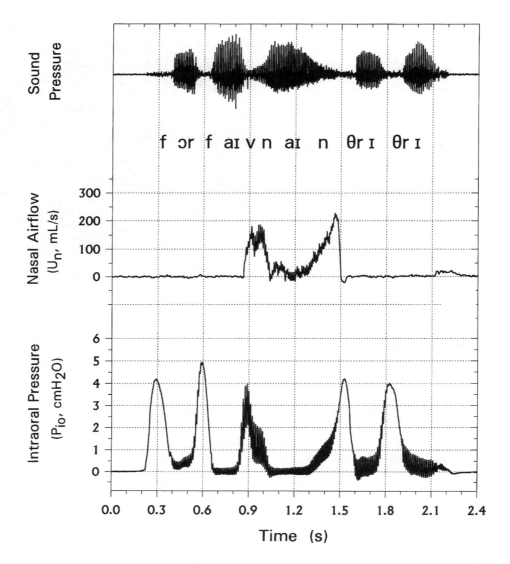

Figure 11–15. An example of simultaneous nasal airflow and intraoral air pressure traces. In this case, a normal speaker said "4, 5, 9, 3, 3." Note that the only significant nasal flow occurred during, and in the immediate vicinity of, "nine."

velopharyngeal incompetence, who was recently fitted with a palatal lift prosthesis. Despite the presence of the obturator, this patient's speech continued to be hypernasal. In a case such as this, the pressure-flow technique may provide insight regarding whether or not the palatal appliance assists velopharyngeal closure. The top pair of traces (A) are associated with the patient's repetition of the syllable /pɑ/. For each of the large pressure peaks (associated with the buildup of plosive consonant pressure), there is a corresponding —and roughly proportional—peak of nasal airflow. If the velopharyngeal port were closed, no transnasal airflow would be expected (as in Figure 11–15). The data,

therefore, suggest that the palatal lift does not allow this patient to achieve velopharyngeal closure. The lower traces (B) are a record of P_{io} and U_n as this patient repeats "Pinocchio" three times. (The intraoral pressure for /k/ does not appear because of the anterior placement of the oral pressure probe.) Note that, as with the previous traces, there is significant nasal airflow associated with each /p/ pressure peak. As expected, each /n/ production is associated with nasal airflow and no substantial buildup of intraoral pressure. What may not be expected, however, is the observation that the nasal flow for /n/ is greater than that for /p/; this, despite the fact that the pressure for /p/ is

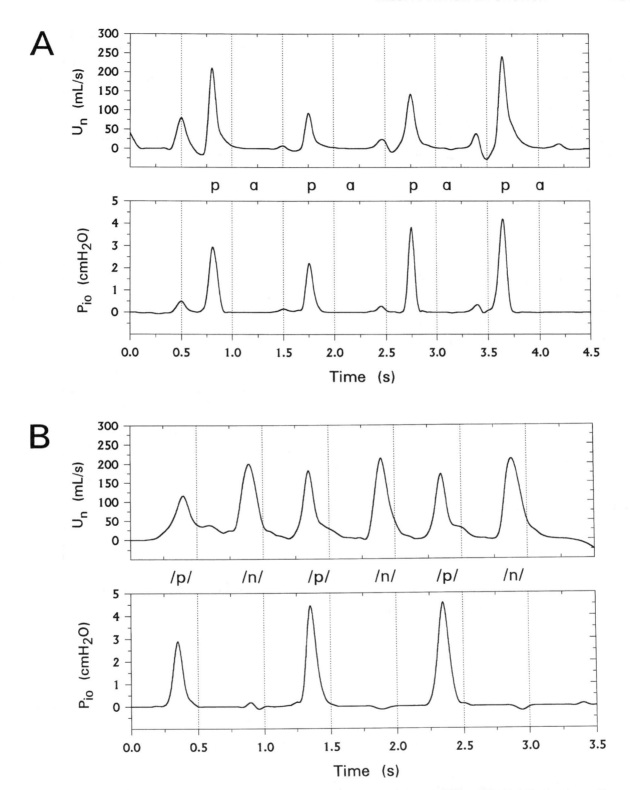

Figure 11–16. Simultaneous nasal airflow (U_n) and intraoral pressure (P_{io}) for a preteen girl with velopharyngeal incompetence speaking with the aid of an obturator. **(A)** Repetition of the syllable /pɑ/. Note the nearly proportional increase in nasal flow with the build-up of intraoral pressure for /p/. **(B)** /p/ and /n/ during repetition of "Pinocchio." As before, there is susbtantial nasal airflow during /p/ production. Assuming a fairly stable oropharyngeal pressure during speech, the fact that nasal flow is greater during /n/ than during /p/ production indicates that the obturator provides at least some benefit to velopharyneal valving.

much higher than the pressure for /n/. There is only one way in which this could happen: the resistance of the velopharyngeal port must be very much higher during the production of /p/ than it is during the production of /n/. That could result only by a significant narrowing of the velopharyngeal orifice during /p/. Thus, although the patient continues to be hypernasal, the pressure-flow traces provide evidence that the obturator does, in fact, benefit this patient's velopharyngeal function.

It has also been shown that abnormal timing characteristics, such as the delay between peak pressure and flow and the duration of the pressure buildup and release, can indicate an inadequate velopharyngeal mechanism (Warren & Mackler, 1968; Netsell, 1969; Netsell & Daniel, 1979; Warren, Dalston, Trier, & Holder, 1985). Clearly, dysarthric speakers may have poor velopharyngeal closure for only a few selected consonants or for a combination of phones, and some may show dysfunction only when the rate of speech or syllables production is changed. Netsell (1969) has proposed a special paradigm for evaluation of velopharyngeal function in such speakers. Intraoral pressure and nasal airflow are observed while the patient produces utterances as shown in Table 11–8. The consonants /t/, /d/, and /n/ provide a contrast of voiceless,

Table 11–8. Test Utterances for the Evaluation of Velopharyngeal Competence in Dysarthria*

Utterance	Testing Condition
/tʌ/	Repetition at rates of 1, 2, 4, and 5 per second
/dʌ/	
/nʌ/	
/ʌtʌd/	Five repetitions of each at a conversational rate
/ʌdʌt/	
/ʌtʌnʌ/	
/ʌdʌdʌ/	
/ʌnʌtʌ/	
/ʌnʌdʌ/	
/ʌndʌntʌn/	
/ʌntʌndʌn/	

*From "Evaluation of Velopharyngeal Function in Dysarthria," by R. Netsell, 1969, *Journal of Speech and Hearing Disorders, 34,* 113–122. Table 1, p. 115. (c) American Speech-Language-Hearing Association, Rockville, MD. Reprinted by permission.

voiced, and nasal productions at a single place of articulation that is not disturbed by a post-molar pressure sensing tube. The neutral vowel also prevents probe tube disruption that might result from the need to achieve more extreme lip or tongue postures. Conversational pitch and loudness are used.

The sensitivity of Netsell's test method as a detector of several different types of problems is illustrated in the output records shown in Figure 11–17, which are taken from Netsell (1969). Difficulty with velar timing is particularly well documented by this technique. Hardy, Netsell, Schweiger, and Morris (1969) have presented a series of case histories that demonstrated the applicability of Netsell's test to children with neuromuscular disorders. Interestingly, the pressure-flow record showed that persistent nasality was associated with residual incompetence of the prosthetically aided velopharyngeal port in cases where lateral X-rays had indicated adequate anteroposterior closure.

Warren (1979) has advocated using the word "hamper" as a target utterance in the aerodynamic assessment of velopharyngeal adequacy. The nasalplosive /mp/ sequence, Warren suggests, is likely to approximate the degree of velopharyngeal closure that occurs in spontaneous speech and therefore may be especially helpful in determining whether a speaker achieves closure quickly enough. Pressure-flow research has since found the "hamper" test utterance to be of value in this regard (Dalston et al., 1988; Minsley, et al., 1988; Dalston, Warren, & Smith, 1990; Laine et al., 1988a, 1988b; Morr, Warren, Dalston, & Smith, 1989; Warren, Dalston, & Mayo, 1993, 1994; Hinton & Warren, 1995; Zajac, 1997; Leeper, Tissington, & Munhall, 1998; Mayo et al., 1998). Dotevall and his coworkers (Dotevall, Lohmander-Agerskov, Almquist, & Bake, 1998) reported similar results when they tested Swedish speakers using three-word phrases that contained /mp/, /nt/, and /ŋk/ blends.

Area of Velopharyngeal Opening

If the pressure difference between the oropharynx and the nasal cavity (ΔP) and the airflow through the nose (U_n) are both known, then the resistance of the velopharyngeal-nasal airway (R_{naw}) is given by $R_{naw} = \Delta P/U_n$. The laws of thermodynamics specify the way in which the resistance of the opening is related to its area. Specifically,

$$\text{Area} = \frac{\text{Flow}}{\sqrt{\frac{2 \times \Delta P}{\text{density}}}}.$$

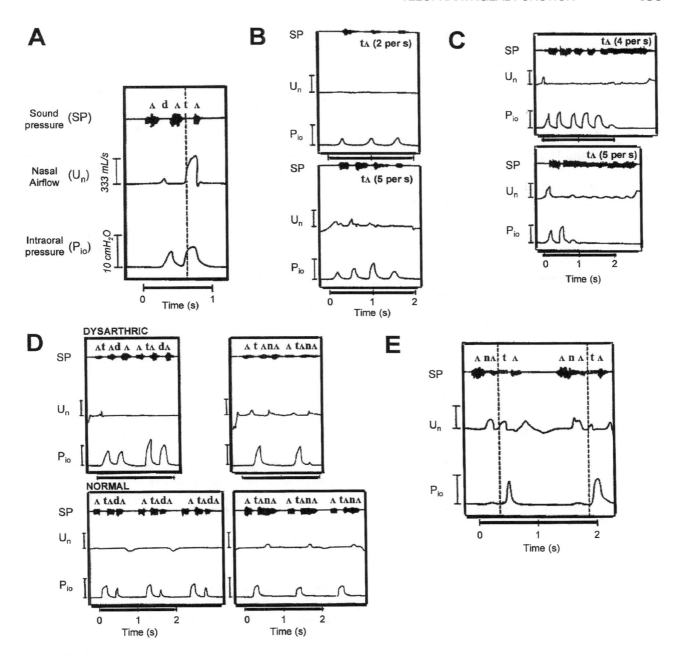

Figure 11-17. Intraoral pressure (P$_{io}$) and nasal airflow (U$_n$) records in dysarthria. (Calibration lines represent 333 mL/s of nasal airflow and 10 cmH$_2$O of intraoral pressure.) **(A)** Dysarthric man repeating /ʊdʊtʊ/, showing premature velopharyngeal opening. **(B)** Dysarthric man repeating /tʌ/ at rates of 2 (upper) and 5 (lower) syllables per second. The lower record shows gradual closure of the velopharyngeal port. **(C)** Dysarthric woman repeating /tʌ/ at rates of 4 (upper) and 5 (lower) syllables per second. The records illustrate gradual opening of the velopharyngeal port. **(D)** Repetitions of /ʊtʊdʊ/ and /ʊtʊnʊ/ by a dysarthric (upper) and normal (lower) woman. The dysarthric speaker uses an inappropriate anticipatory velopharyngeal opening. **(E)** Repetition of /ʌnʌtʌ/ by a dysarthric man showing inappropriate maintenance of velopharyngeal opening. From "Evaluation of Velopharyngeal Function in Dysarthria, by R. Netsell, 1969, *Journal of Speech and Hearing Disorders, 34*, 113–122. Figures 3 through 7, pp. 116–120. (c) American Speech-Language-Hearing Association, Rockville, MD. Used by permission.]

By implication, if the transvelar pressure drop and the nasal airflow are known, it should be possible to calculate the actual area of the velopharyngeal opening.

The equation, however, is valid only for the special case in which there is no turbulence or nonuniformity of flow. To be applicable to estimation of velopharyngeal port size, a correction factor must be introduced to compensate for very real deviations from the ideal case. Warren and DuBois (1964) have used a physical model of the oral and nasal pathways to determine the required value of such a correction factor.[6] They found that under different conditions of flow, pressure, and orifice size, the value varied from 0.59 to 0.72 (when pressure is measured in dynes/cm². Using a mean value of 0.65, they felt, would provide an estimate sufficiently accurate for most purposes. This corresponds to a correction factor of 0.0073 when oropharyngeal and nasal pressures are measured in cmH_2O (Lubker, 1969). The area of the velopharyngeal opening, then, is estimated by a hydrokinetic equation[7] of the form:

$$Area = \frac{U}{0.0073\sqrt{\dfrac{2 \times P_0 - P_n}{\rho}}},$$

where U_n = nasal airflow in mL/s;
P_o = oropharyngeal pressure in cmH_2O;
P_n = nasal pressure in cmH_2O; and
ρ = density of air = 0.001 g/cm^3.

Assuming a constant air density of 0.001 g/cm^3, the equation above can be simplifed to:

$$Area = \frac{U_n}{10.22\sqrt{P_o - P_n}}.$$

When tested on the physical model, the hydrokinetic equation was found to produce an error of about 9% when orifice size was about 120 mm², and of about 8% with an orifice size of 2.4 mm². Further testing on models has since been done by Lubker (1969) and by Smith and Weinberg (1980), both of whom found it to be a valid estimator. The latter study reported a mean accuracy of about 5% for airflows of 50 to more than 400 mL/s, but the error reached as much as 20% with some flow-orifice size combinations. It is difficult to achieve a good estimate of a large velopharyngeal area if airflow is low, since ΔP then becomes too small to measure accurately. Estimation reliability appears to be adequate (Warren & DuBois, 1964; Smith & Weinberg, 1980).

As described, the measurement procedure does not take account of nasal resistance. It therefore misestimates the velopharyngeal orifice area. What it really provides is a measure of the *equivalent area* of the nasal-velopharyngeal airway. Where necessary, a better estimate can be achieved by correcting for the contribution of the nasal cavity (see Warren and DuBois, 1964).[8]

In an attempt to accommodate clinical implementation, Moon and Weinberg (1985) provide a graph (Figure 11–18) derived from the hydrokinetic equation that allows a quick area estimate from individual pressure-flow data. To use the graph method, a patient might be instructed to produce a series of /pɑ/ or /pi/ syllables. If, for example, the measured ΔP is 1 cmH_2O and the nasal airflow is 180 mL/s, the velopharyngeal area would be estimated by identifying the pressure on the vertical axis, finding where the 1-cmH_2O line intersects with the 180-mL/s diagonal line, and then reading down to find the corresponding area along the horizontal axis. In this example, the estimated area would be 20 mm². Moon and Weinberg also provide a second graph to allow area estimation from nasal airway resistance and nasal flow values.

Warren and his colleagues (Warren, Dalston, & Dalston, 1989; Warren, Dalston, Morr, Hairfield, & Smith, 1989) have categorized the adequacy of closure on the basis of velopharyngeal area estimates for the /mp/ segment in "hamper":

- ■ Adequate Closure: less than 5 mm²
- ■ Adequate/Borderline Closure: 5 to 9 mm²
- ■ Borderline/Inadequate Closure: 10 to 19 mm²
- ■ Inadequate Closure: 20 mm² or greater

They based this categorization scheme on perceptual evidence and aerodynamic data derived from normal

---

[6]Müller and Brown (1980, p. 328) argue strongly and persuasively for great caution in the choice of a correction factor. They point out its dependence on the user's assumptions about the geometry of the patient's velopharyngeal port—assumptions that might not be valid.

[7]Derivation of the equation and validation methods are presented in Warren and DuBois (1964). Further aerodynamic implications are explored in Warren and Devereux (1966).

[8]Note that the Warren-DuBois method can also be used to estimate the equivalent area of oral articulatory constrictions. See Hixon (1966), Claypoole et al. (1974), and Smith, Allen, Warren, and Hall (1978).

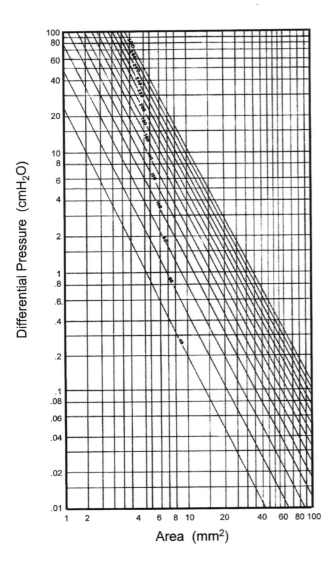

Figure 11-18. A logarithmic graph plotting oral-nasal differential pressure and the area of velopharyngeal opening as a function of the nasal airflow rate (diagonal lines, in increments of 20 mL/s; lower left, flow = 40 mL/s; upper right, flow = 300 mL/s). The orifice area can be estimated by finding the point where a patient's flow and pressure lines intersect. From "Two Simplified Methods for Estimating Velopharyngeal Orifice Area," by J.B. Moon and B. Weinberg, 1985, *Cleft Palate Journal, 22*, 1–10. Figure 4, p. 5. Reprinted with permission.

individuals and from cleft palate speakers who demonstrated varying degrees of velopharyngeal dysfunction. But, regardless of category, the hydrokinetic equation method of area estimation may be most helpful as a means of assessing the success of therapeutic intervention (Hogan, 1973).

Andreassen, Smith, and Guyette (1991) evaluated nasal airflow, differential oral-nasal pressure, and esti-mated velopharyngeal orifice areas in 20 normal men and women who produced a series of selected nasal and nonnasal test syllables. In their study, the pressure-flow characteristics of the /mp/ sequence in "hamper" and of several CV syllables were assessed. For the /p/ segment and the nonnasal syllables, Andreassen and her coworkers measured the nasal flow rate and derived a velopharyngeal area estimate at peak differential pressure, whereas for the nasal utterances, differential pressures and area estimates were obtained at peak nasal flow. Their summary data (Table 11–9) provide a basis of comparison when assessing patients with known or suspected velopharyngeal impairment.

Still, one is confronted yet again with the difference between the *perception* of nasality and the physiological correlates of nasalization. While Warren (1964b) and Warren and Mackler (1968) suggested that velopharyngeal orifice areas greater than 20 mm^2 are associated with perceived hypernasality, and areas over 100 mm^2 with extreme hypernasality, no clear and direct correspondence between the two has been demonstrated. Warren et al. (1994) found a moderate correlation between hypernasality ratings and velopharyngeal orifice size ($r = .66$). They concluded that the duration of velopharyngeal opening and closing gestures often play an important role in perceived speech nasality.

Aerodynamic Bridge Method

For cases in which no invasiveness can be tolerated, the rather novel method proposed by Hixon, Bless, and Netsell (1976) can be used. A specially designed three-tube glass model that simulates the speaker's oral, nasal, and pharyngeal airways is employed in a manner that represents the aerodynamic equivalent of bridge-balancing (see Chapter 2, "Analog Electronics"). Continuously variable shutter valves are installed at the model's equivalent of the nasal, oral, laryngeal, and velopharyngeal openings to permit the size of these ports to be adjusted. A nose mask couples the patient's airway to a hard-walled tube, the other end of which is connected to the nasal port of the model. A sidearm at the tube's midpoint connects it to a generator of oscillatory airflow (made of a series of loudspeakers driven by a sinewave power generator). Identical pneumotachograph and pressure transducer systems are attached to the patient's mouth and to the oral port of the model. When the oscillatory airflow generator is turned on, equal signals are applied to both halves of an aerodynamic bridge. The shutter valves at the model's oral, nasal, and laryngeal ports are preadjusted to resistances typical of these structures (the authors suggest 0.5, 2.0, and 75

Table 11-9. Oral-Nasal Differential Pressure (ΔP, in cmH$_2$O), Nasal Airflow (U$_n$, in mL/s), and Estimated Velopharyngeal Orifice Area (A$_{vp}$, in mm^2) for Utterances Produced by Normal English-Speaking Adults*

Utterance	ΔP Mean (SD)	ΔP Range	U$_n$ Mean (SD)	U$_n$ Range	Estimated A$_{vp}$ Mean (SD)	Estimated A$_{vp}$ Range
Men						
/fi/	6.25 (1.93)	4.03–10.03	4.2 (4.6)	0.4–15.4	0.2 (0.2)	0.0–0.6
/pi/	6.68 (1.31)	4.79–9.49	4.0 (4.3)	0.0–13.1	0.2 (0.2)	0.0–0.5
/pɑ/	6.44 (1.52)	4.32–9.64	17.8 (30.0)	2.7–101.6	0.8 (1.3)	0.1–4.5
/p/ in "hamper"	6.03 (1.19)	4.41–8.29	30.0 (16.5)	2.6–51.3	1.4 (1.0)	0.3–3.0
/mi/	0.26 (0.17)	0.09–0.59	151.5 (33.0)	97.8–212.1	37.2 (9.3)	21.4–50.8
/mɑ/	0.13 (0.10)	0.00–0.36	179.7 (34.4)	108.6–222.9	54.1 (15.2)	38.4–78.4
/m/ in "hamper"	0.97 (0.38)	0.34–1.55	287.1 (66.6)	192.5–377.3	34.4 (11.4)	17.0–52.6
Women						
/fi/	6.51 (1.15)	4.34–8.14	1.6 (1.9)	0.0–6.2	0.1 (0.1)	0.0–0.4
/pi/	6.50 (1.11)	5.17–9.09	2.0 (1.5)	0.0–5.0	0.1 (0.1)	0.0–0.2
/pɑ/	6.07 (1.10)	4.66–8.55	6.7 (8.2)	0.0–28.5	0.3 (0.3)	0.0–1.2
/p/ in "hamper"	5.69 (1.64)	3.41–8.83 (10.9)	12.2 (0.4)	0.0–37.2	0.6	0.0–1.3
/mi/	0.29 (0.13)	0.13–0.55	136.3 (42.1)	75.1–196.0	30.7 (8.0)	20.7–47.8
/mɑ/	0.19 (0.09)	0.09–0.29	164.7 (50.0)	114.0–242.9	48.3 (20.7)	27.5–91.8
/m/ in "hamper"	0.75 (0.35)	0.23–1.42	211.1 (71.6)	82.1–288.8	30.1 (16.8)	13.2–65.6

*Subjects were 10 men and 10 women, 20 to 36 years of age (mean = 28 years); all normal speakers of a midwestern dialect of American English. Speakers repeated CV syllables using a conversational pitch and loudness at a rate of approximately 3 syllables/s; The word "hamper" was repeated three times. Flow and area data have been rounded to the nearest 0.1.

Data from "Pressure-flow Measurements for Selected Oral and Nasal Sound Segments Produced by Normal Adults," by M.L. Andreassen, B.E. Smith, and T.W. Guyette, 1991, *Cleft Palate—Craniofacial Journal, 28,* 398–406. Tables 1–6 (pp. 400–402).

cmH$_2$O/LPS, respectively). Any difference in the magnitude of the sinewave outputs of the two oral pneumotachographs should then be due to an inequality of the velopharyngeal port area of the model and the patient. The two outputs can be equated by adjusting the velopharyngeal shutter valve of the model to change the balance of the bridge, until the balance meter is centered or nulled.

Actual measurement is done by impressing the forced oscillatory flow on the airway while the patient sustains a voiced continuant sound. The size of the model's velopharyngeal opening is adjusted until there is no difference in the flow signal from the two pneumotachographs. When this balance condition is achieved, the patient stops phonating and the area of the velopharyngeal shutter-valve is measured. This area is an estimate of the patient's velopharyngeal port area.

Unfortunately the method is associated with a number of drawbacks that severely limit its clinical utility. For one thing, the aerodynamic bridge procedure will not permit tracking of running speech. Also, like the hydrokinetic equation method, the method really generates an estimate of the equivalent area of the nasal-pharyngeal combination. There are clearly obvious restrictions on patient performance: A single phone has to be sustained long enough for the tester to achieve a balance condition—and the prolongation must be stable.

VELAR MOVEMENT

Although velopharyngeal closure involves more than a simple velar movement, this particular aspect is often important to the clinician, especially in cases of paralysis or higher CNS dysfunction. A number of means are available for transduction of structural displacement in general (see Chapter 12, "Speech Movements") and several have been tried on the soft palate. None has found widespread acceptance for this purpose, however. Further work might lead to an instrument of everyday practicality. This section describes the several velar-motion transduction techniques that have some currency in the speech literature.

Strain Gauge Systems

Bonded strain gauges can be mounted on special supports and anchored in the oral cavity in such a way as to transduce movements of the velum. Moller, Martin, and Christiansen (1971) and Christiansen and Moller (1971) reported on the use of such a system, one that they found to be accurate and reliable. It consisted of a thin (0.01 inch thick) steel beam on which the gauges were mounted. A fine spring wire extended from the beam and rested on the center line of the velum, whose movement thus deformed the strain gauges. The entire unit was anchored in place by an orthodontic band that fit around the maxillary second molar.

When correctly fitted, this kind of transducer does not interfere significantly with articulation, and its frequency response is at least adequate for tracking the velar movements of speech (Hixon, 1972). While such a device is clearly useful for real-time biofeedback in managing the "sluggish" velum (Moller, Path, Werth, & Christiansen, 1973), the difficulty in achieving identical placements of the sensing wire at different test sessions seriously limits its usefulness for documenting long-term changes of velar function.

Electromagnetic Articulography

Electromagnetic articulography uses a specially designed magnetometer system to track articulator movement (Schönle et al., 1987; Schönle, 1988; Engelke & Schönle, 1991; Perkell et al., 1992). Also known as *electromagnetic midsagittal articulometry* (*EMMA*), the technique is addressed in greater detail in Chapter 12 ("Speech Movements"). In devices such as the commerically available *Articulograph AG100* (Carstens Medizinelektronik, Lenglern, Germany), three helmet-mounted transmitter (generator) coils produce alternating magnetic fields that induce a current in small, light-weight sensor (transducer) coils that are attached to the articulators of interest. (Fine wires connect the sensor coils to the receiver electronics.) The strength of the alternating signal induced in the sensor coils will be inversely proportional to the cube of their distance from the transmitter coils. For accurate articulator movement data, the sensor coils must be positioned so that they are parallel to the midline axis of the transmitters on the helmet. As such, most inductive magnetic-field systems are designed to be able to detect and, to a certain extent, to correct for transitory coil misalignment that may result from articulatory movement or from postural adjustment (Perkell et al., 1992; Schönle et al., 1987; Engelke, Müller, & Petersen, 1995).

To track velar movement, an adhesive or an atraumatic suture is used to attach a sensor coil to the midline of the velum—usually to the inferior (oral) surface via a transoral approach (Katz et al., 1990; Engelke, Schönle, & Engelke, 1990; Engelke & Schönle, 1991; Engelke & Hoch, 1994). One or more additional sensor coils are then fixed to bony references, such as between the upper incisors and the bridge of the nose, to allow assessment of velar displacement relative to the position of the speaker's maxilla and to assist in the control of head posture and movement (Perkell et al., 1992; Engelke, Bruns et al., 1996; Engelke, Hoch et al., 1996; Rouco & Recasens, 1996). Electromagnetic articulography appears to hold promise as an assessment and therapeutic tool. Nonetheless, while it may provide movement data that are comparable to those of other established techniques, magnetometric studies of velar displacement in normal and abnormal speakers remain rare.

Photodetection

The intensity of light transmitted through the velopharyngeal port or reflected from the velar surface can also serve as an indicator of velar motion. Ohala (1971) constructed a photodetector system, called the *Nasograph*, that consisted of a highly compressible 4-mm diameter polyethylene tube containing a miniature lamp and a more proximal photodetector. (The device is also described in Abbs and Watkin, 1976, and in Krakow and Huffman, 1993.) The tube is inserted pernasally—far enough to place the light source below and the detector above the velopharyngeal port. As the velopharyngeal port narrows, the tube becomes increasingly pinched. As this occurs, the amount of light transmitted to the detector diminishes and its output falls accordingly. Unfortunately there appears to be no easy way to calibrate the nasograph system and, therefore, it can be used to provide only a relative measure of oronasal coupling (Ohala, 1971; Clumeck, 1976).

Dalston (1982) described another photodetection scheme that places a light source below and a light detector above the velopharyngeal port. Referring to his system as a"modified Nasograph,"Dalston's device replaces the original compressible tube with a probe that consists of two optically-shielded light-transmitting fibers: A 0.51-mm diameter fiber to provide continuous illumination, and a 0.76-mm diameter fiber to serve as a photodetector pickup. The two fibers are bonded so that the light-emitting end of the light-source fiber is maintained 30 mm beyond the pickup end of the photodetector fiber. The bundled fibers are then inserted pernasally until the end of the light-source fiber lies approximately 5 mm below the resting level of the velum. The confounding influence of ambient light is minimized by performing the procedure in a darkened room. Keefe and Dalston (1989) reported that because only the 0.76 mm photodetector fiber must pass through the velopharynx and because the weight of the light-emitting probe resting on the velum is less than one gram, the placement of the instrument is unlikely to interfere with velopharyngeal activity in any meaningful way.

Dalston (1982) found the photodetector data to be reliable, and obtained a high correlation ($r = .91$) between velopharyngeal area estimated by the hydrokinetic equation method of Warren and DuBois (1964) and the output of his photodector system. There also appears to be fairly good correspondence between photodetector output and the determination of velopharyngeal port dimensions by means of cineradiographic (Zimmermann et al., 1987) and nasopharyngoscopic (Karnell, Seaver, & Dalston, 1988) techniques.

Moon and Lagu (1987) described another photodetector system that, instead of optical fibers, uses a small light-emitting diode (LED) and a miniature photodetector attached to small teflon-coated wires that serve as a guide and electrical connection to exterior electronics. As with the original Nasograph placement, the light source is positioned below and the detector above the velopharyngeal port. (The LED is oriented so that it directs light upward toward the velopharyngeal port.) According to Moon and Lagu, this low-cost system provides for improved linearity and reduced sensitivity to ambient light. Specifically, the light emitted from the source diode is modulated at a rate of 10 kHz.

The raw photodetector output (influenced by LED and ambient light) is then filtered to extract the 10-kHz (LED) component of the signal.

Assuming fixed light source and detector positions relative to the velopharyngeal orifice (Covello, Karnell, & Seaver, 1992), photodetector systems allow continuous monitoring of velopharyngeal port area during running speech. Furthermore, because such systems have been shown to have a relatively good frequency response (rise times of 4 and 8 ms have been reported for the Moon and Lagu [1987] and Dalston [1982] systems, respectively), they can be used to great advantage in studies of velopharyngeal timing (Dalston & Keefe, 1987, 1988; Dalston, 1989; Keefe & Dalston, 1989).

In contrast to the type of photodetection systems just described, Condax, Acson, Miki, and Sakoda (1976) used a *photoreflective* system for their phonetic research. In this case, a probe containing two fiberoptic bundles is inserted into the nasal cavity. One bundle shines a beam of light posteriorly onto the nasal surface of the velum, while the other bundle conveys reflected light back to an external photodetector. Elevation of the velum from its rest (open) position results in increased reflection from its superior (nasal) surface and hence a greater output from the phototransducer. Although this system does not require placing a probe through the velopharyngeal orifice, it is not very amenable to accurate calibration, thereby limiting its applicability. In particular, photoreflection techniques are plagued by two significant problems: (1) the difficulty of probe positioning and (2) the difficulty in accounting for the variability in light reflection that may be due to the accumulation and distribution of mucus on the velum or on the walls of the nasopharynx. Despite these limitations, however, a similar device, the *Velograph* of Künzel (1977, 1978, 1979a, 1979b) has been used successfully to provide feedback of velar motion in therapy (Künzel, 1982).

The Velotrace

The *Velotrace* is a mechanical device, developed by Horiguchi and Bell-Berti (1987), that tracks velar position over time. The instrument (shown schematically in Figure 11–19), inserted through the nose, consists of three major parts: (1) a curved 30-mm long internal lever that rests on the superior (nasal) surface of the velum, (2) a 60-mm long external lever, and (3) a 150-mm long set of support- and pushrods that carry and connect the internal and external levers. When the internal lever is raised by the elevation of the velum, the pushrod causes the external lever to move toward the subject. Conversely, when the internal lever is low-

A

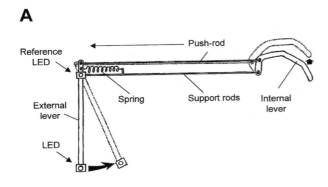

B

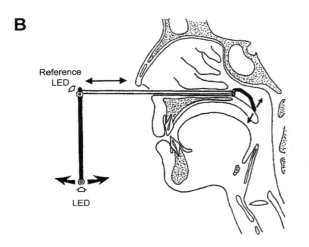

Figure 11–19. **(A)** A schematic illustration of the Velotrace. **(B)** The Velotrace shown positioned in the nasal cavity with its internal lever resting on the nasal surface of the velum. Velar displacement will result in a proportional movement (swing) of the LED placed at the proximal end of the external lever. Both **A** and **B** from "The Velotrace: A Device for Monitoring Velar Position," by S. Horiguchi and F. Bell-Berti, 1987, *Cleft Palate Journal, 24,* 104–111. Figures 1 and 2, p. 105. Reprinted with permission.

ered by a downward movement of the velum, the external lever moves away from the subject. A spring is included in the system to allow the internal lever to respond more rapidly to velar depression and to improve the frequency response of the device in general. The device also provides amplification; because the external lever is longer, its displacement (swing) will be greater than the displacement of the shorter internal lever.

Following application of a topical anesthetic and decongestant to the nasal mucosa, the Velotrace is inserted through the more patent of the patient's nasal passages until the tip of the internal lever rests on the superior surface of the velum. The fulcrum of the internal lever and much of the support rod is made to rest

on the floor of the nasal cavity. A headband and brace are used to stabilize the device once optimal positioning is determined.

Relative velar position is tracked by monitoring the movement of the external lever. This is done with an optoelectronic system that tracks the position of an infrared LED at the end of the external lever relative to a reference LED placed at the fulcrum (Bell-Berti & Krakow, 1991; Kollia et al., 1995), although the position of the external lever can be monitored using a number of different transduction schemes. However, although Velotrace output compares well with fiberoptic and cinefluorographic data regarding vertical velar displacement (Horiguchi & Bell-Berti, 1987), calibration has proven to be difficult. For one thing, positioning of the device cannot be exact. A one-size Velotrace will not fit all patients equally—and placement is bound to vary as a consequence of anatomical differences among speakers. Also, because the tip of the internal lever is not firmly attached to the velar mucosa, the precise tracking point may change as the velum moves.

Although the dimensions of the Velotrace are similar to many standard nasendoscopes, it is an inflexible device. As such, its clinical application is limited to those patients without significant nasal airway impairment who can tolerate the procedure. However, when used with speakers for whom the procedure is appropriate, the Velotrace can offer a useful means of describing the pattern, timing, and coordination of velar movement during speech and swallowing (Bell-Berti & Krakow, 1991; Bell-Berti, 1993; Kollia, Gracco, & Harris, 1995).

Acoustic Reflection

Acoustic rhinometry, as described earlier, uses the acoustic reflection of an impulse signal that has been injected into the nose to map the cross-sectional geometry of the nasal cavity. Since the technique allows area measurement for distances up to about 20 cm from the nosepiece (Hilberg et al., 1989; Hilberg, Lyholm, Michelsen, Pedersen, & Jacobsen, 1998), Dalston (1992) suggested that measuring the reflection of nasally introduced acoustic impulses might provide a useful means of monitoring velopharyngeal activity by tracking changes in epipharyngeal volume. Two preliminary investigations have since been conducted to determine the feasibility of using acoustic reflection in this manner.

Seaver and his colleagues (Seaver, Karnell, Gasparaitis, & Corey, 1995) compared nasal airway distance-by-area functions from two normal men "during rest while not breathing" (open velopharyngeal port) and compared them to those obtained while "sustaining a 'quiet' /f/" (closed velopharyngeal port). When the functions were compared (Figure 11–20), they were essentially identical over the distance of the nasal cavity but began to diverge at a distance that videofluorographic imaging suggested corresponded to the point where the velum elevated above the palatal plane. The X-ray and acoustic data were also in agreement regarding the point of maximum velar elevation. Based on the reflection data alone, however, it was not possible to determine where (or if) velopharyngeal closure occurred.

Kunkel, Wahlmann, and Wagner (1998) conducted a similar study with 29 cleft palate patients and 31 speakers without velopharyngeal pathology. They compared area-distance functions obtained at the end of a quiet expiration with those obtained while the subjects sustained a static vocal tract posture in which intraoral pressure was maintained, but not released, for

an isolated production of /k/. Kunkel and his coworkers found good correspondence between the change in epipharyngeal volume determined through what they called **acoustic pharyngometry** and what was observed separately via nasendoscopy. Although the change in epipharyngeal volume was found to be significantly lower in the adult cleft palate speakers compared with the adult controls, there was a substantial amount of overlap between the two groups. They concluded that the technique, while seemingly inadequate for differentiating normal from abnormal velopharyngeal mobility, may nonetheless prove a useful index for monitoring therapeutic progress.

Although reflection measurements take only 8 ms to complete, it is not possible as yet to continuously track airway volume since a quiescent period is required to allow for the adequate decay of any residual acoustic energy (Hamilton, McRae, Phillips, & Jones, 1995). Perhaps a more crucial limitation is that the "speaker" must be silent during the assessment of cavity dimensions since speech sounds will interfere with the reflection of the acoustic impulse. With further refinement of the instrument and the technique, however, "acoustic pharyngometry" might represent a valuable research and clinical tool that provides a quick and noninvasive assessment of velar mobility.

REFERENCES

Abbs, J. H., & Watkin, K. L. (1976). Instrumentation for the study of speech physiology. In N. J. Lass (Ed.), *Contemporary issues in experimental phonetics* (pp. 41–75). New York: Academic Press.

Abramson, A., Nye, P., Henderson, J., & Marshall, C. (1981). Vowel height and the perception of consonantal nasality. *Journal of the Acoustical Society of America, 70*, 329–338.

Accordi, M., Croatto-Accordi, D., & Cassin, F. (1981). Possibilità e limiti dell'indagine spettrografica nella valutazione della rinolalia aperta. *Acta Phoniatrica Latina, 3*, 25–31.

Åkefeldt, A., Åkefeldt, B., & Gillberg, C. (1997). Voice, speech and language characteristics of children with Prader-Willi syndrome. *Journal of Intellectual Disability Research, 41*, 302–311.

Ali, L., Gallagher, T., Goldstein, J., & Daniloff, R. (1971). Perception of coarticulated nasality. *Journal of the Acoustical Society of America, 49*, 538–540.

Allison, D. L., & Leeper, H. A., Jr. (1990). A comparison of noninvasive procedures to assess nasal airway resistance. *Cleft Palate Journal, 27*, 40–44.

Anderson, R. T. (1996). Nasometric values for normal Spanish-speaking females: A preliminary report. *Cleft Palate—Craniofacial Journal, 33*, 333–336.

Andreassen, M. L., Leeper, H. A., & MacRae, D. L. (1991). Changes in vocal resonance and nasalization following adenoidectomy in normal children: Preliminary findings. *Journal of Otolaryngology, 20*, 237–242.

Andreassen, M. L., Leeper, H. A., MacRae, D. L., & Nicholson, I. R. (1994). Aerodynamic, acoustic, and perceptual changes following adenoidectomy. *Cleft Palate—Craniofacial Journal, 31*, 263–270.

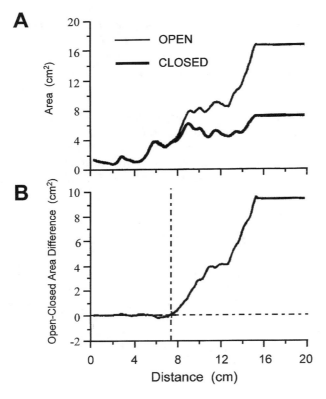

Figure 11–20. Acoustic rhinograms (area-by-distance portraits) for a normal subject. **(A)** Superimposed rhinograms obtained with the velopharyngeal port open and closed. The functions diverge at the entrance to the nasopharynx. **(B)** A "difference" rhinogram derived by subtracting the "closed" from the "open" portraits above. (See also Figure 11–12.) Both **A** and **B** from "Acoustic Rhinometric Measurements of Changes in Velar Positioning," by E.J. Seaver, M.P. Karnell, A. Gasparaitis, and J. Corey, 1995, *Cleft Palate—Craniofacial Journal, 32*, 49–54. Figure 4, p. 51. Reprinted with permission.

Andreassen, M. L., Smith, B. E., & Guyette, T. W. (1991). Pressure-flow measurements for selected oral and nasal sound segments produced by normal adults. *Cleft Palate—Craniofacial Journal, 28,* 398–406.

Austin, C. E., & Foreman, J. C. (1994). Acoustic rhinometry compared with posterior rhinomanometry in the measurement of histamine- and bradykinin-induced changes in nasal airway patency. *British Journal of Clinical Pharmacology, 37,* 33–37.

Awan, S. N. (1996). Development of a low-cost nasalance acquisition system. In T. W. Powell (Ed.), *Pathologies of speech and language: Contributions of clinical phonetics and linguistics* (pp. 211–217). New Orleans, LA: International Clinical Phonetics and Linguistics Association.

Awan, S. N. (1998). Analysis of nasalance: NasalView (the Nasalance Acquisition System). In W. Ziegler & K. Deger (Eds.), *Clinical phonetics and linguistics* (pp. 518–527). London, UK: Whurr Publishers.

Awan, S., Bressman, T., Sader, R., Busch, R., & Horch, H. (1998, November). *Clinical assessment of hypernasality using the NasalView system.* Presentation at the annual convention of the American Speech-Language-Hearing Association. San Antonio, TX.

Baer, T., Gore, J. C., Boyce, S., & Nye, P. W. (1987). Application of MRI to the analysis of speech production. *Magnetic Resonance Imaging, 5,* 1–7.

Baer, T., Gore, J. C., Gracco, L. C., & Nye, P. W. (1991). Analysis of vocal tract shape and dimensions using magnetic resonance imaging: Vowels. *Journal of the Acoustical Society of America, 90,* 799–828.

Baken, R. J., & Orlikoff, R. F. (1987). Phonatory response to step-function changes in supraglottal pressure. In T. Baer, C. Sasaki, & K. S. Harris (Eds.), *Laryngeal function in phonation and respiration* (pp. 273–290). Boston, MA: College-Hill Press.

Barnes, I. J., & Morris, H. L. (1967). Interrelationships among oral breath pressure ratios and articulation skills for individuals with cleft palate. *Journal of Speech and Hearing Research, 10,* 506–514.

Basmajian, J. V., & Dutta, C. R. (1961). Electromyography of the pharyngeal constrictors and levator palati in man. *Anatomical Record, 139,* 561–563.

Beddor, P. S. (1993). The perception of nasal vowels. In M. K. Huffman & R. A. Krakow (Eds.), *Phonetics and phonology, Volume 5: Nasals, nasalization, and the velum* (pp. 171–196). San Diego, CA: Academic Press.

Beddor, P. S., & Strange, W. (1982). Cross-language study of perception of the oral-nasal distinction. *Journal of the Acoustical Society of America, 71,* 1551–1561.

Bell, A. M. (1890). The "nasal twang." *Modern Language Notes, 5,* 150–152.

Bell-Berti, F. (1976). An electromyographic study of velopharyngeal function in speech. *Journal of Speech and Hearing Research, 19,* 225–240.

Bell-Berti, F. (1980). Velopharyngeal function: A spatial-temporal model. In N. J. Lass (Ed.), *Advances in basic research and practice* (Vol. 4, pp. 291–316). New York: Academic Press.

Bell-Berti, F. (1993). Understanding velic motor control: Studies of segmental context. In M. K. Huffman & R. A. Krakow (Eds.), *Phonetics and phonology, Volume 5: Nasals, nasalization, and the velum* (pp. 63–85). San Diego, CA: Academic Press.

Bell-Berti, F., Baer, T., Harris, K. S., & Niimi, S. (1979). Coarticulatory effects of vowel quality on velar function. *Phonetica, 36,* 187–193.

Bell-Berti, F., & Krakow, R. A. (1991). Anticipatory velar lowering: A coproduction account. *Journal of the Acoustical Society of America, 90,* 112–123.

Benguerel, A.-P., Hirose, H., Sawashima, M., & Ushijima, T. (1977a). Velar coarticulation in French: A fiberoptic study. *Journal of Phonetics, 5,* 149–158.

Benguerel, A.-P., Hirose, H., Sawashima, M., & Ushijima, T. (1977b). Velar coarticulation in French: An electromyographic study. *Journal of Phonetics, 5,* 159–167.

Berkinshaw, E. R., Spalding, P. M., & Vig, P. S. (1987). The effect of methodology on the determination of nasal resistance. *American Journal of Orthodontics and Dentofacial Orthopedics, 92,* 329–335.

Bernthal, J. E., & Beukelman, D. R. (1977). The effect of changes in velopharyngeal orifice area on vowel intensity. *Cleft Palate Journal, 14,* 63–77.

Björk, L., & Nylén, B. O. (1961). Cineradiography with synchronized sound spectrum analysis. *Plastic and Reconstructive Surgery, 27,* 397–412.

Blackfield, H., Miller, E., Owsely, J., & Lawson, L. (1962). Cinefluorographic evaluation of patients with velopharyngeal dysfunction in the absence of overt cleft palate. *Plastic and Reconstructive Surgery, 30,* 441–451.

Bloomer, H. (1953). Observation of palatopharyngeal movements in speech and deglutition. *Journal of Speech and Hearing Disorders, 18,* 230–246.

Bloomer, H., & Peterson, G. (1955). A spectrographic study of hypernasality. *Cleft Palate Bulletin, 5,* 5–6.

Bradford, L. J., Brooks, A. R., & Shelton, R. L. (1964). Clinical judgment of hypernasality in cleft palate children. *Cleft Palate Journal, 1,* 329–335.

Bradley, D. P. (1989). Congenital and acquired velopharyngeal inadequacy. In K. R. Bzoch (Ed.), *Communicative disorders related to cleft lip and palate* (3rd ed., pp. 106–122). Boston, MA: College-Hill Press.

Brancewicz, T. M., & Reich, A. R. (1989). Speech rate reduction and "nasality" in normal speakers. *Journal of Speech and Hearing Research, 32,* 837–848.

Broadbent, T. R., & Swinyard, C. A. (1959). The dynamic pharyngeal flap: Its selective use and electromyographic evaluation. *Plastic and Reconstructive Surgery, 23,* 301–312.

Broms, P., Ivarsson, A., & Jonson, B. (1982). Rhinomanometry I: Simple equipment. *Acta Otolaryngologica, 93,* 455–460.

Broms, P., Jonson, B., & Lamm, C. J. (1982). Rhinomanometry II: A system for numerical description of nasal airway resistance. *Acta Otolaryngologica, 94,* 157–168.

Brunner, M., Stellzig, A., Decker, W., Strate, B., Komposch, G., Wirth, G., & Verres, R. (1994). Video-Feedback-Therapie mit dem flexiblen Nasopharyngoskop: Einflussmöglichkeiten auf den velopharyngealen Verschluss und Lautbildungsfehler bei Spaltpatienten. *Fortschritte der Kieferorthopädie, 55,* 197–201.

Buck, M. (1954). Post-operative velo-pharyngeal movements in cleft palate cases. *Journal of Speech and Hearing Disorders, 19,* 288–294.

Buenting, J. E., Dalston, R. M., & Drake, A. F. (1994). Nasal cavity area in term infants determined by acoustic rhinometry. *Laryngoscope, 104,* 1439–1445.

Bzoch, K. R. (1968). Variations in velopharyngeal valving: The factor of vowel changes. *Cleft Palate Journal, 5,* 211–218.

Bzoch, K. R. (1970). Assessment: Radiographic techniques. *ASHA Reports, 5,* 248–270.

Bzoch, K. R. (1989). Measurement and assessment of categorical aspects of cleft palate speech. In K. R. Bzoch (Ed.), *Communicative disorders related to cleft lip and palate,* (3rd ed. pp. 137–173). Boston, MA: College-Hill Press.

Calnan, J., & Renfrew, C. E. (1961). Blowing tests and speech. *British Journal of Plastic Surgery, 13,* 340–346.

Carrell, J. A. (1952). A cinefluorographic technique for the sutdy of velopharyngeal closure. *Journal of Speech and Hearing Disorders, 17,* 224–228.

Cass, L. J. (1967). Measurement of total respiratory and nasal air-flow resistance. *Journal of the American Medical Association, 199,* 396–398.

Chase, R. A. (1960). An objective evaluation of palatopharyngeal competence. *Plastic and Reconstructive Surgery, 26,* 23–29.

Christiansen, R. L., & Moller, K. T. (1971). Instrumentation for recording velar movement. *American Journal of Orthodontics, 59,* 448–455.

Clarke, W. M. (1975). The measurement of the oral and nasal sound pressure levels of speech. *Journal of Phonetics, 3,* 257–262.

Clarke, W. M. (1978). The relationship between subjective measures of nasality and measures of the oral and nasal sound pressure ratio. *Language and Speech, 21,* 69–75.

Claypoole, W. H., Warren, D. W., & Bradley, D. P. (1974). The effect of cleft palate on oral port constriction during fricative productions. *Cleft Palate Journal, 11,* 95–104.

Clumeck, H. (1976). Patterns of soft palate movements in six languages. *Journal of Phonetics, 5,* 149–158.

Cockcroft, D. W., MacCormack, D. W., Tarlo, S. M., Hargreave, F. E., & Pengelly, L. D. (1979). Nasal airway resistance. *American Review of Respiratory Disease, 119,* 921–926.

Cohn, A. C. (1993). The status of nasalized continuants. In M. K. Huffman & R. A. Krakow (Eds.), *Phonetics and phonology, Volume 5: Nasals, nasalization, and the velum* (pp. 329–367). San Diego, CA: Academic Press.

Cohn, E. R., Garver, K. L., Metz, H. C., McWilliams, B. J., Skolnick, M. L., & Garrett, W. S. (1982). Velopharyngeal incompetence in a patient with multifocal eosinophilic granuloma (Hand-Schüller-Christian disease). *Journal of Speech and Hearing Disorders, 47,* 320–323.

Colton, R. H., & Cooker, H. S. (1968). Perceived nasality in the speech of the deaf. *Journal of Speech and Hearing Research, 11,* 553–559.

Colyar, T. C., & Christensen, J. M. (1980). Nasalance patterns in esophageal speech. *Journal of Communication Disorders, 13,* 43–48.

Condax, I. D., Acson, V., Miki, C. C., & Sakoda, K. K. (1976). A technique for monitoring velic action by means of a photo-electric nasal probe: Application to French. *Journal of Phonetics, 4,* 173–181.

Condax, I. D., Howard, I., Ikranagara, K., Lin, Y. C., Crosetti, J., & Yount, D. E. (1974). A new technique for demonstrating velic opening: Application to Sudanese. *Journal of Phonetics, 2,* 297–301.

Connell, J. T. (1982). Rhinometry: Measurement of nasal patency. *Annals of Allergy, 49,* 179–185.

Cooper, F. S. (1965). Research techniques and instrumentation: EMG. *ASHA Reports, 1,* 153–168.

Corey, J. P., Gungor, A., Nelson, R., Fredberg, J., & Lai, V. (1997). A comparison of the nasal cross-sectional areas and volumes obtained with acoustic rhinometry and magnetic resonance imaging. *Otolaryngology—Head and Neck Surgery, 117,* 349–354.

Corey, J. P., Kemker, B. J., Nelson, R., & Gungor, A. (1997). Evaluation of the nasal cavity by acoustic rhinometry in normal and allergic subjects. *Otolaryngology—Head and Neck Surgery, 117,* 22–28.

Counihan, D. T. (1972). Oral and nasal sound pressure measures. In K. R. Bzoch (Ed.), *Communicative disorders related to cleft lip and palate* (pp. 186–193). Boston, MA: Little, Brown.

Counihan, D. T., & Culligan, W. L. (1970). Reliability and dispersion of nasality ratings. *Cleft Palate Journal, 19,* 1–8.

Covello, L. V., Karnell, M. P., & Seaver, E. J. (1992). Videoendoscopy and photodetection: Linearity of a new integrated system. *Cleft Palate—Craniofacial Journal, 29,* 168–173.

Craig, A. B., Dvorak, M., & McIlreath, F. J. (1965). Resistance to airflow through the nose. *Annals of Otology, Rhinology and Laryngology, 74,* 589–603.

Croatto, L., Cinotti, A., Moschi, P., & Toti-Zattoni, A. (1980). Il contributo xeroradiografico nello studio dell'insufficienza velo-faringea. *Acta Phoniatrica Latina, 2,* 31–50.

Curtis, J. F. (1968). Acoustics of speech production and nasalization. In D. C. Spriestersbach & D. Sherman (Eds.), *Cleft palate and communication* (pp. 27–60). New York: Academic Press.

Curtis, J. F. (1970). The acoustics of nasalized speech. *Cleft Palate Journal, 7,* 380–396.

Dalston, R. M. (1982). Photodetector assessment of velopharyngeal activity. *Cleft Palate Journal, 19,* 1–8.

Dalston, R. M. (1989). Using simultaneous photodetection and nasometry to monitor velopharyngeal behavior during speech. *Journal of Speech and Hearing Research, 32,* 195–202.

Dalston, R. M. (1992). Acoustic assessment of the nasal airway. *Cleft Palate—Craniofacial Journal, 29,* 520–526.

Dalston, R. M., & Keefe, M. J. (1987). The use of a microcomputer in monitoring and modifying velopharyngeal movements. *Journal for Computer Users in Speech and Hearing, 3,* 159–169.

Dalston, R. M., & Keefe, M. J. (1988). Digital, labial and velopharyngeal reaction times in normal speakers. *Cleft Palate Journal, 25,* 203–209.

Dalston, R. M., Neiman, G. S., & González Landa, G. (1993). Nasometric sensitivity and specificity: A cross-dialect and cross-culture study. *Cleft Palate—Craniofacial Journal, 30,* 285–291.

Dalston, R. M., & Seaver, E. J. (1990). Nasometric and photo-transductive measurements of reaction times among normal adult speakers. *Cleft Palate Journal, 27,* 61–67.

Dalston, R. M., & Seaver, E. J. (1992). Relative values of standardized passages in the nasometric assessment of patients with velopharyngeal impairment. *Cleft Palate—Craniofacial Journal, 29,* 17–21.

Dalston, R. M., & Warren, D. W. (1986). Comparison of Tonar II, pressure-flow, and listener judgments of hypernasality in the assessment of velopharyngeal function. *Cleft Palate Journal, 23,* 108–115.

Dalston, R. M., Warren, D. W., & Dalston, E. T. (1991a). A preliminary investigation concerning the use of nasometry in identifying patients with hyponasality and/or nasal airway impairment. *Journal of Speech and Hearing Research, 34,* 11–18.

Dalston, R. M., Warren, D. W., & Dalston, E. T. (1991b). The identification of nasal obstruction through clinical judgments of hyponasality and nasometric assessment of speech acoustics. *American Journal of Orthodontics and Dentofacial Orthopedics, 100,* 59–65.

Dalston, R. M., Warren, D. W., & Dalston, E. T. (1991c). Use of nasometry as a diagnostic tool for identifying patients with velopharyngeal impairment. *Cleft Palate—Craniofacial Journal, 28,* 184–188.

Dalston, R. M., Warren, D. W., Morr, K. E., & Smith, L. R. (1988). Intraoral pressure and its relationship to velopharyngeal inadequacy. *Cleft Palate Journal, 25,* 210–219.

Dalston, R. M., Warren, D. W., & Smith, L. R. (1990). The aerodynamic characteristics of speech produced by normal speakers and cleft palate speakers with adequate velopharyngeal function. *Cleft Palate Journal, 27,* 393–399.

Dang, J., Honda, K., & Suzuki, H. (1994). Morphological and acoustical analysis of the nasal and paranasal cavities. *Journal of the Acoustical Society of America, 96,* 2088–2100.

D'Antonio, L. L., Achauer, B. M., & Vander Kam, V. M. (1993). Results of a survey of cleft palate teams concerning the use of nasendoscopy. *Cleft Palate—Craniofacial Journal, 30,* 35–39.

D'Antonio, L. L., Chait, D., Lotz, W. K., & Netsell, R. (1986). Pediatric videonasoendoscopy for speech and voice evaluation. *Otolaryngology—Head and Neck Surgery, 94,* 578–583.

D'Antonio, L. L., Muntz, H. R., Marsh, J. L., Grames, L. M., & Backensto-Marsh, R. (1988). Practical application of flexible fiberoptic nasopharyngoscopy for evaluating velopharyngeal function. *Plastic and Reconstructive Surgery, 82,* 611–618.

Darley, F. L., Aronson, A., & Brown, J. (1969). Clusters of deviant speech dimensions in the dysarthrias. *Journal of Speech and Hearing Research, 12,* 462–496.

Davies, H. J. (1978). Measurement of nasal patency using a Vitalograph. *Clinical Allergy, 8,* 517–523.

Dejonckere, P. H. (1984). L'oscillographie oronasale. *Bulletin d'Audiophonologie, 17,* 207–218.

de Jong, K. J. (1997). Labiovelar compensation in back vowels. *Journal of the Acoustical Society of America, 101,* 2221–2233.

Delattre, P. (1954). Les attributs acoustiques de la nasalité vocalique et consonantique. *Studia Linguistica, 8,* 103–109.

Delattre, P. (1955). La nasalité vocalique en français et en anglais. *French Review, 39,* 92–109.

Dickson, D. R. (1962). An acoustic study of nasality. *Journal of Speech and Hearing Research, 5,* 103–111.

Dickson, S., Barron, S., & McGlone, R. E. (1978). Aerodynamic studies of cleft-palate speech. *Journal of Speech and Hearing Disorders, 43,* 160–167.

Di Girolamo, M., Corsetti, A., Laghi, A., Ferone, E., Iannicelli, E., Rossi, M., Pavone, P., & Passariello, R. (1996). Valutazione con Risonanza Magnetica dei movimenti della laringe e della cavità faringo-buccale durante la fonazione. *La Radiologia Medica, 92,* 33–40.

Dillenschneider, E., Zaleski, T., & Grenier, G. F. (1973). Étude sonagraphique de la nasalité dans le cas d'insuffisance palatovélaire. *Journal Français d'Otorhinolaryngologie, 22,* 201–202.

Djupesland, P. G., Kaastad, E., & Franzen, G. (1997). Acoustic rhinometry in the evaluation of congenital choanal malformations. *International Journal of Pediatric Otorhinolaryngology, 41,* 319–337.

Djupesland, P. G., & Lyholm, B. (1997). Nasal airway dimensions in term neonates measured by continuous wide-band noise acoustic rhinometry. *Acta Otolaryngologica, 117,* 424–432.

Dotevall, H., Lohmander-Agerskov, A., Almquist, S.-Å., & Bake, B. (1998). Aerodynamic assessment of velopharyngeal function during normal speech containing different places of articulation. *Folia Phoniatrica et Logopaedica, 50,* 53–63.

Dunn, H. K. (1950). The calculation of vowel resonances, and an electrical vocal tract. *Journal of the Acoustical Society of America, 22,* 740–753.

Dworkin, J. P. (1991). *Motor speech disorders: A treatment guide* (pp. 41–83). St. Louis, MO: Mosby.

Eisenbach, C. R., II, & Williams, W. N. (1984). Comparing the unaided visual exam to lateral cinefluorography in estimating several parameters of velopharyngeal function. *Journal of Speech and Hearing Disorders, 49,* 136–139.

Elbrønd, O., Hilberg, O., & Felding, J. U. (1991). Acoustic rhinometry: A new method to evaluate the geometry of the nasal cavity and the epipharynx. *American Journal of Rhinology, 5,* 7–9.

Ellis, R. E., Flack, F. C., Curle, H. J., & Selley, W. G. (1978). A system for assessment of nasal airflow during speech. *British Journal of Disorders of Communication, 13,* 31–40.

Emanuel, F. W., & Counihan, D. T. (1970). Some characteristics of oral and nasal air flow during plosive consonant production. *Cleft Palate Journal, 7,* 249–260.

Enderby, P. (1986). Relationships between dysarthria groups. *British Journal of Disorders of Communication, 21,* 189–197.

Engelke, W., Bruns, T., Striebeck, M., & Hoch, G. (1996). Midsagittal velar kinematics during production of VCV sequences. *Cleft Palate—Craniofacial Journal, 33,* 236–244.

Engelke, W., & Hoch, G. (1994). Simultane elektromagnetische Artikulographie und Videoendoskopie. Ein kasuistischer Beitrag zur objektiven Diagnostik des velopharyngealen Sphinkters. *Fortschritte der Kieferorthopädie, 55,* 297–303.

Engelke, W., Hoch, G., Bruns, T., & Striebeck, M. (1996). Simultaneous evaluation of articulatory velopharyngeal function under different dynamic conditions with EMA and videoendoscopy. *Folia Phoniatrica et Logopaedica, 48,* 65–77.

Engelke, W., Müller, C., & Petersen, C. (1995). Physiologie oropharyngealer Schluckbewegungen. *Sprache, Stimme, Gehör, 19,* 105–113.

Engelke, W., & Schönle, P. W. (1991). Elektromagnetische Artikulographie: Eine neue Methode zur Untersuchung von Bewegungsfunktionen des Gaumensegels. *Folia Phoniatrica, 43,* 147–152.

Engelke, W., Schönle, P. W., & Engelke, D. (1990). 2 objektive Verfahren zur Untersuchung motorischer Funktionen nach Eingriffen an Zunge und Velum. *Deutsche Zeitschrift fur Mund-, Kiefer-, und Gesichts-Chirurgie, 14,* 348–358.

Fairbanks, G. (1960). *Voice and articulation drillbook.* New York: Harper.

Farnetani, E. (1979). Foni nasali e nasalizzazione. *Acta Phoniatrica Latina, 1,* 30–57.

Feng, G., & Castelli, E. (1996). Some acoustic features of nasal and nasalized vowels: A target for vowel nasalization. *Journal of the Acoustical Society of America, 99,* 3694–3706.

Finck, C., Gaspard, M., & Melon, J. (1987). Evaluation fonctionnelle d'une insuffisance vélaire par rhinomanométrie antérieure. *Folia Phoniatrica, 39,* 192–195.

Fisher, E. W., Daly, N. J., Morris, D. P., & Lund, V. J. (1994). Experimental studies of the resolution of acoustic rhinometry in vivo. *Acta Otolaryngologica, 114,* 647–650.

Fisher, E. W., Morris, D. P., Biemans, J. M. A., Palmer, C. R., & Lund, V. J. (1995). Practical aspects of acoustic rhinometry: Problems and solutions. *Rhinology, 33,* 219–223.

Flege, J. E. (1988). Anticipatory and carry-over nasal coarticulation in the speech of children and adults. *Journal of Speech and Hearing Research, 31,* 525–536.

Fletcher, S. G. (1970). Theory and instrumentation for quantitative measurement of nasality. *Cleft Palate Journal, 7,* 601–609.

Fletcher, S. G. (1972). Contingencies for bioelectronic modification of nasality. *Journal of Speech and Hearing Disorders, 37,* 329–346.

Fletcher, S. G. (1973). *Manual for measurement and modification of nasality with TONAR II.* Birmingham, AL: University of Alabama.

Fletcher, S. G. (1976). "Nasalance" vs. listener judgments of nasality. *Cleft Palate Journal, 13,* 31–44.

Fletcher, S. G. (1978). *Diagnosing speech disorders from cleft palate.* New York: Grune & Stratton.

Fletcher, S. G., Adams, L. E., & McCutcheon, M. J. (1989). Cleft palate speech assessment through oral-nasal acoustic measures. In K. R. Bzoch (Ed.), *Communicative disorders related to cleft lip and palate* (3rd ed., pp. 246–257). Boston, MA: College-Hill Press.

Fletcher, S. G., & Bishop, M. E. (1970). Measurement of nasality with TONAR. *Cleft Palate Journal, 7,* 610–621.

Fletcher, S. G., & Daly, D. A. (1976). Nasality in utterances of hearing-impaired speakers. *Journal of Communication Disorders, 9,* 63–73.

Fletcher, S. G., & Higgins, J. M. (1980). Performance of children with severe to profound auditory impairment in instrumentally guided reduction of nasal resonance. *Journal of Speech and Hearing Disorders, 45,* 181–194.

Fletcher, S. G., Sooudi, I., & Frost, S. D. (1974). Quantitative and graphic analysis of prosthetic treatment for "nasalance" in speech. *Journal of Prosthetic Dentistry, 32,* 284–291.

Fox, D. R., & Johns, D. (1970). Predicting velopharyngeal closure with a modified tongue-anchor technique. *Journal of Speech and Hearing Disorders, 35,* 248–251.

Fritzell, B. (1963). An electromyographic study of the movements of the soft palate in speech. *Folia Phoniatrica, 15,* 307–311.

Fritzell, B. (1969). A combined electromyographic and cineradiographic study: Activity of the levator and palatoglossus muscles in relation to velar movements. *Acta Otolaryngologica,* Suppl. 250, 1–81.

Fritzell, B. (1979). Electromyography in the study of the velopharyngeal function—A review. *Folia Phoniatrica, 31,* 93–102.

Fritzell, B., & Kotby, N. M. (1976). Observations on thyroarytenoid and palatal levator activation for speech. *Folia Phoniatrica, 28,* 1–7.

Fujimura, O. (1960). Spectra of nasalized vowels. *Quarterly Progress Report of the Research Laboratory of Electronics* (MIT), *15,* 214–218.

Fujimura, O. (1962). Analysis of nasal consonants. *Journal of the Acoustical Society of America, 34,* 1865–1875.

Fujimura, O. (1990). Methods and goals of speech production research. *Language and Speech, 33,* 195–258.

Fujimura, O., Kiritani, S., & Ishida, H. (1973). Computer-controlled radiography for observation of movements of articulatory and other human organs. *Computers in Biology and Medicine, 3,* 371–384.

Garber, S. R., Burzynski, C. M., Vale, C., & Nelson, R. (1979). The use of visual feedback to control vocal intensity and nasalization. *Journal of Communication Disorders, 12,* 399–410.

Garber, S. R., & Moller, K. T. (1979). The effects of feedback filtering on nasality in normal and hypernasal speakers. *Journal of Speech and Hearing Research, 22,* 321–333.

Garnier, S., Gallego, S., Collet, L., & Berger-Vachon, C. (1996). Spectral and cepstral properties of vowels as a means for characterizing velopharyngeal impairment in children. *Cleft Palate—Craniofacial Journal, 33,* 507–512.

Gilain, L., Coste, A., Ricolfi, F., Dahan, E., Marliac, D., Peynegre, R., Harf, A., & Louis, B. (1997). Nasal cavity geometry measured by acoustic rhinometry and computed tomography. *Archives of Otolaryngology—Head and Neck Surgery, 123,* 401–405.

Gilbert, H. R., & Ferrand, C. T. (1987). A respirometric technique to evaluate velopharyngeal function in speakers with cleft palate, with and without prostheses. *Journal of Speech and Hearing Research, 30,* 268–275.

Gilbert, H. R., & Hoodin, R. B. (1984). Effect of speaking rate on nasal airflow in hearing-impaired speakers. *Folia Phoniatrica, 36,* 183–189.

Glaser, E. R., & Shprintzen, R. J. (1979). *See-Scape:* Instrument and manual (review). *Cleft Palate Journal, 16,* 213–214.

Glass, P., & Teller, F. F. (1969). Assessment of dynamics of nasopharyngeal air flow. *American Review of Respiratory Disease, 99,* 437–439.

Gonay, P. (1972). Effet du nasonnement sur les formants vocaliques. *Acta Oto-Rhino-Laryngologica Belgica, 26,* 757–770.

González Landa, G., Santos Terrón, M. J., Miro-Viar, J. L., & Sánchez-Ruiz, I. (1990). Insuficiencia velofaríngea postadenoidectomia en niños con fisuras velopalatinas. *Acta Otorrinolaringologica Española, 41,* 159–161.

Grymer, L. F. (1995). Reduction rhinoplasty and nasal patency: Change in the cross-sectional area of the nose evaluated by acoustic rhinometry. *Laryngoscope, 105,* 429–431.

Grymer, L. F., Hilberg, O., Elbrvnd, O., & Pedersen, O. F. (1989). Acoustic rhinometry: Evaluation of the nasal cavity with septal deviations, before and after septoplasty. *Laryngoscope, 99,* 1180–1187.

Haapanen, M.-L. (1991a). A simple clinical method of evaluating perceived hypernasality. *Folia Phoniatrica, 43,* 122–132.

Haapanen, M.-L. (1991b). Nasalance scores in normal Finnish speech. *Folia Phoniatrica, 43,* 197–203.

Haapanen, M.-L., & Somer, M. (1993). Velocardiofacial syndrome: Analysis of phoniatric and other clinical findings. *Folia Phoniatrica, 45,* 239–246.

Hagerty, R. F., Hill, M. J., Pettit, H. S., & Kane, J. J. (1958a). Posterior pharyngeal wall movement in normals. *Journal of Speech and Hearing Research, 1,* 203–210.

Hagerty, R. F., Hill, M. J., Pettit, H. S., & Kane, J. J. (1958b). Soft palate movements in normals. *Journal of Speech and Hearing Research, 1,* 325–330.

Hamilton, J. W., McRae, R. D., & Jones, A. S. (1997). The magnitude of random errors in acoustic rhinometry and re-interpretation of the acoustic profile. *Clinical Otolaryngology, 22,* 408–413.

Hamilton, J. W., McRae, R. D., Phillips, D. E., & Jones, A. S. (1995). The accuracy of acoustic rhinometry using a pulse train signal. *Clinical Otolaryngology, 20,* 279–282.

Hamilton, L. H. (1979). Nasal airway resistance: Its measurement and regulation. *Physiologist, 22,* 43–49.

Hanson, M. L. (1964). A study of velopharyngeal competence in children with repaired cleft palates. *Cleft Palate Journal, 1,* 217–231.

Hardin, M. A., Van Demark, D. R., & Morris, H. L. (1990). Long-term speech results of cleft palate speakers with marginal velopharyngeal competence. *Journal of Communication Disorders, 23,* 401–416.

Hardin, M. A., Van Demark, D. R., Morris, H. L., & Payne, M. M. (1992). Correspondence between nasalance scores and listener judgments of hypernasality and hyponasality. *Cleft Palate—Craniofacial Journal, 29,* 346–351.

Hardy, J. C. (1965). Air flow and air pressure studies. *ASHA Reports, 1,* 141–152.

Hardy, J. C. (1967). Techniques of measuring intraoral air pressure and rate of air flow. *Journal of Speech and Hearing Research, 10,* 650–654.

Hardy, J. C., & Arkebauer, H. J. (1966). Development of a test for velopharyngeal competence during speech. *Cleft Palate Journal, 3,* 6–21.

Hardy, J. C., Netsell, R. Schweiger, J. W., & Morris, H. L. (1969). Management of velopharyngeal dysfunction in cerebral palsy. *Journal of Speech and Hearing Disorders, 34,* 123–137.

Harrington, R. (1944). A study of the mechanism of velopharyngeal closure. *Journal of Speech and Hearing Disorders, 9,* 325–345.

Harrington, R. (1946). A note on a lingua-velar relationship. *Journal of Speech and Hearing Disorders, 11,* 25.

Harris, K. S., Schvey, M., & Lysaught, G. (1962). Component gestures in the production of oral and nasal stops. *Journal of the Acoustical Society of America, 34,* 743.

Hasegawa, M., Kern, E. G., & O'Brien, P. C. (1979). Dynamic changes of nasal resistance. *Annals of Otolaryngology, 88,* 66–71.

Hattori, S., Yamamoto, K., & Fujimura, O. (1958). Nasalization of vowels in relation to nasals. *Journal of the Acoustical Society of America, 30,* 267–274.

Hawkins, C. F., & Swisher, W. E. (1978). Evaluation of a real-time ultrasound scanner in assessing lateral pharyngeal wall motion during speech. *Cleft Palate Journal, 15,* 161–166.

Hawkins, S., & Stevens, K. N. (1985). Acoustic and perceptual correlates of the non-nasal—nasal distinction for vowels. *Journal of the Acoustical Society of America, 77,* 1560–1575.

Heppt, W., Westrich, M., Strate, B., & Mohring, L. (1991). Nasalanz: Ein neuer Begriff der objektiven Nasalitätsanalyse. *Laryngo-Rhino-Otologie, 70,* 208–213.

Hering, R., Hoppe, W., & Kraft, E. (1965). Über electromyographische Untersuchungen von Patienten mit Gaumenspalten. *Stoma, 18,* 24–36.

Hess, D. A. (1959). Pitch, intensity and cleft palate voice quality. *Journal of Speech and Hearing Research, 2,* 113–125.

Hess, D. A. (1976). A new experimental approach to assessment of velopharyngeal adequacy: Nasal manometric bleed testing. *Journal of Speech and Hearing Disorders, 41,* 427–443.

Hess, D. A., & McDonald, E. T. (1960). Consonantal nasal pressure in cleft palate speakers. *Journal of Speech and Hearing Research, 3,* 201–211.

Hibi, S. R., Bless, D. M., Hirano, M., & Yoshida, T. (1988). Distortions of videofiberoscopy imaging: Reconsideration and correction. *Journal of Voice, 2,* 168–175.

Hilberg, O., Grymer, L. F., Pedersen, O. F., & Elbrvnd, O. (1990). Turbinate hypertrophy. Evaluation of the nasal cavity by acoustic rhinometry. *Archives of Otolaryngology—Head and Neck Surgery, 116,* 283–289.

Hilberg, O., Jackson, A. C., Swift, D. L., & Pedersen, O. F. (1989). Acoustic rhinometry: Evaluation of nasal cavity geometry by acoustic reflection. *Journal of Applied Physiology, 66,* 295–303.

Hilberg, O., Jensen, F. T., & Pedersen, O. F. (1993). Nasal airway geometry: Comparison between acoustic reflections and magnetic resonance scanning. *Journal of Applied Physiology, 75,* 2811–2819.

Hilberg, O., Lyholm, B., Michelsen, A., Pedersen, O. F., & Jacobsen, O. (1998). Acoustic reflections during rhinometry: Spatial resolution and sound loss. *Journal of Applied Physiology, 84,* 1030–1039.

Hinton, V. A., & Warren, D. W. (1995). Relationships between integrated oral-nasal differential pressure and velopharyngeal closure. *Cleft Palate—Craniofacial Journal, 32,* 307–310.

Hirano, M., Takeuchi, Y., & Hiroto, I. (1966). Intranasal sound pressure during utterance of speech sounds. *Folia Phoniatrica, 18,* 369–381.

Hixon, T. J. (1966). Turbulent noise sources for speech. *Folia Phoniatrica, 18,* 168–182.

Hixon, T. J. (1972). Some new techniques for measuring the biomechanical events of speech production: One laboratory's experiences. *ASHA Reports, 7,* 68–103.

Hixon, T. J., Bless, D. M., & Netsell, R. (1976). A new technique for measuring velopharyngeal orifice area during sustained phonation: An application of aerodynamic forced oscillation principles. *Journal of Speech and Hearing Research, 19,* 601–607.

Hixon, T. J., Saxman, J. H., & McQueen, H. D. (1967). A respirometric technique for evaluating velopharyngeal competence during speech. *Folia Phoniatrica, 19,* 203–219.

Hogan, V. M. (1973). A clarification of the surgical goals in cleft palate speech and the introduction of the lateral port control (L.P.C.) pharyngeal flap. *Cleft Palate Journal, 10,* 331–345.

Hoit, J. D., Watson, P. J., Hixon, K. E., McMahon, P., & Johnson, C. L. (1994). Age and velopharyngeal function during speech production. *Journal of Speech and Hearing Research, 37,* 295–302.

Hong, K. H., Kwon, S. H., & Jung, S. S. (1997). The assessment of nasality with a nasometer and sound spectrography in patients with nasal polyposis. *Otolaryngology—Head and Neck Surgery, 117,* 343–348.

Honjo, I., & Isshiki, N. (1971). Pharyngeal stop in cleft palate speech. *Folia Phoniatrica, 23,* 325–354.

Hoodin, R. B., & Gilbert, H. R. (1989). Parkinsonian dysarthria: An aerodynamic and perceptual description of velopharyngeal closure for speech. *Folia Phoniatrica, 41,* 249–258.

Horiguchi, S., & Bell-Berti, F. (1987). The Velotrace: A device for monitoring velar position. *Cleft Palate Journal, 24,* 104–111.

Horii, Y. (1980). An accelerometric approach to nasality measurement: A preliminary report. *Cleft Palate Journal, 17,* 254–261.

Horii, Y. (1983). An accelerometric measure as a physical correlate of perceived hypernasality in speech. *Journal of Speech and Hearing Research, 26,* 476–480.

Horii, Y. (1987). A simplified accelerometer method of nasality measurement. *ASHA, 29,* 123.

Horii, Y. (1990). Comment. *Cleft Palate Journal, 27,* 270–274.

Horii, Y., & Lang, J. E. (1981). Distributional analysis of an index of nasal coupling (HONC) in simulated hypernasal speech. *Cleft Palate Journal, 18,* 279–285.

Horii, Y., & Monroe, N. (1983). Auditory and visual feedback of nasalization using a modified accelerometric method. *Journal of Speech and Hearing Research, 26,* 472–475.

House, A. S. (1957). Analog studies of nasal consonants. *Journal of Speech and Hearing Disorders, 22,* 190–204.

House, A. S., & Stevens, K. N. (1956). Analog studies of the nasalization of vowels. *Journal of Speech and Hearing Disorders, 21,* 218–232.

Hultzen, L. S. (1942). Apparatus for demonstrating nasality. *Journal of Speech Disorders, 7,* 5–6.

Hutchinson, J. M., Robinson, K. L., & Nerbonne, M. A. (1978). Patterns of nasalance in a sample of normal gerontologic subjects. *Journal of Communication Disorders, 11,* 469–481.

Hutters, B., & Brvndsted, K. (1992). A simple nasal anemometer for clinical purposes. *European Journal of Disorders of Communication, 27,* 101–119.

Hyde, S. R. (1968). Nose trumpet: Apparatus for separating the oral and nasal outputs in speech. *Nature, 219,* 763–765.

Ibuki, K., Karnell, M. P., & Morris, H. L. (1983). Reliability of the nasopharyngeal fiberscope (NPF) for assessing velopharyngeal function. *Cleft Palate Journal, 20,* 97–104.

Iglesias, A., Kuehn, D. P., & Morris, H. L. (1980). Simultaneous assessment of pharyngeal wall and velar displacement for selected speech sounds. *Journal of Speech and Hearing Research, 23,* 429–446.

Ingelstedt, S., Jonson, B., & Rundcrantz, H. (1969). A clinical method for determination of nasal airway resistance. *Acta Otolaryngologica, 68,* 189–200.

Isshiki, N., Honjow, I., & Morimoto, M. (1968). Effects of velopharyngeal incompetence upon speech. *Cleft Palate Journal, 5,* 297–310.

Itoh, M., Sasanuma, S., Hirose, H., Yoshiyoka, H., & Sawashima, M. (1983). Velar movements during speech in two Wernicke aphasia patients. *Brain and Language, 19,* 283–292.

Itoh, M., Sasanuma, S., & Ushijima, T. (1979). Velar movements during speech in a patient with apraxia of speech. *Brain and Language, 7,* 227–239.

Jäger, L., Günther, E., Gauger, J., Nitz, W., Kastenbauer, E., & Reiser, M. (1996). Funktionelle MRT des Pharynx bei obstruktiver Schlafapnoe (OSA) mit schnellen 2D-FLASH-Sequenzen. *Radiologe, 36,* 245–253.

Jones, D. L. (1991). Velopharyngeal function and dysfunction. *Clinics in Communication Disorders, 1*(3), 19–25.

Jones, D. L., Folkins, J. W., & Morris, H. L. (1990). Speech production time and judgments of disordered nasalization in speakers with cleft palate. *Journal of Speech and Hearing Research, 33,* 458–466.

Kahane, J. C. (1979). Pathophysiological effects of Möbius syndrome on speech and hearing. *Archives of Otolaryngology, 105,* 29–34.

Kantner, C. E. (1947). The rationale of blowing exercises for patients with repaired cleft palates. *Journal of Speech and Hearing Disorders, 12,* 281–286.

Karling, J., Larson, O., Leanderson, R., Galyas, K., & de Serpa-Leitão, A. (1993). NORAM—An instrument used in the assessment of hypernasality: A clinical investigation. *Cleft Palate—Craniofacial Journal, 30,* 135–140.

Karling, J., Lohmander, A., de Serpa-Leitão, A., Galyas, K., & Larson, O. (1985). NORAM: Calibration and operational advice for measuring nasality in cleft palate patients. *Scandinavian Journal of Plastic and Reconstructive Surgery, 19,* 261–267.

Karnell, M. P. (1994). *Videoendoscopy: From velopharynx to larynx.* San Diego, CA: Singular Publishing Group.

Karnell, M. P. (1995). Nasometric discrimination of hypernasality and turbulent nasal airflow. *Cleft Palate—Craniofacial Journal, 32,* 145–148.

Karnell, M. P. (1998). Videoendoscopic evaluation of swallowing. *Phonoscope, 1,* 209–216.

Karnell, M. P., Folkins, J. W., & Morris, H. L. (1985). Relationships between the perception of nasalization and speech movements in speakers with cleft palate. *Journal of Speech and Hearing Research, 28,* 63–72.

Karnell, M. P., Linville, R. N., & Edwards, B. A. (1988). Variations in velar position over time: A nasal videoendoscopic study. *Journal of Speech and Hearing Research, 31,* 417–424.

Karnell, M. P., & Seaver, E. J., III. (1990). Measurement problems in estimating velopharyngeal function. In J. Bardach & H. L. Morris (Eds.), *Multidisciplinary management of cleft lip and palate* (pp. 776–786). Philadelphia, PA: W. B. Saunders.

Karnell, M. P., Seaver, E. J., & Dalston, R. M. (1988). A comparison of photodetector and endoscopic evaluations of velopharyngeal function. *Journal of Speech and Hearing Research, 31,* 503–510.

Kase, Y., Hilberg, O., & Pedersen, O. F. (1994). Posture and nasal patency: Evaluation by acoustic rhinometry. *Acta Otolaryngologica, 114,* 70–74.

Kastner, C. U., Putnam, A. H. B., & Shelton, R. L. (1985). Custom-fabricated masks for aeromechanical measures. *Cleft Palate Journal, 22,* 197–204.

Katz, W., Machetanz, J., Orth, U., & Schönle, P. (1990). A kinematic analysis of anticipatory coarticulation in the speech of anterior aphasic subjects using electromagnetic articulography. *Brain and Language, 38,* 555–575.

Kavanaugh, J. L., Fee, E. J., Kalinowski, J., Doyle, P. C., & Leeper, H. A. (1994). Nasometric values for three dialectal groups within the Atlantic Provinces of Canada. *Journal of Speech-Language Pathology and Audiology, 18,* 7–13.

Kawano, M., Isshiki, N., Honjo, I., Kojima, H., Kurata, K., Tanokuchi, F., Kido, N., & Isobe, M. (1997). Recent progress in treating patients with cleft palate. *Folia Phoniatrica et Logopaedica, 49,* 117–138.

Keefe, M. J., & Dalston, R. M. (1989). An analysis of velopharyngeal timing in normal adult speakers using a microcomputer based photodetector system. *Journal of Speech and Hearing Research, 32,* 39–48.

Kelleher, R. E., Webster, R. C., Coffey, R. J., & Quigley, L. F., Jr. (1960). Nasal and oral air flow in normal and cleft palate speech; Velocity and volume studies using warm-wire flow meter and two-channel recorder. *Cleft Palate Bulletin, 10,* 66.

Kelsey, C. A., Minifie, F. D., & Hixon, T. J. (1969). Applications of ultrasound in speech research. *Journal of Speech and Hearing Research, 12,* 546–575.

Kent, R. D., Carney, P. J., & Severeid, L. R. (1974). Velar movement and timing: Evaluation of a model for binary control. *Journal of Speech and Hearing Research, 17,* 470–488.

Kent, R. D., Liss, J., & Philips, B. J. (1989). Acoustic analysis of velopharyngeal dysfunction in speech. In K. R. Bzoch (Ed.), *Communicative disorders related to cleft lip and palate* (3rd ed., pp. 258–270). Boston, MA: College-Hill Press.

Kern, E. B. (1973). Rhinomanometry. *Otolaryngologic Clinics of North America, 6,* 863–874.

Kim, Y.-K., Kang, J.-H., & Yoon, K.-S. (1998). Acoustic rhinometric evaluation of nasal cavity and nasopharynx after adenoidectomy and tonsillectomy. *International Journal of Pediatric Otorhinolaryngology, 44,* 215–220.

Kiritani, S., Itoh, K., & Fujimura, O. (1975). Tongue-pellet tracking by a computer-controlled x-ray microbeam system. *Journal of the Acoustical Society of America, 57,* 1516–1520.

Kleppe, S. A., Katayama, K. M., Shipley, K. G., & Foushee, D. R. (1990). The speech and language characteristics of children with Prader-Willi syndrome. *Journal of Speech and Hearing Disorders, 55,* 300–309.

Kollia, H. B., Gracco, V. L., & Harris, K. S. (1995). Articulatory organization of mandibular, labial, and velar movements during speech. *Journal of the Acoustical Society of America, 98,* 1313–1324.

Kortekangas, A. E. (1972). Significance of anterior and posterior technique in rhinomanometry. *Acta Otolaryngologica, 73,* 218–221.

Kotby, N., Abdel Haleem, E. K., Hegazi, M., Safe, I., & Zaki, M. (1997). Aspects of assessment and management of velopharyngeal dysfunction in developing countries. *Folia Phoniatrica et Logopaedica, 49,* 139–146.

Krakow, R. A., & Huffman, M. K. (1993). Instruments and techniques for investigating nasalization and velopharyngeal function in the laboratory: An introduction. In M. K. Huffman & R. A. Krakow (Eds.), *Phonetics and phonology, Volume 5: Nasals, nasalization, and the velum* (pp. 3–59). San Diego, CA: Academic Press.

Kuehn, D. P. (1976). A cineradiographic investigation of velar movement variables in two normals. *Cleft Palate Journal, 13,* 88–103.

Kuehn, D. P., & Dolan, K. D. (1975). A tomographic technique of assessing lateral pharyngeal wall displacement. *Cleft Palate Journal, 12,* 200–209.

Kuehn, D. P., Folkins, J. W., & Cutting, C. B. (1982). Relationships between muscle activity and velar position. *Cleft Palate Journal, 19,* 25–35.

Kuehn, D. P., Folkins, J. W., & Linville, R. N. (1988). An electromyographic study of the musculus uvulae. *Cleft Palate Journal, 25,* 348–355.

Kuehn, D. P., & Moon, J. B. (1994). Levator veli palatini muscle activity in relation to intraoral air pressure variation. *Journal of Speech and Hearing Research, 37,* 1260–1270.

Kuehn, D. P., & Moon, J. B. (1998). Velopharyngeal closure force and levator veli palatini activation levels in varying phonetic contexts. *Journal of Speech, Language, and Hearing Research, 41,* 51–62.

Kumlien, J., & Schiratzki, H. (1979). Methodological aspects of rhinomanometry. *Rhinology, 17,* 107–114.

Kunkel, M., & Hochban, W. (1994a). Acoustic rhinometry: A new diagnostic procedure—Experimental and clinical experience. *International Journal of Oral and Maxillofacial Surgery, 23,* 409–412.

Kunkel, M., & Hochban, W. (1994b). Acoustic rhinometry: Rationale and perspectives. *Journal of Craniomaxillofacial Surgery, 22,* 244–249.

Kunkel, M., Wahlmann, U., & Wagner, W. (1997). Nasal airway in cleft-palate patients: Acoustic rhinometric data. *Journal of Craniomaxillofacial Surgery, 25,* 270–274.

Kunkel, M., Wahlmann, U., & Wagner, W. (1998). Objective, noninvasive evaluation of velopharyngeal function in cleft and noncleft patients. *Cleft Palate—Craniofacial Journal, 35,* 35–39.

Künzel, H. J. (1977). Photoelektrische Untersuchungen zur Velumhöhe bei Vokalen: Erste Anwendung des Velographen. *Phonetica, 34,* 352–370.

Künzel, H. J. (1978). Reproducibility of electromyographic and velographic measurements of the velopharyngeal closure mechanism. *Journal of Phonetics, 6,* 345–351.

Künzel, H. J. (1979a). Röntgenvideographische Evaluierung eines photoelektrischen Verfahrens zur Registrierung der Velumhöhe beim sprechen. *Folia Phoniatrica, 31,* 153–166.

Künzel, H. J. (1979b). Some observations on velar movement in plosives. *Phonetica, 36,* 384–404.

Künzel, H. J. (1982). First applications of a biofeedback device for the therapy of velopharyngeal incompetence. *Folia Phoniatrica, 34,* 92–100.

Ladefoged, P., & Maddieson, I. (1996). *The sounds of the world's languages* (pp. 102–136). Cambridge, MA: Blackwell.

Lai, V. W. S., & Corey, J. P. (1993). The objective assessment of nasal patency. *Ear, Nose and Throat Journal, 72,* 395–400.

Laine, T., Warren, D. W., Dalston, R. M., & Morr, K. E. (1988a). Intraoral pressure, nasal pressure and airflow rate in cleft palate speech. *Journal of Speech and Hearing Research, 31,* 432–437.

Laine, T., Warren, D. W., Dalston, R. M., & Morr, K. E. (1988b). Screening of velopharyngeal closure based on nasal airflow rate measurements. *Cleft Palate Journal, 25,* 220–225.

LaPine, P. R., Stewart, M. G., Settle, S. V., & Brandow, M. (1992). Examining the effects of amplification on the nasalance ratios of hearing-impaired children. *Folia Phoniatrica, 44,* 185–193.

LaPine, P. R., Stewart, M. G., & Tatchell, J. (1991). Application of nasometry to speech samples of hearing-impaired children. *Perceptual and Motor Skills, 73,* 467–475.

Larson, P. L., & Hamlet, S. L. (1987). Coarticulation effects on the nasalization of vowels using nasal/voice amplitude ratio instrumentation. *Cleft Palate Journal, 24,* 286–290.

Leder, S. B., Ross, D. A., Briskin, K. B., & Sasaki, C. T. (1997). A prospective, double-blind, randomized study on the use of a topical anesthetic, vasoconstrictor, and placebo during transnasal flexible fiberoptic endoscopy. *Journal of Speech and Hearing Research, 40,* 1352–1357.

Leder, S. B., & Spitzer, J. B. (1990). A perceptual evaluation of the speech of adventitiously deaf adult males. *Ear and Hearing, 11,* 169–175.

Leeper, H. A., Tissington, M. L., & Munhall, K. G. (1998). Temporal characteristics of velopharyngeal function in children. *Cleft Palate—Craniofacial Journal, 35,* 215–221.

Lenders, G. E., Pentz, S., Brunner, M., & Pirsig, W. (1994). Follow-up of patients with inverted papilloma of the nasal cavities: Computer tomography, video-endoscopy, acoustic rhinometry? *Rhinology, 32,* 167–172.

Lenders, G. E., & Pirsig, W. (1990). Diagnostic value of acoustic rhinometry: Patients with allergic and vasomotor rhinitis compared with normal controls. *Rhinology, 28,* 5–16.

Li, C. H., & Lundervold, A. (1958). Electromyographic study of cleft palate. *Plastic and Reconstructive Surgery, 21,* 427–432.

Lintz, L. B., & Sherman, D. (1961). Phonetic elements and perception of nasality. *Journal of Speech and Hearing Research, 4,* 381–396.

Lippmann, R. P. (1981). Detecting nasalization using a low-cost miniature accelerometer. *Journal of Speech and Hearing Research, 24,* 314–317.

Litzaw, L. L., & Dalston, R. M. (1992). The effect of gender upon nasalance scores among normal adult speakers. *Journal of Communication Disorders, 25,* 55–64.

Lohmander-Agerskov, A., Dotevall, H., Lith, A., & Söderpalm, E. (1996). Speech and velopharyngeal function in children with an open residual cleft in the hard palate, and the influence of temporary covering. *Cleft Palate—Craniofacial Journal, 33,* 324–332.

Lotz, W. K., D'Antonio, L. L., Chait, D. H., & Netsell, R. W. (1993). Successful nasoendoscopic and aerodynamic examinations of children with speech/voice disorders. *International Journal of Pediatric Otorhinolaryngology, 26,* 165–172.

Lotz, W. K., Shaugnessy, A. L., & Netsell, R. (1981, November). *Velopharyngeal and nasal cavity resistance during speech production.* Paper presented at the annual convention of the American Speech-Language-Hearing Association.

Lubker, J. F. (1968). An electromyographic-cinefluorographic investigation of velar function during normal speech production. *Cleft Palate Journal, 5,* 1–18.

Lubker, J. F. (1969). Velopharyngeal orifice area: A replication of analog experiments. *Journal of Speech and Hearing Research, 12,* 210–218.

Lubker, J. F. (1970). Aerodynamic and ultrasonic assessment techniques in speech-dentofacial research. *ASHA Reports, 5,* 207–223.

Lubker, J. F., & Moll, K. L. (1965). Simultaneous oral-nasal air flow measurements and cinefluorographic observations during speech production. *Cleft Palate Journal, 2,* 257–272.

Lubker, J. F., & Schweiger, J. W. (1969). Nasal airflow as an index of success of prosthetic management of cleft palate. *Journal of Dental Research, 48,* 368–375.

Lubker, J. F., Schweiger, J. W., & Morris, H. L. (1970). Nasal airflow characteristics during speech in prosthetically managed cleft palate speakers. *Journal of Speech and Hearing Research, 13,* 326–338.

Machida, J. (1967). Air flow rate and articulatory movement during speech. *Cleft Palate Journal, 4,* 240–248.

MacKay, I. R. A., & Kummer, A. W. (1994). *Simplified nasometric assessment procedures: The MacKay-Kummer SNAP Test.* Lincoln Park, NJ: Kay Elemetrics Corp.

MacKenzie-Stepner, K., Witzel, M. A., Stringer, D. A., & Laskin, R. (1987). Velopharyngeal insufficiency due to hypertrophic tonsils: A report of two cases. *International Journal of Pediatric Otorhinolaryngology, 14,* 57–63.

Maddieson, I., & Ladefoged, P. (1993). Phonetics of partially nasal consonants. In M. K. Huffman & R. A. Krakow (Eds.), *Phonetics and phonology, Volume 5: Nasals, nasalization, and the velum* (pp. 251–301). San Diego, CA: Academic Press.

Maeda, S. (1993). Acoustics of vowel nasalization and articulatory shifts in French nasal vowels. In M. K. Huffman & R. A. Krakow (Eds.), *Phonetics and phonology, Volume 5: Nasals, nasalization, and the velum* (pp. 147–167). San Diego, CA: Academic Press.

Malm, L. (1997a). Measurement of nasal patency. *Allergy, 52* (Suppl. 40), 19–23.

Malm, L. (1997b). Assessment and staging of nasal polyposis. *Acta Otolaryngologica, 117,* 465–467.

Massengill, R., Jr. (1966). Early diagnosis of abnormal palatal mobility by the use of cinefluorography. *Folia Phoniatrica, 18,* 256–260.

Massengill, R., Jr. (1972). *Hypernasality.* Springfield, IL: Charles C Thomas.

Massengill, R., Jr., & Brooks, R. (1973). A study of the velopharyngeal mechanism in 143 repaired cleft palate patients during production of the vowel /i/, the plosive /p/, and a /s/ sentence. *Folia Phoniatrica, 25,* 312–322.

Massengill, R., Jr., & Bryson, M. (1967). A study of velopharyngeal function as related to perceived nasality of vowels, utilizing a cinefluorographic television monitor. *Folia Phoniatrica, 19,* 45–52.

Massengill, R., Jr., Quinn, G., Barry, W. F., Jr., & Pickrell, K. (1966). The development of rotational cinefluorography and its application to speech research. *Journal of Speech and Hearing Research, 9,* 256–265.

Matthies, M. L., Perkell, J. S., & Williams, M. J. (1991). Methods for longitudinal measures of speech nasality in cochlear implant patients. *Journal of the Acoustical Society of America, 89,* 1960(A).

Mayo, R., Floyd, L. A., Warren, D. W., Dalston, R. M., & Mayo, C. M. (1996). Nasalance and nasal area values: Cross-racial study. *Cleft Palate—Craniofacial Journal, 33,* 143–149.

Mayo, R., Warren, D. W., & Zajac, D. J. (1998). Intraoral pressure and velopharyngeal function. *Cleft Palate—Craniofacial Journal, 35,* 299–303.

McCabe, R., & Bradley, D. (1973). Pre- and post-articulation therapy assessment. *Language, Speech, and Hearing Services in Schools, 4,* 13–32.

McCaffrey, T. V., & Kern, E. B. (1979). Clinical evaluation of nasal obstruction. A study of 1,000 patients. *Archives of Otolaryngology, 105,* 542–545.

McClean, M. (1973). Forward coarticulation of velar movements at marked junctural boundaries. *Journal of Speech and Hearing Research, 16,* 286–296.

McDonald, E. T., & Koepp-Baker, H. (1951). Cleft palate speech: An integration of research and clinical observation. *Journal of Speech and Hearing Disorders, 16,* 9–20.

McGowan, J. C., III, Hatabu, H., Yousem, D. M., Randall, P., & Kressel, H. Y. (1992). Evaluation of soft palate function with MRI: Application to the cleft palate patient. *Journal of Computer Assisted Tomography, 16,* 877–882.

McHenry, M. A. (1997). The effect of increased vocal effort on estimated velopharyngeal orifice area. *American Journal of Speech-Language Pathology, 6*(4), 55–61.

McKerns, D., & Bzoch, K. R. (1970). Variations in velopharyngeal valving: The factor of sex. *Cleft Palate Journal, 7,* 652–662.

McWilliams, B. J. (1954). Some factors in the intelligibility of cleft-palate speech. *Journal of Speech and Hearing Disorders, 19,* 524–527.

McWilliams, B. J., & Bradley, D. P. (1965). Rating of velopharyngeal closure during blowing and speech. *Cleft Palate Journal, 2,* 46–55.

McWilliams, B. J., Glaser, E. R., Philips, B. J., Lawrence, C., Lavorato, A. S., Eery, B. C., & Skolnick, M. L. (1981). A comparative study of four methods of evaluating velopharyngeal adequacy. *Plastic and Reconstructive Surgery, 68,* 1–9.

McWilliams, B. J., Morris, H. L., & Shelton, R. L. (1990). *Cleft palate speech* (2nd ed., pp. 163–196). Philadelphia, PA: B. C. Decker.

McWillams, B. J., & Witzel, M. A. (1994). Cleft palate. In G. H. Shames, E. H. Wiig, & W. A. Secord (Eds.), *Human communication disorders: An introduction* (4th ed., pp. 438–479). New York: Merrill.

Miles, K. A. (1989). Ultrasound demonstration of vocal cord movements. *British Journal of Radiology, 62,* 871–872.

Min, Y-G., & Jang, Y. J. (1995). Measurements of cross-sectional area of the nasal cavity by acoustic rhinometry and CT scanning. *Laryngoscope, 105,* 757–759.

Minifie, F. D., Hixon, T. J., Kelsey, C. A., & Woodhouse, R. J. (1970). Lateral pharyngeal wall movement during speech production. *Journal of Speech and Hearing Research, 13,* 584–594.

Minsley, G. E., Warren, D. W., & Hinton, V. (1988). Maintenance of intraoral pressure during speech after maxillary resection. *Journal of the Acoustical Society of America, 83,* 820–824.

Miyazaki, T., Matsuya, T., & Yamaoka, M. (1975). Fiberscopic methods for assessment of velopharyngeal closure during various activities. *Cleft Palate Journal, 12,* 107–114.

Moll, K. L. (1960). Cinefluorographic techniques in speech research. *Journal of Speech and Hearing Research, 3,* 227–241.

Moll, K. L. (1962). Velopharyngeal closure on vowels. *Journal of Speech and Hearing Research, 5,* 30–37.

Moll, K. L. (1964). 'Objective' measures of nasality. *Cleft Palate Journal, 1,* 371–374.

Moll, K. L. (1965a). A cinefluorographic study of velopharyngeal function in normals during various activities. *Cleft Palate Journal, 2,* 112–122.

Moll, K. L. (1965b). Photographic and radiographic procedures in speech research. *ASHA Reports, 1,* 129–139.

Moll, K. L., & Daniloff, R. G. (1971). Investigation of the timing of velar movements during speech. *Journal of the Acoustical Society of America, 50,* 678–684.

Moll, K. L., & Shriner, T. H. (1967). Preliminary investigation of a new concept of velar activity during speech. *Cleft Palate Journal, 4,* 58–69.

Moller, K. T. (1991). An approach to evaluation of velopharyngeal adequacy for speech. *Clinics in Communication Disorders, 1*(1), 61–75.

Moller, K. T., Martin, R. R., & Christiansen, R. L. (1971). A technique for recording velar movement. *Cleft Palate Journal, 8,* 263–276.

Moller, K. T., Path, M., Werth, L. J., & Christiansen, R. L. (1973). The modification of velar movement. *Journal of Speeech and Hearing Disorders, 38,* 323–334.

Montague, J. C., & Hollien, H. (1973). Perceived voice quality disorders in Down's syndrome children. *Journal of Communication Disorders, 6,* 76–87.

Moon, J. (1990). The influence of nasal patency on accelerometric transduction of nasal bone vibration. *Cleft Palate Journal, 27,* 266–270.

Moon, J. B., & Lagu, R. K. (1987). Development of a second-generation phototransducer for the assessment of velopharyngeal inadequacy. *Cleft Palate Journal, 24,* 240–243.

Moon, J. B., & Smith, W. L. (1987). Application of cine computed tomography to the assessment of velopharyngeal form and function. *Cleft Palate Journal, 24,* 226–232.

Moon, J. B., & Weinberg, B. (1985). Two simplified methods for estimating velopharyngeal orifice area. *Cleft Palate Journal, 22,* 1–10.

Moore, C. A. (1992). The correspondence of vocal tract resonance with volumes obtained from magnetic resonance images. *Journal of Speech and Hearing Research, 35,* 1009–1023.

Moore, W. H., Jr., & Sommers, R. K. (1974). Oral manometer ratios: Some clinical and research implications. *Cleft Palate Journal, 11,* 50–61.

Moran, M. J. (1986). Identification of Down's syndrome adults from prolonged vowel samples. *Journal of Communication Disorders, 19,* 387–394.

Morr, K. E., Warren, D. W., Dalston, R. M., & Smith, L. R. (1989). Screening of velopharyngeal inadequacy by differential pressure measurements. *Cleft Palate Journal, 26,* 42–45.

Morris, H. L. (1966). The oral manometer as a diagnostic tool in clinical speech pathology. *Journal of Speech and Hearing Disorders, 31,* 362–369.

Morris, H. L. (1968). Etiological bases for speech problems. In D. C. Spriestersbach & D. Sherman (Eds.), *Cleft palate and communication* (pp. 119–168). New York: Academic Press.

Morris, H. L. (1984). Marginal velopharyngeal incompetence. In H. Winitz (Ed.), *Treating articulation disorders: For clinicians by clinicians* (pp. 211–222). Baltimore, MD: University Park Press.

Morris, H. L., & Smith, J. K. (1962). A multiple approach for evaluating velopharyngeal competency. *Journal of Speech and Hearing Disorders, 27,* 218–226.

Morris, H. L., Spriestersbach, D. C., & Darley, F. L. (1961). An articulation test for assessing competency of velopharyngeal closure. *Journal of Speech and Hearing Research, 4,* 48–55.

Moser, H. M. (1942). Diagnostic and clinical procedures in rhinolalia. *Journal of Speech and Hearing Disorders, 7,* 1–4.

Mra, Z., Sussman, J. E., & Fenwick, J. (1998). HONC measures in 4- to 6-year old children. *Cleft Palate—Craniofacial Journal, 35,* 408–414.

Mueller, P. B. (1971). Parkinson's disease: Motor-speech behavior in a selected group of patients. *Folia Phoniatrica, 23,* 333–346.

Müller, E. M., & Brown, W. S., Jr. (1980). Variations in the supraglottal air pressure waveform and their articulatory interpretation. In N. J. Lass (Ed.), *Speech and language: Advances in basic research and practice* (Vol. 4, pp. 317–389). New York: Academic Press.

Muntz, H. (1992). Navigation of the nose with flexible fiberoptic endoscopy. *Cleft Palate—Craniofacial Journal, 29,* 507–510.

Naito, K., & Iwata, S. (1997). Current advances in rhinomanometry. *European Archives of Otorhinolaryngology, 254,* 309–312.

Nellis, J. L., Neiman, G. S., & Lehman, J. A. (1992). Comparison of Nasometer and listener judgments of nasality in the assessment of velopharyngeal function after pharyngeal flap surgery. *Cleft Palate—Craniofacial Journal, 29,* 157–163.

Netsell, R. (1969). Evaluation of velopharyngeal function in dysarthria. *Journal of Speech and Hearing Disorders, 34,* 113–122.

Netsell, R., & Daniel, B. (1979). Dysarthria in adults: Physiologic approach to rehabilitation. *Archives of Physical Medicine and Rehabilitation, 60,* 502–508.

Newcombe, R. G., O'Neill, G., Tolley, N. S., & Montgomery, P. (1997). Characterization of nasal airflow. *Clinical Otolaryngology, 22,* 414–418.

Nichols, A. C. (1999). Nasalance statistics for two Mexican populations. *Cleft Palate—Craniofacial Journal, 36,* 243–247.

Niimi, S., Bell-Berti, F., & Harris, K. S. (1982). Dynamic aspects of velopharyngeal closure. *Folia Phoniatrica, 34,* 246–257.

Noll, J. D., Hawkins, M. W., & Weinberg, B. (1977). Performance of normal six- and seven-year-old males on oral manometer tasks. *Cleft Palate Journal, 14,* 200–205.

Ohala, J. J. (1971). Monitoring soft palate movements in speech. *Journal of the Acoustical Society of America, 50,* 140(A).

Oluwole, M., Gardiner, Q., & White, P. S. (1997). The naso-oral index: A more valid measure than peak flow rate? *Clinical Otolaryngology, 22,* 346–349.

Ostry, D. J., & Munhall, K. G. (1994). Control of jaw orientation and position in mastication and speech. *Journal of Neurophysiology, 71,* 1528–1545.

Pallanch, J. F., McCaffrey, T. V., & Kern, E. B. (1985). Normal nasal resistance. *Otolaryngology—Head and Neck Surgery, 93,* 778–785.

Parker, A. J., Clarke, P. M., Dawes, P. J., & Maw, A. R. (1990). A comparison of active anterior rhinomanometry and nasometry in the objective assessment of nasal obstruction. *Rhinology, 28,* 47–53.

Parker, A. J., Maw, A. R., & Szallasi, F. (1989). An objective method of assessing nasality: A possible aid in the selection for adenoidectomy. *Clinical Otolaryngology, 14,* 161–166.

Pedersen, O. F., Berkowitz, R., Yamagiwa, M., & Hilberg, O. (1994). Nasal cavity dimensions in the newborn measured by acoustic reflections. *Laryngoscope, 104,* 1023–1028.

Perkell, J. S., Cohen, M. H., Svirsky, M. A., Matthies, M. L., Garabieta, I., & Jackson, M. T. T. (1992). Electromagnetic midsagittal articulometer systems for transducing speech articulatory movements. *Journal of the Acoustical Society of America, 92,* 3078–3096.

Peterson-Falzone, S. (1988). Speech disorders related to craniofacial structural defects. In N. J. Lass, L. McReynolds, J. Northern, & D. Yoder (Eds.), *Handbook of speech-language pathology and audiology.* Philadelphia, PA: B. C. Decker.

Pickett, J. M. (1980). *The sounds of speech communication* (pp. 121–132). Austin, TX: Pro-Ed.

Pigott, R. W. (1969). The nasendoscopic appearance of the normal palatopharyngeal valve. *Plastic and Reconstructive Surgery, 43,* 19–24.

Pigott, R. W., Bensen, J. F., & White, F. D. (1969). Nasendoscopy in the diagnosis of velopharyngeal incompetence. *Plastic and Reconstructive Surgery, 43,* 141–147.

Pigott, R. W., & Makepeace, A. P. (1982). Some characteristics of endoscopic and radiological systems used in elaboration of the diagnosis of velopharyngeal incompetence. *British Journal of Plastic Surgery, 35,* 19–32.

Pinborough-Zimmerman, J., Canady, C., Yamashiro, D. K., & Morales, L., Jr. (1998). Articulation and nasality changes resulting from sustained palatal fistula obturation. *Cleft Palate—Craniofacial Journal, 35,* 81–87.

Pitzner, J. C., & Morris, H. L. (1966). Articulation skills and adequacy of breath pressure ratios of children with cleft palate. *Journal of Speech and Hearing Disorders, 31,* 26–40.

Plante, F., Berger-Vachon, C., & Kauffmann, I. (1993). Acoustic discrimination of velar impairment in children. *Folia Phoniatrica, 45,* 112–119.

Plattner, J., Weinberg, B., & Horii, Y. (1980). Performance of normal speakers on an index of velopharyngeal function. *Cleft Palate Journal, 17,* 205–215.

Polgar, G., & Kong, G. P. (1965). The nasal resistance of newborn infants. *Journal of Pediatrics, 67,* 557–567.

Powers, G. R. (1962). Cinefluorographic investigation of articulatory movements of selected individuals with cleft palates. *Journal of Speech and Hearing Research, 5,* 59–69.

Principato, J. J., & Wolf, P. (1985). Pediatric nasal resistance. *Laryngoscope, 95,* 1067–1069.

Quigley, L. F., Jr., Shiere, F. R., Webster, R. C., & Cobb, C. M. (1964). Measuring palatopharyngeal competence with the nasal anemometer. *Cleft Palate Journal, 1,* 304–314.

Quigley, L. F., Jr., Webster, R. C., Coffey, R. J., Kelleher, R. E., & Grant, H. P. (1963). Velocity and volume measurements of nasal and oral airflow in normal and cleft palate speech, utilizing a warm-wire flowmeter and two-channel recorder. *Journal of Dental Research, 42,* 1520–1527.

Redenbaugh, M. A., & Reich, A. R. (1985). Correspondence between an accelerometric nasal/voice ratio and listeners' direct magnitude estimations of hypernasality. *Journal of Speech and Hearing Research, 28,* 273–281.

Reich, A. R., & Redenbaugh, M. A. (1985). Relation between nasal/voice accelerometric values and interval estimates of hypernasality. *Cleft Palate Journal, 22,* 237–241.

Riechelmann, H., Rheinheimer, M. C., & Wolfensberger, M. (1993). Acoustic rhinometry in pre-school children. *Clinical Otolaryngology, 18,* 272–277.

Riski, J. E., Hoke, J. A., & Dolan, E. A. (1989). The role of pressure flow and endoscopic assessment in successful palatal obturator revision. *Cleft Palate Journal, 26,* 56–62.

Roithmann, R., Cole, P., Chapnik, J., Bareto, S. M., Szalai, J. P., & Zamel, N. (1994). Acoustic rhinometry, rhinomanometry, and the sensation of nasal patency: A correlative study. *Journal of Otolaryngology, 23,* 454–458.

Roithmann, R., Cole, P., Chapnik, J., Shpirer, I., Hoffstein, V., & Zamel, N. (1995). Acoustic rhinometry in the evaluation of nasal obstruction. *Laryngoscope, 105,* 275–281.

Roithmann, R., Shpirer, I., Cole, P., Chapnik, J., Szalai, J. P., & Zamel, N. (1997). The role of acoustic rhinometry in nasal provocation testing. *Ear, Nose and Throat Journal, 76,* 747–750.

Rouco, A., & Recasens, D. (1996). Reliability of electromagnetic midsagittal articulometry and electropalatography data acquired simultaneously. *Journal of the Acoustical Society of America, 100,* 3384–3389.

Ruscello, D. M., Shuster, L. I., & Sandwisch, A. (1991). Modification of context-specific nasal emission. *Journal of Speech and Hearing Research, 34,* 27– 32.

Ryan, W. J., & Hawkins, C. F. (1976). Ultrasonic measurement of lateral pharyngeal wall movement at the velopharyngeal port. *Cleft Palate Journal, 13,* 156–164.

Santos Terrón, M. J., González Landa, G., & Sánchez-Ruiz, I. (1991). Patrones normales del Nasometer en niños de habla Castellana. *Revista Española de Foniatrica, 4,* 71–75.

Sapienza, C. M., Brown, W. S., Williams, W. N., Wharton, P. W., & Turner, G. E. (1996). Respiratory and laryngeal function associated with experimental coupling of the oral and nasal cavities. *Cleft Palate—Craniofacial Journal, 33,* 118–126.

Sawashima, M. (1977). Fiberoptic observation of the larynx and other speech organs. In M. Sawashima & F. S. Cooper (Eds.), *Dynamic aspects of speech production* (pp. 31–46). Tokyo: University of Tokyo Press.

Sawashima, M., & Honda, K. (1987). An airway interruption method for estimating expiratory air pressure during phonation. In T. Baer, C., Sasaki, & K. S. Harris (Eds.), *Laryngeal function in phonation and respiration* (pp. 439–447). Boston, MA: College-Hill Press.

Sawashima, M., Honda, K., Kiritani, S., Sekimoto, S., Ogawa, S., & Shirai, K. (1984). Further works on the airway interruption method of measuring expiratory air pressure during phonation. *Annual Bulletin of the Research Institute for Logopedics and Phoniatrics, 18,* 19–26.

Sawashima, M., Kiritani, S., Sekimoto, S., Horiguchi, S., Okafuji, K., & Shirai, K. (1983). The airway interruption technique for measuring expiratory air pressure during phonation. *Annual Bulletin of the Research Institute for Logopedics and Phoniatrics, 17,* 23–32.

Sawashima, M., & Ushijima, T. (1971). Use of the fiberscope in speech research. *Annual Bulletin of the Research Institute of Logopedics and Phoniatrics, 5,* 25–34.

Sawashima, M., & Ushijima, T. (1972). The use of the fiberscope in speech research. In J. Hirschberg, G. Szépe, & E. Vass-Kovács (Eds.), *Papers in interdisciplinary speech research* (pp. 229–231). Budapest: Adadémiai Kiadó.

Scadding, G. K., Darby, Y. C., & Austin, C. E. (1994). Acoustic rhinometry compared with anterior rhinomanometry in the assessment of the response to nasal allergen challenge. *Clinical Otolaryngology, 19,* 451–454.

Scarsellone, J. M., Rochet, A. P., & Wolfaardt, J. F. (1999). The influence of dentures on nasalance values in speech. *Cleft Palate—Craniofacial Journal, 36,* 51–56.

Schönle, P. W. (1988). *Elektromagnetische Artikulographie.* Berlin: Springer-Verlag.

Schönle, P. W., Gräbe, K., Wenig, P., Höhne, J., Schrader, J., & Conrad, B. (1987). Electromagnetic articulography: Use of alternating magnetic fields for tracking movements of multiple points inside and outside the vocal tract. *Brain and Language, 31,* 26–35.

Schwartz, M. F. (1968a). Relative intra-nasal sound intensities of vowels. *Speech Monographs, 35,* 196–200.

Schwartz, M. F. (1968b). Acoustics of normal and nasal vowel production. *Cleft Palate Journal, 5,* 125–138.

Schwartz, M. F. (1972). Acoustic measures of nasalization and nasality. In K. R. Bzoch (Ed.), *Communicative disorders related to cleft lip and palate* (pp. 194–200). Boston, MA: Little, Brown.

Schwartz, M. F. (1975). Developing a direct, objective measure of velopharyngeal inadequacy. *Clinics in Plastic Surgery, 2,* 305–308.

Seaver, E. J., & Dalston, R. M. (1990). Using simultaneous nasometry and standard audio recordings to detect the acoustic onsets and offsets of speech. *Journal of Speech and Hearing Research, 33,* 358–362.

Seaver, E. J., Dalston, R. M., Leeper, H. A., & Adams, L. E. (1991). A study of nasometric values for normal nasal resonance. *Journal of Speech and Hearing Research, 34,* 715–721.

Seaver, E. J., Karnell, M. P., Gasparaitis, A., & Corey, J. (1995). Acoustic rhinometric measurements of changes in velar positioning. *Cleft Palate—Craniofacial Journal, 32,* 49–54.

Seaver, E. J., III, & Kuehn, D. P. (1980). A cineradiographic and electomyographic investigation of velar positioning in nonnasal speech. *Journal of Speech and Hearing Research, 17,* 216–226.

Sedlácková, E. (1967). The syndrome of the congenital shortened velum and the dual innervation of the soft palate. *Folia Phoniatrica, 19,* 441–443.

Selley, W. G., Zananiri, M-C., Ellis, R. E., & Flack, F. C. (1987). The effect of tongue position on division of airflow in the presence of velopharyngeal defects. *British Journal of Plastic Surgery, 40,* 377–383.

Shaw, N., & Gilbert, H. R. (1982). A respirometric technique for evaluating velopharyngeal closure in children. *Journal of Speech and Hearing Research, 25,* 476–480.

Shelton, D. M., & Eiser, N. M. (1992). Evaluation of active anterior and posterior rhinomanometry in normal subjects. *Clinical Otolaryngology, 17,* 178–182.

Shelton, R. L., Jr., Beaumont, K., Trier, W. C., & Furr, M. L. (1978). Videoendoscopic feedback in training velopharyngeal closure. *Cleft Palate Journal, 15,* 6–12.

Shelton, R. L., Jr., & Blank, J. L. (1984). Oronasal fistulas, intraoral air pressure and nasal air flow during speech. *Cleft Palate Journal, 21,* 91–99.

Shelton, R. L., Jr., Brooks, A. R., & Youngstrom, K. A. (1964). Articulation and patterns of palatopharyngeal closure. *Journal of Speech and Hearing Disorders, 29,* 390–408.

Shelton, R. L., Jr., Brooks, A. R., & Youngstrom, K. A. (1965). Clinical assessment of palatopharyngeal closure. *Journal of Speech and Hearing Disorders, 30,* 37–43.

Shelton, R. L., Jr., Harris, K. S., Sholes, G. N., & Dooley, P. M. (1970). Study of nonspeech voluntary palate movements by scaling and electromyographic techniques. In J. Bosma (Ed.), *Second symposium on oral sensation and perception* (pp. 432–441). Springfield, IL: Charles C Thomas.

Shelton, R. L., Jr., Knox, A. W., Arndt, W. B., Jr., & Elbert, M. (1967). The relationship between nasality score values and oral and nasal sound pressure level. *Journal of Speech and Hearing Research, 10,* 549–557.

Shelton, R. L., Jr., Paesani, A., McClelland, K., & Bradfield, S. S. (1975). Panendoscopic feedback in the study of voluntary velopharyngeal movements. *Journal of Speech and Hearing Disorders, 40,* 232–244.

Shelton, R. L., Jr., & Trier, W. C. (1976). Issues involved in the evaluation of velopharyngeal closure. *Cleft Palate Journal, 17,* 127–137.

Shemen, L., & Hamburg, R. (1997). Preoperative and postoperative nasal septal surgery assessment with acoustic rhinometry. *Otolaryngology—Head and Neck Surgery, 117,* 338–342.

Sherman, D. (1954). The merits of backward playing of connected speech in the scaling of voice quality disorders. *Journal of Speech and Hearing Disorders, 19,* 312–321.

Sherman, D., & Goodwin, F. (1954). Pitch level and nasality. *Journal of Speech and Hearing Disorders, 19,* 423–428.

Shprintzen, R. J. (1989). Nasopharyngoscopy. In K. R. Bzoch (Ed.), *Communicative disorders related to cleft lip and palate* (3rd ed., pp. 211–229). Boston, MA: College-Hill Press.

Shprintzen, R. J., Goldberg, R. B., Lewin, M. J., Sidoti, E. J., Berkman, M. D., Argamaso, R. V., & Young, D. (1978). A new syndrome involving cleft palate, cardiac anomalies, typical facies, and learning disabilities. *Cleft Palate Journal, 15,* 56–62.

Shprintzen, R. J., Goldberg, R. B., Young, D., & Wolford, L. (1981). The velo-cario-facial syndrome: A clinical genetic analysis. *Pediatrics, 67,* 167–172.

Shprintzen, R. J., McCall, G. N., Skolnick, M. L., & Lencione, R. M. (1975). Selective movement of the lateral aspects of the pharyngeal walls during velopharyngeal closure for speech, blowing, and whistling in normals. *Cleft Palate Journal, 12,* 51–58.

Siegel-Sadewitz, V. L., & Shprintzen, R. J. (1982). Nasopharyngoscopy of the normal velopharyngeal sphincter: An experiment of biofeedback. *Cleft Palate Journal, 19,* 194–200.

Skolnick, M. L. (1970). Videofluoroscopic examination of the velopharyngeal portal during phonation in lateral and base projections—A new technique for studying the mechanics of closure. *Cleft Palate Journal, 7,* 803–816.

Skolnick, M. L., & McCall, G. N. (1972). Velopharyngeal competence and incompetence following pharyngeal flap surgery: Video-fluoroscopic study in multiple projections. *Cleft Palate Journal, 9,* 1–12.

Skolnick, M. L., McCall, G. N., & Barnes, M. (1973). The sphincteric mechanism of velopharyngeal closure. *Cleft Palate Journal, 10,* 286–305.

Skolnick, M. L., Zagzebski, J. A., & Watkin, K. L. (1975). Two-dimensional ultrasonic demonstration of lateral pharyngeal wall movement in real time—A preliminary report. *Cleft Palate Journal, 12,* 299–303.

Smith, B. E., Fiala, K. J., & Guyette, T. W. (1989). Partitioning model nasal airway resistance into its nasal cavity and velopharyngeal components. *Cleft Palate Journal, 26,* 327–330.

Smith, B. E., & Guyette, T. W. (1996). Pressure-flow differences in performance during production of the CV syllables /pi/ and /pɑ/. *Cleft Palate—Craniofacial Journal, 33,* 74–76.

Smith, B. E., Skef, Z., Cohen, M., & Dorf, D. S. (1985). Aerodynamic assessment of the results of pharyngeal flap surgery: A preliminary investigation. *Plastic and Reconstructive Surgery, 76,* 402–408.

Smith, B. E., & Weinberg, B. (1980). Prediction of velopharyngeal orifice areas during steady flow conditions and during aerodynamic stimulation of voiceless stop consonants. *Cleft Palate Journal, 17,* 277–282.

Smith, H. Z., Allen, G. D., Warren, D. W., & Hall, D. J. (1978). The consistency of the pressure-flow technique for assessing oral port size. *Journal of the Acoustical Society of America, 64,* 1203–1206.

Solé, M.-J. (1995). Spatio-temporal patterns of velopharyngeal action in phonetic and phonological nasalization. *Language and Speech, 38,* 1–23.

Solomon, W. R., & Stohrer, A. W. (1965). Considerations in the measurement of nasal patency. *Annals of Otology, Rhinology and Laryngology, 74,* 978–990.

Sparks, S. N. (1984). *Birth defects and speech-language disorders.* San Diego, CA: College-Hill Press.

Spriestersbach, D. C. (1955). Assessing nasal quality in cleft palate speech of children. *Journal of Speech and Hearing Disorders, 20,* 266–270.

Spriestersbach, D. C. (1965). The effects of orofacial anomalies on the speech process. *ASHA Reports, 1,* 111–128.

Spriestersbach, D. C., Darley, F. L., & Rouse, V. (1956). Articulation of a group of children with cleft lips and palates. *Journal of Speech and Hearing Disorders, 21,* 436–445.

Spriestersbach, D. C., & Powers, G. R. (1959a). Nasality in isolated vowels and connected speech of cleft palate speakers. *Journal of Speech and Hearing Research, 2,* 40–45.

Spriestersbach, D. C., & Powers, G. R. (1959b). Articulation skills, velopharyngeal closure, and oral breath pressure of children with cleft palates. *Journal of Speech and Hearing Research, 2,* 318–325.

Stellzig, A., Heppt, W., & Komposch, G. (1994). Das Nasometer: Ein Instrument zur objektivierung der Hyperrhinophonie bei LKG-Patienten. *Fortschritte der Kieferorthopädie, 55,* 176–180.

Stevens, K. N., Fant, G., & Hawkins, S. (1987). Some acoustical and perceptual correlates of nasal vowels. In R. Channon, & L. Shockey (Eds.), *Festschrift für Ilse Lehiste* (pp. 241–254). Dordrecht, The Netherlands: Floris.

Stevens, K. N., Kalikow, D. N., & Willemain, T. R. (1975). A miniature accelerometer for detecting glottal waveforms and nasalization. *Journal of Speech and Hearing Research, 18,* 594–599.

Stevens, K. N., Nickerson, R. S., Boothroyd, A., & Rollins, A. M. (1976). Assessment of nasalization in the speech of deaf children. *Journal of Speech and Hearing Research, 19,* 393–416.

Stone, M. (1990). A three-dimensional model of tongue movement based on ultrasound and x-ray microbeam data. *Journal of the Acoustical Society of America, 87,* 2207–2217.

Stone, M. (1996). Instrumentation for the study of speech physiology. In N. J. Lass (Ed.), *Principles of experimental phonetics* (pp. 495–524). St. Louis, MO: Mosby–Year Book.

Stone, M., & Vatikiotis-Bateson, E. (1995). Coarticulation effects on tongue, jaw, and palate behavior. *Journal of Phonetics, 23,* 81–100.

Stringer, D. A., & Witzel, M. A. (1985). Waters projection for evaluation of lateral pharyngeal wall movement in speech disorders. *American Journal of Radiology, 145,* 409–410.

Stringer, D. A., & Witzel, M. A. (1986). Velopharyngeal insufficiency on videofluoroscopy: Comparison of projections. *American Journal of Radiology, 146,* 15–19.

Stringer, D. A., & Witzel, M. A. (1989). Comparison of multi-view videofluoroscopy and nasopharyngoscopy in the assessment of velopharyngeal insufficiency. *Cleft Palate Journal, 26,* 88–92.

Subtelny, J., Kho, G., McCormack, R. M., & Subtelny, J. D. (1969). Multidimensional analysis of bilabial stop and nasal consonants—Cineradiographic and pressure-flow analysis. *Cleft Palate Journal, 6,* 263–289.

Subtelny, J., Koepp-Baker, H., & Subtelny, J. D. (1961). Palatal function and cleft palate speech. *Journal of Speech and Hearing Disorders, 26,* 213–224.

Subtelny, J., Li, W., Whitehead, R., & Subtelny, J. D. (1989). Cephalometric and cineradiographic study of deviant resonance in hearing-impaired speakers. *Journal of Speech and Hearing Disorders, 54,* 249–265.

Subtelny, J., McCormack, R. M., Subtelny, J. D., Worth, J. H., Cramer, L. M., Runyon, J. C., & Rosenblum, R. M. (1968). Synchronous recording of speech with associated physiologic pressure flow dynamics: Instrumentation and procedures. *Cleft Palate Journal, 5,* 93–116.

Sussman, J. E. (1995). HONC measures in men and women: Validity and variability. *Cleft Palate—Craniofacial Journal, 32,* 37–48.

Tarnóczy, T. (1948). Resonance data concerning nasals, laterals, and trills. *Word, 4,* 71–77.

Tatchell, J. A., Stewart, M. G., & LaPine, P. R. (1991). Nasalance measurements in hearing-impaired children. *Journal of Communication Disorders, 24,* 275–285.

Taub, S. (1966a). The Taub oral panendoscope: A new technique. *Cleft Palate Journal, 3,* 328–346.

Taub, S. (1966b). Oral panendoscope for direct observation and audiovisual recording of velopharyngeal areas during phonation. *Transactions of the American Academy of Ophthalmology and Otolaryngology,* Sept-Oct, 855–857.

Theodoros, D. G., Murdoch, B. E., Stokes, P. D., & Chenery, H. (1993). Hypernasality in dysarthric speakers following severe closed head injury: A perceptual and instrumental analysis. *Brain Injury, 7,* 59–69.

Theodoros, D. G., Murdoch, B. E., & Thompson, E. C. (1995). Hypernasality in Parkinson disease: A perceptual and physiological analysis. *Journal of Medical Speech-Language Pathology, 3,* 73–84.

Thompson, A. E., & Hixon, T. J. (1979). Nasal air flow during normal speech production. *Cleft Palate Journal, 16,* 412–420.

Thompson, E. C., & Murdoch, B. E. (1995). Disorders of nasality in subjects with upper motor neuron type dysarthria following cerebrovascular accident. *Journal of Communication Disorders, 28,* 261–276.

Till, J. A., Jafari, M., & Law-Till, C. B. (1994). Accelerometric difference index for subjects with normal and hypernasal speech. In J. A. Till, K. M. Yorkston, & D. R. Beukelman (Eds.), *Motor speech disorders: Advances in assessment and treatment* (pp. 119–133). Baltimore, MD: Paul H. Brookes.

Titze, I. R. (1980). Comments on the myoelastic-aerodynamic theory of phonation. *Journal of Speech and Hearing Research, 23,* 495–510.

Titze, I. R. (1985). Mechanisms of sustained oscillation of the vocal folds. In I. R. Titze & R. C. Scherer (Eds.), *Vocal fold physiology: Biomechanics, acoustics and phonatory control* (pp. 349–357). Denver, CO: Denver Center for the Performing Arts.

Tomkinson, A., & Eccles, R. (1995). Errors arising in cross-sectional area estimation by acoustic rhinometry produced by breathing during measurement. *Rhinology, 33,* 138–140.

Tonndorf, J. (1958). A note on the measurement of nasal flow resistance. *Annals of Otology, Rhinology and Laryngology, 67,* 984–990.

Trost, J. E. (1981). Articulatory additions to the classical description of the speech of persons with cleft palate. *Cleft Palate Journal, 18,* 193–203.

Ushijima, T., Sawashima, M., Hirose, H., Abe, M., & Harada, T. (1976). A kinesiological aspect of myasthenia gravis: An electromyographic study of velar movements during speech. *Annual Bulletin of the Research Institute of Logopedics and Phoniatrics, 10,* 225–232.

Vaissière, J. (1988). Prediction of velum movement from phonological specifications. *Phonetica, 45,* 122–139.

Vallino-Napoli, L. D., & Montgomery, A. A. (1997). Examination of the standard deviation of mean nasalance scores in subjects with cleft palate: Implications for clinical use. *Cleft Palate—Craniofacial Journal, 34,* 512–519.

Van Demark, D. R. (1966). A factor analysis of the speech of children with cleft palate. *Cleft Palate Journal, 3,* 159–170.

Van Demark, D. R. (1970). A comparison of the results of pressure articulation testing in various contexts for subjects with cleft palates. *Journal of Speech and Hearing Research, 13,* 741–754.

Van Demark, D. R. (1971). Articulation changes in the therapy process. *Cleft Palate Journal, 8,* 159–165.

Van Demark, D. R. (1974). Assessment of articulation for children with cleft palate. *Cleft Palate Journal, 11,* 200–208.

Van Demark, D. R. (1979). Predictability of velopharyngeal incompetency. *Cleft Palate Journal, 16,* 429–435.

Van Demark, D. R. (1997). Diagnostic value of articulation tests with individuals having clefts. *Folia Phoniatrica et Logopaedica, 49,* 147–157.

Van Demark, D. R., & Hardin, M. A. (1985). Longitudinal evaluation of articulation and velopharyngeal competence of patients with pharyngeal flaps. *Cleft Palate Journal, 22,* 163–172.

Van Demark, D. R., & Morris, H. L. (1977). A preliminary study of the predictive value of the IPAT. *Cleft Palate Journal, 14,* 124–130.

Van Demark, D. R., Morris, H. L., & VandeHaar, C. (1979). Patterns of articulation abilities in speakers with cleft palate. *Cleft Palate Journal, 16,* 230–239.

Van Demark, D. R., & Swickard, S. L. (1980). A preschool articulation test to assess velopharyngeal competency: Normative data. *Cleft Palate Journal, 17,* 175–179.

van den Berg, Jw. (1956). Direct and indirect determination of the mean subglottic pressure. *Folia Phoniatrica, 8,* 1–24.

van Doorn, J., & Purcell, A. (1998). Nasalance levels in the speech of normal Australian children. *Cleft Palate—Craniofacial Journal, 35,* 287–292.

van Hattum, R. J. (1958). Articulation and nasality in cleft palate speakers. *Journal of Speech and Hearing Research, 1,* 383–387.

Vealey, J., Bailey, C., II, & Belknap, L. II. (1965). Rheadeik: To detect the escape of nasal air during speech. *Journal of Speech and Hearing Disorders, 30,* 82–84.

Vig, P. S., & Zajac, D. J. (1993). Age and gender effects on nasal respiratory function in normal subjects. *Cleft Palate—Craniofacial Journal, 30,* 279–284.

Warren, D. W. (1964a). Velopharyngeal orifice size and upper pharyngeal pressure-flow patterns in cleft palate speech: A preliminary study. *Plastic and Reconstructive Surgery, 34,* 15–26.

Warren, D. W. (1964b). Velopharyngeal orifice size and upper pharyngeal pressure-flow patterns in normal speech. *Plastic and Reconstructive Surgery, 33,* 148–161.

Warren, D. W. (1967). Nasal emission of air and velopharyngeal function. *Cleft Palate Journal, 16,* 279–285.

Warren, D. W. (1979). Perci: A method for rating palatal efficiency. *Cleft Palate Journal, 16,* 279–285.

Warren, D. W. (1984). A quantitative technique for assessing nasal airway impairment. *American Journal of Orthodontics and Dentofacial Orthopedics, 86,* 306–314.

Warren, D. W. (1989). Aerodynamic assessment of velopharyngeal performance. In K. R. Bzoch (Ed.), *Communicative disorders related to cleft lip and palate* (3rd ed., pp. 230–245). Boston, MA: College-Hill Press.

Warren, D. W., Dalston, R. M., & Dalston, E. T. (1989). Maintaining speech pressures in the presence of velopharyngeal impairment. *Cleft Palate Journal, 27,* 53–58.

Warren, D. W., Dalston, R. M., & Mayo, R. (1993). Aerodynamics of nasalization. In M. K. Huffman & R. A. Krakow (Eds.), *Phonetics and phonology, Volume 5: Nasals, nasalization, and the velum* (pp. 119–146). San Diego, CA: Academic Press.

Warren, D. W., Dalston, R. M., & Mayo, R. (1994). Hypernasality and velopharyngeal impairment. *Cleft Palate—Craniofacial Journal, 31,* 257–262.

Warren, D. W., Dalston, R. M., Morr, K. E., Hairfield, W. M., & Smith, L. R. (1989). The speech regulating system: Temporal and aerodynamic responses to velopharyngeal inadequacy. *Journal of Speech and Hearing Research, 32,* 566–575.

Warren, D. W., Dalston, R. M., Trier, W. C., & Holder, M. B. (1985). A pressure-flow technique for quantifying temporal patterns of palatopharyngeal closure. *Cleft Palate Journal, 22,* 11–19.

Warren, D. W., & Devereux, J. L. (1966). An analog study of cleft palate speech. *Cleft Palate Journal, 6,* 134–140.

Warren, D. W., Duany, L. F., & Fischer, N. D. (1969). Nasal pathway resistance in normal and cleft lip and palate subjects. *Cleft Palate Journal, 6,* 134–140.

Warren, D. W., & DuBois, A. B. (1964). A pressure-flow technique for measuring velopharyngeal orifice area during continuous speech flow. *Cleft Palate Journal, 1,* 52–71.

Warren, D. W., Hinton, V. A., Pillsbury, H. C., & Hairfield, W. M. (1987). Effects of size of the nasal airway on airflow rate. *Archives of Otolaryngology, 113,* 405–408.

Warren, D. W., & Mackler, S. B. (1968). Duration of oral port constriction in normal and cleft palate speech. *Journal of Speech and Hearing Research, 11,* 391–401.

Warren, D. W., & Ryon, W. E. (1967). Oral port constriction, nasal resistance, and respiratory aspects of cleft palate speech: An analog study. *Cleft Palate Journal, 4,* 38–46.

Warren, D. W., Wood, M. T., & Bradley, D. P. (1969). Respiratory volumes in normal and cleft palate speech. *Cleft Palate Journal, 6,* 449–460.

Watterson, T., & Emanuel, F. (1981). Observed effects of velopharyngeal orifice size on vowel identification and vowel nasality. *Cleft Palate Journal, 18,* 271–278.

Watterson, T., Hinton, J., & McFarlane, S. C. (1996). Novel stimuli for obtaining nasalance measures from young children. *Cleft Palate—Craniofacial Journal, 33,* 67–73.

Watterson, T., Lewis, K. E., & Deutsch, C. (1998). Nasalance and nasality in low pressure and high pressure speech. *Cleft Palate—Craniofacial Journal, 35,* 293–298.

Watterson, T., Lewis, K. E., & Foley-Homan, N. (1999). Effect of stimulus length on nasalance scores. *Cleft Palate—Craniofacial Journal, 36,* 243–247.

Watterson, T., McFarlane, S. C., & Wright, D. S. (1993). The relationship between nasalance and nasality in children with cleft palate. *Journal of Communication Disorders, 26,* 13–28.

Watterson, T., York, S. L., & McFarlane, S. C. (1994). Effects of vocal loudness on nasalance measures. *Journal of Communication Disorders, 27,* 257–262.

Weatherley-White, R. C. A., Dersch, W. C., & Anderson, R. M. (1964). Objective measurement of nasality in cleft palate patients: A preliminary report. *Cleft Palate Journal, 1,* 120–124.

Wein, B., Drobnitzky, M., Klajman, S., & Angerstein, W. (1991). Evaluation of functional positions of tongue and soft palate with MR imaging: Initial clinical results. *Journal of Magnetic Resonance Imaging, 1,* 381–383.

Weinberg, B., & Shanks, J. C. (1971). The relationship between three oral breath pressure ratios and ratings of severity of nasality for talkers with cleft palate. *Cleft Palate Journal, 8,* 251–256.

Wells, C. G. (1971). *Cleft palate and its associated speech disorders.* New York: McGraw-Hill.

West, R. W., & Ansberry, M. (1968). *The rehabilitation of speech* (4th ed.). New York: Harper & Row.

Westbury, J. (1991). The significance and measurement of head position during speech production experiments using the x-ray microbeam system. *Journal of the Acoustical Society of America, 89,* 1782–1791.

Whalen, D. H. (1990). Intrinsic velar height in supine vowels. *Journal of the Acoustical Society of America, 88* (Suppl. 1), S54.

Williams, R. G., Eccles, R., & Hutchings, H. (1990). The relationship between nasalance and nasal resistance to airflow. *Acta Otolaryngologica, 110,* 443–449.

Williams, R. G., Preece, M., Rhys, R., & Eccles, R. (1992). The effect of adenoid and tonsil surgery on nasalance. *Clinical Otolaryngology, 17,* 136–140.

Williams, W. N. (1989). Radiographic assessment of velopharyngeal function for speech. In K. R. Bzoch (Ed.) , *Communicative disorders related to cleft lip and palate* (3rd ed., pp. 195–210). Boston, MA: College-Hill Press.

Williams, W. N., & Eisenbach, C. R., II. (1981). Assessing VP function: The lateral still technique vs. cinefluorography. *Cleft Palate Journal, 18,* 45–50.

Willis, C. R., & Stutz, M. L. (1972). The clinical use of the Taub oral panendoscope in the observation of velopharyngeal function. *Journal of Speech and Hearing Disorders, 37,* 495–502.

Witzel, M. A., & Posnick, J. C. (1989). Patterns and location of velopharyngeal valving problems: Atypical findings on video nasopharyngoscopy. *Cleft Palate Journal, 26,* 63–67.

Witzel, M. A., Tobe, J., & Salyer, K. (1988a). The use of nasopharyngoscopy biofeedback therapy in the correction of inconsistent velopharyngeal closure. *International Journal of Pediatric Otorhinolaryngology, 15,* 137–142.

Witzel, M. A., Tobe, J., & Salyer, K. (1988b). The use of videonasopharyngoscopy for biofeedback therapy in adults after pharyngeal flap surgery. *Cleft Palate Journal, 26,* 129–134.

Woisard, V., Puech, M., Yardeni, E., Percodani, J., Serrano, E., & Pessey, J. J. (1998). Evaluation of some velar functions before and after surgical treatment of snoring. *Folia Phoniatrica et Logopaedica, 50,* 10–18.

Worth, J. H., Runyon, J. C., & Subtelny, J. D. (1968). Integrating flowmeter for measuring unimpaired oral and nasal flow. *IEEE Transactions on Bio-Medical Engineering, 15,* 196–200.

Yamagiwa, M., Hilberg, O., Pedersen, O. F., & Lundqvist, G. R. (1990). Evaluation of the effect of localized skin cooling on nasal airway volume by acoustic rhinometry. *American Review of Respiratory Disease, 141,* 1050–1054.

Yamawaki, Y., Nishimura, Y., & Suzuki, Y. (1996). Velopharyngeal closure and the longus capitis muscle. *Acta Otolaryngologica, 116,* 774–777.

Yamawaki, Y., Nishimura, Y., Suzuki, Y., Sawada, M., & Yamawaki, S. (1997). Rapid magetic resonance imaging for assessment of velopharyngeal muscle movement on phonation. *American Journal of Otolaryngology, 18,* 210–213.

Yokoyama, M., Yamanaka, N., Ishii, H., Tamaki, K., Yoshikawa, A., & Morita, R. (1996). Evaluation of the pharyngeal airway in obstructive sleep apnea: Study by ultrafast MR imaging. *Acta Otolaryngologica,* Suppl. 523, 242–244.

Yules, R. B., Josephson, J. B., & Chase, R. A. (1969). A dehypernasality trainer. *Behavior Research Methods and Instrumentation, 1,* 160.

Zajac, D. J. (1997). Velopharyngeal function in young and older adult speakers: Evidence from aerodynamic studies. *Journal of the Acoustical Society of America, 102,* 1846–1852.

Zajac, D. J., Lutz, R., & Mayo, R. (1996). Microphone sensitivity as a source of variation in nasalance scores. *Journal of Speech and Hearing Research, 39,* 1228–1231.

Zajac, D. J., & Mayo, R. (1996). Aerodynamic and temporal aspects of velopharyngeal function in normal speakers. *Journal of Speech and Hearing Research, 39,* 1199–1207.

Zajac, D. J., Mayo, R., Kataoka, R. (1998). Nasal coarticulation in normal speakers: A re-examination of the effects of gender. *Journal of Speech, Language, and Hearing Research, 41,* 503–510.

Zajac, D. J., Mayo, R., Kataoka, R., & Kuo, J. Y. (1996). Aerodynamic and acoustic characteristics of a speaker with turbulent nasal emission: A case report. *Cleft Palate—Craniofacial Journal, 33,* 440–444.

Zemlin, W. R., & Fant, G. (1972). The effect of a velopharyngeal shunt upon vocal tract damping times: An analog study. *Speech Transmission Laboratory Quarterly Progress and Status Report, 4,* 6–10.

Ziegler, W., & von Cramon, D. (1986). Timing deficits in apraxia of speech. *European Archives of Psychiatry and Neurological Sciences, 236,* 44–49.

Zimmerman, G., Dalston, R. M., Brown, C., Folkins, J. W., Linville, R. N., & Seaver, E. J. (1987). Comparison of cineradiographic and photodetection techniques for assessing velopharyngeal function during speech. *Journal of Speech and Hearing Research, 30,* 564–569.

Zimmerman, G. N., Karnell, M. P., & Rettaliata, P. (1984). Articulatory coordination and the clinical profile of two cleft palate speakers. *Journal of Phonetics, 12,* 297–306.

Zwitman, D. H., Gyepes, M. T., & Sample, F. (1973). The submentovertical projection in the radiographic analysis of velopharyngeal dynamics. *Journal of Speech and Hearing Disorders, 38,* 473–477.

Zwitman, D. H., Gyepes, M. T., & Ward, P. H. (1976). Assessment of velar and lateral wall movement by oral telescope and radiographic examination in patients with velopharyngeal inadequacy and in normal subjects. *Journal of Speech and Hearing Disorders, 41,* 381–389.

Zwitman, D. H., Sonderman, J. C., & Ward, P. H. (1974). Variations in velopharyngeal closure assessed by endoscopy. *Journal of Speech and Hearing Disorders, 39,* 366–372.

12

Speech Movements

Speech sounds are produced by speech movements. Abnormal sounds are made by abnormal movements —of the chest wall, larynx, pharynx, palate, tongue, or facial structures. The diagnosis of speech disorders is, at base, the process of determining which movements are inadequate, in what ways, and under what circumstances. Often that determination is based on correlates of motor behavior—air pressure, sound intensity, airflow rates, and the like. But it is frequently useful, and sometimes necessary, to monitor the movements themselves. Given that much of the speech system is not readily accessible and that important movements can be very small and extremely fast, the problems involved in observing important movements are often not simple. Other chapters have considered special aspects of speech motor behavior, such as vocal-fold displacement or velopharyngeal closure. This chapter is concerned primarily with articulatory and chest-wall movements in a more general sense.

Of the many possible ways of monitoring the position of speech structures, only a few will be discussed here. The focus will be on those that are relatively innocuous, practicable in the clinical setting, and likely to be cost effective. Obtaining valid and reliable information about the movements of the organs of speech and using that information to design a course of therapy demands a firm understanding the mechanisms of motor behavior in general and of speech motor control in particular. The literature in this area is extensive, but good overviews, at various levels of sophistication, have been prepared by Fujimura (1990), Smith (1992), Abbs (1996), and Kent, Adams, and Turner (1996).

ELECTROMYOGRAPHY

Biological Principles

The structural unit of muscular activity is the muscle fiber, which contracts when appropriately excited. If it is not held at a fixed length it becomes shorter, but its overall tension (the force with which it pulls on the structures to which it is attached) remains relatively constant. Hence muscle contraction that results in length change is called *isotonic*. On the other hand, if muscle shortening is prevented (for example, by simultaneous contraction of opposing muscles), an *isometric* contraction occurs and muscle tension rises significantly. Many muscle actions are a combination of isometric and isotonic contraction. Muscle fibers are capable of contraction only: elongation to precontractile length must be effected by an external force, such as an opposing muscle.

Contraction is controlled by *motoneurons*, each of which synapses on many individual muscle fibers. If a motoneuron is activated, it stimulates *all* of the muscle fibers that it innervates, making them *all* contract. This minimal unit of muscle action—a motoneuron and all of its associated muscle fibers—was named a *motor unit* by Liddell and Sherrington (1925). The number of muscle fibers in a motor unit varies widely. Muscles that are capable of only gross motor control have many muscle fibers per motoneuron (large motor units). The average motor unit in gastrocnemius, for instance, has more than 1,700 muscle fibers (Buchthal & Schmalbruch, 1980). On the other hand, muscles that can be controlled very precisely have very small motor units. The cricothyroid motor unit size has been calculated to be between about 30 and 165 (Faaborg-Andersen, 1957; English & Blevins, 1969). Anatomically, the motor unit is not an isolated entity. Its muscle fibers are dispersed throughout a large region of the gross muscle mass. Muscle fibers lying next to each other are very likely to be members of quite different motor units. The effect of this dispersion is that a single motoneuron does not stimulate a localized contraction somewhere in a muscle, but rather it causes some small amount of contraction throughout the muscle.

Synaptic transmission from a motoneuron causes a wave of electrical activity to sweep along each of the muscle fibers in its motor unit. The electrical wave is associated with the chemical actions of contraction. If it shows electrical activity, a muscle fiber must be contracting. Similarly, if a muscle fiber is contracting, there must be electrical activity. The magnitude of the electrical wave (called a *muscle action potential* or *MAP*) is several tens of millivolts at the muscle itself. It is strong enough to cause an electrical disruption in the muscle fiber's environment up to a distance of several centimeters with rapidly diminishing strength. The force of a muscle's contraction is increased by more frequent synaptic stimulation of each motor unit and by activating a greater number of motor units (Akazawa & Fujii, 1981; Sussman, MacNeilage, & Powers, 1977).

The detection and recording of MAPs is called *electromyography* (*EMG*). It was developed by neurophysiologists (for example, Ardrian & Bronk, 1929; Smith, 1934; Denny-Brown, 1949) and was quickly applied to the study and evaluation of muscle and nerve pathology (Weddell, Feinstein, & Pattle, 1944; see Basmajian & De Luca, 1985, for a thorough review). By the 1950s, electromyographic investigation of speech activity was well under way (Faaborg-Andersen, 1957; Sawashima, Sato, Funasaka, & Totsuka, 1958; Draper, Ladefoged, & Whitteridge, 1959, 1960). Brief reviews of EMG in various areas of speech research have been published by Cooper (1965), Fromkin and Ladefoged

(1966), Harris (1970, 1981), Gay and Harris (1971), Fritzell (1979), Kennedy and Abbs (1979), Pinelli (1992), and Gentil and Moore (1997).

While electromyography reveals a great deal about muscle activity, it provides very little information about structural movement. A muscle contracts in a context of many other opposing or augmenting forces. The precontractile status of the muscle, the activity of its antagonists, and the loading upon it are all significant. So are the biomechanical properties of the larger tissue matrix in which muscle activation occurs. In short, the electromyogram shows the magnitude of a single force vector among the great many that might be acting simultaneously. It is only rarely possible to conclude that a given movement is causally related to particular MAPs. It is to clarify causal relationships that researchers frequently monitor both motion and EMG simultaneously (Lubker, 1968; Fritzell, 1969; Lubker & Parris, 1970; Abbs, 1973a, 1973b; Sussman, Mac-Neilage, & Hanson, 1973; Gay, Ushijima, Hirose, & Cooper, 1974; Hirose, Kiritani, Ushijima, & Sawashima, 1978; McClean, Goldsmith, & Cerf, 1984; Smith, Moore, McFarland, & Weber, 1985; Kempster, Preston, Mack, & Larson, 1987; Folkins, Linville, Garrett, & Brown, 1988; Moore, Smith, & Ringel, 1988; Shaiman, 1989; Walker, Donofrio, Harpold, & Ferrell, 1990; Gentil, 1992; Brancatisano, Engel, & Loring, 1993; van Lieshout, Hulstijn, & Peters, 1996; Ostry, Gribble, Levin, & Feldman, 1997).

Instrumentation

EMG ELECTRODES

Muscle action potentials are detected by conductors, called *electrodes*, placed in the region of the electrical disturbance. Although such electrodes might seem to be simple devices, subject only to straightforward and obvious design principles, this is far from the case. A great many criteria must be satisfied for precision work. The models of electrical behavior at the electrode-to-tissue junction are quite complex (Geddes, 1972; Cobbold, 1992) and well beyond the scope of this discussion. For the present purposes, electrodes can be divided into two comprehensive classes: (1) intramuscular and (2) surface. Aside from pragmatic considerations, the choice between the two types (and among the subcategories within each) depends on the kind of information needed.

Electrodes are used in pairs with a differential amplifier (see Chapter 4, "General-Purpose Tools"). The EMG signal is the difference in the voltages seen by the two electrodes. All of the tissue between them con-

tributes to this difference. The smaller the electrodes and the closer they are to each other, the smaller the volume of muscle tissue contributing to the net electrical input. Moving the electrodes as close as possible to the muscle fibers to be observed also limits the sampled tissue volume. If the electrodes can be made small enough and if they can be kept very close together, it is possible to observe the electrical response of a single muscle fiber. This information is needed by the research physiologist and the physician who must diagnose neuromuscular disorders. Intramuscular electrodes allow them to limit the volume of muscle being observed to a sufficiently small size. Speech clinicians, however, are almost never interested in the response of a single muscle fiber. What matters to them is the behavior of the muscle as an integral structure. For their purposes, then, fairly large electrodes that are not in intimate contact with the muscle mass can often be very useful if certain limitations are understood.

No matter what kind of electrode system is decided on, at least three important criteria must be met. The electrodes:

1. must not interfere with or alter normal motor function;

2. must be able to move with the muscle without generating spurious signals (movement artifacts); and

3. must be usable in confined areas, such as the oral cavity.

Intramuscular Electrodes

Intramuscular electrodes are used when it is important that the volume of muscle being sampled is kept small or when the activity of only one of several muscles in an overlapping arrangement is to be examined.

Needle Electrodes

Originally, intramuscular electrodes were of the needle type. *Monopolar needle electrodes* (Figure 12–1A) simply use the bare tip of a needle as an electrode. Two monopolar needles are inserted into the muscle for recording of the electrical activity in the zone between them. Inserting an insulated wire into the needle so that only its end is exposed creates a *concentric electrode* (Figure 12–1B). The needle and the wire serve as electrodes in this arrangement, and the sampled region is the zone between their exposed tips. If two insulated wires are carried in the needle, the resulting *bipolar electrode* (Figure 12–1C) samples the region between their bare ends while the shaft of the needle serves as a shield to screen out electrical interference.

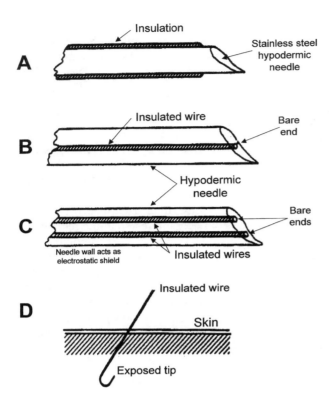

Figure 12–1. Electrodes for electromyography (EMG): **(A)** Monopolar needle; **(B)** Concentric monopolar; **(C)** Bipolar; and **(D)** hooked wire. From *Transducers for Biomedical Measurements: Principles and Applications*, by R. S. C. Cobbold, 1974, New York: John Wiley and Sons. Figure 10.14, p. 438. ©1974 John Wiley and Sons, Inc. Reprinted by permission.

Although needle electrodes have been used successfully to investigate the behavior of the larynx (Fink, Basek, & Epanchin, 1956; Zenker & Zenker, 1960; Buchthal & Faaborg-Andersen, 1964; Faaborg-Andersen, 1965; Hiroto, Hirano, Toyozumi, & Shin, 1967; Rea, Templer, & Davis, 1978; Koufman & Walker, 1998), pharynx and velopharyngeal port (Basmajian & Dutta, 1961), and facial muscles (Leanderson, Persson, & Öhman, 1971) among others, they are not ideally suited to examination of speech behavior. Their rigidity and large size may restrict muscle activity. Shear forces acting on them, when muscles move beneath the skin, cause needle displacement that produces electrical artifacts and significant patient discomfort.

Hooked-wire Electrodes

To circumvent the problems of needle conductors, Basmajian and Stecko (1962) developed what are known as hooked-wire electrodes. They are made (Figure 12–1D) by passing a loop of extremely fine insulated wire through a hypodermic needle. The insulation is removed from the loop, the bare wire is cut, and the two free ends are folded back over the needle tip. After sterilization, the needle is inserted into the muscle and then withdrawn, leaving the wire ends hooked on the muscle fibers. The hypodermic needle is slipped off the trailing wires, which remain the only thing penetrating the skin. Their presence produces very little discomfort, and they are much less prone to displacement by muscle activity. After testing, a fairly gentle tug removes the wire electrodes from the muscle.

Hooked wires have become the electrodes of choice for examining the speech musculature. Techniques have been developed for inserting them into almost all of the muscles of the vocal tract (Hirose, 1971, 1977; Bole & Lesser, 1966; Shipp, Deutsch, & Robertson, 1968; Shipp, Fishman, Morrissey, & McGlone, 1970; Dedo & Hall, 1969; Hirano & Ohala, 1969; Hirose, Gay, Strome, & Sawashima, 1971; Gay, Strome, Hirose, & Sawashima, 1972; Minifie, Abbs, Tarlow, & Kwaterski, 1974; Blair, Berry, & Briant, 1977; Kuehn, Folkins, & Cutting, 1982; Perlman, Luschei, & Du Mond, 1989; Kotby et al., 1992).

Because the tip of an intramuscular electrode cannot be seen, special verification procedures must be followed to prove that it is where it is supposed to be and that it is not picking up signals from surrounding muscles. In general, placement verification is done by observing the electromyographic output during maneuvers that are known to require contraction of the target muscle in relative isolation from those around it. Unfortunately, articulatory actions are very complex, and there is a serious paucity of information upon which to make unequivocal placement verifications for many muscles (Blair & Smith, 1986). Therefore, the tester will often need to fall back on a somewhat subjective, but accurately informed, judgment of placement made against a firm background knowledge of vocal-tract structure and function. Some suggested tests of electrode placement are provided by Shipp and his colleagues (1968, 1970), Hirose (1971), Kennedy and Abbs (1979), and O'Dwyer, Quinn, Guitar, Andrews, and Neilson (1981).

Surface Electrodes

Completely noninvasive, surface electrodes are a viable alternative for some purposes. Attached to the skin, they detect electrical activity in a fairly large volume under them. This makes them too nonspecific for most research purposes (see, for example, Eblen, 1963). They can provide signals very similar to those of intramuscular electrodes, however, only if the muscle being sampled is close to the surface[1] and clearly separate from nearby muscles (for example, Netsell, Daniel, & Celesia, 1975; Abbs & Watkin, 1976; McClean, 1987; Hough & Klich, 1998). The vigorous speech movements of many vocal-tract structures makes firm attachment of the electrodes to the skin or mucous membrane imperative. Any movement of the electrode relative to the skin surface will produce artifacts in the output signal. Electrodes have been specially designed to facilitate cementing them to the skin (Cole, Konopacki, & Abbs, 1983). But beyond using chemical adhesives, there are two relatively simple and harmless ways of achieving firm electrode placement:

1. Workers at Haskins Laboratories (Harris, Rosov, Cooper, & Lysaught, 1964; Cooper, 1965) made surface electrodes out of hollow silver jewelry beads. A bead is cut in half and fitted with a side tube that is connected by plastic tubing to a vacuum manifold. A stranded wire connected to the electrode passes through the vacuum tube to the vacuum chamber, where it is connected to the input leads from the amplifier. The vacuum inside the hemispheric electrode keeps it firmly in place. Electrodes of this type can be made sufficiently small and unobtrusive to be used successfully even on the surface of the tongue (MacNeilage & Sholes, 1964; Huntington, Harris, & Sholes, 1968).

2. Surface electrodes can also be painted on the skin. An acceptable conductive paint can be made by suspending 10 g of silver powder in 10 g of Duco cement thinned with a few milliliters of acetone. A drop of this mixture is applied at the chosen site and allowed to dry. The bared end of a very thin wire is laid on the spot of silver, and another drop of conductive liquid applied. This is allowed to harden into a silver and wire "sandwich." The wire is connected to the EMG amplifier (Allen, Lubker, & Harrison, 1972). Complete specifications for this method are provided by Hollis and Harrison (1970). Allen, Lubker, and Turner (1973) have also suggested that a very simple surface electrode can be made by simply attaching a loop of bare copper wire to the skin with a quick-setting cyanoacrylate cement.

The Processing and Display of Electromyograms

EMG signals are very small—ranging from 200 μV or less to about 1 mV. Very high amplifier gain (on the order of 10,000) is often needed to get an output of sufficient amplitude for recording. Furthermore, the input impedance of the amplifier must be as high as possible (well into the megohm range) to avoid electrical loading of the electrodes (see Chapter 4, "General-Purpose Tools"). The combination of a very small signal and very high input impedance makes the system susceptible to noise. The electrode wires that go to the amplifier act as antennas, picking up stray electromagnetic radiation. Because the wires must be kept as short as possible, it is common practice to put a preamplifier very close to the subject and to use its output as the signal to the EMG amplifier itself. Noise reduction is also facilitated by using differential amplifiers with high ($\geq$100 dB) common-mode rejection ratios (see Chapter 4, "General-Purpose Tools"). (Portable multichannel surface EMG systems that incorporate ultrahigh-impedance amplifiers are available currently from several manufacturers such as DelSys in Boston, MA.)

The appearance of the electromyogram will depend on the volume of muscle "seen" by the electrodes and the nature of the task being examined. If the active region between the electrodes is very small (as with intramuscular bipolar electrodes), individual muscle action potentials may be recorded, especially if the muscle is not very active (Figure 12–2A). The frequency of the "spikes" of electrical activity can range up to more than 40 per second, making the "raw" electromyogram during a speech event look like the one shown in Figure 12–2B. Note that the frequency of the spikes changes from a relatively quiescent resting rate to a much higher rate. The number of spikes per second is a direct measure of the degree of muscle activation.

Normal muscle contraction is actually the result of the excitation of many motor units. Because the fibers belonging to a given motor unit are widely dispersed, the several muscle fibers lying between the electrodes are very likely to be members of different motor units, and their firing will, therefore, be asynchronous. Most often the EMG signal is the sum of the electrical actions occurring at quasi-random times with respect

---

[1]Some specialized "surface" electrodes have been designed to record from muscles deep within body cavities. Hixon, Siebens, and Minifie (1969), for instance, designed such an electrode for the diaphragm, and Lat'ovka, Sram, and Sedlácek (1984) have described a bipolar electrode that can be placed within the larynx.

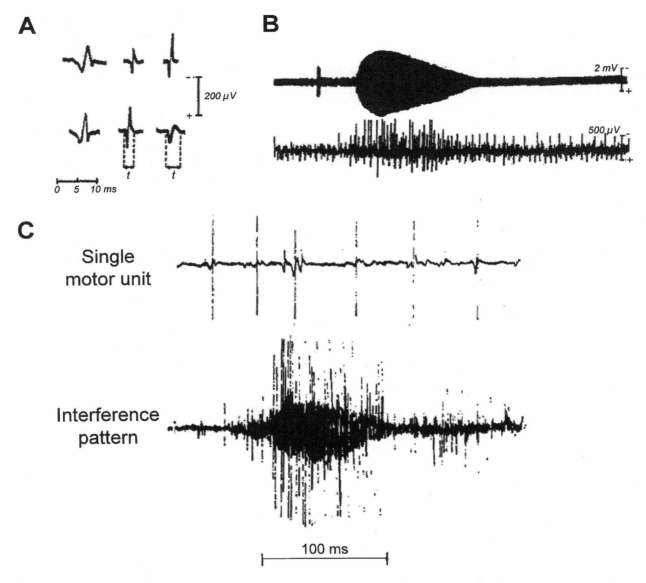

Figure 12–2. Electromyographic signals. **(A)** Single motor unit potentials; **(B)** Rapid sequence of "spikes." Note the change in impulse frequency, indicating a change in the level of muscle excitation; **(C)** EMG interference pattern, resulting from the superimposition of many random spikes. From "Instrumentation for the Study of Speech Physiology," by J. H. Abbs and K. I. Watkins, 1976, In N. J. Lass (Ed.), *Contemporary Issues in Experimental Phonetics* (pp. 41–75). New York: Academic Press. Figure 2.4, p. 45. Reprinted by permission.

to each other. This kind of summation results in an ***interference pattern*** (often colloquially referred to as ***hash***), as shown in Figure 12–2C. Surface electrodes always yield such a pattern because they are influenced by many motor units in the comparatively enormous muscle volume they sample.

Most often, EMG signals are rectified and integrated for analysis. This is the best way of demonstrating the "amount" of electrical activity, and it has been found (Lippold, 1952; Bigland & Lippold, 1954) that the amplitude of the integrated signal is directly proportional to the force of an isometric contraction. The optimal averaging time (RC time constant) will vary with the muscle being observed and the task being evaluated. Fromkin and Ladefoged (1966) point out that it should be relatively long with respect to the interval between electrical spikes, but short compared to the rate of change of activity in the muscle. The longer the averaging time, the more individual MAPs are leveled to create a smooth curve showing electrical activity over time. However, the smoothing also levels the peaks and troughs that indicate muscle activity and quiescence, such that the finer details of EMG changes over time are lost in this averaging. Figure 12–3 clearly shows the loss of temporal resolution as the averaging time is increased, causing the peaks of EMG activity to be very poorly demonstrated in the resulting record.

There is a certain "capriciousness" in the very complex muscle activity of speech. Minor differences in muscle activation occur from one repetition of an utterance to the next. These variations may interfere with an accurate assessment of what a given muscle actually does during a speech task. To mitigate this problem, some laboratories have developed special computer averaging techniques (Cooper, 1965; Fromkin & Ladefoged, 1966; Hirose, 1971; Port, 1971; Gay & Harris, 1971; Kewley-Port, 1973, 1977; Boemke, Gerull, & Hippel, 1992). Basically the technique involves sampling many repetitions of the same utterance. The EMG data are stored in a computer and are temporally aligned at some reference point chosen by the user. The values for each of the samples at each point in time are averaged to produce a final output in which events that are present in every one of the samples are emphasized, but those that are unique are de-emphasized. Figure 12–4 illustrates the results achieved by this kind of averaging process.

BIOFEEDBACK

Clinically, surface electromyography has shown promise as a tool for providing biofeedback of speech motor performance or of the overall level of muscle activity at a particular site (Booker, Rubow, & Coleman, 1969; De Luca, LeFever, & Stulen, 1979; McCarthy & De Luca, 1985; Milutinovic, Last'ovka, Vohradník, & Janosevic, 1988; Redenbaugh & Reich, 1989). Often the patient is provided with an auditory signal whose frequency varies with the amplitude of the EMG voltage (for example, Netsell & Daniel, 1979). The patient, of course, is instructed to control the audible tone (in ways specified by the therapist) by means of muscle control. Biofeedback has been successfully used to reduce facial hypertonicity (Netsell & Cleeland, 1973; Finley, Niman, Standley, & Ender, 1976; Finley, Niman, Standley, & Wansley, 1977; Hand, Burns, & Ireland, 1979; Rubow, Rosenbek, Collins, & Selesia, 1984), to increase labial muscle activity after neural anastomosis (Daniel & Guitar, 1978), to normalize perilaryngeal muscle tension in hyperfunctional voice disorders (Lyndes, 1975; Prosek Montgomery, Walden, & Schwartz, 1978; Stemple, Weiler, Whitehead, & Komray, 1980; Allen, Bernstein, & Chait, 1991; Watson, Allen, & Allen, 1993), and to reduce stuttering (Guitar,

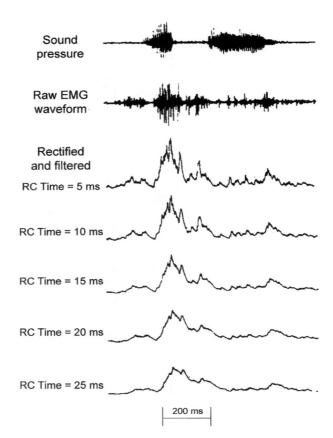

Sound pressure

Raw EMG waveform

Rectified and filtered

RC Time = 5 ms

RC Time = 10 ms

RC Time = 15 ms

RC Time = 20 ms

RC Time = 25 ms

| 200 ms |

Figure 12–3. Rectified and averaged EMG rescores of the utterance /æpæ/, with averaging time increasing from top to bottom. From "Instrumentation for the Study of Speech Physiology," by J. H. Abbs and K. L. Watkin, 1976. In N. J. Lass (Ed.), *Contemporary Issues in Experimental Phonetics* (pp. 41–75). New York: Academic Press. Figure 2.7, p. 53. Reprinted by permission.

1975; Hanna, Wilfling, & McNeil, 1975; Manschreck, Kalotkin, & Jacobson, 1980; Craig & Cleary, 1982; St. Louis, Clausell, Thompson, & Rife, 1982; Craig et al., 1996).

VOCAL TRACT IMAGING

Various imaging techniques have been used to describe articulator shape, position, and movement without the need for direct contact. They offer the advantage of allowing the observation of the vocal tract and articulatory behavior without significantly altering normal movement patterns. However, deriving movement data can be a slow and painstaking process that often requires a frame-by-frame analysis of many sequential images.

Average EMG signals

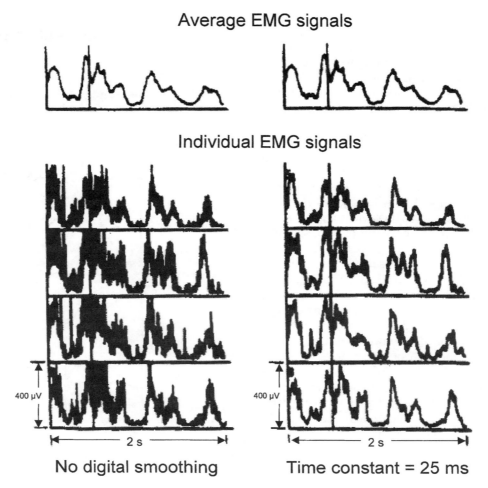

Individual EMG signals

400 µV

2 s

No digital smoothing

400 µV

2 s

Time constant = 25 ms

Figure 12–4. EMG averaging. The top trace represents the average of a total of 10 EMG recordings made during repetitions of a single utterance. (Only 4 of the 10 EMGs are shown here.) The "line-up point" is shown by the vertical line which corresponds to the offset of voicing during the utterance. Averaging of both "raw" (left) and smoothed (right, time constant = 25 ms) are displayed. From "EMG Signal Processing for Speech Research," by D. Kewley-Port, 1977, *Haskins Laboratories Status Report on Speech Research*, *SR*−50, 123–146. Figure 4, p. 140. Reprinted by permission.

Radiographic Techniques

Less than two years after Roentgen discovered the X-ray, Scheier (1897) published a radiographic study of the speech organs. In fact, much of our early understanding about the behavior of the tongue and pharynx during speech production has come from X-ray studies (see MacMillan and Kelemen, 1952, or Subtelny, 1961, for a review) and have continued to be used in the study of speech that is both normal (Moll, 1960, 1965; Sonninen, 1968; Kent & Netsell, 1971; Kent, 1972; Kent & Moll, 1972; Wood, 1979; Hashimoto & Sasaki, 1982; Badin, 1991; Sonninen & Hurme, 1998) and abnormal (Fletcher, Shelton, Smith, & Bosma, 1960; Massengill, 1966; Lubker & Morris,

1968; Tye-Murray, 1987, 1991; Subtelney, Li, Whitehead, & Subtelny, 1989).

X-rays are a form of high-frequency electromagnetic radiation with wavelengths between those of ultraviolet light and gamma rays. Unlike waves within the visible spectrum, X-rays can pass through many materials including almost all bodily tissues. If an X-ray beam is projected through the body, it will be differentially absorbed by the tissues; the proportion absorbed being directly related to the density of the structures through which the beam passes. Because the density, thickness, and composition of tissues will differ from one another, they may be separately resolved in a "shadow" image or *radiogram*. To make a lateral X-ray image of the vocal tract, the X-ray beam is projected from the side of the head to a recording plate positioned on the other side. Likewise, a frontal X-ray can be obtained by projecting a beam through the patient's head from the front to a plate positioned directly behind. The recording plate actually consists of a special cartridge. Inside the cartridge are image-intensifying screens that are composed of fluorescent crystals. These crystals absorb the residual X-ray beam energy causing them to fluoresce, thereby exposing a sheet of photographic film. Alternatively, the residual X-ray energy can be greatly amplified (gains of 1,000 to 3,000 are typical) and projected on a photosensitive fluorescent screen in a procedure known as *fluoroscopy*.

The assessment of speech structure and function using radiographic methods has certain inherent limitations. Of course the hazards of overexposure to radiation are well known (Whalen & Balter, 1984) and the associated health risk alone has severely curtailed the collection of large quantities of data with conventional X-rays. It is also unfortunate that improving radiogram image contrast generally requires an increase in the radiation dose delivered to the patient. Furthermore, soft tissues (such as the tongue and velum) are often difficult to distinguish in an X-ray image because they may be faint or obscured by the far more dense bony structures of the head and neck. *Xeroradiography*, a technique where the radiogram is developed using a powder on an electrically charged plate, may improve soft tissue contrast by emphasizing the edges of structures, but it is a slow process that requires more radiation than ordinary X-rays produced using photographic film. Alternatively, a contrast medium such as a barium sulfate paste (McClean, 1973) or a radioopaque marker such as a gold chain or a series of pellets (Alfonso & Baer, 1982; Weismer & Bunton, 1999) can be used to help identify soft tissue borders. Marking the midline of the tongue in this manner may, in fact, be critically important since the tongue is often grooved during speech. Thus the superior border on the two-dimensional radiogram may represent a lateral edge rather than the midline of the tongue (Fujimura, 1990; Stone, 1991).

MOTION FLUOROGRAPHY

Both *cinefluorography* and *videofluorography*, the recording of radiographic images on motion picture film and videotape, respectively, allow the observation and assessment of articulatory movement during speech and nonspeech tasks (Carrell, 1952; McWilliams & Bradley, 1964; McWilliams & Girdany, 1964; Skolnick, 1970; Subtelny, Oya, & Subtelny, 1972; Kuehn & Tomblin, 1977; Zimmermann, 1980a, 1980b; Folkins, 1981; Zimmermann & Hanley, 1983; Subtelny et al., 1989; Laukkanen, Takalo, Vilkman, Nummen-

ranta, & Lipponen, 1999). However, as valuable as cinefluorographic studies may be to the researcher and clinician, and despite continuing efforts to develop digital radiographic techniques that hold the promise of greater ease, image quality, and versatility (Brady, 1984; Rieppo & Rowlands, 1997; Yaffe & Rowlands, 1997; Zhao et al., 1997), the cumulative radiation dose associated with continuous X-ray exposure obviates the collection of more than just a few, brief speech samples. Although videofluorography generally requires less radiation, image resolution is generally poorer than that of motion picture film. Furthermore, the videotape frame rate is slower than that of motion picture films, so fewer images are obtained per second.

COMPUTED TOMOGRAPHY

Computed tomography (*CT*), also known as *computerized axial tomography* (*CAT*), uses X-rays to produce an image of a thin section (slice) of the body. To produce a section through the vocal tract, the CT scanner rotates around the head and neck passing fine X-ray beams through the tissues at multiple angles. A computer then produces a matrix of numeric data for the entire section that was perpendicular to the CT scanner. Each number within the matrix represents the degree of X-ray absorption associated with a single, localized "volume element," or *voxel*. The depth of the voxel corresponds to the thickness of the cross-section, which can be as thin as 2 mm. Display devices typically portray each small voxel as a two-dimensional "picture element," or *pixel*, that represents beam absorption—and thus tissue density—at that location with a gray scale. A display of the corresponding pixel matrix creates the final CT image (see Takahashi, 1982, or Morgan, 1983, for good overviews of CT principles and techniques). Because the scanner can be oriented in a variety of ways with respect to the structures of interest, sagittal, frontal, oblique, and transverse "tomogram" sections are possible.

In a CT image, bone appears white and airspaces appear black, whereas soft tissues, such as the tongue and velum, appear in varying shades of gray. Because digital summation of a series of scans is used to construct a composite image, CT scans provide sharper edges that provide better definition of soft tissue than is typical of standard X-rays (Kiritani, Tateno, Linuma, & Sawashima, 1977; Gamsu, Mark, & Webb, 1981; Gamsu, Webb, Shallit, & Moss, 1981; Hanafee, 1983; Sundberg, Johansson, Wilbrand, & Ytterbergh, 1987; Friedrich, Kainz, Schneider, & Anderhuber, 1989). Three-dimensional images can be constructed by combining multiple sections. The latest generation of CT scanners can complete several scans per second, making the observation of speech movement possible. But, like all radiographic techniques, CT imaging exposes the patient to the hazardous risk of ionizing radiation. This has seriously restricted its clinical and research application, especially with the development of other, less potentially harmful, imaging techniques.

Ultrasonography

The term *ultrasound* refers to any sound pressure signal above the range of human hearing. Technically, ultrasound waves can range from 20 kHz to 20 MHz, but clinical untrasound general uses a frequency above 1 MHz. An ultrasound signal can be passed into the body from a special transducer in contact with the body surface. The ultrasound transducer consists of a piezoelectric crystal that is deformed by the application of an electric current. The crystal then behaves much as a tuning fork, causing the propagation of sound waves. The sound waves travel in a straight line, penetrating the structural layers as they go. For instance, the beam of ultrasound from a transducer applied to the neck just over the thyroid ala would pass through the skin, underlying fat, fascia, muscle, thyroid cartilage, and vocal folds, finally reaching the airspace of the glottis. Each of these tissues has different acoustic transmissive properties: Some pass the ultrasound with relative ease, while others are comparatively poor ultrasound conductors. It is a general principle of physics that part of a beam of energy will be reflected at the interface between two substances of differing transmissive properties. Every time the beam crosses the border between different tissues, part of the sound energy is reflected back toward the source while the remainder of the beam continues on until the next interface, when another portion is reflected and the remainder continues. Air is an extremely poor conductor of the ultrasound, so that when an airspace is encountered, almost all of the ultrasound energy is reflected, and the transmission is effectively ended. Therefore, ultrasound is not particularly useful for observing the velum, but can be profitably employed for the study of those structures that are adjacent to an airspace, such as the upper surface of the tongue, the vocal folds, and the lateral pharyngeal walls (Ueda, Yano, & Okuno, 1993). Bone can obscure the soft tissue beyond it. When the ultrasound encounters a bone, much of the acoustic energy is reflected, creating a dark shadow in that region. Thus, because the palate and teeth do not appear in ultrasound images, the position of the tongue cannot be studied relative to them. Furthermore, care must be taken to avoid, as far as possible, structures such as the jaw and hyoid bone when imaging the tongue, pharynx, and larynx. It is also important to maintain good contact between the transducer and the skin. To increase acoustic coupling, an acoustic gel is usually applied to the surface of the patient's skin and to the transducer.

The ultrasound reflections are a series of echoes. In *pulse-echo ultrasound*, the crystal used to generate the sound waves also receives the echoes, transducing the acoustic energy back into electrical energy. The longer it takes for an echo to be received, the further from the transducer its reflecting interface between tissues must be. It is a simple matter, then, to determine how deep under the surface the various tissue layers are: we need only time the returning echoes. Since the anatomy of a body region is generally well known, it is a fairly simple matter to associate given echoes with the boundaries between specific structures. At the intensities used in clinical work, ultrasound has no apparent injurious effects. (A good overview of ultrasonography and body-imaging instrumentation is available in Henrick, Hykes, and Starchman, 1995).

There are two major forms of ultrasound display. In the *A-mode*, a beam begins sweeping across a display screen when the ultrasound is pulsed into the tissue. Echoes show as spikes along the screen's horizontal axis. The position of a spike along the horizontal line, therefore, corresponds to the distance of the reflecting interface from the body surface, while the height of the spike indicates the strength of the echo and the amount of acoustic-transmissive difference between the tissues being traversed. The A-mode display is one-dimensional, provides limited information, and is difficult to interpret. It is not, therefore, the preferred display format. Displays using the *B-mode* (also known as the *brightness-mode*) cause the line being drawn on the screen to vary in brightness according to the strength of the echoes. If the transducer rotates slightly as rapidly repeated pulses are sent into the tissue, the echoes from an entire sector can be detected. When the many B-mode lines are drawn next to each other on the display screen in a sequence that corresponds to the transducer position at the time each one was generated, a two-dimensional black and white "picture" of the tissues is built up. Since the entire scanning process can be repeated very rapidly, it is possible to produce many complete sector scans every second, and thereby produce a "motion picture" of activity within the body. Such images have become increasingly familiar to everyone, thanks to their widespread application in cardiology and especially in obstetrics, where they are used to evaluate the status of the fetus in utero.

Minifie, Kelsey, Zagzebski, and King (1971) used pulse-echo ultrasound to visualize the longitudinal contour of the dorsal surface of the tongue. An ultrasound transducer was moved along the anterior midline of the neck and underside of the jaw, from the level of the larynx to the mental symphsis. Transverse contours were generated by moving the transducer under the jaw along the coronal axis. A complete scan required about 3 s, during which the patient had to maintain a stable articulatory position. While the results were clear and impressive, only static positions could be visualized, and there was some discrepancy between the ultrasound and simultaneous X-ray measures taken.

A different system has been devised by Schuette, Shawker, and Whitehouse (1978) and applied to the observation of tongue structure and movement by Sonies and her coworkers (Sonies, Shawker, Hall, Gerber, & Leighton, 1981; Sonies, 1982; Shawker, Sonies, Stone, & Baum, 1983; Morrish, Stone, Sonies, Kurtz, & Shawker, 1984; Morrish, Stone, Shawker, & Sonies, 1985; Shawker & Sonies, 1984; Sonies, Baum, & Shawker, 1984; Shawker, Sonies, & Stone, 1984; Sonies, Baum, & Shawker, 1984; Sonies, Stone, & Shawker, 1984; Stone, Morrish, Sonies, & Shawker, 1987). The transducing crystal is scanned across the structures being observed by rotating it, rather than sliding it along the surface. The rotation is done by a motor, covers a moderately wide angle, and is repeated at least 30 times per second. The transducer scans are synchronized with a monitor on which the ultrasound echoes are displayed after digital processing. Soft-tissue structures are delineated quite clearly (Figure 12–5). Recently, Stone and Davis (1995) have designed a special support system that serves both to stabilize the patient's head and to fix the ultrasound transducer so that mandibular movement exerts little, if any, influence on tongue-movement imaging. Additionally, mathematical methods for describing the configuration of the tongue based on ultrasound data have been developed (Keller & Ostry, 1983; Stone, Sonies, Shawker, Weiss, & Nadel, 1983; Morrish et al., 1984; Unser & Stone, 1992).

Beyond probing the larynx (discussed in Chapter 10, "Laryngeal Function") and the tongue (Munhall, 1985; Ostry & Munhall, 1985; Leidig, Koppenburg, & Bacher, 1987; Koppenburg, Leidig, Bacher, & Dawsch-Neumann, 1988; Stone, Shawker, Talbot, & Rich, 1988; Lenz, Bongers, Ozdoba, & Skalej, 1989; Hirai, Tanaka, Koshino, & Yajima, 1991; Müssig, 1992; Schliephake, Schmelzeisen, Schönweiler, Schneller, & Altenbernd 1998), pulse-echo ultrasound has been used with moderate success to track position changes of the pharyngeal wall (Kelsey, Hixon, & Minifie, 1969; Kelsey, Woodhouse, & Minifie, 1969; Ryan & Hawkins, 1976; Hawkins & Swisher, 1978; Parush & Ostry, 1986, 1993) —in one case by using a 20-transducer array to visualize a significant length of the structure (Skolnick, Zagzebski, & Watkin, 1975).

Transmission* (*M-* or *TM-mode*) *ultrasound measures distance by determining the time required for an ultrasound pulse to travel through a structure from a transmitter to a receiver. The technique, therefore, observes only the small area under the probe. This can be an advantage if the distance between two well-defined points is desired. Watkin and Zagzebski (1973), for example, used transmission ultrasound to determine the displacement of a point on the tongue by cementing a very small receiver to the tongue and placing the transmitter under the jaw. The pulse-transit time in this arrangement is a direct correlate of the height of the receiver above the transmitter. Although carefully tracking the orientation of the receiver to the transmitter will assist in identifying

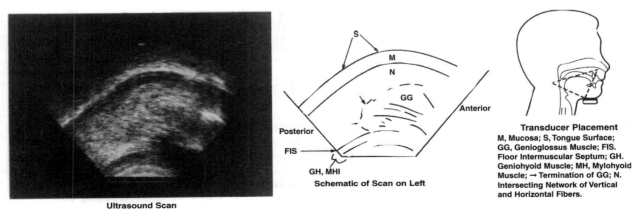

Ultrasound Scan

MIDLINE SAGITTAL SCAN OF MID-TONGUE

Figure 12–5. Ultrasound visualization of the tongue in the midsagittal plane. (Illustration courtesy of Dr. B. Sonies, Bethesda, MD.)

the relative position of the tongue-surface receiver (Kaburagi & Honda, 1994; Stone & Davis, 1995), there remains another problem with this method. The ultrasound transmission path must not have any airspaces in it, or the pulse will be almost completely reflected (Keller, 1987a, 1987b; Kwok, Wiegand, Channin, & Wiegand, 1994). This means, of course, that tongue-tip tracking is not likely to be feasible unless a copious amount of food, drink, or saliva is present or the tip happens to rest on the floor of the mouth.

Despite the limitations of ultrasound imaging, the use of B- and M-mode displays has been found to be useful in the construction of three-dimensional representations of tongue-surface movement (Wein et al., 1988; Böckler, Wein, & Klajman, 1989; Watkin & Rubin, 1989; Stone, 1990; Wein, Angerstein, & Klajman, 1993). The advantage of ultrasound is that it involves no discomfort for the patient and presents minimal, if any, health hazard. In addition, data collection is rapid, the equipment is less expensive than most other imaging equipment, and some ultrasound units are portable. Ultrasound displays have been used to provide visual feedback in articulation therapy with some success (Shawker & Sonies, 1985; Wein, Böckler, Klajman, & Willmes, 1990; Wein, Böckler, Kla-

jman, & Obrebowski, 1991; Wein, Drobnitzky, & Klajman, 1990).

Magnetic Resonance Imaging

Magnetic resonance imaging (*MRI*) is a recently developed technique that produces cross-sectional images by means of *nuclear magnetic resonance* (*NMR*), that is, by using the magnetic properities of the protons within atomic nuclei (James, 1983; Young, 1984). In particular, MRI exploits the magnetic resonance of hydrogen atoms whose nuclei contain a single proton. Hydrogen is abundant in water (H_2O) that, in turn, is abundant to varying degress in body tissue. (Fat and bone marrow are also high in hydrogen content.) To produce an MR image, sometimes called an *NMR tomogram*, the patient is placed within a strong and uniform magnetic field (ranging from 800 to 20,000 gauss[2]) that is created and maintained by electromagnets in the MRI scanner. As schematized in Figure 12–6a, hydrogen protons normally spin about an axis whose orientation is random. This spin causes the nucleus to generate a dipolar magnetic field around itself. The scanner forces an alignment of the spin axes along the direction of the poles of the applied magnetic

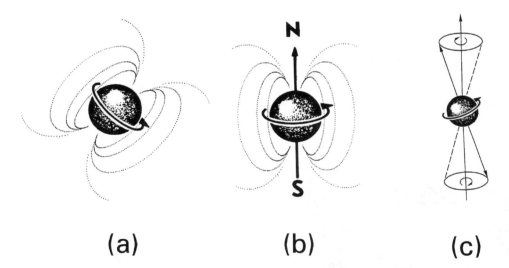

(a)   **(b)**   **(c)**

Figure 12–6. The behavior of hydrogen protons during MRI scanning. **(a)** The spin of hydrogen protons, organized in a random orientation, that causes the nucleus to generate a dipolar magnetic field around itself. **(b)** The forced alignment of the spin axes along the direction of the poles of the applied static magnetic field. **(c)** Precession of the nucleus after a brief pulse knocks it out of magnetic alignment. As it realigns, the nucleus emits a radio frequency signal. These signals are used to create an image based on the density of hydrogen that varies by type of body tissue.

---

[2]By comparison, the strength of the earth's magetic field ranges from about 0.3 gauss (G) at the equator to almost ± 0.7 G at the magnetic poles. One G is defined as the strength of a magnetic field 1 cm from a wire carrying a 5-amp current. The SI unit for magnetic field strength is the tesla (T); 1 T = 10,000 G.

field (Figure 12–6b). The application of a brief pulse (at a radio frequency equal to the resonant frequency of the hydrogen nuclei), knocks—or more correctly, flips—the protons out of alignment and causes their axes of rotation to wobble in a manner known as *precession* (Figure 12–6c). Precession is analogous to the spinning of a top: at first it will revolve about its axis, but as it slows down it will begin to totter in a rotation about its axis. The precession quickly decays as the axes of rotation realign themselves with the static magnetic field. But as this occurs, the energy that had been absorbed from the pulse is emitted by the hydrogen nuclei as small-amplitude (MR) signals of the same resonant radio frequency. These MR signals are detected by a receiving coil (tuned to the appropriate frequency) and are subsequently analyzed by computer.

To select a particular section, a relatively weak magnetic field "gradient" is superimposed on the main magnetic field across the particular axis of interest. Thus, in the presence of the field gradient, hydrogen nuclei at each distant point will be exposed to a different magnetic-field strength. Since protons will precess at a rate proportional to their particular magnetic field, those at different points along the gradient will precess at frequencies that are location specific. Tuning the radio frequency of the pulse causes it to excite only those nuclei in a particular layer of the magnetic field. The intensity of the received MR signal then becomes a direct measure of the hydrogen content[3] (and thus of tissue type) along this plane, while the frequency of the signal can be used to locate the exact position of the hydrogen within the plane. The orientation and thickness (generally ≥3 mm) of the imaged section can be selected arbitrarily. Using a method known as "spin warp," a matrix of data is established whereby each element represents an MR signal from a localized voxel within the imaged section. As with computed tomography, a two-dimensional display of the corresponding pixel array creates the final image and, since each image is stored directly in the computer as a matrix of numbers, three-dimensional imaging is also possible (Figure 12–7). According to several researchers, MRI represents the best available technique for obtaining data on static vocal tract shapes (Rokkaku, Hashimoto, Imaizumi, Niimi, & Kiritani, 1986; Baer, Gore, Boyce, & Nye, 1987; Baer, Gore, Gracco, & Nye, 1991; Lakshminarayanan, Lee, & McCutcheon, 1991; Greenwood, Goodyear, & Martin, 1992; Moore, 1992; Sulter et al., 1992; Dang, Honda, & Suzuki, 1994; Narayanan, Alwan, & Haker, 1995; Story, Titze, & Hoffman, 1996, 1998; Dang & Honda, 1997; Ong & Stone, 1998).

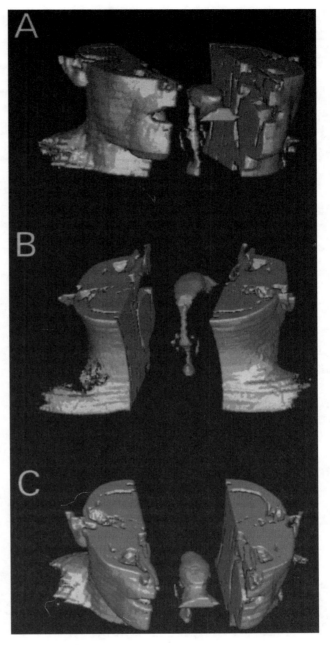

Figure 12–7. Three-dimensional reconstructions of the vocal tract based on MRI data viewed at oblique angles from **(A)** in front, **(B)** behind, and **(C)** above the speaker. (Images courtesy of Dr. B. Story, Denver, CO.)

For the most part, MRI offers unequaled soft-tissue contrast. The technique is noninvasive, unobtrusive, and because it uses low-energy nonionizing radiation, is associated with no known health hazards

---

[3]Tissues are also distinguished on the basis of the time it takes for the decay of both the precessional wobble (relaxation time, T1) and the net magnetization of the tissue perpendicular to the poles of the static field (relaxation time, T2). See Young (1984) for an excellent review of basic NMR principles.

(Roth, 1984; Young, 1984). Although claustrophobic reactions to the small confined space within the core of the NMR electromagnet are not uncommon among patients, "open" MRI units are becoming available. Unfortunately, to make the units serviceable for non-ambulatory patients, they require the patient to maintain a supine body position that may potentially alter articulatory behavior. Despite this limitation, MRI has been found to be an effective means of imaging the structure and position of the tongue, larynx, pharynx, and velum (Lufkin, Larsson, & Hanafee, 1983; Christianson, Lufkin, & Hanafee, 1987; Cha & Patten, 1989; McKenna, Jabor, Lufkin, & Hanafee, 1990; Wein, Drobnitzky, Klajman, & Angerstein, 1991; McGowan, Hatabu, Yousem, Randall, & Kressel, 1992; Niitsu et al., 1994; Watanabe, Arasaki, Nagata, & Shouji, 1994).

The major limitation of the technique, however, has been the amount of time it takes to acquire an image—which can range from a few seconds to several minutes. During this time, the speaker is constrained to maintain a stable vocal tract configuration. For instance, to obtain a 5-mm section through a speaker's vocal tract, Baer and his coworkers (1991), required the subject to produce selected vowels "in a monotone for about 15 s between brief inspirations, and to continue doing so throughout the 3.4 min required for image acquisition." Moore (1992) obtained vocal tract sections 3 mm thick while his speakers maintained each of several vowels, /s/, and /ʒ/ for several "comfortable" 15- to 20-s intervals over the 6 minutes it took to complete the scan, briefly pausing the imaging process each time the speakers inhaled between productions.

Advancements in MRI techniques have substantially decreased image acquisition time, however. Thus, in recent studies of fricative and liquid consonants, Narayanan, Alwan, and Haker (1995, 1997) were able to image 3-mm sections in just 3.2 seconds, allowing multiple images to be obtained for each sustained consonant production. More importantly, however, is the fact that so-called *ultrafast MR imaging* (Hennig, Nauerth, & Friedburg, 1986; Pykett & Rzedzian, 1987; Ordidge et al., 1988; Haase, Matthaei, Bartkowski, Dühmke, & Leibfritz, 1989; McKinnon, 1993; Debatin & McKinnon, 1998), made possible by such techniques as *echo-planar imaging* (*EPI*), *rapid acquisition and relaxation enhancement* (*RARE*), and *fast low-angle shot* (*FLASH*), are allowing clinicians and researchers their first opportunity to use MRI to track movement dynamics (Hagen, Haase, Matthaei, & Henrich, 1990; di Girolamo et al., 1996; Jäger et al., 1996; Yokoyama et al., 1996). For instance, Yamawaki, Nishimura, Suzuki, Sawada, and Yamawaki (1997) assessed velopharyngeal muscle movement using 4-mm thick sections obtained at a rate of 2.8 per second, whereas Foucart, Carpentier, Pajoni, Rabischong, and Pharaboz (1998) have obtained sequential 1-cm sagittal head and neck sections, acquired every 0.2 s, to evaluate swallowing. Efforts to decrease imaging time without losing resolution or increasing signal noise continue (Zhou et al., 1998), and are likely to render dynamic MRI an important and unique imaging tool.

ARTICULATORY CONTACT

Linguapalatal Contact

Information on the exact location of articulatory tongue-palate contact can be derived using a technique known as *palatography*. Various forms of palatography date from the latter part of the 19th century, and were used in many of the important early studies of normal and disordered speech (Rousselot, 1897–1901; Scripture, 1902; Stetson, 1928; Gumpertz, 1931; Moses, 1939).[4] Although interest in palatography had waned, the technique has enjoyed substantial worldwide revival over the past decade or so. This has been due to the fact that it is a moderately simple procedure that, with certain limitations, can provide a great deal of information about the precise location and timing of articulatory contacts that can be of inestimable value to the speech clinician (see, for example, Hardcastle and Morgan, 1982, and Hardcastle and Gibbon, 1997).

Palatographic methods may be classed as direct or indirect, according to whether an artificial palate is used. In both cases, the contact surface is coated with a powder (such as talc, flour, or a mixture of powdered charcoal and cocoa) that is wiped away by lingual contact. The need for the powder can be obviated by more recent electronic devices that sense tongue contact with metallic points on the surface of an artificial palate.

DIRECT PALATOGRAPHY

For *direct palatography*, a powder is dusted onto the patient's hard palate and velum. The test utterance is then produced and the "wipe-off pattern" assessed, since the powder will have been removed wherever there was tongue contact. Although direct palatography is simple, fast, and inexpensive, permanently

---

[4]The history of palatography is sketched by Moses (1940, 1964) and by Abercrombie (1957). Marchal (1988a) reviews the development of palatography and provides descriptive summaries of the various methods and systems available.

recording the results can be quite complicated. The easiest way is to insert a moderately large mirror into the mouth and to photograph its reflection of the palate (see, for instance, Dart, 1998). However, the angle at which the photograph is taken (which can vary significantly from one trial to another) can cause distortion of the image. To minimize this problem, Ladefoged (1957) described a simple arrangement of mirrors that assures a relatively constant camera angle. Nonetheless, the photograph does not depict depth. However, for cases in which the vertical dimension is important, Ladefoged (1957) and Bloomer (1943) have suggested methods of generating contour lines of the palate. In addition, Witting (1953) has proposed a method for numerically describing the contact pattern.

INDIRECT PALATOGRAPHY

For *indirect palatography*, an artificial palate is formed on a plaster cast of the patient's mouth. Although generally made of acrylic, Judson and Weaver (1965, p. 160) provide instructions for forming a metal-foil palate. Just

before use, the artificial palate is coated with a powder that contrasts with the base material. It is carefully fitted over the patient's palate, the test utterance is produced, and the plate is removed and examined. A permanent record in this case can be made by sketching the contact areas on an outline of the palate (Figure 12–8) or by photographing the plate. The artificial palate can be cleaned and reused as often as necessary.

Indirect palatography has a number of obvious drawbacks. The presence of the artificial palate might change articulatory patterns in unknown ways. Then too, it is not usually possible to extend the prosthesis very far over the velum withoug eliciting gagging. Therefore, linguavelar contacts cannot usually be detected with the technique. Most important from a practical point of view, however, is the fact that construction of the plate is an expensive and time-consuming process. On the other hand, the method has two significant advantages. First, the vertical dimension of the tongue contact is accurately shown. Second, the ability to remove the pattern from the mouth makes sketching and undistorted photography easier.

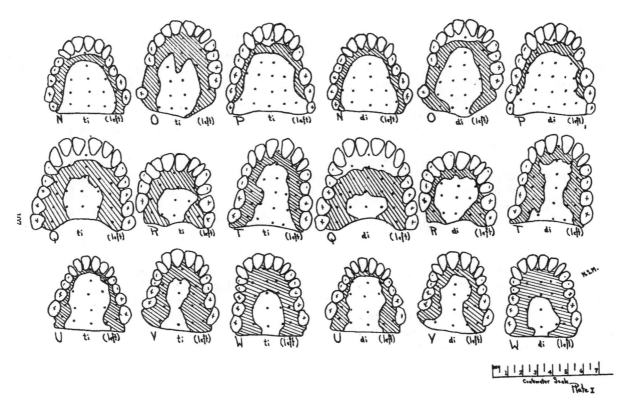

Figure 12–8. Specimen palatograms. From "Palatography and Speech Improvement," by E. R. Moses, Jr., 1939, *Journal of Speech Disorders*, *4*, 103–114. Plate I, p. 107. ©American Speech-Language-Hearing Association, Rockville, MD. Reprinted by permission.

Electropalatography

Electropalatography (EPG), also called *palatometry*, uses a special artificial palate made of a thin acrylic in which is embedded an array of silver or gold electrodes that detect tongue contact. These "electropalates" are typically custom-molded to fit the speaker (Heath, Ferman, & Mollard, 1980) with each electrode connected to its own thin wire. Bundled, these wires pass behind the back molars on each side of the electropalate and exit at the corners of the mouth. Electrical detection offers significant advantages, quite beyond the convenience of not having to bother with powder coatings. The electrodes are always ready and they don't need to be prepared after each contact. This makes it possible to observe and record entire series of different contact patterns during running speech, which permits the determination of the exact temporal duration and sequencing of many articulatory events. As such, EPG has been referred to both as *continuous* (Kydd & Belt, 1964; Rome, 1964) and as *dynamic* (Fujimura, Shibata, Kiritani, Shimada, & Satta, 1968; Fujii, 1970; Harley, 1972; Miyawaki, 1972; Tatsumi, 1972; Palmer, 1973; Fletcher, McCutcheon, & Wolf, 1975; Kiritani, Kakita, & Shibata, 1977; Michi, Suzuki, Yamashita, & Imai, 1986) *palatography*.

Instrumentation

Although several different electropalatographs have been described (Kuzmin, 1962; Kydd & Belt, 1964; Rome, 1964; Fujimura et al., 1968; Kozhevnikov et al., 1968; Hardcastle, 1970, 1972; Fletcher et al., 1975; Kiritani, Kakita, & Shibata, 1977; Autessere & Teston, 1979; Hardcastle, Jones, Knight, Trudgeon, & Calder, 1989; Clayton, 1992; Jones & Hardcastle, 1995), they all depend on the same basic principle: the tongue serves as a conductor that connects an electrical signal from a "sending" to a "receiving" electrode. In the early electropalatographs, the electrodes were arranged in sending and receiving pairs such that tongue contact connected the members of each pair. More recent instruments employ Kydd and Belt's (1964) modification that improves reliability and provides for greater spatial resolution.

At present three commercial EPG systems are available. In addition to a unit produced by the Rion Company in Japan (Fujimura, Tatsumi, & Kagaya, 1973; Shibata et al., 1978; Michi et al., 1986), are the *Reading Electropalatograph* (Millgrant Wells Ltd., Rugby, England), developed by Hardcastle and his colleagues, largely at Reading University and Queen Margaret College in Edinburgh, and the *Palatometer* (Kay Elemetrics, Lincoln Park, NJ), developed in collaboration

with Fletcher and his coworkers at the University of Alabama. In these systems, each palatal electrode is a receiver. The sending "electrode" is the tongue itself. This is arranged by connecting the patient to a imperceptibly small current via an electrode usually held in the patient's hand or attached to his wrist. The entire oral region will then conduct the signal so that when an electrically isolated pseudoplate electrode is touched by the tongue, the curcuit is completed (Figure 12–9B). A high-input-impedance amplifier is provided for each electrode. The electropalate is scanned, and linguapalatal contact data are acquired at a rate of 100 times per second. The data are often recorded by computer and displayed in real-time in the form of diagrams showing the arrangement of electrodes on the artificial palate with an indication of which ones are presently in contact with the tongue. Examples of such diagrams, known as *electropalatograms*, are shown in Figure 12–10.

At present, there is no standard number or arrangement of palate electrodes. The pseudopalate that accompanies the Reading electopalatograph attaches to the teeth of the patient and includes 64 electrodes arranged in 8 lateral rows (Figure 12–9A). The Palatometer electropalate, on the other hand, is formed to cover the patient's teeth (which helps to hold the transducer array in place). It contains 96 electrodes in a less linear configuration that includes not only the palate but the inner, lingual side of the teeth.

As with any form of indirect palatography, EPG shares the problems of possible interference with articulation (Hamlet & Stone, 1976, 1978; Hamlet, Cullison, & Stone, 1979; Likeman & Ferman, 1987; McFarland, Baum, & Chabot, 1996; Baum & McFarland, 1997) and the expense of artificial palates, which can be substantial. There is also a limited ability to detect posterior palatal and linguavelar contact, although Suzuki and Michi (1986) have addressed this problem by constructing an artificial velum that consists of a soft flexible latex sheet fitted with 36 electrodes. Although these authors claim to be able to derive accurate contact data without significant discomfort or restriction of velar movement, the validity and feasibility of "dynamic velopalatography" remains to be determined.

Application

Phoneticians have made extensive use of EPG to document the contact pattern and timing of palatal speech sounds in order to provide some insight into the dynamics of linguapalatal occlusion and tongue grooving during running speech (Fletcher, 1989; Hardcastle & Morgan Barry, 1989; Fletcher & Newman, 1991;

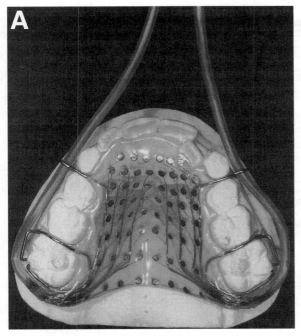

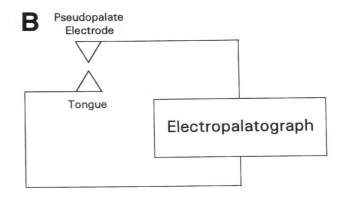

Figure 12–9. (A) The Reading Electropalate, attached to a cast of the upper teeth and palate. (Photograph courtesy of Dr. W. J. Hardcastle, Edinburgh, UK.) **(B)** A schematic illustration of an electropalatograph system. When the tongue contacts an electrode on the pseudopalate, current will follow along the path shown. Typically, the speaker is electrically connected to the electropalatograph by means of an electrode held in the hand or attached to the wrist.

Recasens, 1990, 1991a, 1991b; Farnetani & Faber, 1992; Stone, Faber, Raphael, & Shawker, 1992; Gibbon, Hardcastle, & Nicolaidis, 1993; Recasens, Fontdevila, Pallarès, 1993; Connell, 1995; Recasens, Pallarès, & Fontdevila, 1995; Byrd, 1996; Stone & Lundberg, 1996; Pandeli, Eska, Ball, & Rahilly, 1997). There has been particularly aggressive application of the technique in the study of coarticulatory processes and allophonic variation in speakers of numerous languages, including French (Marchal, 1987, 1988b; Fougeron & Keating, 1997), Castilian Spanish (Recasens, 1984a, 1984b, 1984c), German (Kohler, 1976), Italian (Farnetani, Vagges, & Magno-Caldognetto, 1985; Farnetani & Recasens, 1993), Greek (Nicolaidis, 1994), Swedish (Lundqvist, Karlsson, Lindblad, & Rehnberg, 1995), Hindi (Dixit, 1990; Dixit & Flege, 1991), Tamil (McDonough & Johnson, 1997), Swahili (Hayward, Omar, & Goesche, 1989), Japanese (Fujimura, Tatsumi, & Kagaya, 1973; Miyawaki, Kiritani, Tatsumi, & Fujimura, 1974; Sawashima & Kiritani, 1985), as well as American (Miyawaki, 1972; Dagenais, Lorendo, & McCutcheon, 1994; Byrd & Tan, 1996), Irish (Pandeli et al., 1997), and British (Butcher & Weiher, 1976; Hard-castle & Roach, 1979; Gartenberg, 1984; Hardcastle, 1985; Butcher, 1989; Wright & Kerswill, 1989; Barry, 1992; Gibbon et al., 1993) English.

There have been several recent suggestions regarding means to categorize or otherwise quantify the electropalatogram (Sudo, Kiritani, & Sawashima 1983; Engstrand, 1989; Marchal & Espesser, 1989; Recasens, 1990, 1991a; Fletcher, 1993; Recasens et al., 1993; Fontdevila, Pallarès, & Recasens, 1994a, 1994b; Byrd, Flemming, Mueller, & Tan, 1995; Chiu, Shadle, & Carter, 1995; Holst, Warren, & Nolan, 1995; Nguyen, 1995; McDonough & Johnson, 1997). Hardcastle, Gibbon, and Nicolaidis (1991), for example, have proposed a measure of linguapalatal contact designed to reflect the location of the main concentration of contacted palate electrodes. The measure, called the *center of gravity (COG) index*, gives progressively higher weighting to more anterior electrodes:

$$COG = \frac{\begin{array}{c}[N_{r8}(0.5) + N_{r7}(1.5) + N_{r6}(2.5) + N_{r5}(3.5) + \\ N_{r4}(4.5) + N_{r3}(5.5) + N_{r2}(6.5) + N_{r1}(7.5)]\end{array}}{\Sigma N}$$

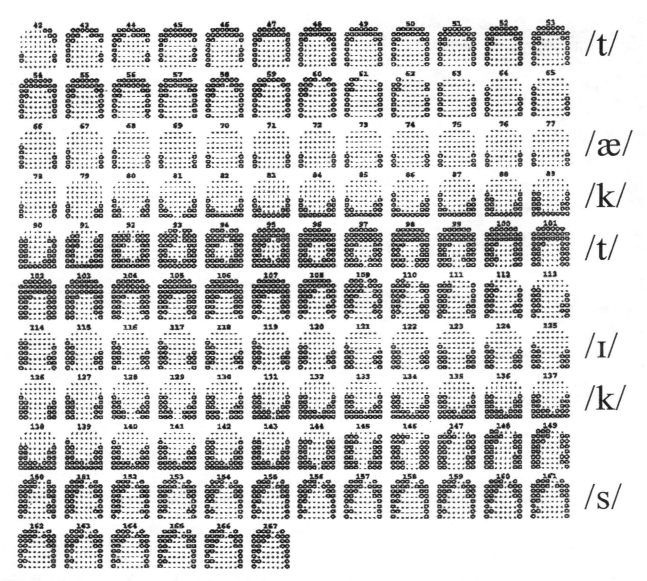

Figure 12–10. Electropalatographic contact patterns obtained every 10 ms while a speaker said the word "tactics." The sequence begins at the upper left. (Illustration courtesy of Dr. W. J. Hardcastle, Edinburgh, UK.)

where N_{r8} is the number of contacted electrodes in row 8 (the most posterior alignment of electrodes), N_{r7} is the number of contacted electrodes in row 7, and so on through N_{r1} (the first, most anterior row of palate sensors), and where ΣN is the total number of contacted electrodes on the pseudopalate. The COG index will vary between 0 and 7.5 depending on the number and location of contacted electrodes. Wakumoto, Issacson, and their colleagues (1996), for instance, calculated COGs for the EPG frames around the area of maximum constriction, converting the scores to percentages (so that a COG of 7.5 = 100%). Unfortunately,

the COG index can only be applied to data obtained from the Reading Electropalatograph that uses an artificial palate with electrodes positioned in 8 relatively straight rows. Furthermore, although Wakumoto, Issacson, et al. (1996) found the COG index to provide "a useful single measure estimating overall anterior/posterior changes in articulatory patterns," the clinical utility of the index (or of any other EPG measure) has not yet been established.

Although some work has also been directed toward phoneme and word recognition based on EPG patterns (Fujii, 1970; Fletcher, 1990; Byrd, 1994, 1995), many users of the technique stress the importance of ancillary speech data in the interpretation of articulatory behavior. That is due largely to the fact that, while electopalatography provides information about the beginning and end of linguapalatal contact, the technique does not record any information about articulator movement before that contact is made. Byrd and her colleagues (1995) quite correctly point out that "because EPG instrumentation only measures contact, inferences about the complete gestural trajectory, tongue shape, articulator velocity, or time of innervation are hazardous or impossible" (p. 822). Thus it is not uncommon for investigators to combine palatographic records with various acoustic (Flege, Fletcher, & Homiedan, 1988; Hoole, Ziegler, Hartmann, & Hardcastle, 1989) and aerodynamic (Hardcastle & Clark, 1981) measures, with displays that depict articulator

movement (Hoole, Nguyen-Trong, & Hardcastle, 1993; Lundqvist et al., 1995), and with ultrasound (Stone et al., 1992; Stone & Lundberg, 1996) and MRI (Alwan, Narayanan, & Haker, 1997; Narayanan et al., 1997) imaging. Commercially available software, such as *Phonédit* (S.Q. Lab, Aix en Provence, France) or that which accompanies the Palatometer and Reading EPGs, allows users to display the electropalatogram with one or more simultaneously obtained signals. For example, in the display shown in Figure 12–11, a cursor may be placed within the microphone signal or associated sound spectrogram and the corresponding electropalatogram (above right) indicates the pattern of linguapalatal contact at that instant. In this case, contact is shown prior to the release of /t/ in the phrase "you wished to know" from the Grandfather passage (Darley, Aronson, & Brown, 1975).

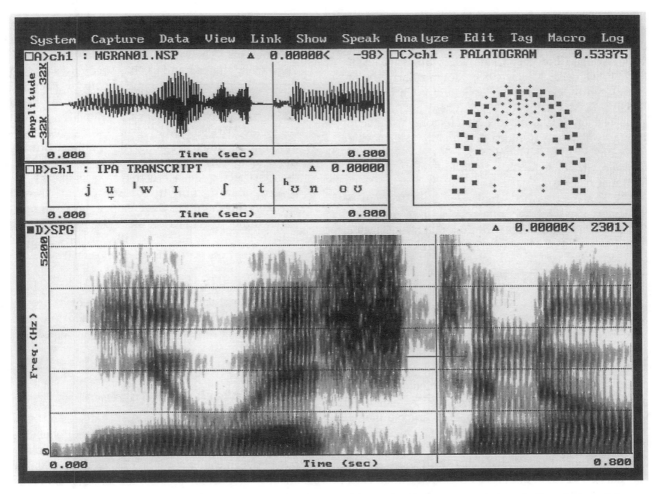

Figure 12–11. A palatographic display obtained with the Kay Elemetrics Palatometer system. In the electropalatogram (**C**, upper right) the squares indicate which of the 96 electrodes are in contact with the tongue. This palatogram corresponds to oral occlusion for /t/ in the phrase "you wished to know" at the point indicated by the vertical line drawn through the sound pressure waveform (**A**, upper left) and corresponding wide-band spectrogram (**D**, below).

Especially with the ability to tie contact data to other speech and voice measures (Dew, Glaister, & Roach, 1989), EPG has been found to be useful in the assessment of a number of different communication disorders (McGlone & Proffit, 1973; Pawlowski, 1975; Hardcastle & Morgan, 1982; Fletcher, 1985; Gibbon & Hardcastle, 1987, 1989; Hardcastle, Morgan Barry, & Clark, 1987; Gibbon, 1990; Gibbon, Hardcastle, & Moore, 1990; Dagenais & Critz-Crosby, 1991; Hardcastle, Gibbon, & Jones, 1991; Yamashita & Michi, 1991; Yamashita, Michi, Imai, Suzuki, & Yoshida, 1992; Hamilton, 1993; Howard, 1993; Morgan Barry, 1993, 1995a; Gibbon, Dent, & Hardcastle, 1993; Dagenais, Critz-Crosby, & Adams, 1994; Dent, Gibbon, & Hardcastle, 1995; Gibbon, Hardcastle, & Dent, 1995; Hardcastle, Gibbon, & Scobbie, 1995; Howard & Pickstone, 1995; Howard & Varley, 1995a; Suzuki et al., 1995; Whitehill, Stokes, Hardcastle, & Gibbon, 1995; Friel, 1998; Parsloe, 1998; Gibbon, 1999). Palatographic data have been used to describe the articulatory abilities and adaptations of stutterers (Harrington, 1987; Wood, 1995; Forster & Hardcastle, 1998), dyspraxics (Hardcastle, Morgan Barry, & Clark, 1985; Sugishita et al., 1987; Edwards & Miller, 1989; Morgan Barry, 1995b, 1995c), and esophageal speakers (Christensen, Fletcher, & McCutcheon, 1992). There has also been some use of EPG data to evaluate tongue behavior during swallowing (Ohkiba & Hanada, 1989; Jack & Gibbon, 1995; Chi-Fishman & Stone, 1996; Chi-Fishman, Stone, & McCall, 1998; Reinicke, Obijou, & Trankmann, 1998).

Several reports have indicated that EPG can be particularly helpful when assessing the functional changes that follow surgery of the oral cavity (Barry & Timmermann, 1985; Fletcher, 1988; Suzuki, 1989; Imai & Michi, 1992; Wakumoto, Ohno, et al., 1996; Wakumoto, Issacson, et al., 1996), and there are many overviews of how EPG may be used effectively as a feedback and therapy tool (Morgan Barry, 1989; Hardcastle, Gibbon, & Jones, 1991; Dent, Gibbon, & Hardcastle, 1992; Michi, Yamashita, Imai, Suzuki, & Yoshida, 1993; Dagenais, 1995; Howard, 1995; Hardcastle & Gibbon, 1997). Electropalatography has been employed in efforts to assist accent reduction (Gibbon, Hardcastle, & Suzuki, 1991; Gibbon & Suzuki, 1991) and to improve the articulation of hearing-impaired (Fletcher & Hasegawa, 1983; Fletcher, Dagenais, & Critz-Crosby, 1991a; Dagenais, Critz-Crosby, Fletcher, & McCutcheon, 1994; Crawford, 1995; Parsloe, 1998), cleft palate (Michi et al., 1986; Michi, Yamashita, Imai, & Ohno, 1991; Dent, Gibbon, & Hardcastle, 1992; Whitehill, Stokes, & Yonnie, 1996), dysarthric, and apraxic (Goldstein, Ziegler, Vogel, & Hoole, 1994; Howard & Varley, 1995b; Morgan Barry, 1995d) children and adults. However, as useful as EPG may be in clinical practice, any clinician employing the technique to assist articulation assessment and therapy should keep the following caveats in mind:

1. An acoustically-acceptable speech sound can result from many different tongue placements. And, while there is great variability even among normal speakers in the contact patterns used to produce a given phone (Moses, 1939; Shohara & Hanson, 1941), the contact pattern of a consonant will be altered additionally as the vowel environment changes and as jaw position alters the distance and orientation of the tongue and palate (Butcher, 1989; Stone et al., 1992; Recasens et al., 1995. Indeed, the contact pattern is subject to significant *random* variation. Therefore, requiring a patient to match a clinician's electropalatogram precisely, or seeking an invariant tongue contact for a phoneme in all contexts, constitutes a misuse of the technique.

2. Hamlet, Bunnell, and Struntz (1986) pointed out an important bias that may affect the interpretation of palatograms. "The lateral, midsaggital view of the vocal tract," they remind us, "has become a standard format for illustrating tongue activity in speech." Because of this, we tend to be poorly informed about contact patterns near the lateral margins of the palate. We also tend to assume that contact patterns are symmetrical about the midline. Studies (for example, Marchal and Espesser, 1989) have demonstrated quite clearly that there is likely to be considerable asymmetry of contact in normal speakers. Furthermore there is likely to be temporal asymmetry: contact on one side may be established before contact on the other. Neither asymmetry necessarily signals abnormality.

It would seem, then, that electropalatography is likely to be of maximal value for the assessment of grossly abnormal articulation or for tracking patient progress in approximating a more normal articulatory position and constriction.

Interlabial Contact

Unlike contact made between the vocal folds, the velum and pharyngeal wall, and the tongue and palate, contact between the lips can be observed directly. The production of bilabial plosive consonants, however, depends on the speaker's ability to not only approximate the lips, but to generate *interlabial contact pressures* that are sufficient to contain the intraoral air pressures that are necessary to produce the release burst (Malécot, 1966; Lubker & Parris, 1970). An impaired ability to generate or to maintain interlabial pressures can lead to an inappropriate release of air, thereby distorting the manner of articulation (Weismer, 1984; Forrest, Weismer, & Turner, 1989).

The maximum voluntary closing force generated by the upper or lower lip has been assessed in normal and abnormal speakers using a load-sensitive cantilever system (Barlow & Rath, 1985; Barlow & Netsell, 1986; Barlow & Burton, 1990; Wood, Hughes, Hayes, & Wolfe, 1992; Amerman, 1993; Langmore & Lehman, 1994; McHenry, Minton, & Wilson, 1994). However, recent technologic advances have resulted in the development of very small and exceptionally thin (1 to 2 mm) pressure and load-cell sensors (Lindman & Moore, 1990), that are now commercially available (Entran Devices, Fairfield, NJ). Their size and sensitivity are such that the transducer may be placed on the speaker's lip to measure interlabial contact pressure during speech production without significantly interfering with articulatory behavior (Hinton & Luschei, 1992). These pressure transducers are sealed, self-contained devices that are composed of four semiconductor strain gauges that are bonded to a thin circular diaphragm (see "Strain Gauges," this chapter). The diameter of the diaphragm sensor is typically 3 to 5 mm which must be completely occluded by the lips to derive an accurate pressure measurement. It is assumed that the force of occlusion acts evenly over the entire interlabial surface; an assumption that can be tested when multiple lip-contact transducers are used. Included with the transducer is a module designed to compensate for temperature changes that are likely to occur during speech as a consequence of the tissue contact on one side of the sensor and the air that flows past the other side.

For controlled speech tasks it has been found that the average peak interlabial pressure for the consonant /p/ tends to fall between 1 and 3 kPa, which represents roughly 10% of the typical speakers' maximum capacity to generate pressure between sealed lips (Hinton, 1996; Hinton & Arokiasamy, 1997; Thompson, Murdoch, & Stokes, 1997). Unfortunately, since there are no data regarding the interlabial contact pressures used by abnormal speakers, the clinical utility of the technique or measure has yet to be demonstrated.

Exploiting technology originally developed to provide tactile sensors for robots, Umemori, Sugawara, Kawauchi, and Mitani (1996) describe a *pressure-distribution sensor* (**PDS**) that they designed to measure lip-sealing force, interlabial contact area, and the distribution of contact pressure (Figure 12–12a). Their transducer consists of a disposable sensor cartridge, less than 2-mm thick, that is placed between the patient's lips and positioned to ensure contact with both angles of the mouth. Inside the cartridge is a thin

light-conducting plate and, in close proximity, a sheet of silicone rubber. On the surface of the sheet facing the plate is a grid of pyramidal projections. As the lip applies force to the cartridge in the vicinity of a particular projection, the contact made between it and the plate increases in a manner that is proportional to the $2/3$ power of the applied pressure. A fiberoptic light source illuminates the plate, but light is detected by a photosensitive film (also within the cartridge) only at points where the plate and sheet make contact. The result is a topographical representation of the interlabial contact pattern and the distribution of pressure across the area of contact (Figure 12–12b).

Although Umemori et al. (1996) claim that the PDS can be used to "measure lip sealing force under any functional conditions," their purpose was to assess maximal lip-sealing force and contact area prior to and following orthognathic surgery. Clearly the instrument is in the initial stages of development and may require a fair amount of adaptation and refinement before it is suitable for the assessment of lip behavior during speech tasks. Of course, a major consideration is the fact that the technique requires the placement of a horizontal cartridge in the patient's mouth, thus precluding tissue contact between the lips and potentially interfering in a consequential way with speech articulation. The uniqueness of the data, however, will probably warrant further development of such optical-pressure techniques.

ARTICULATOR MOVEMENT

Instrumental measurement of the motion of the organs of speech is not difficult in theory. In principle, any of a fairly large selection of transduction and recording techniques could be used and, in fact, have been. No matter what transduction system is assembled and implemented, it must meet certain criteria. The validity of the information gathered will depend on the system's physical characteristics and on the patient's response to the instrumentation. It should be obvious that the measurement system should not expose the patient to significant risk, nor should it cause any change in speech function. It should also be acceptable to the patient in a psychological sense. From the mechanical and electrical point of view, the measurement apparatus must have a response to motion that is, if not linear, then at least governed by some invariant mathematical function. It should be adequately sensitive to motion, without being too sensitive. Many speech movements are small, and there must be adequate gain to detect them unambiguously. At the same time, the very slight physiological tremor that is a normal aspect of muscle contraction should be

A

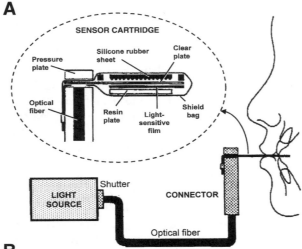

Figure 12–12. (A) Schematic diagram of the lip pressure-distribution sensor (PDS). **(B)** Lip-contact displays obtained with the PDS system before, and then one year following, orthognathic surgery. Original color Illustrations adapted from "A Pressure-Distribution Sensor (PDS) for Evaluation of Lip Functions," by M. Umemori, J. Sugawara, M. Kawauchi, and H. Mitani, 1986, *American Journal of Orthodontics and Dentofacial Orthopedics*, *109*, 473–480. Figure 2, p. 474, and Figure 8, p. 478. Used by permission.

B

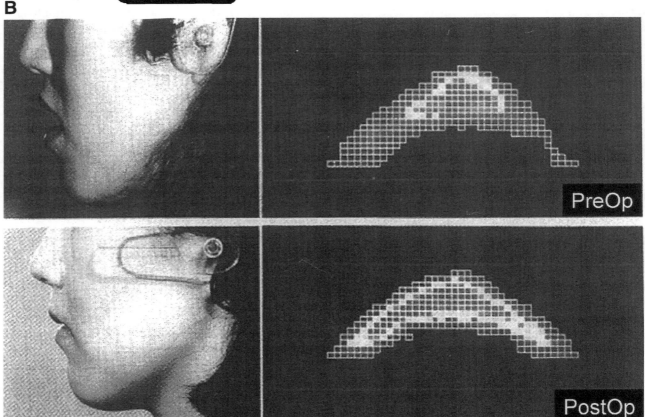

ignored: it constitutes noise in the output. Also, the gain must not be so great as to overdrive the system when a fairly large movement occurs.

Frequency response is another critical variable. Speech structures can move at velocities of several tens of centimeters per second, and acceleration can exceed 500 cm/s/s. The measurement system's bandwidth must extend high enough to track such movements without distortion. At the other end of the scale, the frequency response obviously must extend down to 0 Hz (DC) in order to capture static postures. The system must also be appropriately damped. This means that it must be able to follow rapid changes in signal level with minimal overshoot (in terms of voltage in the electronic elements). As shown in Figure 12–13, over-damped systems are sluggish in their response to sudden change (A), whereas underdamped systems tend to oscillate or "ring" (B). More complete consideration of mechanical and electrical criteria for measurement of physical events is provided by Abbs and Watkin (1976), Geddes and Baker (1989), and Cobbold (1992).

In general, tracking movements of the tongue is more difficult than the more freely-accessible motion of the lip or jaw. It is here that the theoretical ease of obtaining an adequate record meets the structural realities of the human body. The bases of the difficulty are readily apparent. First, the complex muscular arrangement of the tongue allows an almost infinite variety of movements. Second, tongue displacements can be very rapid. Stetson (1951) claimed to have observed tongue-tip trills at a rate of over 30 per second. Finally, the tongue acts in a very confined space, almost totally enclosed. Except for the most anterior portion, it is not directly observable, by eye or by instrument, from outside. Monitoring its behavior by inserting transducers into the vocal tract entails the very real possibility that articulatory behavior will be changed.

Strain-Gauge Systems

Strain gauges are an obvious choice for transducing structural movement. Several investigators have described strain-gauge systems for measuring lip and jaw motion. Almost all use a single basic configuration. Strain gauges are mounted on a flexible metal strip that is anchored at one end to a stable support (Figure 12–14A) to form a cantilever. Movement of the free end of the cantilever bends the metal strip, causing tension in the strain gauge mounted on the convex surface and compression of the one on the concave surface (Figure 12–14B). Wiring the strain gauges together with two other resistors to form a Wheatstone bridge (see Chapter 2, "Analog Electronics"), as shown in Figure 12–14C, creates a very sensitive displacement detector. To track the movement of the lips or mandible, the free end of the cantilever is attached in some way to an appropriate place on the subject's face. With a modified design, however, strain gauges can also be used to evaluate the force of articulatory dis-

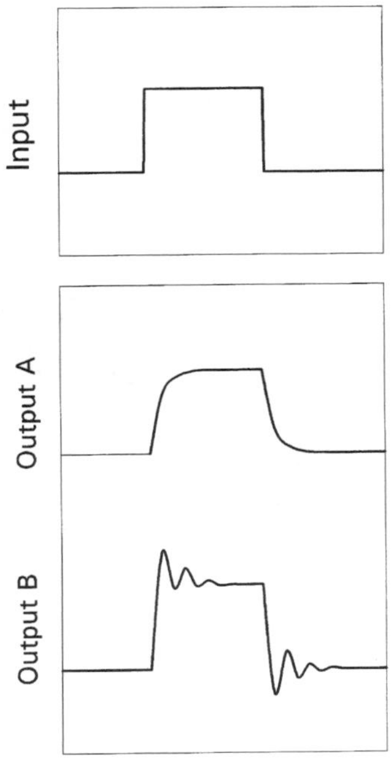

Figure 12–13. The effects of damping. Output A represents the response of an overdamped system to a square wave input. The output changes only slowly after a sudden change in the input signal. Output B represents the response of an underdamped system to the same square-wave input. The system response is very fast, but unstable. There is considerable overshoot, and oscillation (called "ringing") occurs as the output settles down to a final value.

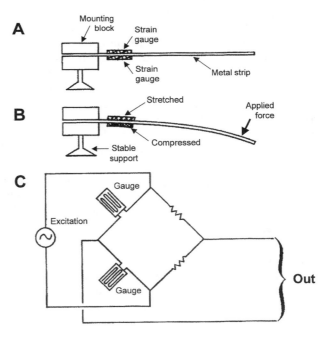

Figure 12–14. Strain gauge displacement transducers. **(A)** A cantilever system. (The gauges are shown proportionally much thicker than they would actually be.) **(B)** Deformation of the upper and lower gauges by a force applied to the end of the cantilever. **(C)** Arrangement of the gauges in a Wheatstone bridge.

placement, which might be useful in the assessment of motor impairments (see "Interlabial Contact," this chapter, and Barlow and Abbs, 1983, for a more complete description).

A number of factors must be taken into account in designing such a transducer. Most important among them is the *loading factor*, the force required to bend the metal strip, which acts as a spring. If too much force is needed, the spring will cause the soft tissue to be deformed. The point at which the transducer is attached will then not move in the same way as the rest of the surrounding structures, and an inaccurate measure will result. In extreme cases, articulatory gestures may be distorted. Minimizing the loading factor is achieved by reducing the stiffness of the cantilever. The dynamic response of the transducer is also important. Accurate transduction requires that the cantilever's mechanical characteristics give it a resonant frequency well above the highest-frequency components of the movement being measured. This objective is accomplished by minimizing the mass of the transducer system. Fortunately, strain gauges are inherently sensitive devices, and so obtaining adequate sensitivity requires no special design precautions (Abbs, 1973a, 1973b, Abbs & Netsell, 1973; Folkins & Abbs, 1975, 1976; Abbs, Folkins, & Sivarajan, 1976; McClean, 1977). Also, using two gauges as shown assures a high degree of temperature stability.

Even with carefully designed transducers, some tissue deformation due to loading is bound to occur. The question is whether the problem is likely to be a serious one for the clinician. Kuehn, Reich, and Jordan (1980) found that jaw displacement determined with strain-gauge measures and from cineradiographic images differed by anywhere from 0.67 to 2.31 mm in the superior-inferior direction and from 0.52 to 1.28 mm in the anterior-posterior plane. Furthermore, the timing of the transducer signal was often slightly out of phase with mandibular movement. The error was not systematically related to the nature of the speech task and was apparently due to soft-tissue loading. The minimum discrepancies found by Kuehn and his colleagues are probably acceptable in the clinical setting, although the maximal errors may not be. The final judgment must be made in the context of the information required. It is probably wise, however, to pay close attention to relevant design factors when assembling a strain-gauge system. Abbs and Gilbert (1973) and Müller and Abbs (1979) provide excellent guidance in this regard.

Although simple phosphor-bronze cantilevers can serve quite adequately, and have been used successfully by researchers (Sussman & Smith, 1970a, 1970b, 1971; Sussman et al., 1973), Müller and Abbs (1979) have described a superior transducer (shown schemat-

ically in Figure 12–15) that has been proven to be quite reliable in numerous studies (Folkins, 1981; Folkins & Linville, 1983; Abbs, Gracco, & Cole, 1984; Gracco & Abbs, 1985; Folkins & Canty, 1986; Folkins et al., 1988; Robin, Bean, & Folkins, 1989; McClean, Kroll, & Loftus, 1990; Adams, 1994; Gracco, 1994; Shaiman, Adams, & Kimelman, 1997; Dromey & Ramig, 1998a, 1998b). The basic cantilever (Figure 12–15A) is made of a tapered piece of stainless steel with a thickness of about 1.25 mm, upon which the strain gauges are mounted. A relatively rigid stainless steel wire extends from distal end of the cantilever and attaches to the

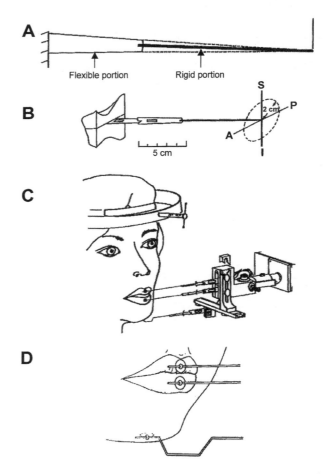

Figure 12–15. The strain gauge transducer of Abbs and his coworkers. **(A)** Basic cantilever design. **(B)** Two-dimensional transducer. **(C)** Mounting of the transducers for measurement. **(D)** Mylar disk/glass bead attachment technique. From "Strain Gauge Tranduction of Lip and Jaw Motion in the Midsagittal Plane: Refinement of a Prototype System," by E. M. Müller and J. H. Abbs, 1979, *Journal of the Acoustical Society of America, 65,* 481–486. Figures 2 and 3, p. 483; Figures 5 and 6, p. 484. Reprinted by permission.

patient, as discussed later in this section. The rigidity of the wire forces most of the bending to occur in the area where the gauges are placed. This arrangement creates an effective increase in length without adding significant mass and, at the same time, preserves sensitivity.

A single cantilever can only transduce motion in one plane—either vertical or horizontal. But lip and jaw movements are complex and certainly not restricted to a single direction. An ingenious modification of their transducer system allowed Abbs and his coworkers to track movements in two dimensions simultaneously. As shown in Figure 12–15B and 12–15C, they mounted the first flexible sheet to the end of another sheet at a 90° angle. Each cantilever can bend in only one direction (across its thickness), therefore each responds only in a single sensitive plane. The rod, however, is free to move in both planes. A pair of strain gauges on each of the segments monitors each of the directions separately.

The transducer system can be attached to the patient by adhesive-taping a small plate soldered to the end of the wire to the appropriate part of the face. But any side-to-side facial movement can distort the output. An alternative attachment scheme (Müller & Abbs, 1979) minimizes this problem (Figure 12–15D). A small jewelry bead is cemented to a flexible plastic disc that can be attached to the skin with double-surfaced adhesive tape. The wire is held in a hole drilled through the bead. The hole is somewhat larger than the wire's diameter so the wire can slide back and forth in case of side-to-side motion. All in all, the Abbs strain-gauge system is reasonably simple and inexpensive to assemble.

Obviously, any externally anchored measurement system imposes the requirement that the position of the transducer remain absolutely constant with respect to the head. Abbs and Stivers (1978) devised a special cephalostat (head holder) that fixes the head in one position while the transducers are mounted on a separate stable support near the subject's face. A very simple system that is better suited to clinical purposes (especially with younger children) is the one described by Sussman and Smith (1970a, 1970b) and by Hixon (1972) that is shown in Figure 12–16A. A somewhat more elaborate head-mount (Figure 12–16B) that permits several transducers to be used on different facial regions has been designed of lightweight tubular aluminum (Barlow, Cole, & Abbs, 1983). The transducers are clamped to a vertical rod that is suspended from an adjustable head band. In this way, the relative position of the transducer is kept constant with respect to the face, while the patient is afforded some degree of mobility.

An example of speech movement data from the work of Shaiman and her colleagues (1997) is shown in Figure 12–17. They used a head-mounted strain-gauge system to track anteroposterior movements of the upper lip in a study of lip protrusion. As is possible with all displacement data, the lip movement trace can be differentiated (see Chapter 2, "Analog Electronics") to yield velocity (rate of change in position) data, while differentiating the resulting velocity trace provides acceleration (rate of change in speed) data.

Optical Transduction Systems

Researchers in the fields concerned with limb movement and locomotion have often attached small, bright light sources to various body parts and tracked their trajectories using television, motion pictures, or more sophisticated computer techniques (see, for example, Grieve, Miller, Mitchelson, Paul, & Smith, 1975; Costigan, Wyss, Deluzio, & Li, 1992; Gabriel, 1997). McCutcheon, Fletcher, and Hasegawa (1977) attached small reflectors (0.5-mm glass beads) to fleshpoints on the lip and jaw. When the speaker's face was brightly lit, each reflector acted as an effective light source. Digital circuits associated with a television system were able to detect the reflectors with a spatial resolution of up to 0.3 mm and to track them at speeds up to 45 cm/s. Sonoda and Wanishi (1982) developed an instrument that allows simultaneous real-time tracking of 8 different points on the lips and jaw. The light sources used were very small *light-emitting diodes* (*LEDs*) that served as point sources of infrared illumination. The heart of the instrument is a special rectangular optoelectronic detector that produces small currents at its electrodes in response to a spot of light shining on it. Requiring relatively simple electronics, the detector's characteristics inherently provide the means for determining exactly where, in two dimensions, the spot shone on it. For use, the LEDs are attached to the fleshpoints of interest on the face and the detector (with a lens system) is set up about 50 cm away facing the speaker. The outputs are analog voltages of the position of each of the LEDs that can then be monitored and recorded.[5] The temporal resolution of the Sonoda and Wanishi system is 4 ms, while spatial resolution is on the order of 0.05 to 0.01 mm.

---

[5]Coelho and his colleagues (Coelho, Gracco, Fourakis, Rossetti, & Oshima, 1994) provide a case example in which a similar optical system was used to assess the repetitive jaw and lip movements of a dysarthric patient.

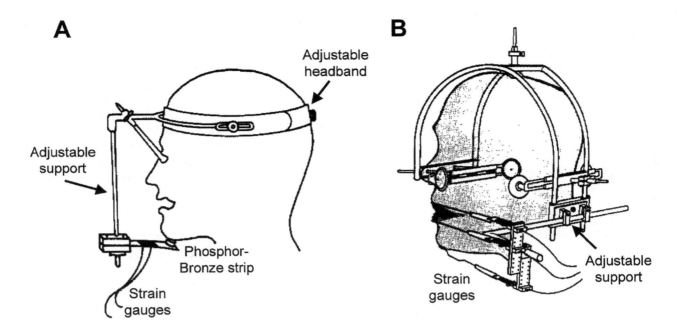

Figure 12–16. **(A)** Headband support for lip and jaw motion transducers. From "Some New Techniques for Measuring the Biomechanical Events of Speech Production: One Laboratory's Experiences," by T. J. Hixon, 1972, *ASHA Reports, 7,* 68–103. Figure 7, p. 83. Reprinted by permission. **(B)** A lightweight aluminum head-mount that supports several transducers that may be positioned to allow tracking of different facial regions. Adapted from "A New Head-mounted Lip-jaw Movement Transduction System for the Study of Motor Speech Disorders," by S. M. Barlow, K. J. Cole, and J. H. Abbs, 1983, *Journal of Speech and Hearing Research, 26,* 283–288. Figure 1, p. 284.

Technologic advances have led to the development of optoelectrical systems that allow the three-dimensional real-time tracking of multiple fleshpoints. Although they can be fairly expensive, there are now a number of systems that are commercially available, including the **ELITE** (Bioengineering Technology & Systems, Milan, Italy; Superfluo Inc., Los Angeles, CA) and **SELSPOT II** (Selcom AB, Partille, Sweden), that allow relatively straightforward acquisition, storage, and analysis of kinematic data (Ferrigno & Pedotti, 1985; Ackermann, Hertrich, & Scharf, 1995; Story, Alfonso, & Harris, 1996; Ackermann, Hertrich, Daum, Scharf, & Spieker, 1997; Ackermann, Konczak, & Hertrich, 1997; Hertrich & Ackermann, 1997; Konczak, Ackermann, Hertrick, Spieker, & Dichgans, 1997). The optoelectric tracking system that is currently most common in speech movement research, however, is the **Optotrak** (Northern Digital Inc., Waterloo, Ontario, Canada). It uses a set of small semiconductor chips that are placed on the surface of the speaker's

face to track movement (Vatikiotis-Bateson & Ostry, 1995). Each chip emits a synchronized infrared signal, while special sets of infrared-sensitive detectors (each with a lens and special signal-processing circuitry) tracks the movement of the markers in three-dimensional space. The current system allows up to 256 chips (fleshpoints) to be tracked at one time. However, as the chips may become uncomfortably warm after a few minutes of use, the length of time data may be collected can be limited.[6]

Several studies have used the Optotrak system to describe normal jaw and lip movement during speech and chewing tasks (McFarland & Lund, 1995; Vatikiotis-Bateson & Ostry, 1995; Dusek, Simmons, Buschang, & al-Hashimi, 1996; Ostry, Gribble, & Gracco, 1996; Ostry, Vatikiotis-Bateson, & Gribble, 1997; Smith & Goffman, 1998; Wohlert & Smith, 1998). Guiard-Marigny and Ostry (1997) have recently developed software that uses kinematic data to generate graphical three-dimensional reconstructions of jaw

---

[6]Borghese and his coworkers (Borghese, Ferrigno, Redolfi, & Pedotti, 1997) have recently described a system that uses passive markers to track the lips and jaw in three dimensions.

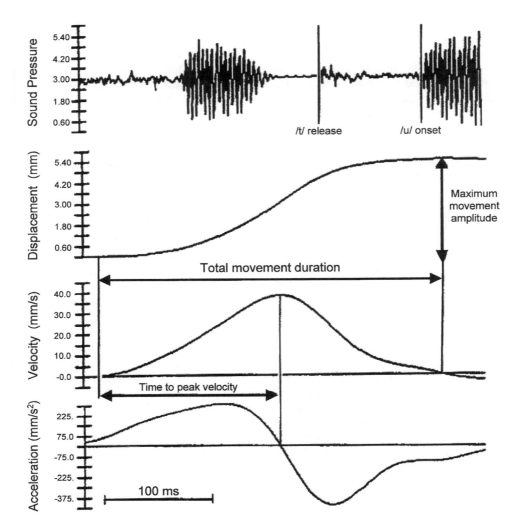

Figure 12–17. Protrusion of the upper lip during the utterance "see two." Displacement data may be differentiated to determine movement velocity (speed of displacement) while acceleration can be tracked by differentiating the velocity. From "Velocity Profiles of Lip Protrusion Across Changes in Speaking Rate," by S. Shaiman, S. G. Adams, and M. D. Z. Kimelman, 1997, *Journal of Speech, Language, and Hearing Research*, *40*, 144–158. Figure 1, p. 147. ©American Speech-Language-Hearing Association, Rockville, MD. Reprinted by permission.

movement. Such displays may be useful for the modelling of normal and abnormal speech movement and for providing visual biofeedback to patients.

While the lips and jaw are readily accessible, an accurate kinematic assessment of structures within the vocal tract can be quite problematic. Various appliances, consisting of metal rods or wires that extend out from the face and support external LEDs, have been used to track the movement of the velum and the mandible during speech and nonspeech tasks (Horiguchi & Bell-Berti, 1987; Edwards & Harris, 1990; Bell-Berti &

Krakow, 1991; Siegler, Hayes, Nocolella, & Fielding, 1991; Kollia, Gracco, & Harris, 1995; Ostry et al., 1996, 1997). By attaching these appliances to the structures of interest, the external movement of these appliances, and thus of the LEDs, allows relatively easy optoelectric tracking of articulatory displacement. The difficulty, however, involves assuring a firm and consistent attachment to each structure, stabilizing the appliance (Kelso, Tuller, Vatikiotis-Bateson, & Fowler, 1984; Kelso, Vatikiotis-Bateson, Saltzman, & Kay, 1985), and accurately calibrating such systems (see "The Velotrace," Chapter 11).

THE GLOSSOMETER AND THE OPTOPALATOGRAPH

Tongue motion has been transduced optically by a reflected-light detector devised by Chuang and Wang (1978). It takes advantage of the fact that the intensity of a reflected beam of light diminishes inversely with the length of the light's path. Small LED light sources and photosensitive detectors were arranged from front to back along the midline of an artificial palate, as shown in Figure 12–18. The light reaching each detector from its associated source is inversely proportional to the distance of the reflecting surface of the tongue from the artificial palate. Because of several characteristics in the physics of the situation (discussed in detail by the authors), the intensity-to-distance relationship is not linear, but the voltage outputs can be linearized by means that are not very elaborate, assuming that extreme precision is not necessary.

Fletcher, McCutcheon, and their coworkers (Fletcher, 1983; McCutcheon, Smith, Stilwell, & Fletcher, 1984) developed an improved system designed specifically for clinical and research use. Referring to the technique as *glossometry*, the "glossometer" has been used with some success to describe normal vowel production (Flege, Fletcher, McCutcheon, & Smith, 1986; Flege, 1989; Fletcher, McCutcheon, Smith, & Smith, 1989) and to improve vowel production by profoundly hearing-impaired speakers by providing visual cues regarding tongue position and posture (Fletcher, Dagenais, & Critz-Crosby, 1991b).

However, like the Chuang and Wang (1978) system, the physical dimensions of the LED-photosensor pair require the artificial palate to be substantially thicker than those used in the typical electropalate. Consequently, in order to minimize interference with articulation, the four sensor pairs are placed only along the midline of the palate and posterior to the alveolar ridge.

Wrench and his colleagues at Queen Margaret College in Edinburgh have developed a prototype (Figure 12–19) for an improved optoelectric tongue-tracking system (Wrench, McIntosh, & Hardcastle, 1996, 1997). Called the *Optopalatograph*, it employs an artifical palate that is similar in thickness to those used in the Reading Electropalatograph system (generally 0.5–2 mm) and is thus less obstructive of articulatory movement. The reduction in the depth of the artificial palate is made possible by placing both the light source and photodectors outside of the speaker's mouth. Light is transmitted by pairs of thin plastic optical fibers: one conducts light from a series of pulsed LEDs, the other transmits reflected light to the remote photodector. Besides allowing for a thinner artificial palate, this design permits multiple receiver-transmitter pairs to be placed over much of the surface of the palate. At present, between 8 and 20 fiberoptic pairs may be included on the "optopalate" to provide real-time three-dimensional tracking of tongue motion. It can be expected that optoelectric tracking of tongue movement will become an increasingly important research and clinical tool.

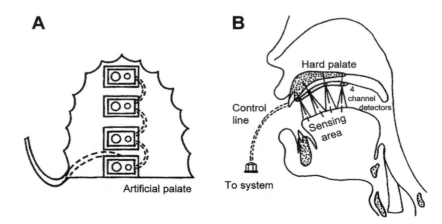

Figure 12–18. An optical scanning system to transduce tongue motion. **(A)** Arrangement of the light sources and photodetectors on an artificial (opto)palate. **(B)** The system in place. From "Use of Optical Distance Sensing to Track Tongue Motion," by C. K. Chuang and W. C. Y. Wang, 1978, *Journal of Speech and Hearing Research, 21,* 482–496. Figure 2, p. 486 and Figure 6, p. 490. ©American Speech-Language-Hearing Association, Rockville, MD. Reprinted by permission.

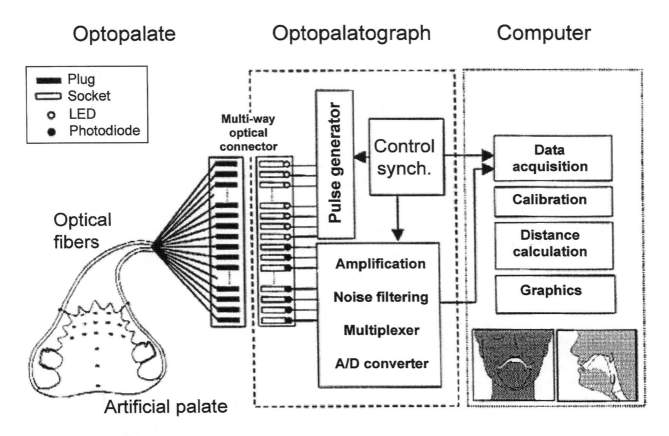

Figure 12–19. Block diagram of a prototype optopalatograph system. (Illustration courtesy of Dr. A. Wrench, Edinburgh, UK.)

Capacitative Transduction Systems

The capacitance, C, of a pair of electrodes is $C = k(A/d)$, where A is the area of the electrodes facing each other, d is the distance between them, and k is the dielectric constant (a measure of insulating ability) of the medium separating them (see Chapter 2, "Analog Electronics"). In a given situation, the area of the electrodes (assuming they do not slide past each other) and the dielectric constant are both unchanging. This being the case, $C \propto 1/d$. That is, capacitance is inversely proportional to the distance separating the capacitor plates. If the plates are attached to body structures, it should be possible to transduce the distance between them by applying high-frequency signals and determining the inter-plate capacitance with appropriate circuitry.

In fact, this principle has been applied to the measurement of speech-organ movement. Mansell and Allen (1970), for instance, attached a small plate to one lip and mounted the other on a separate support a fixed distance away. Intraoral capacitance techniques have been developed by Cole (1972) and by Hillix, Fry, and Hershman (1965). The latter's system employs a silicone-coated plate fixed to the palate. On the plate are two active elements of copper foil, one for the anterior, and the other for the posterior half of the palate. The capacitance between either of the palatal plates and the tongue varies inversely with the distance between them. In theory, it is, therefore, possible to achieve simultaneous measures of front and back tongue position. In practice, however, the output is very nonlinear, changing only slightly until the tongue-palate distance is less than 6 mm, after which the output change is very rapid.

Any advantage offered by capacitative transduction is more than offset by very serious limitations—the nonlinearity of the output, the inconvenience of being able to monitor only very small areas, and the near impossibility of achieving a calibration in terms of absolute distances. For reasons involving fundamental electronic theory, several of the problems will likely prove very refractory. The availability of alternate transduction methods thus makes it very unlikely that capacitative transduction will be intensively developed.

Electromagnetic Articulography

In addition to being able to monitor chest-wall movement (see "Magnetometry," this chapter), magnetometers can be used to track the displacement of structures both within and outside the vocal tract. The technique has come to be known as either *electromagnetic articulography* (**EMA**) or *electromagnetic midsagittal articulometry* (**EMMA**). In its earliest incarnation, Hixon (1971a, 1971b, 1972) used a single generator (transmitter) coil, driven at 1530 Hz, that was attached just under the speaker's chin, and two sensor coils, one on the forehead and the other on the back of the neck. The voltage induced in either of the sensors is inversely proportional to the cube of its distance from the generator. Therefore, as the mandible moves, the distance of the generator coil from one or both of the sensors changes, and the sensor's outputs vary accordingly. With this arrangement, both vertical and horizontal movements of the mandible in the sagittal plane can be transduced. Although the cubic nature of the magnetometer's voltage transfer function means that the voltage analog produced is a nonlinear function of distance, the nonlinearity grows less significant as the change in distance becomes a smaller proportion of the total separation of the coils. Thus, despite the nonlinearity of its output, such a system provides an excellent display of relative motion.

Hixon (1972) suggested that tongue motion might also be tracked by placing a small sensor coil on the surface of the tongue to transduce its distance from a generator under the jaw. A system very similar to this was, in fact, tried by Perkell and Oka (1980), and there are now several sophisticated instruments available that may be used to track multiple fleshpoints on the tongue, jaw, lips, and velum simultaneously (Schönle et al., 1983; Branderud, 1985; Schönle et al., 1987; Schönle, 1988; Schönle, Müller & Wenig, 1989; Schulman, 1989; Tuller, Shao, & Kelso, 1990; Engelke & Schönle, 1991; Perkell et al., 1992; van Lieshout, Peters, & Hulstijn, 1994; Horn et al., 1997; Löfqvist & Gracco, 1997; Guenther et al., 1999). Among the commercial systems currently marketed are the *Movetrack* (Botronic, Hägersten, Sweden) and the *Articulograph AG100* (Carstens Medizinelektronik, Lenglern, Germany). Instead of a single generator coil attached to the subject's jaw, the Movetrack and Articulograph (Figure 12–20) systems employ two and three generator coils, respectively, that are supported by a specially designed helmet or headmount.[7] Oriented in fixed positions along the sagittal plane, each coil generates its own high-frequency alternating magnetic field. A set of small, lightweight sensor coils is attached to the articulators of interest, usually with a temporary adhesive designed for use on surface epithelium and mucosal tissue. The voltage induced in these sensor coils will vary as a consequence of their distance from each generator coil. Since each generator coil is driven at a different frequency in overlapping magnetic fields, the position of each sensor coil can be precisely determined (van der Giet, 1977).

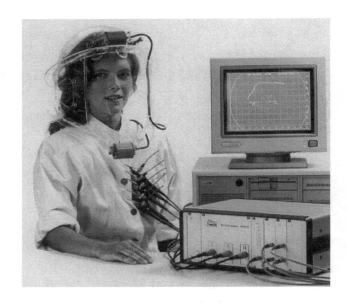

Figure 12–20. The Carstens Articulograph AG100 system. Three generator coils are held in fixed positions along the sagittal plane by means of a head helmet (one is in the vicinity of the forehead, another is near the chin, and a third—not visible in this view—is positioned behind the head of the speaker). Thin wires lead from a set of small sensor coils attached at midline to the speaker's articulators to the articulograph unit. The voltage induced in the sensor coils will vary as a function of their distance from the generator coils. (Photograph courtesy of Carstens Medizinelektronik GmbH, Lenglern, Germany.)

---

[7]See Perkell et al. (1992) or Hoole and Nguyen (1996) for a detailed discussion of the relative benefits and limitations of two- and three-generator-coil systems.

As many as 15 (Articulograph) to 28 (Movetrack) fleshpoints may currently be tracked in this manner. Given their ability to contort and deform, soft-tissue articulators will often require several coils to best gauge position and movement. In assessing tongue motion, for instance, the manufacturer of the Articulograph recommends attaching 5 sensor coils to the midline, each spaced approximately 1 cm apart, the first located roughly 1 cm from the tongue tip. At the very least, one coil should be placed near the tip and another toward the back of the tongue. In addition to soft-tissue fleshpoints, it is often helpful to fix one or more sensor coils to bony references, such as between the upper incisors, the forehead, or the bridge of the nose. But regardless of where the sensor coils are placed, it is imperative that they are positioned so that they remain parallel to the midline axis. Although EMA systems using a trio of generator coils are able quite often to detect and, to a degree, to correct for transitory misalignment of the sensor coils (Perkell et al., 1992; Schönle et al., 1987; Engelke, Müller, & Petersen, 1995; Hoole & Nguyen, 1996), when the coils move out of the midsagittal plane due to rotation or lateral displacement of the articulators, it is likely that the accuracy of movement transduction will be affected.

Although costly, EMA systems are convenient in that they are easily set up and require no head restraint. They may also be used simultaneously with pressure-flow, electroglottographic, and palatographic instruments (see Rouco & Recasens, 1996) to yield a substantial amount of potentially useful data. It remains unknown, however, to what extent the placement of the sensor coils or the fine wires that connect them to the electronics may affect speech movement behavior. This may be a particular concern when sensors are attached to the velum or to the articulating surfaces of the tongue. Nonetheless, there have been a number of studies that have used EMA techniques successfully to describe normal articulatory processes and to help establish models of speech behavior (Engelke, Schönle, Kring, & Richter, 1989; Schulman, 1989; Hoole et al., 1993; Maurer, Gröne, Landis, Hoch, & Schönle, 1993; Nguyen, Hoole, & Marchal, 1994; Engelke et al., 1995; Engelke, Bruns, Striebeck, & Hoch, 1996; Kaburagi & Honda, 1996; Svirsky et al., 1997). Several studies have also found EMA to provide useful and reliable documentation of abnormal articulatory function (Engelke, Engelke, & Schwestka, 1990; Engelke, Schönle, & Engelke, 1990; Katz, Machetanz, Orth, & Schönle, 1990; Schönle, Hoch, & Gröne, 1991; Ackermann, Gröne, Hoch, & Schönle, 1993; Engelke & Hoch, 1994; Katz & Verma, 1994; Engelke, Hoch, Bruns, & Striebeck, 1996; van Lieshout et al., 1996; Alfonso & van Lieshout, 1997), including abnormal timing patterns and inadequate movement coordination.

Despite the fact that no significant health risk from exposure to alternating magnetic fields (from such sources as high-tension power lines, cellular telephones, computer monitors, and hair dryers) can be documented, public and professional concern remains equivocal on the issue. In general, EMA systems are considered safe due to the use of low-strength magnetic fields (in the microtesla range) driven at high frequencies and to the relatively short amount of time subjects are exposed to the field. It would appear, then, that if electromagnetic articulography poses anything more than a negligible health risk, it is not likely to be greater than that offered by any number of household or occupational sources of electromagnetic-field exposure. However, it is advisable to avoid using this technique with those having cardiac pacemakers or other electronic implants. It would also behoove the user to check the specifications of their particular EMA system against the maximum exposure levels recommended by the appropriate federal or local regulating agency.

Radar Tracking

Holzrichter, Burnett, Ng, and Lea (1998) have described the application of radar technology to the noninvasive tracking of speech articulatory movements. **Radar**, an acronym for "*ra*dio *d*etecting *a*nd *r*anging," involves emitting short pulses of electromagnetic energy and then detecting the pulses that have been reflected from objects in their path. The amount of time it takes to receive the pulse after transmission and the direction from which it returns can be used to measure the distance to and location of the reflecting object. To assess the displacement of various articulators during speech production, Holzrichter et al. (1998) used low-power 2.3-GHz electromagnetic waves pulsed at a rate of 2 MHz. By directing the radar sensor upward from under the chin of the speaker, they obtained jaw, tongue, and velar movement data that at least appear to be comparable to other established movement-transduction techniques. (They have also described the tracking of vocal-fold movement by directing the sensor toward the laryngeal prominence.)

Radar tracking is attractive because it is safe, noninvasive, and can be made relatively inexpensive. As a new application to the demanding task of assessing articulator movement, however, a great deal of development and refinement of technique will clearly be needed. At present, with so few speakers studied and in the absence of established calibration methods that have been shown to be both accurate and reliable, data interpretation remains difficult and uncertain at best. Nonetheless, as work progresses, the use of radar tracking techniques to assess articulatory posture and movement may well be on the relatively near clinical horizon.

X-ray Microbeam

As discussed in Chapter 11 "Velopharyngeal Function", the **X-ray microbeam** system (Fujimura, Kiritani, & Ishida, 1973; Kiritani, Itoh, & Fujimura, 1975; Fujimura, 1990; Stone, 1990; Westbury, 1991; Ostry & Munhall, 1994; de Jong, 1997; Hashi, Westbury, & Honda, 1998), like EMA, can be used to track a large number of midsagittal fleshpoints during speech production. These fleshpoints are marked with 2- to 3-mm radio-opaque pellets attached by means of an adhesive or atraumatic suture. Because sophisticated computer control allows a very thin X-ray beam to be used, the subject is exposed to a relatively low radiation level. Unfortunately, while speech researchers have made good use of X-ray microbeam data, the expense of the system—and the fact that patients are exposed to at least some level of ionizing radiation—will doubtlessly preclude any major clinical application of the technique.

DIADOCHOKINESIS

The evaluation of diadochokinesis—the ability to perform rapid repetitions of relatively simple patterns of oppositional contractions—has long been part of the standard speech evaluation. The rationale for such testing rests on the assumption that it provides insight into the adequacy of the patient's neuromotor maturation and integration. In that they provide an acoustic index of the speed of articulatory movement and positioning, diadochokinetic tests are typically viewed as screens for neurologic disability.

There has always been considerable controversy about the value of diadochokinetic tests as diagnostic or prognostic indicators. Early studies of individuals frequently included such non-oral diadochokinetic tasks as finger tapping (for example, Heltman & Peacher, 1943; Strother & Kriegman, 1943). While there may be a common timing mechanism underlying such tasks and speech (Albright, 1948; Tingley & Allen, 1975; Konczak et al., 1997), both research and professional experience showed them to be of little value to speech clinicians. They have largely been abandoned.

Diadochokinetic rates for nonspeech movements of the articulators were also commonly determined, on the assumption that they represented a simpler motor substrate upon which speech movements were built (Fairbanks & Spriestersbach, 1950; Westlake, 1951, 1952; Evans, 1952). However, a number of studies (Heltman & Peacher, 1943; Irwin, 1957; Hixon & Hardy, 1964) have established that the relationship is at best very weak and that diadochokinetic rates for spoken syllables are generally significantly greater than for analogous nonspeech movements. Current practice thus limits diadochokinetic tests to spoken material.

Although it is a fairly simple test, there is no single standardized procedure for eliciting the diadochokinetic performance or, for that matter, for measuring the repetition rate. Generally, the patient is simply instructed that, when told to begin, he is to repeat the test utterance as rapidly as possible and for as long as possible at comfortable pitch and loudness. It is common for the tester to demonstrate the task and to elicit at least one practice trial to be sure the patient correctly understands the instructions.

Rate Measurement

Although appealing, the temptation to simply listen with a stopwatch, counting the patient's syllables "live," is best resisted. It is very difficult to count accurately at the speed that is usually required. Although special electronic counter circuits have been used (for example, Irwin & Becklund, 1953), it is now easy enough to measure repetition rate with a computer display of acoustic data. It is usually a simple matter to count the number of peaks per unit time on a time trace of relative speech intensity. Nonetheless, a decision must be made about what is to be counted. (The notes to Table 12–1 give just some of the alternatives.) Some prefer to count all syllables for the first 5 seconds. Others begin counting from the 2nd second, thereby allowing for an onset adjustment period. Still others take a 2-s sample from the middle of the syllable train. Whatever the sample, rate is usually expressed as the mean number of utterances per second.[8] Obviously, in addition to assessing the adequacy of the rate, it is important for the clinician to evaluate articulatory precision and rate variability during the

---

[8]An alternative is to determine the time it takes to produce a given number of repetitions of the test utterance (Fletcher, 1972; Allen, 1974). While there is no standard number of repetitions for the so-called *time-by-count method*, it is important to determine that the patient is capable of producing the chosen number of syllables on a single breath.

Table 12–1. Diadochokinetic Rates (syllables/s) for /pʌ/, /tʌ/, /kʌ/, and /pʌtəkə/ for Normal Speakers

Subjects			Maximum Syllable Repetition Rate			
Age	Sex	N	Mean	(SD)	Range‡	Source*
			/pʌ/			
5	M/F	12	4.22	—	—	1
6	M/F	10	4.48	—	—	1
6	M	30	3.49	(0.383)	2.51–4.47	2
6	F	30	3.67	(0.419)	2.60–4.74	2
6	M/F	24	4.2	—	—	3
7	M	20	4.34	(0.589)	2.72–5.92	2
7	F	20	4.38	(0.501)	3.00–5.76	2
7	M/F	24	4.2	—	—	3
8	M/F	24	4.8	—	—	3
7–9	M/F	8	4.70	—	—	1
9	M	20	4.56	(0.407)	3.44–5.68	2
9	F	20	4.40	(0.499)	3.03–5.77	2
9	M	10	4.8	(0.49)	—	4
9	F	10	4.4	(0.47)	—	4
9	M/F	24	5.0	—	—	3
10	M	10	4.9	(0.64)	—	4
10	F	10	4.7	(0.76)	—	4
10	M/F	24	5.4	—	—	3
11	M	24	4.80	(0.476)	3.49–6.11	2
11	F	20	4.88	(0.239)	4.22–5.54	2
11	M	10	5.5	(0.64)	—	4
11	F	10	5.2	(0.52)	—	4
11	M/F	24	5.6	—	—	3
12	M/F	24	5.9	—	—	3
13	M	20	5.17	(0.643)	3.40–6.94	2
13	F	20	5.44	(0.417)	4.29–6.59	2
13	M/F	24	6.1	—	—	3
15	M	20	5.86	(0.611)	4.18–7.54	2
15	F	20	5.44	(0.477)	4.13–6.75	2
19–28	M	20	6.0	(0.66)	—	5
18–26	F	25	5.9	(0.35)	—	5
18–28	M	10	6.59	(0.41)	—	6
18–28	F	10	6.67	(0.61)	—	6
18–39	M	28	7.0	(1.0)	5.4–9.4	7
18–38	F	31	6.9	(0.6)	5.8–7.8	7
25.7†	M/F	40	7.0	—	—	8
~30	M	8	7.1	(0.8)	6.2–8.9	9
25–55	M/F	10	7.1	(0.7)	—	10
20–72	M	67	6.5	—	4.5–7.5	11
20–72	F	58	6.1	—	4.6–8.6	11
47†	M	25	6.6	—	—	12
47†	F	25	6.0	—	—	12
~52†	M/F	20	6.6	(0.9)	—	13
50–65	M/F	30	6.4	—	—	14
65–76	M	10	6.0	(0.82)	—	5
65–76	F	12	6.7	(0.93)	—	5
67–88	M	10	6.35	(0.74)	—	6
67–88	F	10	6.09	(0.60)	—	6
68–89	M	27	5.4	(1.2)	2.8–8.2	7
66–93	F	30	5.0	(1.2)	1.3–7.0	7

(Continued)

Table 12–1. Diadochokinetic Rates (syllables/s) for /pʌ/, /tʌ/, /kʌ/, and /pʌtəkə/ for Normal Speakers (*continued*)

	Subjects			Maximum Syllable Repetition Rate			
Age	**Sex**	**N**	**Mean**	**(SD)**	**Range‡**		**Source***
			/tʌ/				
5	M/F	12	4.17	—	—		1
6	M/F	10	4.49	—	—		1
6	M	30	3.33	(0.365)	2.40–4.26		2
6	F	30	3.51	(0.423)	2.41–4.61		2
6	M/F	24	4.1	—	—		3
7	M	20	4.14	(0.422)	2.98–5.30		2
7	F	20	4.33	(0.518)	2.90–5.76		2
7	M/F	24	4.1	—	—		3
8	M/F	24	4.5	—	—		3
7–9	M/F	8	4.66	—	—		1
7–12	M/F	45	5.8	(0.75)	—		15
9	M	20	4.49	(0.484)	3.16–5.82		2
9	F	20	4.32	(0.503)	2.93–5.71		2
9	M	10	4.6	(0.50)	—		4
9	F	10	4.5	(0.65)	—		4
9	M/F	24	4.9	—	—		3
10	M	10	5.0	(0.98)	—		4
10	F	10	4.9	(0.82)	—		4
10	M/F	24	5.3	—	—		3
11	M	20	4.75	(0.537)	3.27–6.23		2
11	F	20	4.84	(0.490)	3.49–6.19		2
11	M	10	5.5	(0.99)	—		4
11	F	10	4.9	(0.47)	—		4
11	M/F	24	5.6	—	—		3
12	M/F	24	5.7	—	—		3
13	M	20	5.09	(0.660)	3.27–6.91		2
13	F	20	5.22	(0.581)	3.62–6.82		2
13	M/F	24	6.1	—	—		3
15	M	20	5.44	(0.604)	4.11–7.43		2
15	F	20	5.38	(0.541)	3.89–6.87		2
19–28	M	20	6.0	(0.96)	—		5
18–26	F	25	5.8	(0.37)	—		5
18–28	M	10	6.63	(0.73)	—		6
18–28	F	10	6.61	(0.43)	—		6
18–39	M	28	6.9	(1.1)	4.2–9.4		7
18–38	F	31	6.8	(1.0)	4.8–8.4		7
25.7†	M/F	40	7.1	—	—		8
~30	M	8	7.1	(0.9)	6.2–8.9		9
25–55	M/F	10	7.1	(0.8)	—		10
20–72	M	67	6.5	—	4.4–8.2		11
20–72	F	58	6.0	—	4.3–8.5		11
47†	M	25	6.5	—	—		12
47†	F	25	6.0	—	—		12
~52†	M/F	20	6.4	(1.0)	—		13
50–65	M/F	30	6.1	—	—		14
65–76	M	10	5.8	(0.69)	—		5
65–76	F	12	6.5	(0.44)	—		5
67–88	M	10	6.20	(0.62)	—		6
67–88	F	10	5.73	(0.90)	—		6
68–89	M	27	5.3	(1.0)	3.0–6.8		7
66–93	F	30	4.8	(1.1)	2.2–6.8		7

(*Continued*)

Subjects			Maximum Syllable Repetition Rate			
Age	**Sex**	**N**	**Mean**	**(SD)**	**Range[‡]**	**Source[*]**
			/kʌ/			
5	M/F	12	3.85	—	—	1
6	M/F	10	4.26	—	—	1
6	M	30	3.18	(0.319)	2.37–3.99	2
6	F	30	3.28	(0.392)	2.28–4.28	2
6	M/F	24	3.6	—	—	3
7	M	20	4.02	(0.402)	2.91–5.13	2
7	F	20	3.88	(0.408)	2.76–5.00	2
7	M/F	24	3.8	—	—	3
8	M/F	24	4.2	—	—	3
7–9	M/F	8	4.16	—	—	1
7–12	M/F	46	5.3	(0.72)	—	15
9	M	20	4.19	(0.519)	2.76–5.62	2
9	F	20	3.94	(0.450)	`2.70–5.18)	2
9	M	10	4.2	(0.51)	—	4
9	F	10	4.1	(0.53)	—	4
9	M/F	24	4.3	—	—	3
10	M	10	4.6	(0.92)	—	4
10	F	10	4.4	(0.53)	—	4
10	M/F	24	4.6	—	—	3
11	M	20	4.52	(0.578)	2.93–6.11	2
11	F	20	4.46	(0.446)	3.32–5.69	2
11	M	10	4.9	(0.44)	—	4
11	F	10	4.6	(0.55)	—	4
11	M/F	24	5.0	—	—	3
12	M/F	24	5.1	—	—	3
13	M	20	4.84	(0.639)	3.08–6.60	2
13	F	20	4.76	(0.498)	3.39–6.42	2
13	M/F	24	5.4	—	—	3
15	M	20	5.27	(0.733)	3.25–7.29	2
15	F	20	5.00	(0.517)	3.58–6.42	2
19–28	M	20	5.4	(0.54)	—	5
18–26	F	25	5.2	(0.60)	—	5
18–28	M	10	6.07	(0.45)	—	6
18–28	F	10	6.34	(0.55)	—	6
18–39	M	28	6.2	(0.8)	5.0–8.2	7
18–38	F	31	6.2	(0.8)	4.6–8.2	7
25.7[†]	M/F	40	6.2	—	—	8
~30	M	8	6.6	(0.8)	5.2–7.8	9
20–72	M	67	6.1	—	4.4–7.5	10
20–72	F	58	5.7	—	4.3–7.9	10
25–55	M/F	10	6.2	(0.8)	—	11
47[†]	M	25	6.0	—	—	12
47[†]	F	25	5.6	—	—	12
~52[†]	M/F	20	6.0	(0.8)	—	13
50–65	M/F	30	5.7	—	—	14
65–76	M	10	5.8	(0.62)	—	5
65–76	F	12	5.9	(0.83)	—	5
67–88	M	10	5.77	(0.64)	—	6
67–88	F	10	5.35	(0.72)	—	6
68–89	M	27	4.9	(1.0)	2.6–6.8	7
66–93	F	30	4.4	(1.1)	2.2–6.4	7

(*Continued*)

Table 12–1. Diadochokinetic Rates (syllables/s) for /pʌ/, /tʌ/, /kʌ/, and /pʌtəkə/ for Normal Speakers (*continued*)

Subjects			Maximum Syllable Repetition Rate			
Age	Sex	N	Mean	(SD)	Range‡	Source*
			/pʌtəkə/			
5	M/F	12	3.43	—	—	1
6	M/F	10	3.80	—	—	1
7–9	M/F	8	3.85	—	—	1
9	M	10	4.3	(0.68)	—	4
9	F	10	4.8	(0.72)	—	4
10	M	10	5.0	(0.80)	—	4
10	F	10	5.0	(0.47)	—	4
11	M	10	5.0	(0.54)	—	4
11	F	10	5.3	(0.58)	—	4
11	M/F	20	6.12	(1.11)	—	16a
11	M/F	20	5.98	(1.23)	—	16b
18–39	M	28	5.8	(1.0)	4.0–8.2	7
18–38	F	31	6.3	(0.9)	3.8–7.8	7
~52†	M/F	20	6.9	(0.9)	—	13
68–89	M	26	4.4	(1.3)	2.4–7.0	7
66–93	F	30	3.6	(1.3)	1.4–6.2	7

†Mean age.

‡95% confidence limits.

Sources:

1. Yoss and Darley, 1974. Specific testing procedure not given. Compared with a group of dyspraxic children.

2. Irwin and Becklund, 1953. Special counter system ("Sylrater"). "Three trials of about 5 s each were . . . given for each test. The peak or maximum rate for each subject for each test item was recorded."

3. Fletcher, 1972. Original data collected using the time-by-count method: A stopwatch was used to determine the number of seconds required to repeat the syllable 20 times. Data converted to syllables per second. For standard deviations, see original source.

4. Blomquist, 1950. Subjects were schoolchildren told to repeat test syllable "as rapidly and as regularly as possible, then to do it again, then a third time." Spectrogram used to calculate mean number of repetitions in the 2.35 s displayed for each sample. Three of the four repetitions were analyzed for each child.

5. Kreul, 1972. "Each diadochokinetic movement was demonstrated with standard instructions, and the subjects were instructed to produce the sounds 'just as rapidly as you can, keeping the sounds clear and distinct'." Single trial for each subject. Data are the number of sounds, to the nearest half, produced in a 2-s sample.

6. Amerman and Parnell, 1982. Mean age of the "young adult" and "older adult" speakers was 23 and 74 years, respectively. Twenty repetitions of each syllable were elicited using the following instructions: "I want you to produce these syllables as rapidly as you can, keeping each one clear and distinct. I will need quite a few repetitions from you so just keep going until I stop you. Please take an adequate amount of air before you begin. You will need to repeat the syllables without pausing to take another breath once you begin" (pp. 58–59). Audio samples were taped-recorded after one practice trial; Measurement from a wide-band spectrogram and corresponding relative speech amplitude trace.

7. Ptacek, Sander, Maloney, and Jackson, 1966. Subjects were asked "to take a deep breath and produce the sounds as rapidly as possible until stopped by the examiner" after demonstration of the task. Seven-second samples, first and last seconds excluded from count, resulting in data based on mean repetition rate in 5 s.

8. Lundeen, 1950. Two 3-s practice sessions. Data are based on middle 5 s of a 7-s sample.

9. Sigurd, 1973. Eight men (3 American, 2 British, 1 German, 1 Swedish, and 1 Korean), "about 30 years" of age "with some dispersion." Speakers were "linguists with some training in phonetics" who were instructed to repeat /pa/, /ta/, and /ka/ (among several other Ca syllables) as rapidly as possible using "English or American pronunciation." "The initial and final parts of the [syllable] strings were generally disregarded because the initial part often included an acceleration phase and the final part a retardation phase . . . Normally a segment including 10 syllables (periods) was measured" (pp. 376–377). Mean, SD, and range data derived from individual repetition rates reported by the author in Table 1 (p. 375).

10. Dworkin, Aronson, and Mulder, 1980. Mean age of the men and women was 38.5 ± 13 years and 37.0 ± 11 years, respectively. Subjects were instructed to repeat syllables "as rapidly, evenly, and as long as possible." Three trials obtained, but only the first was used in the analysis. Average data represent the median value. Compared with a group of patients with amyotrophic lateral sclerosis.

(*Continued*)

11. Tiffany, 1980. Subjects were instructed to repeat the syllables on one breath for at least 6 s. Each was told that "vowels may be indefinite—the easiest you can produce—but should be voiced." Data represents "best performance" from multiple trials.

12. Dworkin and Aronson, 1986. Three trials were tape recorded and analyzed from display of acoustic signal on strip-chart recorder. Comparison made with several patients with different types of dysarthria.

13. LaPointe, Case, and Duane, 1994. Specific testing procedure not given. Seven men and 13 women, "free of neurological disease or history," served as age-matched control subjects for a group of 70 patients diagnosed with spasmodic torticollis (mean age = 52.2 years).

14. Portnoy and Aronson, 1982. Subjects were instructed to repeat syllables "on one uninterrupted breath, as rapidly, regularly, and as long as possible." Samples were tape recorded and analyzed later using analogy and digital instrumentation. Compared with groups of spastic and ataxic dysarthic adults of similar age.

15. Dworkin, 1978. Scores reported in article are number of repetitions per 3 s; Data in this table converted to repetitions per second. Compared with a group of children who "lisp."

16. Fletcher and Meldrun, 1968. Sixth-grade schoolchildren selected from a pool of 210 students *(a)* Twenty students with the relatively shortest lingual frenulum ("limited lingual freedom" group); *(b)* Twenty students with the relatively longest lingual frenulum ("greater lingual freedom" group). The difference between groups was not significant for this utterance.

task (Shanks, 1970; Tatsumi, Sasanuma, Hirose, & Kiritani, 1979; Amerman & Parnell, 1982; Portnoy & Aronson, 1982; Gentil, 1990; Wolff, Michel, & Ovrut, 1990; Rosenfield, Viswanath, Herbrich, & Nudelman, 1991; Hartman & Abbs, 1992; Ackermann, Hertrich, & Hehr, 1995; Ackermann, Konczak, & Hertrich, 1997).

EXPECTED RESULTS

Testing is most often done for the syllables /pʌ/, /tʌ/, and /kʌ/, and for /pʌtəkə/. Table 12–1 summarizes some of the data available for these four utterances. In general, both the age of the speaker and the nature of the syllable will influence the maximal repetition rate. Figure 12–21 is a graphic representation of the data in Table 12–1 showing the overall effect of syllable type and speaker age. Although many other mono- and multisyllabic syllables have been used for clinical and research purposes, data for such utterances are quite limited.[9] Selected syllables have also been used to assess the ability of the larynx to produce rapid and regular abductory-adductory adjustments (for example, Rodriquez, Ford, Bless, & Harmon, 1994). Much of the available information for these types of syllables is summarized in Table 12–2. Details regarding how the samples were elicited and the specific measurement techniques used are provided in the accompanying notes.

Speech diadochokinetic rates have been found to be slower than normal in a wide range of speech disorders. The effect has been verified not only in cases of

neuropathology (for example, Platt, Andrews, Young, & Quinn, 1980; Kent et al. 1991; Hartman & Abbs, 1992; Wit, Maassen, Gabreëls, & Thoonen, 1993; Cannito, Ege, Ahmed, & Wagner, 1994; Leeper, Millard, Bandur, & Hudson, 1996), but in cases of "functional" dyslalia as well (for example, McNutt, 1977; Dworkin, 1978; Hale et al. 1992). Table 12–3 provides a sample of the available data.

CHEST-WALL MOVEMENT

The *chest wall* is defined by the physiologist to include the rib cage, diaphragm, abdominal contents, and anterior abdominal wall. Its movements store a volume of air for speech and pressurize it to an appropriate level. All of the acoustic energy radiated in the speech signal derives from that pressurization. The ventilatory system is the power generator for speech, and the chest wall is the motor that drives that generator.

A general review of the structure and function of the chest wall will not be attempted here. Good basic summaries have been prepared by Hixon (1973), Daniloff, Shuckers, and Feth (1980), and Zemlin (1998). More advanced consideration of breathing for speech is available in Bouhuys (1968), Wyke (1974), Hixon (1982), Weismer (1985), and Hixon and colleagues (1987). A number of points do need to be emphasized, however, because failure to keep them in mind has often led to significant confusion and erroneous impressions of the quality of chest-wall function during speech production.

---

[9]There have also been diadochokinetic tests of isolated consonants (for example, Canning & Rose, 1974), but it remains unclear how these productions may be compared with true CV syllable repetition rates (see Kent, Kent, and Rosenbek, 1987).

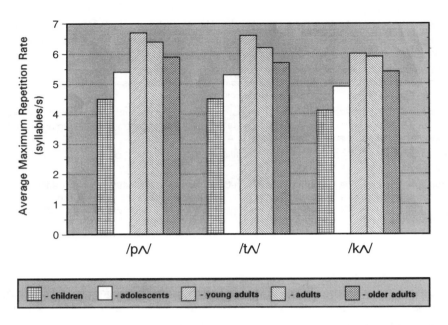

Figure 12–21. Average diadochokinetic rates for the syllables /pʌ/, /tʌ/, and /kʌ/ for normal speakers of different ages. (Data derived from Table 12–1.)

Most important, perhaps, is the fact that the chest wall is a two-part system with what the physiologists call *two degrees of freedom* of movement (Konno & Mead, 1967). One part is the rib cage, which is the primary wall of the thorax itself. The other part includes the diaphragm, which forms the "floor" of the thorax and the "roof" of the abdomen. Each part is independently movable. The muscles of the rib cage act to enlarge or diminish the size of the thorax by increasing the anteroposterior and, to a lesser extent, the transverse diameter of the enclosed space (Agostoni, Mognoni, Torri, & Saracino, 1965; Konno & Mead, 1967). The diaphragm is dome-shaped. Its contraction causes it to flatten, which results in an increase in the height of the thoracic space as well as elevation and spreading of the ribs. At the same time, flattening of the diaphragm also displaces the visceral structures that lie just under it. (Hence, the abdomen's contents are considered part of the chest wall.) The displaced visceral volume appears as a bulge of the anterior abdominal wall, the only resilient region of the abdominal enclosure. The abdominal bulge has the same volume as that added to the thorax by diaphragmatic movement. The diaphragm, like any other muscle, cannot return to its precontraction position by its own power—something else must push it back into its original domed shape. The restorative force is pro-

vided by the anterior abdominal muscles that have been protruded. Their contraction forces the viscera back against the diaphragm, thereby returning it to its original dome-shaped condition. This, of course, reduces the volume of the thorax again. Enlargement of the thorax results in a decrease of the pressure of the gas within it (see "Boyle's Law," Chapter 9). If the airway is patent, outside air at the relatively higher atmospheric pressure will flow along the pressure gradient into the lungs. (Note that the lungs fill because the thorax enlarges; the thorax does not enlarge to accommodate the increasing size of the lungs or the increasing volume of air.) Any action that enlarges the thoracic space can be said to be *inspiratory*, while any action that decreases thoracic size can be called *expiratory*.

Thoracic volume can be increased by movement of the rib cage *or* by movement of the diaphragm (which shows as abdominal motion). Since the rib cage muscles and the diaphragm-abdomen can function independently, it is clear that one set could be acting to enlarge the rib cage, while the other operates to diminish its size. The net change in the lung volume is the sum of the actions of the two chest-wall components. If the rib cage is enlarging while the diaphragm contracts, then both parts are contributing to inspiration. However, if the muscles of the rib cage cause a

Table 12–2. Normal Diadochokinetic Rates (syllables/s) for Utterances Requiring Laryngeal Articulation

Subjects			Maximum Syllable Repetition Rate			
Age	Sex	N	Mean	(SD)	Range	Source*
			/hʌ/			
20–39	F	40	5.46	(0.57)	—	1
40–59	F	40	5.72	—	—	1
60–80	F	40	5.54	(0.75)	—	1
57[†]	M	17	5.6	(1.3)	1.8–6.6	2
			/ʌ/			
18–39	M	28	5.1	(1.0)	2.6–7.0	3
18–38	F	31	5.3	(0.8)	3.0–6.8	3
68–89	M	26	4.1	(0.9)	2.6–6.0	3
66–93	F	30	3.9	(1.3)	1.8–6.6	3
			/i/			
19–28	M	20	4.7	(0.67)	—	4
18–26	F	25	4.9	(0.57)	—	4
65–76	M	10	4.8	(0.63)	—	4
65–76	F	12	5.1	(0.86)	—	4

[†]Median.

Sources:

1. Shanks, 1970. Subjects instructed to repeat syllable as rapidly as possible at a comfortable pitch and loudness. Three 5-s practice trials were followed by three tape-recorded trials of 5 s each. First 3 s of each sample were written by a graphic vocal recorder. The "number of peaks present on 9 [3s, 3 trials] one-second intervals of the tracings was counted to establish the rate of syllable repetition per second."

2. Canter, 1965. Measurement of graphic readout. Comparison with Parkinson disease patients. Subjects repeated the syllable /ha/. Subjects' average age and syllable repetition rate represented by the median.

3. Ptacek, Sander, Maloney, and Jackson, 1966. See note, Table 12–1.

4. Kreul, 1972. See note, Table 12–1.

decrease in its size at the same time that the diaphragm is contracting, the net flow of air will be inspiratory if the diaphragmatic displacement causes a greater volume change than the rib-cage muscles do, but the net flow will be expiratory if the rib-cage contraction makes a greater contribution to the thoracic volume change than the diaphragm does. The critical point here is that *there is no way of knowing whether inspiration or expiration is in progress by watching only the rib cage or the abdomen*. Both parts must be observed, and their relative contribution to thoracic volume change must be known before any observation of ventilatory movement can inform the observer about which ventilatory phase is occurring.

Movements of the chest-wall system are frequently very small, but even small changes can have a meaningful effect on the lung volume or the lung pressure. Furthermore, these small changes occur in a very massive structure, one that is very difficult to see all at once in its entirety. Worse, the movement can be very rapid, on the order of 100 ms or so (Baken, Cavallo, & Weissman, 1979; Baken & Cavallo, 1981), making assessment by simple visual observation still more difficult, and less reliable. Therefore, there is a need for monitoring instrumentation that can accurately show what the system is doing in a way that can be easily followed by the observer.

Table 12–3. Diadochokinetic Rates (syllables/s) for Speakers with Various Communication Disorders

Diagnosis	Age	Sex	N	Syllable	Mean	(SD or Range)	Source*
Functional misarticulation	5	M/F	12	/pʌ/	3.94[†]	—	1
				/tʌ/	3.76[†]	—	1
				/kʌ/	3.50[†]	—	1
	6	M/F	10	/pʌ/	4.34	—	1
				/tʌ/	4.02[†]	—	1
				/kʌ/	3.64[†]	—	1
	7–9	M/F	8	/pʌ/	3.86[†]	—	1
				/tʌ/	3.81[†]	—	1
				/kʌ/	3.48	—	1
("lispers")	7–12	M/F	45	/tʌ/	5.3[†]	(0.75)	2
				/dʌ/	5.2[†]	(0.79)	2
				/kʌ/	4.6[†]	(0.69)	2
				/gʌ/	4.5[†]	(0.62)	2
Cerebral Palsy	4–16	?	50	/dʌ/	2.33	(0.96)	3
Dysarthria							
(spastic)	57	M/F	30	/pʌ/	4.6[‡][†]	—	4
				/tʌ/	4.2[‡][†]	—	4
				/kʌ/	3.5[‡][†]	—	4
(ataxic)	57	M/F	30	/pʌ/	3.8[‡][†]	—	4
				/tʌ/	3.9[‡][†]	—	4
				/kʌ/	3.4[‡][†]	—	4
	57	M/F	5	/pʌ/	4.4	(1.22)	5
				/tʌ/	4.1	(1.13)	5
				/kʌ/	3.5	(1.04)	5
Parkinsonism	56[‡]	M	17	/bʌ/	5.4[‡]	(0–7.4)	6
				/dʌ/	4.8[‡]	(0–7.8)	6
				/gɑ/	3.6[‡]	(0–7.6)	6
				/hʌ/	3.4[‡]	(0–5.6)	6
	56	M/F	23	/pʌ/	6.2	(1.01)	7
				/tʌ/	6.1	(0.82)	7
				/kʌ/	5.4	(0.88)	7
Amyotrophic lateral sclerosis	57	M	11	/pʌ/	4.5[†]	(2.3–6.6)	8
				/tʌ/	4.2[†]	(2.0–6.4)	8
				/kʌ/	4.0[†]	(1.8–6.2)	8
	62	F	8	/pʌ/	3.7[†]	(0.0–6.4)	8
				/tʌ/	3.5[†]	(0.0–6.4)	8
				/kʌ/	3.2[†]	(0.0–6.4)	8
(bulbar)	53–74	M/F	5	/ɑ/	2.34	(0.63)	9
				/hɑ/	5.19	(1.23)	9
(nonbulbar)	35–75	M/F	7	/ɑ/	2.35	(0.57)	9
				/hɑ/	5.69	(1.22)	9
Spasmodic torticollis	52	M	70	/pʌ/	5.08[†]	(1.1)	10
				/tʌ/	4.83[†]	(1.2)	10
				/kʌ/	4.47[†]	(1.1)	10
				/pʌtʌkʌ/	4.79[†]	(1.3)	10
Hearing impairment							
(moderate–severe)	16.9	M/F	7	/pʌ/	4.5	—	11
				/tʌ/	4.3	—	11
				/kʌ/	4.2	—	11
(severe)	17.8	M/F	13	/pʌ/	4.3	—	11
				/tʌ/	3.9	—	11
				/kʌ/	3.5	—	11
(profound)	17.5	M/F	10	/pʌ/	3.0	—	11
				/tʌ/	2.8	—	11
				/kʌ/	2.5	—	11

(Continued)

†Significantly lower than normals tested in same study.

‡Median.

Sources:

1. Yoss and Darley, 1974. Subjects had normal hearing IQ>90, language development no more than 6 months below chronologic age, and no apparent organic etiology.

2. Dworkin, 1978. Scores reported in article are number of repetitions per 3 s; Data in this table converted to repetitions per second.

3. Hixon and Hardy, 1964. Patients include 25 spastic quadriplegics and 25 athetoid paraplegics; Range of involvement from mild to severe. Mean age of patients was 10 years, 6 months. Data converted from reported number of repetitions per 10 s. Score is mean of three trials of each task.

4. Portnoy and Aronson, 1982. Patients were between 50 and 65 years of age; 30 spastic speakers [22M, 8 F] and 30 ataxic speakers [21M, 9 F].

5. Dworkin and Aronson, 1986. All five ataxic patients had cerebellar disease. Mean and SD calculated for individual subject data provided in Table 1 (p. 119).

6. Canter, 1965. No surgery or drugs within 48 hours of testing. "Measures of articulatory diadochokineses were correlated with clarity of articulation: (p. 223).

7. Kreul, 1972. Surgical patients ranging from 36 to 71 years of age. Three trials per task, 2-s sample.

8. Dworkin, Aronson, and Mulder, 1980. Group of patients, ranging in age from 20 to 77 years, "who had the dysarthria of ALS, with both flaccid and spastic components, representing various degrees of speech impairment" (pp. 829–830). The women's maximal syllable repetition rates were significantly lower than those of the men.

9. Leeper, Millard, Bandur, and Hudson, 1996. five ALS patients [4M, 1F] with "classically defined bulbar symptoms . . . i.e., harsh voice, strained-strangled voice, imprecision of consonants, hypernasality . . . i.e., weakness of legs, arms, chest muscles, vocal roughness, slow speech rate." Three trials per task, 5-s sample; Data in this table are from the second test session; Rates rounded to the nearest 0.01.

10. LaPointe, Case, and Duane, 1994. Twenty-five men and 45 women diagnosed with spasmodic torticollis. Several trials were elicited, usually 3, and "the optimal of the multiple attempts was used."

11. Robb, Hughes, and Frese, 1985. Prelingual high-school students at a state school for the deaf. Original data collected using the time-by-count method, recorded as the time required for subjects to produce 20 repetitions of the syllable. Data in this table converted to syllables per second.

The Bellows Pneumograph

For many years, the prime means of monitoring chest-wall motion was with a pneumatic device called the *bellows pneumograph*. Essentially an accordion-pleated tube, it is strapped around the rib cage and abdomen. As chest-wall enlargement occurs, the bellows becomes longer, and hence the volume of the air space within it increases. This causes the pressure in the bellows to drop. A rubber hose attached to the pneumograph couples the change in its air pressure to a pressure transducer (see, for example, Isshiki and Snidecor, 1965, or Snidecor and Isshiki, 1965) or to a pneumatic linkage system that drives a pen that draws a chart record of ventilatory motion.

This system continues to be employed in *polygraphs* (so-called "lie detectors"). Although it may be adequate for that purpose, the bellows pneumograph does not meet the transduction needs of the speech pathologist. Often, no electrical output is provided and thus recording the breathing data or displaying them along with other variables is difficult. More important is the very poor frequency response of this kind of system and the significant loading of the chest wall that it

might represent. While electronic secondary transducers have been incorporated into bellows pneumographs (thus solving some display and data-storage problems), the other limitations are inherent in the physics of the system and are largely irreducible. The bellows pneumograph, then, is not the transducer of choice.

Mercury Strain Gauges

Whitney (1949) constructed an elastic strain gauge by filling the narrow bore of a rubber tube with mercury. As the tube is stretched, the increase in the length of the mercury column and the decrease in its cross-sectional area cause a moderately large change in its electrical resistance. At relatively low AC frequencies, it behaves as an essentially pure resistance, without significant reactance. Therefore, its resistance is easily determined by making it one arm of a Wheatstone bridge (see Chapter 2, "Analog Electronics"). These *mercury strain gauges* (also known as *Whitney gauges*) are thin, lightweight, very flexible, non-loading, and inexpensive.

Movements of the chest wall can be recorded by taping mercury strain gauges across the anterior hemi-circumference of the rib cage and abdomen (Baken, 1977; Baken et al., 1979; Baken & Cavallo, 1981; Baken, McManus, & Cavallo, 1983; Cavallo & Baken, 1985; van Lieshout et al., 1996). The gauges can be used with very simple circuitry. Normally all that is required is an oscillator of some sort and a resistance bridge with an amplifier at its output (Baken & Matz, 1973). If, for any reason, extreme sensitivity is required, a special imped-ance-matching bridge can be used (Elsner, Eagan, & Andersen, 1959). Frequency response is more than adequate for tracking the ventilatory movements of speech and resolution of a fraction of a milimeter is easily achieved. This means of measuring chest-wall behavior is attractive because it is unencumbering and essentially free of risk. It is easy to use: the strain gauges can be attached with ordinary adhesive tape. A mercury strain gauge system can be inexpensively built by almost any technician using gauges available from Parks Medical Electronics (Aloha, Oregon).

The Strain-Gauge Belt Pneumograph

Borrowing upon the strain-gauge technology described earlier (see Strain-Gauge Systems, this chapter), Murdoch, Chenery, Bowler, and Ingram (1989) described the construction of a strain-gauge belt pneumograph. Murdoch and his colleagues have since employed this system in a number of studies conducted at the University of Queensland, Australia, to track circumferential changes in the rib cage and abdomen in a few normal—and in several diverse pop-ulations of abnormal—speakers (Murdoch, Killin, & McCaul, 1989; Murdoch, Chenery, Stokes, & Hardcas-tle, 1991; Murdoch, Theodoros, Stokes, & Chenery, 1993; Manifold & Murdoch, 1993; Murdoch & Hud-son-Tennent, 1993; Theodoros, Murdoch, & Stokes, 1995; Thompson, Murdoch, & Theodoros, 1997). The transducer, shown schematically in Figure 12–22, con-sists of an easily-deformable "bridge" made of thin brass to which are attached two foil strain gauges. Vel-cro attachments at both ends of the transducer couple it to an elastic strap that is wrapped around the speaker's rib cage or abdomen. Circumferential changes will act to induce deformation of the metallic bridge, which is then registered by the pair of strain gauges.

Unfortunately, the linearity and frequency response of the strain-gauge belt pneumograph are largely unknown and remain to be tested. The elasti-cized straps must be secure enough to accurately con-vey changes in torso circumference to the transducer,

but not so tight as to restrict or otherwise alter chest-wall behavior. It is important also to restrict the speaker's arm movements or postural adjustments during recording and to monitor continually for any slippage of the pneumograph belts or attachments.

Magnetometry

The coupling between the two coils of a transformer is inversely proportional to the cube of the distance sep-arating them if the axes of the coils are parallel. There-fore, if a constant AC signal is applied to one coil, the voltage induced in the other will vary as a function of the distance between them. The electromagnetic field created by current flow in a coil easily penetrates non-metallic materials. Thus, if a signal-carrying coil is attached to the body wall, a voltage will be induced in another coil on the other side of the body. The magni-tude of the induced voltage will be inversely related to the distance straight through the body that separates them.

This principle was exploited by Mead and his col-leagues (Mead, Peterson, Grimby, & Mead, 1967), whose measurement system is schematized in Figure 12–23. For each part of the chest wall a pair of identi-cal coils is used. One coil of each pair (the generator) is driven by an oscillator and produces an alternating electromagnetic field. The body offers negligible resis-tance to the passage of the electromagnetic radiation,

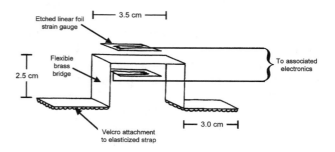

Figure 12–22. Schematic illustration of the strain-gauge belt pneumograph used by Murdoch and his colleagues to transduce rib cage and abdominal movement. The trans-ducer is made of a flexible brass bridge to which are attached etched foil strain gauges. Adapted from "Respira-tory Function in Parkinson's Subjects Exhibiting a Per-ceptible Speech Deficit: A Kinematic and Spirometric Analysis," by B. E. Murdoch, H. J. Chenery, S. Bowler, and J. C. L. Ingram, 1989, *Journal of Speech and Hearing Dis-orders, 54,* 610–626. Figure 2, p. 614. ©American Speech-Language-Hearing Association, Rockville, MD. Used by permission.

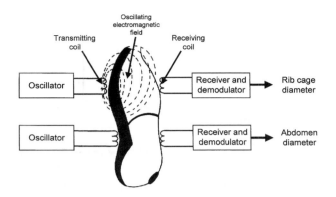

Figure 12–23. Magnetometry for detecting chest-wall movements. Two pairs of coils are used: A pair for the rib cage and another pair for the abdomen. One coil in each pair is a "transmitter" that generates and oscillating electromagnetic field that passes through the body. The other coil serves as a "receiver" that transduces the magnetic energy to an electrical signal. The strength of the magnetic field diminishes in a regular way with distance, so changes in the distance between the two coils results in changes in the strength of the detected signal.

which induces an alternating voltage in the other coil (the sensor). That voltage diminishes proportional to the cube of the body diameter, but, if the change in distance between the coils is small compared to the total distance (which is indeed generally the case with breathing motions), the voltage change closely approximates linearity. The distance measurement can, therefore, be quite accurate (Bancroft, 1978; Stagg, Goldman, & Newsom-Davis, 1978).

Two pairs of coils can be used, one for each chest-wall component, if the two generators are driven at different, and nonharmonic, frequencies. While each sensor will pick up both generator signals, filtering in the detection circuit (see Chapter 2, "Analog Electronics") will pass only one frequency for each sensor. This system has been used extensively in research on the ventilatory mechanics of speech by Hixon and his coworkers (Hixon, 1972; Hixon, Goldman, & Mead, 1973; Hixon, Mead, & Goldman, 1976; Forner & Hixon, 1977; Hoit & Hixon, 1986, 1987; Hoit, Hixon, Altman, & Morgan, 1989; Hoit, Hixon, Watson, & Morgan, 1990; Solomon & Hixon, 1993). The magnetome-

ter system is very simple to use and can provide a clean stable output if the coils are firmly attached to the body wall (usually with double-faced tape). Since a parallel orientation of the generator and sensor coils must be maintained, arm movements and any twisting, extension, or flexion of the spine must be minimized. Although Rolfe (1971) describes the successful application of magnetometry as an apnea monitor for premature infants, debate continues regarding the potential (but as yet unproven) harmful effects of exposure to electromagnetic radiation. Most likely, magnetometry poses no signficant risk to most patients but, as with electromagnetic articulography, it is probably best avoided by patients with electronic implants such as pacemakers. Magnetometers are available commercially from GMG Scientific (Burlington, MA).

Impedance Plethysmography

Body parts offer resistance to the flow of electrical current. The magnitude of that resistance depends on the geometry of the structure and its tissue composition. It is easy to see that, as it expands and contracts, the resistance of the thorax is likely to alter significantly. The changes reflect not only a change in rib-cage shape, but variation in composition caused by the accretion and loss of intrathoracic air. When an electrical current is passed through the thorax, its resistance (which can be measured by any of a number of standard techniques) does indeed change across the breathing cycle.[10] Researchers have used this method primarily in an attempt to find a way of monitoring lung volume without invasion or encumbrance of the airway (Goldensohn & Zablow, 1959; Geddes, Hoff, Hickman, Hinds, & Baker, 1962; Geddes, Hoff, Hickman, & Moore, 1962; Allison, Holmes, & Nyboer, 1964; Kubicek, Kinnen, & Edin, 1964; Khalafalla, 1970; Geddes & Baker, 1989; Jedeikin & Olsfanger, 1990).

There are a great many problems with impedance plethysmography. The relationship between the resistance and actual dimensional change is unknown, for instance. Evan more important, from a practical point of view, is the fact that the speaker must be part of a live electrical circuit. The risks, with properly designed equipment, are not major, but they are nonetheless necessary. Better means of monitoring are available.

---

[10]The theoretical bases of this phenomenon are considered in some detail by Pacela (1966) and Allison (1970).

Inductance Plethysmography

The *respiratory inductive plethysmograph*, available commercially as the **Respitrace** (Ambulatory Monitoring, Ardsley, NY) and as the **Respigraph** (Non-Invasive Monitoring Systems, Miami Beach, FL), uses a rather unusual transduction principle. The inductance of a coil of wire depends on a number of factors, one of which is its diameter. If a wire is wrapped around the torso, the inductance of the single-turn coil it forms will change according to the circumference of the loop. If this single coil can be made stretchable so that it can change size with body movement, then its inductance will always be an analog of the instantaneous torso size.

It is easy to put this inductive change to practical use. There are many oscillator circuits in which the frequency of oscillation is determined by the value of an inductor. If the inductor is the loop around the chest wall, then the frequency of oscillation will be an analog of chest-wall circumference. Put another way, the size of that part of the chest wall within the wire loop is automatically encoded in a frequency-modulated signal. Standard frequency-demodulation techniques can be used to retrieve a DC voltage that represents chest-wall size (Milledge & Stott, 1977; Cohn, Watson, Weisshaut, Stott, & Sackner, 1978, 1982; Sackner, 1980; Sackner, Nixon, Davis, Atkins, & Sackner, 1980; Watson, 1980; Tobin et al., 1983; Cohen, Panescu, Booske, Webster, & Tompkins, 1994; Carry, Baconnier, Eberhard, Cotte, & Benchetrit, 1997).

In the Respitrace, the inductive transducer is a zig-zag of wire attached to an elastic band (Figure 12–24). It is fitted around the rib cage or abdomen, forming the wire into an expandable loop. (The transducers can be stabilized on the subject by an overfitting elastic-mesh vest.) The loop is connected to a miniature oscillator that is also carried on the subject. The output of the oscillator is connected by a cable to the demodulating circuitry that produces a voltage output representing the size (cross-sectional area) of the body enclosed by the transducing loop. In practice, of course, two transducers are used: one for the rib cage and the other for the abdomen. Issues regarding calibration are addressed in Chapter 9 ("Airflow and Volume"), as well as in Chadha et al. (1982).

Like the EMA systems described earlier, inductance plethysmography does expose the user to alternating electromagnetic fields, but it, too, is considered safe as reflected in its wide application in monitoring the respiratory movements of neonates (Stick, Ellis, LeSouëf, & Sly, 1992; Warren & Alderson, 1994; Warren, Horan, & Robertson, 1997), infants (Warren &

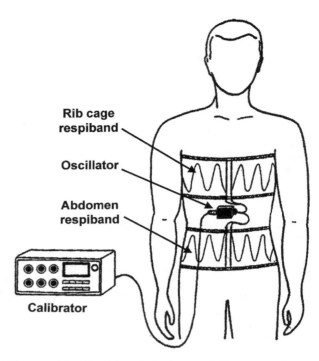

Figure 12–24. Using inductance plethysmography to transduce chest-wall movements. A schematic illustration of the Respitrace system is shown. A zig-zag of wire attached to an elastic "respiband" encircles the speaker's rib cage while another is fit to the abdomen. Each loop of wire is connected to an oscillator which is connected by a cable to the demodulating circuitry (within the "calibration box") that produces a voltage output proportional to the cross-sectional area of those parts of the body enclosed by the inductive loop. (Illustration courtesy of Ambulatory Monitoring, Inc., Ardsley, NY.)

Alderson, 1986; Boliek, Hixon, Watson, & Morgan, 1996; Selbie et al., 1997), and children (Tabachnik, Muller, Toye, & Levison, 1981; Boliek, Hixon, Watson, & Morgan, 1997). Perhaps partly due to its commercial availability, the technique has also been used extensively by a number of clinicians and researchers to study chest-wall kinematics and ventilation during normal and abnormal speech production (Loudon, Lee, & Holcomb, 1988; Russell & Stathopoulos, 1988; Warren, Morr, Rochet, & Dalston, 1989; LaBlance & Rutherford, 1991; Lane, Perkell, Svirsky, & Webster, 1991; Sperry & Klich, 1992; Lee, Loudon, Jacobson, & Stuebing, 1993; Sperry, Hillman, & Perkell, 1994; Winkworth, Davis, Ellis, & Adams, 1994; Winkworth, Davis, Adams, & Ellis, 1995; Boliek et al., 1996, 1997; Story et al., 1996; Dromey & Ramig, 1998a, 1998b; Iwarsson & Sundberg, 1998; Lane et al., 1998).

The Display of Kinematic Chest-Wall Data

Figure 12–25 illustrates a record of chest-wall behavior during reading by a normal man. In addition to the rib cage and abdomen traces are simultaneous signals from a probe microphone and a face-mask and pneumotachograph system (see Chapter 9, "Airflow and Volume"). The airflow data are helpful in interpreting the chest-wall movement record, while the acoustic signal helps tie behavior to specific speech events. The specific details of normal chest-wall kinematics will naturally vary according to the nature of the speech task. Figure 12–25 is typical, however, in its essential characteristics. Inspirations are rapid and are accomplished by cooperative inspiratory motions of both the rib cage and abdomen. Although the rib cage and abdomen both contribute to the speech expirations, note that they do not move in quite the same way. Abdominal motions are less "smooth" than rib-cage movements. This is because the abdominal system is used to adjust pressure and to meet the requirements of word stress and the like. Careful inspection of the chest-wall traces will show also that the rib cage and abdomen do not begin expiratory movements simultaneously. This so-called *prephonatory asynchrony* is normal and may be related to the way in which the chest wall is adjusted for speech (Baken et al., 1979, 1983;

Baken & Cavallo, 1981; Cavallo & Baken, 1985). Typically, the abdomen begins contraction about 100 ms before the rib cage does, and the pattern is seen in very young children and singers, as well as in untrained adult speakers (Wilder & Baken, 1974; Gould & Okamura, 1974).

Another means of displaying and analyzing chest-wall behavior is with a ***relative motion*** (or ***volume-volume***) ***diagram***, such as shown in Figure 12–26. The volume displacement of the rib cage is tracked by measuring the change in its anteroposterior diameter, circumference, or hemicircumference using any of the techniques described previously. This change is plotted along the vertical axis of the diagram. The volume displacement of the diaphragm-abdomen, determined by measuring the change in abdominal dimensions, is plotted on the horizontal axis. Each point on the chart describes the volume displacement of one chest-wall component relative to that of the other. The "isopleth" shown in the figure represents a somewhat idealized version of the trace that would be made by a subject performing an isovolume maneuver (see "Chest-Wall Movement: Calibration," Chapter 9). For this maneuver, the subject inflates or deflates her lungs to a given volume (selected by the tester and determined by means of a spirometer), closes the airway at the glottis to prevent the intake or loss of air, and shifts volume back and forth between her rib cage and abdomen. The

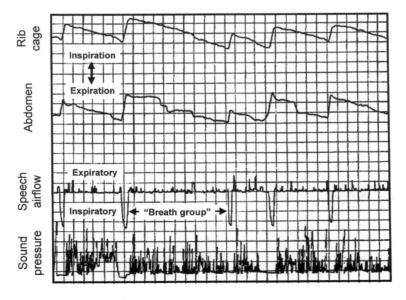

Figure 12–25. A record of normal ventilatory movements during reading. From top to bottom the traces are: rib cage hemicircumference, abdominal hemicircumference, airflow, and sound pressure.

gain of the rib-cage and abdomen transducer channels are adjusted to achieve a −1 isopleth slope. With this adjustment, equal changes in rib cage or abdomen size correspond to an equal change in lung volume. (This is equivalent to adjusting a summing amplifier to reflect no net lung-volume change.) Isovolume maneuvers are typically conducted at 20%-increments of the subject's vital capacity and at her functional residual capacity (FRC). Once the chart is calibrated in this manner, lung volume (the relative combined volume displacement of the rib cage and abdomen) will be shown increasing diagonally upward and to the right along a diagonal "z" axis (Hixon et al., 1973, 1976; Hixon, 1982; Hixon & Putnam, 1983).

The curved "relaxation characteristic" may be obtained by having the speaker adjust her lung volume to a prescribed level and, with her glottis sealed, simply relax her ventilatory muscles. In Figure 12–26, the relaxation characteristic is shown from 0% of the vital capacity (the speaker's RV, or residual volume) to 100% of the vital capacity (that is, TLC, the speaker's total lung capacity). Examples of normal chest-wall kinematic data from Hixon, Goldman, and Mead (1973) for various speech activities are shown in Figure 12–27. Volume data are shown relative to this speaker's relaxation characteristic and the isopleth representing 40% of the speaker's vital capacity, which is at approximately his FRC. It is of particular note that, despite the type of utterance, rarely do they extend below FRC and all are produced to the left of the relaxation characteristic; that is, the abdomen is smaller and the rib cage is larger compared with the passive relaxation characteristics at corresponding lung volumes.

Displays of this sort have been used in a number of studies where the relative contribution of the rib cage and abdomen to lung volume change is a concern (Forner & Hixon, 1977; Hixon, Putnam, & Sharp, 1983; Hoit & Hixon, 1986, 1987; Hodge & Rochet, 1989; Hoit et al., 1989, 1990; Murdoch, Killin, & McCaul, 1989; Murdoch, Chenery et al., 1989; Murdoch et al., 1991; Stathopoulos, Hoit, Hixon, Watson, & Solomon, 1991; Manifold & Murdoch, 1993; Murdoch & Hudson-Tennent, 1993; Solomon & Hixon, 1993; Winkworth et al., 1995). However, while serving this purpose, relative volume charts provide no information about the timing and duration of speech events and do not allow the direct comparison of kinematic data with other physiologic or acoustic signals.

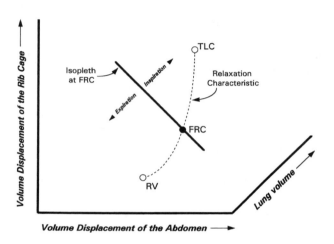

Figure 12–26. A volume-volume diagram to record the relative contribution of the rib cage and diaphragm-abdomen to lung volume change. [TLC = total lung capacity; FRC = functional residual capacity; RV = residual volume.]

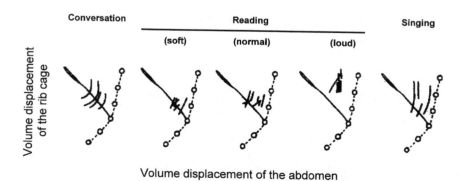

Figure 12–27. Relative motion diagrams for a single normal speaker during conversation, reading, and singing. Diagrams extracted from "Kinematics of the Chest Wall During Speech Production: Volume Displacement of the Rib Cage, Abdomen, and Lung," by T. J. Hixon, M. D. Goldman, and J. Mead, 1973, *Journal of Speech and Hearing Research, 16,* 78–115. Figure 7, p. 94 (speaker TH in upright posture). ©American Speech-Language-Hearing Association, Rockville, MD. Used by permission.

REFERENCES

Abbs, J. H. (1973a). The influence of gamma motor system on jaw movement during speech. *Journal of Speech and Hearing Research, 16*, 175–200.

Abbs, J. H. (1973b). Some mechanical properties of lower lip movement during speech. *Phonetica, 28*, 65–75.

Abbs, J. H. (1996). Mechanisms of speech motor execution and control. In N. J. Lass (Ed.), *Principles of experimental phonetics* (pp. 93–111). St. Louis, MO: Mosby.

Abbs, J. H., Folkins, J. W., & Sivarajan, M. (1976). Motor impairment following blockage of the infraorbital nerve. *Journal of Speech and Hearing Research, 19*, 19–35.

Abbs, J. H., & Gilbert, B. N. (1973). A strain gage transduction system for lip and jaw motion in two dimensions: Design criteria and calibration data. *Journal of Speech and Hearing Research, 16*, 248–256.

Abbs, J. H., Gracco, V. L., & Cole, K. J. (1984). Control of multi-movement coordination: Sensorimotor mechanisms in speech motor programming. *Journal of Motor Behavior, 16*, 195–231.

Abbs, J. H., & Netsell, R. (1973). An interpretation of jaw acceleration during speech. *Journal of Speech and Hearing Research, 16*, 421–425.

Abbs, J. H., & Stivers, D. (1978). A new cephalostat for speech physiology research. *Journal of the Acoustical Society of America, 64*, 1174–1175.

Abbs, J. H., & Watkin, K. L. (1976). Instrumentation for the study of speech physiology. In N. J. Lass (Ed.), *Contemporary issues in experimental phonetics* (pp. 41–75). New York: Academic Press.

Abercrombie, D. (1957). Direct palatography. *Zeitschrift für Phonetik, 10*, 21–25.

Ackermann, H., Gröne, B. F., Hoch, G., & Schönle, P. W. (1993). Speech freezing in Parkinson's disease: A kinematic analysis of orofacial movements by means of electromagnetic articulography. *Folia Phoniatrica, 45*, 84–89.

Ackermann, H., Hertrich, I., Daum, I., Scharf, G., & Spieker, S. (1997). Kinematic analysis of articulatory movements in central motor disorders. *Movement Disorders, 12*, 1019–1027.

Ackermann, H., Hertrich, I., & Hehr, T. (1995). Oral diadochokinesis in neurological dysarthrias. *Folia Phoniatrica et Logopaedica, 47*, 15–23.

Ackermann, H., Hertrich, I., & Scharf, G. (1995). Kinematic analysis of lower lip movements in ataxic dysarthria. *Journal of Speech and Hearing Research, 38*, 1252–1259.

Ackermann, H., Konczak, J., & Hertrich, I. (1997). The temporal control of repetitive articulatory movements in Parkinson's disease. *Brain and Language, 56*, 312–319.

Adams, S. G. (1994). Accelerating speech in a case of hypokinetic dysarthria: Descriptions and treatment. In J. A. Till, K. M. Yorkston, & D. R. Beukelman (Eds.), *Motor speech disorders: Advances in assessment and treatment* (pp. 213–228). Baltimore, MD: Paul H. Brookes.

Agostoni, E., Mognoni, R., Torri, G., & Saracino, F. (1965). Relation between changes of rib cage circumference and lung volume. *Journal of Applied Physiology, 20*, 1179–1186.

Akazawa, K., & Fujii, K. (1981). Physical properties of muscular tissue: Determination of firing rate, number, and size of motor units. In K. N. Stevens & M. Hirano (Eds.), *Vocal fold physiology* (pp. 61–81). Tokyo, Japan: University of Tokyo Press.

Albright, R. W. (1948). The motor abilities of speakers with good and poor articulation. *Speech Monographs, 15*, 164–172.

Alfonso, P. J., & Baer, T. (1982). Dynamics of vowel articulation. *Language and Speech, 25*, 151–173.

Alfonso, P. J., & van Lieshout, P. H. H. M. (1997). Spatial and temporal variability in obstruent gestural spectification by stutterers and controls: Comparisons across sessions. In W. Hulstijn, H. F. M. Peters, & P. H. H. M. van Lieshout (Eds.), *Speech production: Motor control, brain research and fluency disorders* (pp. 151–160). Amsterdam, The Netherlands: Elsevier Science.

Allen, G. D. (1974). On counting to twenty: An aid to measuring diadochokinetic syllable rate. *Journal of Speech and Hearing Disorders, 39*, 110–111.

Allen, G. D., Lubker, J. F., & Harrison, E., Jr. (1972). New paint-on electrodes for surface electromyography. *Journal of the Acoustical Society of America, 52*, 124.

Allen, G. D., Lubker, J. F., & Turner, D. T. (1973). Adhesion to mucous membrane for electromyography. *Journal of Dental Research, 52*, 391.

Allen, K. D., Bernstein, B., & Chait, D. H. (1991). EMG biofeedback treatment of pediatric hyperfunctional dysphonia. *Journal of Behavioral Therapy and Experimental Psychiatry, 22*, 91–101.

Allison, R. D. (1970). Bioelectric impedance measurements—Introduction to basic factors in impedance plethysmography. In R. D. Allison (Ed.), *Basic factors in bioelectric impedance measurements of cardiac output, lung volumes, and the cerebral circulation* (pp. 1–70). Pittsburgh, PA: Instrument Society of America.

Allison, R. D., Holmes, E. L., & Nyboer, J. (1964). Volumetric dynamics of respiration as measured by electrical impedance plethysmography. *Journal of Applied Physiology, 19*, 166–172.

Alwan, A., Narayanan, S., & Haker, K. (1997). Toward articulatory-acoustic models for liquid approximants based on MRI and EPG data: Part II. The rhotics. *Journal of the Acoustical Society of America, 101*, 1078–1089.

Amerman, J. D. (1993). A maximum-force-dependent protocol for assessing labial force control. *Journal of Speech and Hearing Research, 36*, 460–465.

Amerman, J. D., & Parnell, M. M. (1982). Oral motor precision in older adults. *Journal of the National Student Speech-Language-Hearing Association, 10*, 55–66.

Ardrian, E. D., & Bronk, D. W. (1929). The discharge of the impulses in motor nerve fibers: II. The frequency of discharge in reflex and voluntary contractions. *Journal of Physiology, 67*, 119–151.

Autessere, D., & Teston, B. (1979). Description of an electropalatographic system. In H. Hollien & P. Hollien (Eds.), *Current issues in the phonetic sciences* (pp. 407–422). Amsterdam, The Netherlands: John Benjamins B.V.

Badin, P. (1991). Fricative consonants: Acoustic and x-ray measurements. *Journal of Phonetics, 19*, 397–408.

Baer, T., Gore, J. C., Boyce, S., & Nye, P. W. (1987). Application of MRI to the analysis of speech production. *Magnetic Resonance Imaging, 5*, 1–7.

Baer, T., Gore, J. C., Gracco, L. C., & Nye, P. W. (1991). Analysis of vocal tract shape and dimensions using magnetic resonance imaging: Vowels. *Journal of the Acoustical Society of America, 90*, 799–828.

Baken, R. J. (1977). Estimation of lung volume change from torso hemicircumferences. *Journal of Speech and Hearing Research, 20*, 808–812.

Baken, R. J., & Cavallo, S. A. (1981). Prephonatory chest wall posturing. *Folia Phoniatrica, 33*, 193–203.

Baken, R. J., Cavallo, S. A., & Weissman, K. L. (1979). Chest wall movements prior to phonation. *Journal of Speech and Hearing Research, 22*, 862–872.

Baken, R. J., & Matz, B. J. (1973). A portable impedance pneumograph. *Human Communication, 2*, 28–35.

Baken, R. J., McManus, D. A., & Cavallo, S. A. (1983). Prephonatory chest wall posturing in stutterers. *Journal of Speech and Hearing Research, 26,* 444–450.

Bancroft, J. C. (1978, November). *A quantitative evaluation of magnetometers with lung volume estimates.* Paper presented at the annual convention of the American Speech and Hearing Association.

Barlow, S. M., & Abbs, J. H. (1983). Force transducers for the evaluation of labial, lingual, and mandibular motor impairments. *Journal of Speech and Hearing Research, 26,* 616–621.

Barlow, S. M., & Burton, M. K. (1990). Ramp-and-hold force control in the upper and lower lips: Developing new neuromotor assessment applications in traumatically brain injured adults. *Journal of Speech and Hearing Research, 33,* 660–675.

Barlow, S. M., Cole, K. J., & Abbs, J. H. (1983). A new head-mounted lip-jaw movement transduction system for the study of motor speech disorders. *Journal of Speech and Hearing Research, 26,* 283–288.

Barlow, S. M., & Netsell, R. (1986). Differential fine force control of the upper and lower lips. *Journal of Speech and Hearing Research, 29,* 163–169.

Barlow, S. M., & Rath, E. M. (1985). Maximum voluntary closing forces in the upper and lower lips of humans. *Journal of Speech and Hearing Research, 28,* 373–376.

Barry, M. C. (1992). Palatalisation, assimilation and gestural weakening in connected speech. *Speech Communication, 11,* 393–400.

Barry, M. C., & Timmermann, G. (1985). Mispronunciations and compensatory movements of tongue-operated patients. *British Journal of Disorders of Communication, 20,* 81–90.

Basmajian, J.V., & De Luca, C. J. (1985). *Muscles alive: Their functions revealed by electromyography* (5th ed.). Baltimore, MD: Williams & Wilkins.

Basmajian, J.V., & Dutta, C. R. (1961). Electromyography of the pharyngeal constrictors and levator palati in man. *Anatomical Record, 139,* 561–563.

Basmajian, J.V., & Stecko, G. (1962). A new bipolar electrode for electromyography. *Journal of Applied Physiology, 17,* 849.

Baum, S. R., & McFarland, D. H. (1997). The development of speech adaptation to an artificial palate. *Journal of the Acoustical Society of America, 102,* 2353–2359.

Bell-Berti, F., & Krakow, R. A. (1991). Anticipatory velar lowering: A coproduction account. *Journal of the Acoustical Society of America, 90,* 112–123.

Bigland, B., & Lippold, O. C. J. (1954). The relation between force velocity and integrated electrical activity in human muscles. *Journal of Physiology, 123,* 214–224.

Blair, C., & Smith, A. (1986). EMG recording in human lip muscles: Can single muscles be isolated? *Journal of Speech and Hearing Research, 29,* 256–266.

Blair, R. L., Berry, H., & Briant, T. D. R. (1977). Laryngeal electromyography—Techniques, applications and a review of personal experience. *Journal of Otolaryngology, 6,* 496–504.

Blomquist, B. L. (1950). Diadochokinetic movements of nine-, ten-, and eleven-year-old children. *Journal of Speech and Hearing Disorders, 15,* 159–164.

Bloomer, H. (1943). A palatograph for contour mapping of the palate. *Journal of the American Dental Association, 30,* 1053–1057.

Böckler, R., Wein, B., & Klajman, S. (1989). Ultraschalluntersuchung der aktiven und passiven Beweglichkeit der Zunge. *Folia Phoniatrica, 41,* 277–282.

Boemke, W., Gerull, G., & Hippel, K. (1992). Zur Elektromyographie des Larynx mit Hautoberflächenelektroden. *Folia Phoniatrica, 44,* 222–230.

Bole, C. T., II, & Lesser, M. A. (1966). Electromyography of the genioglossus muscles in man. *Journal of Applied Physiology, 21,* 1695–1698.

Boliek, C. A., Hixon, T. J., Watson, P. J., & Morgan, W. J. (1996). Vocalization and breathing during the first year of life. *Journal of Voice, 10,* 1–22.

Boliek, C. A., Hixon, T. J., Watson, P. J., & Morgan, W. J. (1997). Vocalization and breathing during the second and third years of life. *Journal of Voice, 11,* 373–390.

Booker, H. E., Rubow, R. T., & Coleman, P. J. (1969). Simplified feedback in neuromuscular retraining: An automated approach using electromyographic signals. *Archives of Physical Medicine and Rehabilitation, 50,* 621–625.

Borghese, N. A., Ferrigno, G., Redolfi, M., & Pedotti, A. (1997). Automatic integrated analysis of jaw and lip movement in speech production. *Journal of the Acoustical Society of America, 101,* 482–487.

Bouhuys, A. (Ed.). (1968). *Sound production in man. Annals of the New York Academy of Sciences* (Vol. 155). New York: New York Academy of Sciences.

Brady, W. R. (1984). *Digital radiography.* New York: Raven Press.

Brancatisano, A., Engel, L. A., & Loring, S. H. (1993). Lung volume and effectiveness of inspiratory muscles. *Journal of Applied Physiology, 74,* 688–694.

Branderud, P. (1985). Movetrack—A movement tracking system. *Phonetic experimental research at the Institute of Linguistics, University of Stockholm (PERILUS), IV,* 20–29.

Buchthal, F., & Faaborg-Andersen, K. (1964). Electromyography of laryngeal and respiratory muscles: Correlation with phonation and respiration. *Annals of Otology, Rhinology, and Laryngology, 73,* 118–123.

Buchthal, F., & Schmalbruch, H. (1980). Motor units of mammalian muscles. *Physiological Review, 60,* 90–142.

Butcher, A. (1989). Measuring coarticulation and variability in tongue contact patterns. *Clinical Linguistics and Phonetics, 3,* 39–47.

Butcher, A., & Weiher, E. (1976). An electropalatographic investigation of coarticulation in VCV sequences. *Journal of Phonetics, 4,* 59–74.

Byrd, D. (1994). Palatogram reading as a phonetic skill: A short tutorial. *Journal of the International Phonetic Association, 24,* 21–34.

Byrd, D. (1995). Palatogram reading as a phonetic skill: The answer to issue 24(1)'s EPG "mystery" sentence. *Journal of the International Phonetic Association, 25,* 65–70.

Byrd, D. (1996). Influences on articulatory timing in consonant sequences. *Journal of Phonetics, 24,* 209–244.

Byrd, D., Flemming, E., Mueller, C. A., & Tan, C. C. (1995). Using regions and indices in EPG data reduction. *Journal of Speech and Hearing Research, 38,* 821–827.

Byrd, D., & Tan, C. C. (1996). Saying consonant clusters quickly. *Journal of Phonetics, 24,* 263–282.

Canning, B. A., & Rose, M. F. (1974). Clinical measurements of the speed of tongue and lip movements in British children with normal speech. *British Journal of Disorders of Communication, 9,* 45–50.

Cannito, M. P., Ege, P., Ahmed, F., & Wagner, S. (1994). Diadochokinesis for complex trisyllables in individuals with spasmodic dysphonia and nondisabled subjects. In J. A. Till, K. M. Yorkston, & D. R. Beukelman (Eds.), *Motor speech disorders: Advances in assessment and treatment* (pp. 91–100). Baltimore, MD: Paul H. Brookes.

Canter, G. J. (1965). Speech characteristics of patients with Parkinson's disease: III. Articulation, diadochokinesis, and overall speech adequacy. *Journal of Speech and Hearing Disorders, 30,* 217–224.

Carrell, J. (1952). A cinefluorographic technique for the study of velopharyngeal closure. *Journal of Speech and Hearing Disorders, 17,* 224–228.

Carry, P.Y., Baconnier, P., Eberhard, A., Cotte, P., & Benchetrit, G. (1997). Evaluation of respiratory inductive plethysmography: Accuracy for analysis of respiratory waveforms. *Chest, 111,* 910–915.

Cavallo, S. A., & Baken, R. J. (1985). Prephonatory laryngeal and chest wall dynamics. *Journal of Speech and Hearing Research, 28,* 79–87.

Cha, C., & Patten, B. (1989). Amyotrophic lateral sclerosis: Abnormalities of the tongue on magnetic resonance imaging. *Annals of Neurology, 25,* 468–472.

Chadha, T., Watson, H., Birch, S., Jenouri, G., Schneider, A., Cohn, M., & Sackner, M. (1982). Validation of respiratory inductive plethysmography using different calibration procedures. *American Review of Respiratory Disease, 125,* 644–649.

Chi-Fishman, G., & Stone, M. (1996). A new application for electropalatography: Swallowing. *Dysphagia, 11,* 239–247.

Chi-Fishman, G., Stone, M., & McCall, G. N. (1998). Lingual action in normal sequential swallowing. *Journal of Speech, Language, and Hearing Research, 41,* 771–785.

Chiu, W. S., Shadle, C. H., & Carter, J. N. (1995). Quantitative measures of the palate using enhanced electropalatography. *European Journal of Disorders of Communication, 30,* 149–160.

Christensen, J. M., Fletcher, S. G., & McCutcheon, M. J. (1992). Esophageal speaker articulation of /s,z/: A dynamic palatometric assessment. *Journal of Communication Disorders, 25,* 65–76.

Christianson, R., Lufkin, R., & Hanafee, W. (1987). Normal magnetic resonance imaging anatomy of the tongue, oropharynx, hypopharynx, and larynx. *Dysphagia, 1,* 119–127.

Chuang, C. K., & Wang, W. S.-Y. (1978). Use of optical distance sensing to track tongue motion. *Journal of Speech and Hearing Research, 21,* 482–496.

Clayton, C. J. (1992). An intra-oral access device. *Journal of Medical Engineering Technology, 16,* 204–209.

Cobbold, R. S. C. (1992). *Transducers for biomedical measurements: Principles and applications* (2nd ed.). New York: John Wiley.

Coelho, C. A., Gracco, V. L., Fourakis, M., Rossetti, M., & Oshima, K. (1994). Application of instrumental techniques in the assessment of dysarthria: A case study. In J. A. Till, K. M. Yorkston, & D. R. Beukelman (Eds.), *Motor speech disorders: Advances in assessment and treatment* (pp. 103–117). Baltimore, MD: Paul H. Brookes.

Cohen, K. P., Panescu, D., Booske, J. H., Webster, J. G., & Tompkins, W. J. (1994). Design of an inductive plethysmograph for ventilation measurement. *Physiological Measurement, 15,* 217–229.

Cohn, M. A., Rao, A. S., Broudy, M., Birch, S., Watson, H., Atkins, N., Davis, B., Stott, F. D., & Sackner, M. A. (1982). The respiratory inductive plethysmograph: A new noninvasive monitor of respiration. *Bulletin Européen de Physiopathologie Respiratoire, 18,* 643–658.

Cohn, M. A., Watson, H., Weisshaut, R., Stott, F., & Sackner, M. A. (1978). A transducer for non-invasive monitoring of respiration. In F. D. Stott, E. B. Raftery, P. Sleight, & L. Goulding (Eds.), *Proceedings of the Second International Symposium on Ambulatory Monitoring* (pp. 119–128). New York: Academic Press.

Cole, K. J., Konopacki, R. A., & Abbs, J. H. (1983). A miniature electrode for surface electromyography during speech. *Journal of the Acoustical Society of America, 74,* 1362–1366.

Cole, R. M. (1972). Electrical capacitance measures of oropharyngeal functions. In K. R. Bzoch (Ed.), *Communicative disorders related to cleft lip and palate* (pp. 172–177). Boston, MA: College-Hill Press.

Connell, B. (1995). Some articulatory characteristics of the tap. In J. Windsor Lewis (Ed.), *Studies in general and English phonetics* (pp. 39–48). London, UK: Routledge.

Cooper, F. S. (1965). Research techniques and instrumentation. *ASHA Reports, 1,* 153–168.

Costigan, P. A., Wyss, U. P., Deluzio, K. J., & Li, J. (1992). Semiautomatic three-dimensional knee motion assessment system. *Medical and Biological Engineering and Computing, 30,* 343–350.

Craig, A. R., & Cleary, P. J. (1982). Reduction of stuttering by young male stutterers using EMG feedback. *Biofeedback and Self-Regulation, 7,* 241–255.

Craig, A., Hancock, K., Change, E., McCready, C., Shepley, A., McCaul, A., Costello, D., Harding, S., Kehren, R., Masel, C., & Reilly, K. (1996). A controlled clinical trial for stuttering in persons aged 9 to 14 years. *Journal of Speech and Hearing Research, 39,* 808–826.

Crawford, R. (1995). Teaching voiced velar stops to profoundly deaf children using EPG: Two case studies. *Clinical Linguistics and Phonetics, 9,* 255–270.

Dagenais, P. A. (1995). Electropalatography in the treatment of articulation/phonological disorders. *Journal of Communication Disorders, 28,* 303–329.

Dagenais, P. A., & Critz-Crosby, P. (1991). Consonant lingual-palatal contacts produced by normal-hearing and hearing impaired children. *Journal of Speech and Hearing Research, 34,* 1423–1435.

Dagenais, P. A., Critz-Crosby, P., & Adams, J. B. (1994). Defining and remediating persistent lateral lisps in children using electropalatography: Preliminary findings. *American Journal of Speech-Language Pathology, 3*(3), 67–76.

Dagenais, P. A., Critz-Crosby, P., Fletcher, S. G., & McCutcheon, M. J. (1994). Comparing abilities of children with profound hearing impairments to learn consonants using electropalatography or traditional aural-oral techniques. *Journal of Speech and Hearing Research, 37,* 687–699.

Dagenais, P. A., Lorendo, L. C., & McCutcheon, M. J. (1994). A study of voicing and context effects upon consonant lingua-palatal contact patterns. *Journal of Phonetics, 22,* 225–238.

Dang, J., & Honda, K. (1997). Acoustic characteristics of the piriform fossa in models and humans. *Journal of the Acoustical Society of America, 101,* 456–465.

Dang, J., Honda, K., & Suzuki, H. (1994). Morphological and acoustical analysis of the nasal and paranasal cavities. *Journal of the Acoustical Society of America, 96,* 2088–2100.

Daniel, B., & Guitar, B. (1978). EMG feedback and recovery of facial and speech gestures following neural anastomosis. *Journal of Speech and Hearing Disorders, 43,* 9–20.

Daniloff, R., Shuckers, G., & Feth, L. (1980). *The physiology of speech and hearing: An introduction.* Englewood Cliffs, NJ: Prentice-Hall.

Darley, F. L., Aronson, A. E., & Brown, J. R. (1975). *Motor speech disorders.* Philadelphia, PA: W. B. Saunders.

Dart, S. N. (1998). Comparing French and English coronal consonant articulation. *Journal of Phonetics, 26,* 71–94.

Debatin, J. F., & McKinnon, G. C. (1998). *Ultrafast MRI: Techniques and applications.* New York: Springer-Verlag.

Dedo, H. H., & Hall, W. N. (1969). Electrodes in laryngeal electromyography: Reliability comparison. *Annals of Otorhinolaryngology, 78,* 172–179.

de Jong, K. J. (1997). Labiovelar compensation in back vowels. *Journal of the Acoustical Society of America, 101,* 2221–2233.

De Luca, C. J., LeFever, R. S., & Stulen, F. B. (1979). Pasteless electrode for clinical use. *Medical and Biological Engineering and Computing, 17,* 387–390.

Denny-Brown, D. (1949). Interpretation of the electromyogram. *Archives of Neurology and Psychiatry, 61,* 99–128.

Dent, H., Gibbon, F. E., & Hardcastle, W. J. (1992). Inhibiting an abnormal lingual pattern in a cleft palate child using electropalatography (EPG). In M. M. Leahy & J. L. Kallen (Eds.), *Interdisciplinary perspectives in speech and language pathology* (pp. 211–221). Dublin, Ireland: Trinity College.

Dent, H., Gibbon, F. E., & Hardcastle, W. J. (1995). The application of electropalatography (EPG) to the remediation of speech disorders in school-aged children and young adults. *European Journal of Disorders of Communication, 30,* 264–277.

Dew, A. M., Glaister, N., & Roach, P. J. (1989). Combining displays of EPG and automatic segmentation of speech for clinical purposes. *Clinical Linguistics and Phonetics, 3,* 71–80.

Di Girolamo, M., Corsetti, A., Laghi, A., Ferone, E., Iannicelli, E., Rossi, M., Pavone, P., & Passariello, R. (1996). Valutazione con Risonanza Magnetica dei movimenti della laringe e della cavità faringo-buccale durante la fonazione. *Radiologia Medica, 92,* 33–40.

Dixit, R. P. (1990). Linguotectal contact patterns in the dental and retroflex stops of Hindi. *Journal of Phonetics, 18,* 189–201.

Dixit, R. P., & Flege, J. E. (1991). Vowel context, rate and loudness effects on linguopalatal contact patterns in Hindi retroflex /t/. *Journal of Phonetics, 19,* 213–229.

Draper, M. H., Ladefoged, P., & Whitteridge, D. (1959). Respiratory muscles in speech. *Journal of Speech and Hearing Research, 2,* 16–27.

Draper, M. H., Ladefoged, P., & Whitteridge, D. (1960). Expiratory pressures and air flow during speech. *British Medical Journal, 18,* 1837–1843.

Dromey, C., & Ramig, L. O. (1998a). The effect of lung volume on selected phonatory and articulatory variables. *Journal of Speech, Language, and Hearing Research, 41,* 491–502.

Dromey, C., & Ramig, L. O. (1998b). Intentional changes in sound pressure and rate: Their impact on measures of respiration, phonation, and articulation. *Journal of Speech, Language, and Hearing Research, 41,* 1003–1018.

Dusek, M., Simmons, J., Buschang, P. H., & al-Hashimi, I. (1996). Masticatory function in patients with xerostomia. *Gerodontology, 13,* 3–8.

Dworkin, J. P. (1978). Protrusive lingual force and lingual diadochokinetic rates: A comparative analysis between normal and lisping speakers. *Language, Speech, and Hearing Services in Schools, 9,* 8–16.

Dworkin, J. P., & Aronson, A. E. (1986). Tongue strength and alternate motion rates in normal and dysarthric subjects. *Journal of Communication Disorders, 19,* 115–132.

Dworkin, J. P., Aronson, A. E., & Mulder, D. W. (1980). Tongue force in normals and in dysarthric patients with amyotrophic lateral sclerosis. *Journal of Speech and Hearing Research, 23,* 828–837.

Eblen, R. E., Jr. (1963). Limitations on use of surface electromyography in studies of speech breathing. *Journal of Speech and Hearing Research, 6,* 3–18.

Edwards, J., & Harris, K. S. (1990). Rotation and translation of the jaw during speech. *Journal of Speech and Hearing Research, 33,* 550–562.

Edwards, S., & Miller, N. (1989). Using EPG to investigate speech errors and motor agility in a dyspraxic patient. *Clinical Linguistics and Phonetics, 3,* 111–126.

Elsner, R. W., Eagan, C. J., & Andersen, S. (1959). Impedance matching circuit for the mercury strain gauge. *Journal of Applied Physiology, 14,* 871–872.

Engelke, W., Bruns, T., Striebeck, M., & Hoch, G. (1996). Midsagittal velar kinematics during production of VCV sequences. *Cleft Palate—Craniofacial Journal, 33,* 236–244.

Engelke, W., Engelke, D., & Schwestka, R. (1990). Zur klinischen und Instrumentellen Untersuchung motorischer Zungenfunktion. *Deutsche Zahnärztliche Zeitschrift, 45,* 11–16.

Engelke, W., & Hoch, G. (1994). Simultane elektromagnetische Artikulographie und Videoendoskopie. Ein kasuistischer Beitrag zur objektiven Diagnostik des velopharyngealen Sphinkters. *Fortschritte der Kieferorthopädie, 55,* 297–303.

Engelke, W., Hoch, G., Bruns, T., & Striebeck, M. (1996). Simultaneous evaluation of articulatory velopharyngeal function under different dynamic conditions with EMA and videoendoscopy. *Folia Phoniatrica et Logopaedica, 48,* 65–77.

Engelke, W., Müller, C., & Petersen, C. (1995). Physiologie oropharyngealer Schluckbewegungen. *Sprache, Stimme, Gehör, 19,* 105–113.

Engelke, W., & Schönle, P. W. (1991). Elektromagnetische Artikulographie: Eine neue Methode zur Untersuchung von Bewegungsfunktionen des Gaumensegels. *Folia Phoniatrica, 43,* 147–152.

Engelke, W., Schönle, P. W., & Engelke, D. (1990). 2 objektive Verfahren zur Untersuchung motorischer Funktionen nach Eingriffen an Zunge und Velum. *Deutsche Zeitschrift fur Mund-, Kiefer-, und Gesichts-Chirurgie, 14,* 348–358.

Engelke, W., Schönle, P. W., Kring, R. A., & Richter, C. (1989). Zur Untersuchung orofazialer Bewegungsfunktionen mit der elektromagnetischen Articulographie. *Deutsche Zahnärztliche Zeitschrift, 44,* 618–622.

English, D. T., & Blevins, C. E. (1969). Motor units of laryngeal muscles. *Archives of Otolaryngology, 89,* 778–784.

Engstrand, O. (1989). Towards an electropalatographic specification of consonant articulation in Swedish. *Phonetic experimental research at the Institute of Linguistics, University of Stockholm (PERILUS), X,* 115–156.

Evans, M. (1952). Efficiency is the goal in cerebral palsied speech. *Crippled Child, 29,* 19–21.

Faaborg-Andersen, K. (1957). Electromyographic investigation of intrinsic laryngeal muscles in humans. *Acta Physiologica Scandinavica, 41* (Suppl. 140), 1–147.

Faaborg-Andersen, K. (1965). Electromyography of laryngeal muscles in humans: Tecnics and results. *Current Problems in Phoniatrics and Logopedics, 3,* 1–72.

Fairbanks, G., & Spriestersbach, D. C. (1950). A study of minor organic deviations in "functional" disorders of articulation: 1. Rate of movement of oral structures. *Journal of Speech and Hearing Disorders, 15,* 60–69.

Farnetani, E., & Faber, A. (1992). Tongue-jaw coordination in vowel production: Isolated words vs. connected speech. *Speech Communication, 11,* 411–419.

Farnetani, E., & Recasens, D. (1993). Anticipatory consonant-to-vowel coarticulation in the production of VCV sequences in Italian. *Language and Speech, 36,* 279–302.

Farnetani, E., Vagges, K., & Magno-Caldognetto, E. (1985). Coarticulation in Italian /VtV/ sequences: A palatographic study. *Phonetica, 42,* 78–99.

Ferrigno, G., & Pedotti, A. (1985). ELITE: A digital dedicated hardware system for movement analysis via real-time TV signal processing. *IEEE Transactions on Biomedical Engineering, 32,* 943–950.

Fink, B. R., Basek, M., & Epanchin, V. (1956). The mechanism of opening of the human larynx. *Laryngoscope, 66,* 410–425.

Finley, W., Niman, C., Standley, J., & Ender, P. (1976). Frontal EMG biofeedback: Training of athetoid cerebral palsy patients. *Biofeedback and Self-Regulation, 1,* 169–182.

Finley, W., Niman, C., Standley, J., & Wansley, R. A. (1977). Electrophysiologic behaviour modification of frontal EMG in cerebral-palsied children. *Biofeedback and Self-Regulation, 2,* 59–79.

Flege, J. E. (1989). Differences in inventory size affect the location but not the precision of tongue positioning in vowel production. *Language and Speech, 32,* 123–147.

Flege, J. E., Fletcher, S. G., & Homiedan, A. (1988). Compensating for a bite block in /s/ and /t/ production: Palatographic, acoustic, and perceptual data. *Journal of the Acoustical Society of America, 83,* 212–228.

Flege, J. E., Fletcher, S. G., McCutcheon, M. J., & Smith, S. C. (1986). The physiological specification of American English vowels. *Language and Speech, 29,* 361–388.

Fletcher, S. G. (1972). Time-by-count measurement of diadochokinetic syllable rate. *Journal of Speech and Hearing Research, 15,* 763–770.

Fletcher, S. G. (1983). New prospects for speech by the hearing impaired. In N. J. Lass (Ed.), *Speech and language: Advances in basic research and clinical practice* (pp. 1–42). New York: Academic Press.

Fletcher, S. G. (1985). Speech production and oral motor skill in an adult with an unrepaired palatal cleft. *Journal of Speech and Hearing Disorders, 50,* 254–261.

Fletcher, S. G. (1988). Speech production following partial glossectomy. *Journal of Speech and Hearing Disorders, 53,* 232–238.

Fletcher, S. G. (1989). Palatometric specification of stop, affricate and sibilant sounds. *Journal of Speech and Hearing Research, 32,* 736–748.

Fletcher, S. G. (1990). Recognition of words from palatometric displays. *Clinical Linguistics and Phonetics, 4,* 9–24.

Fletcher, S. G. (1992). *Articulation: A physiological approach.* San Diego, CA: Singular Publishing Group.

Fletcher, S. G. (1993). Jaw position in vowel production and perception. *Journal of Medical Speech-Language Pathology, 1,* 171–189.

Fletcher, S. G., Dagenais, P. A., & Critz-Crosby, P. (1991a). Teaching consonants to profoundly hearing-impaired speakers using palatometry. *Journal of Speech and Hearing Research, 34,* 929–942.

Fletcher, S. G., Dagenais, P. A., & Critz-Crosby, P. (1991b). Teaching vowels to profoundly hearing-impaired speakers using glossometry. *Journal of Speech and Hearing Research, 34,* 943–956.

Fletcher, S. G., & Hasegawa, A. (1983). Speech modification by a deaf child through dynamic orometric modeling and feedback. *Journal of Speech and Hearing Disorders, 48,* 178–185.

Fletcher, S. G., McCutcheon, M. J., Smith, S. C., & Smith, W. H. (1989). Glossometric measurements in vowel production and modification. *Clinical Linguistics and Phonetics, 3,* 358–375.

Fletcher, S. G., McCutcheon, M., & Wolf, M. (1975). Dynamic palatometry. *Journal of Speech and Hearing Research, 18,* 812–819.

Fletcher, S. G., & Meldrun, J. R. (1968). Lingual function and relative length of the lingual frenulum. *Journal of Speech and Hearing Research, 11,* 382–390.

Fletcher, S. G., & Newman, D. (1991). [s] and [ʃ] as a function of linguapalatal contact place and sibilant groove width. *Journal of the Acoustical Society of America, 89,* 850–858.

Fletcher, S. G., Shelton, R. L., Jr., Smith, C. C. & Bosma, J. F. (1960). Radiography in speech pathology. *Journal of Speech and Hearing Disorders, 25,* 135–144.

Folkins, J. W. (1981). Muscle activity for jaw closing during speech. *Journal of Speech and Hearing Research, 24,* 601–615.

Folkins, J. W., & Abbs, J. H. (1975). Lip and jaw motor control during speech: Responses to resistive loading of the jaw. *Journal of Speech and Hearing Research, 18,* 207–220.

Folkins, J. W., & Abbs, J. H. (1976). Additional observations on responses to resistive loading of the jaw. *Journal of Speech and Hearing Research, 19,* 820–821.

Folkins, J. W., & Canty, J. L. (1986). Movements of the upper and lower lips during speech: Interactions between lips with the jaw fixed at different positions. *Journal of Speech and Hearing Research, 29,* 348–356.

Folkins, J. W., & Linville, R. N. (1983). The effects of varying lower-lip displacement on upper-lip movements: Implications for the coordination of speech movements. *Journal of Speech and Hearing Research, 26,* 209–217.

Folkins, J. W., Linville, R. N., Garrett, J. D., & Brown, C. K. (1988). Interactions in the labial musculature during speech. *Journal of Speech and Hearing Research, 31,* 253–264.

Fontdevila, J., Pallarès, M. D., & Recasens, D. (1994a). The contact index method of electropalatographic data reduction. *Journal of Phonetics, 22,* 141–154.

Fontdevila, J., Pallarès, M. D., & Recasens, D. (1994b). Electropalatographic data collected with and without a face mask. *Journal of Speech and Hearing Research, 37,* 806–812.

Forner, L. L., & Hixon, T. J. (1977). Respiratory kinematics in profoundly hearing-impaired speakers. *Journal of Speech and Hearing Research, 19,* 373–408.

Forrest, K., Weismer, G., & Turner, G. S. (1989). Kinematic, acoustic, and perceptual analyses of connected speech produced by parkinsonian and normal geriatric adults. *Journal of the Acoustical Society of America, 85,* 2608–2622.

Forster, C., & Hardcastle, W. (1998). An electropalatographic (EPG) study of the speech of two stuttering subjects. *International Journal of Language and Communication Disorders, 33,* 358–363.

Foucart, J. M., Carpentier, P., Pajoni, D., Rabischong, P., & Pharaboz, C. (1998). Kinetic magnetic resonance imaging analysis of swallowing: A new approach to pharyngeal function. *Surgical and Radiologic Anatomy, 20,* 53–55.

Fougeron, C., & Keating, P. A. (1997). Variations in velic and lingual articulation depending on prosodic position: Results for 2 French speakers. *UCLA Working Papers in Phonetics, 92,* 88–96.

Friedrich, G., Kainz, J., Schneider, G. H., & Anderhuber, F. (1989). Die Computertomographie des Larynx in der Stimmdiagnostik: Untersuchungen zur Methodik und Massgenauigkeit. *Folia Phoniatrica, 41,* 283–291.

Friel, S. (1998). When is a /k/ not a [k]? EPG as a diagnostic and therapeutic tool for abnormal velar stops. *International Journal of Language and Communication Disorders, 33,* 439–444.

Fritzell, B. (1969). A combined electromyographic and cineradiographic study: Activity of the levator and palatoglossus muscles in relation to velar movements. *Acta Otolaryngologica,* Suppl. 250, 1–81.

Fritzell, B. (1979). Electromyography in the study of velopharyngeal function: A review. *Folia Phoniatrica, 31,* 93–102.

Fromkin, V., & Ladefoged, P. (1966). Electromyography in speech research. *Phonetica, 15,* 219–242.

Fujii, I. (1970). Phoneme identification with dynamic palatography. *Annual Bulletin of the Research Institute of Logopedics and Phoniatrics, 3,* 67–68.

Fujimura, O. (1990). Methods and goals of speech production research. *Language and Speech, 33,* 195–258.

Fujimura, O., Kiritani, S., & Ishida, H. (1973). Computer-controlled radiography for observation of movements of articulatory and other human organs. *Computers in Biology and Medicine, 3,* 371–384.

Fujimura, O., Shibata, S., Kiritani, S., Shimada, Z., & Satta, C. (1968). A study of dynamic palatography. *Proceedings of the Sixth International Congress on Acoustics,* 21–24.

Fujimura, O., Tatsumi, I. F., & Kagaya, R. (1973). Computational processing of palatographic patterns. *Journal of Phonetics, 1,* 47–54.

Gabriel, D. A. (1997). Shoulder and elbow activity in goal-directed arm movements. *Experimental Brain Research, 116,* 359–366.

Gamsu, G., Mark, A., & Webb, W. R. (1981). Computed tomography of normal larynx during quiet breathing and phonation. *Journal of Computer Assisted Tomography, 5,* 353–360.

Gamsu, G., Webb, W. R., Shallit, J. B., & Moss, A. A. (1981). Computed tomography in carcinoma of the larynx and pyriform sinuses—The value of phonation CT. *American Journal of Radiology, 136,* 577–585.

Gartenberg, R. D. (1984). An electropalatographic investigation of allophonic variation in English /l/ articulations. *Speech Research Laboratory Work in Progress* (University of Reading), *4,* 135–157.

Gay, T., & Harris, K. (1971). Some recent developments in the use of electromyography in speech research. *Journal of Speech and Hearing Research, 14,* 241–246.

Gay, T., Strome, M., Hirose, H., & Sawashima, M. (1972). Electromyography of the intrinsic laryngeal muscles during phonation. *Annals of Otology, Rhinology and Laryngology, 81,* 401–409.

Gay, T., Ushijima, T., Hirose, H., & Cooper, F. S. (1974). Effect of speaking rate on labial consonant-vowel articulation. *Journal of Phonetics, 2,* 47–63.

Geddes, L. A. (1972). *Electrodes and the measurement of bioelectric events.* New York: John Wiley.

Geddes, L. A., & Baker, L. E. (1989). *Principles of applied biomedical instrumentation* (3rd ed.). New York: John Wiley.

Geddes, L. A., Hoff, H. E., Hickman, D. M., Hinds, M., & Baker, L. (1962). Recording respiration and the electrocardiogram with common electrodes. *Aerospace Medicine, 33,* 891.

Geddes, L. A., Hoff, H. E., Hickman, D. M., & Moore, A. G. (1962). The impedance pneumograph. *Aerospace Medicine, 33,* 28–33.

Gentil, M. (1990). Acoustic characteristics of speech in Friedreich's disease. *Folia Phoniatrica, 42,* 125–134.

Gentil, M. (1992). Variability of motor strategies. *Brain and Language, 42,* 30–37.

Gentil, M., & Moore, W. H., Jr. (1997). Electromyography. In M. J. Ball & C. Code (Eds.), *Instrumental clinical phonetics* (pp. 64–86). London, UK: Whurr Publishers.

Gibbon, F. (1990). Lingual activity in two speech-disordered children's attempts to produce velar and alveolar stop consonants: Evidence from electropalatographic (EPG) data. *British Journal of Disorders of Communication, 25,* 329–340.

Gibbon, F. E. (1999). Undifferentiated lingual gestures in children with articulation/phonological disorders. *Journal of Speech, Language, and Hearing Research, 42,* 382–397.

Gibbon, F. E., Dent, H., & Hardcastle, W. J. (1993). Diagnosis and therapy of abnormal alveolar stops in a speech disordered child using electropalatography. *Clinical Linguistics and Phonetics, 7,* 247–267.

Gibbon, F. E., & Hardcastle, W. J. (1987). An articulatory description and treatment of "lateral /s/" using electropalatography: A case study. *British Journal of Disorders of Communication, 22,* 203–217.

Gibbon, F. E., & Hardcastle, W. J. (1989). Deviant articulation in a cleft palate child following late repair of the hard palate: A description and remediation procedure using electropalatography (EPG). *Clinical Linguistics and Phonetics, 3,* 93–110.

Gibbon, F., Hardcastle, W. J., & Dent, H. (1995). A study of obstruent sounds in school-age children with speech disorders using electropalatography (EPG). *European Journal of Disorders of Communication, 30,* 213–225.

Gibbon, F., Hardcastle, W. J., & Moore, A. (1990). Modifying abnormal tongue patterns in an older child using electropalatography. *Child Language Teaching and Therapy, 6,* 227–245.

Gibbon, F., Hardcastle, W. J., & Nicolaidis, K. (1993). Temporal and spatial aspects of lingual coarticulation in /kl/ sequences: A cross-linguistic investigation. *Language and Speech, 36,* 261–277.

Gibbon, F. E., Hardcastle, W. J., & Suzuki, H. (1991). An electropalatographic study of the /r/, /l/ distinction for Japanese learners of English. *Computer Assisted Language Learning, 4,* 153–171.

Goldensohn, E. S., & Zablow, L. (1959). An electrical impedance spirometer. *Journal of Applied Physiology, 14,* 463–464.

Goldstein, P., Ziegler, W., Vogel, M., & Hoole, P. (1994). Combined palatal-lift and EPG-feedback therapy in dysarthria: A case study. *Clinical Linguistics and Phonetics, 8,* 201–218.

Gould, W. J., & Okamura, H. (1974). Respiratory training of the singer. *Folia Phoniatrica, 26,* 275–286.

Gracco, V. L. (1994). Some organizational characteristics of speech movement control. *Journal of Speech and Hearing Research, 37,* 4–27.

Gracco, V. L., & Abbs, J. H. (1985). Dynamic control of the perioral system during speech: Kinematic analyses of autogenic and nonautogenic sensorimotor processes. *Journal of Neurophysiology, 54,* 418–432.

Greenwood, A. R., Goodyear, C. C., & Martin, P. A. (1992). Measurement of vocal tract shapes using magnetic resonance imaging. *Proceedings of the IEEE, 139,* 553–560.

Grieve, D. W., Miller, D. I., Mitchelson, D., Paul, J. P., & Smith, A. J. (1975). *Techniques for the analysis of human movement.* Princeton, NJ: Princeton Book Company.

Guenther, F. H., Espy-Wilson, C. Y., Boyce, S. E., Matthies, M. L., Zandipour, M., & Perkell, J. S. (1999). Articulatory tradeoffs reduce acoustic variability during American English /r/ production. *Journal of the Acoustical Society of America, 105,* 2854–2865.

Guiard-Marigny, T., & Ostry, D. J. (1997). A system for three-dimensional visualization of human jaw motion in speech. *Journal of Speech, Language, and Hearing Research, 40,* 1118–1121.

Guitar, B. (1975). Reduction of stuttering frequency using analog electromyographic feedback. *Journal of Speech and Hearing Research, 18,* 672–685.

Gumpertz, F. (1931). Palatographische Untersuchungen an Stammlern mit Hilfe eines neuen künstlichen Gaumens. *Monatschriften Ohrenheilkeit,* 1095–1116.

Haase, A., Matthaei, D., Bartkowski, R., Dühmke, E., & Leibfritz, D. (1989). Inversion recovery snapshot FLASH MR imaging. *Journal of Computer Assisted Tomography, 13,* 1036–1040.

Hagen, R., Haase, A., Matthaei, D., & Henrich, D. (1990). Oropharyngeale Funktionsdiagnostik mit der FLASH-MR-Tomographie. *HNO, 38,* 421–425.

Hale, S. T., Kellum, G. D., Richardson, J. F., Messer, S. C., Gross, A. M., & Sisakun, S. (1992). Oral motor control, posturing, and myofunctional variables in 8-year-olds. *Journal of Speech and Hearing Research, 35,* 1203–1208.

Hamilton, C. (1993). Investigation of articulatory patterns of young adults with Down's syndrome using electropalatography. *Down's Syndrome: Research and Practice, 1,* 15–28.

Hamlet, S. L., Bunnell, H. T., & Struntz, B. (1986). Articulatory asymmetries. *Journal of the Acoustical Society of America, 79,* 1164–1169.

Hamlet, S. L., Cullison, B. L., & Stone, M. L. (1979). Physiological control of sibilant duration: Insights afforded by speech compensation to dental prostheses. *Journal of the Acoustical Society of America, 65,* 1276–1285.

Hamlet, S., & Stone, M. (1976). Compensatory vowel characteristics resulting from the presence of different types of experimental dental prostheses. *Journal of Phonetics, 4,* 199–218.

Hamlet, S., & Stone, M. (1978). Compensatory alveolar consonant production induced by wearing a dental prosthesis. *Journal of Phonetics, 6,* 227–248.

Hanafee, W. N. (1983). Conventional versus computed tomography in laryngeal lesions. In J. T. Littleton & M. L. Durizch (Eds.), *Sectional imaging methods: A comparison* (pp. 297–306). Baltimore, MD: University Park Press.

Hand, C. R., Burns, M. O., & Ireland, E. (1979). Treatment of hypertonicity in muscles of lip retraction. *Biofeedback and Self-Regulation, 4,* 171–181.

Hanna, R., Wilfling, F., & McNeil, B. (1975). A biofeedback treatment for stuttering. *Journal of Speech and Hearing Disorders, 40,* 270–273.

Hardcastle, W. (1970). Electropalatography in speech research. *University of Essex Language Centre Occasional Papers, 9,* 54–64.

Hardcastle, W. J. (1972). The use of electropalatography in phonetic research. *Phonetica, 25,* 197–215.

Hardcastle, W. J. (1985). Some phonetic and syntactic constraints on lingual coarticulation during /kl/ sequences. *Speech Communication, 4,* 247–263.

Hardcastle, W. J., & Clark, J. E. (1981). Articulatory, aerodynamic and acoustic properties of lingual fricatives in English. *Speech Research Laboratory Work in Progress* (University of Reading), *3,* 51–78.

Hardcastle, W. J., & Gibbon, F. E. (1997). Electropalatography and its clinical applications. In M. J. Ball & C. Code (Eds.), *Instrumental clinical phonetics* (pp. 149–193). London, UK: Whurr Publishers.

Hardcastle, W. J., Gibbon, F. E., & Jones, W. (1991). Visual display of tongue-palate contact: Electropalatography in the assessment and remediation of speech disorders. *British Journal of Disorders of Communication, 26,* 41–74.

Hardcastle, W. J., Gibbon, F. E., & Nicolaidis, W. (1991). EPG data reduction methods and their implications for studies of lingual coarticulation. *Journal of Phonetics, 19,* 251–266.

Hardcastle, W. J., Gibbon, F. E., & Scobbie, J. (1995). Phonetic and phonological aspects of English affricate production in children with speech disorders. *Phonetica, 52,* 242–250.

Hardcastle, W. J., Jones, W., Knight, C., Trudgeon, A., & Calder, G. (1989). New developments in electropalatography: A state-of-the-art report. *Clinical Linguistics and Phonetics, 3,* 1–38.

Hardcastle, W. J., & Morgan, R. A. (1982). An instrumental investigation of articulation disorders in children. *British Journal of Disorders of Communication, 17,* 47–65.

Hardcastle, W. J., & Morgan Barry, R. A. (1989). Articulatory and perceptual factors in /l/ vocalisation in English. *Journal of the International Phonetic Association, 15,* 3–17.

Hardcastle, W. J., Morgan Barry, R. A., & Clark, C. J. (1985). Articulatory and voicing characteristics of adult dysarthric and verbal dyspraxic speakers: An instrumental study. *British Journal of Disorders of Communication, 20,* 249–270.

Hardcastle, W. J., Morgan Barry, R. A., & Clark, C. J. (1987). An instrumental study of lingual activity in articulation-disordered children. *Journal of Speech and Hearing Research, 30,* 171–184.

Hardcastle, W. J., & Roach, P. (1979). An instrumental investigation of coarticulation in stop consonant sequences. In H. Hollien & P. Hollien (Eds.), *Current issues in the phonetic sciences* (pp. 531–540). Amsterdam, The Netherlands: John Benjamins B.V.

Harley, W. T. (1972). Dynamic palatography: A study of lingua-palatal contacts during the production of selected consonant sounds. *Journal of Prosthetic Dentistry, 27,* 364–376.

Harrington, J. M. (1987). Coarticulation and stuttering: an acoustic and electropalatographic study. In H. Peters & W. Hulstijn (Eds.), *Speech motor dynamics in stuttering* (pp. 381–392). New York: Springer-Verlag.

Harris, K. S. (1970). Physiological measures of speech movements: EMG and fiberoptic studies. *ASHA Reports, 5,* 271–282.

Harris, K. S. (1981). Electromyography as a technique for laryngeal investigation. *ASHA Reports, 11,* 70–87.

Harris, K. S., Rosov, R., Cooper, F. S., & Lysaught, G. F. (1964). A multiple suction electrode system. *Electroencephalography and Clinical Neurophysiology, 17,* 698–700.

Hartman, D. E., & Abbs, J. H. (1992). Dysarthria associated with focal unilateral upper motor neuron lesion. *European Journal of Disorders of Communication, 27,* 187–196.

Hashi, M., Westbury, J. R., & Honda, K. (1998). Vowel posture normalization. *Journal of the Acoustical Society of America, 104,* 2426–2437.

Hashimoto, K., & Sasaki, K. (1982). On the relationship between the shape and position of the tongue for vowels. *Journal of Phonetics, 10,* 291–299.

Hawkins, C. F., & Swisher, W. E. (1978). Evaluation of a real-time ultrasound scanner in assessing lateral pharyngeal wall motion during speech. *Cleft Palate Journal, 15,* 161–166.

Hayward, K. M., Omar, Y. A., & Goesche, M. (1989). Dental and alveolar stops in KiMvita Swahili: An electropalatographic study. *African Languages and Cultures, 2,* 51–72.

Heath, M. R., Ferman, A. M., & Mollard, R. (1980). Electropalatography: Thermo-formed pseudopalates and the use of three dimensional display. *Journal of Biomedical Engineering, 2,* 145–147.

Heltman, H. J., & Peacher, G. M. (1943). Misarticulation and diadochokinesis in the spastic paralytic. *Journal of Speech Disorders, 8,* 137–145.

Hennig, J., Nauerth, A., & Friedburg, H. (1986). RARE imaging: A fast imaging method for clinical MR. *Magnetic Resonance in Medicine, 3,* 823–833.

Henrick, W. R., Hykes, D. L., & Starchman, D. E. (Eds.). (1995). *Ultrasound physics and instrumentation* (3rd ed.). St. Louis, MO: Mosby.

Hertrich, I., & Ackermann, H. (1997). Articulatory control of phonological vowel length contrasts: Kinematic analysis of labial gestures. *Journal of the Acoustical Society of America, 102,* 523–536.

Hillix, W. A., Fry, M. N., & Hershman, R. L. (1965). Computer recognition of spoken digits based on six nonacoustic measures. *Journal of the Acoustical Society of America, 38,* 790–796.

Hinton, V. A. (1996). Interlabial pressure during production of bilabial phones. *Journal of Phonetics, 24,* 337–349.

Hinton, V. A., & Arokiasamy, W. M. C. (1997). Maximum interlabial pressures in normal speakers. *Journal of Speech, Language, and Hearing Research, 40,* 400–404.

Hinton, V. A., & Luschei, E. S. (1992). Validation of a modern minature transducer for measurement of interlabial contact pressure during speech. *Journal of Speech and Hearing Research, 35,* 245–251.

Hirai, T., Tanaka, O., Koshino, H., & Yajima, T. (1991). Ultrasound observations of tongue motor behavior. *Journal of Prosthetic Dentistry, 65,* 840–844.

Hirano, M., & Ohala, J. (1969). Use of hooked-wire electrodes for electromyography of the intrinsic laryngeal muscles. *Journal of Speech and Hearing Research, 12,* 362–373.

Hirose, H. (1971). Electromyography of the articulatory muscles: Current instrumentation and technique. *Haskins Laboratories Status Report on Speech Research, SR 25/26,* 73–86.

Hirose, H. (1977). Electromyography of the larynx and other speech organs. In M. Sawashima & F. S. Cooper (Eds.),

Dynamic aspects of speech production (pp. 49–67). Tokyo, Japan: University of Tokyo Press.

Hirose, H., Gay, T., Strome, M., & Sawashima, M. (1971). Electrode insertion technique for laryngeal electromyography. *Journal of the Acoustical Society of America, 50,* 1449–1450.

Hirose, H., Kiritani, S., Ushijima, T., & Sawashima, M. (1978). Analysis of abnormal articulatory dynamics in two dysarthric patients. *Journal of Speech and Hearing Disorders, 43,* 96–105.

Hiroto, I., Hirano, M., Toyozumi, Y., & Shin, T. (1967). Electromyographic investigation of the intrinsic laryngeal muscles related to speech sounds. *Annals of Otology, Rhinology, and Laryngology, 76,* 861–872.

Hixon, T. J. (1971a). Magnetometer recording of jaw movements during speech. *Journal of the Acoustical Society of America, 49,* 104.

Hixon, T. J. (1971b). An electromagnetic method for transducing jaw movements during speech. *Journal of the Acoustical Society of America, 49,* 603–606.

Hixon, T. J. (1972). Some new techniques for measuring the biomechanical events of speech production: One laboratory's experiences. *ASHA Reports, 7,* 68–103.

Hixon, T. J. (1973). Respiratory function in speech. In F. D. Minifie, T. J. Hixon, & F. Williams (Eds.), *Normal aspects of speech, hearing, and language* (pp. 73–125). Englewood Cliffs, NJ: Prentice-Hall.

Hixon, T. J. (1982). Speech breathing kinematics and mechanism inferences therefrom. In S. Grillner, B. Lindblom, J. Lubker, & A. Persson (Eds.), *Speech motor control* (pp. 75–93). Oxford, UK: Pergamon Press.

Hixon, T. J. & colleagues (1987). *Respiratory function in speech and song.* San Diego, CA: College-Hill Press.

Hixon, T. J., Goldman, M. D., & Mead, J. (1973). Kinematics of the chest wall during speech production: Volume displacement of the rib cage, abdomen, and lung. *Journal of Speech and Hearing Research, 16,* 78–115.

Hixon, T. J., & Hardy, J. C. (1964). Restricted mobility of the speech articulators in cerebral palsy. *Journal of Speech and Hearing Disorders, 29,* 293–306.

Hixon, T. J., Mead, J., & Goldman, M. D. (1976). Dynamics of the chest wall during speech production: Function of the thorax, rib cage, diaphragm, and abdomen. *Journal of Speech and Hearing Research, 19,* 297–356.

Hixon, T. J., & Putnam, A. H. B. (1983). Voice disorders in relation to respiratory kinematics. *Seminars in Speech and Language, 4,* 217–231.

Hixon, T. J., Putnam, A. H. B., & Sharp, J. T. (1983). Speech production with flaccid paralysis of the rib cage, diaphragm, and abdomen. *Journal of Speech and Hearing Disorders, 48,* 315–327.

Hixon, T. J., Siebens, A. A., & Minifie, F. D. (1969). An EMG electrode for the diaphragm. *Journal of the Acoustical Society of America, 46,* 1588–1590.

Hodge, M. M., & Rochet, A. P. (1989). Characteristics of speech breathing in young women. *Journal of Speech and Hearing Research, 32,* 466–480.

Hoit, J. D., & Hixon, T. J. (1986). Body type and speech breathing. *Journal of Speech and Hearing Research, 29,* 313–324.

Hoit, J. D., & Hixon, T. J. (1987). Age and speech breathing. *Journal of Speech and Hearing Research, 30,* 351–366.

Hoit, J. D., Hixon, T. J., Altman, M. E., & Morgan, W. J. (1989). Speech breathing in women. *Journal of Speech and Hearing Research, 32,* 353–365.

Hoit, J. D., Hixon, T. J., Watson, P. J., & Morgan, W. J. (1990). Speech breathing in children and adolescents. *Journal of Speech and Hearing Research, 33,* 51–69.

Hollis, L. I., & Harrison, E. (1970). An improved surface electrode for monitoring myopotentials. *American Journal of Occupational Therapy, 24,* 28–30.

Holst, T., Warren, P., & Nolan, F. (1995). Categorising [s], [ʃ] and intermediate electropalatographic patterns: Neural networks and other approaches. *European Journal of Disorders of Communication, 30,* 161–174.

Holzrichter, J. F., Burnett, G. C., Ng, L. C., & Lea, W. A. (1998). Speech articulator measurements using low power EM-wave sensors. *Journal of the Acoustical Society of America, 103,* 622–625.

Hoole, P., & Nguyen, N. (1996). Electromagnetic articulography in coarticulation research. In W. J. Hardcastle & N. Hewlett (Eds.), *Instrumental studies of coarticulation.* London, UK: Cambridge University Press.

Hoole, P., Nguyen-Trong, N., & Hardcastle, W. (1993). A comparative investigation of coarticulation in fricatives: Electropalatographic, electromagnetic, and acoustic data. *Language and Speech, 36,* 235–260.

Hoole, P., Ziegler, W., Hartmann, E., & Hardcastle, W. (1989). Parallel electropalatographic and acoustic measures of fricatives. *Clinical Linguistics and Phonetics, 3,* 59–69.

Horiguchi, S., & Bell-Berti, F. (1987). The Velotrace: A device for monitoring velar position. *Cleft Palate Journal, 24,* 104–111.

Horn, H., Göz, G., Bacher, M., Müllauer, M., Kretschmar, J., & Axmann-Krcmar, D. (1997). Reliability of electromagnetic articulography recording during speaking sequences. *European Journal of Orthodontics, 19,* 647–655.

Hough, M. S., & Klich, R. J. (1998). Lip EMG activity during vowel production in apraxia of speech: Phrase context and word length effects. *Journal of Speech, Language, and Hearing Research, 41,* 786–801.

Howard, S. (1993). Articulatory constraints on a phonological system: A case study of cleft palate speech. *Clinical Linguistics and Phonetics, 7,* 299–317.

Howard, S. (1995). Intransigent articulation disorder: Using electropalatography to assess and remediate misarticulated fricatives. In M. Perkins & S. Howard (Eds.), *Case studies in clinical linguistics* (pp. 39–64). San Diego, CA: Singular Publishing Group.

Howard, S., & Pickstone, C. (1995). Cleft palate: perceptual and instrumental analyses of a phonological system. In M. Perkins & S. Howard (Eds.), *Case studies in clinical linguistics* (pp. 65–90). San Diego, CA: Singular Publishing Group.

Howard, S., & Varley, R. (1995a). Acquired speech disorder: differential diagnosis using perceptual and instrumental analyses. In M. Perkins & S. Howard (Eds.), *Case studies in clinical linguistics* (pp. 212–244). San Diego, CA: Singular Publishing Group.

Howard, S., & Varley, R. (1995b). Using electropalatography to treat severe acquired apraxia of speech. *European Journal of Disorders of Communication, 30,* 246–255.

Huntington, D. A., Harris, K. S., & Sholes, G. N. (1968). An electromyographic study of consonant articulation in hearing-impaired and normal speakers. *Journal of Speech and Hearing Research, 11,* 147–158.

Imai, S., & Michi, K. (1992). Articulatory function after resection of the tongue and floor of the mouth: Palatometric and perceptual evaluation. *Journal of Speech and Hearing Research, 35,* 68–78.

Irwin, J. V., & Becklund, O. (1953). Norms for maximum repetitive rates for certain sounds established with the Sylrater. *Journal of Speech and Hearing Disorders, 18,* 149–160.

Irwin, O. (1957). Correct status of a third set of consonants in the speech of cerebral palsied children. *Cerebral Palsy Review, 18,* 17–20.

Isshiki, N., & Snidecor, J. C. (1965). Air intake and usage in esophageal speech. *Acta Oto-Laryngologica, 59*, 559–573.

Iwarsson, J., & Sundberg, J. (1998). Effects of lung volume on vertical larynx position during phonation. *Journal of Voice, 12*, 159–165.

Jack, F., & Gibbon, F. (1995). Electropalatography in the study of tongue movement during eating and swallowing (a novel procedure for measuring texture-related behaviour). *International Journal of Food Science Technology, 30*, 415–423.

Jäger, L., Günther, E., Gauger, J., Nitz, W., Kastenbauer, E., & Reiser, M. (1996). Funktionelle MRT des Pharynx bei obstruktiver Schlafapnoe (OSA) mit schnellen 2D-FLASH-Sequenzen. *Radiologe, 36*, 245–253.

James, A. E., Jr. (1983). Computed tomographic imaging by nuclear magnetic resonance. In J. T. Littleton & M. L. Durizch (Eds.), *Sectional imaging methods: A comparison* (pp. 67–79). Baltimore, MD: University Park Press.

Jedeikin, R., & Olsfanger, D. (1990). The AR – 8800—A new impedance pneumograph (plethysmograph) respiratory monitor. *Biomedical Instrumentation and Technology, 24*, 127–129.

Jones, W., & Hardcastle, W. J. (1995). New developments in EPG3 software. *European Journal of Disorders of Communication, 30*, 183–192.

Judson, L. S., & Weaver, A. T. (1965). *Voice science* (2nd ed.). New York: Appleton-Century-Crofts.

Kaburagi, T., & Honda, M. (1994). An ultrasonic method for monitoring tongue shape and the position of a fixed point on the tongue surface. *Journal of the Acoustical Society of America, 95*, 2268–2270.

Kaburagi, T., & Honda, M. (1996). A model of articulator trajectory formation based on the motor tasks of vocal-tract shapes. *Journal of the Acoustical Society of America, 99*, 3154–3170.

Katz, W., Machetanz, J., Orth, U., & Schönle, P. (1990). A kinematic analysis of anticipatory coarticulation in the speech of anterior aphasic subjects using electromagnetic articulography. *Brain and Language, 38*, 555–575.

Katz, W. F., & Verma, S. (1994). Kinematic evidence for compensatory articulation by normal and nonfluent aphasic speakers. *Brain and Language, 47*, 357–360.

Keller, E. (1987a). Factors underlying tongue articulation in speech. *Journal of Speech and Hearing Research, 30*, 223–229.

Keller, E. (1987b). Mesures ultrasoniques des mouvements du dos de la langue en production de la parole: Aspects cliniques. *Folia Phoniatrica, 39*, 51–60.

Keller, E., & Ostry, D. J. (1983). Computerized measurement of tongue dorsum movements with pulsed-echo ultrasound. *Journal of the Acoustical Society of America, 73*, 1309–1315.

Kelsey, C. A., Hixon, T. J., & Minifie, F. D. (1969). Ultrasonic measurement of lateral wall displacement. *IEEE Transactions on Bio-Medical Engineering, BME – 16*, 143–147.

Kelsey, C. A., Woodhouse, R. J., & Minifie, F. D. (1969). Ultrasonic observations of coarticulation in the pharynx. *Journal of the Acoustical Society of America, 46*, 1016–1018.

Kelso, J. A. S., Tuller, B., Vatikiotis-Bateson, E., & Fowler, C. A. (1984). Functionally specific articulatory cooperation following jaw perturbations during speech: Evidence for coordinative structures. *Journal of the Experimental Psychology: Human Perception and Performance, 10*, 812–832.

Kelso, J. A. S., Vatikiotis-Bateson, E., Saltzman, E. L., & Kay, B. (1985). A qualitative dynamic analysis of reiterant speech production: Phase portraits, kinematics, and dynamic modeling. *Journal of the Acoustical Society of America, 77*, 266–280.

Kempster, G., Preston, J., Mack, R., & Larson, C. (1987). A preliminary investigation relating laryngeal muscle activity to changes in EGG waveforms. In T. Baer, C. Sasaki, & K. S. Harris (Eds.), *Laryngeal function in phonation and respiration* (pp. 339–348). San Diego: Singular Publishing Group.

Kennedy, J. G., III, & Abbs, J. H. (1979). Anatomical studies of the perioral motor system: Foundation for studies in speech physiology. In N. J. Lass (Ed.), *Speech and language: Advances in basic research and practice* (pp. 211–270). New York: Academic Press.

Kent, R. D. (1972). Some considerations in the cinefluorographic analysis of tongue movement during speech. *Phonetica, 26*, 16–32.

Kent, R. D., Adams, S. G., & Turner, G. S. (1996). Models of speech production. In N. J. Lass (Ed.), *Principles of experimental phonetics* (pp. 3–45). St. Louis, MO: Mosby.

Kent, R. D., Kent, J. F., & Rosenbek, J. C. (1987). Maximum performance tests of speech production. *Journal of Speech and Hearing Disorders, 52*, 367–387.

Kent, R. D., & Moll, K. L. (1972). Cinefluorographic analyses of selected lingual consonants. *Journal of Speech and Hearing Research, 15*, 453–473.

Kent, R. D., & Netsell, R. (1971). Effects of stress contrasts on certain articulatory parameters. *Phonetica, 24*, 23–44.

Kent, R. D., Sufit, R. L., Rosenbek, J. C., Kent, J. F., Weismer, G., Martin, R. E., & Brooks, B. R. (1991). Speech deterioration in amyotrophic lateral sclerosis: A case study. *Journal of Speech and Hearing Research, 34*, 1269–1275.

Kewley-Port, D. (1973). Computer processing of EMG signals at Haskins Laboratories. *Haskins Laboratories Status Report on Speech Research, SR – 33*, 173–184.

Kewley-Port, D. (1977). EMG signal processing for speech research. *Haskins Laboratories Status Report on Speech Research, SR – 50*, 123–146.

Khalafalla, A. S. (1970). Thoracic impedance measurement of respiration. In R. D. Allison (Ed.), *Basic factors in bioelectric impedance measurements of cardiac output, lung volumes, and the cerebral circulation* (pp. 52–77). Pittsburgh, PA: Instrument Society of America.

Kiritani, S., Itoh, K., & Fujimura, O. (1975). Tongue-pellet tracking by a computer-controlled x-ray microbeam system. *Journal of the Acoustical Society of America, 57*, 1516–1520.

Kiritani, S., Kakita, K., & Shibata, S. (1977). Dynamic palatography. In M. Sawashima & F. S. Cooper (Eds.), *Dynamic aspects of speech production* (pp. 159–168). Tokyo, Japan: University of Tokyo Press.

Kiritani, S., Tateno, Y., Iinuma, T., & Sawashima, M. (1977). Computer tomography of the vocal tract. In M. Sawashima & F. S. Cooper (Eds.), *Dynamic aspects of speech production* (pp. 203–206). Tokyo, Japan: University of Tokyo Press.

Kohler, K. (1976). The instability of word-final alveolar plosives in German: An electropalatographic investigation. *Phonetica, 33*, 1–30.

Kollia, H. B., Gracco, V. L., & Harris, K. S. (1995). Articulatory organization of mandibular, labial, and velar movements during speech. *Journal of the Acoustical Society of America, 98*, 1313–1324.

Konczak, J., Ackermann, H., Hertrich, I., Spieker, S., & Dichgans, J. (1997). Control of repetitive lip and finger movements in Parkinson's disease: Influence of external timing signals and simultaneous execution on motor performance. *Movement Disorders, 12*, 665–676.

Konno, K., & Mead, J. (1967). Measurement of the separate volume changes of rib cage and abdomen during breathing. *Journal of Applied Physiology, 22*, 407–422.

Koppenburg, P., Leidig, E., Bacher, M., & Dausch-Neumann, D. (1988). Die Darstellung von Lage und Beweglichkeit der Zunge bei Neugeborenen mit oralen Spaltefehlbildungen durch transorale Ultraschallsonographie. *Deutsche Zahnärztliche Zeitschrift, 43*, 806–809.

Kotby, M. N., Fadly, E., Madkour, O., Barakah, M., Khidr, A., Alloush, T., & Saleh, M. (1992). Electromyography and neruography in neurolaryngology. *Journal of Voice, 6*, 159–187.

Koufman, J. A., & Walker, F. O. (1998). Laryngeal electromyography in clinical practice: Indications, techniques, and interpretation. *Phonoscope, 1*, 57–70.

Kozhevnikov, V. A., Granstrem, M. P., Kuzmin, Y. I., Shupliakov, V. S., Vencov, A. V., Borozdin, A. N., Gerasimov, A. A., & Zhukov, S. J. (1968). System of devices for articulatory and acoustic study of continuous speech. *Zeitschrift für Phonetik, 21*, 123–128.

Kreul, E. J. (1972). Neuromuscular control examination (NMC) for parkinsonism: Vowel prolongations and diadochokinetic and reading rates. *Journal of Speech and Hearing Research, 15*, 72–83.

Kubicek, W. G., Kinnen, E., & Edin, A. (1964). Calibration of an impedance pneumograph. *Journal of Applied Physiology, 19*, 557–560.

Kuehn, D. P., Folkins, J. W., & Cutting, C. B. (1982). Relationships between muscle activity and velar position. *Cleft Palate Journal, 19*, 325–335.

Kuehn, D. P., Reich, A. R., & Jordan, J. E. (1980). A cineradiographic study of chin marker positioning: Implications for the strain gauge transduction of jaw movement. *Journal of the Acoustical Society of America, 67*, 1825–1827.

Kuehn, D. P., & Tomblin, J. B. (1977). A cineradiographic investigation of children's w/r substitutions. *Journal of Speech and Hearing Disorders, 42*, 462–473.

Kuzmin, Y. I. (1962). Mobile palatography as a tool for acoustic study of speech sounds. *Proceedings of the Fourth International Congress of Acoustics* (G35). Copenhagen, Denmark.

Kwok, W., Wiegand, L., Channin, D. S., & Wiegand, D. A. (1994). Development of the bi-directional ultrasound system for base of tongue imaging. *Computers in Biology and Medicine, 24*, 295–304.

Kydd, W. L., & Belt, D. A. (1964). Continuous palatography. *Journal of Speech and Hearing Disorders, 29*, 489–492.

LaBlance, G. R., & Rutherford, D. R. (1991). Respiratory dynamics and speech intelligibility in speakers with generalized dystonia. *Journal of Communication Disorders, 24*, 141–156.

Ladefoged, P. (1957). Use of palatography. *Journal of Speech and Hearing Disorders, 22*, 764–774.

Lakshminarayanan, A., Lee, S., & McCutcheon, M. (1991). MR imaging of the vocal tract during vowel production. *Journal of Magnetic Resonance Imaging, 1*, 71–76.

Lane, H., Perkell, J., Svirsky, M., & Webster, J. (1991). Changes in speech breathing following cochlear implant in postlingually deafened adults. *Journal of Speech and Hearing Research, 34*, 526–533.

Lane, H., Perkell, J., Wozniak, J., Manzella, J., Guiod, P., Matthies, M., MacCollin, M., & Vick, J. (1998). The effect of changes in hearing status on speech sound level and speech breathing: A study conducted with cochlear implant users and NF–2 patients. *Journal of the Acoustical Society of America, 104*, 3059–3069.

Langmore, S. E., & Lehman, M. E. (1994). Physiologic deficits in the orofacial system underlying dysarthria in amyotrophic lateral sclerosis. *Journal of Speech and Hearing Research, 37*, 28–37.

LaPointe, L. L., Case, J. L., & Duane, D. D. (1994). Perceptual-acoustic speech and voice characteristics of subjects with spasmodic torticollis. In J. A. Till, K. M. Yorkston, & D. R. Beukelman (Eds.), *Motor speech disorders: Advances in assessment and treatment* (pp. 57–64). Baltimore, MD: Paul H. Brookes.

Lastovka, M. Šram, F., & Sedláček, K. (1984). Elektromyographie bie funktionelle Dysphonien mit Hilfe der Oberflächenelektrode. *Folia Phoniatrica, 36*, 284–288.

Laukkanen, A.-M., Takalo, R., Vilkman, E., Nummenranta, J., & Lipponen, T. (1999). Simultaneous videofluorographic and dual-channel electroglottographic registration of the vertical laryngeal position in various phonatory tasks. *Journal of Voice, 13*, 60–71.

Leanderson, R., Persson, A., & Öhman, S. (1971). Electromyographic studies of facial muscle activity in speech. *Acta Otolaryngologica, 72*, 361–369.

Lee, L., Loudon, R. G., Jacobson, B. H., & Stuebing, R. (1993). Speech breathing in patients with lung disease. *American Review of Respiratory Disease, 147*, 1199–1206.

Leeper, H. A., Millard, K. M., Bandur, D. L., & Hudson, A. J. (1996). An investigation of deterioration of vocal function in subgroups of individuals with ALS. *Journal of Medical Speech-Language Pathology, 4*, 163–181.

Leidig, E., Koppenburg, P., & Bacher, M. (1987). Sonographische Darstellung der Zungenbeweglichkeit bei Neugeborenen mit Kiefer-Gaumen-Spalte. *Ultraschall in der Medizin, 8*, 189–191.

Lenz, M., Bongers, H., Ozdoba, C., & Skalej, M. (1989). Klinische Wertigkeit der Computertomographie beim pratherapeutischen T-Staging von orofazialen Tumoren. *Rofo Fortschritte auf dem Gebiete der Röntgenstrahlen und der neuen bildgebenden Verfahren, 151*, 138–144.

Liddell, E. G. T., and Sherrington, C. S. (1925). Recruitment and some other features of reflex inhibition. *Proceedings of the Royal Society, 97B*, 488–503.

Likeman, P. R., & Ferman, A. M. (1987). An investigation of the accommodation of the tongue to a dental appliance using electropalatography. *Journal of Dentistry, 15*, 249–252.

Lindman, D. E., & Moore, R. N. (1990). Measurement of intraoral muscle forces during functional exercises. *American Journal of Orthodontics and Dentofacial Orthopedics, 97*, 289–300.

Lippold, O. C. J. (1952). The relation between integrated action potentials in a human muscle and its isometric tension. *Journal of Physiology, 117*, 492–499.

Löfqvist, A., & Gracco, V. L. (1997). Lip and jaw kinematics in bilabial stop consonant production. *Journal of Speech, Language, and Hearing Research, 40*, 877–893.

Loudon, R. G., Lee, L., & Holcomb, B. J. (1988). Volumes and breathing patterns during speech in healthy and asthmatic subjects. *Journal of Speech and Hearing Research, 31*, 219–227.

Lubker, J. F. (1968). An electromyographic-cinefluorographic investigation of velar function during normal speech production. *Cleft Palate Journal, 5*, 1–18.

Lubker, J. F., & Morris, H. (1968). Predicting cineflurographic measures of velopharyngeal opening from lateral still x-ray films. *Journal of Speech and Hearing Research, 11*, 747–753.

Lubker, J. F., & Parris, P. J. (1970). Simultaneous measurements of intraoral pressure, force of labial contact, and labial electromyographic activity during production of the stop consonant cognates /p/ and /b/. *Journal of the Acoustical Society of America, 47*, 625–633.

Lufkin, R., Larsson, S., & Hanafee, W. (1983). Work in progress: NMR anatomy of the larynx and tongue base. *Radiology, 148*, 173–175.

Lundeen, D. J. (1950). The relationship of diadochokinesis to various speech sounds. *Journal of Speech and Hearing Disorders, 15*, 54–59.

Lundqvist, S., Karlsson, S., Lindblad, P., & Rehnberg, I. (1995). An electropalatographic and optoelectric analysis of Swedish [s] production. *Acta Odontologica Scandinavica, 53*, 372–380.

Lyndes, K. O. (1975). The application of biofeedback to functional dysphonia. *Journal of Biofeedback, 2,* 12–15.

MacMillan, A. S., & Kelemen, G. (1952). Radiography of the supraglottic speech organs. *Archives of Otolaryngology, 55,* 671–685.

MacNeilage, P. F., & Sholes, G. N. (1964). An electromyographic study of the tongue during vowel production. *Journal of Speech and Hearing Research, 7,* 209–232.

Malécot, A. (1966). Mechanical pressure as an index of "force of articulation." *Phonetica, 14,* 169–180.

Manifold, J. A., & Murdoch, B. E. (1993). Speech breathing in young adults: Effect of body type. *Journal of Speech and Hearing Research, 36,* 657–671.

Manschreck, T. C., Kalotkin, M., & Jacobson, A. M. (1980). Utility of electromyographic biological feedback in chronic stuttering: A clinical study with follow-up. *Perceptual and Motor Skills, 51,* 535–540.

Mansell, R., & Allen, R. (1970). A first report on the development of a capacitance transducer for the measurement of lip-excursion. *University of Essex Language Centre Occasional Papers, 9,* 88–115.

Marchal, A. (1987). Des clics en français? *Phonetica, 44,* 30–37.

Marchal, A. (1988a). *La palatographie.* Paris: Editions du Centre National de la Recherche Scientifique.

Marchal, A. (1988b). Coproduction: Evidence from EPG data. *Speech Communication, 7,* 287–295.

Marchal, A., & Espesser, R. (1989). L'asymetrie des appuis linguo-palatins. *Journal d'Acoustique, 2,* 53–57.

Massengill, R. (1966). Early diagnosis of abnormal palatal mobility by the use of cinefluorography. *Folia Phoniatrica, 18,* 256–260.

Maurer, D., Gröne, B. F., Landis, T., Hoch, G., & Schönle, P. W. (1993). Re-examination of the relationship between the vocal tract and the vowel sound with electromagnetic articulography (EMA) in vocalizations. *Journal of Clinical Linguistics and Phonetics, 7,* 129–143.

McCarthy, C., & De Luca, C. J. (1985). A myofeedback instrument for clinical use. *Journal for Rehabilitation Research and Development, 21,* 39–44.

McClean, M. (1973). Forward coarticulation of velar movements at marked junctural boundaries. *Journal of Speech and Hearing Research, 16,* 286–296.

McClean, M. (1977). Effects of auditory masking on lip movements for speech. *Journal of Speech and Hearing Research, 20,* 731–741.

McClean, M. D. (1987). Surface EMG recording of the perioral reflexes: Preliminary observations on stutterers and nonstutterers. *Journal of Speech and Hearing Research, 30,* 283–287.

McClean, M., Goldsmith, H., & Cerf, A. (1984). Lower-lip EMG and displacement during bilabial disfluencies in adult stutterers. *Journal of Speech and Hearing Research, 27,* 342–349.

McClean, M. D., Kroll, R. M., & Loftus, N. S. (1990). Kinematic analysis of lip closure in stutterers' fluent speech. *Journal of Speech and Hearing Research, 33,* 755–760.

McCutcheon, M. J., Fletcher, S. G., & Hasegawa, A. (1977). Video-scanning system for measurement of lip and jaw motion. *Journal of the Acoustical Society of America, 61,* 1051–1055.

McCutcheon, M. J., Smith, S. C., Stilwell, D. J., & Fletcher, S. G. (1984). Measurement of tongue position during speech using optical transducers. In L. C. Sheppard (Ed.), *Proceedings of the Third Southern Biomedical Engineering Conference* (pp. 152–155). Oxford, UK: Pergamon Press.

McDonough, J., & Johnson, K. (1997). Tamil liquids: An investigation into the basis of the contrast among five liquids in a dialect of Tamil. *Journal of the International Phonetic Association, 27,* 1–26.

McFarland, D. H., Baum, S. R., & Chabot, C. (1996). Speech compensation to structural modifications of the oral cavity. *Journal of the Acoustical Society of America, 100,* 1093–1104.

McFarland, D. H., & Lund, J. P. (1995). Modification of mastication and respiration during swallowing in the adult human. *Journal of Neurophysiology, 74,* 1509–1517.

McGlone, R. E., & Proffit, W. R. (1973). Patterns of tongue contact in normal and lisping speakers. *Journal of Speech and Hearing Research, 16,* 456–473.

McGowan, J. C., III, Hatabu, H., Yousem, D. M., Randall, P., & Kressel, H. Y. (1992). Evaluation of soft palate function with MRI: Application to the cleft palate patient. *Journal of Computer Assisted Tomography, 16,* 877–882.

McHenry, M. A., Minton, J. T., III, & Wilson, R. L. (1994). Increasing the efficiency of articulatory force testing of adults with traumatic brain injury. In J. A. Till, K. M. Yorkston, & D. R. Beukelman (Eds.), *Motor speech disorders: Advances in assessment and treatment* (pp. 135–146). Baltimore, MD: Paul H. Brookes.

McKenna, K., Jabour, B., Lufkin, R., & Hanafee, W. (1990). Magnetic resonance imaging of the tongue and oropharynx. *Topics in Magnetic Resonance Imaging, 2,* 49–59.

McKinnon, G. C. (1993). Ultrafast interleaved gradient echo-planar imaging on a standard scanner. *Magnetic Resonance in Medicine, 30,* 690–616.

McNutt, J. C. (1977). Oral sensory and motor behaviors of children with /s/ or /r/ misarticulations. *Journal of Speech and Hearing Research, 20,* 694–703.

McWilliams, B. J., & Bradley, D. (1964). A rating scale for evaluation of video tape recorded x-ray studies. *Cleft Palate Journal, 1,* 88–94.

McWilliams, B. J., & Girdany, B. (1964). The use of Televex in cleft palate research. *Cleft Palate Journal, 1,* 398–401.

Mead, J., Peterson, N., Grimby, G., & Mead, J. (1967). Pulmonary ventilation measured from body surface movements. *Science, 156,* 1383–1384.

Michi, K., Suzuki, N., Yamashita, Y., & Imai, S. (1986). Visual training and correction of articulation disorders by use of dynamic palatography: Serial observation in a case of cleft palate. *Journal of Speech and Hearing Disorders, 51,* 226–238.

Michi, K., Yamashita, Y., Imai, S., & Ohno, K. (1991). Results of treatment of speech disorders in cleft palate patients: Patients obtaining adequate velopharyngeal function. In G. Pfeifer (Ed.), *Craniofacial abnormalities and clefts of the lip, alveolus, and palate* (pp. 419–423). New York: Thieme Medical Publishers.

Michi, K., Yamashita, Y., Imai, S., Suzuki, N., & Yoshida, H. (1993). Role of visual feedback treatment for defective /s/ sounds in patients with cleft palate. *Journal of Speech and Hearing Research, 36,* 277–285.

Milledge, J. S., & Stott, F. D. (1977). Inductive plethysmography —A new respiratory transducer. *Journal of Physiology, 267,* 4P–5P.

Milutinovic, Z., Lat'ovka, M., Vohradník, M., & Jansevic, S. (1988). EMG study of hyperkinetic phonation using surface electrodes. *Folia Phoniatrica, 40,* 21–30.

Minifie, F. D., Abbs, J. H., Tarlow, A., & Kwaterski, M. (1974). EMG activity within the pharynx during speech production. *Journal of Speech and Hearing Research, 17,* 497–504.

Minifie, F. D., Kelsey, C. A., Zagzebski, J. A., & King, T. W. (1971). Ultrasonic scans of the dorsal surface of the tongue. *Journal of the Acoustical Society of America, 49,* 1857–1860.

Miyawaki, K. (1972). A preliminary study of American English /r/ by use of dynamic palatography. *Annual Bulletin of the Research Institute of Logopedics and Phoniatrics, 6,* 19–24.

Miyawaki, K., Kiritani, S., Tatsumi, I., & Fujimura, O. (1974). Palatographic observation of VCV articulations in Japanese.

Annual Bulletin of the Research Institute of Logopedics and Phoniatrics, 8, 51–58.

Moll, K. L. (1960). Cinefluorographic techniques in speech research. *Journal of Speech and Hearing Research, 3,* 227–241.

Moll, K. L. (1965). Photographic and radiographic procedures in speech research. *ASHA Reports, 1,* 129–139.

Moore, C. A. (1992). The correspondence of vocal tract images with volumes obtained from magnetic resonance images. *Journal of Speech and Hearing Research, 35,* 1009–1023.

Moore, C. A., Smith, A., & Ringel, R. L. (1988). Task-specific organization of activity in human jaw muscles. *Journal of Speech and Hearing Research, 31,* 670–680.

Morgan, C. L. (1983). *Basic principles of computed tomography.* Baltimore, MD: University Park Press.

Morgan Barry, R. A. (1989). EPG from square one: An overview of electropalatography as an aid to therapy. *Clinical Linguistics and Phonetics, 3,* 81–91.

Morgan Barry, R. (1993). Measuring segmental timing in pathological speech using electropalatography. *Clinical Linguistics and Phonetics, 7,* 275–283.

Morgan Barry, R. (1995a). Acquired dysarthria: A segmental phonological, prosodic and electropalatographic investigation of intelligibility. In M. Perkins & S. Howard (Eds.), *Case studies in clinical linguistics* (pp. 181–211). San Diego, CA: Singular Publishing Group.

Morgan Barry, R. (1995b). The relationship between dysarthria and verbal dyspraxia in children: A comparative study using profiling and instrumental analyses. *Clinical Linguistics and Phonetics, 9,* 277–309.

Morgan Barry, R. (1995c). A comparative study of the relationship between dysarthria and verbal dyspraxia in adults and children. *Clinical Linguistics and Phonetics, 9,* 311–332.

Morgan Barry, R. A. (1995d). EPG treatment of a child with the Worster-Drought syndrome. *European Journal of Disorders of Communication, 30,* 256–263.

Morrish, K. A., Stone, M. L., Shawker, T. H., & Sonies, B. C. (1985). Distinguishability of tongue shape during vowel production. *Journal of Phonetics, 13,* 189–203.

Morrish, K. A., Stone, M. L., Sonies, B. C., Kurtz, D., & Shawker, T. H. (1984). Characterization of tongue shape. *Ultrasonic Imaging, 6,* 37–47.

Moses, E. R., Jr. (1939). Palatography and speech improvement. *Journal of Speech Disorders, 4,* 103–114.

Moses, E. R., Jr. (1940). A brief history of palatography. *Quarterly Journal of Speech, 26.*

Moses, E. R., Jr. (1964). *Phonetics: History and interpretation.* Englewood Cliffs, NJ: Prentice-Hall.

Müller, E. M., & Abbs, J. H. (1979). Strain gauge tranduction of lip and jaw motion in the midsagittal plane: Refinement of a prototype system. *Journal of the Acoustical Society of America, 65,* 481–486.

Munhall, K. G. (1985). An examination of intra-articulator relative timing. *Journal of the Acoustical Society of America, 78,* 1548–1553.

Murdoch, B. E., Chenery, H. J., Bowler, S., & Ingram, J. C. L. (1989). Respiratory function in Parkinson's subjects exhibiting a perceptible speech deficit: A kinematic and spirometric analysis. *Journal of Speech and Hearing Disorders, 54,* 610–626.

Murdoch, B. E., Chenery, H. J., Stokes, P. D., & Hardcastle, W. J. (1991). Respiratory kinematics in speakers with cerebellar disease. *Journal of Speech and Hearing Research, 34,* 768–780.

Murdoch, B. E., & Hudson-Tennent, L. J. (1993). Speech breathing anomalies in children with dysarthria following treatment for posterior fossa tumors. *Journal of Medical Speech-Language Pathology, 1,* 107–119.

Murdoch, B. E., Killin, H., & McCaul, A. (1989). A kinematic analysis of respiratory function in a group of stutterers pre- and posttreatment. *Journal of Fluency Disorders, 14,* 323–350.

Murdoch, B. E., Theodoros, D. G., Stokes, P. D., & Chenery, H. J. (1993). Abnormal patterns of speech breathing in dysarthric speakers following severe closed head injury. *Brain Injury, 7,* 295–308.

Müssig, D. (1992). Die Sonographie—Ein Diagnostisches Mittel zur dynamischen Funktionsanalyse der Zunge. *Fortschritte Kieferorthopadie, 54,* 17–26.

Narayanan, S. S., Alwan, A. A., & Haker, K. (1995). An articulatory study of fricative consonants using magnetic resonance imaging. *Journal of the Acoustical Society of America, 98,* 1325–1347.

Narayanan, S. S., Alwan, A. A., & Haker, K. (1997). Toward articulatory-acoustic models for liquid approximants based on MRI and EPG data: Part I. The laterals. *Journal of the Acoustical Society of America, 101,* 1064–1077.

Netsell, R., & Cleeland, C. (1973). Modification of lip hypertonia in dysarthria using EMG feedback. *Journal of Speech and Hearing Disorders, 38,* 131–140.

Netsell, R., & Daniel, B. (1979). Dysarthria in adults: Physiologic approach to rehabilitation. *Archives of Physical Medicine and Rehabilitation, 60,* 502–508.

Netsell, R., Daniel, B., & Celesia, G. G. (1975). Acceleration and weakness in parkinsonian dysarthria. *Journal of Speech and Hearing Disorders, 40,* 170–178.

Nguyen, N. (1995). EPG bidimensional data reduction. *Eurpoean Journal of Disorders of Communication, 30,* 175–182.

Nguyen, N., Hoole, P., & Marchal, A. (1994). Regenerating the spectral shapes of [s] and [ʃ] from a limited set of articulatory parameters. *Journal of the Acoustical Society of America, 96,* 33–39.

Nicolaidis, K. (1994). Aspects of lingual articulation in Greek: An electropalatographic study. In I. Philippaki-Warburton, K. Nicolaidis, & M. Sifianou (Eds.), *Themes in Greek linguistics* (pp. 225–232). Amsterdam, The Netherlands: John Benjamins B.V.

Niitsu, M., Kumada, M., Campeau, N. G., Niimi, S., Riederer, S. J., & Itai, Y. (1994). Tongue displacement: Visualization with rapid tagged magnetization prepared MR imaging. *Radiology, 191,* 578–580.

O'Dwyer, N. J., Quinn, P. T., Guitar, B. E., Andrews, G., & Neilson, P. D. (1981). Procedures for verification of electrode placement in EMG studies of orofacial and mandibular muscles. *Journal of Speech and Hearing Research, 24,* 273–288.

Ohkiba, T., & Hanada, K. (1989). Adaptive functional changes in the swallowing pattern of the tonue following expansion of the maxillary dental arch in subjects with and without cleft palate. *Cleft Palate Journal, 26,* 21–30.

Ong, D., & Stone, M. (1998). Three dimensional vocal tract shapes in /r/ and /l/: A study of MRI, ultrasound, electropalatography, and acoustics. *Phonoscope, 1,* 1–13.

Ordidge, R. J., Coxon, R., Howseman, A., Chapman, B., Turner, R., Stehling, M., & Mansfield, P. (1988). Snapshot head imaging at 0.5 T using the echo planar technique. *Magnetic Resonance in Medicine, 10,* 563–571.

Ostry, D. J., Gribble, P. L., & Gracco, V. L. (1996). Coarticulation of jaw movements in speech production: Is context sensitivity in speech kinematics centrally planned? *Journal of Neuroscience, 16,* 1570–1579.

Ostry, D. J., Gribble, P. L., Levin, M. F., & Feldman, A. G. (1997). Phasic and tonic stretch reflexes in muscles with few muscle spindles: Human jaw-opener muscles. *Experimental Brain Research, 116,* 299–308.

Ostry, D. J., & Munhall, K. G. (1985). Control of rate and duration of speech movements. *Journal of the Acoustical Society of America, 77,* 640–648.

Ostry, D. J., & Munhall, K. G. (1994). Control of jaw orientation and position in mastication and speech. *Journal of Neurophysiology, 71,* 1528–1545.

Ostry, D. J., Vatikiotis-Bateson, E., & Gribble, P. L. (1997). An examination of the degrees of freedom of human jaw motion in speech and mastication. *Journal of Speech, Language, and Hearing Research, 40,* 1341–1351.

Pacela, A. F. (1966). Impedance pneumography—A survey of instrumental techniques. *Medical and Biological Engineering, 4,* 1–15.

Palmer, J. (1973). Dynamic palatometry. *Phonetica, 28,* 76–85.

Pandeli, H., Eska, J. F., Ball, M. J., & Rahilly, J. (1997). Problems of phonetic transcription: The case of the Hiberno-English slit-t. *Journal of the International Phonetic Association, 27,* 65–75.

Parsloe, R. (1998). Use of the speech pattern audiometer and the electropalatograph to explore the speech production/perception relationship in a profoundly deaf child. *International Journal of Language and Communication Disorders, 33,* 109–121.

Parush, A., & Ostry, D. J. (1986). Superior lateral pharyngeal wall movements in speech. *Journal of the Acoustical Society of America, 80,* 749–756.

Parush, A., & Ostry, D. J. (1993). Lower pharyngeal wall coarticulation in VCV syllables. *Journal of the Acoustical Society of America, 94,* 715–722.

Pawlowski, Z. (1975). Elektropalatografia (EPG). Badania doswiadczalne i kliniczne. *Otolaryngologia Polska, 29,* 265–273.

Perkell, J. S., Cohen, M. H., Svirsky, M. A., Matthies, M. L., Garabieta, I., & Jackson, M. T. T. (1992). Electromagnetic midsagittal articulometer systems for transducing speech articulatory movements. *Journal of the Acoustical Society of America, 92,* 3078–3096.

Perkell, J. S., & Oka, D. (1980). Use of an alternating magnetic field device to track midsagittal plane movements of multiple points inside the vocal tract. *Journal of the Acoustical Society of America, 67,* S92.

Perlman, A. L., Luschei, E. S., & Du Mond, C. E. (1989). Electrical activity from the superior pharyngeal constrictor during reflexive and nonreflexive tasks. *Journal of Speech and Hearing Research, 32,* 749–754.

Pinelli, P. (1992). Neurophysiology in the science of speech. *Current Opinion in Neurology and Neurosurgery, 5,* 744–755.

Platt, L. J., Andrews, G., Young, M., & Quinn, P. T. (1980). Dysarthria of adult cerebral palsy: I. Intelligibility and articulatory impairment. *Journal of Speech and Hearing Research, 23,* 28–40.

Port, D. K. (1971). The EMG data system. *Haskins Laboratories Status Report on Speech Research, SR 25/26,* 67–72.

Portnoy, R. A, & Aronson, A. E. (1982). Diadochokinetic syllable rate and regularity in normal and in spastic and ataxic dysarthric subjects. *Journal of Speech and Hearing Disorders, 47,* 324–328.

Prosek, R. A., Montgomery, A. A., Walden, B. E., & Schwartz, D. M. (1978). EMG biofeedback in the treatment of hyperfunctional voice disorders. *Journal of Speech and Hearing Disorders, 43,* 282–294.

Ptacek, P. H., Sander, E. K., Maloney, W. H., & Jackson, C. C. (1966). Phonatory and related changes with advanced age. *Journal of Speech and Hearing Research, 9,* 353–360.

Pykett, I. L., & Rzedzian, R. R. (1987). Instant images of the body by magnetic resonance. *Magnetic Resonance in Medicine, 5,* 110–115.

Rea, J. L., Templer, J. W., & Davis, W. E. (1978). Design and testing of a new electrode for laryngeal electromyography. *Archives of Otolaryngology, 104,* 685–686.

Recasens, D. (1984a). Vowel-to-vowel coarticulation in Catalan VCV sequences. *Journal of the Acoustical Society of America, 76,* 1624–1635.

Recasens, D. (1984b). Timing constraints and coarticulation: Alveolo-palatals and sequences of alveolar + [j] in Catalan. *Phonetica, 41,* 125–139.

Recasens, D. (1984c). V-to-C coarticulation in Catalan VCV sequences: An articulatory and acoustic study. *Journal of Phonetics, 12,* 61–73.

Recasens, D. (1990). The articulatory characteristics of palatal consonants. *Journal of Phonetics, 18,* 267–280.

Recasens, D. (1991a). An electropalatographic and acoustic study of consonant-to-vowel coarticulation. *Journal of Phonetics, 19,* 177–192.

Recasens, D. (1991b). On the production characteristics of apicoalveolar taps and trills. *Journal of Phonetics, 19,* 267–280.

Recasens, D., Fontdevila, J., & Pallarès, M. D. (1993). An electropalatographic study of stop consonant clusters. *Speech Communication, 12,* 335–355.

Recasens, D., Pallarès, M. D., & Fontdevila, J. (1995). Coarticulatory variability and articulatory-acoustic correlations for consonants. *European Journal of Disorders of Communication, 30,* 203–212.

Redenbaugh, M. A., & Reich, A. R. (1989). Surface EMG and related measures in normal and vocally hyperfunctional speakers. *Journal of Speech and Hearing Disorders, 54,* 68–73.

Reinicke, C., Obijou, N., & Trankmann, J. (1998). The palatal shape of upper removable appliances: Influence of the tongue position in swallowing. *Journal of Orofacial Orthopedics, 59,* 202–207.

Rieppo, P. K., & Rowlands, J. A. (1997). X-ray imaging with amorphous selenium: Theoretical feasibility of the liquid crystal light valve for radiography. *Medical Physics, 24,* 1279–1291.

Robb, M. P., Hughes, M. C., & Frese, D. J. (1985). Oral diadochokinesis in hearing-impaired adolescents. *Journal of Communication Disorders, 18,* 79–89.

Robin, D. A., Bean, C., & Folkins, J. W. (1989). Lip movement in apraxia of speech. *Journal of Speech and Hearing Research, 32,* 512–523.

Rodriquez, A. A., Ford, C. N., Bless, D. M., & Harmon, R. L. (1994). Electromyographic assessment of spasmodic dysphonia patients prior to botulinum toxin injection. *Electromyography and Clinical Neurophysiology, 34,* 403–407.

Rokkaku, M., Hashimoto, K., Imaizumi, S., Niimi, S., & Kiritani, S. (1986). Measurements of the three-dimensional shape of the vocal tract based on the magnetic resonance imaging technique. *Annual Bulletin of the Research Institute of Logopedics and Phoniatrics, 20,* 47–54.

Rolfe, P. (1971). A magnetometer respiration monitor for use with premature babies. *Bio-Medical Engineering, 6,* 402–404.

Rome, J. A. (1964). An artificial palate for continous analysis of speech. *Quarterly Progress Report, Research Laboratory of Electronics* (MIT), *74,* 190–191.

Rosenfield, D. B., Viswanath, N., Herbrich, K. E., & Nudelman, H. B. (1991). Evaluation of the speech motor control system in amyotrophic lateral sclerosis. *Journal of Voice, 5,* 224–230.

Roth, K. (1984). *NMR-tomography and -spectroscopy in medicine: An introduction.* New York: Springer-Verlag.

Rouco, A., & Recasens, D. (1996). Reliability of electromagnetic midsagittal articulometry and electropalatography data acquired simultaneously. *Journal of the Acoustical Society of America, 100,* 3384–3389.

Rousselot, P. J. (1897–1901). *Principes de phonétique expérimentale* (Vol. 1). Paris, France: Welter.

Rubow, R. T., Rosenbek, J. C., Collins, M., & Celesia, G. C. (1984). Reduction in hemifacial spasm and dysarthria following EMG feedback. *Journal of Speech and Hearing Disorders, 49,* 26–33.

Ryan, W. J., & Hawkins, C. F. (1976). Ultrasonic measurement of lateral pharyneal wall movement at the velopharyngeal port. *Cleft Palate Journal, 13,* 156–164.

Sackner, J. D., Nixon, A. J., Davis, B., Atkins, N., & Sackner, M. A. (1980). Non-invasive measurement of ventilation during exercise using a respiratory inductive plethysmograph. *American Review of Respiratory Disease, 122,* 867–871.

Sackner, M. A. (1980). Monitoring of ventilation without a physical connection to the airway. In M. A. Sackner (Ed.), *Diagnostic techniques in pulmonary disease* (Part I, pp. 503–537). New York: Marcel Dekker.

Sawashima, M., & Kiritani, S. (1985). Electropalatographic patterns of Japanese /d/ and /r/ in intervocalic position. *Annual Bulletin of the Research Institute of Logopedics and Phoniatrics, 19,* 1–6.

Sawashima, M., Sato, M., Funasaka, S., & Totsuka, G. (1958). Electromyographic study of the human larynx and its clinical application. *Japanese Journal of Otology, 61,* 1357–1364.

Scheier, M. (1897). Über die Verwertung der Röntgenstrahlen in der Rhino-Laryngologie. *Archiv für Laryngologie und Rhinologie, 6,* 57–66.

Schliephake, H., Schmelzeisen, R., Schönweiler, R., Schneller, T., & Altenbernd, C. (1998). Speech, deglutition and life quality after intraoral tumour resection: A prospective study. *International Journal of Oral and Maxillofacial Surgery, 27,* 99–105.

Schönle, P. W. (1988). *Elektromagnetische Artikulographie.* Berlin, Germany: Springer-Verlag.

Schönle, P. W., Gräbe, K., Wenig, P., Höhne, J., Schrader, J., & Conrad, B. (1987). Electromagnetic articulography: Use of alternating magnetic fields for tracking movements of multiple points inside and outside the vocal tract. *Brain and Language, 31,* 26–35.

Schönle, P. W., Hoch, G., & Gröne, B. (1991). A motor physiological approach to disorders of fluency with electromagnetic articulography. In H. R. Peters, W. Hulstijn, & C. W. Starkweather (Eds.), *Speech motor control and stuttering* (pp. 243–248). Amsterdam, The Netherlands: Elsevier.

Schönle, P. W., Müller, C., & Wenig, P. (1989). Echtzeitanalyse von orofacialen Bewegungen mit Hilfe der elektromagnetische Articulographie. *Biomedizinische Technik, 34,* 126–130.

Schönle, P. W., Wenig, P., Schrader, J., Gräber, K., Bröckmann, E., & Conrad, B. (1983). Ein elektromagnetisches Verfahren zur simultanen Registrierung von Bewegungen im Bereich des Lippen-, Unterkiefer- und Zugensystems. *Biomedizinische Technik, 28,* 263–267.

Schuette, W. H., Shawker, T. H., & Whitehouse, W. C. (1978). An integrated television and real-time ultrasonic imaging system. *Journal of Clinical Ultrasound, 6,* 271–272.

Schulman, R. (1989). Articulatory dynamics of loud and normal speech. *Journal of the Acoustical Society of America, 85,* 295–312.

Scripture, E. W. (1902). *The elements of experimental phonetics.* New York: Scribner's.

Selbie, R. D., Fletcher, M., Arestis, N., White, R., Duncan, A., Helms, P., & Duffty, P. (1997). Respiratory function parameters in infants using inductive plethysmography. *Medical Engineering and Physics, 19,* 501–511.

Shaiman, S. (1989). Kinematic and electromyographic responses to perturbation of the jaw. *Journal of the Acoustical Society of America, 86,* 78–88.

Shaiman, S., Adams, S. G., & Kimelman, M. D. Z. (1997). Velocity profiles of lip protrusion across changes in speaking rate. *Journal of Speech, Language, and Hearing Research, 40,* 144–158.

Shanks, S. J. (1970). Effect of aging upon rapid syllable repetition. *Perceptual and Motor Skills, 30,* 687–690.

Shawker, T. H., & Sonies, B. C. (1984). Tongue movement during speech: A real-time ultrasound evaluation. *Journal of Clinical Ultrasound, 12,* 125–133.

Shawker, T. H., & Sonies, B. C. (1985). Ultrasound biofeedback for speech training: Instrumentation and preliminary results. *Investigative Radiology, 20,* 90–93.

Shawker, T. H., Sonies, B. C., & Stone, M. L. (1984). Soft tissue anatomy of the tongue and floor of the mouth: An ultrasound demonstration. *Brain and Language, 21,* 335–350.

Shawker, T. H., Sonies, B., Stone, M., & Baum, B. J. (1983). Real-time ultrasound visualization of tongue movement during swallowing. *Journal of Clinical Ultrasound, 11,* 485–490.

Shibata, S., Ino, A., Yamashita, S., Hiki, S., Kiritani, S., & Sawashima, M. (1978). A new portable type unit for electropalatography. *Annual Bulletin of the Research Institute of Logopedics and Phoniatrics, 12,* 5–10.

Shipp, T., Deatsch, W. W., & Robertson, K. (1968). A technique for electromyographic assessment of deep neck muscle activity. *Laryngoscope, 78,* 418–432.

Shipp, T., Fishman, B. V., Morrissey, P., & McGlone, R. E. (1970). Method and control of laryngeal emg electrode placement in man. *Journal of the Acoustical Society of America, 48,* 429–430.

Shohara, H. H., & Hanson, C. (1941). Palatography as an aid to the improvement of articulatory movements. *Journal of Speech and Hearing Disorders, 6,* 115–124.

Siegler, S., Hayes, R., Nocolella, D., & Fielding, A. (1991). A technique to investigate the three-dimensional kinesiology of the human temporomandibular joint. *Journal of Prosthetic Dentistry, 65,* 833–839.

Sigurd, B. (1973). Maximum rate and minimal duration of repeated syllables. *Language and Speech, 16,* 373–395.

Skolnick, M. L. (1970). Videofluoroscopic examination of the velopharyngeal portal during phonation in lateral and base projections—A new technique for studying the mechanics of closure. *Cleft Palate Journal, 7,* 803–816.

Skolnick, M. L., Zagzebski, J. A., & Watkin, K. L. (1975). Two-dimensional ultrasonic demonstration of lateral pharyngeal wall movement in real time—A preliminary report. *Cleft Palate Journal, 12,* 299–303.

Smith, A. (1992). The control of orofacial movements in speech. *Critical Reviews in Oral Biology and Medicine, 3,* 233–267.

Smith, A., & Goffman, L. (1998). Stability and patterning of speech movement sequences in children and adults. *Journal of Speech, Language, and Hearing Research, 41,* 18–30.

Smith, A., Moore, C. A., McFarland, D. H., & Weber, C. M. (1985). Reflex responses of human lip muscles to mechanical stimulation during speech. *Journal of Motor Behavior, 17,* 148–167.

Smith, C. (1934). Action potentials from single motor units in voluntary contaction. *American Journal of Physiology, 108,* 629–638.

Snidecor, J. C., & Isshiki, N. (1965). Air volume and air flow relationships of six male esophageal speakers. *Journal of Speech and Hearing Disorders, 30,* 205–216.

Solomon, N. P., & Hixon, T. J. (1993). Speech breathing in Parkinson's disease. *Journal of Speech and Hearing Research, 36,* 294–310.

Sonies, B. C. (1982). Oral imaging systems: A review and clinical applications. *Journal of the National Student Speech-Language-Hearing Association, 10,* 30–43.

Sonies, B. C., Baum, B. J., & Shawker, T. H. (1984). Tongue motion in the elderly: Initial *in situ* observations. *Journal of Gerontology, 39,* 279–283.

Sonies, B. C., Shawker, T. H., Hall, T. E., Gerber, L. H., & Leighton, S. B. (1981). Ultrasonic visualization of tongue motion during speech. *Journal of the Acoustical Society of America, 70,* 683–686.

Sonies, B. C., Stone, M. L., & Shawker, T. H. (1984). Speech and swallowing in the elderly. *Gerodontology, 3,* 115–123.

Sonninen, A. (1968). The external frame function in the control of pitch in the human voice. *Annals of the New York Academy of Sciences, 155,* 68–90.

Sonninen, A., & Hurme, P. (1998). Vocal fold strain and vocal pitch in singing: Radiographic observations of singers and nonsingers. *Journal of Voice, 12,* 274–286.

Sonoda, Y., & Wanishi, S. (1982). New optical method for recording lip and jaw movements. *Journal of the Acoustical Society of America, 72,* 700–704.

Sperry, E. E., Hillman, R. E., & Perkell, J. S. (1994). The use of inductance plethysmography to assess respiratory function in a patient with vocal nodules. *Journal of Medical Speech-Language Pathology, 2,* 137–145.

Sperry, E. E., & Klich, R. J. (1992). Speech breathing in senescent and younger women during oral reading. *Journal of Speech and Hearing Research, 35,* 1246–1255.

Stagg, D., Goldman, M., & Newsom-Davis, J. (1978). Computer-aided measurement of breath volume and time components using magnetometers. *Journal of Applied Physiology, 44,* 623–633.

Stathopoulos, E. T., Hoit, J. D., Hixon, T. J., Watson, P. J., & Solomon, N. P. (1991). Respiratory and laryngeal function during whispering. *Journal of Speech and Hearing Research, 34,* 761–767.

Stemple, J. C., Weiler, E., Whitehead, W., & Komray, R. (1980). Electromyographic biofeedback training with patients exhibiting a hyperfunctional voice disorder. *Laryngoscope, 90,* 471–476.

Stetson, R. H. (1928). Motor phonetics. *Archive Néerlandaise de Phonétique Expérimentale, 3,* 1–216.

Stetson, R. H. (1951). *Motor phonetics.* Amsterdam, The Netherlands: North-Holland.

Stick, S. M., Ellis, E., LeSouëf, P. N., & Sly, P. D. (1992). Validation of respiratory inductance plethysmography ("Respitrace") for the measurement of tidal breathing parameters in newborns. *Pediatric Pulmonology, 14,* 187–191.

St. Louis, K., Clausell, P. L., Thompson, M., & Rife, C. C. (1982). Preliminary investigation of EMG biofeedback induced relaxation with a preschool aged stutterer. *Perceptual and Motor Skills, 55,* 195–199.

Stone, M. (1990). A three-dimensional model of tongue movement based on ultrasound and x-ray microbeam data. *Journal of the Acoustical Society of America, 87,* 2207–2217.

Stone, M. (1991). Imaging the tongue and vocal tract. *British Journal of Disorders of Communication, 26,* 11–23.

Stone, M., & Davis, E. P. (1995). A head and transducer support system for making ultrasound images of tongue/jaw movement. *Journal of the Acoustical Society of America, 98,* 3107–3112.

Stone, M., Faber, A., Raphael, L., & Shawker, T. (1992). Cross-sectional tongue shape and linguopalatal contact patterns in [s], [ʃ], and [l]. *Journal of Phonetics, 20,* 253–270.

Stone, M., & Lundberg, A. (1996). Three-dimensional tongue surface shapes of English consonants and vowels. *Journal of the Acoustical Society of America, 99,* 3728–3737.

Stone, M., Morrish, K., Sonies, B., & Shawker, T. (1987). Tongue curvature: A model of shape during vowels. *Folia Phoniatrica, 39,* 302–315.

Stone, M., Shawker, T. H., Talbot, T. L., & Rich, A. H. (1988). Cross-sectional tongue shape during the production of vowels. *Journal of the Acoustical Society of America, 83,* 1586–1596.

Stone, M., Sonies, B. C., Shawker, T. H., Weiss, G., & Nadel, L. (1983). Analysis of real-time ultrasound images of tongue configuration using a grid-digitizing system. *Journal of Phonetics, 11,* 207–218.

Story, B. H., Titze, I. R., & Hoffman, E. A. (1996). Vocal tract area functions from magnetic resonance imaging. *Journal of the Acoustical Society of America, 100,* 537–554.

Story, B. H., Titze, I. R., & Hoffman, E. A. (1998). Vocal tract area functions for an adult female speaker based on volumetric imaging. *Journal of the Acoustical Society of America, 104,* 471–487.

Story, R. S., Alfonso, P. J., & Harris, K. S. (1996). Pre- and post-treatment comparison of the kinematics of the fluent speech of persons who stutter. *Journal of Speech and Hearing Research, 39,* 991–1005.

Strother, C. R., & Kriegman, L. S. (1943). Diadochokinesis in stutterers and non-stutterers. *Journal of Speech Disorders, 8,* 323–335.

Subtelny, J. (1961). Roentgenography applied to the study of speech. In S. Pruzansky (Ed.), *Congenital anomalies of the face and associated structures* (pp. 309–326). Springfield, IL: Charles C Thomas.

Subtelny, J., Li, W., Whitehead, R., & Subtelny, J. D. (1989). Cephalometric and cineradiographic study of deviant resonance in hearing-impaired speakers. *Journal of Speech and Hearing Disorders, 54,* 249–265.

Subtelny, J., Oya, N., & Subtelny, J. D. (1972). Cineradiographic study of sibilants. *Folia Phoniatrica, 24,* 30–50.

Sudo, M., Kiritani, S., & Sawashima, M. (1983). The articulation of Japanese intervocalic /d/ and /r/: An electropalatographic study. *Annual Bulletin of the Research Institute of Logopedics and Phoniatrics, 17,* 55–59.

Sugishita, M., Konno, K., Kabe, S., Yunoki, K., Togashi, O., & Kawamura, M. (1987). Electropalatographic analysis of apraxia of speech in a left hander and in a right hander. *Brain, 110,* 1393–1417.

Sulter, A. M., Miller, D. G., Wolf, R. F., Schutte, H. K., Wit, H. P., & Mooyaart, E. L. (1992). On the relation between the dimensions and resonance characteristics of the vocal tract: A study with MRI. *Magnetic Resonance Imaging, 10,* 365–373.

Sundberg, J., Johansson, C., Wilbrand, H., & Ytterbergh, C. (1987). From sagittal distance to area: A study of transverse vocal tract cross-sectional area. *Phonetica, 44,* 76–90.

Sussman, H. M., MacNeilage, P. F., & Hanson, R. J. (1973). Labial and mandibular dynamics during the production of labial consonants: Preliminary observations. *Journal of Speech and Hearing Research, 16,* 397–420.

Sussman, H. M., MacNeilage, P. F., & Powers, R. K. (1977). Recruitment and discharge patterns of single motor units during speech production. *Journal of Speech and Hearing Research, 20,* 616–630.

Sussman, H. M., & Smith, K. U. (1970a). Transducer for measuring mandibular movements. *Journal of the Acoustical Society of America, 48,* 857–858.

Sussman, H. M., & Smith, K. U. (1970b). Transducer for measuring lip movements during speech. *Journal of the Acoustical Society of America, 48,* 858–860.

Sussman, H. M., & Smith, K. U. (1971). Jaw movements under delayed auditory feedback. *Journal of the Acoustical Society of America, 50,* 685–691.

Suzuki, N. (1989). Clinical applications of EPG to Japanese cleft palate and glossectomy patients. *Clinical Linguistics and Phonetics, 3,* 127–136.

Suzuki, N., Dent, H., Wakumoto, H., Gibbon, F., Michi, K., & Hardcastle, W. J. (1989). A cross-linguistic study of lateral misarticulation using electropalatography (EPG). *European Journal of Disorders of Communication, 30,* 237–245.

Suzuki, N., & Michi, K. (1986). Dynamic velography: A new method for investigating articulatory palatolingual contact. *Folia Phoniatrica, 38,* 356–357.

Svirsky, M. A., Stevens, K. N., Matthies, M. L., Manzella, J., Perkell, J. S., & Wilhelms-Tricarico, R. (1997). Tongue surface displacement during bilabial stops. *Journal of the Acoustical Society of America, 102,* 562–571.

Tabachnik, E., Muller, N., Toye, B., & Levison, H. (1981). Measurement of ventilation in children using the respiratory inductive plethysmograph. *Journal of Pediatrics, 99,* 895–899.

Takahashi, S. (Ed.). (1982). *Illustrated computer tomography: A practical guide to CT interpretations.* New York: Springer-Verlag.

Tatsumi, I. F. (1972). Some computer techniques for dynamic palatography. *Annual Bulletin of the Research Institute of Logopedics and Phoniatrics, 6,* 15–18.

Tatsumi, I. F., Sasanuma, S., Hirose, H., & Kiritani, S. (1979). Acoustic properties of ataxic and parkinsonian speech in syllable repetition tasks. *Annual Bulletin of the Research Institute of Logopedics and Phoniatrics, 13,* 99–104.

Theodoros, D. G., Murdoch, B. E., & Stokes, P. D. (1995). Variability in the perceptual and physiological features of dysarthria following severe closed head injury: An examination of five cases. *Brain Injury, 9,* 671–696.

Thompson, E. C., Murdoch, B. E., & Stokes, P. D. (1997). Interlabial contact pressures during performance of speech and nonspeech tasks in young adults. *Journal of Medical Speech-Language Pathology, 5,* 191–199.

Thompson, E. C., Murdoch, B. E., & Theodoros, D. G. (1997). Variability in upper motor neurone-type dysarthria: An examination of five cases with dysarthria following cerebrovascular accident. *European Journal of Disorders of Communication, 32,* 397–427.

Tiffany, W. (1980). The effects of syllable structure on diadochokinetic and reading rates. *Journal of Speech and Hearing Research, 23,* 894–908.

Tingley, B. M., & Allen, G. D. (1975). Development of speech timing control in children. *Child Development, 46,* 186–194.

Tobin, M. J., Chadha, T. S., Jenouri, G., Birch, S. J., Gazeroglu, H. B., & Sackner, M. A. (1983). Breathing patterns: 1. Normal subjects. *Chest, 84,* 202–205.

Tuller, B., Shao, S., & Kelso, J. A. S. (1990). An evaluation of an alternating magnetic field device for monitoring tongue movements. *Journal of the Acoustical Society of America, 88,* 674–679.

Tye-Murray, N. (1987). Effects of vowel context on the articulatory closure postures of deaf speakers. *Journal of Speech and Hearing Research, 30,* 99–104.

Tye-Murray, N. (1991). The establishment of open articulatory postures by deaf and hearing speakers. *Journal of Speech and Hearing Research, 34,* 453–459.

Ueda, D., Yano, K., & Okuno, A. (1993). Ultrasonic imaging of the tongue, mouth, and vocal cords in normal children: Establishment of basic scanning positions. *Journal of Clinical Ultrasound, 21,* 431–439.

Umemori, M., Sugawara, J., Kawauchi, M., & Mitani, H. (1996). A pressure-distribution sensor (PDS) for evaluation of lip functions. *American Journal of Orthodontics and Dentofacial Orthopedics, 109,* 473–480.

Unser, M., & Stone, M. (1992). Automated detection of the tongue surface in sequences of ultrasound images. *Journal of the Acoustical Society of America, 91,* 3001–3007.

van der Giet, G. (1977). Computer controlled method for measuring articulatory activities. *Journal of the Acoustical Society of America, 61,* 1072–1076.

van Lieshout, P. H. H. M., Hulstijn, W., & Peters, H. F. M. (1996). Speech production in people who stutter: Testing the motor plan assembly hypothesis. *Journal of Speech and Hearing Research, 39,* 76–92.

van Lieshout, P. H. H. M., Peters, H. F. M., & Hulstijn, W. (1994). Articulo-motorisch onderzoek: Een overzicht van technieken met de nadruk of Electro-Magnetische Medio-sagittale Articulografie (EMA). *Stem-, Spraak- en Taalpathologie, 3,* 241–261.

Vatikiotis-Bateson, E., & Ostry, D. J. (1995). An analysis of the dimensionality of jaw motion in speech. *Journal of Phonetics, 23,* 101–117.

Wakumoto, M., Isaacson, K. G., Friel, S., Suzuki, N., Gibbon, F., Nixon, F., Hardcastle, W. J., & Michi, K. (1996). Preliminary study of articulatory reorganisation of fricative consonants following osteotomy. *Folia Phoniatrica et Logopaedica, 48,* 275–289.

Wakumoto, M., Ohno, K., Imai, S., Yamashita, Y., Akizuki, H., & Michi, K. (1996). Analysis of the articulation after glossectomy. *Journal of Oral Rehabilitation, 23,* 764–770.

Walker, F. O., Donofrio, P. D., Harpold, G. J., & Ferrell, W. G. (1990). Sonographic imaging of muscle contraction and fasciculations: A correlation with electromyography. *Muscle and Nerve, 13,* 33–39.

Warren, D. W., Morr, K., Rochet, A., & Dalston, R. (1989). Respiratory response to a decrease in velopharyngeal resistance. *Journal of the Acoustical Society of America, 86,* 917–924.

Warren, R. H., & Alderson, S. H. (1986). Breathing patterns in infants utilizing respiratory inductive plethysmography. *Chest, 89,* 717–722.

Warren, R. H., & Alderson, S. H. (1994). Chest wall motion in neonates utilizing respiratory inductive plethysmography. *Journal of Perinatology, 14,* 101–105.

Warren, R. H., Horan, S. M., & Robertson, P. K. (1997). Chest wall motion in preterm infants using respiratory inductive plethysmography. *European Respiratory Journal, 10,* 2295–2300.

Watanabe, S., Arasaki, K., Nagata, H., & Shouji, S. (1994). Analysis of dysarthria in amyotrophic lateral sclerosis—MRI of the tongue and formant analysis of vowels. *Rinsho Shinkeigaku, 34,* 217–223.

Watkin, K. L., & Rubin, J. M. (1989). Pseudo–three-dimensional reconstruction of ultrasonic images of the tongue. *Journal of the Acoustical Society of America, 85,* 496–499.

Watkin, K. L., & Zagzebski, J. A. (1973). On-line ultrasonic technique for monitoring tongue displacements. *Journal of the Acoustical Society of America, 54,* 544–547.

Watson, H. (1980). The technology of respiratory inductive plethysmography. In F. D. Stott, E. B. Raftery, & L. Goulding (Eds.), *Proceedings of the Third International Symposium on Ambulatory Monitoring* (pp. 537–558). New York: Academic Press.

Watson, T. S., Allen, S. J., & Allen, K. D. (1993). Ventricular fold dysphonia: Application of biofeedback technology to a rare voice disorder. *Behavior Therapy, 24,* 439–446.

Weddell, G., Feinstein, B., & Pattle, R. E. (1944). The electrical activity of voluntary muscle in man under normal and pathological conditions. *Brain, 67,* 178–257.

Wein, B., Alzen, G., Tolxdorff, T., Böckler, R., Klajman, S., & Huber, W. (1988). Computer-sonographische Darstellung der Zungenmotilität mittels Psuedo–3D-Rekonstruktion. *Ultraschall in der Medizin, 9,* 95–97.

Wein, B., Angerstein, W., & Klajman, S. (1993). Suchbewegungen der Zunge bei einer Sprechapraxie: Darstellung mittels Ultraschall und Pseudo–3D-Abbildung. *Nervenarzt, 64,* 143–145.

Wein, B., Böckler, R., Klajman, S., & Obrebowski, A. (1991). Ultrasonografia jezyka w rehabilitacji zaburzen artykulacyjnych. *Otolaryngologia Polska, 45,* 133–140.

Wein, B., Böckler, R., Klajman, S., & Willmes, K. (1990). Computersonographische Darstellung von Zungenformen bei der Bildung der langen Vokale des Deutschen. *Ultraschall in der Medizin, 11,* 100–103.

Wein, B., Drobnitzky, M., & Klajman, S. (1990). Magnetresonanztomographie und Sonographie bie der Lautbildung. *Rofo Fortschritte auf dem Gebiete der Röntgenstrahlen und der neuen bildgebenden Verfahren, 153,* 408–412.

Wein, B., Drobnitzky, M., Klajman, S., & Angerstein, W. (1991). Evaluation of functional positions of tongue and soft palate with MR imaging: Initial clinical results. *Journal of Magnetic Resonance Imaging, 1,* 381–383.

Weismer, G. (1984). Articulatory characteristics of parkinsonian dysarthria: Segmental and phrase-level timing, spirantization, and glottal-supraglottal coordination. In M. R. McNeil, J. C. Rosenbek, & A. E. Aronson (Eds.), *The dysarthrias: Physiology, acoustics, perception, management* (pp. 101–130). San Diego, CA: Singular Publishing Group.

Weismer, G. (1985). Speech breathing: Contemporary views and findings. In R. G. Daniloff (Ed.), *Speech science: Recent advances* (pp. 47–72). San Diego, CA: College-Hill Press.

Weismer, G., & Bunton, K. (1999). Influences of pellet markers on speech production behavior: Acoustical and perceptual measures. *Journal of the Acoustical Society of America, 105,* 2882–2894.

Westbury, J. (1991). The significance and measurement of head position during speech production experiments using the x-ray microbeam system. *Journal of the Acoustical Society of America, 89,* 1782–1791.

Westlake, H. (1951). Muscle training for cerebral palsied speech cases. *Journal of Speech and Hearing Disorders, 16,* 103–109.

Westlake, H. (1952). *A system for developing speech with cerebral palsied children.* Chicago, IL: National Society for Crippled Children and Adults.

Whalen, J. P., & Balter, S. (1984). *Radiation risks in medical imaging.* Chicago, IL: Year Book Medical.

Whitehill, T., Stokes, S., Hardcastle, W. J., & Gibbon, F. (1995). Electropalatographic and perceptual analysis of the speech of Cantonese children with cleft palate. *European Journal of Disorders of Communication, 30,* 193–202.

Whitehill, T. L., Stokes, S. F., & Yonnie, M. Y. (1996). Electropalatography treatment in an adult with late repair of cleft palate. *Cleft Palate—Craniofacial Journal, 33,* 160–168.

Whitney, R. J. (1949). The measurement of changes in human limb-volume by means of a mercury-in-rubber strain gage. *Journal of Physiology, 109,* 5P – 6P.

Wilder, C. N., & Baken, R. J. (1974). Respiratory patterns in infant cry. *Human Communication, 3,* 18–34.

Winkworth, A. L., Davis, P. J., Adams, R. D., & Ellis, E. (1995). Breathing patterns during spontaneous speech. *Journal of Speech and Hearing Research, 38,* 124–144.

Winkworth, A. L., Davis, P. J., Ellis, E. & Adams, R. D. (1994). Variability and consistency in speech breathing during reading: Lung volumes, speech intensity, and linguistic factors. *Journal of Speech and Hearing Research, 37,* 535–556.

Wit, J., Maassen, B., Gabreëls, F. J. M., & Thoonen, G. (1993). Maximum performance tests in children with developmental spastic dysarthria. *Journal of Speech and Hearing Research, 36,* 452–459.

Witting, C. (1953). New techniques of palatography. *Studia Linguistica, 7,* 54–68.

Wohlert, A. B., & Smith, A. (1998). Spatiotemporal stability of lip movements in older adult speakers. *Journal of Speech, Language, and Hearing Research, 41,* 41–50.

Wolff, P. H., Michel, G. F., & Ovrut, M. (1990). The timing of syllable repetitions in developmental dyslexia. *Journal of Speech and Hearing Research, 33,* 281–289.

Wood, L. M., Hughes, J., Hayes, K. C., & Wolfe, D. L. (1992). Reliability of labial closure force measurements in normal subjects and patients with CNS disorders. *Journal of Speech and Hearing Research, 35,* 252–258.

Wood, S. (1979). A radiographic examination of the constriction location for vowels. *European Journal of Disorders of Communication, 30,* 226–236.

Wood, S. (1995). An electropalatographic analysis of stutterers' speech. *European Journal of Disorders of Communication, 30,* 226–236.

Wrench, A. A., McIntosh, A. D., & Hardcastle, W. J. (1996). Optopalatograph (OPG): A new apparatus for speech production analysis. *Proceedings of the International Conference on Spoken Language Processing* (Vol. 3, pp. 1589–1592), Philadelphia, PA.

Wrench, A., McIntosh, A., & Hardcastle, W. (1997). Optopalatograph: Development of a device for measuring tongue movement in 3D. *Proceedings of the Fifth European Conference on Speech Communication Technology* (Vol. 2, pp. 1055–1058), Rhodes, Greece.

Wright, S., & Kerswill, P. (1989). Electropalatography in the study of connected speech processes. *Clinical Linguistics and Phonetics, 3,* 49–57.

Wyke, B. D. (Ed.). (1974). *Ventilatory and phonatory control systems.* New York: Oxford University Press.

Yaffe, M. J., & Rowlands, J. A. (1997). X-ray detectors for digital radiography. *Physics in Medicine and Biology, 42,* 1–39.

Yamashita, Y., & Michi, K. (1991). Misarticulation caused by abnormal lingual-palatal contact in patients with cleft palate with adequate velopharyngeal function. *Cleft Palate—Craniofacial Journal, 28,* 360–366.

Yamashita, Y., Michi, K., Imai, S., Suzuki, N., & Yoshida, H. (1992). Electropalatographic investigation of abnormal lingual-palatal contact patterns in cleft palate patients. *Clinical Linguistics and Phonetics, 6,* 201–217.

Yamawaki, Y., Nishimura, Y., Suzuki, Y., Sawada, M., & Yamawaki, S. (1997). Rapid magnetic resonance imaging for assessment of velopharyngeal muscle movement on phonation. *American Journal of Otolaryngology, 18,* 210–213.

Yokoyama, M., Yamanaka, N., Ishii, H., Tamaki, K., Yoshikawa, A., & Morita, R. (1996). Evaluation of the pharyngeal airway in obstructive sleep apnea: Study by ultrafast MR imaging. *Acta Otolaryngologica,* Suppl. 523, 242–244.

Yoss, K. A., & Darley, F. L. (1974). Developmental apraxia of speech in children with defective articulation. *Journal of Speech and Hearing Research, 17,* 399–416.

Young, S. W. (1984). *Nuclear magnetic resonance imaging: Basic principles.* New York: Raven Press.

Zemlin, W. R. (1998). *Speech and hearing science: Anatomy and physiology* (4th ed.). Boston, MA: Allyn and Bacon.

Zenker, W., & Zenker, A. (1960). Über die Regelung der Stimmlippenspannung durch von aussen eingreifende Mechanismen. *Folia Phoniatrica, 12,* 1–36.

Zhao, W., Blevis, I., Germann, S., Rowlands, J. A., Waechter, D., & Huang, Z. (1997). Digital radiography using active matrix readout of amorphous selenium: Construction and evaluation of a prototype real-time detector. *Medical Physics, 24,* 1834–1843.

Zhou, X., Liang, Z.-P., Gewalt, S. L., Cofer, G. P., Lauterbur, P. C., & Johnson, G. A. (1998). A fast spin echo technique with circular sampling. *Magnetic Resonance in Medicine, 39*, 23–27.

Zimmermann, G. (1980a). Articulatory dynamics of fluent utterances of stutterers and nonstutterers. *Journal of Speech and Hearing Research, 23*, 95–107.

Zimmermann, G. (1980b). Articulatory behaviors associated with stuttering: A cinefluorographic analysis. *Journal of Speech and Hearing Research, 23*, 108–121.

Zimmermann, G., & Hanley, J. M. (1983). A cinefluorographic investigation of repeated fluent productions of stutterers in an adaptation procedure. *Journal of Speech and Hearing Research, 26*, 35–42.

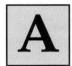

Conversion Tables

MASS OR WEIGHT

Multiply:		by	To get:	
g	grams	3.5275×10^{-2}	oz	ounces
		2.2046×10^{-3}	lb	pounds
kg	kilograms	2.2046	lb	pounds
		35.2739	oz	ounces
oz	ounces	38.3495	g	grams
		2.8349×10^{-2}	kg	kilograms
		6.25×10^{-2}	lb	pounds
lb	pounds	4.5359×10^{2}	g	grams

LENGTH

Multiply:		by	To get:	
m	meters	1×10^{3}	mm	millimeters
		1×10^{2}	cm	centimeters
		39.3700	in	inches
		3.2808	ft	feet
		1.0936	yd	yards
mm	millimeters	1×10^{-3}	m	meters
		1×10^{-1}	cm	centimeters
		3.937×10^{-2}	in	inches
		3.2808×10^{-2}	ft	feet

	Multiply:	*by*		*To get:*
in	inches	1.0936×10^{-3}	yd	yards
		25.4000	mm	millimeters
		2.5400	cm	centimeters
		2.5400×10^{-2}	m	meters
		8.3333×10^{-2}	ft	feet
		2.7777×10^{-2}	yd	yards
yd	yards	9.1440×10^{2}	mm	millimeters
		91.440	cm	centimeters
		0.9144	m	meters

AREA

	Multiply:	*by*		*To get:*
in^2	square inches	6.4516×10^{2}	mm^2	square millimeters
		6.4516	cm^2	square centimeters
		6.4516×10^{-4}	m^2	square meters
mm^2	square millimeters	1.5499×10^{-3}	in^2	square inches
		1×10^{-2}	cm^2	square centimeters
		1×10^{-6}	m^2	square meters
cm^2	square centimeters	0.1549	in^2	square inches
		1×10^{2}	mm^2	square millimeters
		1×10^{-4}	m^2	square meters
m^2	square meters	1.5499×10^{3}	in^2	square inches
		1×10^{6}	mm^2	square millimeters
		1×10^{4}	cm^2	square centimeters

VOLUME

	Multiply:	*by*		*To get:*
mL	milliliters	6.1025×10^{-2}	in^3	cubic inches
		1.0567×10^{-3}	qt	U.S. quarts
L	liters	61.0251	in^3	cubic inches
		1.0567	qt	U.S. quarts
qt	U.S. quarts	0.9463	L	liters
		946.231	mL	milliliters
		57.75	in^3	cubic inches
in^3	cubic inches	1.6387×10^{-2}	L	liters
		16.387	mL	milliliters
		1.7316×10^{-2}	qt	U.S. quarts

ANGLE

Multiply:	by	To get:
rad radians	5.7296	° degrees
° degrees	1.7453×10^{-2}	rad radians

TEMPERATURE

K Kelvin	$= °C + 273.15$
	$= (0.5555 \times °F) + 255.3722$
°F °Fahrenheit	$= 1.8K - 459.67$
	$= (1.8 \times °C) \times 32$
°C centigrade	$= K - 273.15$
	$= (0.5555 \times °F - 17.7777$

PRESSURE

Multiply:	by		To get:
dyn/cm² dynes/cm²	1.00	μb	microbars
	1.0197×10^{-2}	mmH₂O	millimeters of water
	1.0197×10^{-2}	mmH₂O	millimeters of water
	9.8692×10^{-7}	atm	atmospheres
	4.0147×10^{-4}	inH₂O	inches of water
	3.3456×10^{-5}	ftH₂O	feet of water
	2.9530×10^{-5}	inHg	inches of mercury
	1×10^{-4}	kPa	kilopascal
mm H₂O millimeters of water	98.0637	μb	microbars
	7.3554×10^{-2}	mmHg	millimeters of mercury
	9.6781×10^{-5}	atm	atmospheres
	3.9370×10^{-2}	inH₂O	inches of water
	3.2808×10^{-3}	ftH₂O	feet of water
	2.8958×10^{-3}	inHg	inches of mercury
	9.8068×10^{-3}	kPa	kilopascal
mmHg millimeters of mercury	1.3332×10^{-3}	μb	microbar
	13.5955	mmH₂O	millimeters of water
	1.3158	atm	atmospheres
	0.5352	inHg	inches of water
	4.4605×10^{-2}	ftH₂O	feet of water
	3.9369×10^{-2}	inHg	inches of mercury
	0.1333	kPa	kilopascal

Multiply:		by	To get:	
atm	atmospheres	1.0132×10^6	μb	microbar
		1.0333×10^4	mmH$_2$O	millimeters of water
		760	mmHg	millimeters of mercury
		4.0679×10^2	inH$_2$O	inches of water
		33.8995	ftH$_2$O	feet of water
		29.9212	inHg	inches of mercury
inH$_2$O	inches of water	2.4908×10^3	mmH$_2$O	millimeters of water
		1.8683	mmHg	millimeters of mercury
		2.4582×10^{-3}	atm	atmospheres
		8.3333×10^{-2}	ftH$_2$O	feet of water
		$7.3554 \times 10^{-}$	inHg	inches of mercury
		0.2491	kPa	kilopascal
inHg	inches of mercury	3.3864×10^4	μb	microbar
		3.4533×10^2	mmH$_2$O	millimeters of water
		25.4000	mmH$_2$O	millimeters of mercury
		3.3421×10^{-2}	atm	atmospheres
		13.5955	inH$_2$O	inches of water
		1.1329	ftH$_2$O	feet of water
		29.53	kPa	kilopascal
kPa	kilopascal	1×10^4	μb	microbar
		1.0197	mmH$_2$O	millimeters of water
		7.501	mmHg	millimeters of mercury
		0.2491	inH$_2$O	inches of water

B

The Rainbow Passage

When the sunlight strikes raindrops in the air, they act   10

like a prism and form a rainbow. The rainbow is   20

a division of white light into many beautiful colors. These   30

take the shape of a long round arch, with its   40

path high above and its who end apparently beyond the   50

horizon. There is, according to legend, a boiling pot of   60

gold at one end. People look, but no one ever   70

finds it. When a man looks for something beyond his   80

reach his friends say he is looking for the pot   90

of gold at the end of the rainbow.   98

Throughout the centuries men have explained the rainbow in various   108

ways. Some have accepted it as a miracle without physical   118

explanation. To the Hebrews it was a token that there   128

would be no more universal floods. The Greeks used to   138

image that it was a sign from the gods to   148

foretell war or heavy rain. The Norsemen considered the rainbow   158 as a bridge over which the gods passed from earth 168

to their home in the sky. Other men have tried 178

to explain the phenomenon physically. Aristotle thought that the rainbow 188

was caused by reflection of the sun's rays by the 198

rain. Since then physicists have found that it is not 208

reflection, but refraction by the raindrops which causes the rainbow. 218

Many complicated ideas about the rainbow have been formed. The 228

difference in the rainbow depends considerably upon the size of 238

the water drops, and the width of the colored band 248

increases as the size of the drops increases. The actual 258

primary rainbow observed is said to be the effect of 268

superposition of a number of bows. If the red of 278

the second bow falls upon the green of the first, 288

the result is to give a bow with an abnormally 298

wide yellow band, since red and green lights when mixed 308

form yellow. This is a very common type of bow, 318

one showing mainly red and yellow, with little or no 328

green or blue. 331

From Fairbanks, G. (1960). *Voice and Articulation Drillbook* (second ed.). New York: Harper and Bros., p. 127.

Phonemic Analysis of the First Three Sentences
(as spoken by a "General American" speaker)

Total words		51
Total syllables		66
Total phonemes		177

	Number	*Percent*
Front vowels	21	11.8
Back vowels	7	3.9
Central vowels	24	13.6
Diphthongs	16	9.0
Voiced consonants and combinations	71	40.1
Voiceless consonants and combinations	38	21.4
Total voiced elements:		78.4
vowels		29.3
diphthongs		9.0
consonants		40.1

Adapted from "Fundamental Frequency Characteristics of Japanese Asai Speakers," by E. T. Curry, J. C. Snidecor, and N. Isshiki, 1973, *Laryngoscope 38,* 1759–1763. Table I, p.1761. Reprinted by permission.

C

The Grandfather Passage

You wish to know all about my grandfather. Well, he is nearly 93 years old, yet he still thinks as swiftly as ever. He dresses himself in an ancient black frock coat, usually missing several buttons. A long beard clings to his chin, giving those who observe him a pronounced feeling of the utmost respect. When he speaks, his voice is just a bit cracked and quivers a bit. Twice each day, he plays skillfully and with zest upon a small organ. Except in the winter, when the snow or ice prevents, he slowly takes a short walk in the open air each day. We have often urged him to walk more and smoke less, but he always answers, "Banana Oil." Grandfather likes to be modern in his language.

Source: Darley, Aronson, and Brown (1975).

D
The Zoo Passage

Look at this book with us. It's a story about a zoo. That is where bears go. Today it's very cold out of doors, but we see a cloud overhead that's a pretty, white fluffy shape. We hear that straw covers the floor of cages to keep the chill away; yet a deer walks through the trees with her head high. They feed seeds to birds so they're able to fly.

From "Contingencies for Bioelectronic Modification of Nasality" by a S. G. Fletcher, 1972. *Journal of Speech and Hearing Disorders, 37*, 329–346.

Metric (SI) Style Conventions

The internationally accepted version of the metric system is formally known as the Système International d'Unités (International System of Units, SI). It is based on seven *base units*. Those of most interest to professionals in speech communication are

Quantity	Unit name	Unit symbol
length	meter	m
mass	kilogram	kg
time	second	s
electric current	ampere	A

From the base units, a number of officially recognized *derived units* are obtained. These include, for example, units for frequency (hertz, Hz), speed or velocity (meters per second, m/s), force (newton, N), pressure or stress (pascal, Pa), and power (watt, W).

Still other units are officially *accepted* for use with the SI, including the units of time (hour, h; minute, min; and second, s) and volume (liter, L).

Unit names are modified by prefixes that indicate the power of ten by which they are to be multiplied. The standard prefixes, and their symbols, are

Power of ten	Factor	Prefix	Symbol
10^9	1 000 000 000	giga	G
10^6	1 000 000	mega	M
10^3	1 000	kilo	k
10^2	100	hecto	h
10^1	10	deka	da
10^{-1}	0.1	deci	d

Power of ten	Factor	Prefix	Symbol
10^{-2}	0.01	centi	c
10^{-3}	0.001	milli	m
10^{-6}	0.000 001	micro	μ
10^{-9}	0.000 000 001	nano	n

Style conventions:

A unit symbol (such as s) is not an abbreviation and thus is not followed by a period.

Those symbols that represent a proper name have their first letter in upper case (for example, Hz) although the name of the unit itself is not capitalized (for example, hertz).

The spelling of unit names is specific to each language, and thus varies (English kilogram, French kilogramme) but the symbols are invariant.

Pluralization of unit names follows the conventions of the language being used. Thus the singular "henry" (the unit of inductance) is pluralized as "henries" in English. An exception is hertz, whose plural is hertz.

Unit symbols are never pluralized. Thus 3 kg, not 3 kgs.

Complete information concerning SI is available at http://physics.nist/gov/SI

Fundamental Frequencies (Hz) of the Musical (12-interval chromatic) Scale (A = 440 Hz)

NOTE			OCTAVE							
			c^{-3}	c^{-2}	c^{-1}	c^0	c^1	c^2	c^3	c^4
	C		16.35	32.70	65.41	130.81	261.63	523.25	1046.50	2093.00
C#		D_b	17.32	24.65	69.30	138.59	277.18	554.37	1108.73	2217.46
	D		18.35	36.70	73.42	146.83	293.66	587.33	1174.66	2349.32
D#		E_b	19.45	38.89	77.78	155.56	311.13	622.25	1244.51	2489.02
	E		20.60	41.20	82.41	164.81	329.63	659.26	1318.51	2637.02
	F		21.83	43.65	87.31	174.61	349.23	689.46	1396.91	2791.83
F#		G_b	23.12	46.25	92.50	185.00	369.99	739.99	1479.98	2959.96
	A		27.50	55.00	110.00	220.00	440.00	880.00	1760.00	3520.00
A#		B_b	30.87	61.74	123.47	246.96	493.88	987.77	1975.53	3951.07

THE INTERNATIONAL PHONETIC ALPHABET (revised to 1993, updated 1996)

CONSONANTS (PULMONIC)

	Bilabial	Labiodental	Dental	Alveolar	Postalveolar	Retroflex	Palatal	Velar	Uvular	Pharyngeal	Glottal
Plosive	p b			t d		ʈ ɖ	c ɟ	k g	q ɢ		ʔ
Nasal	m	ɱ		n		ɳ	ɲ	ŋ	N		
Trill	ʙ			r					R		
Tap or Flap				ɾ		ɽ					
Fricative	ɸ β	f v	θ ð	s z	ʃ ʒ	ʂ ʐ	ç ʝ	x ɣ	χ ʁ	ħ ʕ	h ɦ
Lateral fricative				ɬ ɮ							
Approximant		ʋ		ɹ		ɻ	j	ɰ			
Lateral approximant				l		ɭ	ʎ	L			

Where symbols appear in pairs, the one to the right represents a voiced consonant. Shaded areas denote articulations judged impossible.

CONSONANTS (NON-PULMONIC)

Clicks		Voiced implosives		Ejectives	
ʘ	Bilabial	ɓ	Bilabial	'	Examples:
ǀ	Dental	ɗ	Dental/alveolar	p'	Bilabial
ǃ	(Post)alveolar	ʄ	Palatal	t'	Dental/alveolar
ǂ	Palatoalveolar	ɠ	Velar	k'	Velar
ǁ	Alveolar lateral	ʛ	Uvular	s'	Alveolar fricative

OTHER SYMBOLS

ʍ	Voiceless labial-velar fricative	ɕ ʑ	Alveolo-palatal fricatives
w	Voiced labial-velar approximant	ɺ	Alveolar lateral flap
ɥ	Voiced labial-palatal approximant	ɧ	Simultaneous ʃ and x
ʜ	Voiceless epiglottal fricative		
ʢ	Voiced epiglottal fricative		Affricates and double articulations can be represented by two symbols joined by a tie bar if necessary. k͡p t͡s
ʡ	Epiglottal plosive		

VOWELS

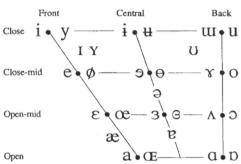

Where symbols appear in pairs, the one to the right represents a rounded vowel.

SUPRASEGMENTALS

ˈ	Primary stress
ˌ	Secondary stress ˌfoʊnəˈtɪʃən
ː	Long eː
ˑ	Half-long eˑ
˘	Extra-short ĕ
ǀ	Minor (foot) group
‖	Major (intonation) group
.	Syllable break ɹi.ækt
‿	Linking (absence of a break)

TONES AND WORD ACCENTS

LEVEL			CONTOUR		
e̋ or ˥	Extra high		ě or ˇ	Rising	
é ˦	High		ê ˆ	Falling	
ē ˧	Mid		e᷄ ˀ	High rising	
è ˨	Low		e᷅ ˀ	Low rising	
ȅ ˩	Extra low		e᷈	Rising-falling	
↓	Downstep		↗	Global rise	
↑	Upstep		↘	Global fall	

DIACRITICS   Diacritics may be placed above a symbol with a descender, e.g. ŋ̊

̥	Voiceless	n̥ d̥	̤	Breathy voiced	b̤ a̤	̪	Dental	t̪ d̪
̬	Voiced	s̬ t̬	̰	Creaky voiced	b̰ a̰	̺	Apical	t̺ d̺
ʰ	Aspirated	tʰ dʰ	̼	Linguolabial	t̼ d̼	̻	Laminal	t̻ d̻
̹	More rounded	ɔ̹	ʷ	Labialized	tʷ dʷ	̃	Nasalized	ẽ
̜	Less rounded	ɔ̜	ʲ	Palatalized	tʲ dʲ	ⁿ	Nasal release	dⁿ
̟	Advanced	u̟	ˠ	Velarized	tˠ dˠ	ˡ	Lateral release	dˡ
̠	Retracted	e̠	ˤ	Pharyngealized	tˤ dˤ	̚	No audible release	d̚
̈	Centralized	ë	̴	Velarized or pharyngealized	ɫ			
̽	Mid-centralized	e̽	̝	Raised	e̝ (ɹ̝ = voiced alveolar fricative)			
̩	Syllabic	n̩	̞	Lowered	e̞ (β̞ = voiced bilabial approximant)			
̯	Non-syllabic	e̯	̘	Advanced Tongue Root	e̘			
˞	Rhoticity	ɚ a˞	̙	Retracted Tongue Root	e̙			

Reprinted courtesy of the International Phonetics Association

A Poor Man's Tour of Physical Quantities and Units[1]

INTRODUCTION

Physical quantities are objective events that can assume numerical values. *Basic quantities* are limited to mass, time, displacement (or length) and electric charge. *Derived quantities* are generated through algebraic combination of basic quantities and other derived quantities. These include velocity, acceleration, pressure, force, work, power, and temperature, as well as the quantities of electricity and electronics (except for electric charge). *Units of measurement*, on the other hand, are standardized amounts of quantities. In most cases, units are named in honor of the individuals whose scientific efforts clarified our understanding of the respective phenomenon. Finally, *values* are specific amounts of units. In the expression, "she was 5 feet, 4 inches tall," feet and inches are units, the numbers 5 and 4 are values, and "tall" denotes the quantity of vertical length.

QUANTITIES AND UNITS

Quantities differ from units. For example, the basic quantity length is defined as the distance between two points. Any particular length can be expressed by a host of units, including inches, centimeters, feet, meters, rods, furlongs, miles, kilometers, etc. Similarly, the derived quantity force (F) is defined by Newton's second law of motion as mass (M) times acceler-

ation (a), whereas, the metric unit for force is defined as the newton (N).

Force (quantity): $F = M * a$
Force (MKS unit): $1 N = 1 kg * 1 m / sec^2$

Although physical quantities are well-standardized, the symbols and abbreviations used to represent them are not. Indeed, they differ considerably among authors, scholarly journals, and scientific or professional disciplines. Symbols for units are formally defined by international standards bodies and are even the subject of treaties among nations. Generally, honorific units (those named in honor of individuals) are written without capitalization (to distinguish the unit from the person); when abbreviated, honorific units are capitalized.

MEASUREMENT SYSTEMS

Physical measurement always requires specification of both a value (i.e., a number representing "how much") and a unit (i.e., "of what"). *Systems of measurement* are formal strategies for indexing amounts of specified physical quantities. Such systems include (1) definitions of quantities, (2) units of measurement—the names we give quantities when we want to be specific, (3) standards of measurement—formally defined reference values for units, and (4)

---

[1]Reprinted courtesy of M. R. Chial

procedures (rules) of measurement for applying standards to specific things or events.

Units of measurement and the physical standards underpinning them become progressively more precise as science and technology develop. In other words, newer standards are capable of accommodating smaller *differences* in the amounts of the quantities measured. Standard units (e.g., the standard second and the standard meter) also are periodically redefined in pursuit of greater objectivity and repeatability. The second originally was standardized as the duration between heartbeats (problem: whose heart and after what activity?). Today, the standard second is defined in terms of atomic events, allowing resolution of time to 10^{-12} seconds (one trillionth of a second, or 1 picosecond).

The most common systems of units are the English system (foot-pound-second or FPS), the early metric system (centimeter-gram-second or CGS), and the *Systeme International d'Unites* (meter-kilogram-second or MKS). All three systems use the same units for the basic quantities of time (the second) and electric charge (the coloumb). Different units are employed for mass. The CGS system uses the gram, the MKS system uses the kilogram, and the FPS system uses the *slug* or *poundal*. The more familiar *pound* is a unit of weight (a force), not a unit of mass. Both metric systems employ a powers-of-ten (decimal) number scheme, whereas the English system is based on doublings, triplings, or other multiples (e.g., 2 cups = 1 pint, 2 pints = 1 quart; 3 feet = 1 yard). Confusions related to the inconsistencies of the English FPS system are among the reasons it is seldom used in science and engineering.

The *Systeme International d'Unites* (abbreviated SI) is the contemporary version of the metric system originally developed by the French Academy of Science in 1791. The SI also is referred to as the *rationalized MKS system*, so-called because both basic and derived units are defined as having unity (1) values, even though derived units may be given new names. *Basic units* and *basic quantities* are not the same (see above). Basic units (see Table 1) are required in the SI to accomplish the goal of unity value for derived units. Note that two of the basic units of the SI are honorific. Those for displacement, mass, time, light intensity and molecular substance are not.

The quantities in Table 1 define the MKS system and also underpin the FPS and CGS systems. Many everyday quantities are missing from Table 1, for example, area, volume, velocity (or speed), and power. These and other *derived quantities* are defined as combinations of the quantities listed in Table 1. The methods by which basic quantities are combined to form derived quantities (and, for that matter, by which derived quantities may be combined to define still other derived quantities) are inherently algebraic. These mathematical methods are based upon known lawful relations of the physical universe and generally are quite simple. Thus, formal systems of measurement constitute a world-view about how the universe and everything in it works. Table 2 lists commonly used derived SI units.

METRIC PREFIXES

A distinct advantage of the SI system is a set of prefixes that can be applied to units to indicate scale of measurement, i.e., to overall size or magnitude of a measured quantity. The most commonly used pre-

Table 1. Base units of measurement in the Systeme International d'Unites (also called the "rationalized MKS system"). Asterisks in the left-hand column designate basic quantities. All other quantities are derived.

Quantity	Unit	Symbol	Physical Definition
*Displacement (Length)	meter	m	distance traveled by light in a vacuum in 1 / 299 792 458 of a second
*Mass	kilogram	kg	mass equal to that of a prototype platinum-iridium cylinder kept in Paris, France
*Time	second	s	duration of 9 192 631 770 periods of radiation of the cesium 133 atom in transition between two states
Electric current	ampere	A	coulomb / s
Temperature	kelvin	K	1 / 273.2 of the triple point of water
Light intensity	candela	cd	directional radiant intensity of 1 / 683 watt per steradian at a monochrome frequency of 540 × 1012 hertz
Molecular substance	mole	mol	amount of substance equal to that of 0.012 kg of carbon-12

Table 2. Some derived units of measurement in the *Systeme International d'Unites*. Many additional derived units are in common use. Basic and derived units of measurement (including those honoring individuals) always are given in lower-case letters when written out in full. Thus, people can be distinguished from the physical units named after them. When abbreviated, units named to honor people are capitalized. Asterisks in the right-hand column designate multiplication.

Quantity	Unit	Symbol	Other Definition	
Area	m^2	m^2	displacement squared	
Volume	m^3	m^3	displacement cubed	
Density	kg / m^3	kg / m^3	mass / unit volume	
Velocity	m / s	m / s	Δ displacement / unit time	
Acceleration	m / s^2	m / s^2	Δ velocity / unit time	
Plane angle	radian	rad	2π rad = 360°	
Angular velocity	rad / s	ω	2π rad / s = 360° / s	
Solid angle	steradian	sr	(complex)	
Energy	joule	J	$kg * m^2 / s^2$	= N * m
Force	newton	N	$kg * m / s^2$	= J / m
Pressure or stress	pascal	Pa	$(kg * m / s^2) / m^2$	$= N / m^2$
Power	watt	W	$kg * m^2 / s^3$	= J / s
Electric charge	coulomb	C	A * s	
Electric potential (emf)	volt	V	$kg * m^2 / s^3 * A = J / A * s$	= W / A
Electric resistance	ohm	Ω	$kg * m^2 / s^3 * A^2$	= V / A
Electric capacitance	farad	F	$A^2 *s^4 / kg * m^2$	= A * s / V
Electric inductance	henry	H	$kg * m^2 / s^2 * A^2$	= V * s / A
Frequency	hertz	Hz	cycle / s	$= s^{-1}$
Magnetic flux	weber	Wb	$kg * m^2 / s^2 * A$	= V * s
Magnetic flux density	telsa	T	$kg / s^2 * A$	$= Wb / m^2$
Luminous flux	lumen	lm	cd * sr	
Customary temperature	degree Celsius	°C	K − 273.15	

fixes are noted in Table 3. Note that prefixes employ a base-10 exponential progression such that prefixes close to the <unit> (i.e., from milli to kilo) are based upon small differences in exponents, while extremely large and extremely small magnitudes are based upon numerically greater differences in exponents. Table 4 gives instructions for converting values expressed with one common prefix to identical values expressed with another common prefix.

STANDARDS ORGANIZATIONS

The SI is but one part of a larger process by which scientific, technical, and professional communities strive to standardize measurements. In the United States, the National Technical Institute (NTI—formerly called the National Bureau of Standards) is responsible for defining and increasing the precision of the physical standards that underpin scientific and commercial measurement. A branch of the US Department of Commerce, the NTI was originally formed to insure that materials and equipment purchased by the federal government (including the military) conformed to consistent standards of measurement.

Other national groups, such as the American National Standards Institute (ANSI) and international groups, such as the International Standards Organization (ISO) and the International Electrotechnical Commission (IEC), are voluntary organizations that exist for the purpose of documenting generally accepted practices for making and reporting measurements. A major goal of these groups is to facilitate communication among scientists, technical workers, and various professionals so as to insure that differences in measurement practices do not cause differences in the meaning of reported data.

Standards published by standards organizations fall into four distinct categories.

(1) **Definition standards** which formally define physical quantities, units, and related concepts,
(2) **Data standards** which precisely define reference quantities for units, for technical instruments, or for technical procedures,
(3) **Instrument standards** which specify the tolerances of devices used to make measurements for different purposes, and

---

Table 3. Metric prefixes. Note the use of capital letters to distinguish among abbreviations for prefixes.

Prefix	Symbol	Power of 10	Numerical Value
exa	E	10^{18}	1 000 000 000 000 000 000
peta	P	10^{15}	1 000 000 000 000 000
tera	T	10^{12}	1 000 000 000 000
giga	G	10^{9}	1 000 000 000
mega	M	10^{6}	1 000 000
kilo	k	10^{3}	1 000
hecto	h	10^{2}	100
deka	da	10^{1}	10
—<unit>—	(none)	10^{0}	1
deci	d	10^{-1}	0.1
centi	c	10^{-2}	0.01
milli	m	10^{-3}	0.001
micro	μ	10^{-6}	0.000 001
nano	n	10^{-9}	0.000 000 001
pico	p	10^{-12}	0.000 000 000 001
femto	f	10^{-15}	0.000 000 000 000 001
atto	a	10^{-18}	0.000 000 000 000 000 001

Table 4. Metric conversions. To convert a unit of measurement expressed with an original value prefix to the same unit expressed with a different value prefix, start by finding the correct cell in the table below. Then move the decimal point of the original value the number of places indicated by the digit in the direction indicated by the arrow. For example, 5 kilometers equals 500,000 centimeters (5⇒ move the decimal 5 spaces to the right); 12.5 milliseconds equals 0.0125 seconds (⇐3 move the decimal 3 spaces to the left).

	Desired Prefix ⇓								
Original Prefix ⇓	*giga*	*mega*	*kilo*	*—(unit)—*	*centi*	*milli*	*micro*	*nano*	*pico*
giga	⇐**0**⇒	3⇒	6⇒	8⇒	11⇒	12⇒	15⇒	18⇒	21⇒
mega	⇐3	⇐**0**⇒	3⇒	6⇒	8⇒	11⇒	12⇒	15⇒	18⇒
kilo	⇐6	⇐3	⇐**0**⇒	3⇒	6⇒	8⇒	11⇒	12⇒	15⇒
—(unit)—	⇐9	⇐6	⇐3	⇐**0**⇒	3⇒	6⇒	8⇒	11⇒	12⇒
centi	⇐10	⇐9	⇐6	⇐3	⇐**0**⇒	3⇒	6⇒	8⇒	11⇒
milli	⇐12	⇐10	⇐9	⇐6	⇐3	⇐**0**⇒	3⇒	6⇒	8⇒
micro	⇐15	⇐12	⇐10	⇐9	⇐6	⇐3	⇐**0**⇒	3⇒	6⇒
nano	⇐18	⇐15	⇐12	⇐10	⇐9	⇐6	⇐3	⇐**0**⇒	3⇒
pico	⇐21	⇐18	⇐15	⇐12	⇐10	⇐9	⇐6	⇐3	⇐**0**⇒

---

(4) **Procedure standards** which detail the steps to be taken in making measurements of interest to the public or particular scientific, technical, or professional groups.

Five groups currently active within ANSI are highly relevant to scientists and clinicians who work with persons who have disorders of speech, language, or hearing. These are designated as ANSI Committee

S1-Acoustics (dealing with the physical measurement of sound), ANSI Committee S2-Vibration (dealing with physical measurement of mechanical events), ANSI Committee S3-Bioacoustics (dealing with the measurement of hearing), ANSI Committee S12-Noise (dealing with the physical measurement of generally unwanted acoustical signals, as well as ways to assess and prevent unwanted effects of such sounds), and ANSI Committee S14-Electroacoustics (dealing with sound recording and reproduction).

Hundreds of other industry, government, and professional groups exist to standardize everything from the size of photographic film, to computer languages, to audiogram symbols, to envelope sizes, to screw threads and wire gauges, to the dimensions of the cardboard cores found in toilet paper, to the speed of audio tapes, to the capacity of CD-audio disks. Some of these eventually become standards endorsed by ANSI, ISO, or both. Others do not. In France, for example, a government agency requires that common baked goods such as croissants be prepared using specified recipes. Non-standardized industries include shoe and clothing manufacturing. If such products were more rigorously standardized, we would have little use for phrases such as "if the shoe fits. . . ."

REFERENCES

Adams, H. (1974). *SI metric units: An introduction* (rev. ed.) Toronto, ON: McGraw-Hill Ryerson, Limited.

Anderson, H. (Ed.). (1989). *A physicist's desk reference: The physics vade mecum* (2nd ed.). New York, NY: American Institute of Physics.

Klein, H. (1974). *The science of measurement: A historical survey.* New York, NY: Simon & Schuster, Inc. Republished (1988) by Dover Publications, Inc.

SELECTED CONVERSION FACTORS

The following material is not intended to encourage you to translate metric measures into the arguably more familiar foot-pound-second (FPS) measures in common use in the United States, but instead to illustrate the complexity of the FPS system and the simplicity of the *Systeme International d'Unites*, even for routine measurement. The superiority of the SI system is particularly evident for dry and liquid volume measurements. The English FPS system employs two entirely different sets of units for such measurements, while the SI uses only one. It is noteworthy that the English FPS system is no longer used in England, or in any of the nations of the former British Commonwealth.

Linear Measure

1 inch = 2.54 centimeters
1 foot = 12 inches = 30.48 centimeters
1 yard = 3 feet = 36 inches = 0.914 4 meters
1 rod = 5.25 yards = 5.029 meters
1 furlong = 40 rods = 201.17 meters
1 statute mile = 5280 feet = 1760 yards = 8 furlongs = 1 609.344 meters
1 league = 3 miles = 4.83 kilometers

1 meter = 39.370 08 inches = 3.280 840 feet = 1.093 613 yards

1 meter = 100 centimeters = 1 000 millimeters = 0.001 kilometers

Square Measure

1 square inch = 6.452 square centimeters
1 square foot = 144 square inches = 929 square centimeters
1 square yard = 9 square feet = 0.836 1 square meters
1 square rod = 30.25 square yards = 25.29 square meters
1 acre = 4 840 square yards = 0.404 7 hectacres
1 square mile = 640 acres = 2.59 square kilometers

1 square meter = 10.763 91 square feet = 1.195 990 square yards

1 square meter = 10 000 square centimeters = 0.000 1 hectacre

Cubic Measure

1 cubic inch = 16.387 cubic centimeters
1 cubic foot = 1 728 cubic inches = 0.028 3 cubic meters
1 cubic yard = 27 cubic feet = 0.764 6 cubic meters
1 cord = 128 cubic feet = 3.625 cubic meters

1 cubic meter = 1 000 liters

Volume or Capacity Dry Measure)

1 bushel = 4 pecks = 32 dry quarts = 64 dry pints = 2 150.42 cubic inches
= 35.239 07 liters = 0.035 239 07 cubic meters

1 liter = 1.816 166 dry pints

1 liter = 1 000 milliliters = 0.001 cubic meters

Volume or Capacity (Liquid Measure)

1 gallon = 4 liquid quarts = 8 liquid pints = 32 gills = 128 liquid ounces = 728 teaspoons = 61 440 minims = 3.785 411 784 liters = 0.003 785 411 784 cubic meters

1 liter = 202.884 136 211 teaspoons = 2.113 376 liquid pints = 0.264 172 05 gallons

1 liter = 1 000 milliliters = 0.001 cubic meters

Nautical Measure

1 fathom = 6 feet = 2 yards = 1.829 meters
1 nautical mile = 1.508 statute miles

60 nautical miles = 1 degree of a great circle of the earth
1 knot = 1 nautical mile per hour (a measure of speed)

1 kilometer = 1 000 meters

Weight

1 avoirdupois pound = 16 avoirdupois ounces = 12 troy ounces = 0.000 5 short tons = 0.000 446 428 6 long tons = 256 avoirdupois drams = 7 000 grains = 0.453 592 37 kilograms

1 kilogram = 15, 432.36 grains = 35.273 96 avoirdupois ounces = 32.150 75 troy ounces = 0.001 102 31 short tons = 0.000 984 2 long tons = 2.204 623 avoirdupois pounds = 2.679 229 troy pounds

1 kilogram = 1 000 grams = 0.001 metric tons

I

Index